Oncogenes
and Viral Genes

CANCER CELLS

COLD SPRING HARBOR LABORATORY
1984

2
Oncogenes and Viral Genes

Edited by

George F. Vande Woude
National Cancer Institute, National Institutes of Health

Arnold J. Levine
State University of New York at Stony Brook

William C. Topp
Cold Spring Harbor Laboratory

James D. Watson
Cold Spring Harbor Laboratory

CANCER CELLS
1 / The Transformed Phenotype
2 / Oncogenes and Viral Genes

Oncogenes and Viral Genes
© 1984 by Cold Spring Harbor Laboratory
Printed in the United States of America
Cover design by Emily Harste

Library of Congress Cataloging in Publication Data

Main entry under title:

Oncogenes and viral genes.

   (Cancer cells series, ISSN 0743-2194 ; v. 2)
   Bibliography: p.
   Includes index.
   1. Oncogenes.   2. Cancer—Genetic aspects.
I. Vande Woude, George F.   II. Cold Spring Harbor
Laboratory.   III. Series.   [DNLM: 1. Cell trans-
formation, Neoplastic.   2. Oncogenes.   3. Oncogenic
viruses.   W1 CA677BG v.2 / QZ 202 0545]
RC268.4.053   1984   616.99'4071   83-26336
ISBN 0-87969-169-7

Cover: Relationship between the amino acid sequence of platelet-
derived growth factor (partial amino acid sequences of peptides
purified from PDGF are shown) and the predicted amino acid sequence of *v-sis.* (Figure courtesy of M.D. Waterfield [ICRF]. Re-
produced, with permission, from *Nature* **304:** 35-39, 1983.)

All Cold Spring Harbor Laboratory publications are available
through booksellers or may be ordered directly from Cold
Spring Harbor Laboratory, Box 100, Cold Spring Harbor, New
York 11724.   SAN 203-6185

Conference Participants

Aaronson, Stuart, NCI, National Institutes of Health, Bethesda, Maryland

Albrecht-Buehler, Guenter, Department of Cell Biology, Northwestern University School of Medicine, Chicago, Illinois

Andersen, Philip, Department of Molecular Biology, Abbott Laboratories, North Chicago, Illinois

Appert, Hubert, Department of Surgery, Medical College of Ohio, Toledo

Arai, Ken-Ichi, DNAX Research Institute, Palo Alto, California

Axelrod, David E., Department of Biological Sciences, Rutgers University, New Brunswick, New Jersey

Baltimore, David, Center for Cancer Research, Massachusetts Institute of Technology, Cambridge

Baluda, Marcel, Department of Pathology, University of California School of Medicine, Los Angeles

Barbacid, Mariano, NCI, National Institutes of Health, Bethesda, Maryland

Barnes, David W., Department of Biological Sciences, University of Pittsburgh, Pennsylvania

Barrett, J. Carl, National Institute of Environmental Health Sciences, Research Triangle Park, North Carolina

Baserga, Renato, Department of Pathology, Temple University School of Medicine, Philadelphia, Pennsylvania

Basilico, Claudio, Department of Pathology, New York University Medical Center, New York

Beemon, Karen, Department of Biology, Johns Hopkins University, Baltimore, Maryland

Belsham, Graham, Department of Biochemistry, National Institute for Medical Research, London, England

Benade, Leonard, Department of Virology, American Type Culture Collection, Rockville, Maryland

Bender, Timothy, NCI, National Navy Medical Center, Bethesda, Maryland

Benjamin, Thomas, Department of Pathology, Harvard Medical School, Boston, Massachusetts

Bennett, David, Department of Viral Oncology, Veteran's Administration Hospital, Salt Lake City, Utah

Bennett, Ellen, Department of Microbiology, McGill University, Montreal, Canada

Blair, Donald, NCI, Frederick Cancer Research Facility, Frederick, Maryland

Blumberg, Peter, NCI, National Institutes of Health, Bethesda, Maryland

Bos, J.L., Department of Medical Biochemistry, Silvius Laboratories, Leiden, The Netherlands

Boschek, C. Bruce, Department of Virology, Justus Liebig University, Giessen, Federal Republic of Germany

Bosselman, Robert, Amgen, Inc., Thousand Oaks, California

Brackenbury, Robert, Rockefeller University, New York, New York

Bravo, Rodrigo, European Molecular Biology Laboratory, Heidelberg, Federal Republic of Germany

Breitman, Martin, Department of Genetics, Hospital for Sick Children, Toronto, Canada

Brenner, Sidney, MRC, Cambridge, England

Brickell, Paul, Department of Biochemistry, Imperial College, London, England

Brugge, Joan, Department of Microbiology, State University of New York, Stony Brook

Butel, Janet S., Department of Virology, Baylor College of Medicine, Houston, Texas

Calberg-Bacq, C.M., Department of General Microbiology, University of Liege, Belgium

Campisi, Judith, Department of Cell Growth and Regulation, Dana-Farber Cancer Institute, Boston, Massachusetts

Canaani, Eli, Department of Immunology, Weizmann Institute of Science, Rehovot, Israel

Carley, William, Department of Cell Biology, Yale University, New Haven, Connecticut

Carroll, Robert B., Department of Pathology, New York University Medical Center, New York

Casnellie, John, Department of Pharmacology, University of Washington, Seattle

Cattoni, Sebastiano, Cancer Center, Columbia University, New York, New York

Celis, Julio, Biostructural Division, Aarhus University, Denmark

Chakrabarti, Sekhar, NCI, National Institutes of Health, Bethesda, Maryland

Chen, Lan-Bo, Dana-Farber Cancer Institute, Boston, Massachusetts

Chen, M.J., Department of Molecular Biology, Smith, Kline and Beckman, Swedeland, Pennsylvania

Chinnadurai, G., Department of Molecular Virology, St. Louis University Medical Center, Missouri

Chipperfield, Randall, Department of Biology, Massachusetts Institute of Technology, Cambridge

Clark, Robin, Cetus Corporation, Emoryville, California

Colby, Wendy W., Department of Molecular Biology, Genetech Inc., San Francisco, California

Cole, John S. III, NCI, National Institutes of Health, Bethesda, Maryland

Cole, Michael, Department of Biochemistry, St. Louis University School of Medicine, Missouri

Conrad, Susan, Department of Molecular Biology, University of California, Berkeley

Cook, Donald N., Department of Microbiology, McGill University, Montreal, Canada

Cooper, Jonathan, Department of Molecular Biology and Virology, Salk Institute, San Diego, California

Courtneidge, Sara, Department of Biochemistry, National Institute for Medical Research, London, England

Covey, Lori, Department of Biological Sciences, Columbia University, New York, New York

Crawford, Lionel, Imperial Cancer Research Fund, London, England

Croce, Carlo M., Wistar Institute, Philadelphia, Pennsylvania

Cuzin, Francois, Biochemistry Center, University of Nice, France

Danos, Olivier, Department of Molecular Biology, Pasteur Institute, Paris, France

Defendi, V., Department of Pathology, New York University Medical Center, New York

Dermer, Gerald, Department of Pathology, University of North Carolina, Chapel Hill

Deuel, Thomas F., Jewish Hospital at Washington University School of Medicine, St. Louis, Missouri

Diamond, Alan M., Dana-Farber Cancer Institute, Boston, Massachusetts

Dickson, Clive, Imperial Cancer Research Fund, London, England

Di Mayorca, G., University Medical and Dental School of New Jersey, Newark

Duesberg, Peter, Department of Molecular Biology, University of California, Berkeley

Dunn, Ashley F., Melbourne Tumor Biology Division, Ludwig Institute for Cancer Research, Victoria, Australia

Eisenmann, Robert, Fred Hutchinson Cancer Research Center, Seattle, Washington

Eva, A., NCI, National Institutes of Health, Bethesda, Maryland

Feramisco, James R., Cold Spring Harbor Laboratory, New York

Fink, Leslie, NCI, National Institutes of Health, Bethesda, Maryland

Fisher, Richard, Biogen Research Corporation, Cambridge, Massachusetts

Franke, Werner, Institute of Cell and Tumor Biology, German Cancer Research Center, Heidelberg, Federal Republic of Germany

Fried, Michael, Imperial Cancer Research Fund, London, England

Friedman, Beth Ann, Dept. of Toxicology, Massachusetts Institute of Technology, Cambridge

Fuchs, Elaine, Department of Biochemistry, University of Chicago, Illinois

Furth, Mark, Department of Molecular Oncogenesis, Memorial Sloan-Kettering Cancer Center, New York, New York

Gallimore, Phillip, Department of Cancer Studies, University of Birmingham, England

Garrels, James, Cold Spring Harbor Laboratory, New York

Gattoni-Cellis, S., Columbia University College of Physicians & Surgeons, New York, New York

Geiger, Benjamin, Department of Chemical Immunology, Weizmann Institute of Science, Rehovot, Israel

Gentry, Lawrence, Department of Viral Oncology, Fred Hutchinson Cancer Research Center, Seattle, Washington

Gernot, Walter, Immunobiology Institute, University of Freiberg, Federal Republic of Germany

Gilmer, Tona M., Department of Microbiology and Immunology, University of North Carolina, Chapel Hill

Goldberg, Allan, Rockefeller University, New York, New York

Gooding, Linda R., Department of Microbiology, Emory University School of Medicine, Atlanta, Georgia

Graesser, Friedrich, Department of Immunobiology, University of Freiburg, Federal Republic of Germany

Gray, Harry, Dana-Farber Cancer Institute, Boston, Massachusetts

Graziani, Y., Department of Pathology, University of Colorado Health Sciences Center, Denver

Green, Howard, Department of Physiology and Biophysics, Harvard University Medical School, Boston, Massachusetts

Greenberg, Michael, Department of Biochemistry, New York University Medical Center, New York

Gross, Ludwik, Veterans Administration Hospital, Bronx, New York

Grosveld, Gerard, Department of Cell Biology and Genetics, Erasmus University, Rotterdam, The Netherlands

Halligan, Brian, Department of Physiological Chemistry, Johns Hopkins University School of Medicine, Baltimore, Maryland

Hanafusa, Hidesaburo, Rockefeller University, New York, New York

Hann, Steve, Fred Hutchinson Cancer Center, Seattle, Washington

Hare, David, Amgen Development, Inc., Boulder, Colorado

Harlow, Edward, Cold Spring Harbor Laboratory, New York

Hassell, John, Department of Microbiology, McGill University, Montreal, Canada

Hawley, Robert, Biological Research Division, Ontario Cancer Institute, Toronto, Canada

Hayday, Adrian C., Center for Cancer Research, Massachusetts Institute of Technology, Cambridge

Hayman, M.J., Imperial Cancer Research Fund, London, England

Hayward, William, Memorial Sloan-Kettering Cancer Center, New York, New York

Herrlich, Peter, Department of Genetics, University of Karlsruhe, Federal Republic of Germany

Hill, M., Institute of Cancerology and Immunogenetics, Villejuif, France

Hillova, Jane, Institute of Cancerology and Immunogenetics, Villejuif, France

Hirschhorn, Ricky R., Department of Pathology, Temple University Health Sciences Center, Philadelphia, Pennsylvania

Hirt, Bernard, Swiss Cancer Institute, Lausanne, Switzerland

Hoffman, Robert, Department of Pediatrics, University of California, San Diego

Hsiao, Wendy, Douglaston, New York

Huang, Jung San, Jewish Hospital at Washington University School of Medicine, St. Louis, Missouri

Hunter, Tony, Salk Institute, San Diego, California

Hyland, Julia K., Department of Pathology, Temple University School of Medicine, Philadelphia, Pennsylvania

Ikawa, Yoji, Riken Institute, Saitama, Japan

Ikegaki, Naohiko, Department of Human Genetics, University of Pennsylvania School of Medicine, Philadelphia

Ip, Stephen, Cambridge Research Laboratory, Massachusetts

Ito, Yoshiaki, NCI, National Institutes of Health, Bethesda, Maryland

Janssen, J.W.G., Department of Experimental Cytology, Netherlands Cancer Institute, Amsterdam

Jenkins, J.R., Marie Curie Memorial Foundation Research Institution, Surrey, England

Jonak, Gerald, DuPont Experimental Station, Wilmington, Delaware

Kakunaga, Takeo, NCI, National Institutes of Health, Bethesda, Maryland

Kamen, Robert, Genetics Institute, Boston, Massachusetts

Kaplan, Paul, Salk Institute, San Diego, California

Khoury, George, NCI, National Institutes of Health, Bethesda, Maryland

Koprowski, Hilary, Department of Anatomy and Biology, Wistar Institute, Philadelphia, Pennsylvania

Kozma, Sara, Institute for Genetics and Toxology, Karlsruhe, Federal Republic of Germany

Kriegler, Michael, Department of Molecular Biology, University of California, Berkeley

Krueger, James, Rockefeller University, New York, New York

Kuehl, Mike, NCI, National Navy Medical Center, Bethesda, Maryland

Land, Hartmut, Massachusetts Institute of Technology, Cambridge

Leder, Philip, Department of Genetics, Harvard University Medical School, Boston, Massachusetts

Lee, William, Department of Medicine, University of California, San Francisco

Lehto, Veli-P., Department of Pathology, University of Helsinki, Finland

Lens, P.F., Department of Chemical Carcinogesis, Netherlands Cancer Institute, Amsterdam

Levine, Arnold J., Department of Microbiology, State University of New York, Stony Brook

Levinson, Arthur, Genentech, Inc., South San Francisco, California

Lewin, Benjamin, *Cell*, Cambridge, Massachusetts

Lewis, C.M., Department of Immunobiology, Glaxo Group Research, Middlesex, England

Linzer, Daniel, Department of Molecular Biology and Genetics, Johns Hopkins University School of Medicine, Baltimore, Maryland

Lipp, Martin, Biochemistry Institute, Ludwig-Maximilians University, Munich, Federal Republic of Germany

Livingston, David M., Dana-Farber Cancer Institute, Boston, Massachusetts

Luciw, Paul, Chiron Corporation, Emeryville, California

Maltzman, Warren, Department of Biological Sciences, Rutgers University, New Brunswick, New Jersey

Maness, Patricia, Department of Biochemistry, University of North Carolina, Chapel Hill

Maniatis, Thomas, Department of Biochemistry and Molecular Biology, Harvard University, Cambridge, Massachusetts

Mannino, Raphael, Department of Microbiology and Immunology, Albany Medical College, New York

Mansfield, Brian, Department of Molecular Biology and Genetics, Johns Hopkins University School of Medicine, Baltimore, Maryland

Mao, Jen-I., Collaborative Research Inc., Lexington, Massachusetts

Marcu, Kenneth, Department of Biochemistry, State University of New York, Stony Brook

Marks, Paul A., Memorial Sloan-Kettering Cancer Center, New York, New York

Martin, G. Steven, Department of Zoology, University of California, Berkeley

Martin, M.A., National Institutes of Health, Bethesda, Maryland

Marx, Jean L., *Science*, Washington, DC

Matsumura, Fumio, Cold Spring Harbor Laboratory, New York

McClain, Kenneth, University of Minneapolis Hospital, Minnesota

McClure, Don, University of California, San Diego

Mendelson, Ella, NCI, National Institutes of Health, Bethesda, Maryland

Mercer, W. Edward, Department of Pathology, Temple University School of Medicine, Philadelphia, Pennsylvania

Mes-Masson, A., Department of Microbiology, McGill University, Montreal, Canada

Miles, Vincent, Amersham International, Amersham, England

Miyatake, Sho, DNAX Research Institute, Palo Alto, California

Moelling, Karin, Department of Molecular Genetics, Max-Planck Institute, Berlin, Federal Republic of Germany

Mroczkowski, B., Department of Biochemistry, Vanderbilt University, Nashville, Tennessee

Murphy, Cheryl, Dana-Farber Cancer Institute, Boston, Massachusetts

Murphy, David, Imperial College, London, England

Nathans, Daniel, Department of Molecular Biology and Genetics, Johns Hopkins University Medical School, Baltimore, Maryland

Nevins, Joseph, Rockefeller University, New York, New York

Newmark, Peter, *Nature*, London, England

Nishizuka, Yasutomi, Department of Biochemistry, Kobe University School of Medicine, Japan

Noda, Makoto, NCI, National Institutes of Health, Bethesda, Maryland

Nunn, Michael, University of California, Berkeley

Nusse, Roel, Netherlands Cancer Institute, Amsterdam

O'Farrell, Minnie, Department of Biology, University of Essex, England

Oren, Moshe, Department of Immunology, Weizmann Institute of Science, Rehovot, Israel

Oroszlan, Stephen, NCI, Frederick Cancer Research Facility, Frederick, Maryland

Osborn, Mary, Department of Biophysical Chemistry, Max-Planck Institute, Goettingen, Federal Republic of Germany

Ozanne, Brad, Department of Microbiology, University of Texas Health Science Center, Dallas

Papas, Takis S., NCI, Frederick Cancer Research Facility, Frederick, Maryland

Parada, Luis, Massachusetts Institute of Technology, Cambridge

Parker, Richard, Department of Microbiology, University of California, San Francisco

Parsons, J.T., Department of Microbiology, University of Virginia, Charlottesville

Patch, Cephas, NCI, National Institutes of Health, Bethesda, Maryland

Pearson, Mark L., NCI-Frederick Cancer Research Facility, Frederick, Maryland

Pellicer, Angel, Department of Pathology, New York University Medical Center, New York

Perucho, M., Department of Biochemistry, State University of New York, Stony Brook

Peters, Gordon, Imperial Cancer Research Fund, London, England

Pipas, James M., Department of Biological Sciences, University of Pittsburgh, Pennsylvania

Radke, Kathryn, Department of Veterinary Medicine, University of California, Davis

Rall, Leslie B., Chiron Corporation, Emeryville, California

Rapp, Ulf, NCI, Frederick Cancer Research Facility, Frederick, Maryland

Reid, Lola, Department of Molecular Pharmacology, Albert Einstein College of Medicine, Bronx, New York

Rein, A., NCI-Frederick Cancer Research Facility, Frederick, Maryland

Reynolds, Fred, NCI, Frederick Cancer Research Facility, Frederick, Maryland

Reynolds, Steven, Department of Tumor Virology, Fred Hutchinson Cancer Research Facility, Seattle, Washington

Rheinwald, James F., Dana-Farber Cancer Institute, Boston, Massachusetts

Rhim, J., NCI, National Institutes of Health, Bethesda, Maryland

Riemen, Mark W., Merck, Sharp and Dohme Research Laboratories, West Point, Pennsylvania

Rigby, P.W.J., Imperial College of Science and Technology, London, England

Rohrschneider, Larry, Fred Hutchinson Cancer Research Facility, Seattle, Washington

Rosner, Marsha, Toxicology, Massachusetts Institute of Technology, Cambridge

Rotter, Varda, Department of Cell Biology, Weizmann Institute of Science, Rehovot, Israel

Rowley, Janet D., Department of Medicine, University of Chicago, Illinois

Ruley, Earl, Cold Spring Harbor Laboratory, New York

Rusch, Harold, McArdle Laboratory, University of Wisconsin, Madison

Sabrin, Ira, Pall Corporation, Glen Cove, New York

Sager, Ruth, Dana-Farber Cancer Institute, Boston, Massachusetts

Saito, Haruo, Cancer Research Center, Massachusetts Institute of Technology, Cambridge

Schecter, Alan, Center for Cancer Research, Massachusetts Institute of Technology, Cambridge

Schlom, Jeffrey, NCI, National Institutes of Health, Bethesda, Maryland

Schneider, C., Imperial Cancer Research Fund, London, England

Schwab, Manfred, University of California, San Francisco

Schwartz, Stephen, Department of Pathology, University of Chicago, Illinois

Sefton, Bart, Salk Institute, San Diego, California

Senger, Donald, Department of Pathology, Beth Israel Hospital, Boston, Massachusetts

Shall, S., Department of Cellular and Molecular Biology, University of Sussex School of Biological Science, Brighton, England

Shalloway, David, Pennsylvania State University, University Park

Sharp, Phillip, Center for Cancer Research, Massachusetts Institute of Technology, Cambridge

Shenk, Thomas, Department of Microbiology, State University of New York, Stony Brook

Sherr, C.J., Department of Human Tumor Cell Biology, St. Jude Children's Hospital, Memphis, Tennessee

Shoyab, Mohammed, NCI, National Institutes of Health, Bethesda, Maryland

Shulman, Marc J., Wellesley Hospital, Toronto, Canada

Siebert, Gary R., Department of Cell Biology, Becton Dickinson Research Center, Research Triangle Park, North Carolina

Smart, John E., Biogen, Inc., Cambridge, Massachusetts

Smith, Alan E., Department of Biochemistry, MRC National Institute of Medical Research, London, England

Snitman, David, Amgen Development, Boulder, Colorado

Spandidos, Demetrios, Beatson Institute for Cancer Research, Glasgow, Scotland

Sporn, Michael, NCI, National Institutes of Health, Bethesda, Maryland

Spurr, N.K., Imperial Cancer Research Fund, London, England

Srinivason, A., NCI, National Institutes of Health, Bethesda, Maryland

Stabinsky, Yizahak, Amgen Development, Inc., Boulder, Colorado

Stephenson, John R., NCI, National Institutes of Health, Bethesda, Maryland

Stern, David, F., Massachusetts Institute of Technology, Cambridge

Stiles, Charles, Dana-Farber Cancer Institute, Boston, Massachusetts

Sun, T.-T., Department of Dermatology and Pharmacology, New York University School of Medicine, New York

Tevethia, Satvir, Department of Microbiology, Pennsylvania State University College of Medicine, Hershey

Tjian, Robert, Department of Biochemistry, University of California, Berkeley

Todaro, George, Oncogen, Inc., Seattle, Washington

Tonegawa, Susumu, Massachusetts Institute of Technology, Cambridge

Iooze, John, EMBO, Heidelberg, Federal Republic of Germany

Tsichlis, Phillip, Fox Chase Cancer Institute, Philadelphia, Pennsylvania

Turek, Lubomir, Department of Pathology, University of Iowa, Iowa City

van der Eb, Alex, Sylvius Laboratories, Leiden, The Netherlands

Vande Woude, George, NCI, Frederick Cancer Research Facility, Frederick, Maryland

Verbeek, Joseph, Geert Girdote Plein Noores, Nymegen, The Netherlands

Verma, Inder M., Department of Molecular Biology and Virology, Salk Institute, San Diego, California

Vincenzo, S., Department of Cell Biology, Sezione Science Microbiologiche, Rome, Italy

Vogt, Peter, Department of Microbiology, University of California, Los Angeles

Wallner-Philipp, Barbara, Biogen, Inc., Cambridge, Massachusetts

Wang, Jean, Massachusetts Institute of Technology, Cambridge

Wang, Lu-Hai, Rockefeller University, New York, New York

Waterfield, M.D., Imperial Cancer Research Fund, London, England

Weber, Klaus, Department of Biophysical Chemistry, Max-Planck Institute, Goettingen, Federal Republic of Germany

Weber, Michael, Department of Microbiology, University of Illinois, Urbana

Weinstein, I.B., Columbia University, New York, New York

Weiss, Robin, Chester Beatty Laboratories, Institute for Cancer Research, London, England

Weissman, Sherman, Yale University School of Medicine, New Haven, Connecticut

Wigler, Michael, Cold Spring Harbor Laboratory, New York

Wilhelmsen, K.C., McArdle Laboratory, University of Wisconsin, Madison

Williams, Lewis T., Massachusetts General Hospital, Boston

Wilsnack, Roger E., Becton Dickinson Research Center, Research Triangle Park, North Carolina

Wirschubsky, Zvi, Department of Tumor Biology, Karolinska Institutet, Stockholm, Sweden

Witte, Owen, Molecular Biology Institute, University of California, Los Angeles

Wolf, David, Department of Cell Biology, Weizmann Institute of Science, Rehovot, Israel

Wong, Tai Wai, Rockefeller University, New York, New York

Wong-Staal, Flossie, NCI, National Institutes of Health, Bethesda, Maryland

Wu, Ying-Jye, Cambridge Research Laboratory, Massachusetts

Yang, Liu, Department of Physiological Chemistry, Johns Hopkins University School of Medicine

Zack, Jerry, Department of Microbiology, University of Texas Health Science Center, Dallas

Zimmer, S., Department of Pathology, University of Kentucky Medical Center, Lexington

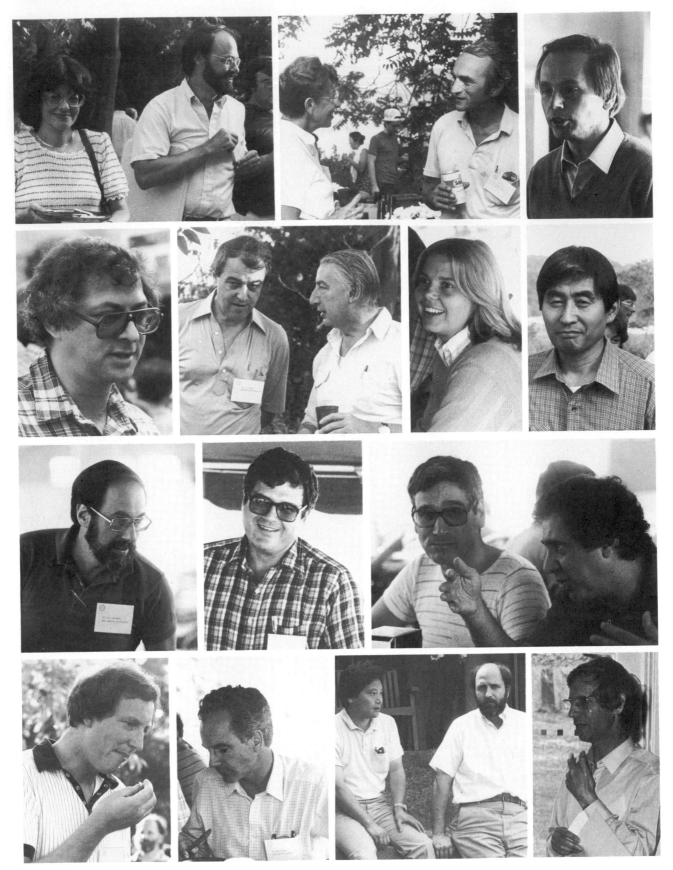

First row: T. Grodzicker, P. Sharp; R. Sanger, F. Cuzin; W. Topp
Second row: A. Levine; G. Di Mayorca, V. Defendi; J. Brugge; H. Hanafusa
Third row: D. Baltimore; G. Vande Woude; R. Weiss, G. Todaro
Fourth row: P. Gallimore; P. Duesberg; Y. Ito, R. Kamen, M. Yaniv

Preface

In a period of just four years we have witnessed a rapid succession of major advances in our understanding of the molecular basis for neoplastic disease. It was not until the late 1970s that a common thread linking viruses with chemical and physical genetic insults began to emerge. We first learned that retroviral proviruses were structurally similar to transposons, a finding which suggested that proviruses, like transposons, could modify expression of the region of the host chromosome into which they insert. Indeed, proviral insertion into a cellular oncogene locus could result in tumorigenesis. More than 15 unique viral oncogenes have since been identified and additional transforming genes have been detected by the DNA transfection assay.

With rapid progress being made on several fronts, we undertook to organize a meeting on The Cancer Cell at Cold Spring Harbor in September 1983 to herald the convergence of several lines of basic cancer research and the unravelling of the mysteries of the transformed cell phenotype through the study of oncogenes and viral genes. In the midst of this intensive meeting, which consisted of three sessions per day for five days and covered many possible (and in some cases impossible) aspects of the cellular and molecular biology of cancer, we learned that, like the multiple viral genes from adenovirus and polyoma virus that are required to effect transformation of primary cells in culture, the *myc* and *ras* oncogenes fall into similar complementation groups. In each case, one gene appears to rescue cells from senescence while the other effects morphological transformation. The merging of cytogenetics and molecular biology was evident in the demonstrations that the breakpoints for nonrandom chromosomal translocations involve oncogenic loci. We were treated to the results of computer searches for homology to the amino acid sequence of human platelet-derived growth factor, which have revealed a striking similarity to the amino acid sequence of the *sis* oncogene. Several chemical carcinogens were shown to activate cellular *ras* oncogenes. It was particularly fitting that, at this meeting where so many new advances were described, Mrs. Albert D. Lasker was honored for her continuous efforts in stimulating support for medical and cancer research.

In organizing this year's Cancer Cell conference, we tried to ensure that all new advances and relevant subjects were suitably covered. We are especially grateful to Earl Ruley, Mike Wigler, Mike Bishop, Howard Temin, Harold Varmus, David Baltimore, and Steve Hughes for their helpful advice and for identifying key research areas. We are also grateful for the financial support that the National Cancer Institute, the American Cancer Society, Fogarty International Center, and Becton-Dickinson and Co. provided for this meeting. These awards offset the expenses of many of our colleagues.

With more than 400 registrants and faced with contiguous meetings, Gladys Kist and her staff were subjected to more than the usual pressures in coordinating arrivals and departures. In spite of this challenge, their cheerful attitude made everyone feel welcome. Herb Parsons is to be commended for providing excellent coverage to the auxiliary viewing areas via closed-circuit color TV and zoom lens accessories.

This was the first in a new series of Cold Spring Harbor meetings focussing on the cancer cell. These meetings supersede the Cold Spring Harbor Conferences on Cell Proliferation, which were held for the last ten years. "Oncogenes and Viral Genes" and its companion volume "The Transformed Phenotype," the first two volumes in the new *Cancer Cells* series, provide an integrated and timely account of the Cancer Cell meeting.

The completion of the first two *Cancer Cells* volumes in an exceptionally short period of time is a major accomplishment for the Publications Department at Cold Spring Harbor. As editors of these volumes, we are especially grateful to Judy Cuddihy, Doug Owen, Karen Sundin, Joan Ebert, and Nancy Ford for their superlative efforts in producing these two volumes in record time.

The Editors

Contents

ras

ONCOGENES AND VIRAL GENES

ADENOVIRUS E1A, E1B

Transforming Activity of the *c-src* Gene

H. Hanafusa,* H. Iba,* T. Takeya,† and F.R. Cross*

*The Rockefeller University, New York, New York 10021
†Institute for Chemical Research, Kyoto University, Kyoto, Japan

Evidence has accumulated indicating that, during their replication cycles, some retroviruses have captured certain cellular genes (proto-oncogenes) into the viral genome and these genes become the viral transforming genes (oncogenes) (Bishop 1983). Whether the cellular genes can function as oncogenes without alterations in the sequence or whether certain mutations are required to gain transforming activity by their gene products are important questions that remain unresolved for many oncogenes.

Earlier studies by the groups of Vande Woude (Oskarsson et al. 1980; Blair et al. 1981) and of Scolnick (DeFeo et al. 1981; Chang et al. 1982) have shown that the elevated expression of *c-mos* and *c-Ha-ras* can lead to 3T3 cell transformation when these *c-onc* sequences were transfected after being linked to viral promoter sequences. On the other hand, transforming genes detected in human tumor cells by 3T3 cell transfection have been demonstrated to belong to a family of the *c-ras* genes that have a mutation at specific sites. These mutations are required for transforming activity (Der et al. 1982; Reddy et al. 1982; Tabin et al. 1982; Taparowsky et al. 1982).

Previously, in studies on the formation of recovered avian sarcoma virus (rASV) in chickens infected with RSV mutants that contain deletions in the *src* gene (Hanafusa et al. 1977; Wang et al. 1978; Karess and Hanafusa 1981; Takeya and Hanafusa 1983), we had demonstrated that the majority of the *src* sequence of Rous sarcoma virus (RSV) can be replaced by the cellular *src* sequence to encode an active transforming protein. Molecular cloning and sequencing of the *c-src* gene and the *v-src* gene of the Schmidt-Ruppin strain of RSV (SR-RSV) and one rASV demonstrated various sequence differences between the *c-src* gene and the transforming *src* genes. To determine whether any of the differences between *v-src*- and *c-src*-coding sequences

are required for transformation, we have constructed plasmids in which varying portions of the *v-src* gene of RSV DNA were replaced by the corresponding portions of the *c-src* gene. When the *v-src* gene was completely replaced by the *c-src* gene, the strong capacity of the *v-src* gene to transform cells was lost. However, mutations that convert the virus carrying the *c-src* gene into a strongly transforming virus take place with a relatively high frequency.

Results and Discussion

Comparison of structures of the *v-src* and *c-src* genes

Fragments of chicken DNA containing the *c-src* gene have been cloned, and the structure of the *c-src* gene was analyzed by restriction enzyme digestion and heteroduplex formation (Parker et al. 1981; Shalloway et al. 1981; Takeya et al. 1981). Later, the nucleotide sequence of the coding regions of the *c-src* locus was determined (Takeya and Hanafusa 1983) and compared with the sequence of the *v-src* gene (Czernilofsky et al. 1980, 1983; Takeya et al. 1982; Takeya and Hanafusa 1982; Schwartz et al. 1983). These results indicated that (1) the *c-src* gene consists of 12 exons, (2) the sequence is quite similar between *c-src* and *v-src* genes, but (3) the last 19 carboxyterminal amino acids of $p60^{c-src}$ are replaced with a new set of 12 amino acids in $p60^{v-src}$. Most of the sequence encoding the carboxyterminal sequence of $p60^{v-src}$ is found about 1 kb downstream from the termination codon of the *c-src* gene.

The comparison of amino acid sequences between $p60^{c-src}$ and $p60^{v-src}$ of SR-RSV and rASV1441 is shown in Figure 1. In addition to the major substitution at the carboxyl termini, there are eight amino acid differences between $p60^{c-src}$ and SR-RSV p60. Five of these eight amino acids unique to SR-RSV are replaced in rASV1441 p60 by the amino acids found in $p60^{c-src}$; three remaining

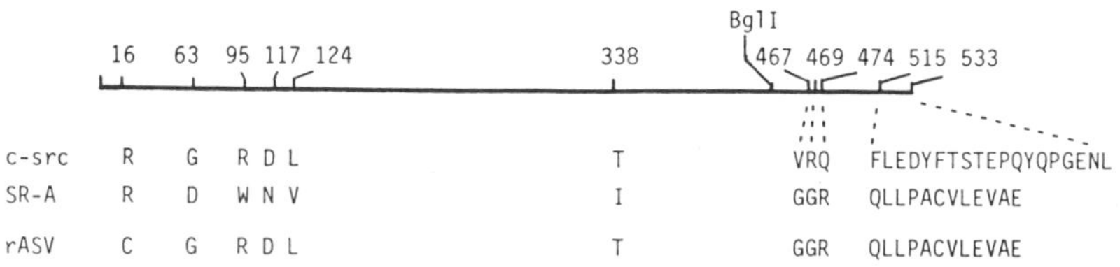

Figure 1 Comparisons of amino acid sequences of p60 products of *c-src*, SR-RSV-A, and rASV1441 (Takeya and Hanafusa 1983). The numbers shown above the line indicate the amino acid positions from the amino terminus. p60 consists of 533 amino acids for *c-src* and 526 amino acids for *v-src*. The position of the *Bgl*I site that was used for construction of chimeric DNAs is indicated.

1

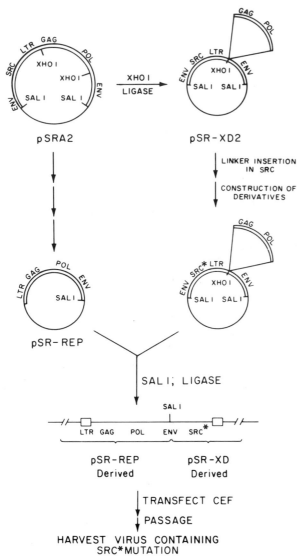

Figure 2 Two subclones, pSR-REP and pSR-XD2, were constructed from pSRA2 (Cross and Hanafusa 1983). Both subclones contain a deletion of the coding regions of SR-RSV, and thus their products of transfection are defective in replication. The ligation of two plasmids produces a structure similar to that of the integrated provirus.

amino acids are common to SR-RSV and rASV because they are located in the carboxyl end, the region that was not deleted in the parent of rASV1441. Thus, these comparisons suggest that the major difference in the amino acid sequence between viral and cellular *src* gene products is in their carboxyl termini, although other differences might also contribute to conformational changes.

Construction of viral DNA containing *c-src* sequences

To examine whether the overexpression of the *c-src* sequence in cells leads to cell transformation, we have

chosen to construct recombinant DNA molecules that can be tested in chicken cells, the natural host cells for RSV and the species from which our *c-src* clone was isolated. Cooper and Okenquist (1978) showed that foci can be formed in chicken embryo fibroblasts (CEF) by transfection with RSV DNA only when it produces infectious virus that can establish new rounds of infection in recipient cultures. Previously, we had constructed two plasmid clones, pSR-XD2 and pSR-REP, as shown in Figure 2 (Cross and Hanafusa 1983). These two plasmids can be ligated together to produce infectious RSV, but neither DNA alone can produce RSV. In this study, parts of the *v-src* gene of pSR-XD2 were substituted with parts of the *c-src* gene and the expression of the recombinants was examined by transfection of CEF after ligation with pSR-REP.

As shown in Figure 1, *Bgl*I cuts at the codon for Glu-432 in the *src* gene between nucleotides 1295 and 1296 (Takeya and Hanafusa 1983). (We use the amino acid and nucleotide numberings of Takeya and Hanafusa 1983.) Therefore, interchange of the *v-src* and *c-src* sequences at the *Bgl*I site conveniently interchanges their major differences, including three amino acid differences at amino acids 467, 469, and 474 (Fig. 1).

The details of the construction of various recombinant DNA molecules will be given elsewhere. Briefly, pN4 is similar to pSR-XD2 except that a *Bgl*II linker (CAGATCTG) was inserted at an *Nru*I site 95 bp downstream from the termination codon of *v-src*. pBB4 (Fig. 3A) is one of the recombinants between *v-src* and *c-src* sequences. The *Bgl*I–*Bgl*II (produced by the linker insertion) fragment of pN4 was replaced by a *Bgl*I–*Sac*I fragment of pRW10, a subclone of *c-src* clone λRCS3 (Takeya and Hanafusa 1982). This *Bgl*I–*Sac*I fragment was derived from the *Bgl*I site equivalent to that in pN4 and a *Sac*I site present 13 bp downstream from the termination codon of *c-src* (Takeya and Hanfusa 1983). The *Sac*I site was modified with a *Bgl*II linker to allow the substitution of this fragment for the *Bgl*I–*Bgl*II fragment of pN4. pTT701 (Fig. 3A)' contains a large *Nco*I–*Bgl*I fragment derived from λRCS3 as a replacement of the equivalent *Nco*I–*Bgl*I fragment in pN4, except that a repeated gp37 sequence was present due to the construction process (T. Takeya and F. Cross, unpubl.). Thus, pBB4 and pTT701 are complementary to each other in terms of the coding sequences before and after the *Bgl*I site. pPB5 is similar to pBB4, but this plasmid contains the *Pst*I–*Sac*I fragment from *c-src* DNA with the *Sac*I site converted to a *Bgl*II site. The *Pst*I site used is present 40 bp upstream of the *v-src* termination codon, just 5′ to the divergence of the *v-src* and *c-src* carboxyl termini. In all of our recombinant virus clones, the *c-src* sequence incorporated ended at the *Sac*I site and, thus, did not contain the sequence encoding most of the *v-src* carboxyl terminus found about 1 kb 3′ to the termination codon (Takeya and Hanafusa 1983).

pTT501 (Fig. 3B) is a construction containing the entire *c-src*-coding sequence and is made by replacing the 3′ end of the pTT701 *src* sequence with the *Bgl*I–*Bgl*II fragment of pBB4. pHB5 (Fig. 3B) is another construct

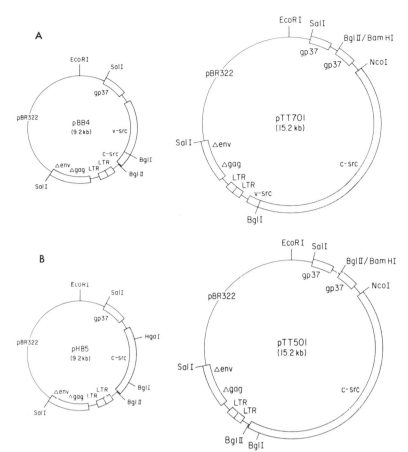

Figure 3 Various plasmids constructed from pSR-XD2 by substituting various parts with corresponding *c-src* sequences.

with a *src* sequence equivalent to the *c-src*-coding region, except that it lacks introns. A *Hga*I site is present 0.25 kb downstream from the initiation codon of the *v-src* sequence. pHB5 was constructed by replacing the *Hga*I–*Bgl*I fragment (1.0 kb) of pBB4 with the equivalent fragment of pTT108 DNA, which contains the rASV1441 *src* sequence (Takeya et al. 1981). (Since pBB4 is derived from pSR-XD2, which originated from SR-RSV-SF [Czernilofsky et al. 1980, 1983], the resulting pHB5 does not contain the point mutation of aspartic acid [position 63; see Fig. 1] in SR-RSV NY.)

Transfection of chicken cells with various DNAs

The constructed plasmid DNAs were cut with *Sal*I, ligated to *Sal*I-cut pSR-REP, and transfected onto CEF according to the procedure of Wigler et al. (1979). Transfected cultures were usually kept in liquid medium, but at each subculture some plates were overlaid with soft agar to maximize the detection of focus formation. Cultures transfected with pN4, pBB4, pPB5, and pTT701 showed morphological changes at approximately similar times, 6–7 days after transfection. Transformation quickly spread, and usually within 9 days the entire culture was transformed. During the same period of time, no morphological changes were detectable in pHB5- and

pTT501-transfected cultures. These cultures showed some focal morphological changes later than 11 days. However, these changes in pHB5 and pTT501 cultures did not spread, and they remained within a small minority of the cells in the cultures continuously up to 25 days when the experiment was terminated.

The success of cotransfection of each DNA with pSR-REP was evaluated by the assay of reverse transcriptase activity in the medium of transfected cultures, which indicates the production of infectious virus. The enzyme activity became detectable in 6–7 days and reached a maximum in 8–9 days in all cultures, including those transfected with pHB5 and pTT501. Therefore, we concluded that in every case cotransfection with pSR-REP was successfully established and infectious virus was spread to the entire culture by 9 days.

Figure 4 shows results of the analysis of proviral DNA in transfected cultures at 9 days after transfection. Total cellular DNA was digested with *Sal*I and *Bgl*II, and after electrophoresis the blot was hybridized with a *v-src* probe. Lanes 1 and 2 show the *Sal*I–*Bgl*II fragments of plasmid pHB5 and pTT501. Their size agreed with the expected values, 8.9 kb and 2.9 kb, respectively. DNA fragments from transfected cultures were run in lanes 4 to 6. The 14.0-kb band present in each lane should be derived

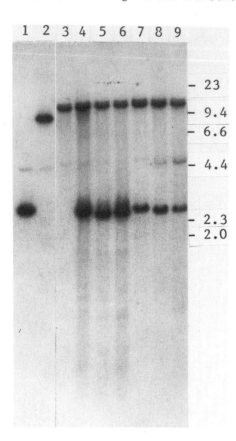

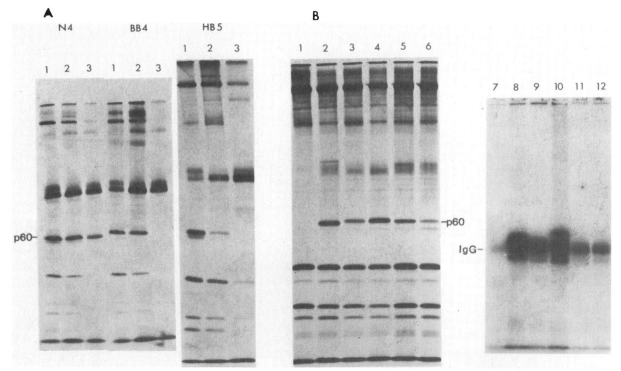

Figure 4 Analysis of proviral DNA in transfected cultures. DNA samples were completely digested with both *Sal*I and *Bgl*II and analyzed by Southern blot hybridization. The probe used for hybridization was a ^{32}P-labeled 0.87-kb *Pvu*II DNA fragment from pTT107 (Takeya et al. 1981), which contains about 60% of the *v-src*-coding sequence. (Lanes *1* and *2*) DNA of plasmid pHB5 and pTT501; (lane *3*) untransfected CEF DNA; (lanes *4–6*) DNA from CEF at 9 days after transfection with pN4, pHB5, and pTT501 together with pSR-REP; (lanes *7–9*) DNA from CEF infected with high titers of viruses NYN4, NYHB5, and NY501. The figures shown at right indicate the size (in kb) of *Hin*dIII-cut λ DNA fragments.

Figure 5 Analysis of proteins extracted from transfected cultures. (*A*) Autoradiogram of immunoprecipitates of extracts from [3H]leucine-labeled cultures infected with NYN4, NYBB4, and NYHB5. Three preparations (lanes *1–3*) of TBR serum were used for immunoprecipitation. (*B*) Autoradiogram of immunoprecipitates of extracts from [3H]leucine-labeled cultures at 9 days after transfection (lanes *1–6*) and that of reaction products of protein kinase assay on these immunoprecipitates (lanes *7–12*): untransfected CEF (lanes *1* and *7*), CEF transfected with pN4 (lanes *2* and *8*), pPB5 (lanes *3* and *9*), pBB4 (lanes *4* and *10*), pHB5 (lanes *5* and *11*), and pTT501 (lanes *6* and *12*).

from the endogenous *c-src* locus, since the same band appeared in lane 3—control untransfected cell DNA. Except for this 14.0-kb band, all cultures contained only one band of 2.9 kb or 2.8 kb, which corresponds to the *Sa*l–*Bgl*II fragments of pN4 and pHB5, respectively, lacking introns. The pTT501-transfected culture also contained the same 2.8-kb DNA, indicating that at this point in the transfection, the introns in the transfected pHB5 or pTT501 DNAs were processed in mRNA and packaged into infectious virions. The vast majority of cultures were infected with virus containing the processed RNA.

The formation of p60^{src} in transfected cultures was analyzed by immunoprecipitation with tumor-bearing rabbit (TBR) serum. Since p60^{src}s expected to be produced by the transfected DNAs are not identical in their amino acid sequences, we first examined the specificity of the immunoprecipitation of p60^{src} products with available TBR sera. The serum used for precipitation of cell extracts from cultures infected with viruses obtained from pN4-, pBB4-, and pHB5-transfected cultures in Figure 5A (lane 3) was known to be incapable of precipitating cellular p60^{c-src}. As seen in Figure 5A, this serum recognized only the *src* protein made by pN4, whereas two other TBR sera (lanes 1 and 2) recognized p60^{src} of all three cultures. Since the differences between pN4 and pBB4 or pHB5 are limited to the *Bgl*I–*Bgl*II fragment, the serum used in lane 3 appears to recognize primarily determinants dependent on the *v-src*-specific carboxyl terminus.

Since the TBR serum used in lane 1 of Figure 5A recognized p60^{src} encoded by all three plasmids, this serum was used for the analysis of p60^{src} in cultures at 9 days after transfection. As seen in Figure 5B, although there were some differences in the amounts precipitated, all transfected cultures contained significant levels of p60^{src}, and this was shown also in the levels of protein kinase activity measured by phosphorylation of IgG (Fig. 5B, lanes 7–12).

These results indicate that all transfected cultures, including those that received pHB5 and pTT501, which showed only limited and focal morphological transformation, were infected to about the same extent by virus containing processed *src* RNA and produced significant levels of p60^{src}, which is an active protein kinase. Therefore, one can conclude that pBB4 and pPB5, which contain 5′ *v-src* and 3′ *c-src*, and pTT701, which contains 5′ *c-src* and 3′ *v-src*, probably transform cells as efficiently as pN4 (wild type). However, plasmids containing the complete *c-src* gene induced cell transformation poorly, if at all, compared with plasmids containing the complete *v-src* gene or a recombinant *src* gene.

Production of transforming virus from transfected cultures

The production of transforming virus in transfected cultures was assayed by titration on CEF. Figure 6 shows a representative result. The titer of transforming virus in pN4-, pBB4-, and pPB5-transfected cultures reached a maximum of about 10^7 ffu/ml 9 days after transfection.

In a separate experiment, a similar result was obtained in pTT701-transfected cultures. On the other hand, the titer of transforming virus was 10–10,000 times lower in pHB5- and pTT501-transfected cultures. Furthermore, no substantial increase in titer was seen after 9 days. As is discussed above, the production of virus, as measured by production of reverse transcriptase in the medium, was approximately the same in all the transfected cultures, and reached a maximum 9 days after transfection.

The morphologies of foci of transformed cells induced by these viruses were different from each other. Basically, foci induced by NYN4, NYBB4, and NYPB5 (viruses recovered from transfection with pN4, pBB4, and pPB5) were similar to each other (although not identical), with transformed cells somewhat spread, whereas NY701, NY501, and NYHB5 produced more compact, smaller foci reminiscent of those of rASVs (Hanafusa et al. 1977).

The few foci seen in pTT501- and pHB5-transfected cultures were sensitive to culture conditions. Foci were nearly undetectable in liquid medium or under a soft agar overlay (3.8%) but were detectable with a hard agar overlay (7.5%). The transformed cells were easily lost in subculture.

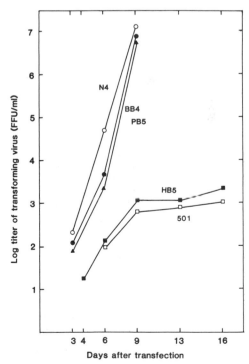

Figure 6 Production of transforming virus from transfected cultures. Culture fluid of cultures at various days after transfection was assayed for transforming virus on fresh CEF. (○) N4; (●) BB4; (▲) PB5; (■) HB5; (□) 501.

Table 1 Effects of Subculture on Focus Formation in NY 501-infected Cultures

	Dilution of virus						
	10^0	10^{-1}	10^{-2}	10^{-3}	10^{-4}	10^{-5}	10^{-6}
Original culture	32[a]	8	1	0	0	0	0
After first subculture	196	228	96	29	7	0	0
After second subculture	276	240	236	118	31	15	0

CEFs were infected with 10-fold serial dilutions of culture fluid obtained from a culture at 9 days after transfection with pTT501. The infected cultures were subcultured at 4-day intervals, and at each subculture one plate was overlaid with agar for counting foci of transformed cells.

[a]Number of foci/plate.

The culture fluid of a pTT501-transfected culture was assayed for transforming virus by infection of fresh CEF. The results are shown in Table 1. The minimum dilution yielding foci before passage, 10^{-2}, contains about 10^3 infectious units (as measured by interference assay). Therefore, the infectious unit/focus-forming unit ratio for this virus is about 10^3, compared with a ratio of about 1 for wild-type SR-RSV. This result confirms the weakly transforming or nontransforming nature of NY501 virus.

The reason for the small number of foci observed in these cultures is under investigation. The kinetics of the appearance of foci on the subculture of plates infected with high dilutions of virus (Table 1) might suggest that these foci represent mutations derived predominantly during passage. However, we cannot rule out the possibility that the pTT501 genome can transform a small minority of clones of CEF.

Passaged viruses from NY501- and NYHB5-infected cultures were assayed for induction of colony formation in soft agar. Colonies resulted that were only slightly smaller than wild-type SR-RSV-induced colonies, and virus recovered from these colonies was highly transforming, with titers comparable to wild-type virus titers. This strong difference from the original NY501 or NYHB5 virus stocks is clear evidence that highly transforming mutants are easily recovered from the pTT501 or pHB5 genomes.

Summary

By transfection of chicken cells with RSV DNA in which various portions of v-src were replaced with corresponding c-src sequences, we found the replacement of v-src either upstream or downstream from the BglI site with c-src sequences did not affect the transforming activity of the resultant virus. However, in cultures transfected with viral DNA in which the src sequence is totally replaced by the c-src sequence, we found the gene product p60[src] is expressed without appreciable transformation of cells. Therefore, we conclude that the c-src product cannot transform chicken cells in the same way the v-src product does. In c-src DNA-transfected cultures, we found the production of weakly transforming viruses. We have not yet determined whether these weakly transforming viruses carry the unaltered c-src gene or a mutated gene. After passage, however, strongly transforming mutant viruses emerged. These results show that after a proto-oncogene is incorporated into a retroviral genome, transforming mutants are rapidly generated, and they can be selected on the basis of their transforming capacity.

Acknowledgments

We are greatly indebted to J. Brugge, R. Erikson, and B. Sefton for supplying us with sera against p60. We thank also R. Williams for excellent technical assistance. The work was supported by Public Health Service grants CA14935 and 18213 from the National Cancer Institute. F.C. is supported by training grant T32AI07233.

References

Bishop, J.M. 1983. Cellular oncogenes and retroviruses. *Annu. Rev. Biochem.* **52:** 301.

Blair, D.G., M.K. Oskarsson, T.G. Wood, W.L. McClements, P.J. Fischinger, and G.F. Vande Woude. 1981. Activation of the transforming potential of a normal cell sequence: A molecular model for oncogenesis. *Science* **212:** 941.

Chang, E.H., M.E. Furth, E.M. Scolnick, and D.R. Lowy. 1982. Tumorigenic transformation of mammalian cells induced by a normal human gene homologous to the oncogene of Harvey murine sarcoma virus. *Nature* **297:** 479.

Cooper, G.M. and S. Okenquist. 1978. Mechanism of transfection of chicken embryo fibroblasts by Rous sarcoma virus DNA. *J. Virol.* **28:** 45.

Cross, F.R. and H. Hanafusa. 1983. Local mutagenesis of Rous sarcoma virus: The major sites of tyrosine and serine phosphorylation of p60[src] are dispensable for transformation. *Cell* **34:** 597.

Czernilofsky, A.P., A.D. Levinson, H.E. Varmus, J.M. Bishop, E. Tischer, and H.M. Goodman. 1980. Nucleotide sequence of an avian sarcoma virus oncogene (src) and proposed amino acid sequence for gene product. *Nature* **287:** 198.

———. 1983. Corrections to the nucleotide sequence of the src gene of Rous sarcoma virus. *Nature* **301:** 736.

DeFeo, D., M.A. Gonda, H.A. Young, E.H. Chang, D.R. Lowy, E.M. Scolnick, and R.W. Ellis. 1981. Analysis of two divergent rat genomic clones homologous to the transforming gene of Harvey murine sarcoma virus. *Proc. Natl. Acad. Sci.* **78:** 3328.

Der, J.C., T.G. Krontiris, and G.M. Cooper. 1982. Transforming genes of human bladder and lung carcinoma cell lines are homologous to the ras genes of Harvey and Kirsten sarcoma viruses. *Proc. Natl. Acad. Sci.* **79:** 3637.

Hanafusa, H., C.C. Halpern, D.L. Buchhagen, and S. Kawai. 1977. Recovery of avian sarcoma virus from tumors induced by transformation-defective mutants. *J. Exp. Med.* **146:** 1735.

Karess, R.E. and H. Hanafusa. 1981. Viral and cellular *src* genes contribute to the structure of recovered avian sarcoma virus transforming protein. *Cell* **24:** 155.

Oskarsson, M., W.L. McClements, D.G. Blair, J.V. Maizel, and G.F. Vande Woude. 1980. Properties of a normal mouse cell DNA sequence (*sarc*) homologous to the *src* sequence of Moloney sarcoma virus. *Science* **207:** 1222.

Parker, R.C., H.E. Varmus, and J.M. Bishop. 1981. Cellular homologue (*c-src*) of the transforming gene of Rous sarcoma virus: Isolation, mapping, and transcriptional analysis of *c-src* and flanking regions. *Proc. Natl. Acad. Sci.* **78:** 5842.

Reddy, E.P., R.K. Reynolds, E. Santos, and M. Barbacid. 1982. A point mutation is responsible for the acquisition of transforming properties by the T24 human bladder carcinoma oncogene. *Nature* **300:** 149.

Schwartz, D.E., R. Tizard, and W. Gilbert. 1983. Nucleotide sequence of Rous sarcoma virus. *Cell* **32:** 853.

Shalloway, D., A.D. Zelenetz, and G.M. Cooper. 1981. Molecular cloning and characterization of the chicken gene homologous to the transforming gene of Rous sarcoma virus. *Cell* **24:** 531.

Tabin, C.J., S.M. Bradley, C.I. Bargmann, R.A. Weinberg, A.G. Papageorge, E.M. Scolnick, R. Dhar, D.R. Lowy, and E.H. Chang. 1982. Mechanism of activation of human oncogene. *Nature* **300:** 143.

Takeya, T. and H. Hanafusa. 1982. DNA sequence of the viral and cellular *src* gene of chicken. II. Comparison of the *src* genes of two strains of avian sarcoma virus and of the cellular homolog. *J. Virol.* **44:** 12.

———. 1983. Structure and sequence of the cellular gene homologous to the RSV *src* gene and the mechanism for generating the transforming virus. *Cell* **32:** 881.

Takeya, T., R.A. Feldman, and H. Hanafusa. 1982. DNA sequence of the viral and cellular *src* gene of chicken. I. The complete nucleotide sequence of an EcoRI fragment of recovered avian sarcoma virus which codes for gp37 and pp60^{src}. *J. Virol.* **44:** 1.

Takeya, T., H. Hanafusa, R.P. Junghans, G. Ju, and A.M. Skalka. 1981. Comparisons between the viral transforming gene (*src*) of recovered avian sarcoma virus and its cellular homolog. *Mol. Cell. Biol.* **1:** 1024.

Taparowsky, E., Y. Suard, O. Fusano, K. Shimizu, M. Goldfarb, and M. Wigler. 1982. Activation of the T24 bladder carcinoma transforming gene is linked to a single amino acid change. *Nature* **300:** 762.

Wang, L.-H., C.C. Halpern, M. Nadel, and H. Hanafusa. 1978. Recombination between viral and cellular sequences generates transforming sarcoma viruses. *Proc. Natl. Acad. Sci.* **75:** 5812.

Wigler, M., A. Pellicer, S. Silverstein, R. Axel, G. Urlaub, and L. Chasin. 1979. DNA-mediated transfer of the adenine phosphoribosyltransferase locus into mammalian cells. *Proc. Natl. Acad. Sci.* **76:** 1373.

c-src and src Homolog Overexpression in Mouse Cells

D. Shalloway, P.M. Coussens, and P. Yaciuk

Molecular and Cell Biology Program, The Pennsylvania State University, University Park, Pennsylvania 16802

The extensive characterization of the biochemical and biological phenotypes associated with v-src transformation has provided us with a molecular overview of at least one mechanism of neoplastic transformation and a data base from which to begin determining the causal factors and relationships involved. The unusual tyrosine kinase activity of pp60^{v-src}, a property shared with other oncogenic proteins and peptide hormone receptors, provides a convenient biochemical "handle" for tracing src activity and appears to be required for transformation (Sefton et al. 1980; Ushiro and Cohen 1980; Beemon 1981; Hunter and Cooper 1981; Reynolds et al. 1981; Ek et al. 1982; Kasuga et al. 1982). The effect of v-src transformation on cellular tyrosine phosphorylation is dramatic: Total cellular phosphotyrosine content increases about eightfold (Hunter and Sefton 1980; Sefton et al. 1980) and the level of phosphotyrosine is significantly enhanced in a large number of proteins (Radke and Martin 1979; Cooper and Hunter 1981; Beemon et al. 1982; Martinez et al. 1982). It seems likely that only a subset of these proteins is directly phosphorylated by pp60^{v-src} and that many proteins are phosphorylated by other cellular kinases which themselves are activated directly or indirectly by pp60^{v-src}. Elucidation of the causal progression of tyrosine kinase activity through the cellular molecular machinery would provide valuable insight into the mechanism of transformation, but the large number of potential direct substrates for the src tyrosine kinase activity complicates such analysis.

One approach to this problem is to compare the tyrosine phosphorylation patterns induced by homologs of pp60^{v-src} to see if the phosphorylation substrates can be segregated into distinguishable subgroups that are coordinately phosphorylated and to see how phosphorylation of these subgroups is correlated with other biological and biochemical parameters of transformation. Transfection of NIH-3T3 cells with recombinant src expression plasmids provides an attractive model system for such comparison: Homologous cells, which differ only because of the expression of single plasmid-coded gene products, can be generated and compared. We have begun such a study by constructing genes coding for a number of closely related homologs of pp60^{v-src} and are investigating their transforming activity and patterns of induced tyrosine phosphorylation.

A natural homolog to consider is pp60^{c-src}, the cellular product of the chicken c-src gene from which v-src was originally derived. Like pp60^{v-src}, pp60^{c-src} has tyrosine kinase activity (Hunter and Sefton 1980) but its prop-

erties have not been well studied because of technical difficulties associated with its low level of expression in normal cells. The extensive conservation of c-src in animal evolution (Shiloh and Weinberg 1981) suggests that it plays an important role in the cell and that transformation due to v-src may result from perturbation of a normal growth or developmental regulatory pathway mediated by c-src. Because pp60^{v-src} is expressed at 10–100-fold higher levels in transformed cells than pp60^{c-src} is expressed in normal cells (Collett et al. 1978; Karess et al. 1979; Opperman et al. 1979), it has not been known whether v-src transformation is the result of the high level of expression, of functional differences between the v-src and c-src proteins, or both.

Comparison between the v-src and c-src sequences shows that the inferred amino acid sequences of the two proteins are very similar except at the immediate carboxyl termini (Takeya and Hanafusa 1982, 1983; Czernilofsky et al. 1983; Schwartz et al. 1983). This is in accord with in vivo recombination studies that show that the endogenous chicken c-src gene can complement deletions in all of v-src genes except possibly for a region of less than 100 nucleotides at the 3′ end of the gene (Karess et al. 1979; L.-H. Wang, pers. comm.). These results suggest that if c-src and v-src functional differences do exist, they derive from structural differences at the carboxyl termini. Accordingly, we have concentrated our investigation on the activities of molecularly cloned recombinant genes that generate pp60^{src} homologs with modified carboxyl termini.

Methods

Plasmids

pCS12.13 (and four other plasmids differing in the location of the SV40 promoter relative to c-src exon number 1) was generated by a multistep cloning procedure. The resultant plasmid contains the DNA segments described in Figure 1 ligated together as follows (proceeding counterclockwise from the top): (1) the c-src HindIII site at location 9.5 kbp (all c-src map locations refer to Fig. 1 in Shalloway et al. [1981]) was filled in with a DNA polymerase Klenow fragment (New England Biolabs) and blunt-end ligated to the filled-in pBR322 EcoRI site; (2) the pBR322 PvuII site was ligated to the PvuII site proximal to the late side of the SV40 origin; (3) the SV40 origin-Ecogpt-SV40 early region-SV40 origin DNA segment is as described for plasmid pSV3-gpt by Mulligan and Berg (1980); (4) the following Ecogpt-

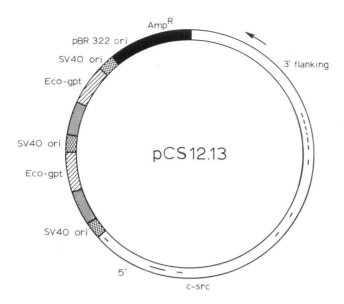

Figure 1 *c-src* expression plasmid pCS12.13. This plasmid (and four others differing in the amount of separation between the SV40 promoter and *c-src* exon number 1) were constructed by a multistep cloning procedure from pBR322, SV40, and bacterial (*Ecogpt*) and chicken *c-src* DNA. Proceeding counterclockwise from the top, they contain DNA sequence from (1) pBR322 (*Eco*RI–*Pvu*II fragment) containing the *amp*^R gene and origin of replication, (2) SV40 origin-*Ecogpt*-SV40 early-region DNA derived from the *Pvu*II–*Bam*HI fragment of pSV2, (3) a direct repeat of the region in (2) except beginning at the *Hpa*II site near the SV40 origin, (4) the SV40 origin region (*Hpa*II–*Hind*III fragment) containing the 72-bp tandem repeat (enhancer) and early promoter, and (5) the chicken *c-src* locus running from a BAL 31-generated location at 3.7 kp to a *Hind*III site at 9.5 kb (see Fig. 1 in Shalloway et al. [1981] for coordinates). The locations of the exons determined by heteroduplex analysis and sequencing are indicated by the lines in the *c-src* region. The SV40 promoter is upstream from exon number 1. Total length ≈ 20.5 kb.

SV40 early region-SV40 origin segment is a direct repeat of that in (3);(5) the *Hind*III site on the early side of the SV40 origin was filled in and ligated to a *Sal*I linker (Collaborative Research); and (6) the *Sal*I site was ligated to a *Sal*I site provided by a linker attached to BAL 31-(Bethesda Research Labs) trimmed *c-src* DNA derived from λ phage λCS3 (Shalloway et al. 1981). (Plasmid pCS1B.13 containing the BAL 31-trimmed, *Sal*I-linked *c-src* DNA was provided by A.D. Zelenetz and G.M. Cooper). Plasmid pCS12.13 was linearized for transfection by cutting at the unique *Pvu*I site in the pBR322 segment or at the unique *Bss*HII site at *c-src* location 6.1 kb (1.3 kb downstream from the *c-src* termination codon).

Plasmid psrc11 (provided by A.D. Zelenetz and G.M. Cooper) is composed of three ligated fragments: (1) the *Pvu*II (site located 33 bp upstream from the *v-src* termination codon)–*Xho*I (site located about 250 bp downstream from the *gag* initiation codon) fragment from cloned Schmidt Ruppin(SR)-RSV-D circular-form DNA which contains a long teminal repeat (LTR) and the 5′ end of *gag* (including the normal splice donor site); (2) the *Sal*I (site located about 700 bp upstream from the *env* termination codon)–*Xho*I (site located about 250 bp downstream from the downstream *gag* initiation codon) fragment from SR-RSV-D DNA containing the 3′ end of *env*, *v-src*, the downstream LTR, and the 5′ end of *gag*; and (3) the pBR322 *Sal*I–*Pvu*II origin and *amp*^R fragment. (See Fig. 5 in Shalloway et al. [1981] for a SR-RSV-D restriction map.) These fragments are ligated together in the order given (*Sal*I and *Xho*I are cross-ligated twice).

Plasmid pRS2 was constructed by replacing the *Bgl*I (site in the *v-src*-coding sequence)–*Bam*HI (site in the pBR322-derived segment) fragment from psrc11 containing the *v-src* 3′ end with the *Bgl*I (site in the *c-src* coding-sequence)–*Bam*HI (*c-src* map location 6.0, about

1.15 kb downstream from the *c-src* termination codon) *c-src* fragment from pCS12.13.

Plasmid pRS3 is identical to pCS12.13 except that the *c-src* region between the *Bgl*I site (*c-src* map location 4.4 kb) and the *Sac*I site (at *c-src* map location 4.9 kb) was replaced by a *Bgl*I–*Sac*I RSV circular-form DNA fragment (excised from psrc11) containing the *v-src* 3′ end and downstream LTR. The *Sac*I site in pCS12.13 is 11 bp downstream from the *c-src* termination codon. It was ligated to the *Sac*I site in the RSV fragment, which is about 120 bp upstream of the *gag*-coding region. The *Bgl*I site used is at the sequence coding for amino acid 431 in both *c-src* and *v-src*.

The structure of the recombinant plasmid was verified by restriction mapping. Plasmid pRS3 was linearized for transfection by cutting at the unique *Bss*HII site at *c-src* location 6.1 kb.

Plasmid RS4 was constructed by replacing the *Pvu*II (site 33 bp upstream from the *v-src* termination codon)–*Bgl*I (site in the *amp*^R gene) psrc11 fragment containing the *v-src* 3′ terminal region and downstream LTR with the *Pvu*II (SV40 sequence location 3509, Tooze [1981])–*Bgl*I (site in the *amp*^R gene) fragment from pSV3 (Mulligan and Berg 1980). This fragment contains the sequence coding for the 3′ end of SV40 T antigen, the early SV40 polyadenylation site, and SV40 sequence up to the SV40 *Eco*RI site.

Tissue culture and biological assays

NIH-3T3 mouse cells and C57BL/6J-3T3 mouse cells (the latter donated by N. Copeland and N. Jenkins) were grown and assayed in Temin's modified Eagle's medium (M.A. Bioproducts) supplemented with 10% calf serum. This medium was supplemented with mycophenolic acid (25 μg/ml), aminopterin (2 μg/ml), xanthine (250 μg/ml), adenine (25 μg/ml), and thymidine (10 μg/ml) to make *Ecogpt*-selective media (Mulligan and Berg 1981).

Transfection of NIH-3T3 cells and C57BL/6J-3T3 cells was initialized by plating cells at a density of 5×10^5 cells/60-mm culture dish. After overnight incubation at 37°C, the cells were inoculated with linearized DNA and treated with 15% glycerol as described by Copeland and Cooper (1979). Media were changed at 2–3-day intervals, and foci of neoplastically transformed cells were counted 12–14 days after exposure to DNA. pCS12.13-transfected cells were selected for *Ecogpt* expression using selective media as described by Mulligan and Berg (1981). Transfected cells were biologically cloned by end-point dilution in multiwell plates.

Colony formation in soft agarose by transfected NIH-3T3 cell lines was assayed by plating 3×10^5 cells in 4 ml of medium containing 0.25% agarose over a base layer of 3 ml of medium containing 0.5% agarose. Colonies were counted after 7–14 days of incubation at 37°C. Photomicrographs were made after 10 days.

In vivo tumorigenicity was assayed by scraping transfected and biologically selected C57BL/6J cells from culture dishes and injecting 6×10^5 cells subcutaneously in the neck region of syngeneic C57BL/6J mice (Jackson Labs). Mice were checked for tumor growth at 3–4-day intervals for 14 weeks. Normal C57BL/6J-3T3 cells are not tumorigenic in this assay.

Immune complex kinase assay

Cell lysis and immune complex kinase assays were performed essentially as described by Collett and Erickson (1978), except that protein A beads (Pharmacia) were substituted for protein A containing *Staphylococcus aureus* and adsorption times were increased to 45 minutes at 4°C. Protein kinase activity was assayed by adding 0.2–1.0 μM [γ-^{32}P]ATP (>400 Ci/mmole; ICN) to the phosphorylation reaction mixture and incubating for 10 minutes at room temperature.

Samples were analyzed by electrophoresis in 10% polyacrylamide gels containing 0.8% *N*,*N*′-methylene-bis-acrylamide using the buffer system described by Laemmli (1970). The phosphorylated IgG heavy chain (IgG-H) was visualized by autoradiography (approximately 12-hr exposure with an intensifying screen).

Phosphoamino acid analysis

Cells were seeded at a density of 3.5×10^6/60-mm plate. After 8–10 hours, the plates were rinsed twice with prewarmed 150 mM NaCl/50 mM Tris-HCl (pH 7.2)/1 mM EDTA solution, and the cells were labeled by adding 2 ml of phosphate-free DMEM (GIBCO) supplemented with 0.5–1.0 mCi/ml [^{32}P]orthophosphate (carrier free, ICN). Labeling was for 12–14 hours. Cell lysis and analysis of total phosphoamino acid content were performed as described by Hunter and Sefton (1980); 1.5×10^6 cpm of each hydrolyzate was used. ^{32}P-labeled phosphoamino acids were visualized by autoradiography with an intensifying screen for 8 hours.

Results

c-src expression plasmids

To investigate the effects of enhanced *c-src* expression, we constructed plasmids in which the SV40 origin region (containing the enhancer and early promoter) was ligated upstream of *c-src* exon number 1 (noncoding) (Parker et al. 1981; Shalloway et al. 1981; Takeya et al. 1981; Swanstrom et al. 1983; Takeya and Hanafusa 1983). Since our preliminary promoter-*c-src* transfection experiments had indicated that *c-src* would not transform NIH-3T3 cells, the *Ecogpt* gene was also included to provide biological selection of stably transfected cells even in the absence of neoplastic transformation. Five plasmids of this type, differing only in the location of the SV40 promoter, were created by a multistep cloning procedure (Fig. 1). No foci were observed in multiple transfection experiments with these plasmids, so genetically transformed cells were isolated using *Ecogpt*-selective media and were analyzed for immune complex phosphorylation of cross-reactive RSV-induced tumor-bearing rabbit (TBR) IgG. Cells expressing *Ecogpt* activity from any of the five plasmids also showed enhanced in vitro kinase activity (ranging from 10- to 100-fold over the endogenous level in NIH-3T3 cells) (Fig. 2, data not shown for one plasmid), suggesting that pp60^{c-src} was being overexpressed. Since plasmid pCS12.13 induced the highest amount of in vitro kinase activity, it was selected for further study. Cells transfected with this plasmid were biologically cloned to generate cell line NIH(pCS12.13).3. Immunoprecipitates from in vivo ^{32}P-labeled NIH(pCS12.13).3 cells using *v-src* TBR sera showed the presence of enhanced levels of a 60-kD phosphoprotein (data not shown) consistent with overexpression of correctly initiated pp60^{c-src}. Since the *c-src* sequence shows that there are at least 30 codons in exons numbers 1 and 2 separating the normal *c-src* initiation codon from any potential upstream initiation codon, we know that a protein initiated at such an inappropriate upstream site would have a molecular weight of greater than 63,000 in contrast with this result.

5′ *c-src*–3′ *v-src* recombinant

The absence of transformation in the pCS12.13-transfected cells strongly suggests that functional differences between pp60^{v-src} and pp60^{c-src} are involved in transformation. To see if the significant structural differences could be localized as well as to verify that the transfected *c-src* sequences were being correctly expressed, the 3′ end of the *c-src* gene in plasmid pCS12.13 was replaced with the corresponding end of the SR-D *v-src* gene to generate plasmid pRS3 (Fig. 3). The replacement took place beginning at a *Bgl*I site (corresponding to amino acid position 431) lying in sequence common to both *v-src* and *c-src*. This site is 15 amino acids downstream from the *src* phosphotyrosine residue and (based on comparison of the SR-A [Takeya and Hanafusa 1982; Czernilofsky et al. 1983] and *c-src* [Takeya and Hanafusa 1983] sequences) results in the exchange of isolated amino acids at positions 467, 469, and 474, and substitution of the 12 amino acids at the carboxyl end of *v-src* for the 19 amino acids at the carboxyl end of *c-src* (Fig. 4). Transfection of this plasmid into NIH-3T3 cells caused efficient focus formation, 10^4 foci/pmole, an enhancement of at least 5×10^3 relative to *c-src* expression

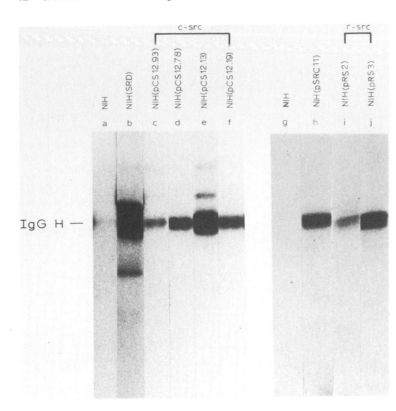

Figure 2 Immune complex kinase assay. Cell lysates were prepared and assayed for in vivo kinase activity as described in Methods. Lysates were prepared from (lane *a*) normal NIH-3T3 mouse cells, (*b*) cells neoplastically transformed with *v-src* DNA, (*c–f*) cells transfected with *c-src* expression plasmids pCS12.93, pCS12.78, pCS12.13, and pCS12.19 and selected for stable *Ecogpt* expression, (*g*) NIH-3T3 cells, and (*h–j*) cells transformed with plasmids psrc11, pRS2, and pRS3. Lanes *a–f* and lanes *g–j* have been cut from autoradiographs from two separate experiments, respectively. The relative amounts of IgG heavy chain (IgG-H) phosphorylation for the two experiments are 0.005:1:0.05:0.1:0.5:0.1 (*a:b:c:d:e:f*) and –:1:0.5:1.4 (*g:h:i:j*).

plasmid pCS12.13 (Table 1). pRS3-transformed cells show high levels of in vitro kinase activity comparable to that found in *v-src*-transformed cells (Fig. 2).

5′ *v-src*–3′ *c-src* recombination
The stimulation of *c-src* focus-forming activity by recombination with the *v-src* 3′ end suggested that *v-src* focus-forming activity would be inhibited by replacement of its 3′ end with the corresponding sequence from *c-src*. To investigate this hypothesis, we created the inverse recombinant pRS2 (Fig. 3) by joining the 5′ end of the SR-D *v-src* gene to the 3′ end of the *c-src* gene at the same *Bgl*I site that was used for the pRS3 construction. This plasmid was made by modifying the *v-src* expression plasmid psrc11 which uses the Rous sarcoma virus (RSV) LTR for transcriptional promotion (Fig. 3). The replacement of the *v-src* 3′ end with the *c-src* 3′ end resulted in the reduction in focus-forming activity by 500-fold (Table 1). However, in contrast to plasmid pCS12.13, a small number of foci were observed. Transformed cells from the one focus analyzed to date express high levels of in vitro kinase activity (Fig. 2). Immunoprecipitates from these cells using TBR sera show the presence of a 60-kD phosphoprotein.

v-src random carboxyterminal homolog
To explore further the role of the specific sequence at the *src* carboxyl terminus, we made a recombinant, pRS4 (Fig. 3), in which the sequence coding for the last nine amino acids of *v-src* was replaced with sequence coding for nine random amino acids. This plasmid was con-

structed by replacing the 3′ end of *v-src* in psrc11 (beginning at a *Pvu*II site 33 bp upstream of the *src* termination codon) with a SV40 DNA fragment that contains the SV40 early polyadenylation sequence. The SV40 sequence is read in an unconventional reading frame so the resultant amino acid sequence is unrelated to any SV40 proteins. The DNA in the region of the recombination was sequenced (data not shown) to verify the construction. A comparison between the predicted *c-src*, *v-src*, and pRS4 recombinant-*src* protein carboxyl termini is shown in Figure 4b. Transfection of plasmid pRS4 induced focus formation with the same frequency as transfection with *v-src* expression plasmid psrc11 (Table 1), indicating the specific *v-src* carboxyl terminus is not required for transforming activity. Transformed cells from these foci express a high level of in vitro kinase activity comparable to that found in *v-src*-transformed cells (data not shown).

Characterization of *c-src* overexpresser cells
The set of homologous mouse cell lines that have been transfected with the *v-src*, *c-src*, and recombinant-*src* (*r-src*) plasmids can now be used for comparison of biological and biochemical parameters, particularly tyrosine phosphorylation substrates. We have begun this investigation by focusing on the NIH(pCS12.13) *c-src* overexpresser cells.

Whereas cells transfected with pCS12.13 do not form foci (Table 1), their morphological characteristics are intermediate between those of normal NIH-3T3 cells and *c-src*-transformed cells (Fig. 5a). Furthermore, they form

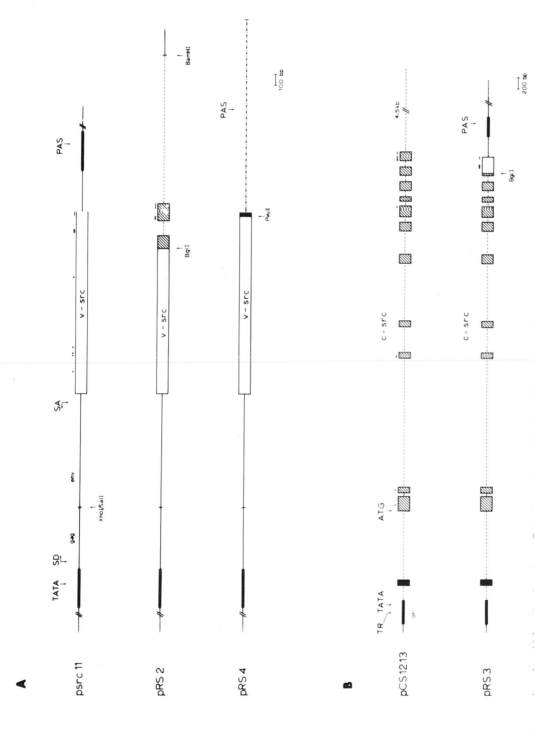

Figure 3 *src* expression plasmid functional regions. Only the coding and eukaryotic control regions of the plasmids are shown. The fragments shown are embedded in pBR322-derived vectors. Plasmids pCS12.13 and pRS3 also contain two copies of the *Ecogpt* selectable marker. (*A*) Plasmids using the RSV LTR promoter: psrc11 uses the LTR, *gag* splice donor, and *src* splice acceptor for the expression of SR-D *v-src*. pRS2 was derived from psrc11 by replacing the sequence downstream from the *v-src Bgl*I site (at the sequence coding for amino acid 431) with the corresponding *c-src* 3′ end including 1.15 kb of downstream flanking sequence. (*B*) Plasmids using the SV40 early promoter: pCS12.13 contains an SV40 enhancer-early promoter upstream from *c-src* exon number 1 (noncoding), the unspliced *c-src* gene, and 4.5 kb of downstream flanking sequence. pRS3 was derived from pCS12.13 by replacing the sequence downstream from the *c-src Bgl*I site with the SR-D *v-src* 3′ end and downstream LTR. Dots or bars above the coding sequence regions specify the locations of differences between *c-src* and SR-A *v-src* inferred amino acid sequences. (SD) Splice donor; (SA) splice acceptor; (PAS) polyadenylation sequence; (TATA) promoter TATA box; (TR) SV40 origin 72-bp tandem repeat sequences. (▨) *c-src* coding; (▨) *v-src* coding; (□) *c-src* noncoding; (▩) random coding; (▬▬) *c-src* control element; (·······) SV 40. (▬▬) pBR322; (▬▬) RSV; (— — —) chicken; (▬▬▬) SV40.

A

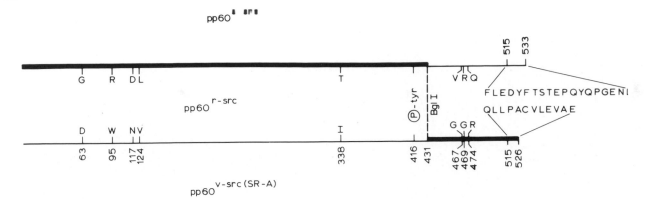

B

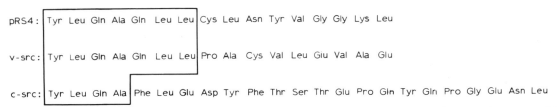

Figure 4 Predicted pp60[r-src] amino acid sequences. (*A*) The positions of the amino acid differences between pp60[c-src] and pp60[v-src] (SR-A) are shown using the one-letter amino acid symbols. The protein sequence coded by pRS3 is indicated by the heavy line; the sequence coded by pRS2 is indicated by the light line. (*B*) Comparison of the predicted amino acid sequences at the carboxyl termini of the proteins encoded by pRS4 *r-src*, *v-src*, and *c-src*. The upstream sequences are identical for pRS4 *r-src* and *v-src* and differ at isolated locations as indicated in *A* for *c-src* and *v-src*.

small colonies in soft agarose with reasonable efficiency (Fig. 5b), a characteristic that is intermediate between that of normal and *v-src*-transformed cells. The in vivo tumorigenicity of *c-src* overexpresser cells in mice has been tested by injecting C57BL/6J mice with syngeneic C57BL/6J-3T3 mouse cells transfected with plasmids pCS12.13 or p*src*11. Although all 15 syngeneic mice injected with 6 × 10⁶ p*src*11-transfected cells/mouse

developed tumors within 7 days, none of the 10 mice injected with pCS12.13-transfected cells developed tumors within 14 weeks.

NIH(pCS12.13).3 cells were labeled in vivo (12–14 hr) with ^{32}P and lysates were analyzed to determine total phosphoamino acid composition (Fig. 6). The *c-src* overexpresser cells have the same level of phosphotyrosine relative to total phosphoamino acids (0.24%) as do the

Table 1 Transformation of NIH-3T3 Cells by *src* Homolog Expression Plasmids

Donor DNA	Expressed protein	Focus-forming activity (foci/pmole DNA)
Carrier DNA	—	—
p*src*11	(*v-src*)	2 × 10⁴
pCS12.13	(*c-src*)	< 2
pRS2	(5′ *v-src*; 3′ *c-src*)	40
pRS3	(5′ *c-src*; 3′ *v-src*)	1 × 10⁴
pRS4	(carboxyterminal *r-src*)	2 × 10⁴

NIH-3T3 mouse cells were transfected with (0.01 μg donor + 20 μg carrier) DNA/60-mm culture plate as described in Methods.

Foci were counted 12–14 days after transfection. A minimum of six cultures (in multiple experiments) was used for each plasmid.

NIH 3T3   NIH(pCS 12.13). 3   NIH(psrc 11)

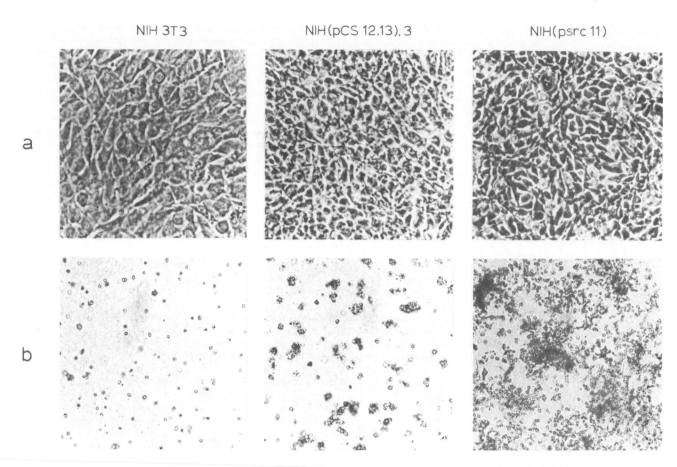

Figure 5 Biological characterization of *c-src* overexpresser cells. NIH-3T3 cells transfected with plasmid pCS12.13 were selected using the *Ecogpt* marker and were biologically cloned by end-point dilution. One of the biological clones, NIH(pCS12.13).3, was selected for further analysis. (*Left to right*) NIH-3T3, NIH(pCS12.13).3, NIH(psrc11) (*v-src*-transformed cells). (*a*) Cell morphology in monolayer culture; (*b*) growth in semisolid medium.

v-src-transformed cells, indicating that high levels of in vivo tyrosine phosphorylation is not a sufficient condition for the appearance of the full complement of *v-src*-transformed growth characteristics.

Discussion

The simplest interpretation of these results is (1) pp60$^{c\text{-}src}$ has less transforming activity than pp60$^{v\text{-}src}$— the proteins are functionally distinct; (2) the structural differences responsible for the functional differences reside near the carboxyl termini of the proteins; (3) there exists at least one significant modification of the pp60$^{v\text{-}src}$ carboxyl terminus that does not reduce transforming activity; (4) enhancement of total cellular phosphotyrosine content is not a sufficient condition for transformation.

Comparison of the focus-forming activities of pCS12.13 and pRS3 (Table 1) shows that the *c-src* 3′ end inhibits focus formation. This is consistent with the results obtained from the study of recovered avian sarcoma viruses which indicate that all but possibly the 3′ end of the endogenous *c-src* gene can be used to generate transformation-competent virus.

The efficient focus formation by pRS3 supports the hypothesis that pCS12.13 is expressing authentic pp60$^{c\text{-}src}$, since both plasmids contain exactly the same promoter system, 5′ end, and 10 out of 11 introns. The molecular weight of the immunoprecipitated pCS12.13 protein (distinguishable from the weight of a protein initiated at the nearest inappropriate Met codon) and its tyrosine kinase activity also indicate that *c-src* is being correctly expressed.

Comparison of the psrc11 and pRS2 focus-forming activities also shows that the *c-src* 3′ end inhibits focus formation. The approximate equality of kinase activity levels in cells transfected with psrc11 compared with pRS3 and in cells transfected with pRS2 compared with pCS12.13 suggests that the differences in promoter systems and splicing requirements do not significantly affect the levels of expression of the respective genes. The moderate enhancement of kinase activity expressed by the clones containing the *v-src* 3′ end (psrc11 and pRS3) or modified 3′ end (pRS4) relative to those containing the *c-src* 3′ end (pCS12.13 and pRS2) may reflect differences in sera cross-reactivity, the specific kinase activities of the proteins, or effects of the downstream flanking sequences. We do not know if suppression of transforming activity by the *c-src* 3′ end is at all associated with its downstream untranslated sequence,

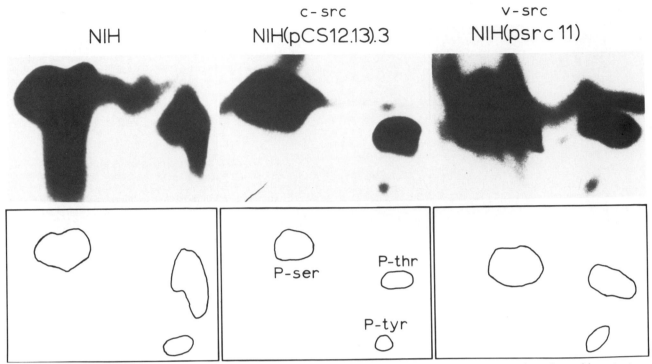

Figure 6 Analysis of whole-cell phosphoamino acid content. ^{32}P-labeled cells were analyzed for phosphoamino acid content as described in Methods. The positions of the radiolabeled phosphoamino acids (*upper figures*) were correlated with the positions of phosphoamino acid standards visualized by ninhydrin staining (*lower figures*). (*a*) Normal NIH-3T3 cells; (*b*) NIH(pCS12.13).3. (*c-src* overexpresser cells); and (*c*) NIH(psrc11) (*v-src*-transformed cells). The phosphotyrosine (total phosphoamino acid) ratio for both NIH(pCS12.13).3 and NIH(psrc11) cells is 0.24% and below background (0.05%) for normal NIH-3T3 cells.

a possibility having precedent in the case of *c-fos*, where it has been found that the 3′ untranslated sequence has an inhibitory effect on transformation (Verma et al., this volume).

We do not understand the reason for the low level of focus formation observed with *r-src* plasmid pRS2 as opposed to the total lack of transformation observed with *c-src* plasmid pCS12.13. It is possible that the isolated mutations between *v-src* and *c-src* in the region upstream from the *Bgl*I recombination site (Fig. 4) play a minor role in enhancing transforming activity. Alternatively, the difference in the amounts of downstream flanking chicken sequence present in the two clones (4.5 kb in pCS12.13, 1.15 kb in pRS2) may be relevant.

The fact that pRS2 is capable of generating a completely transformed phenotype but does so only at a significantly reduced frequency is also puzzling and may imply the involvement in the transformation process of an additional, as yet undetermined, probabilistic factor. This may relate to the differences in *c-src* transforming activity observed between experiments done in chicken (Hanafusa et al., this volume) versus mouse (this paper) or rat (Parker et al., this volume) cells. These cell-specific differences may reflect the fact that viral reinfection is an obligatory intermediate in chicken, but not rodent, cell transfection (Cooper and Okenquist 1978; Copeland et al. 1979) and that plasmids generating replication-competent virus were used in the chicken but not

rodent cell experiments. It is possible that viral replication in the chicken cell experiments amplifies a relatively rare primary event.

The transforming activity of the random carboxyterminal homolog plasmid pRS4, which generates a protein having the same length as pp60^{v-src}, is significant in view of the evident importance of the carboxyl region sequence. By contrast, a similar random carboxyterminal homolog (Ch*dl*300, constructed in Parsons' laboratory [Parsons et., this volume]), which generates a protein having the same length as pp60^{c-src}, does not induce transformation. It will be interesting to determine whether these functional differences reflect the effects of the carboxyterminal lengths, the CH*dl*300 modification of the two leucines immediately upstream from the pRS4 modification, or sequence-specific differences in the random-coded regions.

Investigation of a second biological clone of *c-src* overexpresser cells shows no evidence of high cellular phosphotyrosine levels. Thus, we are not certain at this time of the significance of the NIH(pCS12.13).3 in vivo phosphotyrosine result.

Acknowledgments

We thank T. Kmiecik for sequencing the pRS4 recombination site; P.J. Johnson, M. Wilson, and J.A. Kruper for technical assistance; A.D. Zelenetz and G.M. Cooper for providing plasmids p*src*11 and pCS1B13; J.M. Bishop, J. Brugge, H. Hanafusa, and L. Rohrschneider for TBR sera used in the early phases of these experiments; and G.M. Cooper for helpful discussion.

This investigation was supported by Public Health Service grant number 1RO1CA32317-01, an American Cancer Society Junior Faculty Research Award to D.I. Shalloway, and a generous gift from Dr. E. Shapiro.

References

Beemon, K. 1981. Transforming proteins of some feline and avian sarcoma viruses are related structurally and functionally. *Cell* **24**: 145.

Beemon, K., T. Ryden, and E.A. McNelly. 1982. Transformation by avian sarcoma viruses leads to phosphorylation of multiple cellular proteins on tyrosine residues. *J. Virol.* **42**: 742.

Collett, M.S. and R.L. Erikson. 1978. Protein kinase activity associated with the avian sarcoma virus *src* gene product. *Proc. Natl. Acad. Sci.* **75**: 2021.

Collett, M.S., J.S. Brugge, and R.L. Erikson. 1978. Characterization of a normal avian cell protein related to the avian sarcoma virus transforming gene product. *Cell* **15**: 1363.

Cooper, J.A. and T. Hunter. 1981. Changes in protein phosphorylation in Rous sarcoma virus-transformed chicken embryo cells. *Mol. Cell. Biol.* **1**: 165.

Cooper, G.M. and S. Okenquist. 1978. Mechanism of transfection of chicken embryo fibroblasts by Rous sarcoma virus DNA. *J. Virol.* **28**: 45.

Copeland, N.G. and G.M. Cooper. 1979. Transfection by exogenous and endogenous murine retrovirus DNAs. *Cell* **16**: 347.

Copeland, N.G., A.D. Zelenetz, and G.M. Cooper. 1979. Transformation of NIH/3T3 mouse cells by DNA of Rous sarcoma virus. *Cell* **17**: 993.

Czernilofsky, A.P., A.D. Levinson, H.E. Varmus, J.M. Bishop, E. Tischer, and H. Goodman. 1983. Corrections to the nucleotide sequence of the *src* gene of the Rous sarcoma virus. *Nature* **301**: 736.

Ek, B., B. Westermark, A. Wasteson, and C.-H. Heldin. 1982. Stimulation of tyrosine-specific phosphorylation by platelet-derived growth factor. *Nature* **295**: 419.

Hunter, T. and J.A. Cooper. 1981. Epidermal growth factor induces rapid tyrosine phosphorylation of proteins in A431 human tumor cells. *Cell* **24**: 741.

Hunter, T. and B. Sefton. 1980. Transforming gene product of Rous sarcoma virus phosphorylates tyrosine. *Proc. Natl. Acad. Sci.* **77**: 1311.

Karess, R.E., W.S. Hayward, and H. Hanafusa. 1979. Cellular information in the genome of recovered avian sarcoma virus directs the synthesis of transforming protein. *Proc. Natl. Acad. Sci.* **76**: 3154.

Kasuga, M., F.A. Karlsson, and C.R. Kahn. 1982. Insulin stimulates the phosphorylation of the 95,000-dalton subunit of its own receptor. *Science* **215**: 185.

Laemmli, U.K. 1970. Cleavage of structural proteins during the assembly of the head of bacteriophage T4. *Nature* **227**: 680.

Martinez, R., K.D. Nakamara, and M.J. Weber. 1982. Identification of phosphotyrosine-containing proteins in untransformed and Rous sarcoma virus-transformed chicken embryo fibroblasts. *Mol. Cell. Biol.* **2**: 653.

Mulligan. R.C. and P. Berg. 1980. Expression of a bacterial gene in mammalian cells. *Science* **209**: 1422.

———. 1981. Selection for animal cells that express the *Escherichia coli* gene coding for xanthine-guanine phosphoribosyltransferase. *Proc. Natl. Acad. Sci.* **78**: 2072.

Oppermann, H., A.D. Levinson, H.E. Varmus, L. Levintow, and J.M. Bishop. 1979. Uninfected vertebrate cells contain a protein that is closely related to the product of the avian sarcoma virus transforming gene (*src*). *Proc. Natl. Acad. Sci.* **76**: 1804.

Parker, R.C., H.E. Varmus, and J.M. Bishop. 1981. Cellular homologue (c-*src*) of the transforming gene of Rous sarcoma virus: Isolation, mapping, and transcriptional analysis of c-*src* and flanking regions. *Proc. Natl. Acad. Sci.* **78**: 5842.

Radke, K. and G.S. Martin. 1979. Transformation by Rous sarcoma virus: Effects of *src* gene expression on the synthesis and phosphorylation of cellular polypeptides. *Proc. Natl. Acad. Sci.* **76**: 5212.

Reynolds, F.H., Jr., G.J. Todaro, C. Fryling, and J. Stephenson. 1981. Human transforming growth factors induce tyrosine phosphorylation of EGF receptors. *Nature* **292**: 259.

Schwartz, D.E., R. Tizard, and W. Gilbert. 1983. Nucleotide sequence of Rous sarcoma virus. *Cell* **32**: 853.

Sefton, B.M., T. Hunter, K. Beemon, and W. Eckhart. 1980. Evidence that the phosphorylation of tyrosine is essential for transformation by Rous sarcoma virus. *Cell* **20**: 807.

Shalloway, D., A.D. Zelenetz, and G.M. Cooper. 1981. Molecular cloning and characterization of the chicken gene homologous to the transforming gene of Rous sarcoma virus. *Cell* **24**: 531.

Shiloh, B.-Z. and R.A. Weinberg. 1981. DNA sequences homologous to vertebrate oncogenes are conserved in *Drosophila melanogaster*. *Proc. Natl. Acad. Sci.* **78**: 6789.

Swanstrom, R., R.C. Parker, H.E. Varmus, and J.M. Bishop. 1983. Transduction of a cellular oncogene: The genesis of Rous sarcoma virus. *Proc. Natl. Acad. Sci.* **80**: 2519.

Takeya, T. and H. Hanafusa. 1982. DNA sequence of the viral and cellular *src* gene of chickens. II. Comparison of the *src* genes of two strains of avian sarcoma virus and of the cellular homolog. *J. Virol.* **44**: 12.

———. 1983. Structure and sequence of the cellular gene homologous to the RSV *src* gene and the mechanism for generating the transforming virus. *Cell* **32**: 881.

Takeya, T., H. Hanafusa, R.P. Junghans, G. Ju, and A.M. Skalka. 1981. Comparison between the viral transforming gene (*src*) of recovered avian sarcoma virus and its cellular homolog. *Mol. Cell. Biol.* **1**: 1024.

Tooze, J., ed. 1981. Appendix A. In *Molecular biology of tumor viruses*, 2nd edition, part 2: *DNA tumor viruses*. Cold Spring Harbor Laboratory. Cold Spring Harbor, New York.

Ushiro, H. and S. Cohen. 1980. Identification of phosphotyrosine as a product of epidermal growth factor-activated protein kinase in A-431 cell membranes. *J. Biol. Chem.* **255**: 8363.

Transduction and Alteration of a Cellular Gene (*c-src*) Created an RNA Tumor Virus: The Genesis of Rous Sarcoma Virus

R.C. Parker,* R. Swanstrom,† H.E. Varmus, and J.M. Bishop
Department of Microbiology and Immunology, University of California, School of Medicine, San Francisco, California 94143

The recognition that the transforming genes of RNA tumor viruses evolved from cognates present in normal animal cells posed a central dilemma for researchers: Why do cells that express a normal gene become transformed when a highly related viral gene is expressed? Comparison of the transforming gene of Rous sarcoma virus (RSV), *v-src*, and its cellular progenitor, *c-src*, indicated that the genes were structurally alike, but distinct. Additionally, the protein products they encode, pp60^{v-src} and pp60^{c-src}, although similar can be distinguished by protease mapping (Collett et al. 1979; Oppermann et al. 1979). The cellular protein is present in almost all vertebrate cells studied, however, its intracellular level is usually very low—in the order of 10^4 molecules per cell (Sefton et al. 1982). Cells transformed by RSV, however, usually contain large quantities of pp60^{v-src}.

To understand whether pp60^{v-src} transforms cells because it is qualitatively different from pp60^{c-src} or simply because of its quantitatively higher intracellular level, we isolated clones containing the gene that encodes pp60^{c-src} from a recombinant DNA library representative of the chicken genome (Parker et al. 1981). The clones contain over 30 kb of DNA, including the entire coding region of pp60^{c-src} and an additional gene 3′ of *c-src*. A comparison of the coding regions of *v-src* and *c-src* indicated that the latter, like many eukaryotic genes, contains intervening sequences. At least two introns are present in the 5′ untranslated region of the gene; the most 5′ of these introns is removed by splicing at a site that is 75 nucleotides 5′ of the translational start codon in the mRNA. This splice acceptor site and the 16 nucleotides immediately 5′ of it are present in RSV; this signal is used to form the subgenomic viral RNA that encodes pp60^{v-src}. The 3′ end of *v-src* is very different from the 3′ end of *c-src* and contains 12 amino acids that replace the carboxyterminal 19 amino acids found in pp60^{c-src}. Most of these 12 amino acids, however, are encoded in the chicken genome less than 1 kb 3′ of the pp60^{c-src} stop codon.

The biological effects of elevated intracellular levels of pp60^{c-src} were assessed by subcloning *c-src* into an eukaryotic expression vector and transfecting rat fibroblasts with the plasmid. Levels of pp60^{c-src} that are 10 times greater than those normally found in rat fibroblasts do not morphologically transform the cells, nor do such levels enhance the ability of the cells to grow in soft agar.

Materials and Methods

Cell culture
Rat-2 (R2) cells, a thymidine kinase (TK)-deficient cell line (Topp 1981), were grown in Dulbecco's modified Eagle's medium (DMEM) containing 10% fetal bovine serum, penicillin, streptomycin, and fungizone (psf). All derivatives (RV, RC, RCV) of this line were grown in the above medium that was supplemented with 15 µg/ml of hypoxanthine, 500 µg/ml of thymidine, and 0.4 µg/ml of methotrexate (HMT) or with HMT and 250 µg/ml of G418.

Transfections
The rat fibroblasts were transfected according to established procedures (Wigler et al. 1977).

Soft agar cloning
A 3-ml bottom layer of 0.7% agarose A (Calbiochem) was used as a support in 60-mm dishes. Cells (approximately 10^3–10^4, depending upon the experiment) were seeded in 2 ml of 0.35% agarose and then fed every 4–7 days with 1 ml of 0.35% agarose. The agarose solution contained: DMEM, psf, hypoxanthine (15 µg/ml), thymidine (500 µg/ml), and either 4% or 10% calf serum. Colonies were scored 2 weeks after the initial plating as: −, less than 10 colonies per plate; +, many small colonies per plate; + +, hundreds of small colonies per plate; and + + +, hundreds of large colonies per plate.

Nucleic acids
Techniques involving nucleic acids have been described in previous papers (Parker et al. 1981; Swanstrom et al. 1983).

Results and Discussion

Clones containing *c-src*
Two overlapping clones, λCs1 and λCs2, were isolated from a recombinant DNA library (similar clones were reported by Shalloway et al. [1981] and Takeya et al.

*Present address: Department of Microbiology, College of Physicians and Surgeons of Columbia University, New York, New York 10032.
†Present address: Department of Biochemistry and Nutrition and Cancer Research Center, University of North Carolina, Chapel Hill, North Carolina 27514.

[1981]). These clones span more than 30 kb of the chicken genome and share approximately 4 kb of DNA within *c-src*. One of these clones, λCs2, contains the entire coding region of pp60^{c-src}, and after being subcloned into a plasmid was used to form a heteroduplex with a *v-src*-containing plasmid.

An electron micrograph of the resulting heteroduplex (Fig. 1) revealed that *c-src* contained six introns not present in *v-src*. The first of these introns is in the 5′ untranslated region of the gene. These are not the only introns in *c-src*. While determining the nucleotide sequence of *c-src*, Takeya and Hanafusa found five additional exons and introns that were too small to be detected by electron microscopy (Takeya and Hanafusa 1983).

Stable RNA from *c-src* and surrounding regions

The 30 kb of DNA in λCs1 and λCs2 does not appear to contain any moderately or highly repeated sequences. Accordingly, DNA fragments from these clones seemed suitable as probes in hybridization experiments with cellular RNAs.

Polyadenylated RNA from chicken embryos contained two discrete populations that hybridized to these clones. One population of 3.9 kb hybridized to probes from the *c-src* region of the clones and to *v-src* probes; this appears to be the mRNA that encodes pp60^{c-src}. Both its size and low copy number are consistent with data found in earlier studies using *v-src* as a probe (Spector et al. 1978).

The complexity of this RNA is 2.5 times greater than is needed to encode a 60-kD protein. It remains unclear what percentage of the additional sequences present in the RNA are 5′, and what percentage are 3′, of the gene; it is possible that the transcript extends thousands of bases 3′ of the coding region.

Approximately 5 kb 3′ of the pp60^{c-src} stop codon there is a *Hind*III recognition site. Another *Hind*III site exists 4.7 kb further away from *c-src*. This fragment was used to probe polyadenlylated RNA. It did not hybridize to the 3.9-kb RNA; however, it did hybridize to a 2.0-kb species. This latter RNA is approximately 10-fold more abundant than the *c-src* transcript.

Splicing the 5′ end of *c-src*

To understand the mechanism by which a retrovirus transduced *c-src* to form RSV, we compared the 5′ and 3′ ends of the viral and cellular genes. RNA was isolated from chicken embryo fibroblasts before and after they were infected with RSV.

These RNAs were hybridized to an end-labeled DNA fragment of *v-src*. This fragment was only labeled with ^{32}P at a site 27 nucleotides past the start codon; it extended 242 bases 5′ of the coding region. The RNA:DNA duplexes were digested with S1 nuclease and then denatured; the resulting products were analyzed by polyacrylamide gel electrophoresis and autoradiography (Fig. 2).

The first lane shows the migration of the DNA probe after it was digested with *Pst*I, which cleaves 76 bases 5′ of the start codon. This shortens the labeled fragment from its original size of 269 bp to a final length of 103

bp and provides a size marker for the S1 analysis. Lane 2 also consists of size markers (see legend). Lanes 3 and 4 show the size of the full-length probe in a control experiment with yeast RNA. In the absence of S1, the probe remains intact and migrates as a single large band. However, as shown in lane 4, when the probe is not hybridized to RNA, it is completely digested by S1 leaving no detectable bands. The final control appears in lane 5 and demonstrates that the entire probe is protected from S1 digestion when it is hybridized to virion RNA. RSV virions do not contain subgenomic, spliced RNAs but do hold full-length genomic RNA.

The products after S1 digestion of hybrids between the probe and RNA from RSV infected cells are shown in lane 6. The full-length band is a result of hybridization with genomic RNA, however, the smaller band represents probe that hybridized with the subgenomic, 21S *v-src* mRNA. The size of the fragment indicates that there is a functional splice acceptor site approximately 100 bases away from the labeling site. Since the label was within the coding region of *v-src*, this would locate the splice acceptor site about 75 bases 5′ of the coding region.

Lane 7 shows that a fragment of the same size is protected from S1 digestion by chicken embryo RNA. The low abundance of *c-src* mRNA necessitated our using 100-fold more RNA for this experiment than for the infected cell experiment.

Nucleotide sequence analysis of this region demonstrated that the sequences of the viral and cellular genes are identical for 91 bases preceding the protein start codon. Within these 91 bases, a consensus splice acceptor site (Mount 1982) (TCTGTGTGCTGCAGG) exists that, based upon the S1 results, is used for forming both mRNAs.

This result also proved that RSV contains part of a *c-src* intron (nucleotides 76 to 91 5′ of the start codon), and therefore transduction could not have simply involved recombination between RNA from a retrovirus and *c-src* mRNA (since the latter lacks introns). It seems more likely that an early step in transduction involves DNA:DNA recombination.

Transduction at the 3′ end

The carboxyl dozen amino acids of pp60^{v-src} originated from a part of the chicken genome that is almost 1 kb past the stop codon for pp60^{c-src} (Fig. 3). These 12 amino acids follow 514 amino acids that are very conserved in pp60^{c-src} and pp60^{v-src} (Takeya and Hanafusa 1983). The progenitor of the 3′ end of *v-src* is immediately preceded by a potential splice acceptor site (based upon sequence analysis) and may be part of the 3.9-kb *c-src* mRNA (see above).

As shown by Takeya and Hanafusa (1983), however, *c-src* contains a very poor splice donor signal near the sequences encoding amino acid 514, and it is very unlikely that splicing normally occurs. In fact, our nucleotide sequence analysis of the human *c-src* loci (R.C. Parker et al., in prep.) shows that intron nucleotide sequences at the 3′ end of *src* are not conserved between

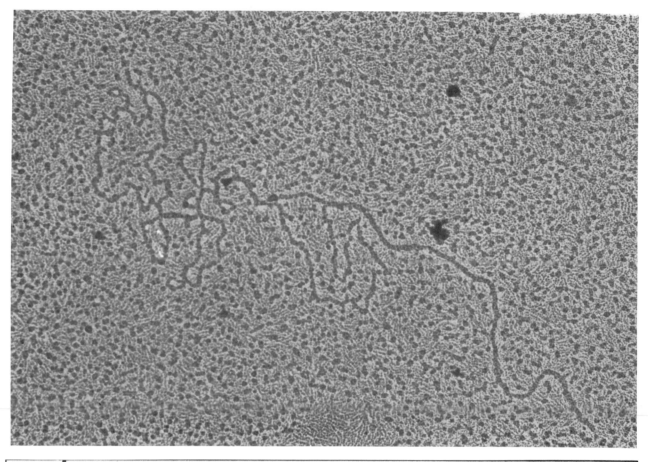

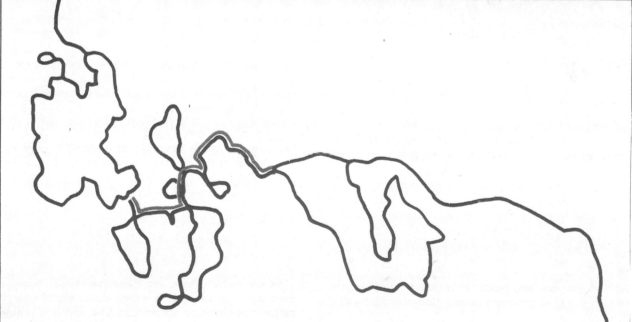

Figure 1 (*Top*) Electron micrograph of a heteroduplex between plasmids containing *v-src* and *c-src*. (*Bottom*) Line drawing depicting the heteroduplex between *v-src* (gray) and *c-src* (black). The black loops represent introns. The lines to the left and the right of the duplex region represent DNA that is part of the plasmids but not part of the *src* heteroduplex. (Reprinted, with permission, from Bishop 1983.)

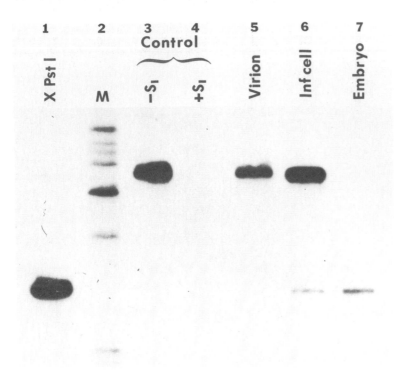

Figure 2 Analysis of DNAs protected from hydrolysis by nuclease S1. (Lane *1*) Marker DNA obtained by cleaving the end-labeled DNA probe with *Pst*I; (lane *2*) marker DNA fragments produced by cleavage of pBR322 with *Hin*f; (lane *3*) DNA hybridized with yeast RNA; (lane *4*) DNA hybridized with yeast RNA and hydrolyzed with nuclease S1; (lane *5*) DNA hybridized with virion RNA of RSV and hydrolyzed with nuclease S1; (lane *6*) DNA hybridized with 5 μg of total RNA from RSV-infected chicken cells after digestion by nuclease S1; (lane *7*) DNA hybridized with 50 μg of polyadenylated RNA from uninfected chicken cells after digestion with nuclease S1.

chickens and humans but that the amino acid-coding region 3' of the poor splice donor site is conserved. The nucleotide sequences allow the inference that neither the chicken nor the human genes would be spliced at this point and both would encode proteins ending after an additional 19 amino acids.

Somehow, transduction of *c-src* to form RSV has replaced the coding region of these 19 amino acids with a sequence located approximately 1 kb away. Since the sequence is preceded by a potential splice site, its presence in *v-src* may be a remnant of an infrequent splicing event. It is also preceded by an 8-bp sequence (underlined in Fig. 3) that is present around amino acid 514, immediately before the *c-src/v-src* divergence. Accordingly, transduction may have involved a DNA:DNA recombination event at the 3' end of the gene, as suggested by Takeya and Hanafusa (1983), in addition to one at the 5' end. A third alternative, that this 8-bp

sequence mediated an RNA:RNA recombination event, is proposed below.

The mechanism of transduction

A simple analysis of *c-src* and *v-src* requires that a transduction model explain four facts: (1) *c-src* contains introns and *v-src* does not; (2) RSV contains part of a *c-src* intron 5' of *v-src* and both genes share a splice acceptor site; (3) the 3' ends of *v-src* and *c-src* are quite different, however, most of the 3' end of *v-src* is derived from the chicken genome; and (4) *v-src* is flanked by a direct repeat of retroviral sequences (Czernilofsky et al. 1980; Schwartz et al. 1983). A more detailed analysis also must explain the presence of an element that resembles a transposon that is present 3' of *v-src* in the Prague-C strain of RSV and 5' of *v-src* in the Schmidt-Ruppin A strain (see Swanstrom et al. 1983).

To explain the four fundamental points, we posit the

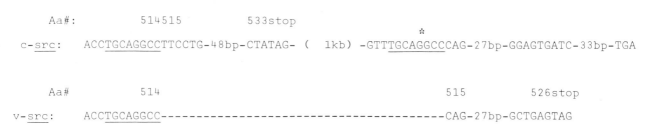

Figure 3 The 3' ends of *c-src* and *v-src*. pp60^*c-src* contains 533 amino acids. An 8-bp repeat is present in the *c-src* locus near the region encoding amino acid 514 and approximately 1 kb after the termination codon (the 8-bp repeat is underlined). A potential splice acceptor site within the 8-bp repeat that is present 3' of the gene is denoted by an asterisk. pp60^*v-src* contains 526 amino acids. The first 514 of these are very similar to those found in the cellular homolog, however, the carboxyl terminus of pp60^*v-src* is encoded by sequences similar to those 3' of the *c-src* gene.

following: (1) infection of a chicken by a retrovirus (the helper); (2) creation of a helper provirus 5' of the c-src locus in the same transcriptional orientation; (3) DNA:DNA recombination joining the provirus to c-src and deleting the right-hand long terminal repeat (LTR) of the provirus, the promoter of c-src, a splice donor site of c-src, and all sequences in between; (4) transcription beginning at the proviral promoter and extending through the viral 5' end, the gag, pol, and env genes, the 3' untranslated region of the virus and through the c-src locus including the remaining portion 5' of the translational start codon, the entire coding region, and kilobases beyond the gene (this will include the region 1 kb past the pp60^{c-src} stop codon that will ultimately encode the 3' end of v-src).

This transcript will be polyadenylated at the site normally used for polyadenylation of c-src mRNA. The transcript will contain all of the retroviral genes and packaging signals, the entire c-src-coding region, and many c-src introns. All of the c-src introns that are flanked by splice donor and acceptor signals will now be removed by splicing. Note that the DNA recombination event removed a 5' c-src splice donor but left a splice acceptor 5' of the gene that is part of RSV.

The final transcript, lacking c-src introns, will contain the 5' end of the helper virus followed by gag, pol, env, 3' untranslated, a splice acceptor site, c-src, and sequences 3' of c-src. This transcript can then be packaged in a virion along with a helper RNA. Packaging of the two molecules in one virion would follow the normal pathway of packaging retroviral dimers. The helper RNA would consist of: 5' end, gag, pol, env, 3' untranslated, and 3' end sequences.

After infection of another cell by this heterodimer, the normal process of reverse transcription would copy the RNA templates into DNA. Transcription of retroviruses begins by copying the 5' end and then the 3' end and then the 3' untranslated sequences. The last two steps would occur on the helper templates. Then the enzyme would have to shift templates and copy the sequences 3' of c-src, followed by c-src, the splice acceptor site, the 3' untranslated region, env, pol, gag, and the 5' end of the virus. This process would form a viral RNA containing c-src (hence now v-src) (1) flanked by a direct repeat (the 3' untranslated region), (2) lacking introns, and (3) containing a splice acceptor site 5' of the gene.

The virus, however, would contain the entire coding region of pp60^{c-src} in addition to sequences 3' of src encoding what we know to be the carboxyl terminus of v-src. At this time, however, the virus would direct the synthesis of pp60^{c-src} and not the protein with the altered carboxyl terminus. As noted above, the sequences encoding that terminus are preceded by an 8-bp sequence that is repeated near the sequences encoding amino acid 514. It seems likely that during subsequent infections, this 8-bp repeat could serve as a site for template jumping by the RNA-dependent DNA polymerase. Such a jump would delete the intervening 1 kb of sequences and join the present end of v-src to the body of the gene.

The selective advantage of such an event need not be an alteration in the transforming capacity of the gene (though, as discussed below, such an alteration in transforming capacity is probably associated with the 3' end). Instead, deletion of the 1 kb would make a smaller retrovirus—one that might fit more easily within the viral envelope. Even without this extra 1 kb of RNA, the genome of RSV is the largest of the avian retroviruses.

Obviously, it is not possible to discern between the three models discussed as to the ontogeny of the 3' end of v-src. It may just as well be the result of a DNA:DNA recombination event, or a rare splicing event, as an RNA-dependent DNA polymerase-mediated RNA recombination event. Regardless of the mechanism by which it occurred, the change at the 3' end is structurally the most dramatic difference between pp60^{c-src} and pp60^{v-src}.

Expression of chicken c-src in rat cells

The chicken c-src gene was cloned into pSV2, a eukaryotic expresssion vector that contains the early promoter of SV40 (Mulligan and Berg 1981). The resulting plasmid, pCS105fA, was capable of directing the synthesis of enzymatically active pp60^{c-src} after transfection of R2 cells with a calcium phosphate precipitate of pCS105fA, salmon sperm carrier DNA, and a plasmid containing the herpes simplex virus tk gene (Wagner et al. 1981).

Colonies of cells were isolated in HMT that expressed both ptk and pCS105fA. One colony, RC, contained approximately 10-fold more pp60^{c-src} than did the parental R2 cells. This elevated level was demonstrated by assaying immunoprecipitable proteins labeled with either [^{35}S]methionine or ^{32}P. The greater quantity of protein resulted in a 10-fold increase in the amount of phosphate transferred from [γ-^{32}P]ATP to the heavy chain of immunoglobulin G in the immune-complex kinase assay. RC cells are not morphologically transformed even though they contain 10 times more pp60^{c-src} than do R2 cells.

Expression of v-src in rat cells

In addition to being able to transform avian cells, RSV can transform rodent cells. A derivative of R2 cells that was morphologically transformed by v-src was prepared by E. Jakobovits. The transformed line, RV, was made by cotransfecting ptk and a plasmid containing v-src linked to a mouse mammary tumor virus promoter.

This cell line, although morphologically transformed, only contains 3.5 times more pp60^{v-src} than rat pp60^{c-src}. This difference was determined by measuring the amounts of immunoprecipitable radioactively labeled proteins. The RV cells contain significantly less pp60^{src} than do the RC cells.

v-src transformation of RC cells

The observation that morphologically normal RC cells contain more pp60^{c-src} than the amount of pp60^{v-src} found in transformed RV cells suggested that the cellular and viral proteins are qualitatively different. The observed difference, however, might be attributable to an unusual clonal line of rat cells that was resistant to src-mediated transformation.

To test this hypothesis, RC cells were transfected with

a precipitate containing pAG60, a plasmid that confers resistance to G418 (Colbère-Garapin et al. 1981), and a plasmid containing RSV DNA. Cells were selected for their ability to grow in the presence of G418; approximately 20% of the colonies were morphologically transformed, indicating that RC cells are not resistant to *src*-mediated transformation. One colony, RCV, was chosen for further study.

Soft agar cloning

The four cell lines were assayed for their ability to grow in soft agar as an additional method of assessing their state of transformation. Cells were plated at two different densities in agarose containing either 4% or 10% calf serum.

As shown in Table 1, the parental R2 cells could grow in 10% calf serum but did not grow as well as in 4% calf serum. The derivative containing high levels of $pp60^{c-src}$ (RC) did not grow in 4% serum and grew poorly in 10%. Its inability to grow in soft agar like its parent may simply be a reflection of the properties of this clone of cells and not be related to the elevated level of $pp60^{c-src}$.

RV cells, the morphologically transformed *v-src* derivative of R2, is capable of growing in either concentration of serum. At the higher concentration, where R2 cells grow, RV cells form more colonies and larger colonies than the parent line. Finally, the RSV DNA-transformed derivative of RC cells, RCV, also grows very well in either 4% or 10% serum. This is in marked contrast to the RC cells.

Summary

The isolation of recombinant DNA clones containing the chicken *c-src* locus has allowed us to study the mechanism by which it was transduced to form RSV, and to characterize some of its biological properties as compared with those of *v-src*. We now know that not only are the viral and cellular proteins structurally different but that those differences are involved in the ability of the viral protein to transform cells. It remains unclear whether the qualitative difference in biological effects can be overcome by a greatly elevated level of $pp60^{c-src}$.

Table 1 Colony Formation in Soft Agar

Cells	Serum	
	4%	10%
R2	+	+ +
RC	−	+
RV	+ + +	+ + +
RCV	+ + +	+ + +

Cells were plated in 0.35% agarose containing either 4% or 10% calf serum; colonies were scored as described in Materials and Methods.

However, it is certain that $pp60^{c-src}$ is not as capable as $pp60^{v-src}$ of transforming cells.

It seems likely that the significant structural change at the 3' end of the genes is responsible for the difference in transforming capacity. Whether the sequences present in *v-src* are involved in this capacity or simply replace inhibitory sequences present in *c-src* is not known but should be easily tested.

It will be far more difficult to ascertain how RSV came to replace the carboxyl terminus of *c-src* with sequences approximately 1 kb downstream. Three models have been suggested, but no method for discerning between them is apparent.

Our data demonstrate that transduction on the 5' side of *c-src* probably involved formation of a provirus followed by a DNA:DNA recombination event. Additionally, we have posited that recombination also involved an RNA:RNA event 3' of *c-src*.

Acknowledgments

We thank G. Mardon for preliminary data. We wish to acknowledge grant support from the American Cancer Society and the National Institutes of Health, and fellowships for R.C.P. from the American Cancer Society (California Division) and the Leukemia Society of America.

References

Bishop, J.M. 1983. Oncogenes and proto-oncogenes. *Hosp. Pract.* **18:** 67.

Colbere-Garapin, F., F. Horodniceanu, P. Kourilsky, and A.-C. Garapin. 1981. A new dominant hybrid selective marker for higher eukaryotic cells. *J. Mol. Biol.* **150:** 1.

Collett, M.S., E. Erikson, A.F. Purchio, J.S. Brugge, and R.L. Erikson. 1979. A normal cell protein similar in structure and function to the avian sarcoma virus transforming gene product. *Proc. Natl. Acad. Sci.* **76:** 3159.

Czernilofsky, A.P., A.D. Levinson, H.E. Varmus, J.M. Bishop, E. Tischer, and H.M. Goodman. 1980. Nucleotide sequence of an avian sarcoma virus oncogene (*src*) and proposed amino acid sequence for gene product. *Nature* **287:** 198.

Mount, S.M. 1982. A catalogue of splice junction sequences. *Nucleic Acids Res.* **10:** 459.

Mulligan, R.C. and P. Berg. 1981. Factors governing expression of a bacterial gene in mammalian cells. *Mol. Cell. Biol.* **1:** 449.

Oppermann, H., A.D. Levinson, H.E. Varmus, L. Levintow, and J.M. Bishop. 1979. Uninfected vertebrate cells contain a protein that is closely related to the product of the avian sarcoma virus transforming gene (*src*). *Proc. Natl. Acad. Sci.* **76:** 1804.

Parker R.C., H.E. Varmus, and J.M. Bishop. 1981. The cellular homologue (*c-src*) of the transforming gene of Rous sarcoma virus: Isolation, mapping and transcriptional analysis of c-src and flanking regions. *Proc. Natl. Acad. Sci.* **78:** 5842.

Schwartz, D.E., R. Tizard, and W. Gilbert. 1983. Nucleotide sequence of Rous sarcoma virus. *Cell* **32:** 853.

Sefton, B.M., T. Patschinsky, C. Berdot, T. Hunter, and T.J. Elliot. 1982. Phosphorylation and metabolism of the transforming protein of Rous sarcoma virus. *J. Virol.* **41:** 813.

Shalloway, D., A.D. Zelentz, and G.M. Cooper. 1981. Molecular cloning and characterization of the chicken gene homologous to the transforming gene of Rous sarcoma virus. *Cell* **24:** 531.

Spector, D., B. Baker, H.E. Varmus, and J.M. Bishop. 1978. Characteristics of cellular RNA related to the transforming gene of avian sarcoma viruses. *Cell* **13:** 371.

Swanstrom, R., R.C. Parker, H.E. Varmus, and J.M. Bishop.

1983. Transduction of a cellular oncogene: The genesis of Rous sarcoma virus. *Proc. Natl. Acad. Sci.* **80:** 2519.

Takeya, T. and H. Hanafusa. 1983. Structure and sequence of the cellular gene homologous to the RSV *src* gene and the mechanism for generating the transforming virus. *Cell* **32:** 881.

Takeya, T., H. Hanafusa, R.P. Junghans, G. Ju, and A.M. Skalka. 1981. Comparison between the viral transforming gene (*src*) of recovered avian sarcoma virus and its cellular homologue. *Mol. Cell. Biol.* **1:** 1024.

Topp, W.C. 1981. Normal rat cell lines deficient in nuclear thymidine kinase. *Virology* **113:** 408.

Wagner, M.J., J.A. Sharp, and W.C. Summers. 1981. Nucleotide sequence of the thymidine kinase gene of herpes simplex virus type 1. *Proc. Natl. Acad. Sci.* **78:** 1441.

Wigler, M., S. Silverstein, L.S. Lee, A. Pellicer, Y.C. Cheng, and R. Axel. 1977. Transfer of purified herpes virus thymidine kinase gene to cultured mouse cells. *Cell* **11:** 223.

Modification of the Activity of the Catalytic Subunit of the cAMP-dependent Protein Kinase by pp60^{src}

Y. Graziani,** J.L. Maller,† Y. Sugimoto,*§ and R.L. Erikson*§

Departments of *Pathology and †Pharmacology, University of Colorado School of Medicine, Denver, Colorado 80262

The transformation of cells by Rous sarcoma virus (RSV) is mediated by the expression of its transforming gene product, pp60^{src}. Thus far, only a single function has been assigned to pp60^{src} that could account for its pleiotropic effect on cells. The molecule apparently is a protein kinase that specifically phosphorylates tyrosine residues in protein substrates (for review, see Erikson et al. 1980b). Since the discovery of tyrosine phosphorylation, considerable effort has been expended in the search for possible substrates of pp60^{src}; however, these studies have not led to the identification of substrates, the phosphorylation of which appears to be crucial for the transformation process. Of those cellular proteins that become phosphorylated on tyrosine as a result of pp60^{src} expression, only a small fraction of the total amount of each protein is phosphorylated, raising the issue of the physiological significance of the phosphorylation observed.

Although much attention has been focused on tyrosine phosphorylation, analysis of specific proteins, such as the ribosomal protein S6 (Decker 1981), reveals that protein phosphorylation on serine residues is also quantitatively altered by pp60^{src} expression. These observations suggest that some effects of pp60^{src} may be mediated by the regulation of a protein kinase and/or a protein phosphatase specific for serine. One obvious candidate is the cAMP-dependent protein kinase, an enzyme known to be involved in the regulation of diverse pathways (for reviews, see Langan 1973; Rubin and Rosen 1975; Krebs and Beavo 1979; Flockhart and Corbin 1982). Consequently, we have carried out in vitro studies on the catalytic subunit of the cAMP-dependent protein kinase and have found that it can be phosphorylated on tyrosine residues by pp60^{src}. Furthermore, we have found that pp60^{src} can alter the enzymatic activity of the catalytic subunit and its regulation by the regulatory subunit (RII). These results suggest a possible explanation for the changes in serine phosphorylation mentioned above. The significance of these findings with regard to cell transformation is discussed.

Materials and Methods

H$_3$^{32}PO$_4$ carrier-free (285 Ci/mg) was purchased from ICN. [γ-^{32}P]ATP (5000–9000 Ci/mmole) was prepared by the method of Johnson and Walseth (1979). Protein kinase inhibitor (PKI) from rabbit skeletal muscle was prepared according to the procedure of Walsh et al. (1971) and was kindly provided by J.G. Foulkes. Glycogen synthase I from rabbit skeletal muscle was prepared as described by Soderling et al. (1970) and stored at −70°C in 50 mM Tris (pH 7.2), 10% sucrose, 15 mM β-mercaptoethanol, and 2 mM EDTA. The synthetic peptide substrate for the cAMP-dependent protein kinase (Kemptide; Leu-Arg-Arg-Ala-Ser-Leu-Gly) was obtained from Boehringer-Mannheim. Calf thymus histone HI was a gift from T.A. Langan (Department of Pharmacology). Glycogen phosphorylase kinase was purified from rabbit skeletal muscle by the method of Hayakawa et al. (1973). Sodium dodecyl sulfate (SDS), α-casein, and molecular-weight markers were from Sigma, bovine serum albumin (BSA) was from Miles Laboratories, ATP and ADP were from P-L Laboratories, and polyethyleneimine (PEI)-cellulose sheets (Macherey-Nagel) were from Brinkmann. cAMP-Sepharose was prepared by the method of Dills et al. (1975).

Purification of pp60^{src} by ion-exchange chromatography will be described elsewhere (Y. Sugimoto et al., in prep.). Briefly, the protocol consisted of sequential use of hydroxylapatite (BioRad), butylagarose (Miles Laboratories), DEAE-Sephacel (Pharmacia), ADP-agarose (P-L Laboratories), and Sephacryl S-200 (Pharmacia) starting with a P100 preparation from RSV-transformed vole cells (Erikson et al. 1980a). By this procedure, pp60^{src} was purified more than 2500-fold with a yield of 20%. The catalytic and regulatory subunits of the cAMP-dependent protein kinase were prepared essentially by the method of Beavo et al. (1974). The purity of these preparations is presented in Figure 1. After 10% SDS-polyacrylamide gel electrophoresis, the catalytic subunit preparation contained one stainable band in the region of M_r = 41,000 as judged by silver staining. A fivefold greater amount of the catalytic subunit preparation (~125 ng of protein) did not reveal any other bands in this gel. As indicated in the same figure, the pp60^{src} preparation (~30 ng protein) revealed a single band in the region of M_r 60,000. The regulatory subunit (RII) of the cAMP-dependent protein kinase consisted of two protein bands of M_r 54,000 and 57,000, which correspond to the phosphorylated (s) and unphosphorylated (f) forms of this protein (Rangel-Aldao and Rosen 1976, 1977; Corbin et al. 1978; Flockhart et al. 1980; Carmichael et al. 1982).

**Y. Graziani is on leave of absence from the Department of Biology, Ben-Gurion University, Beer-Sheva, Israel.

§Present address: The Biological Laboratories, Department of Cellular and Developmental Biology, Harvard University, Cambridge, Massachusetts 02138.

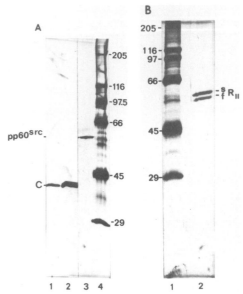

Figure 1 Analysis of catalytic subunit, pp60[src] and regulatory subunit (RII) preparations. (A) Samples of the catalytic subunit preparation containing 25 ng (track 1) or 125 ng (track 2) of protein and a sample of the pp60[src] preparation (~30 ng) (track 3) were resolved by 10% polyacrylamide gel electrophoresis. Commercial markers obtained from Sigma (myosin, M_r 205,000; β-galactosidase, M_r 116,000; phosphorylase B, M_r 97,500; bovine albumin, M_r 66,000; egg albumin, M_r 45,000; and carbonic anhydrase, M_r 29,000) were used for molecular-weight determination (track 4). The gel was stained with silver nitrate according to the procedure of Oakley et al. (1980). The numbers on the right side of the figure indicate the approximate molecular weights $\times$ 10^{-3}. (C) Catalytic subunit. (B) A sample of the regulatory subunit (RII) preparation containing ~100 ng of protein (track 2) was analyzed similarly. Track 1 demonstrates the commercial markers. (RII) Regulatory subunit; (s) slow-moving band of RII; (f) fast-moving band of RII.

Phosphorylation of catalytic subunit of pp60[src]

The phosphorylation of catalytic subunit with pp60[src] was carried out in 25 μl of 10 mM KP$_i$ (pH 7.1), 2.5 mM MgCl$_2$, 1 mM EDTA, 15 mM 2-mercaptoethanol, 20 μM [γ-^{32}P]ATP (approximately 2.5 $\times$ 10^7 cpm of the radiolabeled trinucleotide). The reaction mixtures were incubated at 30°C for 15 minutes and terminated by the addition of 8 μl of 5$\times$ concentrated electrophoresis sample buffer and by heating at 95°C for 1 minute (electrophoresis sample buffer: 70 mM Tris-HCl [pH 6.8], 11% glycerol, 3% SDS, 0.01% bromphenol blue, 5% 2-mercaptoethanol). The products of the reaction were resolved by SDS-polyacrylamide gel electrophoresis and visualized by autoradiography, as previously described (Graziani et al. 1983). The pertinent bands were excised and the radioactivity was quantified by liquid scintillation spectrometry.

Assay of catalytic subunit phosphotransferase activity

The catalytic subunit was incubated with pp60[src] as described above in the presence or absence of 20 μM unlabeled ATP and 2.5 mM MgCl$_2$. When RII was added

to the reaction, 3 μl of various concentrations of this preparation were added and the catalytic and regulatory subunits were allowed to reassociate for 6 minutes at 30°C. Then the various substrates were added in the presence of [γ-^{32}P]ATP and MgCl$_2$ (final concentration of 100 μM and 2.5 mM, respectively, and 4.5 $\times$ 10^6 cpm of the radiolabeled trinucleotide), and the samples were incubated for 5 minutes at 30°C. For determination of the phosphorylation of the Kemptide, 2.5-μl samples of the reaction mixture were spotted onto PEI-cellulose and developed with distilled water. Under these conditions, the positively charged phosphopeptide separates from the negatively charged compounds in the reaction mixture. After autoradiography, the radioactive spots were cut out and the radioactivity was quantified by liquid scintillation spectrometry. Application of different amounts of [γ-^{32}P]ATP onto PEI-cellulose (~2,000–100,000 cpm), and quantification of the radioactivity gave a linear relationship. For determination of phosphorylation of glycogen synthase, glycogen phosphorylase kinase or HI histone, the reactions were terminated by the addition of 8 μl of fivefold concentrated sample buffer, and the proteins were resolved by polyacrylamide gel electrophoresis.

Protein determination

Approximate quantification of the amount of pp60[src] was obtained by silver staining, as described previously (Graziani et al. 1983). Similar determinations were performed with the catalytic subunit. Other protein analyses were carried out according to the procedure of Lowry et al. (1951) or Bradford (1976).

Results

The result of pp60[src] on the regulation of catalytic subunit by RII

The stimulation of cAMP-dependent protein kinase by cAMP is a well-documented phenomenon. cAMP activates this enzyme by dissociation of the regulatory subunits (RI and RII) from the catalytic subunit. Also, the reassociation of the catalytic subunit with its regulatory subunits can be inhibited by cAMP (for reviews see Langan 1973; Rubin and Rosen 1975; Krebs and Beavo 1979).

To assay the activity of the cAMP-dependent protein kinase, we used a synthetic peptide that corresponds in sequence to the phosphorylation site of pig liver pyruvate kinase (Kemp et al. 1977). This peptide lacks tyrosine and, therefore, is useful for determining cAMP-dependent protein kinase activity in the presence of pp60[src], which phosphorylates proteins exclusively on tyrosine residues.

As demonstrated in Figure 2, preincubation of the catalytic subunit (2 μg/ml) with pp60[src] (30 ng/ml) in the presence of 0.1 mg/ml BSA for 15 minutes at 30°C, decreased the ability of RII to regulate the kinase activity of the catalytic subunit in the absence of cAMP. At molar ratios of RII to catalytic subunit between 1:1 and 4:1, the protein kinase activity was five- to tenfold higher in the presence of pp60[src] than in its absence.

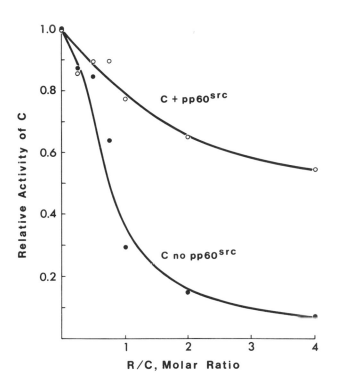

Figure 2 The effect of pp60*src* on the regulation of catalytic subunit by RII. Catalytic subunit (70 ng, 1.7 pmoles) together with 1 ng of pp60*src* (16.7 fmoles) were incubated for 15 min at 30°C in the presence of 0.1 mg/ml BSA, 10 mM KP$_i$ (pH = 7.1), 1 mM EDTA, 15 mM 2-mercaptoethanol in a final volume of 21 µl. After this incubation period, 3 µl of RII at different concentrations were added and the samples were incubated for another 6 min at 30°C. The phosphotransferase activity of the catalytic subunit was initiated by the addition of Mg^{++} (2.5 mM), [γ-^{32}P]ATP (~4.5 × 10^6 cpm), and Kemptide to give a final concentration of both substrates of 100 µM. After 5 min of incubation, samples of 2.5 µl were spotted onto PEI-cellulose and analyzed as described in Materials and Methods. The relative activity of the catalytic subunit was calculated from samples that did not contain RII. The specific activity of the catalytic subunit in the presence or absence of pp60*src* was 2.4 and 1.5 µmole/mg·min, respectively.

Since pp60*src* partially mimics the ability of cAMP to prevent reassociation of the catalytic and regulatory subunits, we measured the amount of cAMP in the pp60*src* preparation. A quantity of pp60*src* tenfold greater than that used for the experiments described above did not contain measurable cAMP (<0.1 pmole/µl). Furthermore, unlike the regulatory subunit, pp60*src* was unable to bind cAMP under the experimental conditions described by Gilman (1970) (data not shown). It should be noted that pp60*src*, unlike cAMP, did not affect the dissociation of the cAMP-dependent protein kinase (data not shown).

The type-II cAMP-dependent protein kinase holoenzyme has a phosphotransferase activity in which the catalytic subunit phosphorylates the regulatory subunit (Rosen and Erlichman 1975). Furthermore, the catalytic subunit is also able to undergo autophosphorylation (Chiu and Tao 1978). Upon examination of the unphosphorylated and phosphorylated bands of RII in silver-stained gels, we observed that the addition of pp60*src* to a mixture of RII and catalytic subunit increased the rate and extent of the conversion of the unphosphorylated band of RII to the phosphorylated one (Fig. 3). Incubation of RII with pp60*src* and ATP in the absence of the catalytic subunit did not result in a change in the distribution between the phosphorylated and unphosphorylated forms (data not shown). When this reaction was carried out in the presence of [γ-^{32}P]ATP, more radiolabeling was found in RII in the presence than in the absence of pp60*src* (Fig. 4A). In addition, four- to fivefold greater radiolabeling of the catalytic subunit occurred under these conditions in the presence of both RII and pp60*src* than in the presence of RII alone (Fig. 4B). It is important to note that the increased phosphorylation of RII in the presence of pp60*src* preceded the phosphorylation of the catalytic subunit.

Phosphorylation of the catalytic subunit with pp60*src*
Because the phosphorylation of both subunits of the cAMP-dependent protein kinase was increased in the presence of pp60*src* (Figs. 3 and 4), we wished to determine whether the purified and separated catalytic or regulatory subunits of the cAMP-dependent protein kinase could be substrates for pp60*src*.

As shown in Figure 5, when the catalytic subunit alone was incubated in the presence of [γ-^{32}P]ATP, one phosphorylated band of M_r 41,000 could be detected. This observation confirms previous studies that demonstrated autophosphorylation of the catalytic subunit in the presence of [γ-^{32}P]ATP (Chiu and Tao 1978). Phosphorylation of pp60*src* under the same conditions revealed radiolabel in the region of M_r 60,000, corresponding to the autophosphorylation of pp60*src* previously described (Collett et al. 1980; Erikson et al. 1980a). When pp60*src* and the catalytic subunit were incubated together, the radiolabeling of both the catalytic subunit and pp60*src* was increased. The phosphorylation of both the catalytic subunit and pp60*src* was linear for 30 minutes. Variation of the pp60*src* concentration at constant catalytic subunit concentration as well as variation of the catalytic subunit concentration at constant pp60*src* concentration resulted in a saturating increase of radiolabeling in both proteins. At a pp60*src* concentration of 150 ng/ml and a catalytic subunit concentration of 2100 ng/ml, a maximum of 0.15 moles of phosphate per mole catalytic subunit and 4–5

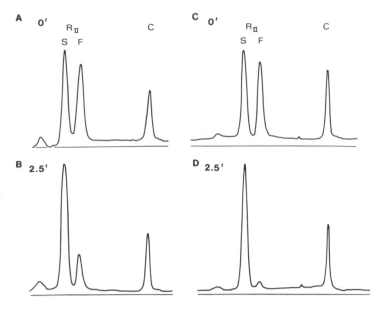

Figure 3 Phosphorylation of RII in the presence of catalytic subunit and pp60[src]. The experiment presented in this figure was performed essentially as described in Fig. 2, except that no BSA was present. After preincubation of the catalytic subunit with pp60[src], 190 ng of RII (3.4 pmoles) were added. After 6 min of incubation, ATP and MgCl₂ (100 μM and 2.5 mM final concentration) were added, the reaction proceeded for 2.5 min and was stopped by addition of 8 μl of fivefold concentrated sample buffer. The proteins were then separated on a 10% acrylamide gel and stained with silver nitrate. The stained bands of phosphorylated (s) and unphosphorylated (f) RII and of the catalytic subunit (C) were scanned with a 4310 Ortec densitometer. (*A,B*) RII + catalytic subunit after incubation for 0 min and 2.5 min with 100 μM ATP, respectively. (*C,D*) RII + catalytic subunit + pp60[src] after incubation for 0 min and 2.5 min with 100 μM ATP, respectively.

moles of phosphate per mole pp60[src] was incorporated. Incubation of RII in the presence of pp60[src] did not result in any phosphorylation of RII (data not shown).

Phosphoamino acid analysis of phosphorylated pp60[src], catalytic, and regulatory subunits

The phosphoamino acid composition of the phosphorylated preparations of pp60[src] and catalytic subunit described above was determined. As shown in Figure 6, autophosphorylated pp60[src] yielded phosphotyrosine; however, when it was phosphorylated in the presence of catalytic subunit, pp60[src] yielded both phosphotyrosine and phosphoserine. Analysis of the autophosphorylated catalytic subunit revealed only phosphoserine residues, whereas the catalytic subunit phosphorylated in the presence of pp60[src] yielded both phosphoserine and phosphotyrosine (track 4), with phosphotyrosine accounting for most of the increased phosphorylation. Therefore, it appears that each protein kinase may serve as a substrate for the other under in vitro conditions. Determination of the phosphoamino acids of RII phos-

phorylated in the presence of catalytic subunit with or without pp60[src] (Figs. 3 and 4) revealed only phosphoserine (data not shown).

The effect of pp60[src] on the activity of catalytic subunit

To evaluate whether phosphorylation of the catalytic subunit by pp60[src] affected its enzymatic activity, the phosphorylation of catalytic subunit and pp60[src] was carried out in the presence of unlabeled ATP for 15 minutes and then [γ-³²P]ATP and the synthetic peptide were added to the reaction mixtures. As shown in Figure 7 (panel A), catalytic subunit preincubated in the presence of pp60[src] caused three- to fivefold greater amounts of radiolabeled phosphate to be incorporated into the peptide than catalytic subunit incubated without pp60[src] (tracks 2 and 4). As expected, no radiolabel was incorporated into the peptide due to the activity of pp60[src] (track 3). The phosphorylation of the peptide demonstrated in tracks 2 and 4 was due to the activity of the catalytic subunit, since PKI, the inhibitor of the catalytic subunit, almost

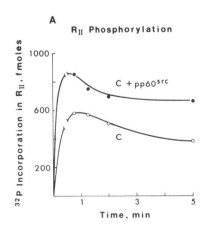

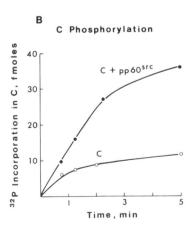

Figure 4 Phosphorylation of the regulatory and catalytic subunits in the presence of pp60[src] and ATP. The incorporation of ³²P into RII (2.0 pmoles) in the presence of catalytic subunit (1 pmole) and in the presence or absence of 16.7 fmoles of pp60[src] was performed as described in Fig. 3, except that [γ-³²P]ATP (100 μM; 3 × 10⁷ cpm per reaction) was used. At the times indicated, the reaction was stopped by the addition of sample buffer and by boiling, and the proteins were separated on a 10% acrylamide gel. The gel was dried and the radioactive bands were localized by autoradiography as described in Materials and Methods. The radiolabeled bands corresponding to the pertinent proteins were excised and counted. (*A*) Labeling of RII. (*B*) Labeling of the catalytic subunit.

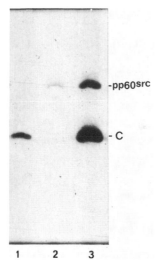

Figure 5 Phosphorylation of catalytic subunit and pp60*src* in the presence of ATP. Phosphotransferase reactions were carried out for 15 min at 30°C in the presence of 20 μM [γ-³²P]ATP as described in Materials and Methods. (Track *1*) Catalytic subunit (70 ng); (track *2*) pp60*src* (1 ng); (track *3*) catalytic subunit (70 ng) and pp60*src* (1 ng.)

completely inhibited the phosphorylation by both catalytic subunit and by catalytic subunit modified by pp60*src* (tracks 5 and 6, respectively). Catalytic subunit incubated at 4°C under the same conditions had phosphorylation activity similar to the catalytic subunit that had been treated with ATP at 30°C (tracks 2 and 7).

In addition, glycogen synthase, a physiological substrate of catalytic subunit, as well as of other protein kinases (Nimmo and Cohen 1974, 1977; Cohen et al. 1982), also was found to be phosphorylated more rapidly by catalytic subunit that had been incubated with pp60*src* (Fig. 7, panel B). A similar high activity of catalytic subunit preincubated with pp60*src* was also observed with glycogen phosphorylase kinase (both α- and β-subunits) and histone HI as substrates (data not shown).

Kinetic properties of catalytic subunit activity modified by pp60*src*

The phosphorylation of catalytic subunit by pp60*src*, as well as the changes in catalytic subunit activity, raised the question of whether the kinetic properties of the catalytic subunit with its substrates had changed. As shown in Figure 8A, incubation of the catalytic subunit with pp60*src* caused an increase of the K_m of ATP for phosphorylation of the synthetic peptide from 14 μM to 72 μM. Furthermore, the V_{max} of ATP for catalytic subunit was 1.25 and 6.25 μmole/min·mg protein, respectively. In addition, at 100 μM concentration of ATP, the K_m of the catalytic subunit for the Kemptide was increased by incubation with pp60*src* (33 μM and 167 μM, respectively) (Fig. 8B). The V_{max} for the peptide after incubation of catalytic subunit in the presence of pp60*src* also increased from 1.1 to 6.3 μmole/min·mg protein (Fig. 8B).

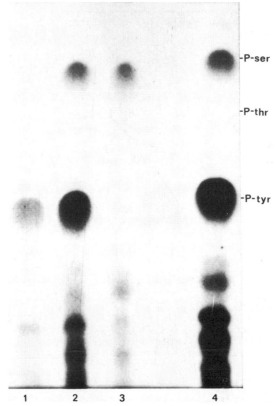

Figure 6 Phosphoamino acid analysis of pp60*src* and the catalytic subunit phosphorylated separately or in a mixture. pp60*src*, catalytic subunit, and a mixture of both preparations were phosphorylated and resolved by 10% SDS-polyacrylamide gel electrophoresis as shown in Fig. 5. The pertinent proteins were eluted from the gels, concentrated by trichloroacetic acid (TCA) precipitation, and subjected to acid hydrolysis as previously described (Collett et al. 1980; Erikson et al. 1980a). The phosphoamino acids were separated by electrophoresis at pH 3.5. Authentic phosphoamino acid markers were included in all samples. (Track *1*) Autophosphorylated pp60*src*; (track *2*) pp60*src* phosphorylated in the presence of catalytic subunit; (track *3*) autophosphorylated catalytic subunit; (track *4*) catalytic subunit phosphorylated in the presence of pp60*src*.

What is the reason for the difference in the catalytic subunit activity in the presence and absence of pp60*src*?

As demonstrated in Figure 9, during incubation of the catalytic subunit (2.0 μg/ml = 0.5 × 10⁻⁷ M) for 45 minutes at 30°C in the absence of BSA, its activity decreased greatly. On the other hand, in the presence of ~30 ng/ml of pp60*src* (0.5 × 10⁻⁹ M), the catalytic subunit activity remained constant. This indicates that the catalytic subunit is more stable in the presence of pp60*src*.

Is the phosphotransferase activity of pp60*src* needed to affect the catalytic subunit activity? To answer this question, the phosphotransferase activity of pp60*src* toward α-casein and the catalytic subunit was compared with its efficiency to affect catalytic subunit phosphotransferase activity toward the Kemptide. Preincubation of pp60*src* at 41°C for 15 minutes abolished more than 95% of its autophosphorylating activity as well as its

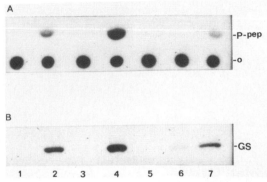

Figure 7 The effect of pp60^{src} on the phosphorylation of the synthetic peptide and glycogen synthase by catalytic subunit. Catalytic subunit (70 ng) was phosphorylated by pp60^{src} (1 ng) in the presence of 20 μM unlabeled ATP under the conditions described in Fig. 5. After 15 min at 30°C, the ATP concentration was raised to 110 μM and the Kemptide (100 μM) and [γ-^{32}P]ATP (3.5 × 10^6 cpm per sample) were added. After incubation for an additional 5 min, 2.5 μl from each tube was analyzed by chromatography on PEI-cellulose as described in Materials and Methods. The reaction was linear with time until 60–70% of the radiolabeled [γ-^{32}P]ATP had been consumed. In the experiment represented here, the consumption of the radiolabeled ATP did not exceed 50%. For phosphorylation of glycogen synthase, similar incubation conditions were used except that glycogen synthase (0.1 mg/ml final concentration) was added to each reaction and the products were resolved by polyacrylamide gel electrophoresis. The specific activity of the catalytic subunit for phosphorylation of the synthetic peptide was 0.76 or 2.6 μmole/mg·min in the absence or presence of pp60^{src}, respectively, and for phosphorylation of glycogen synthase it was 0.10 and 0.24 μmole/mg·min in the absence or presence of pp60^{src}, respectively. (*A*) Phosphorylation of the synthetic peptide; (*B*) phosphorylation of glycogen synthase. (Track *1*) No additions; (track *2*) catalytic subunit; (track *3*) pp60^{src}; (track *4*) catalytic subunit incubated with pp60^{src}; (track *5*) catalytic subunit plus PKI; (track *6*) catalytic subunit incubated with pp60^{src}, plus PKI; (track *7*) catalytic subunit kept at 4°C during the initial 15-min incubation. (P-pep) Synthetic peptide; (GS) glycogen synthase.

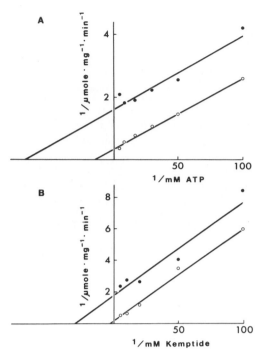

Figure 8 Kinetic parameters of the activity of catalytic subunit incubated in the presence or absence of pp60^{src}. (*A*) Catalytic subunit was incubated with or without pp60^{src} at 30°C for 15 min in the presence of 20 μM ATP. [γ-^{32}P]ATP at various concentrations, 10–200 μM (~3.5 × 10^6 cpm), was added together with 100 μM of the synthetic peptide. After incubation for 5 min at 30°C, 2.5-μl samples were analyzed by chromatography on PEI-cellulose. The K_m of ATP and V_{max} of ATP values were calculated from the reciprocal relationship of the velocity of the reaction and the ATP concentration. (*B*) For determination of the K_m of peptide and V_{max} of peptide values, experiments similar to those described in *A* were performed, except that the [γ-^{32}P]ATP was constant (100 μM) and the concentration of the synthetic peptide varied (10–200 μM). (○) Catalytic subunit incubated in the presence of pp60^{src}; (●) catalytic subunit incubated in the absence of pp60^{src}.

phosphotransferase activity toward both α-casein and the catalytic subunit (data not shown). As Figure 9 illustrates, pp60^{src} incubated at 41°C for 15 minutes still retained its ability to affect the catalytic subunit phosphotransferase activity. On the other hand, boiling for 10 minutes or treatment with trypsin inhibited its ability to maintain the high activity of the catalytic subunit (data not shown).

Are ATP and Mg^{++} needed in the preincubation period with pp60^{src} for the high activity of the catalytic subunit to be maintained? As demonstrated in Table 1, pp60^{src} alone at a concentration of ~30 ng/ml (0.5 × 10^{-9} M) in the reaction mixture was sufficient to cause fivefold higher activity of the catalytic subunit, which was at a concentration of 2 μg/ml (0.5 × 10^{-7} M). The addition to the preincubation mixture of either ATP[Mg] or dATP[Mg], which serve as phosphate donors for pp60^{src} phosphotransferase activity (Richert et al. 1979; Levinson et al. 1980; Graziani et al. 1983), or the addition of the nonphosphorylating trinucleotide analog App(NH)p also resulted in higher catalytic subunit activity. These results indicate that preincubation with ATP is not required for the effect of pp60^{src} on catalytic subunit. In addition, the effect of pp60^{src} on the regulation of catalytic subunit activity by RII (Fig. 2) did not require ATP in the preincubation.

Comparison of the effect of pp60^{src} and BSA on catalytic subunit activity

Since the purification of the catalytic subunit from rabbit skeletal muscle was reported (Beavo et al. 1974), investigators have consistently added BSA at concentrations between 0.1–0.5 mg/ml to maintain the high activity of this enzyme (see, for example, Whitehouse et al. 1983). Therefore, pp60^{src} and highly purified BSA were compared for their ability to preserve high catalytic subunit activity. As shown in Figure 10, pp60^{src} preparations were found to be up to 3000- to 4000-fold more efficient than BSA, on the basis of protein concentration, in sustaining the catalytic subunit activity. Furthermore, even in the presence of 0.1 mg/ml BSA, the activity of the catalytic subunit was 50–80% higher when pp60^{src} was added to the reaction mixture (data not shown).

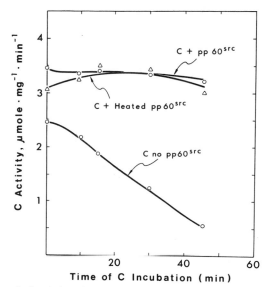

Figure 9 Catalytic subunit activity in the presence of heat-treated pp60*src*. Catalytic subunit (1.7 pmole) was incubated for different times without the addition of unlabeled ATP at 30°C in the absence or in the presence of pp60*src* (16.7 fmole) or in the presence of pp60*src* that had been heated for 15 min at 41°C. At the times indicated, 6 µl of the catalytic subunit substrates (100 µM ATP, 100 µM Kemptide) were added and the phosphotransferase activity was determined

Discussion

In this article, we have demonstrated that the catalytic subunit of cAMP-dependent protein kinase isolated from beef heart can be modified by highly purified pp60*src* (more than 95% of the silver-stainable protein found in M_r 60,000). The modifications of the catalytic subunit by pp60*src* include:

1. Decreased capacity to be regulated by RII (Figs. 2–4).
2. Tyrosine phosphorylation of a protein of M_r 41,000 that comigrates on 10% acrylamide gels with the sil-

ver-stainable band of the catalytic subunit (Figs. 5–6).
3. Modification of its activity toward well-defined physiological and synthetic substrates (Fig. 7).
4. Five- to sevenfold increase of its kinetic parameters (K_m and V_{max}) toward both ATP and the Kemptide (Fig. 8).

That the catalytic subunit of the cAMP-dependent protein kinase is phosphorylated by pp60*src* is indicated by the observation that a homogeneous protein with M_r 41,000 (Fig. 1) (Chiu and Tao 1978), which is autophosphorylated (Fig. 5) on serine residues (Fig. 6), serves as a substrate for pp60*src*, which phosphorylates protein substrates specifically on tyrosine residues (Figs. 5 and 6). That the changes in the activity observed are due to catalytic subunit is indicated by: (1) the homogeneity of the protein with an M_r 41,000 as shown in Fig. 1; (2) the specific inhibition of the phosphotransferase activity by the heat-stable catalytic subunit inhibitor (Fig. 7); and (3) the phosphorylation of serine residues in physiological substrates, consistent with the specificity of catalytic subunit.

Although it it tempting to correlate the increased activity of catalytic subunit with its phosphorylation on tyrosine by pp60*src*, the difference between the stability at 41°C of the phosphotransferase activity of pp60*src* as compared with the stability of the effect of the pp60*src* preparation on the catalytic subunit activity (Fig. 9) indicates that tyrosine phosphorylation may not account for the increased activity of catalytic subunit. Moreover, the phosphorylation of catalytic subunit by pp60*src* in the presence of RII (Fig. 4B) occurred much more slowly than the activation of RII phosphorylation in the presence of pp60*src* (Fig. 4A). The ability of the pp60*src* preparation alone to preserve high activity of the catalytic subunit (Table 1) without ATP during preincubation further indicates that the phosphotransferase activity of pp60*src* may not be involved in the modification of the catalytic subunit activity. However, because of the rapid rate of activation of catalytic subunit by pp60*src*, the absence of

Table 1 The Effect of Mg^{++}, ATP, dATP, and AppNHp on Catalytic Subunit Activity in the Presence of pp60*src*

	S.A. µmole · mg^{-1} · min^{-1}	
	catalytic subunit	catalytic subunit + pp60*src*
KP$_i$ buffer	0.20	1.30
+ 2.5 mM MgCl$_2$	0.25	1.20
+ MgCl$_2$ + 20 µM ATP	0.27	1.26
+ MgCl$_2$ + 20 µM dATP	0.27	1.25
+ MgCl$_2$ + 20 µM AppNHp	0.23	1.18

Catalytic subunit (1.7 pmoles) was incubated in the presence or absence of pp60*src* (16.7 fmoles) for 30 min at 30°C in the presence of different trinucleotides, as indicated. After the preincubation period, [γ-^{32}P]ATP and Kemptide were added, and the phosphotransferase activity of the enzyme was determined.

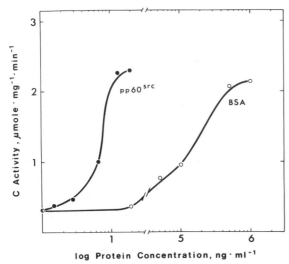

Figure 10 The effect of increasing concentrations of pp60^{src} and of BSA on the catalytic subunit phosphotransferase activity. Catalytic subunit (1.7 pmole) was incubated for 30 min at 30°C as described in Fig. 9 in the presence of increasing concentrations of pp60^{src} or BSA as indicated in the figure, 6 μl of the substrates (100 μM ATP and 100 μM Kemptide final concentration) were added and the reaction was carried out for an additional 5 min. The estimation of the catalytic subunit activity was done as described in Figs. 2 and 7.

ATP during preincubation might not affect the activity change seen with the catalytic subunit (Table 1). Thus, it is not certain whether the effect of pp60^{src} on the catalytic subunit requires ATP.

To date, we have no explanation for the limit of about 0.15 moles of tyrosine phosphate incorporated per mole of catalytic subunit in the presence of pp60^{src}. Several pertinent facts regarding catalytic subunit have been described (Peters et al. 1977) and should be considered in this regard. (1) There are at least three species of catalytic subunit, as judged by isoelectric focusing; (2) it is phosphorylated on serine and threonine; (3) it is prone to aggregation. One or all of these features may limit tyrosine phosphorylation to a fraction of the total population of molecules, and experiments are in progress to examine these questions.

The catalytic subunit is the first example of an enzyme that undergoes an activity change in vitro by incubation with pp60^{src}. Perhaps the most important issue raised by these studies is the possibility that the catalytic subunit may be influenced by pp60^{src} in transformed cells. The increase in both K_m and V_{max} for the catalytic subunit substrates observed here is consistent with a role for the catalytic subunit in the increased serine phosphorylation observed in transformed cells because the intracellular ATP concentration is at least 1 mM and the molar concentration of potential substrates, such as the ribosomal protein S6, is rather high. Such a change in K_m and V_{max} for a substrate may also result in the phosphorylation of an altered spectrum of protein substrates by the catalytic subunit in the transformed cell. The fact

that the activation has uncompetitive kinetics suggests that the modification of catalytic subunit activity is stable.

The molecular mechanism by which pp60^{src} preparations modify the catalytic subunit activity is unclear. The experiments shown in Figure 2 suggest that pp60^{src} partially mimics the effect of cAMP on the reassociation properties of catalytic subunit with its regulatory subunit (RII) in vitro. This effect of cAMP is well documented in the literature (Rangel-Aldao and Rosen 1976, 1977), although the exact mechanism of dissociation/reassociation both in vitro and in vivo is still unclear.

Raising the level of cAMP in cells has been reported to produce diverse effects on cellular growth. Exogenous addition of high levels of dibutyryl-cAMP apparently causes growth arrest and the restoration of more normal properties to certain lines of transformed cells (for review, see Pastan et al. 1975). By contrast, in other instances, moderate increases in cAMP levels have been associated with the stimulation of cell division (Hovi and Vaheri 1973; Schor and Rosengurt 1973). It is beyond the scope of this discussion to resolve such issues, although it seems likely that all the effects of cAMP are mediated via cAMP-dependent protein kinase activity. If the observations reported here are relevant to the transformation of cells by RSV, they must be reconciled with previous results. It is possible that the modification of the catalytic subunit by pp60^{src} mimics moderate increases in the levels of cAMP, producing a stimulation of cell division. Thus, conceivably, transformed cells might have a high level of catalytic subunit activity even in the presence of low cAMP levels. It also seems likely that the changes in K_m and V_{max} reported here will not only change the phosphorylation level of normal substrates by catalytic subunit but could also change the substrate specificity of the enzyme, unlike the addition of cAMP. The results reported here indicate that functional relationships exist between serine and tyrosine protein kinases, and it seems likely that cell transformation alters this network of interactions by mechanisms that remain to be elucidated.

Acknowledgments

We thank Eleanor Erikson for a critical reading of the manuscript. This work was supported by grants from the National Institutes of Health (CA-15823 and CA-21117 to R.L.E. and AM-28353 to J.L.M.), by a grant from the American Cancer Society (CD-187 to J.L.M.), by an award from the American Business Cancer Research Foundation to R.L.E., and, indirectly, by a gift from R.J. Reynolds Industries, Inc., to the Department of Pathology. R.L.E. is an American Cancer Society Professor of Cellular and Developmental Biology. J.L.M. is an Established Investigator of the American Heart Association.

References

Beavo, J.A., P.J. Bechtel, and E.G. Krebs. 1974. Preparation of homogeneous cyclic AMP-dependent protein kinase(s) and its subunits from rabbit skeletal muscle. *Methods Enzymol.* **38:** 299.

Bradford, M.M. 1976. A rapid and sensitive method for quantitation of microgram quantities of protein utilizing the principle of protein dye binding. *Anal. Biochem.* **72**: 248.

Carmichael, D.F., R.L. Geahlen, S.M. Allen, and E.G. Krebs. 1982. Type II regulatory subunit of the cAMP-dependent protein kinase. *J. Biol. Chem.* **257**: 10440.

Chiu, Y.S. and M. Tao. 1978. Autophosphorylation of rabbit skeletal muscle cyclic-AMP-dependent protein kinase I catalytic subunit. *J. Biol. Chem.* **253**: 7145.

Cohen, P., D. Yellowlees, A. Aitken, A. Donella-Deana, B.A. Hemmings, and P.J. Parker. 1982. Separation and characterisation of glycogen synthase kinase 3, glycogen synthase kinase 4 and glycogen synthase kinase 5 from rabbit skeletal muscle. *Eur. J. Biochem.* **124**: 21.

Collett, M.S., A.F. Purchio, and R.L. Erikson. 1980. Avian sarcoma virus-transforming protein, pp60*src* shows protein kinase activity specific for tyrosine. *Nature* **285**: 167.

Corbin, J.D., P.H. Sugden, L. West, D.A. Flockhart, T.M. Lincoln, and D. McCarthy. 1978. Studies on the properties and mode of action of the purified regulatory subunit of bovine heart adenosine 3':5'-monophosphate-dependent protein kinase. *J. Biol. Chem.* **253**: 3997.

Decker, S. 1981. Phosphorylation of ribosomal protein S6 in avian sarcoma virus-transformed chicken embryo fibroblasts. *Proc. Natl. Acad. Sci.* **78**: 1112.

Dills, W.L., J.A. Beavo, P.J. Bechtel, and E.G. Krebs. 1975. Purification of rabbit skeletal muscle protein kinase regulatory subunit using cyclic adenosine-3':5'-monophosphate affinity chromatography. *Biochem. Biophys. Res. Commun.* **62**: 70.

Erickson, R.L., M.S. Collett, E. Erikson, A.F. Purchio, and J.S. Brugge. 1980a. Protein phosphorylation mediated by partially purified avian sarcoma virus transforming-gene product. *Cold Spring Harbor Symp. Quant. Biol.* **44**: 907.

Erikson, R.L., A.F. Purchio, E. Erikson, M.S. Collett, and J.S. Brugge. 1980b. Molecular events in cells transformed by Rous sarcoma virus. *J. Cell. Biol.* **87**: 319.

Flockhart, D.A. and J.D. Corbin. 1982. Regulatory mechanisms in the control of protein kinases. *CRC Crit. Rev. Biochem.* **12**: 133.

Flockhart, D.A., D.M. Watterson, and J.D. Corbin. 1980. Studies on functional domains of the regulatory subunit of bovine heart adenosine 3':5'-monophosphate-dependent protein kinase. *J. Biol. Chem.* **255**: 4435.

Gilman, A.G. 1970. A protein binding assay for adenosine 3':5' cyclic monophosphate. *Proc. Natl. Acad. Sci.* **67**: 305.

Graziani, Y., E. Erikson, and R.L. Erikson. 1983. Characterization of the Rous sarcoma virus transforming gene product. *J. Biol. Chem.* **258**: 6344.

Hayakawa, T., J.P. Penkins, and E.G. Krebs. 1973. Studies on the subunit structure of rabbit skeletal muscle phosphorylase kinase. *Biochemistry* **12**: 574.

Hovi, T. and A. Vaheri. 1973. Cyclic AMP and cyclic GMP enhance growth of chick embryo fibroblasts. *Nat. New Biol.* **245**: 175.

Johnson, R.A. and T.F. Walseth. 1979. The enzymatic preparation of [α-^{32}P]ATP, [α-^{32}P]GTP, [^{32}P]cAMP, and [^{32}P]cGMP, and their use in the assay of adenylate and guanylate cyclases and cyclic nucleotide phosphodiesterases. *Adv. Cyclic Nucleotide Res.* **10**: 135.

Kemp, B.E., D.J. Graves, E. Benjamin, and E.G. Krebs. 1977. Role of multiple basic residues in determining the substrate specificity of cyclic AMP-dependent protein kinase. *J. Biol. Chem.* **252**: 4888.

Krebs, E.G. and J.A. Beavo. 1979. Phosphorylation-dephosphorylation of enzymes. *Annu. Rev. Biochem.* **44**: 923.

Langan, T.A. 1973. Protein kinases and protein kinase substrates. *Adv. Cyclic Nucleotide Res.* **3**: 99.

Levinson, A.D., H. Oppermann, H.E. Varmus, and J.M. Bishop. 1980. The purified product of the transforming gene of avian sarcoma virus phosphorylates tyrosine. *J. Biol. Chem.* **255**: 11973.

Lowry, O.H., N.J. Rosenbrough, A.L. Farr, and R.J. Randall. 1951. Protein measurements with the Folin phenol reagent. *J. Biol. Chem.* **193**: 265.

Nimmo, H.G. and P. Cohen. 1974. Glycogen synthetase kinase 2 (GSK2): The identification of a new protein kinase in skeletal muscle. *FEBS Lett.* **47**: 162.

———. 1977. Hormonal control of protein phosphorylation. *Adv. Cyclic Nucleotide Res.* **8**: 145.

Oakley, B.R., D.R. Kirsh, and N.R. Morris. 1980. A simplified ultra-sensitive silver stain for detecting proteins in polyacrylamide gels. *Anal. Biochem.* **105**: 361.

Pastan, I.H., G.S. Johnson, and W.B. Anderson. 1975. Role of cyclic nucleotides in growth control. *Annu. Rev. Biochem.* **44**: 491.

Peters, A.K., J.G. Demaille, and E.H. Fischer. 1977. Adenosine 3':5'-monophosphate dependent protein kinase from bovine heart. Characterization of the catalytic subunit. *Biochemistry* **16**: 5691.

Rangel-Aldao, R. and O.M. Rosen. 1976. Mechanism of self-phosphorylation of adenosine 3':5' monophosphate-dependent protein kinase from bovine cardiac muscle. *J. Biol. Chem.* **251**: 7526.

———. 1977. Effect of cAMP and ATP on the reassociation of phosphorylated and nonphosphorylated subunits of the cAMP dependent protein kinase from bovine cardiac muscle. *J. Biol. Chem.* **252**: 7140.

Richert, N.D., P.J.A. Davis, and I.H. Pastan. 1979. Characterization of an immune complex kinase in immunoprecipitates of avian sarcoma virus-transformed fibroblasts. *J. Virol.* **31**: 695.

Rosen, O.M. and J. Erlichman. 1975. Reversible autophosphorylation of a cyclic 3':5'-AMP-dependent protein kinase from bovine cardiac muscle. *J. Biol. Chem.* **250**: 7788.

Rubin, C.S. and O.M. Rosen. 1975. Protein phosphorylation. *Annu. Rev. Biochem.* **44**: 831.

Schor, S. and E. Rosengurt. 1973. Enhancement by purine nucleosides and nucleotides of serum-induced DNA synthesis in quiescent 3T3 cells. *J. Cell. Physiol.* **81**: 339.

Soderling, T.R., J.P. Hickenbottom, E.N. Reimann, F.L. Hunkeler, D.A. Walsh, and E.G. Krebs. 1970. Inactivation of glycogen synthetase and activation of phosphorylase kinase by muscle adenosine 3':5'-monophosphate-dependent protein kinases. *J. Biol. Chem.* **245**: 6317.

Walsh, D.A., C.D. Ashby, C. Gonzales, D. Calkins, E.H. Fischer, and E.G. Krebs. 1971. Purification and characterization of a protein inhibitor of adenosine 3',5'-monophosphate-dependent protein kinases. *J. Biol. Chem.* **246**: 1977.

Whitehouse, S., J.R. Feramisco, J.E. Casnellie, E.G. Krebs, and D.A. Walsh. 1983. Studies on the kinetic mechanism of the catalytic subunit of the cAMP-dependent protein kinase. *J. Biol. Chem.* **258**: 3693.

Site-directed Mutagenesis of Rous Sarcoma Virus pp60*src*: Identification of Functional Domains Required for Transformation

J.T. Parsons, D. Bryant,* V. Wilkerson, G. Gilmartin,† and S.J. Parsons

Department of Microbiology, University of Virginia Medical School, Charlottesville, Virginia 22908

Cellular transformation, induced by Rous sarcoma virus (RSV), results from the expression of a single viral gene, the *src* gene (Hanafusa 1977). The *src* gene product pp60*src* is a tyrosine protein kinase that is capable of catalyzing the phosphorylation of a variety of substrates in vitro (Collett and Erikson 1978; Hunter and Sefton 1978; Levinson et al. 1978). In vivo, cellular expression of the *src* gene product results in the tyrosine-specific phosphorylation of several specific cellular proteins (Erikson and Erikson 1980; Radke et al. 1980; Cooper and Hunter 1981; Brugge and Darrow 1982). These unique phosphorylation events, coupled with the intrinsic kinase activity of pp60*src*, indicate that tyrosine-specific phosphorylation of specific cellular target proteins plays a critical role in cellular transformation.

A number of transforming retroviruses, isolated from cats, chickens, and mice, contain genes (oncogenes) that also encode tyrosine protein kinases (Cooper 1982). Nucleotide sequence analysis of several of these viral oncogenes has shown that these oncogenes have amino acid sequence homology with the carboxyterminal half of pp60*src* (Hampe et al. 1982; Kitamura et al. 1982; Shibuya and Hanafusa 1982; Reddy et al. 1983). In addition, the oncogene products of Moloney sarcoma virus (*v-mos*, Barker and Dayhoff 1982), McDonough feline sarcoma virus (*v-fms*, C. Sherr, pers. comm.), and avian erythroblastosis virus (*erb-B*, J.M. Bishop, pers. comm.) exhibit significant amino acid sequence homology with pp60*src*, although these proteins do not appear to function as tyrosine protein kinases. In spite of the considerable evidence involving tyrosine protein kinases in cellular transformation, we remain essentially ignorant about their interactions with cellular target proteins and, possibly, with cellular regulatory factors. In addition, the functional differences between viral tyrosine protein kinases and their normal cellular counterparts (pp60*c-src* in the case of RSV *src*) remain largely obscure.

To delineate the various structural and functional domains of pp60*src*, we have used site-directed mutagenesis to construct a variety of deletion mutations (*dl*), point mutations (*pm*), and insertion mutations (*is*) within the *src* gene of molecularly cloned Prague A (PrA) RSV DNA. Here, we summarize the biological characterization of several such mutants of RSV, we describe the

biochemical analysis of the *src* proteins encoded by individual mutants, and we present a model that attempts to delineate the structural and functional domains of pp60*src*.

Methods of Experimental Procedures

Cells, viruses, and plasmids

Primary chicken embryo fibroblast cultures were prepared and maintained as previously described (Bryant and Parsons 1982). The plasmid pSL102, which contains a permuted RSV genome in pBR322 (Bryant and Parsons 1982), was recloned to yield a plasmid (pJD100) containing a nonpermuted copy of the RSV genome. This plasmid or plasmids containing subgenomic fragments derived from pJD100 were used for mutagenesis experiments. Transfection of chicken embryo cells was carried out as described previously (Bryant and Parsons 1982).

Construction of mutations

The construction of deletion mutations was carried out as described previously (Bryant and Parsons 1982; Gilmartin and Parsons 1983). CH*dl*119 was obtained by BAL 31 exonuclease digestion of plasmid DNA opened at the *Bgl*II restriction site (nucleotides 606–611) in the *src* gene (Schwartz et al. 1982). CH*dl*300 was obtained by BAL 31 digestion of plasmid DNA opened at the *Mst*II restriction site at nucleotide positions 1506–1511 in *src*. CH*dl*121 and CH*dl*120 were obtained by joining plasmid DNAs containing oligonucleotide linkers inserted at defined restriction sites within the *src* gene. The details of these constructions will be presented elsewhere (V.W. Wilkerson and J.T. Parsons, in prep.). Bisulfite mutagenesis at the *Bgl*I restriction site in *src* and subsequent analysis of the mutagenized clones have been described previously (Shortle and Nathans 1978; Bryant and Parsons 1982). Mutations were identified by sequencing a 393-bp *Taq*I–*Pst*I fragment containing the *Bgl*I restriction site. A minimum of 50 bp on either side of *Bgl*I site were sequenced for each mutant. All mutations were confirmed by direct DNA sequencing (Maxam and Gilbert 1980).

Immunoprecipitation and protein kinase assays

Cells were labeled with [35S]methionine or 32P; and immunoprecipitated as described previously (Parsons et al. 1983). Protein kinase assays were performed as described earlier (Bryant and Parsons 1982, 1983), except

---

*Current address: Oncogen, Seattle, Washington 98121.

†Current address: Institut für Molekularbiologie II, Universitat Zurich, Zurich, Switzerland.

that the reaction buffer contained 20 mM PIPES (pH 7.0) and 10 mM MnCl$_2$.

Results

Structural alterations within the aminoterminal half of pp60^{src}

We have used several site-specific mutagenesis techniques to isolate mutants containing deletions within the 5′-terminal half of the *src* gene sequence. Three of these mutants (CH*dl*121, *ts*CH*dl*119, *ts*CH*dl*120) have been characterized in some detail (Bryant and Parsons 1982; Table 1). The genome of *ts*CH*dl*119 contains an inphase deletion of 162 nucleotides and encodes a structurally altered *src* protein pp53^{src} containing a deletion of Leu-173 to Val-227. The mutation (168 bp) within *ts*CH*dl*-120 is similar to that of *ts*CH*dl*119, and results in the deletion of Arg-169 to Gln-225. Both mutants exhibited a similar phenotype upon infection of chicken embryo cells. Infected cells grown at 35°C were indistinguishable from wild-type PrA RSV-infected cells. However, upon shift of the cultures to 41°C, the cell morphology was altered and resembled that of normal cells. Immune complexes containing pp53^{src} isolated from either *ts*-CH*dl*119- or *ts*CH*dl*120-infected cells grown at 41°C exhibited only 40–50% less tyrosine-specific kinase activity than immune complexes isolated from mutant-infected cells grown at 35°C. In vivo ^{32}P-labeling experiments have shown that *ts*CH*dl*119-infected cells grown at 41°C exhibited only a 40% reduction in total cellular phosphotyrosine labeling and a similar 40% reduction in the amount of the phosphotyrosine-labeled 34K protein (Cooper et al. 1983). These data indicate that *ts*CH*dl*119 or *ts*CH*dl*120-infected cells grown at the nonpermissive temperature exhibit a normal morphology, yet retain substantial levels of tyrosine protein kinase activity.

The genome of CH*dl*121 contains an inphase deletion of 251 bp, resulting in the deletion of sequences encoding Gly-82 to Arg-165. Chicken embryo cells infected with CH*dl*121 have a normal morphology, yet contain high levels of a structurally altered *src* protein, pp50^{src}. Immune complexes isolated from CH*dl*121 cells contained readily detectable levels of tyrosine protein kinase activity (approximately 40% of wild type), indicating that the large deletion of aminoterminal sequences does not totally inactivate the kinase activity of the mutant protein.

Single amino acid changes within a highly conserved structural domain of pp60^{src}

Several regions of the *src* protein appear to be highly conserved among tyrosine protein kinases, in particular the amino acid sequences corresponding to residues 427–433 and 443–449. We have previously shown that the alteration of Ala-433 to Thr results in the generation of an enzymatically altered form of pp60^{src} (Bryant and Parsons 1983). We have continued to explore the role of these highly conserved amino acid sequences in pp60^{src} function, isolating mutants of RSV that encode *src* proteins with single amino acid substitutions within one of

the highly conserved regions that spans residues 427–433. Point mutations within the *src* gene were obtained using previously described techniques of sodium bisulfite mutagenesis within a short sequence defined by a *BglI* restriction site. Analysis of individual mutagenized plasmids by *BglI* restriction enzyme analysis, direct DNA sequencing, and transfection of chicken embryo cells resulted in the identification of the point mutations listed in Table 1. The mutant CH*pm*26 contains a single C → T change, altering the codon for Ala-430 (GCC) to Val (GTC); CH*pm*9 contains a single C → T change, altering the codon for Pro-431 (CCC) to Ser (TCC); CH*pm*6 contains two G → A alterations, changing the codon for Glu-432 (GAG) to Lys (AAA); and CH*pm*65 contains a single G → A change, altering the codon for Ala-433 (GCA) to Thr (ACA). CH*pm*59 contains a G → A change in the third base of the codon for Glu-432 and therefore does not alter the amino acid sequence at this position. Transfection of chicken embryo cells with mutagenized plasmid DNAs showed that *pm*26, *pm*9, *pm*6, and *pm*65 were defective for transformation, whereas *pm*59 readily transformed chicken cells.

To confirm that cells infected with the individual mutants contained elevated levels of *src* protein, infected cells were labeled with [^{35}S]methionine, and cell extracts were prepared and immunoprecipitated with rabbit antisera to bacterial p60^{src} (anti-p60^{src}) (Gilmer and Erikson 1982). Analysis of immunoprecipitates (Fig. 1) showed that both PrA RSV-infected cells and cells infected with individual mutants synthesized similar levels of *src* protein. Figure 1 also shows that immunoprecipitates from cells infected with the transformation-defective mutants contained significantly reduced levels of the pp60^{src}-associated protein p90. This protein and a second cellular protein, p50, are associated with soluble pp60^{src} (Brugge et al. 1981; Opperman et al. 1981). Although the role of the p90-p50-pp60^{src} complex in cellular transformation is still unclear, it would appear that the above mutant pp60^{src} proteins either do not associate with p90 and p50, or that the complex is unstable in mutant infected cells.

To define the functional defects in the mutant *src* gene products, we have examined the in vitro tyrosine protein kinase activity. Immune complexes were isolated from cells infected with *pm*26, *pm*9, *pm*6, *pm*59, incubated with [γ-^{32}P]ATP, and the level of pp60^{src} autophosphorylation was measured (Fig. 2). Immune complexes from cells infected with each of the transformation-defective mutants exhibited significantly decreased, but detectable, levels of protein kinase activity when compared with immune complexes from wild-type RSV- or *pm*59-infected cells (Fig. 2). Similar levels of protein kinase activity were observed when casein or the peptide angiotensin II were used as substrates for phosphorylation. Therefore, the structural alterations induced by the single amino acid changes at residues 430–433 result in an alteration of tyrosine protein kinase activity in vitro. We have also determined that the decreased kinase activity of the transformation-defective mutants observed in vitro was paralleled by a decrease in tyrosine

Table 1 Summary of Site-directed Mutants in the *src* Gene of RSV

Mutant	Position of mutation in amino acid sequence	Morphology of infected cells 35°C	Morphology of infected cells 41°C	Apparent M_r of mutant protein	Kinase activity autophosphorylation 35°C	Kinase activity autophosphorylation 41°C	Kinase activity 34K 35°C	Kinase activity 34K 41°C
CH*dl*119	deletion Leu-173→Val-227	tfo⁺	tfo⁻	54,000	+	+	+	+
CH*dl*120	deletion Arg-169→Gln-225	tfo⁺	tfo⁻	54,000	+	+	N.D.ᵇ	
CH*dl*121	deletion Gly-82→Arg-169	tfo⁻		50,000	+		N.D.	
CH*is*333	4-amino-acid insertion after Val-111	tfo⁺		60,000	+		N.D.	
CH*pm*26	Ala-439→Val	tfo⁻		60,000	−		−	
CH*pm*9	Pro-431→Ser	tfo⁻		60,000	−		−	
CH*pm*6	Glu-432→Lys	tfo⁻		60,000	−		−	
CH*pm*1, -7, -65	Ala-433→Thr	tfo⁻		60,000	−		−	
CH*pm*59	Glu-432 (3rd base change)	tfo⁺		60,000	+		+	
CH*dl*300	deletion Glu 504→Arg-506	tfo⁻		57,000–60,000	−		−	
CH*is*1511	3-amino-acid insertion after Glu-504 (frameshift)	tfo⁻		58,000–60,000	−		−	
CH*is*1545	2-amino-acid insertion after Gln-515 (frameshift)	tfo⁻		58,000–60,000	−		−	
CH-VC-15	amino acids 1–431 from *v-src* amino acids 432–533 from *c-src*	tfoᵃ		61,000	+		N.D.	

ᵃCells exhibit an altered morphology, however distinct from PrA-infected cells.
ᵇN.D., not done.

phosphorylation in vivo of the cellular 34K protein, which is rapidly phosphorylated on tyrosine in response to transformation by RSV (Radke et al. 1980). The above observations provide additional support for the conclusion that functional protein kinase activity is required for morphological transformation of cells.

Alterations of the carboxyl terminus of pp60ˢʳᶜ
Takeya and Hanafusa (1983) have recently shown that the carboxyterminal 19 amino acids of pp60ᶜ⁻ˢʳᶜ (the cel-

lular homolog of virus-coded pp60ᵛ⁻ˢʳᶜ) were replaced by a new set of 12 amino acids of pp60ᵛ⁻ˢʳᶜ. We have investigated the role of these sequences in the maintenance of functional *src* protein activity, first, by introducing mutations that alter all or part of the terminal 25 amino acids of pp60ˢʳᶜ and, second, by replacing the 3′-terminal nucleotide sequence of *v-src* with the cognate sequence from *c-src*, to generate a hybrid gene product composed of both viral and cellular *src* sequences. Three mutations within the 3′-terminal 71 bp of the *src* gene have been isolated. The mutant CH*dl*300 contains a deletion of 10 bp (1509–1518 within the *src* gene) and

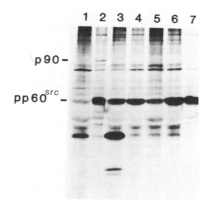

Figure 1 Immunoprecipitation of *src* protein from cells infected with PrA RSV or mutant RSV. Chicken cells infected with PrA RSV or CH*pm*26,-9,-6,-65, or -59 mutants of RSV were labeled with [³⁵S]methionine, harvested, immunoprecipitated with rabbit anti-*src* sera (Gilmer and Erikson 1982), and analyzed by polyacrylamide gel electrophoresis and autoradiography. Molecular weights of the proteins indicated were determined relative to the position of known molecular-weight standards. (Lane *1*) Uninfected cells; (lane *2*) PrA RSV-infected cells; (lane *3*) CH*pm*26-infected cells; (lane *4*) CH*pm*9-infected cells; (lane *5*) CH*pm*6-infected cells; (lane *6*) CH*pm*65-infected cells; (lane *7*) CH*pm*59-infected cells.

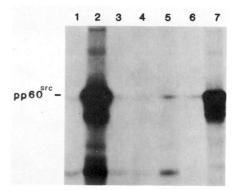

Figure 2 In vitro protein kinase activity of *src* proteins from PrA RSV- and mutant-infected cells. Cells infected with PrA RSV or individual mutant virus (described in Fig. 1) were harvested, immunoprecipitated with rabbit anti-*src* antisera, and assayed for autophosphorylation activity as described in the text. (Lane *1*) Uninfected cells; (lane *2*) PrA RSV-infected cells; (lane *3*) CH*pm*26-infected cells; (lane *4*) CH*pm*9-infected cells; (lane *5*) CH*pm*6-infected cells; (lane *6*) CH*pm*65-infected cells; (lane *7*) CH*pm*59-infected cells.

encodes a *src* protein that contains a deletion of Glu-504 to Arg-506 and terminates with an unrelated amino acid sequence that is generated as a result of a frameshift to an alternative reading frame. The mutation CH*is*1511 was generated by insertion of an 8-bp *Cla*I linker at an *Mst*II site 71 bp from the 3' end of the *src* gene. This insertion-frameshift mutant encodes a *src* protein with 31 amino acids of unrelated sequence at the carboxyl terminus. The third mutation (CH*is*1545) was derived by insertion of an 8-bp *Cla*I linker at a *Pvu*II restriction site, 35 bp from 3' end of the *src* gene. This insertion-frameshift mutant encodes a *src* protein containing only 18 unrelated amino acids at the carboxyl terminus. When transfection of chicken embryo cells was carried out with each of the mutants described above, no morphological transformation was observed, indicating that each of the mutants was transformation defective.

To examine the effects of the structural alteration of the carboxyl terminus of the *src* protein, chicken embryo cells were infected with the mutants CH*dl*300, CH*is*1511, and CH*is*1545, labeled with [^{35}S]methionine, and extracts immunoprecipitated with anti-p60^{src} sera. Figure 3 shows that each of the mutants encodes a 60,000 M_r protein, as expected from the nucleotide sequence analysis. However, additional *src*-related proteins (M_r 58,000–59,000) were detected in each of the mutant-derived immunoprecipitates. The smaller forms of *src* protein likely reflect proteolytic processing of the mutant proteins due to the unrelated carboxyterminal protein sequences. Interestingly, we have not observed cellular p90 in immunoprecipitates from CH*dl*300-, C*his*1511-, or CH*is*1545-infected cell extracts, suggesting that these mutant *src* proteins are unable to form stable complexes with p90.

To determine what effects a structural alteration of the carboxyl terminus has on tyrosine protein kinase activity, cells were infected with mutant or wild-type RSV, labeled with ^{32}P, and extracts were immunoprecipitated with anti-p60^{src} or anti-34K sera. Figure 4 shows that each of the

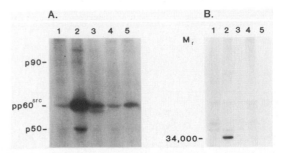

Figure 4 In vivo kinase activity of wild-type or mutant *src* proteins. Chicken cells infected with PrA RSV, CH*dl*300, CH*is*-1511, or CH*is*1545 were labeled with ^{32}P$_i$. Cell lysates were immunoprecipitated with rabbit anti-p60^{src} (*A*) or anti-34K sera (*B*). (Lane *1*) Uninfected cells; (lane *2*) PrA RSV; (lane *3*) CH*dl*300; (lane *4*) CH*dl*1511; (lane *5*) CH*is*1545.

3' mutations encodes a *src* protein with significantly reduced levels of in vivo phosphorylation. Similarly, mutant-infected cells contain a decrease in the level of tyrosine-phosphorylated 34K protein (Fig. 4B). These observations show that alterations of the carboxyterminal sequence of the *src* protein (including only the last 11 amino acids) lead to both the loss of transforming potential and substantial decreases in tyrosine protein kinase activity, and provide evidence that the catalytic domain of pp60^{src} is exquisitely sensitive to structural modifications.

Characterization of *src* proteins containing sequences derived from viral *src* and cellular *src*

The observations that *v-src* and *c-src* genes encode proteins that differ substantially at the carboxyl terminus, as well as our own observation that mutations altering the carboxyterminal residues yielded defective transforming virus, have prompted us to construct a hybrid *src* gene containing nucleotide sequences derived from *v-src* and *c-src* genes. These hybrid *src* gene constructions (to be detailed elsewhere) encode a *src* gene product containing amino acid residues 1–431 of *v-src* and residues 432–533 of *c-src*. Transfection of chicken embryo cells resulted in the synthesis of a 61,000 M_r protein at levels comparable to PrA RSV-infected cells (Table 1). However, virus containing the hybrid *src* gene induced an alteration in cell morphology, readily distinguishable from that induced by wild-type RSV (J.T. Parsons et al., in prep.). The differences in morphological transformation exhibited by *v-c-src* hybrid-infected cells lends further evidence that changes in sequence at the carboxyl terminus influence functional expression of the *src* gene product.

Discussion

The biological and biochemical characterization of RSV mutants containing defined mutations within the *src* gene has led us to propose that the *src* gene product pp60^{src} contains several overlapping functional domains. The organization of these domains is depicted schematically in Figure 5. Considerable evidence has shown that pp60^{src}

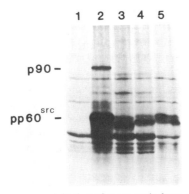

Figure 3 Immunoprecipitation of *src* protein from cells infected with carboxyterminal mutants, CH*dl*300, CH*is*1511, or CH*is*1545. Chicken cells infected with PrA RSV or mutant virus were labeled with [^{35}S]methionine as described in the text. Cells were harvested, lysed, and immunoprecipitated with rabbit anti-p60^{src} sera as described in Fig. 1. (Lane *1*) Uninfected cells; (lane *2*) PrA RSV; (lane *3*) CH*dl*300; (lane *4*) CH*dl*1511; (lane *5*) CH*dl*1545.

FUNCTIONAL DOMAINS OF pp60^{src}

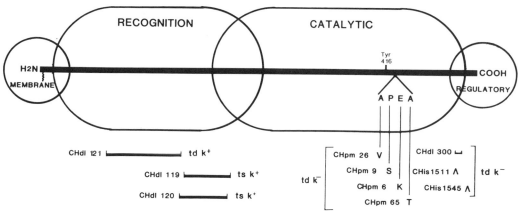

Figure 5 Schematic diagram of the functional domains of pp60^{src}.

is associated with the plasma membrane via an amino-terminal domain (Courtneidge et al. 1980; Levinson et al. 1981; Krueger et al. 1982). The observation that pp60^{src} contains tightly bound lipid (Sefton et al. 1982) suggests that this moiety may be responsible for anchoring the *src* protein in the plasma membrane. Deletion of nucleotide sequences within the 5′ half of the *src* gene has yielded RSV mutants that encode structurally altered forms of *src* protein. In the case of CH*d*l121, the alteration rendered the virus transformation defective, whereas, in mutants CH*d*l119 and CH*d*l120, the sequence alterations yielded virus that was temperature sensitive for morphological transformation. In both instances, the *src* protein encoded by the mutant virus retains substantial protein kinase activity in vitro. Therefore, these viruses appear to represent a class of mutants containing mutations mapping within a functionally important domain of the *src* protein, distinct from the domain specifying the protein kinase activity. Such a recognition domain might specify the interaction of the *src* protein with a specific target protein or set of target proteins. Recently, two mutants of RSV having properties similar to CH*d*l121 and CH*d*l119 have been reported (Kitamura and Yoshida 1983; Mardon and Varmus 1983).

The conservation of amino acid sequences between the carboxyterminal one-half of pp60^{src} and other viral tyrosine protein kinases suggests that this part of pp60^{src} contains a functional catalytic domain or domains necessary for tyrosine protein kinase activity. The isolation of transformation-defective virus containing point mutations, resulting in single amino acid changes within a highly conserved amino acid sequence, would argue that this region of the *src* protein specifies a functional domain whose expression is essential for cellular transformation (Fig. 5). That this functional domain specifies protein kinase activity is indicated by the observation that

these mutants encode *src* proteins with decreased protein kinase activity measured both in vitro and in vivo (Table 1). Therefore, the high degree of amino acid sequence conservation within this part of the *src* protein likely reflects the requirement to preserve the structural integrity of this essential domain.

The carboxyl terminus of the *src* protein is clearly involved in maintaining catalytic activity and, in the case of *c-src*, may play a role in modulating or regulating protein kinase activity. The alteration of the carboxyl terminus of pp60^{v-src} has a deleterious effect on transformation as well as protein kinase activity (Table 1), suggesting that the carboxyterminal portion of pp60^{v-src} is intimately involved in maintaining the overall tertiary structure of the enzymatically active *src* protein. If such structural changes alter pp60^{v-src} activity, what role does the carboxyl terminus of the *c-src* protein play in the specificity or regulation of *c-src* activity? We would like to suggest that a possible functional difference between *v-src* gene product pp60^{v-src} and its cellular counterpart pp60^{c-src} resides within a carboxyterminal regulatory domain (Fig. 5) that is present in pp60^{c-src} but not in pp60^{v-src}. Hence, cellular transformation mediated by pp60^{v-src} results from the "unregulated" expression of protein kinase activity. In contrast, the activity of the cellular *src* protein is likely regulated in normal cells and may be modulated in response to external growth factors. Such a hypothesis would predict the presence of one or more proteins capable of interacting with and modulating the activity of pp60^{c-src}. The search for such proteins is currently in progress in our laboratory, using appropriate hybrid gene constructs.

Acknowledgments

We thank B. Creasy, R. Renaud, and D. McCarley for excellent technical assistance. We wish to thank R. Erikson for providing the anti-34K sera used in this study. D.B. is a postdoctoral fellow of the National Cancer Institute; J.T.P. is a recipient of a Faculty Research Award from the American Cancer Society. This work was supported by Public Health Service grants CA 29243 and CA 27578 from the National Cancer Institute, and grant MV-29 from the American Cancer Society.

References

Barker, W.C. and M.O. Dayhoff. 1982. Viral *src* gene products are related to the catalytic chain of mammalian cAMP-dependent protein kinase. *Proc. Natl. Acad. Sci.* **79:** 2836.

Brugge, J. and D. Darrow. 1982. Rous sarcoma virus-induced phosphorylation of a 50,000 molecular weight cellular protein. *Nature* **295:** 250.

Brugge, J.S., E. Erikson, and R.L. Erikson. 1981. The specific interaction of the Rous sarcoma virus transforming protein pp60^{src} with two cellular proteins. *Cell* **25:** 363.

Bryant, D. and J.T. Parsons. 1982. Site-directed mutagenesis of the *src* gene of Rous sarcoma virus: Construction and characterization of a deletion mutant temperature sensitive for transformation. *J. Virol.* **44:** 683.

————. 1983. Site-directed point mutation in the *src* gene of Rous sarcoma virus results in an inactive *src* gene product. *J. Virol.* **45:** 1211.

Collett, M.S. and R.L. Erikson. 1978. Protein kinase activity associated with the avian sarcoma virus *src* gene product. *Proc. Natl. Acad. Sci.* **75:** 2021.

Cooper, G. 1982. Cellular transforming genes. *Science* **218:** 801.

Cooper, J.A. and T. Hunter. 1981. Changes in protein phosphorylation in Rous sarcoma virus-transformed chicken embryo cells. *Mol. Cell. Biol.* **1:** 165.

Cooper, J., K. Nakamura, T. Hunter, and M.L. Weber. 1983. Phosphotyrosine-containing proteins and expression of transformation parameters in cells infected with partial transformation mutants of Rous sarcoma virus. *J. Virol.* **46:** 15.

Courtneidge, S., A.D. Levinson, and J.M. Bishop. 1980. The protein encoded by the transforming gene of avian sarcoma virus (pp60^{src}) and a homologous protein in normal cells (pp60$^{proto-src}$) are associated with the plasma membrane. *Proc. Natl. Acad. Sci.* **77:** 3783.

Erikson, E. and R.L. Erikson. 1980. Identification of a cellular protein substrate phosphorylated by the avian sarcoma virus-transforming gene product. *Cell* **21:** 829.

Gilmartin, G. and J.T. Parsons. 1983. Identification of transcriptional elements within the long terminal repeat of Rous sarcoma virus. *Mol. Cell. Biol.* **3:** 1834.

Gilmer, T. and R. Erikson. 1982. Development of anti-pp60^{src} serum with antigen produced in *Escherichia coli*. *J. Virol.* **45:** 462.

Hampe, A., I. Laprevotte, F. Galibert, L.A. Fedele, and C.J. Sherr. 1982. Nucleotide sequences of feline retroviral oncogenes (v-*fes*) provide evidence for a family of tyrosine-specific protein kinase genes. *Cell* **30:** 775.

Hanafusa, H. 1977. Cell transformation by RNA tumor viruses. In *Comprehensive virology* (ed. H. Fraenkel-Conrat and R.R. Wagner), vol. 10, p. 401. Plenum Press, New York.

Hunter, T. and B. Sefton. 1978. Transforming gene product of Rous sarcoma virus phosphorylates tyrosine. *Proc. Natl. Acad. Sci.* **77:** 1311.

Kitamura, N. and M. Yoshida. 1983. Small deletion in *src* of Rous sarcoma virus modifying transformation phenotypes: Identification of 207-nucleotide deletion and its smaller product with protein kinase activity. *J. Virol.* **46:** 985.

Kitamura, N., A. Kitamura, K. Toyoshima, Y. Hirayama, and M. Yoshida. 1982. Avian sarcoma virus Y73 genome sequence and structural similarity of its transforming gene product to that of Rous sarcoma virus. *Nature* **297:** 205.

Krueger, J.G., E.A. Garber, A.R. Goldberg, and H. Hanafusa. 1982. Changes in amino-terminal sequences of pp60^{src} lead to decreased membrane association and decreased *in vivo* tumorigenicity. *Cell* **28:** 889.

Levinson, A.D., S.A. Courtneidge, and J.M. Bishop. 1981. Structural and functional domains of the Rous sarcoma virus transforming protein pp60^{src}. *Proc. Natl. Acad. Sci.* **78:** 1624.

Levinson, A.D., H. Oppermann, L. Levintow, H.E. Varmus, and J.M. Bishop. 1978. Evidence that the transforming gene of avian sarcoma virus encodes a protein kinase associated with a phosphoprotein. *Cell* **15:** 561.

Mardon, G. and H.E. Varmus. 1983. Frameshift and intragenic suppressor mutations in a Rous sarcoma provirus suggests *src* encodes two proteins. *Cell* **32:** 871.

Maxam, A.M. and W. Gilbert. 1980. Sequencing end-labeled DNA with base-specific chemical cleavages. *Methods Enzymol.* **65:** 499.

Oppermann, H., A.D. Levinson, L. Levintow, H.E. Varmus, J.M. Bishop, and S. Kawai. 1981. Two proteins that immunoprecipitate with the transforming protein of Rous sarcoma virus. *Virology* **113:** 736.

Parsons, S.J., D. McCarley, C. Ely, D. Benjamin, and J.T. Parsons. 1983. Isolation and partial characterization of a monoclonal antibody to the Rous sarcoma virus transforming protein pp60^{src}. *J. Virol.* **45:** 1190.

Radke, K., T. Gilmore, and G.S. Martin. 1980. Transformation by Rous sarcoma virus: A cellular substrate for transformation-specific protein phosphorylation contains phosphotyrosine. *Cell* **21:** 821.

Reddy, E.P., M.J. Smith, and A. Srinivason. 1983. Nucleotide sequence of Abelson murine leukemia virus genome: Structural similarity of its transforming gene product to other *onc* gene products with tyrosine-specific kinase activity. *Proc. Natl. Acad. Sci.* **80:** 3623.

Schwartz, D., R. Tizard, and W. Gilbert. 1982. The complete nucleotide sequence of the Pr-C strain of Rous sarcoma virus. In *Molecular biology of tumor viruses*, 2nd edition: *RNA tumor viruses* (ed. R. Weiss et al.), p. 1338. Cold Spring Harbor Laboratory, Cold Spring Harbor, New York.

Sefton, B.M., I.S. Trowbridge, and J.A. Cooper. 1982. The transforming proteins of Rous sarcoma virus, Harvey sarcoma virus and Abelson virus contains tightly bound lipid. *Cell* **31:** 465.

Shibuya, M. and H. Hanafusa. 1982. Nucleotide sequence of Fujinami sarcoma virus: Evolutionary relationship of its transforming gene with transforming genes of other sarcoma viruses. *Cell* **30:** 787.

Shortle, D. and D. Nathans. 1978. Local mutagenesis: A method for generating viral mutants with base substitutions in preselected regions of the viral genome. *Proc. Natl. Acad. Sci.* **75:** 1270.

Takeya, T. and H. Hanafusa. 1983. Structure and sequence of the cellular gene homologous to the RSV *src* gene and the mechanism for generating the transforming virus. *Cell* **32:** 881.

Structural and Functional Studies of the Rous Sarcoma Virus Transforming Protein, pp60^{src}

L.A. Lipsich, W. Yonemoto, J.B. Bolen,* M.A. Israel,* and J.S. Brugge

Department of Microbiology, State University of New York at Stony Brook, Stony Brook, New York 11794;
*Pediatric Branch, National Cancer Institute, National Institutes of Health, Bethesda, Maryland 20205

Oncogenic transformation by Rous sarcoma virus (RSV) is mediated by the protein product of a single viral gene, denoted src (for review, see Bishop and Varmus 1982). This gene encodes a protein of M_r 60,000 (pp60^{src}) that functions as a tyrosine-specific phosphotransferase (Brugge and Erikson 1977; Collett and Erikson 1978; Levinson et al. 1978; Purchio et al. 1978; Hunter and Sefton 1980). Studies using cells infected with mutant viruses containing temperature-sensitive defects in the src gene suggest that pp60^{src}-induced transformation involves the phosphorylation of cellular proteins on tyrosine (Sefton et al. 1980). Many candidate substrates have been shown to contain elevated levels of phosphotyrosine in RSV-transformed cells; however, the precise cellular targets that mediate transformation are not known.

The transforming proteins encoded by several other retroviruses have been shown to possess tyrosine-specific protein kinase activity (Feldman and Hanafusa 1980; Pawson et al. 1980; Witte et al. 1980; Blomberg et al. 1981). All of the transforming proteins that carry this function share considerable amino acid homology, especially in the domain surrounding the major tyrosine acceptor of phosphate within pp60^{src} (Hampe et al. 1982; Kitamura et al. 1982; Shibuya and Hanafusa 1982; Takeya et al. 1982; Reddy et al. 1983; Schwartz et al. 1983).

Uninfected cells contain genes homologous to the retroviral transforming genes, and the protein products of several of these genes have been identified (Collett et al. 1978; Oppermann et al. 1979; Rohrschneider et al. 1979; Feldman and Hanafusa 1980). It is not clear whether the mere overproduction of the tyrosine kinase transforming gene products in virus-transformed cells is responsible for oncogenic transformation or whether mutational alteration of the cellular genes is required to confer oncogenicity on these genes.

Analysis of the expression of pp60^{src} and related tyrosine kinases in transformed cells is dependent on the availability of antibody probes that recognize these proteins. The pp60^{src} protein was first identified by immunoprecipitation from transformed cell lysates using serum from rabbits bearing tumors induced by RSV (Brugge and Erikson 1977). This serum, denoted tumor-bearing rabbit (TBR) serum, was useful for the initial characterization of pp60^{src} and for the identification of its associated protein kinase activity. However, there are many drawbacks to the use of this serum. TBR serum is polyspecific, containing antibodies to the RSV-encoded structural proteins as well as to pp60^{src}. In addition, most TBR sera specifically recognize pp60^{src} encoded by the Schmidt-Ruppin (SR) strain of RSV alone and are highly sensitive to denaturation of pp60^{src}. Finally, few sera recognize the cellular homolog of pp60 in avian or mammalian cells and allow phosphorylation of exogenous substrates.

To improve the technology available for the analysis of pp60^{src} and related tyrosine kinases, we have developed a battery of monoclonal antibodies directed against pp60^{src} (Lipsich et al. 1983). Similar reagents have also been isolated by Parsons and co-workers (Parsons et al. 1983 and pers. comm.). These antibodies have proved to be valuable tools for structural and functional studies of pp60^{src}, its cellular homolog, the transforming proteins of tyrosine kinase transforming proteins from related avian sarcoma-inducing retroviruses (PRCII, Yamaguchi 73 [Y73], and UR2 sarcoma viruses), and the protein kinase activity associated with the transforming protein of polyoma virus, a DNA tumor virus. In this report, we will summarize the properties of these monoclonal antibodies and describe two studies that have resulted from the analysis and use of these reagents.

Materials and Methods

Cells and virus

The Prague (PR), subgroup-A strain of RSV was obtained from T. Parsons (University of Virginia); Y73 sarcoma virus from H. Hanafusa (Rockefeller University); PRCII sarcoma virus from K. Beemon (Johns Hopkins University); and UR2 sarcoma virus from P. Balduzzi (Rochester University). RSV-3T3 cells were obtained by infection of BALB-3T3 cells with the SRD strain of RSV using polyethylene glycol (Kawai 1980). Chicken embryo fibroblasts were prepared from virus-free embryos (Spafas, Norwich, Connecticut). Mouse brain tissue was obtained from a 2-month-old BALB-3T3 mouse. Rat-1 cells and polyoma virus dl8-transformed cells were obtained from Y. Ito (National Institutes of Health, Bethesda, Maryland).

Serum

TBR serum was prepared from rabbits bearing tumors induced by the SRD strain of RSV from L. Rohrschneider, as described previously (Brugge and Erikson 1977). Monoclonal antibody to pp19^{gag} was provided by D. Boettiger (University of Pennsylvania Medical School). Monoclonal antibodies to pp60^{src} were prepared from hybridoma cells with spleen cells from a mouse immunized with pp60^{src} produced in Escherichia coli (Gilmer and Erikson 1981). The details for the preparation and characterization of these antibodies are described in Lipsich et al. (1983). Antiserum to mouse immunoglobulin was obtained from Meloy Laboratories (Springfield, Virginia). Hamster tumor serum was obtained from hamsters bearing tumors induced by PyT-54-transformed cells, as described (Takomoto et al. 1966).

Immunoprecipitation and sample analysis

Details for the radiolabeling of cells and immunoprecipitation are described in Brugge and Erikson (1977) with the exception that the RIPA lysis buffer contained 1 mM EDTA. The samples were electrophoresed on 7.5% or 10% SDS-polyacrylamide gels according to Laemmli (1970), as described.

Protease digestion

Immunoprecipitates were incubated with 50 µl of ammonium carbonate containing the indicated concentration of L-1-tosylamido-2-phenylethylchloromethyl ketone (TPCK)-treated trypsin (Worthington Biochemicals, Worthington, Delaware) or chymotrypsin (Sigma Chemical Co., St. Louis, Missouri) for 10 minutes at room temperature. The reaction was terminated by the addition of 100 units of aprotinin (FBA Pharmaceutical, New York) or sample buffer.

Detection of phosphotransferase activity

Autophosphorylation

To phosphorylate immune-complex-bound antigens, the immunoprecipitates were incubated with 50 µl of 10 mM Tris-HCl (pH 7.2), 5 mM $MnCl_2$ using 5 µCi of [γ-^{32}P]ATP for 10 minutes at room temperature.

TBR-IgG

Phosphorylation of IgG was carried out as described for autophosphorylation, except that the reaction was performed at 4°C.

Casein

The reaction was carried out as described in Autophosphorylation except that 10 µg of casein was added to each reaction and was carried out for 20 minutes.

Results and Discussion

Analysis of monoclonal antibodies to pp60^{src}

Figure 1A shows an immunoprecipitation of ^{32}P-labeled lysates of RSV-transformed mouse cells using several of the monoclonal antibodies (mAb) directed against pp60^{src}. The major protein immunoprecipitated from these cells was pp60^{src}. All of the monoclonal antibodies precipitated pp60 from cells infected with either the PR or SR strains of RSV and any of the temperature-sensitive mutant viruses that have been derived in vivo from these viruses. All of the monoclonal antibodies, as well as TBR serum, precipitated a protein of M_r 130,000 from RSV-transformed mouse cells. This protein is not precipitated from uninfected mammalian cells and does not appear to be related to pp60^{src} by partial proteolytic peptide mapping with *Staphylococcus* V8 protease (data not shown). The identity of this protein and the basis for its immunoprecipitation by the monoclonal antibodies is un-

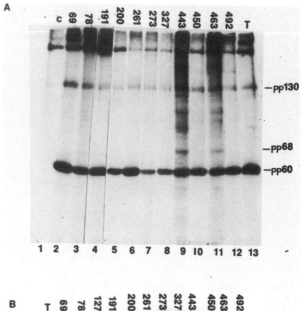

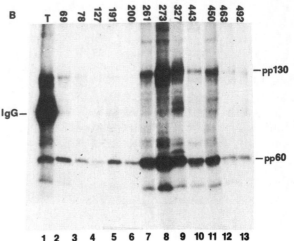

Figure 1 Proteins immunoprecipitated from SR-D 3T3 cells. (*A*) An autoradiogram of a gel containing the proteins immunoprecipitated from a [^{32}P]orthophosphate-labeled SRD-3T3 cell lysate. (Lane *1*) Anti-mouse IgG alone. (Lane *2*) IgG from monoclonal antibodies: 69; (lane *3*) 78; (lane *4*) 191; (lane *5*) 200; (lane *6*) 261; (lane *7*) 273; (lane *8*) 327; (lane *9*) 443; (lane *10*) 450; (lane *11*) 463; (lane *12*) 492; (lane *13*) TBR B antiserum. (*B*) An autoradiogram of a gel representing the phosphorylation of pp60^{src} after immunoprecipitation of unlabeled SR-D 3T3 cells and incubation in the presence of [γ-^{32}P]ATP. (Lane *1*) TBR B antiserum. (Lane *2*) IgG from monoclonal antibodies: 69; (lane *3*) 78; (lane *4*) 127; (lane *5*) 199; (lane *6*) 200; (lane *7*) 261; (lane *8*) 273; (lane *9*) 327; (lane *10*) 443; (lane *11*) 450; (lane *12*) 463; (lane *13*) 492.

der investigation. In addition to these proteins, mAbs 443 and 463 precipitated several other ^{32}P-labeled proteins. The proteins of M_r 68,000 and 19,000 (not detectable on this autoradiogram) are most consistently detected in these immunoprecipitates. These latter proteins were also detected in uninfected avian and mammalian cells (data not shown) and we are presently investigating the possibility that these proteins could represent cellular tyrosine kinases that are recognized by the most highly cross-reactive (see below) monoclonal antibodies.

Figure 1B shows the proteins phosphorylated in vitro after precipitation of RSV-transformed mouse cell lysates with the various monoclonal antibodies. None of the monoclonal antibodies interfered with the autophosphorylation of pp60[src], the major phosphorylated product of these reactions. In this reaction, phosphate was transferred to tyrosine residues within the carboxyl half of pp60[src] (data not shown). The 130K protein detected in Figure 1A was also phosphorylated in vitro. We have found that 130K was exclusively phosphorylated on tyrosine (data not shown). It is not known whether pp60[src] is responsible for the phosphorylation of 130K or if 130K is autophosphorylated in this reaction. A protein of M_r 50,000 was also detected in several reactions (lanes 7–13). This protein is not related to either pp60[src] or pp50, the cellular protein associated in a complex with a small fraction of pp60[src] (data not shown). None of the monoclonal antibodies were phosphorylated in vitro, as observed in the phosphorylation of IBR-specific immunoglobulin (Collett and Erikson 1978; Levinson et al. 1978). Both ATP and GTP served as phosphate donors in this assay (data not shown).

Figure 2A shows the in vitro phosphorylation of the cellular homolog of pp60[src] after precipitation of this protein by the monoclonal antibodies. mAbs 273 and 327 precipitated pp60[c-src] most efficiently; however, all of the mAbs that recognize pp60[v-src] also recognized pp60[c-src]. We have found that this in vitro assay was approximately 10-fold more sensitive for detection of both the cellular and viral forms of pp60 when compared with in vivo labeling with ^{32}P. The cellular homolog of pp60[v-src] was also detected in mouse, rat, and human cells with the mAbs (data not shown).

Figure 2, B, C, and D, shows the phosphorylation of the transforming proteins of Y73, PRCII, and UR2 sarcoma viruses. pp90[yes], the Y73 sarcoma virus-transforming protein (Kawai et al. 1980), was precipitated most efficiently by mAb 261 (lane 8) and pp110[fps] (Neil et al. 1981) and pp68[ros] (Feldman et al. 1982) were precipitated by mAbs 443 and 463 (lanes 10 and 12). The monoclonal antibodies that were negative in this in vitro assay were also negative for the precipitation of the analogous proteins radiolabeled in vivo. We have been unable to detect other tyrosine kinase transforming proteins, i.e., those encoded by Abelson sarcoma virus, or the transforming proteins encoded by either avian erythroblastosis virus or the McDonough strain of feline sarcoma virus. The latter transforming proteins contain a domain with some homology to the tyrosine kinase domain of pp60[src], but have not been shown to possess tyrosine phosphotransferase activity.

The pp60[src]-specific monoclonal antibodies can also provide a rapid monoclonal-bound assay of phosphorylation of exogenous proteins. Figure 3 shows the phosphorylation of casein by the transforming proteins of RSV after precipitation by several of the monoclonal antibodies. None of the monoclonal antibodies interfered with the phosphorylation of casein. The levels of casein phosphorylation directly correlated with the amount of transforming protein precipitated in the reaction. We have also found that other exogenous substrates such as tubulin or angiotensin can also be phosphorylated in this reaction (data not shown). This method should prove useful to assay the phosphorylation of exogenous substrates by mutant forms of pp60 without the laborious purification of this enzyme. It is also possible to assay conditions that can bring about the activation or inhibition of phosphotransferase activity.

To use these monoclonal reagents for structural studies of pp60, it is important to map the antigenic determinants on pp60 that are recognized by these antibodies. This analysis has not been straightforward. To date, we have attempted to map the antibody binding sites on pp60 using either deletion mutants of pp60 generated by in vitro mutagenesis (F. Cross and H. Hanafusa, pers. comm.; or Bryant and Parsons 1982 and pers. comm.) or by the generation of fragments of pp60 by proteolytic digestion in vitro. With the exception of two deleted proteins that we have studied, none of the pp60 molecules with large deletions were recognized by any of the monoclonal antibodies. The two exceptions were pp60[src] encoded by mutant 119 of Bryant and Parsons (1982), which contains a deletion from amino acid 202 to 255, and the 52K cleavage product of pp60, which is generated during cell lysis under certain buffer conditions. All of the monoclonal antibodies recognized both of these mutant src gene products. This indicates that none of the antibodies contained within the region between amino acids 202–255 or the aminoterminal 8K of pp60. The inability of the monoclonal antibodies to precipitate mutant proteins that contain large deletions does not necessarily imply that the monoclonal antibodies bind in the deleted portions of these molecules, since deletions can induce conformational changes in the protein that mask or destroy antigenic determinants. We have recently developed the protein-blotting technique of Symington et al. (1981) for use with the monoclonal antibodies and expect that this assay will be less sensitive to conformational changes brought about by deletion because the procedure involves the use of denatured antigen.

Analysis of the catalytic domain of phosphotransferase activity

One experimental procedure that was designed to map the monoclonal antibody-binding sites on pp60[src] has led to an analysis of structural and functional properties of the catalytic domain of phosphotransferase activity. In this experiment, we attempted to generate proteolytic fragments from different domains of pp60. Figure 4 shows the results of one of the first attempts to produce partial proteolytic digestion products of pp60. Proteolytic digestion with trypsin resulted in the production of a single fragment of M_r 29,000. Digestion of pp60 with either chymotrypsin- or thermolysin-generated fragments with the same electrophoretic mobility as the trypsinized product (Brugge and Darrow 1984). Peptide analysis of this protease-resistant (PTR) fragment indicated that it was derived from the carboxyl half of pp60[src]

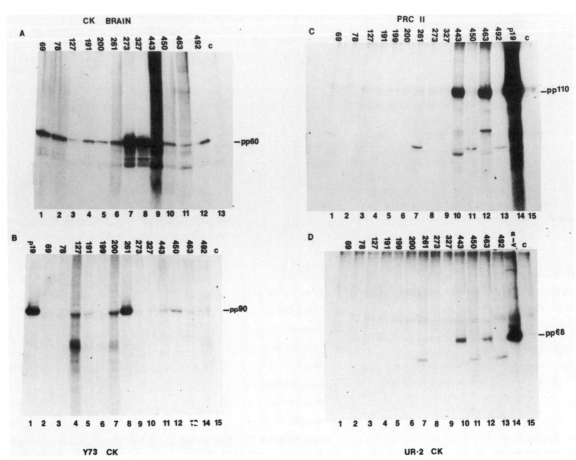

Figure 2 Proteins immunoprecipitated from normal chicken, Y73, PRCII, and UR2 infected cells. (*A*) An autoradiogram of a gel containing the proteins phosphorylated in vitro after immunoprecipitation of a lysate of chicken brain with purified IgG and incubation in the presence of [γ-³²P]ATP. Monoclonal antibodies: (lane *1*) 69; (lane *2*) 78; (lane *3*) 127; (lane *4*) 191; (lane *5*) 200; (lane *6*) 261; (lane *7*) 273; (lane *8*) 327; (lane *9*) 443; (lane *10*) 450; (lane *11*) 463; (lane *12*) 492; (lane *13*) anti-mouse IgG alone. (*B*) An autoradiogram of a gel containing the proteins phosphorylated in vitro after immunoprecipitation from a lysate of Y73-transformed chicken cells and incubation with [γ-³²P]ATP. (Lane *1*) Anti-p19 antibody. Concentrated medium from monoclonal antibodies: (lane *2*) 69; (lane *3*) 78; (lane *4*) 127; (lane *5*) 191; (lane *6*) 199; (lane *7*) 200; (lane *8*) 261; (lane *9*) 273; (lane *10*) 327; (lane *11*) 443; (lane *12*) 450; (lane *13*) 463; (lane *14*) 492; (lane *15*) anti-mouse IgG alone. (*C*) An autoradiogram of a gel containing the proteins phosphorylated in vitro after immunoprecipitation from a lysate of PRCII-transformed chicken cells and incubation with [γ-³²P]ATP. IgG from monoclonal antibodies: (lane *1*) 69; (lane *2*) 78; (lane *3*) 127; (lane *4*) 191; (lane *5*) 199; (lane *6*) 200; (lane *7*) 261; (lane *8*) 273; (lane *9*) 327; (lane *10*) 443; (lane *11*) 450; (lane *12*) 463; (lane *13*) 492; (lane *14*) anti-p19 antibody; (lane *15*) anti-mouse IgG alone. (*D*) An autoradiogram of a gel containing the proteins phosphorylated in vitro after immunoprecipitation from a lysate of UR2-transformed chicken cells and incubation with [γ-³²P]ATP. IgG from monoclonal antibodies: (lane *1*) 69; (lane *2*) 78; (lane *3*) 127; (lane *4*) 191; (lane *5*) 199; (lane *6*) 200; (lane *7*) 261; (lane *8*) 273; (lane *9*) 327; (lane *10*) 443; (lane *11*) 450; (lane *12*) 463; (lane *13*) 492; (lane *14*) TBR antiserum; (lane *15*) anti-mouse IgG alone.

(Brugge and Darrow 1984). Although this PTR fragment did not prove to be useful in mapping the monoclonal antibody binding sites (since none of the monoclonal antibodies recognize this isolated peptide), we have analyzed the phosphotransferase activity of this fragment. Levinson and co-workers (1981) have reported that brief treatment of transformed cell lysates with trypsin results in the generation of a 30K fragment from the carboxy-terminal domain of pp60 that is able to phosphorylate TBR-IgG in the immune-complex, protein kinase assay. Figure 5 shows the phosphorylation of TBR-IgG in the immune-complex, protein kinase assay after treatment with 20 μg/ml of trypsin. In this experiment, the cells were labeled with [³H]lysine to follow the percentage of

pp60 molecules that were resistant to proteolysis. Figure 5A shows that only 20% of the *src* protein molecules were detectable after 10 minutes of incubation with trypsin. Despite this fivefold reduction in pp60^{src}-derived molecules, the trypsin-treated immunoprecipitates incorporated 2.4-fold greater levels of ³²P than the untreated sample.

Since TBR-IgG phosphorylation represents a rather unusual enzyme–substrate interaction, we have also examined the ability of this isolated domain of pp60 to phosphorylate exogenous substrates. In these experiments, pp60^{src} was immunoprecipitated with monoclonal antibody and the immune complex was incubated in the presence of trypsin. Under these conditions, 10–20%

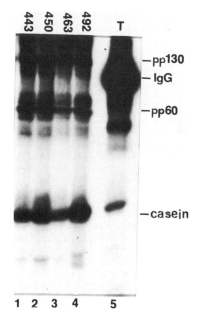

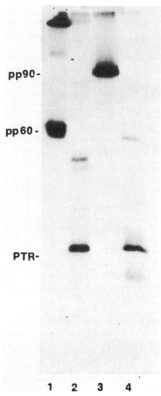

Figure 3 Phosphorylation of casein by pp60^{src} bound to the monoclonal antibodies. The figure is an autoradiogram of a gel representing the phosphorylation of casein after immunoprecipitation of pp60^{src} from SR-D-transformed 3T3 cells and incubation in the presence of 5 μg of casein and [γ-^{32}P]ATP. IgG from monoclonal antibodies: (lane *1*) 443; (lane *2*) 450; (lane *3*) 463; (lane *4*) 492; (lane *5*) TBR B antiserum.

Figure 4 Digestion of the transforming proteins of Rous and Y73 sarcoma viruses with trypsin. RSV-3T3 cells (lanes *1* and *2*) or Y73-transformed chicken cells (lanes *3* and *4*) were immunoprecipitated with TBR serum (lanes *1* and *2*) or monoclonal antibody to p19 (lanes *3* and *4*). The washed immunoprecipitates were incubated with (lanes *2* and *4*) or without (lanes *1* and *3*) 20 μg/ml of trypsin as described in the text.

of pp60 molecules were recovered as the 29K PTR fragment. The levels of phosphorylation of angiotensin and tubulin were unaffected by proteolysis. In the case of the angiotensin phosphorylation reactions, trypsin treatment caused a fivefold stimulation of phosphorylation (Brugge and Darrow 1984). Therefore, in each of the above protein kinase assays, trypsinization did not diminish the phosphotransferase activity of pp60 and indeed appeared to increase the specific activity of this enzyme.

To determine whether the phosphotransferase activity detected in the trypsin-treated immunoprecipitates was associated with the 29K protease-resistant fragment, we subjected the trypsin-solubilized peptide to filtration on a Bio-Gel P-60 column. This analysis demonstrated that all of the detectable phosphotransferase activity eluted as a 29–30K protein (Brugge and Darrow 1984).

The transforming protein of other tyrosine kinase-transforming proteins shares a high degree of homology with pp60 within the regions corresponding to the pp60-derived PTR fragment. To determine whether this portion of other tyrosine kinase-transforming proteins shares structural and functional properties with this domain of pp60, we examined the protease resistance of pp90^{yes}, the transforming protein of the Y73 sarcoma virus. Trypsin treatment of this molecule generated a fragment that comigrated with the PTR fragment of pp60 on polyacrylamide gels (Fig. 4). This peptide was derived from the

carboxyterminal 29 kD of pp90^{yes} and was capable of phosphorylating TBR-IgG, tubulin, and angiotensin (Brugge and Darrow 1984). In contrast to the PTR-fragment of pp60, the PTR pp90^{yes} was autophosphorylated after incubation with [γ-^{32}P]ATP. Weinmaster and co-workers (1983) have reported that treatment of the Fujinami sarcoma virus transforming protein with trypsin results in the production of 45K and 29K peptides that are phosphorylated in an immune-complex, protein kinase assay. These results suggest that the protease-resistant conformation of the catalytic domain of phosphotransferase activity is highly conserved in this class of viral tyrosine kinases.

The isolation of the catalytic domain of phosphotransferase activity provides the means to determine whether any properties of the protein kinase activity of these molecules are dependent on sequences outside of the catalytic domain, i.e., substrate specificity, specific activity, etc. Since cleavage of pp60 resulted in an apparent increase in the specific activity of this enzyme, it is conceivable that sequences in the amino domain of pp60

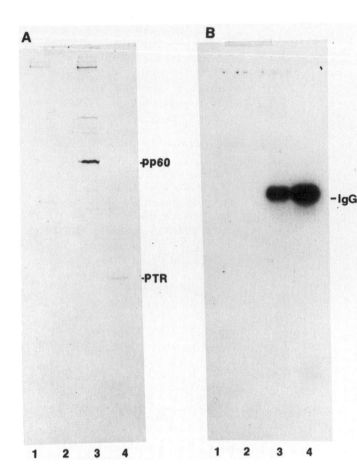

Figure 5 Phosphorylation of TBR-IgG by trypsin-treated pp60[src]. RSV-3T3 cells were labeled with 200 μCi/ml [³H]lysine for 16 hr, lysed, and immunoprecipitated with 5 μl of normal rabbit serum (lanes *1* and *2*) or TBR serum (lanes *3* and *4*). The washed immunoprecipitates were incubated with (lanes *2* and *4*) or without (lanes *1* and *3*) 20 μg/ml trypsin, as described in the text. After the addition of aprotinin, sample buffer was added to one-half of the samples (*A*) and the other samples were adjusted to 10 mM Tris-HCl (pH 7.2) and 5 mM $MgCl_2$ and incubated with 5μCi of [γ-³²]ATP, as described in the text. The reaction was terminated with the addition of electrophoresis sample buffer. The samples were analyzed on 10% gels. The intensity of the pp60[src] band from lane *3* was found by densitometric analysis to be 10-fold greater than the PTR fragment from lane *4*. Since lysine residues are distributed evenly throughout pp60[src], this indicates that approximately 20% of pp60 was resistant to proteolysis.

regulate the enzymatic activity of this enzyme. Indeed, Purchio and co-workers have reported evidence that suggests the possibility that phosphorylation on tyrosine residues in the amino half of pp60 increases the activity of the molecule five- to eightfold (A.F. Purchio et al., in prep.). The analysis of in vitro-derived mutants of pp60 also provided evidence that alterations within the amino domain can affect the catalytic domain of pp60 (Bryant and Parsons 1982; F. Cross and H. Hanafusa, pers. comm.). We have compared several properties of the protein kinase activity of the PTR fragment to those of intact pp60. Both forms of the enzyme were found to phosphorylate specifically tyrosine residues on TBR-IgG, angiotensin, and casein, and both were able to phosphorylate glycerol. No differences were found in the cation requirements of the enzymes and both forms could transfer phosphate from either ATP or GTP to TBR-IgG. Therefore, by the criteria that we have examined thus far, we can distinguish no differences between the properties of the intact molecule and its carboxyl-derived cleavage product.

Interaction of the polyoma virus tumor antigen with the cellular homolog of pp60[src]

The only DNA tumor virus transforming protein that possesses an associated tyrosine kinase activity is the middle T antigen of polyoma virus. Three tumor (T) antigens (small, middle, and large) are encoded within the early region of the polyoma virus genome (Tooze 1981). The expression of middle T antigen is sufficient to produce the fully transformed phenotype in immortalized rodent cells (Treisman et al. 1981), although a complementary function within large T antigen is required for the transformation of primary rodent cells in culture (Rassoulzadegen et al. 1982). In the presence of ATP and Mg⁺⁺, immunoprecipitates containing this antigen allow phosphorylation of middle T antigen (Eckart et al. 1979; Schaffhausen and Benjamin 1979; Smith et al. 1979). There is no evidence to indicate that the kinase activity is intrinsic to the middle T protein. The middle T antigen translated in an in vitro translation system is not active in the kinase assay and middle T antigen expressed in *E. coli* is also not phosphorylated in immunoprecipitates (Schaffhausen and Benjamin 1981). Recently, Courtneidge and Smith (1983) have presented evidence suggesting that middle T is associated with the cellular homolog of pp60. The association of middle T and pp60 raises the question of whether the phosphorylation of middle T is dependent on its interaction with cellular pp60, and it suggests that middle T could be a substrate of cellular kinase activity.

The monoclonal antibodies directed against pp60 are useful reagents to study this interaction because (1) they are monospecific antibodies, (2) they recognize mammalian cellular *src*, and (3) these antibodies allow pp60^{src} to autophosphorylate in vitro. Figure 6A shows the proteins phosphorylated in vitro after immunoprecipitation of a lysate of Rat-1 cells transformed with *dl*8 (Griffin and Maddock 1979), a polyoma virus with a truncated middle T protein (M, 51,000) (Segawa and Ito 1982). The major phosphorylated protein immunoprecipitated with hamster tumor serum was polyoma middle T (lane 5). A faint band that comigrated with pp60$^{c\text{-}src}$ was also detected in this lane. Monoclonal antibody to pp60^{src} (327) immunoprecipitated pp60$^{c\text{-}src}$ from lysates of *dl*8 Rat-1 cells as well as a faster-migrating phosphoprotein that comigrated with polyoma middle T (lane 7). Cellular *src* was also immunoprecipitated and phosphorylated in vitro with mAb 327 from a lysate of rodent brain tissue that was included as a positive control for the immunoprecipitation of mammalian pp60$^{c\text{-}src}$ (lane 3). Control experiments with either hamster normal serum or rabbit anti-mouse serum showed no immunoprecipitation of either middle T or cellular *src* from *dl*8 Rat-1 or rodent brain lysates (lanes 2,4,6,8).

The in vitro-phosphorylated bands in Figure 6A were excised and analyzed by partial proteolytic peptide mapping using the V8 enzyme of *Staphylococcus aureus* (Fig. 6B). The pp60$^{c\text{-}src}$ immunoprecipitated with mAb 327 from rodent brain tissue (lane 3) or *dl*8 Rat-1 cells (lane 2) both contained the phosphorylated V2 fragment, representing the phosphotyrosine-containing carboxyl fragment of pp60$^{c\text{-}src}$. Unfortunately, there were not enough counts in the 60-kD band phosphorylated in vitro in the hamster tumor serum immunoprecipitate to be analyzed and compared with pp60$^{c\text{-}src}$. When the middle T (lane 5) and the monoclonal antibody-immunoprecipitated 51-kD bands (lane 4) were analyzed with V8 protease, it was found that these two maps were identical. This result demonstrates that middle T coimmunoprecipitates with pp60$^{c\text{-}src}$ and confirms the observation of Courtneidge and Smith (1983). The result also shows that middle T can be phosphorylated in vitro after immunoprecipitation with a monoclonal antibody directed against pp60^{src}.

We have also examined mouse embryo fibroblasts productively infected with either wild-type or *dl*8 polyoma virus and polyoma-transformed hamster embryo fibroblasts. In each cell type, mAb 327 coimmunoprecipitated pp60$^{c\text{-}src}$ and polyoma middle T (data not shown). Several monoclonal antibodies that recognize different antigenic sites of pp60^{src} were found to coimmunoprecipitate middle T from polyoma-transformed cell lysates (data not shown). This result indicates that the immunoprecipitation of middle T with monoclonal antibodies directed against pp60^{src} is not due to a single shared antigenic determinant between middle T and cellular *src*. These results further suggest that the basis of the coimmunoprecipitation of the middle T and pp60$^{c\text{-}src}$ is the formation of a complex between these two proteins. Studies are in progress to determine if the association between

A

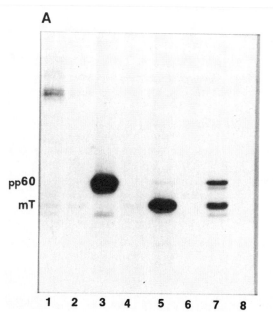

B

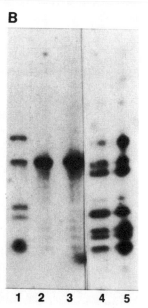

Figure 6 Analysis of the products phosphorylated in vitro after immunoprecipitation of polyoma virus-transformed cells. (*A*) Lysates of rodent brain tissue (lanes *1–4*) or polyoma virus *dl*8-infected Rat-1 cells (lanes *5–8*) were immunoprecipitated with the following antibodies and phosphorylated in vitro. The phosphorylated products were analyzed on a 7.5% SDS-polyacrylamide gel. (Lanes *1* and *5*) hamster tumor serum; (lanes *2* and *6*) hamster normal serum; (lanes *3* and *7*) mAb 327; (lanes *4* and *8*) rabbit anti-mouse IgG. (*B*) The proteins phosphorylated in *A* were excised from the gel and reelectrophoresed in the presence of 100 ng of *S. aureus* V8 protease on 12.5% polyacrylamide gel. (Lane *1*) In vivo [^{32}P]orthophosphate-labeled pp60$^{c\text{-}src}$, digested as a marker; (lane *2*) in vitro-labeled pp60$^{c\text{-}src}$ immunoprecipitated with mAb 327 from a lysate of *dl*8 Rat-1 cells (*A*, lane 7); (lane *3*) in vitro-labeled pp60$^{c\text{-}src}$ immunoprecipitated with mAb 327 from a lysate of rodent brain tissue (*A*, lane 3); (lane *4*) in vitro-labeled 52-kD protein, immunoprecipitated with mAb 327 from a lysate of *dl*8 Rat-1 cells (*A*, lane 7); (lane *5*) in vitro-labeled middle T, immunoprecipitated with hamster tumor serum from a lysate of *dl*8 Rat-1 cells (*A*, lane 5).

pp60^{c-src} and middle T is necessary for transformation by polyoma virus and also to resolve if the interaction between middle T and cellular *src* can alter the qualitative and quantitative functions of pp60^{c-src}.

Acknowledgments

The authors wish to thank Phyllis Leder and Sandi Burns for assistance in the preparation of this manuscript. L.A.L. is a fellow of the Muscular Dystrophy Association. This work was supported by grant CA2795104 from the National Cancer Institute.

References

Bishop, J. and H. Varmus. 1982. Functions and origins of retroviral transforming genes. In *Molecular biology of tumor viruses,* 2nd edition: *RNA tumor viruses* (ed. R. Weiss et al.), p. 999. Cold Spring Harbor Laboratory, Cold Spring Harbor, New York.

Blomberg, J., J.M. Van de Ven, F.H. Reynolds, Jr., R.P. Natewalk, and J.R. Stephenson. 1981. Snyder-Theilen feline sarcoma virus P85 contains a single phosphotyrosine acceptor site recognized by its associated protein kinase. *J. Virol.* **38:** 886.

Brugge, J.S. and D. Darrow. 1984. Analysis of the catalytic domain of phosphotransferase activity of two avian sarcoma virus-transformed proteins. *J. Biol. Chem.* (in press).

Brugge, J.S. and R.L. Erikson. 1977. Identification of a transformation-specific antigen induced by an avian sarcoma virus. *Nature* **269:** 346.

Bryant, D. and T. Parsons. 1982. Site-directed mutagenesis of the *src* gene of Rous sarcoma virus: Construction and characterization of a deletion mutant temperature-sensitive for transformation. *Virology* **44:** 683.

Collett, M.S. and R.L. Erikson. 1978. Protein kinase activity associated with the avian sarcoma virus *src* gene product. *Proc. Natl. Acad. Sci.* **75:** 2021.

Collett, M.S., J.S. Brugge, and R.L. Erikson. 1978. Characterization of a normal avian cell protein related to the avian sarcoma virus transforming gene product. *Cell* **15:** 1363.

Courtneidge, S.A. and A.E. Smith. 1983. Polyoma virus transforming protein associates with the product of the *c-src* cellular gene. *Nature* **303:** 435.

Eckhart, W., M.A. Hutchinson, and T. Hunter. 1979. An activity phosphorylating tyrosine in polyoma T antigen immunoprecipitates. *Cell* **18:** 925.

Feldman, R. and H. Hanafusa. 1980. Characterization of protein kinase activity associated with the transforming gene product of Fujinami sarcoma virus. *Cell* **22:** 757.

Feldman, R.A., L.-H. Wang, H. Hanafusa, and P.C. Balduzzi. 1982. Avian sarcoma virus UR2 encodes a transforming protein which is associated with a unique protein kinase activity. *J. Virol.* **42:** 228.

Gilmer, T. and R.L. Erikson. 1981. Rous sarcoma virus transforming protein, pp60^{src}, expressed *E. coli*, functions as a protein kinase. *Nature* **294:** 771.

Griffin, B. and C. Maddock. 1979. New classes of viable deletion mutants in the early region of polyoma virus. *J. Virol.* **31:** 645.

Hampe, A., I. Laprevotte, F. Galibert, L.A. Fedele, and C.J. Sherr. 1982. Nucleotide sequences of feline retroviral oncogenes (v-fes) provide evidence for a family of tyrosine-specific protein kinase genes. *Cell* **30:** 775.

Hunter, T. and B. Sefton. 1980. Transforming gene product of Rous sarcoma virus phosphorylates tyrosine. *Proc. Natl. Acad. Sci.* **77:** 1311.

Kawai, S. 1980. Transformation of rat cells by fusion-infection with Rous sarcoma virus. *J. Virol.* **34:** 772.

Kawai, S., M. Yoshida, K. Segawa, R. Sugiyama, R. Ishizaki, and K. Toyoshima. 1980. Characterization of Y73, an avian sarcoma virus: A unique transforming gene and its product, a phosphoprotein kinase activity. *Proc. Natl. Acad. Sci.* **77:** 6199.

Kitamura, N., A. Kitamura, K. Toyoshima, Y. Hirayama, and M. Yoshida. 1982. Avian sarcoma virus Y73 genome sequence and structural similarity of its transforming gene product to that of Rous sarcoma virus. *Nature* **297:** 205.

Laemmli, U.K. 1970. Cleavage of structural proteins during the assembly of the head of bacteriophage T4. *Nature* **227:** 680.

Levinson, A.D., S.A. Courtneidge, and J.M. Bishop. 1981. Structural and functional domains of the Rous sarcoma virus-transforming protein (pp60^{src}). *Proc. Natl. Acad. Sci.* **78:** 1624.

Levinson, A.D., H. Oppermann, L. Levintow, H.E. Varmus, and J.B. Bishop. 1978. Evidence that the transforming gene of avian sarcoma virus encodes a protein kinase associated with a phosphoprotein. *Cell* **15:** 561.

Lipsich, L.A., A.J. Lewis, and J.S. Brugge. 1983. Isolation of monoclonal antibodies that recognize the transforming proteins of avian sarcoma viruses. *J. Virol.* **48:** 352.

Neil, J., M.L. Breitman, and P.K. Vogt. 1981. Characterization of a 105,000 molecular weight gag-related phosphoprotein from cells transformed by the defective avian sarcoma virus PRCII. *Virology* **108:** 98.

Oppermann, H., A.D. Levinson, H.E. Varmus, L. Levintow, and J.M. Bishop. 1979. Uninfected vertebrate cells contain a protein that is closely related to the product of the avian sarcoma virus transforming gene (*src*). *Proc. Natl. Acad. Sci.* **76:** 1804.

Parsons, S.J., D.J. McCarley, C.M. Eliy, D.C. Benjamin, and J.T. Parsons. 1983. Isolation and partial characterization of a monoclonal antibody to the Rous sarcoma virus transforming protein pp60^{src}. *J. Virol.* **45:** 1190.

Pawson, T., J. Guyden, T.-H. Kung, K. Radke, T. Gilmore, and G.S. Martin. 1980. A strain of Fujinami sarcoma virus which is temperature-sensitive for protein phosphorylation and cellular transformation. *Cell* **22:** 767.

Purchio, A.F., E. Erikson, J.S. Brugge, and R.L. Erickson. 1978. Identification of a polypeptide encoded by the avian sarcoma virus *src* gene. *Proc. Natl. Acad. Sci.* **75:** 1567.

Rassoulzadegen, M., A. Cowie, A. Carr, N. Glaichenhaus, R. Kamen, and F. Cuzin. 1982. The role of individual polyoma virus early proteins in oncogenic transformation. *Nature* **300:** 713.

Reddy, P.E., M.J. Smith, and A. Srinivason. 1983. Nucleotide sequence of Abelson murine leukemia virus genome: Structural similarity of its transforming gene product to other *onc* gene products with tyrosine-specific kinase activity. *Proc. Natl. Acad. Sci.* **80:** 3623.

Rohrschneider, L.R., R.N. Eisenman, and C.R. Leitch. 1979. Identification of a Rous sarcoma virus transformation-related protein in normal avian and mammalian cells. *Proc. Natl. Acad. Sci.* **76:** 4479.

Schaffhausen, B. and T. Benjamin. 1979. Phosphorylation of polyoma T antigens. *Cell* **18:** 935.

———. 1981. Comparison of two polyoma virus middle-T antigens *in vivo* and *in vitro*. *J. Virol.* **40:** 184.

Schwartz, D., R. Tizard, and W. Gilbert. 1983. Nucleotide sequence of Rous sarcoma virus. *Cell* **32:** 853.

Sefton, B.M., T. Hunter, K. Beemon, and W. Eckhart. 1980. Evidence that the phosphorylation of tyrosine is essential for cellular transformation by Rous sarcoma virus. *Cell* **20:** 807.

Segawa, K. and Y. Ito. 1982. Differential subcellular localization of *in vivo* phosphorylated and nonphosphorylated middle-sized tumor antigen of polyoma virus and its relationship to middle-sized tumor antigen phosphorylating activity *in vitro*. *Proc. Natl. Acad. Sci.* **79:** 6812.

Shibuya, M. and H. Hanafusa. 1982. Nucleotide sequence of Fujinami sarcoma virus: Evolutionary relationship of its transforming gene with the transforming genes of other sarcoma viruses. *Cell* **30:** 787.

Smith, A.E., R. Smith, B. Griffin, and M. Fried. 1979. Protein kinase activity associated with polyoma virus middle-T antigen *in vitro*. *Cell* **18:** 915.

Symington, J., M. Green, and K. Brackmann. 1981. Immunoautoradiographic detection of proteins after electrophoretic transfer from gels to diazo-paper. *Proc. Natl. Acad. Sci.* **78:** 177.

Takeya, T., R.A. Feldman, and H. Hanafusa. 1982. DNA sequence of the viral and cellular *src* gene of chickens. I. Complete nucelotide sequences of an EcoRI fragment of recovered avian sarcoma virus which codes for gp37 and pp60*src*. *J. Virol.* **44:** 1.

Takomoto, K.K., R.A. Malgren, and K. Habel. 1966. Heat labile serum factor required for immunofluorescence of polyoma tumor antigen. *Science* **153:** 1122.

Tooze, J., ed. 1981. *Molecular biology of tumor viruses*, 2nd edition, revised: *DNA tumor viruses*. Cold Spring Harbor Laboratory, Cold Spring Harbor, New York.

Treisman, R., U. Novak, J. Favaloro, and R. Kamen. 1981. Transformation of rat cells by an altered polyoma virus genome expressing only middle-T protein. *Nature* **292:** 595.

Weinmaster, G., E. Hinze, and T. Pawson. 1983. Mapping of multiple phosphorylation sites within the structural and catalytic domains of the Fujinami avian sarcoma virus transforming protein. *J. Virol.* **46:** 29.

Witte, O.N., A. Dasgupta, and D. Baltimore. 1980. Abelson murine leukemia virus protein is phosphorylated *in vitro* to form phosphotyrosine. *Nature* **283:** 826.

Identification of the Active Site of the Transforming Protein of Rous Sarcoma Virus

Mark P. Kamps* † and Bartholomew M. Sefton†

*Department of Chemistry, University of California at San Diego, La Jolla, California 92093
†Molecular Biology and Virology Laboratory, The Salk Institute, San Diego, California 92138

Oncogenic transformation by Rous sarcoma virus (RSV) is induced by the activity of a single viral phosphoprotein, p60^{src} (Purchio et al. 1978), that possesses a protein kinase activity (Collett and Erikson 1978; Levinson et al. 1978) specific for tyrosine residues (Hunter and Sefton 1980). In addition to RSV, five other classes of RNA tumor viruses encode proteins that display tyrosine kinase activity in vitro (Feldman et al. 1980, 1982; Kawai et al. 1980; Pawson et al. 1980; Witte et al. 1980; Naharro et al. 1983). These families have as their prototypes the three avian sarcoma viruses FSV, Y73 virus, and UR2 virus, the Abelson murine leukemia virus, and Gardner-Rasheed feline sarcoma virus. A normal cellular gene homologous to each of these viral transforming genes has been found in chromosomal DNA (Stehelin et al. 1976; Goff et al. 1980; Yoshida et al. 1980; Shibuya et al. 1982). These cellular genes have been conserved throughout speciation, and each is transcribed in at least some specific cell types (Spector et al. 1978; Mueller et al. 1982; Shibuya et al. 1982; Wang and Baltimore 1983). In normal cells, tyrosine kinases are associated with the receptors of growth-promoting peptides such as epidermal growth factor (EGF), platelet-derived growth factor (PDGF), and insulin (Ushiro and Cohen 1980; Nishimura et al. 1982; Kasuga et al. 1983). These observations were the first to link tyrosine kinases with normal cellular growth control and present a compelling argument for the importance of such enzymes, not only as the effectors of viral transformation but also as essential proteins in normal cells.

To phosphorylate proteins on tyrosine, p60^{src} must bind both ATP and a tyrosine-containing substrate at separate locations within its active site. Our interests have focused on locating this ATP-binding site in p60^{src} and identifying specific residues involved in the phosphotransferase reaction. To locate the ATP-binding site, we have used the reactive ATP analog p-fluorosulfonylbenzoyl 5′-adenosine (FSBA) (Pal et al. 1975). FSBA is structurally similar to ATP with the exception that the three phosphates have been replaced by a side chain of equal length that terminates with a chemically reactive sulfonylfluoride group. This group is known to react with the free electron pairs found in serine, threonine, tyrosine, cysteine, lysine and histidine, yielding a covalent linkage between the sulfonylbenzoyladenosine and the participating amino acid. Our findings show that incubation of p60^{src} in an immunoprecipitate with 1.0 mM FSBA eliminates 90% of kinase activity within an hour. Competition studies with other ATP analogs prove that this inactivation occurs within the ATP-binding site. Further studies indicate that Lys-295 is the target of this reaction. It is likely therefore, that Lys-295 is located within the ATP-binding site of p60^{src} and may play an essential role in the enzyme's phosphotransferase activity.

The sequences of four tyrosine protein kinases and of the serine- and threonine-specific, cAMP-dependent protein kinase have been found to have partial homology. When aligned to give maximal homology, all contain a lysine residue in a position homologous to Lys 295 in p60^{src} (Shoji et al. 1981; Barker and Dayhoff 1982; Kitamura et al. 1982; Shibuya and Hanafusa 1982; Reddy et al. 1983; Schwartz et al. 1983). In the case of the catalytic subunit of the cAMP-dependent protein kinase, FSBA has been shown to inactivate the enzyme by reacting with a lysine located in the homologous position to Lys-295 of p60^{src} (Zoller et al. 1981). The observation that equivalent lysines react with FSBA in both p60^{src} and in the catalytic subunit presents convincing evidence that there exist both sequence homology and functional similarity within the active sites of the viral tyrosine protein kinases and the cAMP-dependent serine kinase.

Methods of Experimental Procedures

Labeling with [¹⁴C]FSBA

[¹⁴C]FSBA at 40.0 mCi/mmole was obtained from New England Nuclear. For reaction with p60^{src}, 2.5 μCi were dried and dissolved in 1.2 μl of DMSO. To this solution, 98.8 μl of 10 mM sodium phosphate (pH 6.8) and 5 mM MgCl$_2$ were added with vigorous mixing to give a final concentration of 500 μM [¹⁴C]FSBA. Immunoprecipitates containing p60^{src}, prepared from RSV-transformed chick cells lysed in NP-40 buffer, were resuspended in this solution and incubated 1 hour at 30°C. The immunoprecipitates were subsequently washed four times in 50 mM Tris (pH 7.2), 150 mM NaCl, and 0.1% NP-40 to remove excess [¹⁴C]FSBA. A Tris-buffered solution was used because the amino group of the Tris base also reacts with FSBA and neutralizes its reactive sulfonylfluoride group.

Peptide mapping

Two-dimensional tryptic peptide mapping was performed as described previously (Gibson 1974; Beemon and Hunter 1978). Digestion of specific tryptic peptides with Staphylococcus aureus V8 protease was performed according to the procedure of Patschinsky and Sefton (1981). Electrophoresis was carried out at 1.0 kV for 27 minutes for tryptic maps and for 8 minutes for S. aureus protease maps. In all cases, electrophoresis was from left to right, with the origin on the left and the negative electrode on the right. Chromatography was performed for 6 hours in each case. The chromatography buffer was composed of butanol:pyridine:acetic acid:H_2O (97:75:15:60 [v/v], pH 5.3) and causes hydrophobic peptides to migrate faster than hydrophilic ones.

Gels
All samples were run on 15% low bis-SDS-polyacrylamide gels.

Partial proteolytic mapping
The partial proteolytic mapping procedure of Cleveland et al. (1977) was used. Gel pieces containing the protein of interest were inserted into the wells of the stacking gel and digested with 30 ng of *S. aureus* V8 protease in the stacking gel.

Antisera
p60^{src} was isolated by immunoprecipitation using a tumor-bearing rabbit (TBR) serum that recognizes both p60^{v-src} and p60^{c-src}.

Results and Discussion

FSBA specifically reacts with the ATP-binding site of p60^{src}
In our initial experiments, we used p60^{src} obtained from cells lysed in RIPA buffer. Incubation of such immunoprecipitates for 30 minutes at 30°C in 10 mM sodium phosphate (pH 6.8), 5 mM $MgCl_2$, destroyed greater than 90% of the kinase activity of p60^{src}. This inherent instability made accurate studies of inactivation by FSBA impossible. However, if immunoprecipitates were prepared from cells lysed in NP-40 buffer, which differs from RIPA buffer only in that it lacks both 1% NaDOC and 0.1% SDS (Sefton et al. 1980), the kinase activity of p60^{src} was essentially stable for periods greater than 2 hours of 30°C. Incubation of such NP-40 immunoprecipitates of p60^{src} from Prague (PR)-RSV-C with 1.0 mM FSBA caused inactivation of 90% of the kinase activity (Fig. 1).

Two control experiments demonstrate that this inactivation is due to the reaction of FSBA with the active site of p60^{src}. First, inactivation by 1.0 mM FSBA was blocked by 1.0 mM ADP. This indicates that ADP competes strongly for the same binding site as does FSBA, a result that would not be obtained if this inactivation were due to nonspecific reaction of FSBA with amino acids in p60^{src} outside the ATP-binding site. cAMP, which is less similar in structure to ATP than is ADP, did not block inactivation by FSBA. Second, the kinase activity of p60^{src} was unaffected by incubation with phenylmethylsulfonylfluoride (PMSF), a reagent that contains the same sulfonylfluoride moiety as FSBA but does not possess an adenine ring structure. This demonstrates that the adenosine portion of FSBA is essential for its specific reactivity with p60^{src} and that nonspecific kinase inactivation due to random reaction with amino acids does not contribute significantly to the inactivation ob-

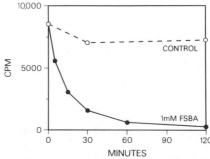

Figure 1 FSBA inactivates the kinase activity of p60^{src}. p60^{src} was obtained by immunoprecipitation using NP-40 buffer containing 2.0 mM EDTA from PR-RSV-C-transformed chick cells. Preincubation was with 1.0 mM FSBA at 30°C in a 10 mM sodium phosphate (pH 7.2), 5 mM magnesium chloride kinase buffer supplemented with 1.2% DMSO. Control samples were incubated solely in kinase buffer and 1.2% DMSO. After preincubation for the indicated times, the samples were washed three times in 0.5 ml of 10 mM sodium phosphate (pH 7.2), 150 mM NaCl, and 0.1% NP-40 detergent and stored on ice. When the preincubations were finished, samples were resuspended in 20 µl of the same kinase buffer containing 2 µCi [^{32}P]ATP and incubated at 30°C for 10 min. ^{32}P incorporated into the Ig heavy chain was analyzed by SDS-polyacrylamide gel electrophoresis and quantified by scintillation counting.

served. It seems clear therefore that FSBA inactivates p60^{src} by reaction with a residue in the ATP-binding site.

p60^{src} can be labeled with [^{14}C]FSBA
If the loss of kinase activity resulting from reaction with FSBA was due to covalent modification of p60^{src}, it should be possible to label p60^{src} with [^{14}C]FSBA. The p60^{src} molecules encoded by Schmidt-Ruppin (SR)-RSV-D and PR-RSV-C were therefore either labeled biosynthetically with [^{35}S]methionine or incubated in vitro with [^{14}C]FSBA and analyzed by SDS-polyacrylamide gel electrophoresis (Fig. 2). Since the immunoprecipitates were prepared in NP-40 buffer so as to retain the ATP-binding activity of p60^{src}, they contained more contaminating proteins than are present in immunoprecipitates prepared with RIPA buffer. These contaminating proteins, however, are useful as controls for the extent of nonspecific labeling. Most of the [^{14}C]FSBA that reacted with proteins in the immunoprecipitate was present on the heavy and light chains of the immunoglobulin (Fig. 2). This was not surprising, as they were present at a 300-fold excess over p60^{src}. Labeling of p60^{src} with FSBA was detectable in the case of PR-RSV-C, which encodes a p60^{src} larger than the immunoglobin heavy chain. Labeling of the p60^{src} protein of SR-RSV-D occurred, but was only apparent after peptide mapping (see below).

[^{14}C]FSBA reacts with the 34K aminoterminal fragment of p60^{src}
To prove that the 60-kD protein labeled with FSBA was p60^{src} and to locate where in the protein the [^{14}C]FSBA

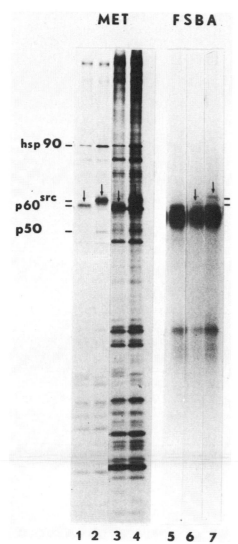

MET   FSBA

hsp 90 —

p60*src* =

p50 —

1 2   3 4   5 6 7

Figure 2 [¹⁴C]FSBA labels p60*src*. p60*src* was isolated with rabbit anti-RSV tumor serum from [³⁵S]methionine-labeled SR-RSV-D- and PR-RSV-C-transformed chick cells using either RIPA buffer or NP-40 buffer for lysis and washing. Unlabeled p60*src* was isolated in parallel in NP-40 buffer and subsequently incubated with 500 μM [¹⁴C]FSBA as described in Methods of Experimental Procedure. All of the samples were analyzed by SDS-polyacrylamide gel electrophoresis on a single gel. Vertical arrows designate the location of p60*src*. (Lane 1) SR-RSV-D p60*src*, [³⁵S]methionine, RIPA buffer; (lane 2) PR-RSV-C p60*src*, [³⁵S]methionine, RIPA buffer; (lane 3) SR-RSV-D p60*src*, [³⁵S]methionine, NP-40 buffer; (lane 4) PR-RSV-C p60*src*, [³⁵S]methionine, NP-40 buffer; (lane 5) control immunoprecipitate, [¹⁴C]FSBA, NP-40 buffer; (lane 6) SR-RSV-D p60*src*, [¹⁴C]FSBA, NP-40 buffer; and (lane 7), PR-RSV-C p60*src*, [¹⁴C]FSBA, NP-40 buffer.

was found, we used the partial proteolytic mapping procedure of Cleveland. In the case of PR-RSV-C, we used the [¹⁴C]FSBA-labeled 60-kD band present uniquely in this immunoprecipitate. For SR-RSV-D, we excised a piece of gel that would contain p60*src*, were it labeled. When digested by *S. aureus* V8 protease, p60*src* is initially cleaved into an aminoterminal 34K fragment that contains three methionine residues and a carboxyter-

minal 26K fragment that contains 10 methionines (Collett et al. 1979). Digestion with *S. aureus* protease released [¹⁴C]FSBA-labeled 34-kD fragments from the p60*src* proteins of both SR-RSV-D and PR-RSV-C (Fig. 3). These labeled fragments certainly arise from p60*src* itself and not from the contaminating, nonspecifically labeled Ig heavy chain, since they differ in apparent molecular weight in precisely the same manner as do the 34-kD aminoterminal fragments of the protein labeled biosynthetically with [³⁵S]methionine. No obvious labeling of the 26K carboxyterminal fragment could be detected. The several radioactive fragments present in each sample labeled with [¹⁴C]FSBA can be ascribed to heavy-chain digestion products. [¹⁴C]FSBA therefore has located the reactive amino acid of the ATP-binding site of p60*src* within the 34K aminoterminal fragment.

With which amino acid does FSBA react?

In the β-subunit of the F1-ATPase, FSBA reacts with a tyrosine (Esch and Allison 1978). In the cAMP-dependent protein kinase, FSBA reacts with a lysine. We examined the possibility that FSBA modified a lysine in p60*src* for two reasons. First, lysines are positively charged

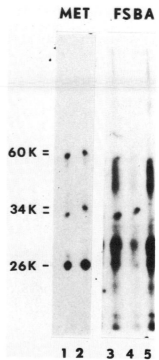

MET   FSBA

60 K =

34 K =

26 K —

1 2   3 4 5

Figure 3 [¹⁴C]FSBA modification occurs within the aminoterminal 34K fragment of p60*src*. Parallel samples from Fig. 2 were excised from the gel and examined by partial digestion using 30 ng of *S. aureus* V8 protease, as described in Methods of Experimental Procedures. A sample from an immunoprecipitate made from uninfected cells with rabbit anti-RSV tumor serum was incubated with FSBA and the Ig heavy chain analyzed in parallel so as to estimate the contribution to the pattern of nonspecifically labeled heavy chain. (Lane 1) [³⁵S]methionine-labeled SR-RSV-D p60*src*; (lane 2) [³⁵S]methionine-labeled PR-RSV-C p60*src*; (lane 3) [¹⁴C]FSBA-labeled SR-RSV-D p60*src*; (lane 4) [¹⁴C]FSBA-labeled PR-RSV-C p60*src*; and (lane 5) [¹⁴C]FSBA-labeled immunoglobulin heavy chain.

(pK$_a$ = 9) at intracellular pH and therefore could serve to stabilize the negative charges of the phosphates of ATP. Second, the positive charge of lysine could provide an electron-withdrawing effect capable of activating the γ-phosphate of ATP for subsequent attack by tyrosine. To determine whether FSBA reacts with a lysine within p60^{src}, we utilized the fact that if any lysine reacted with FSBA it would no longer be recognized as a site for tryptic cleavage. If such a lysine were part of, or adjacent to, a methionine-containing tryptic peptide, modification by FSBA would cause this peptide to disappear from a two-dimensional map of the protein and a new peptide to appear. The new peptide would represent two previously unique tryptic peptides now joined at an FSBA-modified lysine. Therefore, we examined whether the tryptic peptide map of [^{35}S]methionine-labeled p60^{src} would be affected by reaction with FSBA (Fig. 4). To our surprise, two peptides (labeled A and B) were reduced in abundance by reaction with FSBA and two new peptides (labeled A' and B') appeared.

Why were two peptides affected? There are two possible explanations. First, it could indicate the modification of two lysines. Alternatively, it could result from incomplete tryptic digestion in the vicinity of a single modified lysine. To decide between these two possibilities, we digested peptides A and B with *S. aureus* V8 protease, which cleaves after glutamic acid residues, and analyzed the digestion products by two-dimensional peptide mapping (Fig. 5). The two peptides were clearly related. Each yielded two new methionine peptides, one of which, peptide 1, was present in both tryptic peptides.

This eliminates the possibility that two unrelated lysines reacted with FSBA and strongly suggests that A and B originate from a single site within p60^{src} and that the two forms are a result of incomplete digestion. A comparison of *S. aureus* protease digests of tryptic peptides A and A', and tryptic peptides B and B', showed that A shares peptide 2 with A' and that B shares peptide 3 with B' (Fig. 5). This showed that A' is a modified form of A and B' is a modified form of B. Additionally, comparison of the *S. aureus* protease digestion products of tryptic peptide A' with tryptic peptide B' revealed that each contained peptide 4 and consequently they were related to each other. This suggested that the appearance of two new peptides was also the result of incomplete digestion.

The site with which FSBA reacts must therefore be part of or next to a peptide that contains two methionines separated by a glutamic acid residue and is present in the aminoterminal 34 kD of p60^{src}. Which methionine-containing peptide is represented here? There are only three predicted tryptic peptides in the deduced sequence of p60^{src} that contain two methionines. They are peptides 296–315, 358–377, and 479–498. Peptide 358–377 can be eliminated because it contains no glutamic acid residue between the two methionines. Peptide 479–498 can also be eliminated since it is located almost at the carboxyl terminus of p60^{src} and hence cannot be in the aminoterminal 34 kD. Only peptide 296–315 matches the requirements of being contained in the 34 kD aminoterminal fragment and having a glutamic acid residue between two methionines. Figure 6 displays the sequence surrounding this peptide, and at this point the

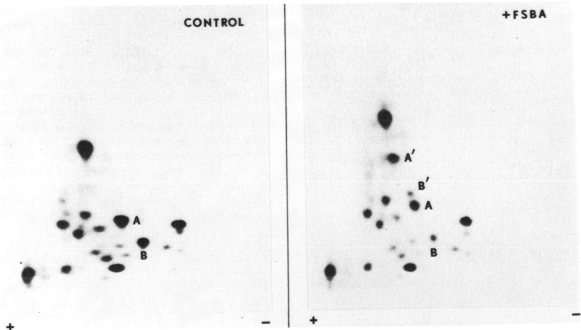

Figure 4 FSBA modification of p60^{src} causes the shift of two tryptic peptides. p60^{src} was isolated by immunoprecipitation from 10^7 PR-RSV-C-transformed chick cells labeled overnight with 2.0 mCi [^{35}S]methionine. Half of the immunoprecipitate was incubated with 1.0 mM FSBA in 10 mM sodium phosphate (pH 6.8), 5 mM MgCl$_2$, and 1.2% DMSO. Tryptic peptides were generated from each preparation and analyzed by two-dimensional mapping, as described in Methods of Experimental Procedure. (Control) Unmodified p60^{src}; (FSBA) FSBA-modified p60^{src}.

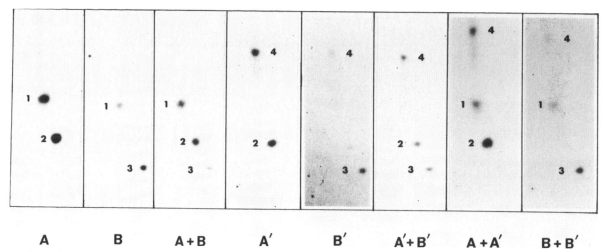

Figure 5 The relationship of peptides A, B, A', and B' is revealed by *S. aureus* protease digestion. Tryptic peptides A, B, A', and B' (see Fig. 4) were eluted and subjected to digestion with *S. aureus* protease. The digestion products were analyzed by two-dimensional mapping as in Fig. 4 except that electrophoresis was for 8 min instead of 27 min.

explanation for the incomplete digestion products becomes clear. Tryptic peptide 296–315 is bordered by a lysine at its carboxyl terminus. Trypsin should cleave p60*src* with equal initial frequencies after Lys-315 and after Lys-316. Removal of Lys-316 from those fragments cleaved initially after this residue will be inefficient, however, because trypsin is known to have difficulty removing the carboxyterminal lysine from a peptide that terminates in Lys-Lys-COOH (Kasper 1975). Conse-

quently, two different peptides containing residues 296–315 will be produced, even in tryptic digests produced by fairly exhaustive digestion. One would consist of residues 296–315, and the second would contain amino acids 296–316.

Which peptide is A and which is B? Peptide 296–316 contains an additional positive charge and therefore will migrate further during electrophoresis and more slowly during chromatography. These are the properties of peptide B, and consequently peptide 296–316 must correspond to this peptide. Therefore, peptide A consists of residues 296–315.

How does reaction with FSBA change the mobilities of these peptides? Examination of the *S. aureus* protease digests of tryptic peptides A, B, A', and B' and the deduced sequences of A and B presented in Figure 6 shows that before reaction with FSBA, A and B share a common aminoterminal *S. aureus* protease peptide, peptide 1, but differ in their carboxyterminal peptides, peptides 2 and 3. After reaction with FSBA, the two carboxyterminal peptides, peptides 2 and 3, remain unchanged but the aminoterminal peptide, peptide 1, is modified and reappears in the form of peptide 4, which is much more hydrophobic and contains less net positive charge. FSBA consequently is reacting either with one of the amino acids between Thr-296 and Glu-305 or alternatively creating a fused peptide by reacting with Lys-295. The simple addition of FSBA to any single amino acid within peptide 296–305 is probably insufficient to account for the large increase seen in the hydrophobicity of peptide 4. Reaction with Lys-295, however, would destroy the positive charge on Lys-295 and result in the addition of the hydrophobic sequence Val-Ala-Ile-Lys(FSBA) to peptide 1. This modification would shift peptide 1 precisely as observed. We believe, therefore, that Lys-295 reacts with FSBA and that the new peptides A' and B' arise from the addition of the sequence Val-Ala-Ile-Lys(FSBA) to their unmodified forms.

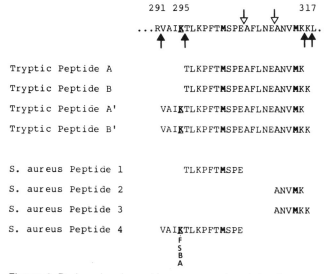

Figure 6 Deduced amino acid sequences of each tryptic peptide and their *S. aureus* V8 protease digestion products. The sequence of p60*src* of PR-RSV-C between residues 291 and 317 is presented here (Schwartz et al. 1983). Lys-295 is underlined. Sites of tryptic cleavage are represented by solid arrows and sites of *S. aureus* cleavage by open arrows.

Summary

We have used the ATP analog, FSBA, to locate the ATP-binding site of p60^{src}. FSBA was found to react with Lys-295 and inactivate the kinase activity of p60^{src} by this covalent modification. It is apparent, therefore, that Lys-295 and the residues that adjoin it comprise part of the active site of p60^{src}. By virtue of its positive charge, Lys-295 itself may function as an essential residue for binding ATP. All four tyrosine protein kinases whose sequences are known, and the cAMP-dependent serine protein kinase, have sequence homology. When aligned, all five proteins contain a lysine at exactly the same position as Lys-295 of p60^{src}. The homologous lysine in the cAMP-dependent protein kinase has been shown also to react with FSBA. Thus, it appears that the ATP-binding region contained within the active sites of both serine and tyrosine kinases is functionally very similar.

Acknowledgments

We thank Susan Taylor for her generous gift of FSBA and for helpful suggestions on ways to approach these experiments. In addition, we thank Tony Hunter for both his donation of [^{14}C]FSBA and for his insights concerning peptide mapping. This work was supported by National Institutes of Health grants CA-14195 and CA-17289.

References

Barker, W.C. and M.O. Dayhoff. 1982. Viral *src* gene products are related to the catalytic chain of mammalian cAMP-dependent protein kinase. *Proc. Natl. Acad. Sci.* **79:** 2836.

Beemon, K. and T. Hunter. 1978. Characterization of Rous sarcoma virus *src* gene products synthesized in vitro. *J. Virol.* **28:** 551.

Cleveland, D.W., S.G. Fischer, M.W. Kirschner, and U.K. Laemmli. 1977. Peptide mapping by limited proteolysis in sodium dodecyl sulfate and analysis by gel electrophoresis. *J. Biol. Chem.* **252:** 1102.

Collett, M.S. and R.L. Erikson. 1978. Protein kinase activity associated with the avian sarcoma virus *src* gene product. *Proc. Natl. Acad. Sci.* **75:** 2021.

Collett, M.S., E. Erikson, and R.L. Erikson. 1979. Structural analysis of the avian sarcoma virus transforming protein: Sites of phosphorylation. *J. Virol.* **29:** 770.

Esch, F.S. and W.S. Allison. 1978. Identification of a tyrosine residue at a nucleotide binding site in the β subunit of the mitochondrial ATPase with p-fluorosulfonyl (^{14}C)-benzoyl-5'-adenosine. *J. Biol. Chem.* **253:** 6100.

Feldman, R.A., T. Hanafusa, and H. Hanafusa. 1980. Characterization of protein kinase activity associated with the transforming gene product of Fujinami sarcoma virus. *Cell* **22:** 757.

Feldman, R.A., L. Wang, H. Hanafusa, and P.C. Balduzzi. 1982. Avian sarcoma virus UR2 encodes a transforming protein which is associated with a unique protein kinase activity. *J. Virol.* **42:** 228.

Gibson, W. 1974. Polyoma virus proteins: A description of the structural proteins of the virion based on polyacrylamide gel electrophoresis and peptide analysis. *Virology* **62:** 319.

Goff, S.P., E. Gilboa, O.N. Witte, and D. Baltimore. 1980. Structure of the Abelson murine leukemia virus genome and the homologous cellular gene: Studies with clones viral DNA. *Cell* **22:** 777.

Hunter, T. and B.M. Sefton. 1980. Transforming gene product of Rous sarcoma virus phosphorylates tyrosine. *Proc. Natl. Acad. Sci.* **77:** 1311.

Kasper, C.B. 1975. Fragmentation of proteins for sequence studies and separation of peptide mixtures. *Mol. Biol. Biochem. Biophys.* **8:** 132.

Kasuga, M., Y. Fujita-Yamaguchi, D.L. Blithe, and C.R. Kahn. 1983. Tryosine-specific protein kinase activity is associated with the purified insulin receptor. *Proc. Natl. Acad. Sci.* **80:** 2137.

Kawai, S., M. Yoshida, K. Segawa, H. Sugiyama, R. Ishizaki, and K. Toyoshima. 1980. Characterization of Y73, an avian sarcoma virus: A unique transforming gene and its product, a phosphopolyprotein with protein kinase activity. *Proc. Natl. Acad. Sci.* **77:** 6199.

Kitamura, N., A. Kitamura, K. Toyoshima, Y. Hirayama, and M. Yoshida. 1982. Avian sarcoma virus Y73 genome sequence and structural similarity of its transforming gene product to that of Rous sarcoma virus. *Nature* **297:** 205.

Levinson, A.D., H. Oppermann, L. Levintow, H.E. Varmus, and J.M. Bishop. 1978. Evidence that the transforming gene of avian sarcoma virus encodes a protein kinase associated with a phosphoprotein. *Cell* **15:** 561.

Mueller, R., D.F. Slamon, J.M. Tremblay, M.J. Cline, and I.M. Verma. 1982. Differential expression of cellular oncogenes during pre- and postnatal development of the mouse. *Nature* **299:** 640.

Naharro, G., C.Y. Dunn, and K.C. Robbins. 1983. Analysis of the primary translational product and integrated DNA of a new feline sarcoma virus, GR-FeSV. *Virology* **125:** 502.

Nishimura, J., J.S. Huang, and T.F. Deuel. 1982. Platelet-derived growth factor stimulates tyrosine-specific protein kinase activity in Swiss mouse 3T3 cell membranes. *Proc. Natl. Acad. Sci.* **79:** 4303.

Pal, P.K., W.J. Wechter, and R.F. Colman. 1975. Affinity labeling of the inhibitory DPNH site of bovine liver glutamate dehydrogenase by 5'-fluorosulfonylbenzoyl adenosine. *J. Biol. Chem.* **250:** 8140.

Patschinsky, T. and B. Sefton. 1981. Evidence that there exist four classes of RNA tumor viruses which encode proteins with associated tyrosine protein kinase activities. *J. Virol.* **39:** 104.

Pawson, T., J. Guyden, T.-H. Kung, K. Radke, T. Gilmore, and G.S. Martin. 1980. A strain of Fujinami sarcoma virus which is temperature-sensitive in protein phosphorylation and cellular transformation. *Cell* **22:** 767.

Purchio, A.F., E. Erikson, J.S. Brugge, and R.L. Erikson. 1978. Identification of a polypeptide encoded by the avian sarcoma virus *src* gene. *Proc. Natl. Acad. Sci.* **75:** 1567.

Reddy, E.P., M.J. Smith, and A. Srinivasan. 1983. Nucleotide sequence of Abelson murine leukemia virus genome: Structural similarity of its transforming gene product to other *onc* gene products with tyrosine-specific kinase activity. *Proc. Natl. Acad. Sci.* **80:** 3623.

Schwartz, D., R. Tizard, and W. Gilbert. 1983. Nucleotide sequence of Rous sarcoma virus. *Cell* **32:** 853.

Sefton, B.M., T. Hunter, and K. Beemon. 1980. Temperature-sensitive transformation by Rous sarcoma virus and temperature-sensitive protein kinase activity. *J. Virol.* **33:** 220.

Shibuya, M. and H. Hanafusa. 1982. Nucleotide sequence of Fujinami sarcoma virus: Evolutionary relationship of its transforming gene with transforming genes of other sarcoma viruses. *Cell* **30:** 787.

Shibuya, M., H. Hanafusa, and P.C. Balduzzi. 1982. Cellular sequences related to three new *onc* genes of avian sarcoma virus (*fps, yes,* and *ros*) and their expression in normal and transformed cells. *J. Virol.* **42:** 143.

Shoji, S., D.C. Parmelee, R.C. Wade, S. Kumar, L.H. Ericsson, K.A. Walsh, H. Neurath, G.L. Long, J.G. Demaille, E.H. Fischer, and K. Titani. 1981. Complete amino acid sequence of the catalytic subunit of bovine cardiac muscle cyclic AMP-dependent protein kinase. *Proc. Natl. Acad. Sci.* **78:** 848.

Spector, D.H., K. Smith, T. Padgett, P. McCombe, D. Roulland-Dussoix, C. Moscovici, H.E. Varmus, and J.M. Bishop. 1978. Uninfected avian cells contain RNA related to the transforming gene of avian sarcoma virus. *Cell* **13:** 371.

Stehelin, D., H.E. Varmus, J.M. Bishop, and P.K. Vogt. 1976. DNA related to the transforming gene(s) of avian sarcoma viruses is present in normal avian DNA. *Nature* **260:** 170.

Ushiro, H. and S. Cohen. 1980. Identification of phosphotyrosine as a product of epidermal growth factor-activated protein kinase in A-431 cell membranes. *J. Biol. Chem.* **255:** 8363.

Wang, J.Y.J. and D. Baltimore. 1983. Cellular RNA homologous to the Abelson murine leukemia virus transforming gene: Expression and relationship to the viral sequence. *Mol. Cell. Biol.* **3:** 773.

Witte, O.N., A. Dasgupta, and D. Baltimore. 1980. The Abelson murine leukemia virus protein is phosphorylated in vitro to form phosphotyrosine. *Nature* **283:** 826.

Yoshida, M., S. Kawai, and K. Toyoshima. 1980. Uninfected avian cells contain structurally unrelated progenitors of viral sarcoma genes. *Nature* **287:** 653.

Zoller, M.J., N.C. Nelson, and S.S. Taylor. 1981. Affinity labeling of cAMP-dependent protein kinase with *p*-fluorosulfonylbenzoyl adenosine. *J. Biol. Chem.* **256:**10837.

Rapid Tyrosine Phosphorylation of a 42,000-Dalton Protein Is a Common Response to Many Mitogens

Tony Hunter and Jonathan A. Cooper

Molecular Biology and Virology Laboratory, The Salk Institute, San Diego, California 92138

The connection between the unrestrained growth of transformed cells and their other phenotypic changes has attracted considerable attention over the past few years. In the case of cells transformed by viruses, a major focus has been the question of whether the unfettered growth is a primary consequence of the action of the relevant viral transforming protein or a secondary response dependent on a chain of events. On the one hand, the transforming protein might interact directly with a normal cellular growth-control pathway. On the other hand, a primary phenotypic change, such as altered cell morphology, might induce continuous cell division.

The molecular mechanism of transformation is best understood for a group of retroviruses whose transforming proteins have a common enzymatic activity, namely the ability to phosphorylate tyrosine residues in other proteins (Hunter and Sefton 1982). Although formal proof is lacking, it is believed that tyrosine phosphorylation of cellular proteins plays a crucial role in transformation by such viruses. These transforming proteins are all encoded, at least in part, by viral sequences that can readily be shown to have arisen from normal cellular genes (Bishop and Varmus 1982). This group of viruses represents five or possibly six cellular genes, which apparently encode tyrosine protein kinases in normal cells (the viral genes and representative viruses are v-src, Rous sarcoma virus [RSV]; v-yes, Y73 virus; v-fps, Fujinami sarcoma virus [FuSV]; v-abl, Abelson murine leukemia virus [Ab-MLV]; v-ros, UR2 virus; v-fgr, Gardner-Rasheed feline sarcoma virus [GR-FeSV]). Despite their common activity, one might question whether these viral transforming proteins all function in the same manner in transformation. From the four genes that have been examined at the nucleotide sequence level, however, it is apparent that the viral protein kinases, and their cellular homologs, are all closely related members of a tyrosine protein kinase family. The four proteins show striking homology in a 30-kD region thought to encompass the catalytic domain (Czernilofsky et al. 1980; Hampe et al. 1982; Kitamura et al. 1982; Shibuya and Hanafusa 1982; Reddy et al. 1983).

Cells transformed by these viruses all show a large increase in the level of phosphotyrosine in total protein, presumably reflecting the intracellular activity of the viral enzymes (Hunter and Sefton 1982). A number of individual proteins containing increased amounts of phosphotyrosine have been identified in appropriate virally transformed cells (Erikson and Erikson 1980; Radke et al. 1980; Cooper and Hunter 1981a,b; Sefton et al. 1981). Several of these prove to be common to cells transformed by members of the six different classes of retrovirus as might be anticipated from their familial relationship. Among these substrates are the cytoskeletal protein vinculin, the glycolytic enzymes, enolase, phosphoglycerate mutase, and lactate dehydrogenase, and a 34–39-kD plasma membrane-associated protein (p36) (Erikson and Erikson 1980; Radke et al. 1980; Sefton et al. 1981; Cooper et al. 1983b). Although the functions of several of these proteins are known, for technical reasons it has not yet been possible to ascertain the effects of tyrosine phosphorylation on these functions. Nevertheless, one can speculate that vinculin phosphorylation may play a role in altered cell morphology, although such modification clearly is not sufficient for complete morphological transformation (Rohrschneider and Rosok 1983). The three glycolytic enzymes are not normally considered to be rate limiting for glycolysis, so it seems unlikely that their phosphorylation in transformed cells is responsible for increased glycolytic flux. The precise function of p36 is unknown, but its association with the cytoplasmic face of the plasma membrane in cultured fibroblasts and its concentration in the terminal web structure of the columnar epithelial cells of the gut suggest that it may be structural (Courtneidge et al. 1983; Greenberg and Edelman 1983; Nigg et al. 1983; Radke et al. 1983; Gould et al. 1984). What effect phosphorylation has on p36 function is unclear.

Since none of these tyrosine protein kinase substrates has an established role in regulating cell growth, one might ask whether there is any evidence that the viral tyrosine protein kinases modulate cell growth directly. Essentially nothing is known about cellular growth-control pathways at the molecular level. Proteins in such pathways are likely to be rare and thus difficult to detect as substrates for the viral tyrosine protein kinases, given the current limitations in detecting less-abundant substrates. Despite this pessimism, however, there are grounds for believing that unrestricted cell growth is a primary consequence of the activity of these viral transforming proteins. The epidermal growth factor (EGF) receptor has an intrinsic tyrosine protein kinase activity, which is activated upon binding EGF (Buhrow et al. 1982). The platelet-derived growth factor (PDGF) and insulin receptors are also tightly associated with tyrosine protein kinases which are activated upon binding their respective growth factors (Ek et al. 1982; Kasuga et al.

1982; Nishimura et al. 1982). The analogous functions of the growth factor receptors and the viral transforming proteins suggest that the viral tyrosine protein kinases might phosphorylate in a constitutive fashion one or more substrates normally modified by the receptor tyrosine protein kinases in the course of mitogenesis. To test this idea, one needs to identify the substrates for the growth factor-activated tyrosine protein kinases and to determine whether there is any overlap with the substrates of the viral tyrosine kinases.

Experimental Procedures

NR-6 3T3 cells (Pruss and Herschmann 1977) were maintained and labeled with [^{32}P]orthophosphate as described (Cooper et al. 1982), or in Dulbecco's modified Eagle's medium containing 3% of the usual phosphate concentration, 1% complete calf serum, and 10 mM HEPES buffer (pH 7.2). Dishes labeled for 2 hours only were incubated in the low-phosphate medium overnight before ^{32}P$_i$ addition. PDGF was kindly supplied by Elaine Raines and Russell Ross (University of Washington, Seattle, Wash.). EGF was the gift of Sue Potter (The Salk Institute, San Diego, Calif.). Tetradecanoyl phorbol acetate (TPA) was from Sigma. ^{32}P-labeled cells were lysed and analyzed by two-dimensional gel electrophoresis, as detailed previously (Cooper et al. 1982). For Figure 3C, a 35-mm dish culture of cells was lysed in 50 μl of 1% SDS, 1% 2-mercaptoethanol, 1 mM EDTA, 10 mM sodium phosphate (pH 7), and incubated at 100°C for 1 minute. It was then diluted with 120 μl *Staphylococcal* nuclease solution (Garrels 1979), incubated with nucleases for 30 seconds at 4°C, lyophilized, and dissolved in 170 μl of sample buffer (Garrels 1979). Hence, it was 1.7-times the volume of parallel dishes, and the exposure time of the gel was increased accordingly. Gels were treated with alkali prior to indirect autoradiography (Cooper and Hunter 1981a). The phosphoamino acid composition of individual spots from untreated two-dimensional gels was determined as described (Cooper et al. 1983a).

Results and Discussion

What are the substrates for the growth factor receptor tyrosine kinases?

Treatment of resting mouse fibroblasts with EGF or PDGF leads to a rapid increase in the level of phosphotyrosine in protein, and a number of newly phosphorylated phosphotyrosine-containing proteins have been identified (Cooper et al. 1982). For example, phosphorylation of several proteins at tyrosine is detectable soon after adding a saturating amount of PDGF (0.83 nM) to quiescent ^{32}P-labeled NR-6 3T3 cells, a line that possesses high numbers of PDGF receptors (Bowen-Pope and Ross 1982). Phosphorylation is slightly increased at 1 minute, maximal at 5–15 minutes, and somewhat reduced by 1 hour (Cooper et al. 1982). This time course approximately parallels the number of PDGF receptors on the cell surface that have bound PDGF, since after 30 min-

utes at 37°C internalization and degradation of PDGF exceeds new binding (Bowen-Pope and Ross 1982). The effect of a 60-minute treatment with PDGF on proteins of NR-6 3T3 cells containing alkali-stable phosphate is shown in Figure 1D compared with the phosphoproteins of control cells (Fig. 1A). Amongst the proteins phosphorylated at increased level, two 42-kD proteins (pp42), two 45-kD proteins (pp45), and one 41-kD protein (pp41) were found to contain phosphotyrosine (Fig. 2 and data not shown). (We have previously described pp42 and pp41 as having molecular weights of 43,000 and 42,000, respectively [Cooper et al. 1982]. We have adopted this new nomenclature to be consistent with that which will be used by Weber et al. and Martin et al. [both this volume], who have detected mitogen-induced tyrosine phosphorylation of proteins of 42 kD apparently identical to pp42.) Phosphorylation of p36 was also slightly, but detectably, increased (Fig. 1). Other proteins phosphorylated at increased levels in PDGF-treated cells (small arrowheads, Fig. 1D) were found not to contain phosphotyrosine (data not shown). With intermediate concentrations of PDGF, intermediate stimulation of phosphorylation was achieved (Fig. 1B,C). Half-maximal phosphorylation was observed with about 0.33 nM PDGF, for all the phosphotyrosine-containing and the nonphosphotyrosine phosphoproteins whose phosphorylation was stimulated by PDGF. An identical concentration dependence was observed after a 5-minute instead of 60-minute exposure to PDGF, except that at all three concentrations of PDGF tested the extent of the induced phosphorylations was greater than at 60 minutes (data not shown). Stimulation of tyrosine phosphorylation of individual proteins shows similar dependence on the concentration of PDGF to both overall phosphorylation of tyrosine in total cell proteins and PDGF binding under these culture conditions (Cooper et al. 1982).

Phosphorylation of proteins homologous to p42 has been detected in other cell types treated with other mitogens (see below). In contrast, phosphorylation of p45 and p41 is not always detected, even in NR-6 3T3 cells incubated with PDGF, whereas the level of pp36 in PDGF-treated NR-6 3T3 cells is insignificant compared with that found in virally transformed cells, suggesting that its phosphorylation is irrelevant to the mitogenic response. For these reasons, we have concentrated on pp42. The two forms of pp42 in mitogen-treated mouse cells were shown to be related to one another by partial proteolysis (Cooper et al. 1984). The more basic form (pp42B) contains approximately equal amounts of phosphotyrosine and phosphoserine (Fig. 2B). The more acidic form (pp42A) contains phosphoserine, phosphothreonine, and phosphotyrosine (Fig. 2A). We do not know how pp42A is related to pp42B, but there are three obvious possibilities. First, pp42A might be the singly phosphorylated form of p42 and pp42B the doubly phosphorylated isomer. Second, pp42A might be derived from pp42B by another type of posttranslational modification. Third, pp42A and

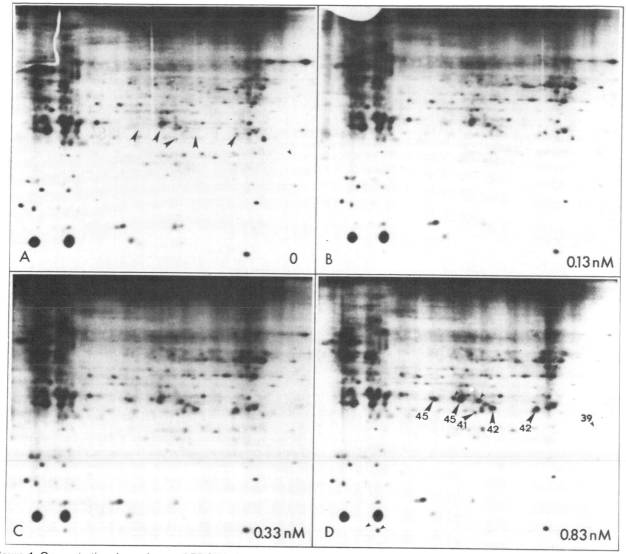

Figure 1 Concentration dependence of PDGF-induced phosphorylations in NR-6 3T3 cells. Quiescent cells were labeled with ³²P for 17 hr. Purified PDGF was added to the labeling medium at a final concentration of 0 nM (*A*), 0.13 nM (*B*), 0.33 nM (*C*), or 0.83 nM (*D*) for a further 1 hr. Autoradiographs (18 hr) of alkali-treated, two-dimensional gels are shown with acidic proteins at the left. Numbers indicate apparent molecular masses. (Large arrowheads) Positions of induced phosphoproteins demonstrated to contain phosphotyrosine; (small arrowheads) positions of other induced phosphoproteins. With the exception of pp36 (labeled '39' in this and subsequent Figures) which was not tested, these other induced phosphoproteins lack phosphotyrosine.

pp42B might be phosphorylated forms of two different but related primary translation products. In the case of another tyrosine protein kinase substrate with multiple-charge isomers, we have been able to determine the relationships between the various forms by measuring their charge separations on two-dimensional gels (Cooper and Hunter 1983). A prerequisite for this type of analysis is identification of the unphosphorylated form(s) of pp42. Our search for this apoprotein has yielded one candidate, but we lack conclusive proof of its identity.

Rapid tyrosine phosphorylation of p42 is induced in cells of several species, including human, rat, mouse, and chicken, treated with EGF and PDGF. The highly conserved nature of this response supports the idea that

p42 is a primary substrate for the growth factor receptor tyrosine kinases and that its phosphorylation is involved in transmission of the mitogenic signal, even though there is no direct evidence for this. If p42 phosphorylation were important for mitogenesis, it is vital to know whether p42 is phosphorylated on tyrosine in appropriate virally transformed cells. pp42B can be detected in chick cells transformed by avian sarcoma viruses of the *src, fps,* and *yes* families (protein *n*; Cooper and Hunter 1981a,b). However, pp42 is not detectable in mammalian cells transformed by the same viruses, even though it is readily seen when the parental cells are treated with EGF or PDGF. Perhaps the threshold level of p42 phosphorylation necessary for growth is below our limit of detection. Until this is resolved, the question of whether the viral

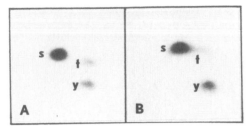

Figure 2 Phosphoamino acids of pp42A (*A*) and pp42B (*B*). NR-6 3T3 cells labeled with 3 mCi $^{32}P_i$ for 18 hr were incubated with 0.83 nM PDGF for 1 hr. Their phosphoproteins were separated by two-dimensional gel electrophoresis and spots corresponding to pp42A and pp42B identified without treating the gels with alkali. These phosphoproteins were extracted and their phosphoamino acids liberated by partial acid hydrolysis, separated by thin-layer electrophoresis, and identified by indirect autoradiography for 15 hr. Marker phosphoserine (s), phosphothreonine (t), and phosphotyrosine (y) were located by staining.

tyrosine kinases abrogate normal growth regulation by intervention at this step must remain open.

p42 is phosphorylated de novo in mitogen-treated cells

To determine the role of pp42 in mitogenesis, we have begun to characterize both the apoprotein (p42) and its phosphorylated derivatives. Initially, it was important to show that p42 is phosphorylated de novo in response to mitogens, since elevated levels of ^{32}P in pp42 in mitogen-treated cells could be due to increased turnover of a phosphoprotein whose phosphate has a long half-life in quiescent cells. This seemed unlikely in view of the long time allowed for $^{32}P_i$ equilibration prior to adding PDGF, but we tested whether increased amounts of pp42 were present in PDGF-treated cells by two-dimensional gel analysis of [^{35}S]methionine-labeled NR-6 3T3 cells. Since phosphorylation of a protein alters its isoelectric point, a phosphoprotein has a different position on a two-dimensional gel from its apoprotein. We found that [^{35}S]methionine-labeled proteins with mobilities identical to pp42A and pp42B were present in PDGF-treated but not in control cells (data not shown). Since ^{32}P-labeled pp42 was detectable following PDGF addition to cells in which protein synthesis was inhibited with emetine (data not shown), we conclude that the effect of PDGF is to induce a de novo phosphorylation.

If p42 is a substrate for tyrosine protein kinases active in PDGF-treated cells, it might also be phosphorylated in lysates of these cells. It was conceivable, therefore, that the increased tyrosine phosphorylation of pp42 observed in samples prepared from PDGF-treated cells (e.g., Fig. 1D) was due to tyrosine protein kinase activity occurring *after* cell lysis. We explored this possibility by varying the conditions of cell lysis in two ways. First, nonradioactive ATP (2 mM) was included in the buffer used to lyse ^{32}P-labeled, PDGF-treated NR-6 3T3 cells. This did not reduce the PDGF-stimulated $^{32}P_i$ incorporation into pp42 detected in this experiment (Fig. 3A,B). Second, cells were lysed in a buffer containing 1% SDS

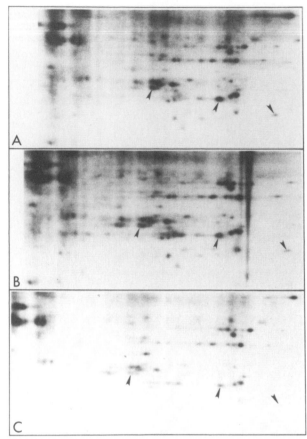

Figure 3 Effect of cell lysis conditions on protein phosphorylation. NR-6 3T3 cells labeled overnight with $^{32}P_i$ and treated for 10 min with PDGF were washed with cold saline. One culture (*A*) was prepared for two-dimensional gel electrophoresis by our standard method. The culture in *B* was prepared similarly, but the lysis buffer contained 2 mM ATP. The culture in *C* was lysed with warm SDS solution and heated at 100°C (Experimental Procedures). (➤) pp45, pp42B, pp36.

and then incubated at 100°C for 1 minute—conditions expected to reduce the activity of both protein kinases and phosphatases. For unknown reasons, this reduced the overall recovery of phosphoproteins, but phosphorylation of pp42 was still readily detected (Fig. 3C) in treated cells but not in control cells analyzed in similar fashion (data not shown). We conclude that the detection of phosphotyrosine in pp42 in response to PDGF is more likely to reflect increased tyrosine protein kinase activity in the intact cell than either increased tyrosine protein kinase activity or decreased phosphotyrosine-protein phosphatase activity following cell lysis.

Serine and threonine phosphorylations induced by PDGF

Since tyrosine protein kinase activity is stimulated when PDGF is added to NR-6 3T3 cell membranes in vitro (Pike et al. 1983), it is possible that elevated tyrosine phosphorylation may precede, and perhaps trigger, increased serine and threonine phosphorylation in the PDGF-treated cell. Even at the shortest time of incubation tested (1 min), however, increased phosphorylation of proteins that contain no phosphotyrosine, as well as of the proteins that do contain phosphotyrosine, has been detected (Cooper et al. 1982). L.T. Williams and A.R. Frackelton (pers. comm.) have found that a 175-kD protein thought to be the PDGF receptor is detectably phosphorylated at tyrosine following exposure of 3T3 cells to PDGF at 4°C. Therefore, we labeled NR-6 3T3 cells with $^{32}P_i$ at 37°C for 18 hours and then lowered the temperature to 4°C. PDGF (0.83 nM) was added to one culture, and incubation continued at 4°C for 2 hours. Phosphorylation of both p42 and p36 were detectably stimulated by PDGF at 4°C (Fig. 4; cf. Fig. 5A, the 37°C control for this experiment). In contrast, increased phosphorylation of four proteins, whose phosphorylation at serine and threonine is induced by PDGF at 37°C (Fig. 1), was not detected (Fig. 4). It is difficult to test whether all phosphorylations at serine and threonine induced by PDGF at 37°C are inhibited at 4°C, since the constitutive level of phosphorylation of proteins at these amino acids is high and only increased slightly by PDGF. However, the dissociation of increased tyrosine phosphorylation from induced phosphorylation of at least some proteins at other amino acids, suggests that tyrosine phosphorylation may be a proximal effect of PDGF binding, whereas serine/threonine phosphorylation may be a more distal one.

Phosphorylation of p42 is induced by other mitogens

Increased tyrosine phosphorylation, at least of p42, is also detectable with other mitogenic agents. In quiescent chick cells, we have found that phosphorylation of pp42A and pp42B is induced by exposure not only to PDGF and EGF but also to serum, the mitogenic protease trypsin, and tumor promoters of both the phorbol ester and indole alkaloid families (Cooper et al. 1984). The list of agents able to induce tyrosine phosphorylation is still lengthening. We are currently reexamining mitogens that did not detectably increase overall tyrosine phosphorylation, looking specifically for the individual pp42 forms. Increased sensitivity is afforded by the observation that many constitutively phosphorylated cell proteins are not detectably labeled after short incubation of cells with $^{32}P_i$ (Fig. 5). Phosphorylations induced by added PDGF are then readily detected over the reduced background of constitutive phosphorylations. pp42 contains a greater fraction of incorporated, alkali-stable ^{32}P after 2 hours of labeling than after 18 hours (Fig. 5), and can even be detected on autoradiographs of alkali-treated, one-dimensional SDS gels as a band whose labeling is increased by PDGF (data not shown). Exposing 3T3 cells labeled for 2 hours with $^{32}P_i$ to PDGF or partially purified fibroblast growth factor (FGF) for 10 minutes stimulates incorporation into pp42 (data not shown). Labeling for longer time periods will be required to show whether this results from an increased extent of phosphorylation rather than increased turnover of phosphate. This is important, because although an increased phosphate content could modulate protein function, it is more difficult to imagine how altered phosphate turnover rate could do so. So far, we have not detected p42 phosphorylation in fibroblasts in response to insulin even though the insulin receptor is reported to be associated with a tyrosine protein kinase that is activated upon binding insulin.

The stimulation of tyrosine phosphorylation by tumor

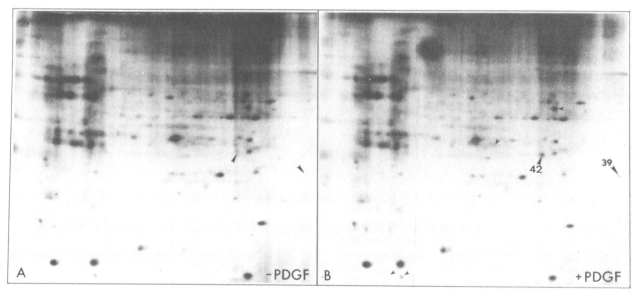

Figure 4 PDGF stimulates p42 phosphorylation at 4°C. NR-6 3T3 cells were labeled with $^{32}P_i$ for 14 hr at 37°C. The medium was made 50 mM in HEPES buffer (pH 7.2) in two cultures which were transferred to a 4°C room. After 10 min to allow temperature equilibration, 0.83 nM PDGF was added to one culture. After a further 2 hr, phosphoproteins of control (A) and PDGF-treated cells (B) were analyzed by two-dimensional gel electrophoresis. Alkali-treated gels were exposed for 14 hr. (Large arrowheads) Positions of pp42B and pp36; (small arrowheads) positions of other phosphoproteins whose phosphorylation was not increased by PDGF at 4°C. Fig. 5A is a parallel culture treated with PDGF at 37°C.

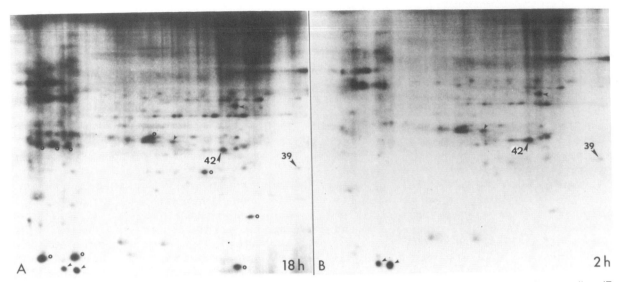

Figure 5 Effect of different durations of ³²P$_i$ labeling. NR-6 3T3 cell cultures were incubated in the low-phosphate medium (Experimental Procedures) for 18 hr. The culture in *A* received ³²P$_i$ at the start of the incubation; the culture in *B* received ³²P$_i$ 16 hr later. Ten min before the end of the labeling period, 0.83 nM PDGF was added to both cultures. Control cultures were not incubated with PDGF (data not shown). Alkali-treated gels were exposed for 14 hr. (Large arrowheads) pp42B and pp36; (small arrowheads) PDGF-induced phosphoproteins that lack phosphotyrosine; (○) phosphoproteins detected after 18 hr label but not after 2 hr.

promoters is interesting because of the implication of a serine/threonine-specific protein kinase, C-kinase, as a receptor for tumor promoters (Castagna et al. 1982; Niedel et al. 1983). Indeed, we have found that incubation of A431 human tumor cells with tumor promoters induces serine and threonine phosphorylation, specifically of the EGF receptor (Cochet et al. 1984). The sites phosphorylated at threonine are those phosphorylated in vitro when purified C-kinase is incubated with membranes from A431 cells. Unfortunately, we have not yet been able to extend these observations to cells for which tumor promoters are mitogenic. In such cells, we anticipated that tumor promoters would increase the activity of a tyrosine protein kinase. Even though stimulation of the tyrosine protein kinase activity of A431 cell EGF receptors by EGF is reduced by tumor promoters (Cochet et al. 1984), we tested whether functional EGF receptors are involved in the stimulation of tyrosine phosphorylation in fibroblasts by tumor promoters. NR-6 3T3 cells lack EGF binding sites (Pruss and Herschmann 1977), but can respond to TPA as a mitogen (Pruss and Herschmann 1977). ³²P-labeled cells were incubated for 10 minutes with either EGF, TPA, or PDGF. Phosphorylation of p42 and p45 and trace phosphorylation of p36 was induced by PDGF (Fig. 6). These phosphorylations were not induced by EGF. Increased phosphorylation of p42 was induced by TPA, suggesting that EGF-binding sites are not needed for this effect (note, however, that it is possible that these cells possess EGF receptors which cannot bind EGF but which can phosphorylate tyrosine). This implies that it is another tyrosine protein kinase that is activated upon phosphorylation by C-kinase. Previous work has shown that there is little change in the activity of pp60$^{c\text{-}src}$ in TPA-treated cells,

at least when measured in the Ig kinase assay (Goldberg et al. 1980). Another possibility is the PDGF receptor kinase. A431 cells lack PDGF receptors, and TPA fails to induce phosphorylation of p42 in these cells. We have not, however, tested the effect of TPA on other cells lacking PDGF receptors to see whether this is a general phenomenon.

Conclusions

Our work on mitogen-stimulated phosphorylation of p42 is supported by similar observations from two other groups. Michael Weber and his colleagues have found that the only detectable increase in tyrosine phosphorylation in quiescent chick cells treated with EGF, PDGF, or TPA was in proteins of 40–45 kD (Nakamura et al. 1983; Weber et al., this volume). Although their analysis was performed on one-dimensional SDS gels by a technique that does not allow resolution of individual proteins, it seems likely that pp42 was in part responsible for the increased tyrosine phosphorylation they observed. Steven Martin and Tom Gilmore have also detected tyrosine phosphorylation of pp42A and pp42B by two-dimensional gel analysis of TPA-treated chick cells (Martin et al., this volume). They showed that this was a rapid effect occurring within 5 minutes and that the dose response was similar to that for other biological effects of TPA on chick cells.

There are clearly large gaps in our knowledge of p42. Apart from proving that p42 phosphorylation is important for mitogenesis, there are several other questions we would like to answer. What is the stoichiometry of p42 phosphorylation and what is the relationship between pp42A and pp42B? What is the turnover rate of phos-

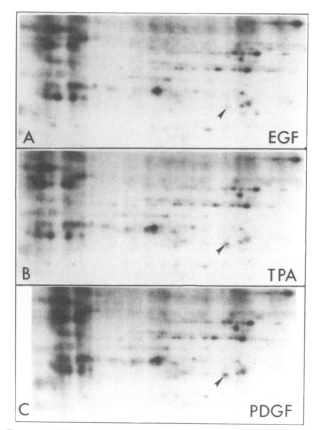

Figure 6 Effect of a tumor promoter on NR-6 3T3 cells. NR-6 3T3 cells were labeled with $^{32}P_i$ for 17 hr and 3.3 nM EGF (*A*), 150 nM TPA (*B*), or 0.83 nM PDGF (*C*) were added for 10 min. The TPA culture also received 0.1% dimethyl sulfoxide, but this solvent alone, or inactive phorbol, did not alter the pattern of 3T3 cell phosphoproteins (data not shown). Alkali-treated two-dimensional gels were exposed for 8 hr. (➤) pp42B.

phate on pp42, i.e., how long does pp42 remain phosphorylated after the external stimulus is withdrawn? Are the serine and threonine phosphorylations of pp42 important? Is p42 normally phosphorylated in growing cells and, if so, is this limited to a particular time in the cell cycle? Is p42 synthesis itself modulated throughout the cell cycle? Is there a critical threshold level of p42 phosphorylation required for growth? Assuming a chain of events leading to mitogenesis in which p42 phosphorylation is an early step, what is the next step in the pathway, i.e., what are the target(s) for pp42? How does phosphorylation of p42 affect its interaction with these targets? Purification of p42 and generation of an antiserum or monoclonal antibody would be enormously helpful in this regard. We have preliminary indications that pp42 is a soluble cytoplasmic protein. Mutant or variant cells conditionally defective in their p42 phosphorylation response would also be very useful.

It is perhaps surprising that p42 tyrosine phosphorylation is induced not only by mitogenic agents that are known to activate tyrosine protein kinases but also by mitogens whose cell-surface receptors are not known to possess tyrosine protein kinase activity. Among these

latter mitogens, FGF is of interest because of its polypeptide nature and potential similarity to EGF and PDGF. As discussed above, tumor promoters bind to and activate the serine/threonine specific Ca^{++}/phospholipid/diacylglycerol-dependent protein kinase, C-kinase. Activation through C-kinase-mediated phosphorylation of an unidentified tyrosine protein kinase would provide a satisfactory explanation for the ability of tumor promoters to induce p42 phosphorylation. Trypsin can potentially interact with many cell-surface proteins including the EGF and PDGF receptors, but any explanation based on activation through proteolysis has to account for the fact that chymotrypsin does not induce p42 phosphorylation (Cooper et al. 1984) nor is it a mitogen for chick cells (Teng and Chen 1975). Regardless of the precise mechanism inducing phosphorylation in each instance, the commonality of the response implies that tyrosine phosphorylation may play a role in mitogenesis.

Even if p42 phosphorylation is necessary for mitogenesis, it is probably not sufficient. In the case of EGF and PDGF, there are several reasons for thinking that the induced tyrosine phosphorylation is not sufficient for subsequent mitogensis. For instance, treatment of cells with a CNBr-cleaved derivative of EGF or a monovalent anti-EGF receptor Fab fragment induces phosphorylation but not cell growth (Schreiber et al. 1981). There is a qualification to this apparent dissociation of phosphorylation from mitogenesis, since the two parameters were measured in different cell types. Second, the maximum phosphorylation response is seen at doses of growth factor that saturate the receptor binding capacity, but are 10-fold higher than those needed to provoke a total mitogenic response. Third, maximal phosphorylation is achieved within a few minutes of adding growth factor, whereas commitment to synthesize DNA requires the continuous presence of growth factor for several hours. This lag could be accounted for by the time required to accumulate a threshold concentration of a regulatory molecule whose synthesis was dependent on continued phosphorylation. Growth factor-induced phosphorylation may be responsible for some of the early growth factor-mediated events such as increased transport and elevation of ornithine decarboxylase activity. It is not clear whether tyrosine phosphorylation is sufficient for all the early events or whether other potentially directly induced effects such as increased ion flux or activation of other protein kinases are needed.

To return to the question with which we started, we cannot yet say whether the viruses encoding tyrosine kinases activate cell growth directly by impinging on a growth control pathway that utilizes tyrosine phosphorylation. Further efforts to determine whether p42 is phosphorylated in virally transformed cells and the identification of new substrates for the growth factor activated tyrosine protein kinases are required.

Acknowledgments

We thank Bart Sefton for his contributions to this study. This work was supported by Public Health Service grants

CA-14195, CA-17096, and CA-28458 awarded by the National Cancer Institute.

References

Bishop, J.M. and H. Varmus. 1982. Functions and origins of retroviral transforming genes. In *Molecular biology of tumor viruses*, 2nd edition: *RNA tumor viruses* (ed. R. Weiss et al.), p. 999. Cold Spring Harbor Laboratory, Cold Spring Harbor, New York.

Bowen-Pope, D.F. and R. Ross. 1982. Platelet-derived growth factor. II. Specific binding to cultured cells. *J. Biol. Chem.* **257**: 5161.

Buhrow, S.A., S. Cohen, and J.V. Staros. 1982. Affinity labeling of the protein kinase associated with the epidermal growth factor receptor in membranes from A431 cells. *J. Biol. Chem.* **257**: 4019.

Castagna, M., Y. Takai, K. Kaibuchi, K. Sano, U. Kikkawa, and Y. Nishizuka. 1982. Direct activation of calcium-activated, phospholipid-dependent protein kinase by tumor-promoting phorbol esters. *J. Biol. Chem.* **257**: 7847.

Cochet, C., G.N. Gill, J. Meisenhelder, J.A. Cooper, and T. Hunter. 1984. Phosphorylation of the EGF receptor by C-kinase. *J. Biol. Chem.* **259**: 2553.

Cooper, J.A. and T. Hunter. 1981a. Changes in protein phosphorylation in Rous sarcoma virus transformed chicken embryo cells. *Mol. Cell. Biol.* **1**: 165.

———. 1981b. Four different classes of retroviruses induce phosphorylation of tyrosine present in similar cellular proteins. *Mol. Cell. Biol.* **1**: 394.

———. 1983. Identification and characterization of cellular targets for tyrosine protein kinases. *J. Biol. Chem.* **258**: 1108.

Cooper, J.A., B.M. Sefton, and T. Hunter. 1983a. Detection and quantification of phosphotyrosine in proteins. *Methods Enzymol.* **99**: 387.

———. 1984. Diverse mitogenic agents induce the phosphorylation of two related 42,000 dalton proteins on tyrosine in quiescent chick cells. *Mol. Cell. Biol.* **4**: 30.

Cooper, J.A., N.A. Reiss, R.J. Schwartz, and T. Hunter. 1983b. Three glycolytic enzymes are phosphorylated on tyrosine in cells transformed by Rous sarcoma virus. *Nature* **302**: 218.

Cooper, J.A., D.F. Bowen-Pope, E. Raines, R. Ross, and T. Hunter. 1982. Similar effects of platelet-derived growth factor and epidermal growth factor on the phosphorylation of tyrosine in cellular proteins. *Cell* **31**: 263.

Courtneidge, S., R. Ralston, L. Alitalo, and J.M. Bishop. 1983. Subcellular location of an abundant substrate (p36) for tyrosine-specific protein kinases. *Mol. Cell. Biol.* **3**: 340.

Czernilofsky, A.P., A.D. Levinson, H.E. Varmus, J.M. Bishop, E. Tischler, and H.M. Goodman. 1980. Nucleotide sequence of an avian sarcoma virus oncogene (*src*) and proposed amino acid sequence for the gene product. *Nature* **287**: 193.

Ek, B., B. Westermark, A. Wasteson, and C.-H. Heldin. 1982. Stimulation of tyrosine-specific phosphorylation by platelet-derived growth factor. *Nature* **295**: 419.

Erikson, E. and R.L. Erikson. 1980. Identification of a cellular protein substrate phosphorylated by the avian sarcoma virus transforming gene product. *Cell* **21**: 829.

Garrels, J.I. 1979. Two-dimensional gel electrophoresis and computer analysis of proteins synthesized by clonal cell lines. *J. Biol. Chem.* **254**: 7961.

Goldberg, A.R., K.B. Delclos, and P.M. Blumberg. 1980. Phorbol ester action is independent of viral and cellular *src* kinase levels. *Science* **208**: 191.

Gould, K.L., J.A. Cooper, and T. Hunter. 1984. The 46,000 dalton tyrosine protein kinase substrate is widespread whereas the 36,000 dalton substrate is only expressed at high levels in certain rodent tissues. *J. Cell Biol.* **98**: 487.

Greenberg, M.E. and G.M. Edelman. 1983. The 34kD-pp60*src*

substrate is located at the plasma membrane in normal and RSV-transformed cells. *Cell* **33**: 767.

Hampe, A., I. Laprevotte, F. Galibert, L.A. Fedele, and C. Scherr. 1982. Nucleotide sequences of feline retroviral oncogenes (*v-fes*) provide evidence for a family of tyrosine-specific protein kinase genes. *Cell* **30**: 775.

Hunter, T. and B.M. Sefton. 1982. Protein kinases and viral transformation. In *Molecular aspects of cellular regulation: The molecular actions of toxins and viruses* (ed. P. Cohen and S. van Heyningen), vol. 2, p. 333. Elsevier/North-Holland, Amsterdam.

Kasuga, M., F.A. Karlsson, and C.R. Kahn. 1982. Insulin stimulates the phosphorylation of the 95,000-dalton subunit of its own receptor. *Science* **215**: 185.

Kitamura, N., A. Kitamura, K. Toyoshima, Y. Hirayama, and M. Yoshida. 1982. Avian sarcoma virus Y73 genome sequence and structural similarity of its transforming gene product to that of Rous sarcoma virus. *Nature* **297**: 205.

Nakamura, K.D., R. Martinez, and M.J. Weber. 1983. Tyrosine phosphorylation of specific proteins following mitogen stimulation of chicken embryo fibroblasts. *Mol. Cell. Biol.* **3**: 380.

Niedel, J.E., L.J. Kuhn, and G.R. Vandenbark. 1983. Phorbol diester receptor copurifies with protein kinase C. *Proc. Natl. Acad. Sci.* **80**: 36.

Nigg, E.A., J.A. Cooper, and T. Hunter. 1983. Immunofluorescent localization of a 39,000-dalton substrate of tyrosine protein kinases to the cytoplasmic surface of the plasma membrane. *J. Cell Biol.* **96**: 1601.

Nishimura, J., J.S. Huang, and T.F. Deuel. 1982. Platelet-derived growth factor stimulates tyrosine-specific protein kinase activity in Swiss mouse 3T3 cell membranes. *Proc. Natl. Acad. Sci.* **79**: 4303.

Pike, L.J., D.F. Bowen-Pope, R. Ross, and E.G. Krebs. 1983. Characterization of platelet-derived growth factor-stimulated phosphorylation in cell membranes. *J. Biol. Chem.* **258**: 9383.

Pruss, R.M. and H.R. Herschmann. 1977. Variants of 3T3 cells lacking mitogenic response to epidermal growth factor. *Proc. Natl. Acad. Sci.* **74**: 3918.

Radke, K., T. Gilmore, and G.S. Martin. 1980. Transformation by Rous sarcoma virus: A cellular substrate for transformation-specific protein phosphorylation contains phosphotyrosine. *Cell* **21**: 821.

Radke, K., V.C. Carter, P. Moss, P. Dehazya, M. Schliwa, and G.S. Martin. 1983. Membrane-association of a 36,000 dalton substrate for tyrosine phosphorylation in chicken embryo fibroblasts transformed by avian sarcoma viruses. *J. Cell. Biol.* **97**: 1601.

Reddy, E.P., M.J. Smith, and A. Srinavasan. 1983. Nucleotide sequence of Abelson murine leukemia virus genome: Structural similarity of its transforming gene products to other *onc* gene products with tyrosine-specific protein kinase activity. *Proc. Natl. Acad. Sci.* **80**: 3623.

Rohrschneider, L.R. and M.J. Rosok. 1983. Transformation parameters and pp60*src* localization in cells infected with partial transformation mutants of Rous sarcoma virus. *Mol. Cell. Biol.* **3**: 731.

Schreiber, A.B., Y. Yarden, and J. Schlessinger. 1981. A non-mitogenic analogue of epidermal growth factor enhances the phosphorylation of endogenous membrane proteins. *Biochem. Biophys. Res. Commun.* **101**: 517.

Sefton, B.M., T. Hunter, E.H. Ball, and S.J. Singer. 1981. Vinculin: A cytoskeletal substrate of the transforming protein of Rous sarcoma virus. *Cell* **24**: 165.

Shibuya, M. and H. Hanafusa. 1982. Nucleotide sequence of Fujinami sarcoma virus: Evolutionary relationship of its transforming gene with transforming genes of other sarcoma viruses. *Cell* **30**: 787.

Teng, N.N.H. and L.B. Chen. 1975. The role of surface protein in cell proliferation as studied with thrombin and other proteases. *Proc. Natl. Acad. Sci.* **72**: 413.

Phosphotyrosine-containing Membrane Proteins in Rous Sarcoma Virus-transformed Cells

C.A. Monteagudo, D.L. Williams, G.A. Crabb, M. Tondravi, and M.J. Weber*
Department of Microbiology, University of Illinois, Urbana, Illinois 61801

The discovery that pp60^{src} has a tyrosine-specific protein kinase activity (Collett and Erikson 1978; Hunter and Sefton 1980) appeared to make possible for the first time the identification of cellular proteins that are primary targets for the oncogenic activity of a transforming protein: Proteins that become phosphorylated on tyrosine during transformation by Rous sarcoma virus (RSV) would be candidate substrates for pp60^{src}, and could play a functional role in oncogenesis. However, it is now clear that numerous proteins become phosphorylated on tyrosine during transformation by RSV (Cooper and Hunter 1981, 1983; Martinez et al. 1982; Weber 1983), and at least some of these phosphorylations are adventitious and are unlikely to play a functionally significant role in transformation (Cooper et al. 1983a; Snyder et al. 1983; Weber 1983). Thus, it is difficult to determine which phosphotyrosine-containing proteins are functionally significant targets for the tyrosine-specific protein kinase activity of pp60^{src} and which are adventitious substrates.

For the following reasons, we suspect that at least some biologically significant targets of pp60^{src} will prove to be plasma membrane proteins: pp60^{src} is to a large extent localized in the plasma membrane (Rohrschneider 1979; Willingham et al. 1979; Courtneidge et al. 1980; Krueger et al. 1980; Krzyzek et al. 1980) and variant forms of pp60^{src} that do not associate with the plasma membrane display decreased tumorigenicity (Krueger et al. 1982). At least some of the phenotypic alterations that characterize transformed cells are manifested by or caused by alterations in the structure or function of the plasma membrane, including changes in hexose transport (Weber 1973), adhesiveness (Weber et al. 1977), and morphology (Ali et al. 1977; Yamada and Olden 1978). Finally, both intercellular communication and the response to mitogenic polypeptide hormones are mediated through plasma membrane receptors.

To identify candidate membrane targets for pp60^{src}, we have analyzed membrane fractions of RSV-transformed cells for proteins phosphorylated on tyrosine. We found that membrane fractions contain a large number of different phosphotyrosine-containing proteins covering a wide span of molecular weights. The complexity of tyrosine phosphorylations in these membrane fractions did not differ greatly from that seen in whole cells or in the cytosol (Martinez et al. 1982). In all these cases, the predominant phosphotyrosine-containing protein was a protein of M_r 36,000 (Radke and Martin 1979; Radke et al. 1980). This protein was enriched in dense plasma membrane fractions.

Although total plasma membrane fractions were similar to whole cells in their profile of phosphotyrosine-containing proteins, glycoproteins isolated by lectin affinity chromatography showed a strikingly different pattern from whole cells. Of the proteins that bind to concanavalin A (ConA), the major glycoprotein phosphorylated on tyrosine was a protein of 93,000 M_r. We speculate that this protein may be a subunit of a hormone receptor that becomes constitutively phosphorylated in transformed cells.

Methods of Experimental Procedure

Cells and cell culture
Chicken embryo fibroblast cell cultures were prepared from 10–11-day embryos (SPAFAS, Roanoke, Ill.) by standard techniques and infected with Schmidt-Ruppin strain sugroup-A RSV (SR-RSV-A) as secondary cultures. Infected secondary cultures were trypsinized and replated at 1.5×10^5 cells/ml in Dulbecco's modified Eagle's medium containing 10% tryptose phosphate broth, 4% calf serum, and 1% heat-inactivated chicken serum (GIBCO, Grand Island, N.Y.). These tertiary cultures were used in all experiments, 2 days after plating.

Radiolabeling
Tertiary cultures were changed to phosphate-free medium with no tryptose phosphate broth, and with 4% calf serum and 1% chicken serum. They were labeled for 10–14 hours with 1 mCi/ml ^{32}P for the cell fractionation experiments, and 3–6 mCi/ml for the lectin chromatography experiments.

Cell fractionation
The procedure of Hay (1974) was used. Cell cultures were rinsed quickly on the plate in ice cold buffer, allowed to swell in ice cold hypotonic buffer for 15 minutes, and were broken with 25–50 strokes in a tight-fitting Dounce homogenizer. Cell breakage was monitored by phase microscopy and was at least 95% complete. The whole-cell homogenate was centrifuged at 1000g to yield a 1000g supernatant (S1) and pellet (P1).

---

*Present address: Department of Microbiology, University of Virginia School of Medicine, Charlottesville, Virginia 22908.

The S1 was centrifuged at 45,000g to yield a 45,000g supernatant (S45) and pellet (P45). The P45 was further separated by equilibrium centrifugation on a 35-ml discontinuous sucrose gradient consisting of 60%, 45%, 35%, 30%, 25%, and 20% sucrose for 14 hours at 70,000g in an SW-27 rotor. The material at the five interfaces was collected, washed by centrifugation, and used for subsequent analysis. The material from the interfaces is referred to as bands I, II, III, IV, and V, with the band-I material having the lowest density (20/25% interface).

Because the cell fractionation procedure required 20 hours to complete, we were concerned that phosphatase activity might affect the results obtained. Incubation of a cell homogenate at 4°C for 25 hours resulted in a 30% decrease in phosphotyrosine content. This decrease in phosphotyrosine content was blocked by 0.1 mM ZnCl$_2$ (Brautigan et al. 1981). Since the decrease in phosphotyrosine was modest, and since the presence of zinc might affect the cell fractionation, we chose to perform the fractionations in the absence of zinc. Note, however, that if the loss of phosphotyrosine was selective some of the data shown in Figures 1–3 in Results could be altered.

NADH-diaphorase was used as a marker for the endoplasmic reticulum, 5′-nucleotidase for the plasma membrane, and lactate dehydrogenase (LDH) for the cytosol. Protein was assayed by the method of Lowry with bovine serum albumin (BSA) as a standard.

Lectin affinity chromatography

After labeling with ^{32}P, cultures were quickly rinsed with cold phosphate-buffered saline and directly lysed in boiling 1% SDS. This stopped all detectable phosphatase activity. The lysates were diluted in a buffered detergent mixture to give a final concentration of 0.5% deoxycholate, 0.5% NP-40, 0.05% SDS, 0.5 mM Tris (pH 7.2), 0.5% Trasylol, 0.5 mM ZnCl$_2$, and 0.5 mM NaF. The detergents in this mixture, at the concentrations used, are compatible with ConA binding (Kahane et al. 1976; Lotan et al. 1977; C.A. Monteagudo and M.J. Weber, unpubl.).

The diluted cell lysates were loaded onto a column of ConA-Sepharose 4B (Sigma, St. Louis, Mo.) which had been equilibrated with the detergent mixture. The column was washed with the detergent mixture, then with 0.4 M mannitol, and the glycoproteins were eluted with 0.4 M α-methylmannoside.

Gel electrophoresis and phosphoamino acid analysis

Phosphoamino acid analysis and identification of phosphotyrosine-containing proteins were performed as described by Martinez et al. (1982) and by Nakamura et al. (1983). Briefly, lysates that were prepared in Laemmli sample buffer were electrophoresed on 1-cm, 10% polyacrylamide tube gels, with dansylated proteins as internal molecular-weight markers. The gels were sliced into approximately 30–120 slices, and the protein from each slice was eluted, trichloracetic acid (TCA)-precipitated, and acid-hydrolyzed, and the phosphoamino

acids were separated by two-dimensional high-voltage paper electrophoresis at pH 1.9 and then at pH 3.5. The phosphoamino acids were located by autoradiography and ninhydrin staining, cut from the paper, and quantitated by scintillation spectrometry.

Results

Cell fractionation

RSV-transformed chicken embryo cells were lysed in hypotonic buffer and fractionated by differential centrifugation and sucrose density gradient centrifugation. Table 1 reveals that the fractionation scheme successfully separated the three marker enzymes, with very little of the cytosol marker, LDH, appearing in the particulate fraction (P45). The P45 was, however, enriched for the membrane markers NADH-diaphorase and 5′-nucleotidase, as well as being enriched equivalently for phosphotyrosine (relative to phosphoserine and threonine).

Fractionation of the P45 on sucrose density gradients separated the plasma membrane marker (5′-nucleotidase) from the endoplasmic reticulum marker (NADH-diaphorase) (Table 1 and Fig. 1). Bands I and II displayed the highest specific activity of 5′-nucleotidase, with band II having the highest amount of the enzyme. The NADH-diaphorase activity was concentrated in band IV. In a separate study, cells were labeled with [^{3}H]uridine to serve as a marker for ribosomes. The majority of the label was found in band V, and most of the rest in band IV (data not shown). On the basis of these assays, we believe that bands I and II are enriched for plasma membranes, band IV for endoplasmic reticulum, and band V for rough endoplasmic reticulum and free ribosomes.

Figure 1 displays the distribution of the marker enzymes and phosphoamino acids through the sucrose gradient fractionation of the P45. The fraction with the largest amount of phosphotyrosine was band III. The phosphotyrosine-containing protein of 36,000 M_r (originally described by Radke and Martin 1979) also appeared predominantly in band III, as determined by immunoprecipitation with antiserum raised against the purified protein (Erikson and Erikson 1980) (Figs. 1 and 2). Note that this membrane band is denser than the bands that contain the bulk of the 5′-nucleotidase. Phosphoserine and phosphothreonine showed the greatest enrichment in the densest regions of the sucrose gradient.

Each of the sucrose gradient bands and the P45 were collected and washed by centrifugation, and the proteins were separated on polyacrylamide tube gels. The gels were cut into approximately 30 slices, and the phosphoamino acid content of the proteins eluted from each slice was determined as described (Martinez et al. 1982; Nakamura et al. 1983). This yielded a profile of phosphoamino acid content as a function of molecular weight for each of the sucrose gradient fractions and the P45. The results are shown in Figure 3. It is clear that phosphotyrosine-containing proteins covering a wide span of molecular weights were found in every band from the sucrose gradient. The most abundant phosphotyrosine-containing protein in the P45 and in bands I–IV of the

Table 1 Marker Enzymes and Phosphoamino Acids in Cell Fractions

Fraction	Marker enzymes (relative specific activity)			Phosphoamino acids (% of total in each fraction)		
	LDH	diaphorase	5′-nucleotidase	p-tyr	p-thr	p-ser
Homogenate	1.0	1.0	1.0	1.2	7.7	91.1
S1	2.2	1.8	1.7	2.4	4.3	93.3
P1	0.1	1.3	0.1	N.D.	N.D.	N.D.
S45	3.3	0.2	0.7	1.2	4.2	94.6
P45	0.1	1.6	1.2	2.7	6.3	90.9
Band I	N.D.[a]	1.7	11.3	5.6	7.5	86.9
Band II	N.D.	1.3	11.3	7.6	6.5	85.9
Band III	N.D.	1.4	4.8	6.4	7.2	86.5
Band IV	N.D.	4.5	1.3	4.3	8.5	87.3
Band V	N.D.	2.6	0.2	1.8	6.1	92.1

[a]N.D. = not determined.

sucrose gradient was the 36,000 M_r protein that we previously showed was the most abundant phosphotyrosine-containing protein in whole cells (Martinez et al. 1982). This peak was most prominent in bands II and III, and was barely detectable in band V, consistent with the results of the immunoprecipitation (Figs. 1 and 2). As a percentage of the phosphotyrosine-containing proteins, the 36,000 M_r protein was enriched approximately two- to fourfold in the membrane fractions, compared with its concentration in whole cells. Two very low M_r protein peaks were also visible and were substantially enriched in the densest fraction, band V.

Lectin affinity chromatography

Since cell fractionation experiments did not reveal unique phosphotyrosine-containing proteins that had not previously been described, we turned to lectin affinity chromatography as a more selective procedure for examining the tyrosine phosphorylation of membrane proteins. Cellular proteins labeled with ^{32}P were chromatographed on a column of ConA-Sepharose and specifically eluted with 0.4 M α-methylmannoside (Fig. 4). The specificity of the elution was demonstrated by the fact that mannitol at 0.4 M or 0.8 M did not elute significant amounts of radioactively labeled protein. α-Methylglucoside at 0.4 M or 0.8 M did not elute any additional radioactive material that was not eluted with 0.4 M α-methylmannoside. However, substantial amounts of radioactivity could be removed from the column with 8 M urea (data not shown). Whether this radioactivity represents very tightly binding glycoproteins or nonspecifically adsorbed material remains to be determined.

The ConA-binding glycoprotein fraction was enriched more than 20-fold for phosphotyrosine, relative to phosphothreonine and phosphoserine: Whereas phosphotyrosine was 0.34% of the total phosphoamino acids in the crude extract in this experiment, phosphotyrosine was 7.44% of the phosphoamino acid in this glycoprotein fraction.

We wished to determine whether the proteins phosphorylated on tyrosine that were isolated by lectin affinity

chromatography displayed the same pattern of M_r distribution seen in whole cells and membrane fractions. Therefore, the ConA-binding glycoprotein fraction was separated by SDS-polyacrylamide gel electrophoresis, the gel was divided into 30 slices, and the phosphoamino acid composition of each slice was determined. The results, shown in Figure 5, reveal a strikingly different profile of phosphoamino acids in this glycoprotein fraction. Particularly noteworthy is the fact that the major peak of phosphotyrosine is at 93 kD. This peak is coincident with peaks of phosphothreonine and phosphoserine. Peaks of phosphotyrosine were also seen at >200,000 M_r, <20,000 M_r, and a broad peak was noted between about 30,000 and 55,000 M_r. A shoulder of phosphotyrosine was also seen at 125,000 M_r. The 125,000 M_r shoulder and the region just above 30,000 M_r have high levels of phosphotyrosine, but low levels of phosphoserine. Thus, even though these regions did not contain the major phosphotyrosine-containing peaks, the phosphotyrosine in these regions constituted as much as 30% of the total phosphoamino acid.

Discussion

Because so many proteins become phosphorylated on tyrosine in RSV-transformed cells (Cooper and Hunter 1981, 1983; Martinez et al. 1982; Weber 1983), it has been extremely difficult to determine what role—if any—these phosphorylations might play in transformation (Nakamura and Weber 1982; Kahn et al. 1982; Cooper et al. 1983a; Rohrschneider and Rosok 1983). Of the numerous proteins known to become phosphorylated on tyrosine during transformation, only five are proteins of known function: pp60^{src}, vinculin, enolase, phosphoglycerate mutase, and LDH. In the case of pp60^{src}, the major tyrosine phosphorylation is unnecessary for transformation and may be adventitious (Snyder et al. 1983). For the other proteins, no biological effect of the phosphorylation has been demonstrated. In particular, phosphorylation of the three glycolytic enzymes (Cooper et al. 1983b) may well be adventitious since these enzymes

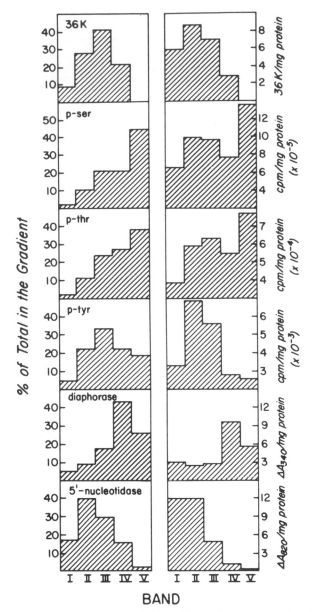

BAND

Figure 1 Distribution of a 36,000 M_r tyrosine-phosphorylated protein, protein-bound phosphoamino acids, and two membrane markers in a P45 fraction separated on a discontinuous sucrose density gradient. The 36,000 M_r protein content was determined by immunoprecipitation of a constant aliquot from each sucrose density gradient band with antiserum against the purified 36,000 M_r protein. The amount of ^{32}P in the protein was quantitated by densitometric scanning of a gel electropherogram of the immunoprecipitate. (Band I) 20/25% interface; (band II) 25/30% interface; (band III) 30/35% interface; (band IV) 35/45% interface; (band V) 45/60% interface.

are not generally believed to be regulatory or rate-limiting for glycolysis. (Note, however, that phosphorylation of enolase and phosphoglycerate mutase did correlate with the rate of hexose transport in cells infected with a panel of partially transforming virus mutants, consistent with the possibility that these phosphorylations play some role in regulating glucose metabolism) (Cooper et al. 1983a).

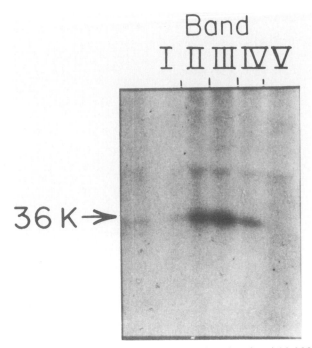

Figure 2 Gel electropherogram of the phosphorylated 36,000 M_r protein immunoprecipitated from aliquots of a P45 fractionated on a discontinuous sucrose density gradient.

In the case of vinculin, phosphorylation correlated with the ability of cells to grow in soft agar (Rohrschneider and Rosok 1983); however, the correlation was based on a small sample of partially transforming mutants, and in any event, the mechanistic relationship between vinculin and growth control is thus far unknown. Thus, even for those proteins that have a known functional identity, the biological significance of their phosphorylation on tyrosine remains obscure at best. The major protein to become phosphorylated on tyrosine in RSV-transformed cells is a protein of 36,000 M_r and of unknown function.

In hopes of identifying cellular proteins whose phosphorylation might play some easily ascertainable role in transformation, we have examined the phosphotyrosine-containing proteins of membrane fractions from RSV-transformed cells. The rationale for this approach was based on our belief that at least some of the functionally significant cellular targets for $pp60^{src}$ activity will prove to be membrane proteins and that membrane fractions would contain fewer phosphotyrosine-containing proteins than whole cells, thus simplifying their analysis.

We were surprised and disappointed to find that membrane fractions from transformed cells prepared by conventional cell fractionation techniques did not yield a less complex pattern of phosphotyrosine-containing proteins than did whole cells. Rather, both plasma membrane fractions and endoplasmic reticulum fractions contained a large number of phosphotyrosine-containing proteins covering a wide range of molecular weights and displayed an overall pattern of phosphotyrosine-containing proteins that was similar to that seen in whole cells.

Some of this complexity could be due to the associ-

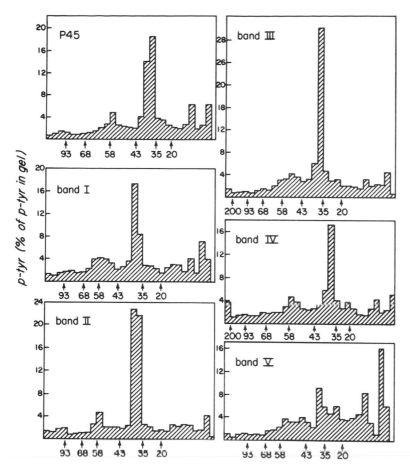

Figure 3 Profile of phosphotyrosine-containing proteins as a function of M_r in particulate fractions from RSV-transformed cell cultures. Cell fractions were electrophoresed on SDS-polyacrylamide tube gels, the gels were cut into approximately 30 slices, and the phosphoamino acid content of the proteins eluted from each slice was determined. The numbers below each profile represent M_r as determined with dansylated protein markers.

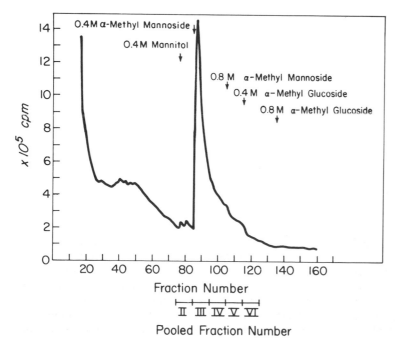

Figure 4 Elution of phosphoproteins from a column of ConA-Sepharose. Cells were labeled with ^{32}P, lysed with detergents, and passed over the lectin column. The column was washed extensively, first with detergents, then with detergents plus 0.4 M mannitol. The glycoprotein fraction was specifically eluted with 0.4 M α-methylmannoside.

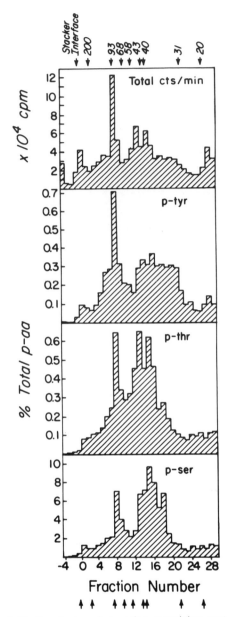

Figure 5 Profile of phosphotyrosine-containing proteins as a function of M_r in the glycoprotein fraction isolated from transformed cells by ConA affinity chromatography. The arrows above and below the figure represent the positions of dansylated protein M_r markers.

did effectively separate the LDH activity from the membrane fractions.

Cell fractionation experiments revealed that much of the 36,000 M_r phosphotyrosine-containing protein was associated preferentially with membrane fractions, in agreement with the findings of Courtneidge et al. (1982), Greenberg and Edelman (1983), and Kaji and Amini (1983). In our work, however, the plasma membrane was subdivided into several fractions of differing density, and the 36,000 M_r protein was found preferentially in fractions that were denser than those containing the bulk of the plasma membrane marker 5′-nucleotidase. This is consistent with observations that this protein is associated with a submembranous filamentous network (Cheng and Chen 1981; Greenberg and Edelman 1983), since protein-rich plasma membrane fractions would display a greater than average density on sucrose gradients.

Isolation of membrane glycoproteins by lectin affinity chromatography yielded a more than 20-fold enrichment for phosphotyrosine and a dramatically different profile of phosphotyrosine-containing proteins, relative to whole cells or membrane fractions. The major peak of phosphotyrosine was at 93,000 M_r and was coincident with a peak of phosphoserine and phosphothreonine. Although we do not yet know the identity of this 93,000 M_r protein, this is approximately the same M_r as has been reported for the β-subunit of the receptor for insulinlike growth factor type I (Czech 1982). In analogy with the β-subunit of the insulin receptor, which has a similar M_r and becomes phosphorylated on tyrosine in response to insulin (Avruch et al. 1982; Kasuga et al. 1982; Petruzzelli et al. 1982), it is likely that the receptor for insulinlike growth factor type I also is susceptible to phosphorylation on tyrosine (Rubin et al. 1983). If, indeed, a receptor for an insulinlike growth factor becomes phosphorylated on tyrosine in RSV-transformed cells, it could help explain the increased growth and glucose transport that characterize these cells.

Acknowledgments

We wish to thank Ricardo Martinez, Ken Nakamura, and Ted McNair for their advice during the course of this work, and Margaret Bruesch for technical assistance. Eleanor and Raymond Erikson generously provided antiserum against the 36,000 M_r protein. This research was supported by U.S. Public Health Service grants CA 12467 and CA 32964.

References

Ali, I.V., V. Mautner, R. Lanza, and R.O. Hynes. 1977. Restoration of normal morphology, adhesion and cytoskeleton in transformed cells by addition of a transformation-specific surface protein. *Cell* **11:** 115.

Avruch, J., R.A. Nemenoff, P.J. Blackshear, M.W. Pierce, and R. Osathanodh. 1982. Insulin-stimulated phosphorylation of the insulin receptor in detergent extracts of human placental membranes. *J. Biol. Chem.* **257:** 15162.

Brautigan, D.L., D.L. Bornstein, and B. Gallis. 1981. Phosphotyrosyl-protein phosphatase: Specific inhibition by Zn^2. *J. Biol. Chem.* **256:** 6519.

Cheng, Y.S. and L.B. Chen. 1981. Detection of phosphoty-

ation of cytoplasmic proteins with the membrane fractions. For example, Cooper and Hunter (1982) have found that the 36,000 M_r protein can fractionate either with membranes or cytosol, depending on how the cells are harvested and lysed. The chemical nature of the association between membranes and these phosphotyrosine-containing proteins is unknown, although, it is clear that the 36,000 M_r protein is not an intrinsic membrane protein (Courtneidge et al. 1982; Greenberg and Edelman 1983). In any event, the association of phosphotyrosine-containing proteins with the membrane cannot be entirely random, since our membrane isolation procedure rosine-containing 34,000-dalton protein in the framework of cells transformed with Rous sarcoma virus. *Proc. Natl. Acad. Sci.* **78**: 2388.

Collett, M.S. and R. Erikson. 1978. Protein kinase activity associated with the avian sarcoma virus *src* gene product. *Proc. Natl. Acad. Sci.* **75**: 2021.

Cooper, J.A. and T. Hunter. 1981. Changes in protein phosphorylation in Rous sarcoma virus-transformed chicken embryo cells. *Mol. Cell. Biol.* **1**: 394.

———. 1982. Discrete primary locations of a tyrosine protein kinase and of three proteins that contain phosphotyrosine in virally transformed chick fibroblasts. *J. Cell Biol.* **94**: 287.

———. 1983. Regulation of cell growth and transformation by tyrosine-specific protein kinases: The search for important cellular substrate proteins. *Curr. Top. Microbiol. Immunol.* **107**: 125.

Cooper, J.A., K.D. Nakamura, T. Hunter, and M.J. Weber. 1983a. Phosphotyrosine-containing proteins and the expression of transformation parameters in cells infected with partial transformation mutants of Rous sarcoma virus. *J. Virol.* **46**: 15.

Cooper, J.A., N.A. Reiss, R.J. Schwartz, and T. Hunter. 1983b. Three glycolytic enzymes are phosphorylated on tyrosine in cells transformed by Rous sarcoma virus. *Nature* **302**: 218.

Courtneidge, S.A., A.D. Levinson, and J.M. Bishop. 1980. The protein encoded by the transforming gene of avian sarcoma virus (pp60^{src}) and a homologous protein in normal cells (pp60$^{proto-src}$) are associated with the plasma membrane. *Proc. Natl. Acad. Sci.* **77**: 3783.

Courtneidge, S.A., R. Ralston, K. Alitalo, and J.M. Bishop. 1982. Subcellular location of an abundant substrate (p36) for tyrosine-specific protein kinases. *Mol. Cell. Biol.* **3**: 340.

Czech, M.P. 1982. Structural and functional homologies in the receptors for insulin and the insulin-like growth factors. *Cell* **31**: 8.

Erikson, E. and R.L. Erikson. 1980. Identification of a cellular protein substrate phosphorylated by the avian sarcoma virus-transforming gene product. *Cell* **21**: 829.

Greenberg, M.E. and G.M. Edelman. 1983. The 34 kd pp60^{src} substrate is located at the inner face of the plasma membrane. *Cell* **33**: 767.

Hay, A.J. 1974. Studies on the formation of the influenza virus envelope. *Virology* **60**: 398.

Hunter, T. and B.M. Sefton. 1980. The transforming gene product of Rous sarcoma virus phosphorylates tyrosine. *Proc. Natl. Acad. Sci.* **77**: 1311.

Kahane, I., H. Furthmayr, and V.T. Marchesi. 1976. Isolation of membrane glycoproteins by affinity chromatography in the presence of detergents. *Biochim. Biophys. Acta* **426**: 464.

Kahn, P., K. Nakamura, S. Shin, R.E. Smith, and M.J. Weber. 1982. Tumorigenicity of partial transformation mutants of Rous sarcoma virus. *J. Virol.* **42**: 602.

Kaji, A. and S. Amini. 1983. Association of pp36, a phosphorylated form of the presumed target for the *src* protein of Rous sarcoma virus, with the membrane of chicken cells transformed by Rous sarcoma virus. *Proc. Natl. Acad. Sci.* **80**: 960.

Kasuga, M., Y. Zick, D.L. Blith, F.A. Karlsson, H.U. Haring, and C.R. Kahn. 1982. Insulin stimulation of phosphorylation of the beta subunit of the insulin receptor. Formation of both phosphoserine and phosphotyrosine. *J. Biol. Chem.* **257**: 9891.

Krueger, J.G., E. Wang, and A.R. Goldberg. 1980. Evidence that the *src* gene product of Rous sarcoma virus is membrane associated. *Virology* **101**: 25.

Krueger, J.G., E.A. Garber, A.R. Goldberg, and H. Hanafusa. 1982. Changes in amino-terminal sequences of pp60^{src} lead to decreased membrane association and decreased *in vivo* tumorigenicity. *Cell* **28**: 889.

Krzyzek, R.A., R.L. Mitchell, A.F. Lau, and A.J. Faras. 1980. Association of pp60^{src} and *src* protein kinase activity with the plasma membrane of nonpermissive and permissive avian sarcoma virus-infected cells. *J. Virol.* **36**: 805.

Lotan, R., G. Beattie, W. Hubbell, and G.L. Nicolson. 1977. Activities of lectins and their immobilized derivatives in detergent solutions. Implications on the use of lectin affinity chromatography for the purification of membrane glycoproteins. *Biochemistry* **16**: 1787.

Martinez, R., K.D. Nakamura, and M.J. Weber. 1982. Identification of phosphotyrosine-containing proteins in untransformed and Rous sarcoma virus-transformed chicken embryo fibroblasts. *Mol. Cell. Biol.* **2**: 653.

Nakamura, K.D. and M.J. Weber. 1982. Phosphorylation of a 36,000 Mr cellular protein in cells infected with partial transformation mutants of Rous sarcoma virus. *Mol. Cell. Biol.* **2**: 147.

Nakamura, K.D., R. Martinez, and M.J. Weber. 1983. Tyrosine phosphorylation of specific proteins after mitogen stimulation of chicken embryo fibroblasts. *Mol. Cell. Biol.* **3**: 380.

Petruzzelli, L.M., S. Ganguly, C.J. Smith, M.H. Cobb, C.H. Rubin, and O.M. Rosen. 1982. Insulin activates a tyrosine-specific protein kinase in extracts of 3T3-L1 adipocytes and human placenta. *Proc. Natl. Acad. Sci.* **79**: 6792.

Radke, K. and G.S. Martin. 1979. Transformation by Rous sarcoma virus: Effects of *src* gene expression on the synthesis and phosphorylation of cellular polypeptides. *Proc. Natl. Acad. Sci.* **76**: 5212.

Radke, K., T. Gilmore, and G.S. Martin. 1980. Transformation by Rous sarcoma virus: A cellular substrate for transformation-specific protein phosphorylation contains phosphotyrosine. *Cell* **21**: 821.

Rohrschneider, L.R. 1979. Immunofluorescence on avian sarcoma virus transformed cells: Localization of the *src* gene product. *Cell* **16**: 11.

Rohrschneider, L.M. and M.J. Rosok. 1983. Transformation parameters and pp60^{src} localization in cells infected with partial transformation mutants of Rous sarcoma virus. *Mol. Cell. Biol.* **3**: 731.

Rubin, J.B., M.A. Shia, and P.F. Pilch. 1983. Stimulation of tyrosine-specific phosphorylation *in vitro* by insulin-like growth factor I. *Nature* **305**: 438.

Snyder, M.A., J.M. Bishop, W.W. Colby, and A.D. Levinson. 1983. Phosphorylation of tyrosine 416 is not required for the transforming properties and kinase activity of pp60^{v-src}. *Cell* **32**: 891.

Weber, M.J. 1973. Hexose transport in normal and in Rous sarcoma virus-transformed cells. *J. Biol. Chem.* **248**: 2978.

———. 1983. Malignant transformation by Rous sarcoma virus: From phosphorylation to phenotype. *Adv. Viral Oncol.* (in press).

Weber, M.J., A.H. Hale, and L. Losasso. 1977. Decreased adherence to the substrate in Rous sarcoma virus-transformed chicken embryo fibroblasts. *Cell* **10**: 45.

Willingham, M.C., G. Jay, and I. Pastan. 1979. Localization of ASV *src* gene product to the plasma membrane of transformed cells by electron microscopic immunocytochemistry. *Cell* **18**: 125.

Yamada, K.M. and K. Olden. 1978. Fibronectins: Adhesive glycoproteins of cell surface and blood. *Nature* **275**: 179.

Subcellular Localization of Viral and Cellular Tyrosyl Protein Kinases

A.R. Goldberg, E.A. Garber, J.G. Krueger, and T.W. Wong

The Rockefeller University, New York, New York 10021

Tyrosyl protein kinase activities have been demonstrated to be associated with or intrinsic to three classes of proteins that include the transforming gene products of several sarcoma-inducing retroviruses, the cellular receptors for growth factors, and the cellular enzymes of normal cells. The relationship and/or interaction among any of these enzymes is unknown.

It is possible that transforming (onc) proteins affect cellular metabolic control points that have unique subcellular localizations. Thus, by determining an onc protein's specific subcellular location, it may be possible to ascertain those cellular proteins with which it interacts and thereby gain new insights into the mechanism of transformation. Investigators from several laboratories using the techniques of immunofluorescence microscopy, electron microscopic immunocytochemistry, and subcellular fractionation have shown that pp60^{src}, the transforming protein encoded by the src gene of Rous sarcoma virus (RSV) in RSV-transformed chicken embryo fibroblasts (CEF), is predominantly associated with the cytoplasmic face of the plasma membrane and specialized portions of the plasma membrane, including adhesion plaques and regions of cell-cell contact (for review, see Krueger et al. 1983a). Available evidence indicates that pp60^{src} behaves as an integral membrane protein (Krueger et al. 1980a,b; Levinson et al. 1981; Garber et al. 1982) and that a hydrophobic aminoterminal domain appears to be responsible for its interaction with the membrane (Krueger et al. 1980a,b; Levinson et al. 1981). Tightly associated lipid may contribute to the protein's hydrophobicity (Sefton et al. 1982; Garber et al. 1983b). Although pp60^{src} is a membrane protein, it is nonetheless synthesized on free polyribosomes (Lee et al. 1979; Purchio et al. 1980). It has been suggested that pp60^{src} is transported through the cytoplasm to the plasma membrane by transiently complexing with two cellular phosphoproteins, pp50 and pp90 (Courtneidge and Bishop 1982; Brugge et al. 1983).

To analyze the function of the aminoterminal membrane-binding domain, we have studied two isolates of recovered avian sarcoma viruses (rASVs), 1702 and 157, which encode pp60^{src} proteins with alterations in the aminoterminal region of the molecule (Karess and Hanafusa 1981). We showed that the rASV 1702 and 157 src proteins differed from wild-type pp60^{src} in their interaction with membranes, displayed a salt-sensitive subcellular distribution, and fractionated as soluble, cytoplasmic proteins under isotonic salt conditions (Krueger et al. 1982). Most interestingly, although cells infected with rASV 1702 or 157 contained high levels of src-specific tyrosine kinase activity and showed a number of the parameters normally associated with transformed cells in culture, their in vivo tumorigenicity was greatly reduced (Krueger et al. 1982). Furthermore, we were unable to detect lipid associated with their src proteins (Garber et al. 1983a).

The src protein encoded by tsNY68 also behaves as a soluble cytoplasmic protein in infected cells maintained at the nonpermissive temperature (41–42°C), and was found almost exclusively in the pp50:pp90 complexed form (Courtneidge and Bishop 1982; Brugge et al. 1983; Garber et al. 1983b). Unlike cells transformed by rASV 157 and 1702, cells infected with tsNY68 do not appear morphologically transformed at the nonpermissive temperature, show lower levels of kinase activity (Collett and Erikson 1978; Levinson et al. 1978), showed reduced in vivo tumorigenicity (Kawai and Hanafusa 1971; Poirier et al. 1982), and show reduced levels of lipid associated with pp60^{src} (Garber et al. 1983a). The first portion of this article will be devoted to a further elucidation of the nature of the interaction of "soluble" src proteins with subcellular structures in rASV 157- and rASV 1702-infected cells and to a clarification of the differences and similarities between these aminoterminally altered pp60^{src} and tsNY68 pp60^{src} species. To that end, we have examined (1) the intracellular localization of these src proteins, (2) the morphology of cells transformed by these viruses using scanning electron microscopy (SEM), and (3) the organization of cytoskeleton, adhesion plaques, and fibronectin in rASV-transformed cells by indirect immunofluorescence microscopy.

The second part of this paper will be concerned with our efforts to identify and characterize tyrosyl protein kinases in normal tissue. Such experiments were made possible by using peptide substrates in vitro that contained tyrosine but lacked serine or threonine (Casnellie et al. 1982; Hunter 1982; Pike et al. 1982; Wong and Goldberg 1983a). We have studied the abundance of tyrosyl protein kinases in rat liver subcellular components by making use of the in vitro phosphorylation of angiotensin peptides (Wong and Goldberg 1983a,b). Our data indicate the presence of as many as three tyrosyl protein kinases in normal tissue.

Methods of Experimental Procedures

Cells and viruses

CEF were grown in monolayer culture and were infected with the Schmidt-Ruppin strain of RSV, subgroup A (SR-

RSV-A), its temperature-sensitive mutant *ts*NY68, or *td* 109-derived rASV isolates 157, 1702, or 3811, as described previously (Karess and Hanafusa 1981; Krueger et al. 1980a, 1982; Garber et al. 1983b).

Antisera

Tumor-bearing rabbit (TBR) serum was obtained as described by Collett and Erikson (1978). Antiserum specific for pp60^{src} was prepared from TBR serum by reaction with an insoluble matrix to which viral structural proteins had been covalently linked. Antiserum prepared in this fashion was monospecific for pp60^{src} (Krueger et al. 1980a) and has been used to localize pp60^{src} in CEF transformed by RSV and *ts*NY68 (Garber et al. 1983b). Goat antisera to chicken fibronectin was obtained from Calbiochem Laboratories.

Indirect immunofluorescence microscopy

Cells that had been grown in monolayer culture on glass coverslips were washed with phosphate-buffered saline (PBS) and fixed at room temperature for 20 minutes in PBS containing 3.5% (w/v) paraformaldehyde. The fixed cells were rinsed with PBS and permeabilized by 5 minutes of treatment with 1% Triton X-100 in PBS. Coverslips were washed twice with 1% glycine (w/v) in PBS, and then were incubated with pp60^{src}-specific serum or rabbit antiserum raised against purified filamin for 1 hour at 37°C in a humid chamber. Coverslips were washed three times with PBS at 37°C and then were incubated for 30 minutes at 37°C in a humid chamber with fluorescein- or rhodamine-conjugated goat anti-rabbit IgG that had been preadsorbed against CEF cells. Coverslips again were washed with PBS at 37°C and were mounted for microscopic analysis. For visualization of the F-actin-containing cytoskeleton, fixed, permeabilized cells were stained with NBD-phallacidin (132 ng/ml) in PBS for 30–60 minutes in a humid chamber at 37°C (Barak et al. 1980). To visualize extracellular fibronectin, a 1:20 dilution of anti-fibronectin serum was incubated with fixed but unpermeabilized cells for 30 minutes at 37°C. After washing with PBS, these cells were incubated with a 1:20 dilution of fluorescein-conjugated rabbit anti-goat IgG for an additional 30 minutes at 37°C. Coverslips were washed with warm PBS and mounted. Mounted coverslips were viewed through 63× oil-immersion objectives with a Zeiss photomicroscope equipped with epifluorescent illumination. All micrographs in this manuscript have a magnification of 316× at the camera photographic plate, but were enlarged during photographic printing to display different cellular details. Photographs were taken on Kodak Tri-X film at ASA 1600.

Scanning electron microscopy

Cells grown on glass coverslips were fixed in half-strength Karnofsky's fixative (2.5% glutaraldehyde, 2% formaldehyde, 0.1 M sodium phosphate [pH 7.4], saturated $CaCl_2$) and postfixed with 2% OsO_4 in 0.1 M sodium phosphate (pH 7.4). Fixed cells were dehydrated through graded alcohols into acetone and were critical-point-dried in liquid CO_2. After coating with Au-Pd, cells were viewed with an accelerating voltage of 25 kV in a JEOL JSM 35 scanning electron microscope, and micrographs were recorded on Polaroid type-55 film.

Preparation of cytoskeleton matrices

Cytoskeleton matrices were prepared by extraction of transformed cells as described by Burr et al. (1980, 1981).

Subcellular fractionation of rat liver

Fractionation of rat liver was as described by Wong and Goldberg (1983b).

Kinase assays

Tyrosyl protein kinase activity was determined by using angiotensin peptides as substrates as described (Wong and Goldberg 1983a,b).

Results

Viral tyrosyl protein kinase localization

We have investigated the interaction of the size-variant *src* proteins with the pp50:pp90 complex (Krueger et al. 1983b). Glycerol gradient sedimentation of extracts from cells infected with either rASV 1702 or rASV 157 showed that the "soluble" *src* proteins of these viruses were distributed between free and pp50:pp90-complexed forms as was demonstrated previously for wild-type RSV pp60^{src}; they were found mostly in free form, with only a small fraction in the complex. Like wild-type RSV pp60^{src}, the rASV 1702 *src* protein was shown by pulse-chase studies to form a transient complex with pp50 and pp90.

Localization of "soluble" *src* proteins—Indirect immunofluorescence microscopy

To investigate whether or not size-variant *src* molecules were transported to specific subcellular sites through interaction with the pp50:pp90 complex, we used indirect immunofluorescence microscopy to determine their localization. Figure 1B shows the staining of pp60^{src} in RSV-transformed CEF. pp60^{src} was observed both in the free cell edge and in cell-cell contact regions when the focal plane was set at approximately midnuclear or midcytoplasmic level. Control CEF showed no reaction with the antisera (Fig. 1A). On occasion we also have observed pp60^{src} in discrete spots near the cell ventral surface. Interference reflection microscopy confirmed that these spots coincide with adhesion plaques, as described by Rohrschneider (1980). We operationally define adhesion plaques as areas of cell-substratum adhesion which are seen by interference reflection microscopy as streaks or dark spots. In CEF transformed by rASV 3811, which encodes a 60-kD *src* protein, we also observed *src* at the free cell edge and occasionally in small, individually occurring adhesion plaques (Fig. 1C). In contrast, rASV 157-transformed CEF, which contain a "soluble" *src* protein, showed pp60^{src} in adhesion plaques which occurred in large peripheral clusters (Fig. 1D) and at regions of cell-cell contact (not shown). Similarly, cells transformed by rASV 1702, also encoding a size-variant "soluble" *src* protein, contained *src* in abundant adhesion plaques which occurred in clusters

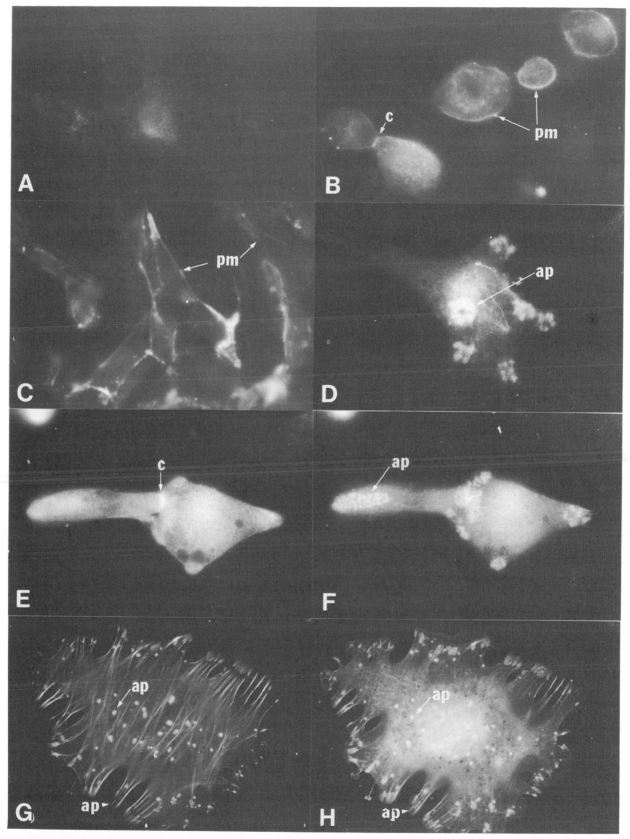

Figure 1 Localization of pp60^{src} in transformed CEF. Antiserum specific for pp60^{src} was reacted with uninfected cells (*A*), SR-RSV-A-transformed cells (*B*), rASV 3811-transformed cells (*C*), rASV 157-transformed cells (*D*), rASV 1702-transformed cells seen at two focal planes (*E,F*), and CU2-transformed cells (*H*). The same cell seen in *H* also was reacted with NBD-phallacidin to show actin-containing structures (*G*). pm, plasma membrane; ap, adhesion plaque; c, region of cell-cell contact.

(Fig. 1F) and at points of cell-cell contact (Fig. 1E). Cells transformed by the RSV CU2 mutant (Anderson et al. 1981) contained large, abundant adhesion plaques as indicated by phallacidin staining (Fig. 1G), and those adhesion plaques also contained pp60[src] (Fig. 1H). pp60[src] encoded by CU2, rASV 1702, or rASV 157 showed striking interaction with adhesion plaques, but not with the free cell edge (Fig. 1D,E,H).

Figure 2 shows paired micrographs of NBD-phallacidin fluorescence and interference reflection patterns in uninfected CEF and in cells transformed by rASV 3811, 157, and 1702. CEF contain actin stress fibers, seen by NBD-phallacidin staining, terminating in streaklike adhesion plaques (Fig. 2A,B), which are areas of close (10–15 nm) cell-substratum contact that appear black in interference micrographs (Izzard and Lochner 1976). CEF transformed by rASV 3811 (Fig. 2C,D) or RSV (not shown) showed fewer and smaller adhesion plaques than uninfected CEF. The remaining adhesion plaques were of two types: (1) streaklike cell-substratum adhesions occurring at the cell periphery and (2) round, punctate adhesions that appeared less dark by interference reflection microscopy and were intensely stained by NBD-phallacidin (Fig. 1C,D). CEF transformed by rASV 157 (Fig. 2E,F) or 1702 (Fig. 2G,H) showed large clusters of punctate adhesion plaques that stained intensely with NBD-phallacidin. More normal-appearing streaklike adhesion plaques were seen only occasionally in CEF transformed by size-variant pp60[src]s. Although CEF transformed by CU2 also contained abundant punctate adhesion plaques, they did not appear in large clusters, and numerous streaklike adhesion plaques were seen by NBD-phallacidin staining (Fig. 1G).

Analysis of transformed CEF by SEM

Using SEM, we examined transformation-related changes in cell morphology and surface topology in CEF transformed by RSV and rASV 1702 and 157. Whereas normal CEF are flat and show a regular, smooth dorsal cell surface (Fig. 3A), RSV-transformed CEF are round and display extensive microvilli similar to those observed previously in *ts*NY68-infected cells at the permissive temperature (Wang and Goldberg 1976). CEF transformed either by rASV 1702 or 157 vary from spindle-form to flat-type morphology. These cells contained large cell-surface blebs and small microvilli which occurred in clusters on the dorsal cell surface (Fig. 3, C–F). Interestingly, the transformation-related cell-surface changes appeared to parallel the localization of pp60[src] in underlying adhesion plaques. We conclude that there is a strong correlation between the localization of the size-variant pp60[src]s in restrictive areas of the plasma membrane with the regional cell-surface changes seen by SEM in cells infected with rASV 1702 or 157.

Expression of extracellular fibronectin

The work of Hynes and Destree (1978) and Singer and Paradiso (1981) indicated that fibronectin on the cell surface interacts with intracellular stress fibers through focal adhesions. Therefore, we examined fibronectin expression and organization on the surface of normal and transformed CEF. Compared with normal CEF (Fig. 4A,B), RSV- and rASV 3811-transformed CEF (Fig. 4, C–F) showed little or no cell-surface fibronectin. In contrast, rASV 1702- and 157-transformed CEF (Fig. 4, G–J) retained cell-surface fibronectin.

Interaction of pp60[src] with cytoskeleton matrix

We also compared the ability of wild-type RSV pp60[src] and rASV 1702 pp60[src] to bind to cytoskeleton matrices. Cytoskeleton matrices were prepared from transformed cells by extraction with CSK buffers (Burr et al. 1980, 1981) containing either Mg^{++} or EDTA and the varying KCl concentrations shown in Table 1. Since rASV 1702 pp60[src] appears to bind to cytoskeleton matrix components primarily via electrostatic interactions, it may interact with adhesion plaques contained in the plasma membrane as a peripheral protein.

Cellular tyrosyl protein kinase localization

Subcellular fractionation

We chose a well-characterized, readily available normal tissue to study the abundance and nature of cellular tyrosyl protein kinases in untransformed cells. Rat liver homogenates were fractionated by differential centrifugation into nuclei, plasma membranes, mitochondria, microsomes, and a high-speed supernatant. Using [Val[5]]angiotensin II as a substrate, and including *p*-nitrophenyl phosphate as a phosphatase inhibitor (Wong and Goldberg 1983a), we assayed each of the fractions for tyrosyl protein kinase activity. Approximately 60% of the recovered kinase activity sedimented with the microsomal fraction and 30–35% was localized to the 100,000*g* supernatant (Table 2). The nuclei, plasma membranes, and mitochondria each contained 1–2% of the total recovered tyrosyl kinase activity.

Chromatography of cytosolic and microsomal tyrosyl protein kinases

Adjustment of the high-speed supernatant to pH 5.0 resulted in the removal of 80% of the proteins from that fraction and enhancement of the specific activity of the tyrosyl kinases by five- to sixfold. The pH 5 fraction was freed of nucleic acid by chromatography on DEAE-Sephacel and was subjected to chromatography on phosphocellulose. The activity eluted from phosphocellulose as a single peak between 0.26 M and 0.32 M NaCl (Fig. 5A). Further purification of the eluted material was effected by gel filtration on a Sephacryl S-200 column. This step (Fig. 5B) resulted in the elution of a minor peak (I) close to the void volume of the column and a major peak (II) possessing a mobility corresponding to a molecular mass of approximately 75 kD (referred to as TPK75).

The microsomal salt-wash fraction purified similarly. Phosphocellulose chromatography and Sephacryl S-200 chromatographic patterns of kinase activity were virtually identical and resulted in the final separation of two ac-

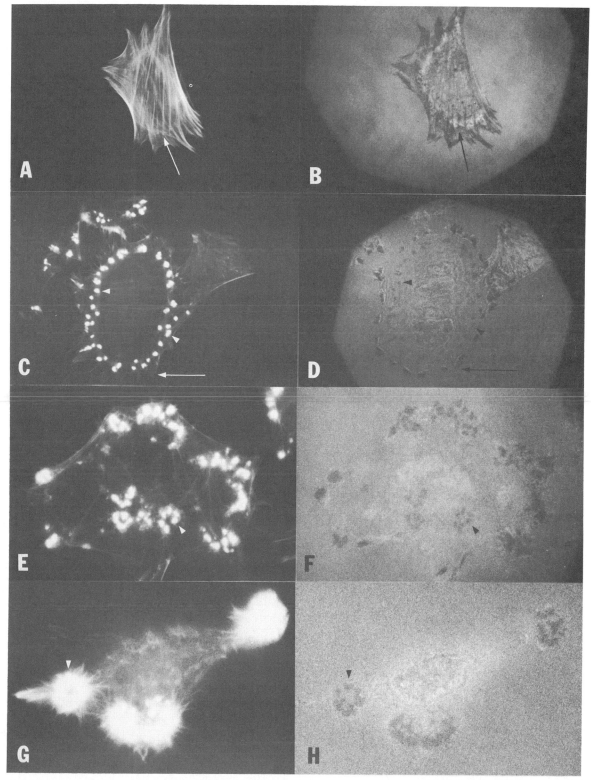

Figure 2 Microscopic analysis of adhesion plaques in rASV-transformed cells. Paired micrographs of actin fluorescence (*left*) and an interference reflection image of the same cell (*right*). The cells are uninfected CEF (*A,B*) and CEF transformed by rASV 3811 (*C,D*), rASV 157 (*E,F*), and rASV 1702 (*G,H*). Arrows indicate normal-appearing streaklike adhesion plaques, whereas arrowheads indicate punctate adhesion plaques occurring only in transformed cells. Focus was set at the ventral cell surface in all micrographs.

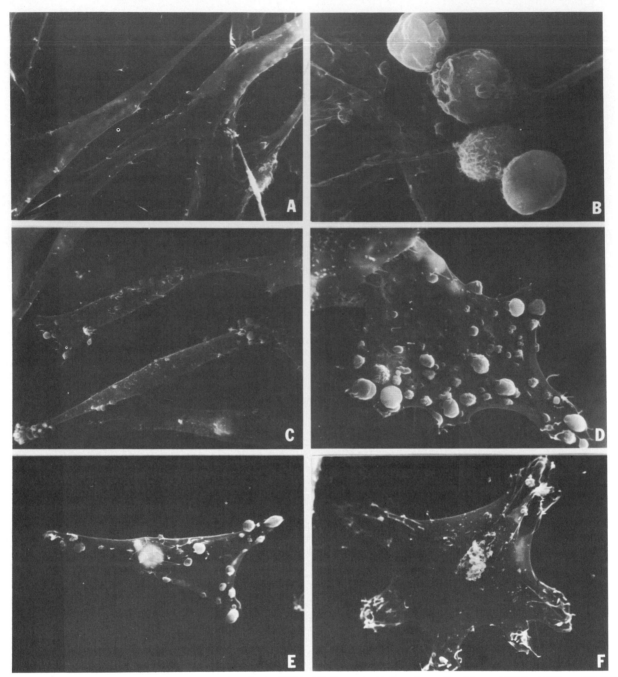

Figure 3 Analysis of RSV- or rASV-transformed cells by SEM. (*A*) Normal chick embryo fibroblasts (CEF), 1900×; (*B*) RSV-transformed CEF, 2600×; (*C*) rASV 1702-transformed CEF, 1600×; (*D*) rASV 1702-transformed CEF, 2600×; (*E*) rASV 157-transformed CEF, 1600×; and (*F*) rASV 157-transformed CEF 2600×.

tivity peaks whose molecular masses were greater than 160 kD and 75 kD (Fig. 5C,D).

To determine if the kinases derived from the cytosol and microsomal salt-wash fraction were identical, we incubated peak fractions with [γ-^{32}P]ATP and MnCl$_2$ and analyzed the reaction products by gel electrophoresis. Figure 6 (lanes 3 and 6) shows that a 75-kD phosphoprotein was the major phosphorylation product of peak II of both the cytosol and the microsome salt wash. Anal-

ysis of the proteins upon extraction from the gel indicated that they contained >95% phosphotyrosine.

Effect of various reagents on kinase activity associated with TPK75

We found that the addition of effectors of cyclic nucleotide-dependent protein kinases (e.g., cAMP or cGMP) had no effect on TPK75 activity (Table 3). Similarly, the growth factors epidermal growth factor (EGF) and in-

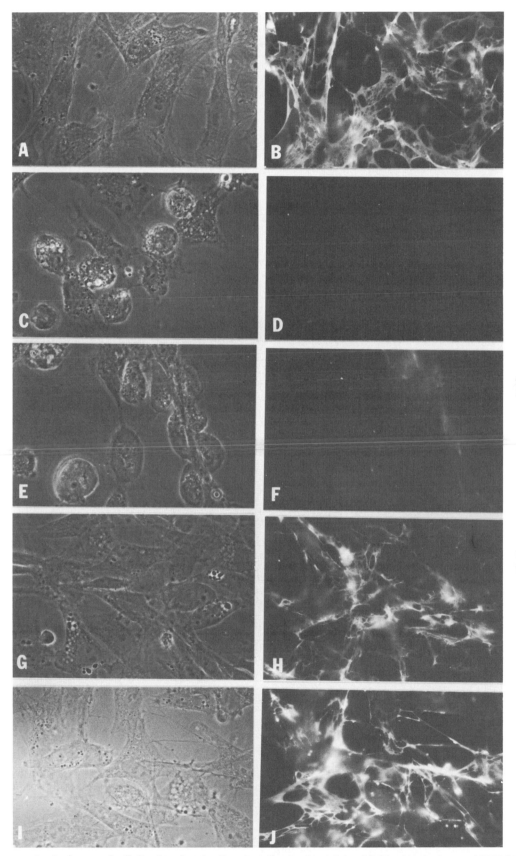

Figure 4 Phase-contrast micrographs (*left column*) and cell-surface fibronectin staining (*right column*) of normal CEF (*A,B*) and CEF transformed by RSV (*C,D*), rASV 3811 (*E,F*), rASV 157 (*G,H*), or rASV 1702 (*I,J*).

Table 1 Binding of pp60[src] to Cytoskeleton Matrices Prepared from SR-A or rASV 1702-transformed Cells by Extraction with CSK Buffer Containing Different Ionic Compositions

	Percent kinase released into supernatant[a]			
	CSK buffer + Mg[++]		CSK buffer + EDTA	
	virus strain			
Extraction buffer	SR-A	1702	SR-A	1702
CSK buffer + 10 mM KCl	7.7	2.7	17.3	41.0
CSK buffer + 100 mM KCl	9.3	10.5	19.6	45.8
CSK buffer + 250 mM KCl	9.8	19.5	23.2	52.1
CSK buffer + 500 mM KCl	10.6	27.8	35.7	76.8

CSK buffer contains 10 mM PIPES (pH 6.8), 1% NP-40, 300 mM sucrose, 2.5 mM MgCl$_2$, or 2.5 mM EDTA.
[a]Remaining pp60[src]-kinase is associated with the cytoskeletal matrix.

sulin did not affect the kinase activity. The thiol reagents *p*-chloromercuribenzoic acid (PCMB) and *N*-ethylmaleimide were among the most potent inhibitors that we assayed.

Discussion

A large number of studies using indirect immunofluorescence microscopy and biochemical cellular fractionation to localize pp60[src] proteins encoded by rASV 1702, rASV 157, and the RSV mutants CU2 and *ts*NY68 have shown altered interaction of these proteins with the cell (Rohrschneider 1980; Courtneidge and Bishop 1982; Krueger et al. 1982; Rohrschneider et al. 1982; Brugge et al. 1983; Garber et al. 1983a,b; Rohrschneider and Rosok 1983). Because all of these viruses have shown decreased tumorigenicity in vivo, the specific nature of these altered subcellular interactions may be particularly important. Table 4, summarizing some of the data from this paper, indicates that decreased tumorigenic potential seems to correlate with the absence of pp60[src] in the free cell edge and with the absence of aminoterminal-bound lipid (Garber et al. 1983a). Furthermore, CEF transformed by rASVs 1702 and 157 (Table 4) and the RSV mutant CU2 (Rohrschneider et al. 1982; Rohrsch-

neider and Rosok 1983) show more abundant pp60[src]-containing adhesion plaques than CEF transformed by other viruses. Thus, interaction of pp60[src] with adhesion plaques does not appear to be related to tumorigenic potential. We also can conclude that the presence of pp60[src] in adhesion plaques is not a sufficient condition to cause loss of extracellular fibronectin. Last, the correlation between focal membrane changes observed by SEM in cells transformed by rASV 1702 or rASV 157 and localization of size-variant pp60[src] protein in discrete membrane regions suggests that pp60[src] may need to be in direct contact with the plasma membrane to effect cellular changes associated with the transformed phenotype. Therefore, the failure of the size-variant *src* proteins to interact with critical plasma membrane regions may explain why infection of CEF with rASV 157 or rASV 1702 results in the production of a partial transformation phenotype. Biochemical properties of size-variant pp60[src] that lead to decreased interaction with membranes in cultured cells also may be responsible for the decreased in vivo potential of these viruses.

To date, investigations of tyrosyl protein kinases in normal cells have been limited to approaches that utilized antibodies directed against viral enzymes (Collett et al. 1978; Oppermann et al. 1979; Mathey-Prevot et al. 1982).

Table 2 Distribution of Tyrosyl Protein Kinase Activity in Rat Liver Subcellular Fractions

| | | | Marker enzyme activity (μmole/min · mg) | | |
Fraction	Protein (mg)	Kinase activity (units/g liver)[a]	5′-nucleotidase	succinate-cytochrome c reductase	glucose-6-phosphatase
Homogenate	2900	77.2		0.084	0.018	0.029
Nuclei	33.6	0.851 (0.8)	0.044	0.017	0.032
Plasma membrane	8.10	2.02 (1.9)	0.607	N.D.[b]	0.023
Mitochondria	171	2.27 (2.2)	0.207	0.292	0.068
Microsomes(P$_{100}$)	150	64.0 (61.4)	0.237	0.031	0.143
Supernatants(S$_{100}$)	940	35.2 (33.8)	0.013	N.D.	0.018

Rat livers (17 g) were homogenized and fractionated as described (Wong and Goldberg 1983b).
[a]Numbers in parentheses are percent of total kinase activity recovered.
[b]N.D., not determined.

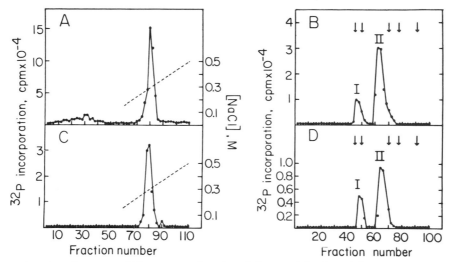

Figure 5 Chromatography of rat liver tyrosyl kinases on phosphocellulose and Sephacryl S-200 columns. (A) Phosphocellulose chromatography of pH 5 fraction (300 mg) prepared from high-speed supernatant as described (Wong and Goldberg 1983b). (B) Sephacryl S-200 chromatography of phosphocellulose column fractions 76–84 (A). (C) Phosphocellulose chromatography of microsomal salt-wash fraction. Microsomal fraction was prepared and extracted with high-salt buffer as described (Wong and Goldberg 1983b). The salt-wash fraction was dialyzed and chromatographed on DEAE-Sephacel and phosphocellulose S-200 chromatography of phosphocellulose column fractions 76–84 (C). Results are shown as radioactivity incorporated into peptide substrate. Arrows in B and D represent elution patterns of dextran blue, aldolase, bovine serum albumin, ovalbumin, and chymotrypsinogen, respectively.

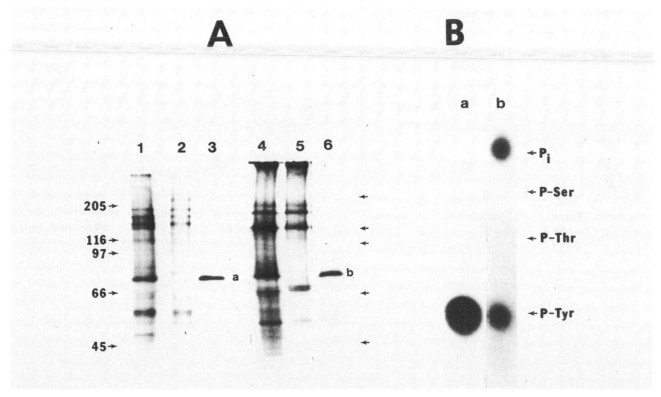

Figure 6 Autoradiogram of a SDS-polyacrylamide gel of in vitro phosphorylation products of rat liver kinase fractions. (A) Partially purified fractions of tyrosyl kinases were incubated in 25-μl reaction mixtures containing 25 mM 2-(N-morpholine)ethanesulfonic acid (pH 6.5), 5 mM $MnCl_2$, 0.1 μM [γ-^{32}P]ATP (7 × 10^6 cpm/pmole), and 10 mM 2-mercaptoethanol, and the reaction products were separated on a 10% gel . (Lanes 1–3) The pH 5 fraction; (lanes 4–6) the microsomal salt-wash fraction. (Lanes 1 and 4) Fractions eluted with 0.26–0.32 M NaCl from phosphocellulose column (Fig. 1A,C); (lanes 2 and 5) products from peak I of Sephacryl S-200 columns (Fig. 1B,D); (lanes 3 and 6) products from peak II of Sephacryl S-200 columns (Fig. 1B,D). Arrows indicate the positions of protein standards whose molecular masses are given in kD. (B) Phosphoamino acid analyses of bands labeled a and b in A. (P-Ser) Phosphoserine; (P-Thr) phosphothreonine; (P-Tyr) phosphotyrosine.

Table 3 Effects of Various Reagents on Tyrosyl Protein Kinase Activity Associated with TPK75

Effector	Concentration	Percent activity
cAMP	100 µM	106
cGMP	100 µM	110
Heat-stable kinase inhibitor	0.8 mg/ml	103
EGF	0.3 µM	107
EGF	3.0 µM	117
Insulin	1.0 µM	102
Insulin	10 µM	113
N-Ethylmaleimide	10 mM	9.6
Iodoacetamide	10 mM	88
TPCK[a]	10 mM	75
TLCK[b]	10 mM	41
PCMB[c]	10 mM	0

Purified TPK75 (0.15 unit) was incubated at 0°C for 10 min with one of the above reagents and the reaction was started by the addition of ATP. Reaction products were separated by paper electrophoresis. Results are expressed as percent of control values determined in reactions that did not contain any of the above reagents.

[a]TPCK, L-1-tosylamido-2-phenylethyl chloromethyl ketone.
[b]TLCK, N-α-tosyl-L-lysine chloromethyl ketone.
[c]PCMB, p-chloromercuribenzoic acid.

Using the tyrosine-containing peptide [Val[5]]angiotensin II as a substrate, we have been able to study the abundance of tyrosyl kinases in rat liver subcellular components. The most abundant of these enzymes, a protein with an apparent molecular mass of 75 kD, was partially purified and characterized. We also identified a tyrosyl kinase with a high molecular mass (160–200 kD) and another that associates tightly with microsomes (Wong and Goldberg 1983b).

The existence of tyrosyl protein kinases in a normal tissue such as rat liver raises questions concerning the role of tyrosine phosphorylation in normal cell metabolism. Studies on the phosphorylation of serine and threonine residues by cyclic-nucleotide-dependent protein kinases suggest a regulatory role for such posttranslational modifications. It is not unreasonable to assume the same importance for phosphorylation of tyrosine residues. Indeed, given the low level of phosphotyrosine in normal cells, it is highly plausible that such a modification is necessary for very fine tuning of carefully regulated metabolic pathways. We have considered three possible mechanisms whereby viral tyrosyl protein kinases might affect cell metabolism: (1) viral tyrosyl kinases might phosphorylate proteins not normally phosphorylated on tyrosine and thereby affect their enzymatic activity in either a negative or positive fashion; (2) viral tyrosyl kinases might overphosphorylate proteins normally containing phosphotyrosine and thereby affect, either negatively or positively, the modulatory role of normal tyrosine phosphorylation; (3) the effect of viral tyrosyl kinases might be a mixture of the first and second possibilities. We plan to try to resolve these possibilities by further studying the normal cell tyrosyl kinases.

Acknowledgments

This research was supported by U.S. Public Health Service grants CA13362 and CA18213 and in part by Biomedical Research Support grant SO7RR07065. T.W.W. was supported by a predoctoral fellowship from the Merinoff Family Cancer Research Fund.

References

Anderson, D.D., R.P. Beckmann, E.H. Harms, K. Nakamura, and M.J. Weber. 1981. Biological properties of "partial" transformation mutants of Rous sarcoma virus and characterization of their pp60*src* kinase. *J. Virol.* **37**: 445.

Barak, L.S., R.R. Yocum, E.A. Nothnagel, and W.W. Webb. 1980. Fluorescence staining of the cytoskeleton in living cells with 7-nitrobenz-2-oxa-1,3-diazolephallacidin. *Proc. Natl. Acad. Sci.* **77**: 980.

Brugge, J.S., W. Yonemoto, and D. Darrow. 1983. Interaction between the Rous sarcoma virus transforming protein and two cellular phosphoproteins: Analysis of the turnover and distribution of this complex. *Mol. Cell. Biol.* **3**: 9.

Burr, J.G., S.R. Lee, and J.M. Buchanan. 1981. In situ phosphorylation of proteins associated with the cytoskeleton of chick embryo fibroblasts. *Cold Spring Harbor Conf. Cell Proliferation* **8**: 1217.

Burr, J.G., G. Dreyfuss, S. Penman, and J.M. Buchanan. 1980. Association of the *src* gene product of Rous sarcoma virus

Table 4 Subcellular Localization of *src* Proteins Encoded by Different Viruses and Some Properties of CEF Transformed by These Viruses

Transforming virus	src localization		Actin stress fibers	Cell-surface fibronectin	Tumor-igenicity
	adhesion plaques	free cell edge			
SR-RSV-A	+	+	−	−	+
rASV 3811	+	+	+	−	+
rASV 1702	+ + +	−	+	+	↓
rASV 157	+ + +	−	+	+	↓
CU 2	+ + +	−	+ +	−	↓
CU 12	−	−	+	+	↓
tsNY68 (37°C)	+	+	−	−	↓
tsNY68 (42°C)	−	−	+ + +	+	

with cytoskeletal structures of chicken embryo fibroblasts. *Proc. Natl. Acad. Sci.* **77**: 3484.

Casnellie, J.E., M.L. Harrison, L.J. Pike, K.E. Hellstrom, and E.G. Krebs. 1982. Phosphorylation of synthetic peptides by a tyrosine protein kinase from the particulate fraction of a lymphoma cell line. *Proc. Natl. Acad. Sci.* **79**: 282.

Collett, M.S. and R.L. Erikson. 1978. Protein kinase activity associated with the avian sarcoma virus *src* gene product. *Proc. Natl. Acad. Sci.* **75**: 2021.

Collett, M.S., J.S. Brugge, and R.L. Erikson. 1978. Characterization of a normal avian sarcoma virus transforming gene product. *Cell* **15**: 1363.

Courtneidge, S.A. and J.M. Bishop. 1982. The transit of pp60^{src} to the plasma membrane. *Proc. Natl. Acad. Sci.* **79**: 7117.

Garber, E.A., J.G. Krueger, and A.R. Goldberg. 1982. Novel localization of pp60^{src} in Rous sarcoma virus-transformed rat and goat cells and in chicken cells transformed by viruses rescued from these mammalian cells. *Virology* **118**: 419.

Garber, E.A., J.G. Krueger, H. Hanafusa, and A.R. Goldberg. 1983a. Temperature-sensitive membrane association of pp60^{src} in tsNY68-infected cells correlates with increased tyrosine phosphorylation of membrane-associated proteins. *Virology* **126**: 73.

———. 1983b. Only membrane-associated RSV *src* proteins have amino-terminally bound lipid. *Nature* **302**: 161.

Hunter, T. 1982. Synthetic peptide substrates for a tyrosine protein kinase. *J. Biol. Chem.* **257**: 4843.

Hynes, R.O. and A.T. Destree. 1978. Relationships between fibronectin (LETS) protein and actin. *Cell* **15**: 875.

Izzard, C.S. and L.R. Lochner. 1976. Cell-to-substrate contacts in living fibroblasts: An interference reflexion study with an evaluation of the technique. *J. Cell Sci.* **21**: 129.

Karess, R.E. and H. Hanafusa. 1981. Viral and cellular *src* genes contribute to the structure of recovered avian sarcoma virus transforming protein. *Cell* **24**: 155.

Kawai, S. and H. Hanafusa. 1971. The effect of temperature on the transformed state of cells infected with a Rous sarcoma virus mutant. *Virology* **46**: 470.

Krueger, J.G., E.A. Garber, and A.R. Goldberg. 1983a. Subcellular localization of pp60^{src} in RSV-transformed cells. *Curr. Top. Microbiol. Immunol.* **107**:51.

Krueger, J.G., E. Wang, and A.R. Goldberg. 1980a. Evidence that the *src* gene product of Rous sarcoma virus is membrane associated. *Virology* **101**: 25.

Krueger, J.G., E.A. Garber, A.R. Goldberg, and H. Hanafusa. 1982. Changes in amino-terminal sequences of pp60^{src} lead to decreased membrane association and decreased *in vivo* tumorigenicity. *Cell* **28**: 889.

Krueger, J.G., E. Wang, E.A. Garber, and A.R. Goldberg. 1980b. Differences in intracellular location of pp60^{src} in rat and chicken cells transformed by Rous sarcoma virus. *Proc. Natl. Acad. Sci.* **77**: 4142.

Krueger, J.G., E.A. Garber, S.S.-M. Chin, H. Hanafusa, and A.R. Goldberg. 1983b. Size-variant rASV pp60^{src}s interact with adhesion plaques as periperal membrane proteins: Effects on cell transformation. *Mol. Cell Biol.* (in press).

Lee, J.S., H.E. Varmus, and J.M. Bishop. 1979. Virus-specific messenger RNAs in permissive cells infected by avian sarcoma virus. *J. Biol. Chem.* **254**: 8015.

Levinson, A.D., S.A. Courtneidge, and J.M. Bishop. 1981. Structural and functional domains of the Rous sarcoma virus transforming protein (pp60^{src}). *Proc. Natl. Acad. Sci.* **78**: 1624.

Levinson, A.D., H. Oppermann, L. Levintow, H.E. Varmus, and J.M. Bishop. 1978. Evidence that the transforming gene of avian sarcoma virus encodes a protein kinase associated with a phosphoprotein. *Cell* **15**: 561.

Mathey-Prevot, B., H. Hanafusa, and S. Kawai. 1982. A cellular protein is immunologically crossreactive with and functionally homologous to the Fujinami sarcoma virus transforming protein. *Cell* **28**: 897.

Oppermann, H., A.D. Levinson, H.E. Varmus, L. Levintow, and J.M. Bishop. 1979. Uninfected vertebrate cells contain a protein that is closely related to the product of the avian sarcoma virus transforming gene (*src*). *Proc. Natl. Acad. Sci.* **76**: 1804.

Pike, L.J., B. Gallis, J.E. Casnellie, P. Bornstein, and E.G. Krebs. 1982. Epidermal growth factor stimulates the phosphorylation of synthetic tyrosine-containing peptides by A431 cell membranes. *Proc. Natl. Acad. Sci.* **79**: 1443.

Poirier, F., D. Lawrence, P. Vigier, and P. Jullien. 1982. A ts mutant of Schmidt Ruppin strain of Rous sarcoma virus restricted at 39.5° for the morphological transformation and the tumorigenicity of chicken embryo fibroblasts. *Int. J. Cancer* **29**: 69.

Purchio, A.F., S. Jonanovich, and R.L. Erikson. 1980. Sites of synthesis of viral proteins in avian sarcoma virus-infected chicken cells. *J. Virol.* **35**: 629.

Rohrschneider, L.R. 1980. Adhesion plaques of Rous sarcoma virus-transformed cells contain the *src* gene product. *Proc. Natl. Acad. Sci.* **77**: 3514.

Rohrschneider, L.R. and M.J. Rosok. 1983. Transformation parameters and pp60^{src} localization in cells infected with partial transformation mutants of Rous sarcoma virus. *Mol. Cell. Biol.* **3**: 731.

Rohrschneider, L.R., M. Rosok, and K. Shriver. 1982. Mechanism of transformation by Rous sarcoma virus: Events within adhesion plaques. *Cold Spring Harbor Symp. Quant. Biol.* **46**: 953.

Sefton, B.M., I.S. Trowbridge, J.A. Cooper, and E.M. Scolnick. 1982. The transforming proteins of Rous sarcoma virus, Harvey sarcoma virus, and Abelson virus contain tightly bound lipid. *Cell* **31**: 465.

Singer, I. and P.R. Paradiso. 1981. A transmembrane relationship between fibronectin and vinculin (130 kd protein): Serium modulation in normal and transformed hamster fibroblasts. *Cell* **24**: 481.

Wang, E. and A.R. Goldberg. 1976. Changes in microfilament organization and surface topography upon transformation of chick embryo fibroblasts with Rous sarcoma virus. *Proc. Natl. Acad. Sci.* **73**: 4065.

Wong, T.W. and A.R. Goldberg. 1983a. *In vitro* phosphorylation of angiotensin analogs by tyrosyl protein kinases. *J. Biol. Chem.* **258**: 1022.

———. 1983b. Tyrosyl protein kinases in normal rat liver: Identification and partial characterization. *Proc. Natl. Acad. Sci.* **80**: 2529.

The Role of Protein Phosphorylation at Tyrosine in Transformation and Mitogenesis

G.S. Martin, K. Radke,* C. Carter, P. Moss, P. Dehazya, and T. Gilmore
Department of Zoology, University of California, Berkeley, California 94720

Malignant transformation of cells by several distinct avian and mammalian retroviruses is mediated by viral transforming proteins with associated tyrosine-specific protein kinase activity (Hunter et al., this volume). Cells transformed by Rous, Fujinami, PRCII, and Y73 avian sarcoma viruses (ASV), by Abelson murine leukemia virus, and by the Snyder-Theilen (ST)- and Gardner-Arnstein (GA)- strains of feline sarcoma virus all show increases in the phosphotyrosine content of cellular proteins. In addition, the plasma membrane receptors for growth factors such as epidermal growth factor (EGF) and platelet-derived growth factor (PDGF) are associated with tyrosine-specific protein kinase activity (Ushiro and Cohen 1980; Ek et al. 1982). These growth factors, and others such as the somatomedin multiplication stimulating activity (MSA), induce phosphorylation of certain cellular polypeptides at tyrosine in vivo (Cooper et al. 1982; Nakamura et al. 1983). Recently, it has been shown that the sequence of human PDGF is closely related to that of the product of the simian sarcoma virus *sis* gene (see Waterfield et al.; Robbins et al.; both this volume). These and other observations have led to the hypothesis that malignant transformation by viruses and mitogenesis by growth factors both involve the phosphorylation of cellular polypeptides whose normal functions involve the control of growth and the maintenance of structure.

Using a variety of different techniques, a number of groups have now identified several different polypeptides that become phosphorylated at tyrosine in retrovirus-transformed or growth factor-stimulated cells. The first of these to be identified is a 36K protein of unknown function that can also be phosphorylated by pp60[src] in vitro (Radke and Martin 1979; Erikson and Erikson 1980; Radke et al. 1980). The cytoskeletal protein vinculin is phosphorylated at tyrosine in certain retrovirus-transformed cells (Sefton et al. 1981). Three enzymes in the glycolytic pathway, enolase, phosphoglycerate mutase, and lactate dehydrogenase, also become phosphorylated at tyrosine in retrovirus-transformed cells (Cooper et al. 1983b). A 50K protein containing phosphotyrosine is found to be complexed to the viral transforming protein in a number of different ASV-transformed cells; the phosphorylation of this protein at tyrosine is dependent on the expression of a viral transforming protein, although

it is not temperature dependent in cells infected by temperature-sensitive mutants (Brugge and Darrow 1982; Gilmore et al. 1982). Finally, two related 42K phosphoproteins appear in retrovirus-transformed and mitogen-stimulated cells (Cooper and Hunter 1981; Cooper et al. 1982; Nakamura et al. 1983); these proteins are discussed in more detail below.

These findings raise a number of basic and as yet unanswered questions. If uninfected cells contain a number of different tyrosine-specific protein kinases, are the proteins that become phosphorylated in retrovirus-transformed cells phosphorylated directly by the viral protein kinases, or by cellular kinases activated by the viral transforming proteins? Is the phosphorylation of cellular proteins at tyrosine required for transformation? Do the substrates identified to date play some role in transformation, or is their phosphorylation adventitious (see discussion in Cooper et al. 1983a)? One possible approach to these questions is to examine individual substrates to determine if they are directly phosphorylated by the viral kinases in subcellular fractions and if tyrosine phosphorylation affects their function. We have chosen to characterize the 36K protein, both because of its abundance and because it has been shown to act as a substrate for tyrosine phosphorylation in vitro. Another approach involves a comparison of the polypeptides phosphorylated in response to different viruses or growth factors. Here we describe tyrosine-specific protein phosphorylation induced in cells exposed to the tumor promoter phorbol ester or transformed by avian erythroblastosis virus (AEV), two agents that were not previously known to activate tyrosine phosphorylation.

Materials and Methods

The procedures used in this study are reported in full elsewhere as noted briefly below. Purification of the 36K protein was as described by Erikson and Erikson (1980). The preparation of antibody to the 36K protein, cell fractionation procedures, and methods for immunofluorescence microscopy are described in Radke et al. (1983). To examine the in vitro phosphorylation of the 36K protein in membrane preparations from uninfected or virus-transformed chicken embryo fibroblasts (CEF), P100 fractions were prepared using a modification of the method of Courtneidge et al. (1980); the P100 fractions (100 μg protein per 50-μl reaction mixture) were incubated at 30°C in 50 mm Tris-HCl (pH7.2), 10 mm MgCl$_2$,

*Present address: Department of Surgery, School of Veterinary Medicine, University of California, Davis, California 95616.

and 10 mM NaF containing 320 μM [γ-^{32}P]ATP (specific activity 50 Ci/mmole). The membranes were solubilized in RIPA buffer and the 36K protein isolated by immuno- precipitation as described by Radke et al. (1983). Pro- cedures for SDS-polyacrylamide gel electrophoresis and for two-dimensional polyacrylamide gel electrophoresis (2D-PAGE) were as described by Radke and Martin (1979) and Radke et al. (1980). For analysis by 2D- PAGE, samples were separated in the first dimension by isoelectric focusing pH 6–8, and in the second di- mension by electrophoresis on SDS-polyacrylamide gels containing 15% acrylamide and 0.09% methylene bis- acrylamide. To enrich for phosphoproteins containing phosphotyrosine, dried gels were incubated in 1 M KOH at 55°C for 2 hours, neutralized in 10% acetic acid/10% isopropanol, and dried again (Cooper and Hunter 1981).

Results

The 36K substrate: Cellular localization and in vitro phosphorylation

As an initial step in characterizing the 36K protein, we have examined its intracellular location using cell frac- tionation and immunocytochemical techniques. Subcel- lular fractions were prepared from transformed CEF by differential centrifugation, followed by isopycnic banding of the particulate material on sucrose gradients. Individ- ual fractions were then analyzed for their content of 36K protein by immunoprecipitating [^{35}S]methionine-labeled protein from each fraction, using a rabbit antibody pre- pared against the protein purified by the method of Er- ikson and Erikson (1980). The 36K protein was found mainly in the postnuclear particulate fraction, although a significant amount was usually also found in the nuclear fraction. When the high-speed particulate fraction was subfractionated on a discontinuous sucrose gra- dient, the majority of the 36K protein was found at the 20%/35% interface, along with the plasma membrane marker 5'-nucleotidase (Table 1; see also Courtneidge et al. 1983; Greenberg et al., this volume). If postnuclear supernatants were treated with increasing concentra- tions of salt prior to the high-speed centrifugation step, it was found that increasing quantities of the 36K protein were solubilized. These results indicate that the 36K protein is associated with light-density membranes, probably the plasma membrane, but is not an integral membrane protein: It might be a peripheral membrane

protein or might be connected indirectly to the plasma membrane via cytoskeletal elements.

To explore further the location of the 36K protein, we used the anti-36K serum for indirect immunofluores- cence staining of uninfected or virally transformed CEF. A reticular pattern of fluorescence was observed both in uninfected cells (Fig. 1A) and in RSV-transformed cells (Fig. 2A,C); neither preimmune serum (Fig. 1C) nor anti-36K serum blocked with purified protein (Fig. 1D) gave significant levels of fluorescence. The reticular staining was excluded from regions containing actin fil- aments. This exclusion of 36K staining from actin fila- ments can be seen by comparison of panel A in Figure 1 with panel B in the same figure: In A, the 36K staining is visualized with a fluorescein-conjugated second an- tibody, whereas in B the same cell has been stained with rhodamine-conjugated phalloidin, a drug that binds spe- cifically to polymerized (F) actin. When the cells were briefly extracted with Brij 58 prior to fixation, patchy ag- gregations of fluorescence were observed with the anti- 36K serum (Fig. 1E), whereas prior treatment with Triton X-100 abolished staining almost completely (Fig. 1F). Thus, the structures that contain the 36K protein are unstable when the plasma membrane is solubilized by detergent. The reticular pattern of staining was also ob- served in RSV-transformed cells (Fig. 2A,C); however, because the antibody does not discriminate between phosphorylated and nonphosphorylated forms, and be- cause only 10–15% of the protein is phosphorylated in transformed cells, we cannot exclude the possibility that the phosphorylated form has an altered location in trans- formed cells.

Recently, it has been shown that nonerythroid cells contain cytoskeletal proteins related structurally and functionally to spectrin, the cytoskeletal protein that is found, with actin and other proteins, in a network un- derneath the erythrocyte plasma membrane (Branton et al. 1981). The pattern of immunofluorescent staining of the 36K protein is strikingly similar to that described for nonerythroid spectrin in fibroblasts (Levine and Willard 1981; Burridge et al. 1982). In particular, when fibro- blasts are stained with anti-brain spectrin antibody, a reticular or mottled pattern that is excluded from stress fibers is observed. We have compared the staining pat- terns of the 36K protein and fibroblast spectrin directly in CEF, using an antiserum against pig brain spectrin kindly provided by K. Burridge (University of North Car- olina Medical School), and have found that they do in-

Table 1 Fractionation of the 36K Protein from a P150 Fraction by Centrifugation on Discontinuous Sucrose Gradients

| Sucrose interface | Percentage of total recovered | | | |
	36K	protein	5'-nucleotidase	NADH-diaphorase
20%/35%	84 (80–88)[a]	40	69 (61–93)[a]	27
35%/40%	13 (10–16)	14	19 (5–29)	27
40%/50%	3 (2–4)	46	12 (1–16)	46

[a]Average and range for three experiments.

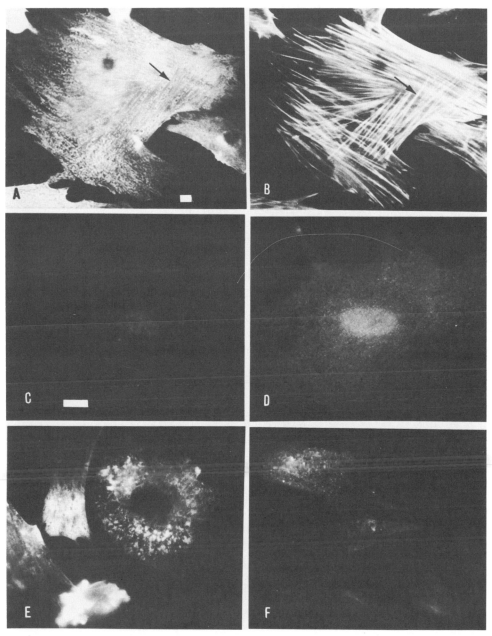

Figure 1 Immunofluorescent staining of the 36K protein in uninfected CEF. (*A–D*) CEF growing on glass coverslips were fixed with para-formaldehyde and permeabilized with 0.1% Triton X-100. (*A,B*) Cells were treated sequentially with the anti-36K rabbit serum, with FITC-conjugated second antibody, and with rhodamine-conjugated phalloidin. Cells in the same field were photographed in the same focal plane with barrier filters appropriate to show 36K staining (*A*) and F actin staining (*B*). (*C*) Cells were treated with preimmune rabbit serum and with FITC-conjugated second antibody. (*D*) Cells were treated with anti-36K serum that had been preincubated with 6.4 μg of purified 36K protein; the cells were then incubated with FITC-conjugated second antibody. (*E–F*) CEF growing on glass coverslips were extracted at room temperature with buffer containing 0.2% Brij 58 (5 min) (*E*) or 0.1% Triton X-100 (1 min) (*F*) before fixation with paraformaldehyde; the fixed cells were treated with anti-36K serum and FITC-conjugated second antibody. Photographs were taken with a 40× objective (*A,B,F*) or with a 63× oil objective (*C,D,E*). Bar, 10 μm.

deed have a very similar, although not identical, distribution (not shown). These observations suggest that the 36K protein may play a structural role, since the spectrin-actin cortex that is located on the inside of erythrocyte membranes contributes structural support to those membranes (Branton et al. 1981). Modification of a fraction of the 36K protein by phosphorylation might then

have a significant effect on the organization of the cell cortex.

The finding that the 36K protein and pp60^{src} are both present in membrane fractions has allowed us to examine the phosphorylation of these proteins in situ in isolated membranes. When [γ-^{32}P]ATP is added to membrane preparations prepared from CEF, it is rapidly hydrolyzed

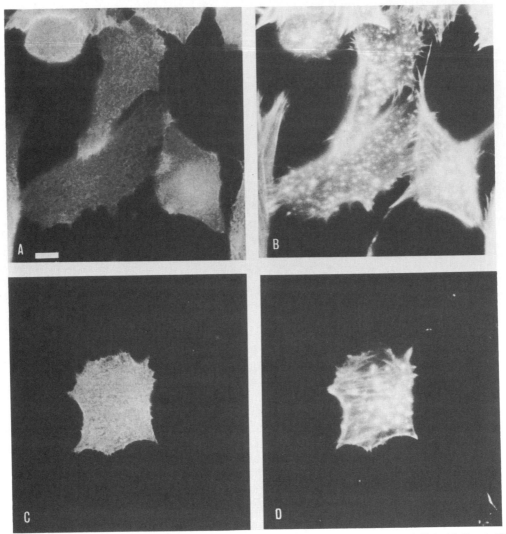

Figure 2 Immunofluorescent staining of the 36K protein in RSV-transformed CEF. Cells transformed with Schmidt-Ruppin RSV-A were fixed and stained as described for uninfected cells in the legend to Fig. 1, A and B. Photographs are shown of 36K immunofluorescence (*A,C*) and F-actin immunofluorescence (*B,D*). Relatively flat (*A,B*) and rounder (*C,D*) cells were photographed with a 63× objective. Bar, 10 μm.

by membrane ATPases. However, if high concentrations of ATP (320 μM) are used, the ATP concentration remains above the reported K_m for pp60^{src} (approximately 14 μM; see Levinson et al. 1980) for several minutes. Under these conditions, when membranes from RSV-transformed cells are used, the phosphorylation of pp60^{src} is linear for at least 1 minute and the phosphorylation of the 36K protein is linear for at least 4 minutes. It is therefore possible to quantitate the reaction rates in these preparations. In membranes from uninfected cells, the 36K protein is phosphorylated at low levels on serine. In contrast, in membranes from transformed cells, the 36K protein is phosphorylated at considerably higher levels, primarily on tyrosine. When tumor-bearing rabbit (TBR) serum containing anti-pp60^{src} antibody is added to the reaction mixture, the tyrosine phosphorylation of the 36K protein is inhibited almost completely (Fig. 3). These results support the hypothesis that the 36K protein is a substrate for direct phosphorylation by pp60^{src}.

However, we cannot exclude the possibility that other kinases may phosphorylate the 36K in vivo but are not detectable in these preparations (for example, because they are not membrane associated).

The 36K protein thus represents a useful model for examining the interactions between viral transforming proteins and their cellular substrates. We do not yet know if its phosphorylation is necessary for cell transformation. However, it is possible that it plays a significant role in the organization of the cell cortex, and further characterization of this protein may provide additional information about membrane–cytoskeletal interactions at the cell periphery and the structural alterations that accompany transformation.

Protein phosphorylation at tyrosine induced by phorbol ester and diacylglycerol

The phorbol ester 12-O-tetradecanoyl-phorbol-13-acetate (TPA) is an efficient tumor promoter in vivo. In vitro, TPA

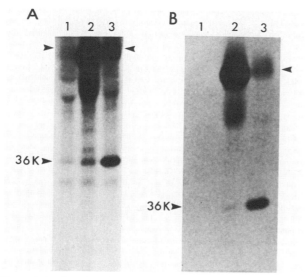

Figure 3 In vitro phosphorylation of the 36K protein in membrane preparations from uninfected and virus-transformed CEF. (*A*) Membrane preparations from uninfected CEF (lane *1*) or RSV-transformed CEF (lanes *2,3*) were incubated at 0°C for 30 min in the absence (lanes *1,3*) or the presence (lane *2*) of excess TBR serum. After the preincubation, the membranes were incubated at 30°C with [γ-^{32}P]ATP as described in Materials and Methods; the 36K protein was immunoprecipitated and examined by SDS gel electrophoresis and autoradiography. The positions of the 36K protein and of pp60^{src} (which is also present in these immunoprecipitates) are indicated by arrowheads. (*B*) After the initial autoradiographic exposure, the gel was incubated with alkali to hydrolyze phosphoserine residues (Cooper and Hunter 1981), neutralized, dried, and reexposed to film. Tracks *1–3* are identical to those in *A*.

activates the Ca^{++}- and phospholipid-dependent protein kinase, kinase C (Castagna et al. 1982; Niedel et al. 1983). This activation is believed to reflect the structural similarity between TPA and diacylglycerol, the endogenous protein kinase C activator which is produced in vivo by hydrolysis of phosphatidyl-inositol (for review, see Nishizuka 1983). Protein kinase C phosphorylates protein substrates at serine and threonine residues in vitro (Castagna et al. 1982). The effects of TPA on cultured fibroblasts, such as enhanced hexose uptake, disruption of actin stress fibers, and growth stimulation, are very similar to those induced by ASV transforming proteins and by peptide growth factors such as epidermal growth factor (EGF), platelet-derived growth factor (PDGF), or MSA. These observations suggested that some of the effects of TPA in vivo may be mediated by protein phosphorylation at tyrosine residues. A 42K polypeptide was previously shown to be phosphorylated at tyrosine in CEF transformed by ASV (Cooper and Hunter 1981) and in cells stimulated by EGF, PDGF, or MSA (Cooper et al. 1982; Nakamura et al. 1983; this polypeptide is referred to as 43K or spot n in Cooper and Hunter 1981). We show here that this polypeptide also becomes phosphorylated at tyrosine in cells treated with TPA. Furthermore, exogenously added diacylglycerol likewise stimulates the phosphorylation of this protein at tyrosine.

To compare the effects of TPA and EGF on tyrosine-specific phosphorylation, CEF were prelabeled for 6 hours with [^{32}P]orthophosphate in serum- and phosphate-free medium, to equilibrate the radiolabel in the ATP pool, and then treated with 50 ng/ml TPA or with 500 ng/ml EGF. At 1 hour after the treatment, radiolabeled phosphoproteins were analyzed by 2D-PAGE and autoradiography; to enrich for phosphoproteins containing phosphotyrosine, the gels were treated with alkali as described by Cooper and Hunter (1981). As shown in Figure 4, two 42K phosphoproteins (indicated as spots a and b in the figures) were detected in TPA- and EGF-treated CEF. Untreated cultures, cultures treated with dimethylsulfoxide (the solvent used for TPA), or cultures treated with the biologically inactive phorbol ester 4-α-phorbol-12,13-didecanoate, showed only low levels of phosphorylation of these proteins. The phosphorylation appears to occur de novo; analysis of TPA-treated cultures prelabeled with [^{35}S]methionine showed the appearance of spots in the positions of the 42K phosphoproteins. Partial proteolytic digestion of [^{32}P]orthophosphate- and [^{35}S]methionine-labeled proteins with *Staphylococcus aureus* protease V8 indicated that the 42K phosphoproteins were the same as those that appear in ASV-transformed CEF (Cooper and Hunter 1981)(not shown). Mapping by partial proteolysis also indicated that the two 42K polypeptides (spots a and b) are related to each other (not shown; J. Cooper, pers. comm.), suggesting that the more acidic spot probably represents a more highly phosphorylated species of the same polypeptide present in the less acidic spot.

To determine the phosphoamino acid content of these polypeptides, the 42K phosphoproteins from TPA-treated cells were excised from the alkali-treated gels and subjected to partial acid hydrolysis. Both were found to contain phosphotyrosine as their major phosphoamino acid, plus minor amounts of phosphoserine and phosphothreonine; it is possible that these phosphoproteins may contain significant amounts of phosphoserine and phosphothreonine that are lost during the alkali hydrolysis.

The phosphoproteins appear rapidly after TPA treatment: Phosphorylation is detectable after 5 minutes of treatment and maximal phosphorylation occurs by 15 minutes. Phosphorylation, although considerably diminished, is still detectable after 6 hours. The phosphorylation of these polypeptides is half-maximal at 2.5 ng/ml and near maximal at 5 ng/ml. The doses of TPA required to produce these effects are similar to those required to induce morphological changes, enhanced hexose uptake, or stimulation of DNA synthesis (Blumberg 1980).

TPA induces a variety of rapid responses in platelets, and exogenously added diacylglycerol induces the same effects (Kaibuchi et al. 1982; Rink et al. 1983). To determine if diacylglycerol can also induce tyrosine phosphorylation in fibroblasts, we examined the effects of 200 μg/ml 1-oleoyl-2-acetyl-glycerol on the phosphorylation of the 42K protein. As shown in Figure 5, diacylglycerol also induces the appearance of the 42K phosphoproteins. The relatively high concentration of diacylglycerol needed to produce this effect perhaps reflects the rapidity with which the exogenously added compound is metabolized; in contrast, TPA intercalates into the lipid bilayer and is metabolized only very slowly.

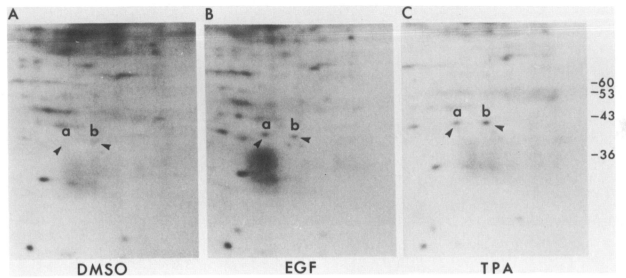

Figure 4 Analysis of radiolabeled phosphoproteins in EGF- or TPA-treated CEF by 2D-PAGE. Secondary cultures of CEF were seeded at 10^6 cells/35-mm dish. On day 3 after plating, the cells were prelabeled for 6 hr with 0.33 mCi [^{32}P]orthophosphate in 1 ml of serum- and phosphate-free medium. Cultures were then treated with either DMSO (final concentration, 0.005%) (*A*), EGF (final concentration 500 ng/ml) (*B*), or TPA (final concentration, 50 ng/ml) (*C*). After 1 hr, the cells were lysed and the samples analyzed by 2D-PAGE as described in Materials and Methods. The gels were treated with alkali as described by Cooper and Hunter (1981) to enrich for phosphoproteins containing phosphotyrosine. A section of the autoradiogram is shown above, the acidic end of the first dimension is to the left and the basic end to the right. Molecular-weight markers ($\times 10^{-3}$) are shown at the right of the figure. Arrowheads indicate the 42K phosphoproteins, designated a and b in the figure.

The tyrosine phosphorylation of the 42K protein represents a rapid response to the binding of TPA to its receptors. A variety of membrane receptors with intrinsic or associated tyrosine kinase activity have been identified, including those for EGF (Ushiro and Cohen 1980), PDGF (Ek et al. 1982), and insulin (Kasuga et al. 1982). However, the only known receptor for TPA is protein kinase C (Castagna et al. 1982; Niedel et al. 1983); since kinase C is a serine/threonine-specific kinase, it seems unlikely that the 42K protein is directly phosphorylated by this enzyme. It is possible that TPA and diacylglycerol may interact with kinases other than kinase C, and that a tyrosine kinase may be directly activated by these agents. Alternatively, the activation of protein kinase C by TPA or diacylglycerol may result in the activation, directly or indirectly, of one or more tyrosine-specific kinases. Since the identity of the kinase that phosphorylates the 42K protein is not known, it is not as yet possible to distinguish between these possibilities.

Protein phosphorylation at tyrosine induced by AEV

The genome of AEV includes two genes of cellular origin, *erb-A* and *erb-B* (reviewed in Graf and Beug 1983). Genetic analysis using mutants generated in vitro indicates that the major transforming gene is *erb-B*; the product of this gene is a membrane-associated glycoprotein (Hayman et al. 1983; Privalsky et al. 1983). Studies using temperature-sensitive mutants suggest that transport of this protein to the plasma membrane may be required for transformation (Hayman et al., this volume). As yet, no tyrosine-specific protein kinase activity has been detected in immunoprecipitates of the *erb-B* gene product. However the amino acid sequence of this protein (as deduced from the DNA sequence) does have some homology to that of pp60^{src} (M. Privalsky and R. Ralston, pers. comm.).

We reported some time ago that the 36K protein shows an enhanced level of phosphorylation in AEV-infected fibroblasts (Radke and Martin 1979). This observation, and the homology of *erb-B* to *src*, suggested that AEV might induce tyrosine-specific phosphorylation in vivo. We therefore examined the ^{32}P-labeled phosphoproteins of AEV-transformed CEF by 2D-PAGE, using alkali digestion to enrich for phosphotyrosine-containing phosphoproteins (Cooper and Hunter 1981). The results are shown in Figure 6; the spots corresponding to specific polypeptides are labeled as described by

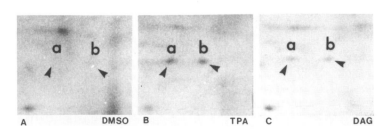

Figure 5 Stimulation of phosphorylation of the 42K polypeptide by diacylglycerol. Prelabeled CEF were exposed for 15 min to 0.4% DMSO plus 4 μg/ml bovine serum albumin (BSA)(*A*); 50 ng/ml TPA (*B*); 200 μg/ml 1-oleoyl-2-acetyl glycerol (kindly provided by Roger Tsien) plus 0.4% DMSO and 4 μg/ml BSA (*C*). Phosphoproteins were analyzed as described in the legend to Fig. 4; only the relevant portions of the autoradiograms are shown.

Cooper and Hunter (1981), except that the two forms of the 42K protein are indicated as spots a and b. Of the spots showing either de novo or increased tyrosine phosphorylation in RSV-transformed fibroblasts, spots p (the 36K protein) and spots a and b (the two forms of the 42K protein) show de novo phosphorylation in AEV-transformed fibroblasts; spots k and m show increased tyrosine phosphorylation in AEV-transformed fibroblasts, whereas spots l and q (enolase and phosphoglycerate mutase, respectively; see Cooper et al. 1983b) do not show enhanced phosphorylation. Phosphoaminoacid analysis of spots eluted from the gels confirmed that these polypeptides contained phosphotyrosine.

Thus, protein phosphorylation at tyrosine is induced by AEV in vivo. It is possible that the *erb-B* gene product is itself a tyrosine-specific protein kinase, and that its activity is not detectable in immunoprecipitates, either because the immunoprecipitating antibody blocks the catalytic activity or because appropriate substrates are not available. Alternatively the *erb-B* product might induce the phosphorylation of the 36K and 42K proteins by activating a cellular enzyme. Analysis of tyrosine-specific phosphorylation in vitro using membrane preparations from AEV-transformed cells may help to distinguish between these alternatives.

Discussion

The results discussed above indicate that the phosphorylation of the 36K protein in membranes from RSV-transformed cells, and probably also in vivo, is largely due to a direct interaction with pp60[src]. This may also be true of some of the other phosphotyrosine-containing proteins in ASV-transformed cells. Tyrosine-specific phosphorylation of the 42K protein is observed in CEF stimulated in a variety of ways, including ASV transformation, trypsin treatment (Hunter et al., this volume), and exposure to phorbol esters (see above). This suggests that this phosphorylation might be important in some pathway leading to cell growth or transformation. How could such a role for these cellular substrates in growth regulation or transformation be demonstrated directly?

It has not as yet been possible to correlate the phosphorylation of specific cellular substrates with specific phenotypic changes (see Cooper et al. 1983a). However, it is conceivable that if the pathways that involve tyrosine phosphorylation are as complex as those involved in metabolic regulation, it may not be possible to make such simple correlations. These pathways may be redundant, in the sense that a given result may be achieved by a variety of different pathways. A precedent for such a situation is provided by the enzymes involved in the regulation of glycogen metabolism; the cAMP-dependent kinase phosphorylates phosphorylase kinase, glycogen synthase, and an inhibitor of phosphoprotein phosphatase-1. Phosphorylase kinase is also regulated by Ca^{++}, so that glycogen breakdown and synthesis can be regulated by multiple pathways. If the same redundancy is observed in the pathways involved in transformation, phosphorylation of any one substrate

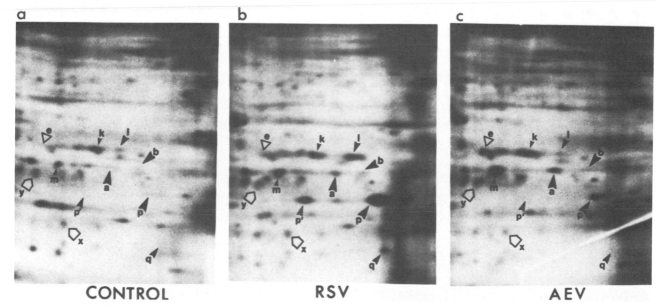

Figure 6 Radiolabeled phosphoproteins of uninfected and virus-transformed CEF. Cells were labeled for 18 hr with [^{32}P]orthophosphate in phosphate-free medium containing 4% calf serum and 1% chick serum, and the radiolabeled phosphoproteins analyzed as described in the legend to Fig. 4. (*a*) Uninfected CEF; (*b*) RSV-transformed CEF; (*c*) AEV-transformed CEF. The phosphoproteins which show de novo phosphorylation in both RSV- and AEV-transformed cells (p, a, and b) are indicated by large solid arrowheads; those showing de novo phosphorylation only in RSV-transformed CEF (l and q) are indicated by intermediate solid arrowheads; those showing increased phosphorylation in both RSV- and AEV-transformed cells (k and m) are indicated by small solid arrowheads; spot e, a phosphoserine-containing polypeptide that appears in AEV-transformed cells is indicated by an open arrowhead. Phosphoproteins x and y are reference spots whose intensity of labeling does not appear to be affected by transformation by RSV or AEV. The letters used to indicate individual phosphoproteins are those used by Cooper and Hunter (1981), with the exception of the 42K phosphoproteins (spots a and b, see text).

may not be an essential requirement for transformation. It is also possible that some phosphorylations are "silent" and are not involved in transformation; such "silent" phosphorylations that do not appear to affect protein function in any obvious way occur on a number of metabolic enzymes, e.g., ATP-citrate lyase (Cohen 1982).

Given these complexities, how can the physiological significance of these phosphorylations be assessed? The finding that high levels of *c-src* expression are not sufficient to transform (see Hanafusa et al.; Parker et al.; Shalloway et al.; all this volume) suggests that it may be possible to identify significant differences between viral and cellular products, either in substrate specificity or in cellular localization (or both). Indeed we have recently observed (J. Young and G.S. Martin, unpubl.) that *v-fps* and *c-fps* products behave differently in cell fractionation experiments, and thus may have different cellular localizations. The ideal tool to examine the mechanism by which phosphorylation leads to transformation would be a set of cellular mutants in which these regulatory pathways have been altered. For example, one could attempt to isolate nontransformable revertants of sarcoma virus-transformed cells in which the transforming protein remains functional but the susceptibility of the cell to its enzymatic activity has been altered; however, if there are multiple physiologically significant substrates, and if the pathways are functionally redundant, the isolation of such mutants may not be easy. Alternatively, one could look for cellular suppressors of viral mutations, e.g., cellular mutations with which a *ts* virus gives temperature-independent transformation. A different type of genetic analysis for tyrosine kinase function may become possible if unicellular microorganisms contain this type of enzyme. We have recently observed (G.S. Martin et al., unpubl.) that acid hydrolysates of ^{32}P-labeled yeast phosphoproteins contain phosphotyrosine. If this indeed represents the result of tyrosine protein kinase activity, then it may be possible to analyze the role of these enzymes in the cell cycle using the powerful techniques for molecular genetic analysis that are available in yeast.

Acknowledgments

We thank K. Burridge for providing antiserum against pig brain spectrin; T. Weiland for rhodamine-conjugated phalloidin; R. Tsien for the gift of synthetic diacylglycerol and for stimulating discussions; M. Schliwa for encouragement and for advice about immunofluorescence; S. Courtneidge, M. Weber, B. Sefton, J.A. Cooper, and T. Hunter for communicating results prior to publication; and M. Namba and D. Schleske for excellent technical assistance.

This work was supported by National Institutes of Health grant CA-17542 and a grant from the University of California Cancer Research Co-ordinating Committee. P.M. and V.C.C. were fellows of the Leukemia Society of America. K.R. was supported in part by a Senior Fellowship from the American Cancer Society, California Division. P.D., K.R., and T.G. were supported in part by NIH training grant CA-09141.

References

Blumberg, P.M. 1980. In vitro studies on the mode of action of the phorbol esters, potent tumor promoters. *CRC Crit. Rev. Toxicol.* **8:** 153.

Branton, D., C.M. Cohen, and J. Tyler. 1981. Interaction of cytoskeletal proteins on the human erythrocyte membrane. *Cell* **24:** 24.

Brugge, J. and D. Darrow. 1982. Rous sarcoma virus-induced phosphorylation of a 50,000 molecular weight cellular protein. *Nature* **295:** 250.

Burridge, K., T. Kelly, and P. Mangeat. 1982. Nonerythrocyte spectrins: Actin membrane attachment proteins occurring in many cell types. *J. Cell Biol.* **95:** 478.

Castagna, M., Y. Takai, K. Kaibuchi, K. Sano, W. Kiddawa, and Y. Nishizuka. 1982. Direct activation of calcium activated, phospholipid-dependent protein kinase by tumor promoting phorbol esters. *J. Biol. Chem.* **257:** 7847.

Cohen, P. 1982. The role of protein phosphorylation in neural and hormonal control of cellular activity. *Nature* **296:** 613.

Cooper, J.A. and T. Hunter. 1981. Changes in protein phosphorylation in Rous sarcoma virus-transformed chicken embryo cells. *Mol. Cell. Biol.* **1:** 165.

Cooper, J.A., K.D. Nakamura, T. Hunter, and M.J. Weber. 1983a. Phosphotyrosine-containing proteins and expression of transformation parameters in cells infected with partial transformation mutants of Rous sarcoma virus. *J. Virol.* **46:** 15.

Cooper, J.A., N.A. Reiss, R.J. Schwartz, and T. Hunter. 1983b. Three glycolytic enzymes are phosphorylated at tyrosine in cells transformed by Rous sarcoma virus. *Nature* **302:** 218.

Cooper, J.A., D.F. Bowen-Pope, E. Raines, R. Ross, and T. Hunter. 1982. Similar effects of platelet-derived growth factor and epidermal growth factor on the phosphorylation of tyrosine in proteins. *Cell* **31:** 263.

Courtneidge, S.A., A.D. Levinson, and J.M. Bishop. 1980. The protein encoded by the transforming gene of avian sarcoma virus (pp60^{src}) and a homologous protein in normal cells (pp60$^{proto-src}$) are associated with the plasma membrane. *Proc. Natl. Acad. Sci.* **77:** 3783.

Courtneidge, S.A., R. Ralston, K. Alitalo, and J.M. Bishop. 1983. Subcellular location of an abundant substrate (p36) for tyrosine-specific protein kinases. *Mol. Cell. Biol.* **3:** 340.

Ek, B., B. Westermark, A. Wasteson, and C.-H. Heldin. 1982. Stimulation of tyrosine phosphorylation by platelet-derived growth factor. *Nature* **295:** 419.

Erikson, E. and R. Erikson. 1980. Identification of a cellular protein substrate phosphorylated by the avian sarcoma virus transforming gene product. *Cell* **21:** 829.

Gilmore, T., K. Radke, and G.S. Martin. 1982. Tyrosine phosphorylation of a 50K cellular polypeptide associated with the Rous sarcoma virus transforming protein pp60^{src}. *Mol. Cell. Biol.* **2:** 199.

Graf, T. and H. Beug. 1983. Role of the v-erbA and v-erbB oncogenes of avian erythroblastosis virus in erythroid cell transformation. *Cell* **34:** 7.

Hayman, M.J., G.M. Ramsay, K. Savin, G. Kitchener, T. Graf, and H. Beug. 1983. Identification and characterization of the avian erythroblastosis virus erbB product as a membrane glycoprotein. *Cell* **32:** 579.

Kaibuchi, K., K. Sano, M. Hoshijima, Y. Takai, and Y. Nishizuka. 1982. Phosphatidylinositol turnover in platelet activation; calcium mobilization and protein phosphorylation. *Cell Calcium* **3:** 323.

Kasuga, M., Y. Zick, D.L. Blithe, M. Crettaz, and C.R. Kahn. 1982. Insulin stimulates the tyrosine phosphorylation of the insulin receptor in a cell free system. *Nature* **298:** 667.

Levine, J. and M. Willard. 1981. Fodrin: Axonally transported polypeptides associated with the internal periphery of many cells. *J. Cell Biol.* **90:** 631.

Levinson, A.D., H. Oppermann, H.E. Varmus, and J.M. Bishop. 1980. The purified product of the transforming gene of avian sarcoma virus phosphorylates tyrosine. *J. Biol. Chem.* **255:** 11973.

Nakamura, K.D., R. Martinez, and M.J. Weber. 1983. Tyrosine phosphorylation of specific proteins after mitogen stimulation of chicken embryo fibroblasts. *Mol. Cell. Biol.* **3:** 380.

Niedel, J.E., L.J. Kuhn, and G.R. Vanderbark. 1983. Phorbol diester receptor copurifies with protein kinase C. *Proc. Natl. Acad. Sci.* **80:** 36.

Nishizuka, Y. 1983. Phospholipid degradation and signal translation for protein phosphorylation. *Trends Biochem. Sci.* **8:** 13.

Privalsky, M.L., L. Sealy, J.M. Bishop, J.P. McGrath, and A.D. Levinson. 1983. The product of the avian erythroblastosis virus erbB locus is a glycoprotein. *Cell* **32:** 1257.

Radke, K. and G.S. Martin. 1979. Transformation by Rous sarcoma virus: Effects of src gene expression on the synthesis and phosphorylation of cellular polypeptides. *Proc. Natl. Acad. Sci.* **76:** 5212.

Radke, K., T. Gilmore, and G.S. Martin. 1980. Transformation by Rous sarcoma virus: A cellular substrate for transformation-specific protein phosphorylation contains phosphotyrosine. *Cell* **21:** 821.

Radke, K., V.C. Carter, P. Moss, P. Dehazya, M. Schliwa, and G.S. Martin. 1983. Membrane association of a 36,000-dalton substrate for tyrosine phosphorylation in chicken embryo fibroblasts transformed by avian sarcoma viruses. *J. Cell Biol.* **97:** 1601.

Rink, T.J., A. Sanchez, and T.J. Hallam. 1983. Diacylglycerol and phorbol ester stimulate secretion without raising cytoplasmic free calcium in human platelets. *Nature* **305:** 317.

Sefton, B., T. Hunter, E.H. Ball, and S.J. Singer. 1981. Vinculin: A cytoskeletal target of the transforming protein of Rous sarcoma virus. *Cell* **24:** 165.

Ushiro, H. and S.J. Cohen. 1980. Identification of phosphotyrosine as a product of epidermal growth-factor activated protein kinase in A431 cell membranes. *J. Biol. Chem.* **255:** 8363.

Subcellular Localization and Tissue Distribution of the 34,000-Dalton Tyrosine Kinase Substrate

M.E. Greenberg, R. Brackenbury, and G.M. Edelman
The Rockefeller University, New York, New York 10021

In recent years, substantial progress has been made towards elucidating the mechanisms regulating the growth and division of normal cells and the alterations in cell growth that occur as a consequence of viral transformation. Many retroviruses cause transformation through the action of a single gene product (for review, see Bishop and Varmus 1982) and several of these virally coded transforming proteins have been found to possess tyrosine kinase activity (for review, see Hunter and Sefton 1982). Other experiments suggest that tyrosine kinases may play a role in the response of normal cells to growth factors. For example, the cell-surface receptors for epidermal growth factor (EGF), insulin, and platelet-derived growth factor (PDGF) are all associated with a growth factor-stimulated tyrosine kinase activity (Carpenter et al. 1979; Ek et al. 1982; Kasuga et al. 1982; Petruzzelli et al. 1982). Clearly, the identification and characterization of the substrates of these tyrosine kinases would enhance our understanding of the biochemical mechanisms by which cell growth is regulated.

One potential target of the retroviral transforming proteins is a 34-kD protein that is phosphorylated at a tyrosine residue in cells transformed by Rous sarcoma virus (RSV) but not in normal cells (Erikson and Erikson 1980; Radke et al. 1980; Cooper and Hunter 1981a). This 34-kD protein was purified and shown to be phosphorylated in vitro by the RSV transforming protein, pp60[src], at the same site that is phosphorylated in vivo (Erikson and Erikson 1980) suggesting that the 34-kD protein is a direct target of the pp60[src] kinase. Phosphorylation of the 34-kD protein on tyrosine has also been correlated with the transforming activity of several other retroviruses (Pawson et al. 1980; Cooper and Hunter 1981b; Erikson et al. 1981b), although recent experiments indicate that one RNA tumor virus that encodes a tyrosine kinase is able to transform lymphoid cells without stimulating phosphorylation of the 34-kD protein (Sefton et al. 1983). Phosphorylation of the 34-kD protein was also enhanced when epidermoid carcinoma A-431 cells were treated with EGF (Erikson et al. 1981a; Hunter and Cooper 1981), however, stimulation of normal fibroblasts with EGF or PDGF was not accompanied by increased 34-kD protein phosphorylation (Cooper et al. 1982; Decker 1982; Nakamura et al. 1983).

The combined data suggest that the 34-kD protein may be involved in the response of cells to growth signals under some conditions, but its specific function is unknown. In an effort to gain some insight into the function of this protein in normal cells, we have prepared monoclonal antibodies against a preparation of partially purified 34-kD protein (Greenberg and Edelman 1983a). We have used these antibodies to affinity purify the 34-kD protein and to study its subcellular localization in normal and virally transformed cells (Greenberg and Edelman 1983b) and its tissue distribution (Greenberg et al. 1984).

Results and Discussion

Characterization of antibodies to the 34-kD tyrosine kinase substrate

The monoclonal antibody used in these studies was raised against partially purified 34-kD protein prepared following the protocol of Erikson and Erikson (1980). Several criteria were used to establish that the protein recognized by the monoclonal antibody is identical to the 34-kD pp60[src] substrate previously studied by other workers (Erikson and Erikson 1980; Radke et al. 1980; Cooper and Hunter 1981a). The antibody immunoprecipitates a 34-kD protein from normal and transformed chick embryo fibroblasts (CEF) (Fig. 1A, lanes 1 and 2). Phosphoamino acid analysis of $^{32}PO_4$-labeled 34-kD protein extracted under conditions (lysis in boiling SDS) designed to inactivate kinases and phosphatases showed that the protein is phosphorylated at a tyrosine residue in transformed cells, but not in normal cells (Fig. 1B, compare top and bottom). The 34-kD phosphoprotein recognized by the monoclonal antibody has an isoelectric point of 7.5, as previously described for the pp60[src] substrate. Finally, rabbit antisera (kindly provided by Dr. Raymond Erikson) raised against the originally identified 34-kD tyrosine kinase substrate (Erikson et al. 1981b), recognize the 34-kD protein obtained by affinity chromatography (Greenberg and Edelman 1983a) using the monoclonal antibody employed in this study.

Immunoaffinity purification of the 34-kD protein

Rapid procedures were developed for purifying the 34-kD protein from a number of chicken tissues including brain, liver, skin, and gizzard using a monoclonal antibody affinity column (Greenberg and Edelman 1983a). Although all these tissues contained detectable amounts of the protein, the largest amount, by at least fivefold, was obtained from CEF grown in culture. Chicken gizzards, which can be obtained in large quantitites, were

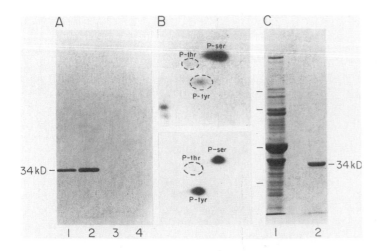

Figure 1 Characterization of monoclonal antibodies to the 34-kD protein. (*A*) Normal (lanes *1* and *3*) or RSV-transformed (lanes *2* and *4*) CEF were labeled with [³H]leucine, and extracts were immunoprecipitated with monoclonal anti-34-kD protein antibodies (lanes *1* and *2*) or a control monoclonal antibody (lanes *3* and *4*). (*B*) Phosphoamino acid analysis of the 34-kD protein. ³²PO₄³⁻ labeled 34-kD protein immunoprecipitated from extracts of normal (*top panel*) or RSV-transformed (*bottom panel*) CEF was eluted from gels and hydrolyzed. Phosphoamino acids were separated by two-dimensional, thin-layer electrophoresis as described (Greenberg and Edelman 1983a). Radioactive amino acids were visualized by autoradiography; the positions of unlabeled marker amino acids are indicated. (*C*) SDS-polyacrylamide gel analysis of the affinity purification of the 34-kD protein. (Lane *1*) Crude cell homogenate; (lane *2*) affinity-purified 34-kD protein. The protein bands were visualized by staining with Coomassie brilliant blue.

also a useful source for affinity purification of the 34-kD protein. CEF or gizzards were homogenized in the presence of EDTA and the extracts fractionated on DEAE-cellulose to remove actin, which binds nonspecifically to the affinity column. The unbound fraction was applied to the affinity column, and elution at high pH gave milligram quantities of an apparently homogeneous preparation of the 34-kD protein (Fig. 1C, lane 2). It was possible to purify the 34-kD protein from CEF by a one-step protocol (Greenberg and Edelman 1983a), inasmuch as the fibroblasts contain significantly less actin than chicken gizzards.

The affinity purification of the 34-kD protein has several advantages. Since the monoclonal antibody-antigen complex could be disrupted under fairly mild conditions, the affinity purification should help to preserve biological activities that might be lost under less rapid or harsher procedures. In addition, extraction and purification of the 34-kD protein in the absence of detergent will facilitate cell microinjection experiments as well as other biological studies.

Subcellular localization of the 34-kD tyrosine kinase substrate

Using the monoclonal antibody and a rabbit antibody raised against affinity-purified 34-kD protein, we have found by both subcellular fractionation and immunofluorescence studies (Greenberg and Edelman 1983b) that the 34-kD protein is primarily localized at the inner surface of the plasma membrane in both normal and RSV-transformed CEF. These results are in agreement with the findings of several other laboratories (Amini and Kaji 1983; Courtneidge et al. 1983; Nigg et al. 1983; Radke et al. 1983).

For the subcellular fractionation experiments, CEF were disrupted in hypotonic salt, separated into soluble and particulate fractions, and the membrane-containing pellet fractionated on a discontinuous sucrose gradient as shown in Table 1. The specific amount of the 34-kD protein was highest in the plasma membrane-containing fractions. The distribution of the 34-kD protein closely paralleled that of the plasma membrane marker enzyme 5′-nucleotidase as well as the pp60^{src} kinase, and was

Table 1 Fractionation of SR-RSV-A-transformed CEF Membranes on a Discontinuous Sucrose Gradient

Sucrose/sucrose interface	Specific activity (units/mg protein)[a]			
	34-kD protein	5′-nucleotidase	pp60^{src} kinase	NADH-diaphorase
20–25%	18.1	24.50	23.0	12.0
25–30%	10.9	7.80	21.0	4.2
30–35%	6.9	5.30	13.2	21.0
35–45%	1.7	1.70	5.3	38.0
45–60%	1.1	0.87	3.4	26.0

[a]34-kD protein, units/mg are expressed as counts per minute (cpm) × 10⁻⁴ [³H]leucine-labeled 34-kD protein immunoprecipitated, under conditions of antibody excess, from a gradient fraction per mg protein. 5′-Nucleotidase, the specific activity equals the number of micromoles × 10⁻² of phosphate released per hour per mg of protein. pp60^{src} kinase, the specific activity is expressed as cpm × 10⁻³ ³²PO₄³⁻ transferred to immune complex IgG per mg of protein. NADH-diaphorase, the specific activity is expressed as micromoles × 10² NADH oxidized per minute per mg of protein. The recovery of total protein from the gradient was 78%, 34-kD protein recovery was 100%, 5′-nucleotidase recovery was 69%, pp60^{src} activity recovery was 50%, and NADH-diaphorase recovery was 100%. (Data taken from Greenberg and Edelman 1983b.)

distinct from that of the endoplasmic reticulum marker NADH-diaphorase (Table 1) and the cytoplasmic enzyme lactate dehydrogenase (LDH) (not shown). Additional fractionation experiments indicated that the 34-kD protein is not an intrinsic membrane protein (Greenberg and Edelman 1983b). A significant proportion of this protein (44%) was solubilized by 1 mM EDTA and it was almost completely extracted (87%) by 0.5 M NaCl. The ionic detergents deoxycholate and SDS released a substantial fraction of the 34-kD protein from membranes whereas the nonionic detergent NP-40 was not an effective method of extraction.

The nature of the association of the 34-kD protein with the plasma membrane was further analyzed by a variety of immunofluorescence staining experiments. Fluorescence staining results similar to those discussed here have also been obtained in other laboratories (Nigg et al. 1983; Radke et al. 1983). The 34-kD protein is not exposed on the outside surface of the cell since no staining of CEF with anti-34-kD protein antibodies (monoclonal or polyclonal) was detected if the cells were not permeabilized prior to staining. When CEF were fixed with formaldehyde, permeabilized with Triton X-100, and stained by indirect immunofluorescence with the monoclonal antibody, a diffuse, sometimes reticular staining pattern was seen throughout the cell (Fig. 2a). The staining of RSV-transformed CEF with the anti-34-kD protein monoclonal antibody was similar to that seen with normal CEF, although in the well-rounded cells the pattern was more diffuse than reticular. This most likely reflects the difficulty of detecting the reticular pattern in round cells rather than an actual change in the subcellular distribution of the 34-kD protein. Reticular staining was observed in the flatter cells of the transformed cell population. No staining of normal or transformed CEF was detected using a control monoclonal antibody (Fig. 2b). If CEF were extracted with a detergent containing cytoskeletal extraction buffer (CSK) prior to fixation, a procedure that solubilizes cytoplasmic proteins but few membrane and cytoskeletal components (Lenk and Penman 1979), the 34-kD protein was observed by fluorescence staining to be associated with a cagelike structure (Fig. 2c). Although the actual staining pattern most likely results from a redistribution of membrane and cytoskeletal components during the permeabilization procedure, several aspects of this staining pattern suggested that the 34-kD protein is primarily associated with the plasma membrane. The 34-kD staining (Fig. 2c) was found in a double immunofluorescence staining experiment to be virtually identical to the staining obtained with an antibody to α-spectrin (Fig. 2d). α-Spectrin is an actin-binding protein that is known to be present at the inner surface of the plasma membrane (Levine and Willard 1981; Burridge et al. 1982; Repasky et al. 1982). In CSK buffer-extracted cells, the 34-kD protein was localized primarily in two distinct focal planes corresponding to the free and attached surfaces of the cell, further suggesting that this protein is plasma membrane associated. In addition, in staining experiments with thin, frozen sections of CEF, the 34-kD protein was concentrated at the edge of the cell, whereas actin was located throughout the cytoplasm (Greenberg and Edelman 1983b).

The significance of the reticular staining pattern observed in formaldehyde-fixed cells has not been established. This pattern and the cagelike structure detected in the CSK buffer-extracted cells may reflect the interaction of the 34-kD protein with other membrane components to form a complex of proteins associated with the plasma membrane. The similarity of the staining patterns of α-spectrin and the 34-kD protein raises the possibility that these two proteins may interact or that the 34-kD protein, like α-spectrin, may be involved structurally in anchoring cytoskeletal proteins to the membrane. Measurements of the amount of the 34-kD protein in a cell (Erikson and Erikson 1980; Radke et al. 1980; Cooper and Hunter 1983) established that it is a major cell protein (approximately 0.3% of total cell protein) and are consistent with the idea that the 34-kD protein might play a structural role in cytoskeletal–plasma membrane interactions. An association of the 34-kD protein with the cytoskeleton has previously been suggested (Cheng and Chen 1981).

It is significant that in addition to the 34-kD protein, pp60[src] (Willingham et al. 1979; Courtneidge et al. 1980; Krueger et al. 1980) and vinculin, another of its substrates (Geiger 1979; Burridge and Feramisco 1980; Sefton et al. 1981), are located at the inner face of the plasma membrane. This common intracellular localization is consistent with the hypothesis that the 34-kD protein and vinculin are direct targets of the pp60[src] kinase. Experiments using temperature-sensitive src mutants (Radke and Martin 1979) established that the phosphorylation of the 34-kD protein is an early event in transformation. This fact, coupled with the observation that the 34-kD protein is plasma membrane associated, suggests that some of the early pp60[src]-induced changes in the plasma membrane such as increased membrane ruffling, changes in cell shape, or disruption of the cytoskeleton (Edelman and Yahara 1976) may be mediated via phosphorylation of the 34-kD protein.

Expression of the 34-kD protein during growth and differentiation

Previous studies on the role of the 34-kD protein in cell growth have focused on changes in its phosphotyrosine content. To test whether the function of the 34-kD protein might be regulated by controlling its level of expression as well as its state of phosphorylation, we used the specific antibodies to examine its expression in cells and tissues at different stages of growth or differentiation.

Cells of 14-day embryonic chicken forebrain grown in tissue culture contain two differentiated cell types: postmitotic neuronal cells and glial cells, which express a differentiated phenotype but retain the capacity to divide in culture. Striking results were obtained when these forebrain cells were stained with the anti-34-kD protein monoclonal antibody. The 34-kD protein was present in the actively dividing glial cells but was absent from the nondividing differentiated neuronal cells (Fig. 2e,f). However, additional experiments indicated that expres-

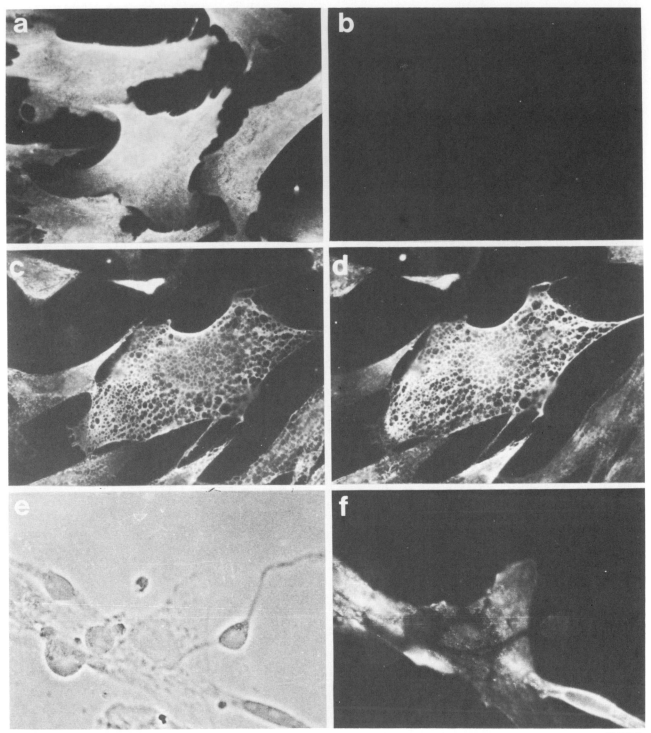

Figure 2 Immunofluorescence staining of CEF with anti-34-kD protein monoclonal antibody. Cells were fixed with 3.7% formaldehyde, permeabilized with Triton X-100, and stained with anti-34-kD monoclonal antibody (*a,f*) or a control antibody (*b*). CSK buffer-extracted CEF were compared in a double-immunofluorescence experiment (*c,d*), anti-34-kD protein monoclonal antibody visualized with fluorescein-conjugated goat antibody to mouse IgG (*c*); and rabbit anti-spectrin antibody visualized with rhodamine-conjugated goat antibody to rabbit IgG (*d*). Chicken embryonic forebrain cells stained with the anti-34-kD protein monoclonal antibody were visualized by phase contrast illumination (*e*) or indirect immunofluorescence staining (*f*).

sion of the 34-kD protein did not correlate with the growth state of these cells since the protein was not detected in extracts of actively dividing neuronal cells from 5–10-day embryos. Therefore, the differential expression of the 34-kD protein in neuronal and glial cells appears to reflect their state of differentiation.

The observation that neuronal cells did not contain the 34-kD protein was surprising because Poirier et al. (1982) have reported that transformed neuroretinal cells express substantial amounts of the 34-kD protein. We found by immunoblotting that extracts of cultured neuroretinal cells from 6-day embryos contained low amounts of the 34-kD protein (Fig. 3A, lane 1), however, within 2–3 days after RSV infection, the transformed cell extracts contain a significant amount of this tyrosine kinase substrate (Fig. 3A, lane 3). When neuroretinal cells were infected with a transformation-defective RSV (*td*107) containing a deletion in the *src* gene, expression of the 34-kD protein was not enhanced (Fig. 3A, lane 2), indicating that pp60*src* is required to activate expression of the 34-kD protein in these cells. These experiments suggest that in particular differentiated cell types such as neuronal cells, pp60*src* and other tyrosine kinases may exert their transforming effect by first turning on the expression of substrate proteins and then by altering their state of phosphorylation.

Tissue distribution of the 34-kD protein

An alternative to the hypothesis that the 34-kD protein functions in the regulation of growth signals in particular differentiated cell types is the possibility that this protein is involved in membrane functions such as secretion, movement, formation of cell–cell junctions, or transport.

To investigate these possibilities, we have studied the distribution of the 34-kD protein in a range of tissues of the embryonic and adult chicken. The tissue distribution was determined, using the anti-34-kD protein antibody, by three methods: (1) immunoblotting of extracted tissues, (2) fluorescence staining of thin frozen sections, and (3) peroxidase anti-peroxidase (PAP) staining of paraffin-embedded tissue sections. The results of these studies have been reported in detail (Greenberg et al. 1984).

Anti-34-kD protein antibody immunoblots of detergent extracts of various chicken organs are shown in Figure 3B. The 34-kD protein was found to be present in many, but not all, tissues of the chick. Significant quantities of the protein were detected in skin, intestine, lung, and spleen, but very little protein was present in skeletal muscle, liver, kidney, or brain. The immunoblotting also demonstrated that in all tissues examined, the anti-34-kD protein antibodies uniquely recognized the 34-kD protein.

Staining of tissue sections established that the 34 kD protein was present in a variety of cells including epithelial cells of the skin, gastrointestinal and respiratory tracts, as well as in fibroblasts and chondrocytes of connective tissue and mature cartilage, and endothelial cells of blood vessels. The 34-kD protein was also found in subpopulations of cells in thymus, spleen, bone marrow, and bursa. The protein was not detected in cardiac, skeletal, or smooth muscle cells, nor in epithelial cells of liver, kidney, or pancreas. The detailed tissue specificity of the 34-kD protein was not easily categorized and did not compellingly suggest a particular function for the protein. However, the identification of tissues that did not contain the 34-kD protein suggested that it is not involved in an essential metabolic process of all cells, nor can it be a necessary component of the processes of cell growth and division, secretion, protein synthesis, transport within a cell and across membranes, or formation of cell–cell junctions. Cells that exhibited mitotic figures after histological processing were often devoid of the 34-kD protein, and many cells that are actively involved in secretion such as those of the liver, adrenals, kidney, and pancreas do not contain detectable amounts of the 34-kD protein. In addition, cells that are known to form intercellular junctions and adhere tightly to each other, including lens epithelia and a variety of glandular epithelia, do not synthesize this protein.

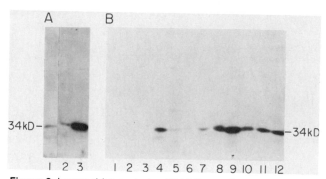

Figure 3 Immunoblot analysis of 34-kD protein content of cultured neuroretinal cells (*A*) and of various organs of adult chicken (*B*). Detergent extracts of cells or tissues were prepared, fractionated on an 8.5% SDS-polyacrylamide gel, transferred to nitrocellulose, and blotted with rabbit anti-34-kD protein antibodies followed by ^{125}I-labeled protein A. The 34-kD protein was visualized by autoradiography. (*A*) (Lane 1) Noninfected neuroretinal cells; (lane 2) neuroretinal cells infected with the transformation defective mutant *td*107; (lane 3) cells infected with Schmidt-Ruppin RSV strain A. (*B*) Extracts blotted were heart (lane 1), brain (lane 2), bone marrow (lane 3), spleen (lane 4), liver (lane 5), pancreas (lane 6), kidney (lane 7), skin (lane 8), intestine (lane 9), adipose tissue (lane 10), CEF fibroblasts (lane 11), and gizzard (lane 12).

Changes in the distribution of the 34-kD protein during tissue maturation

A major finding of this study is that significant changes in the distribution of the 34-kD protein occur during the differentiation or maturation of several tissues. For example by the PAP method, the most rapidly dividing cells in the chicken tongue (Fig. 4C,D), the basal epithelial cells of the stratum germinativum, were lightly stained with the anti-34-kD protein antibody while the second layer, the stratum spinosum, which is composed of the more differentiated prickly cells and is undergoing the process of keratinization, was intensely stained. The flat-

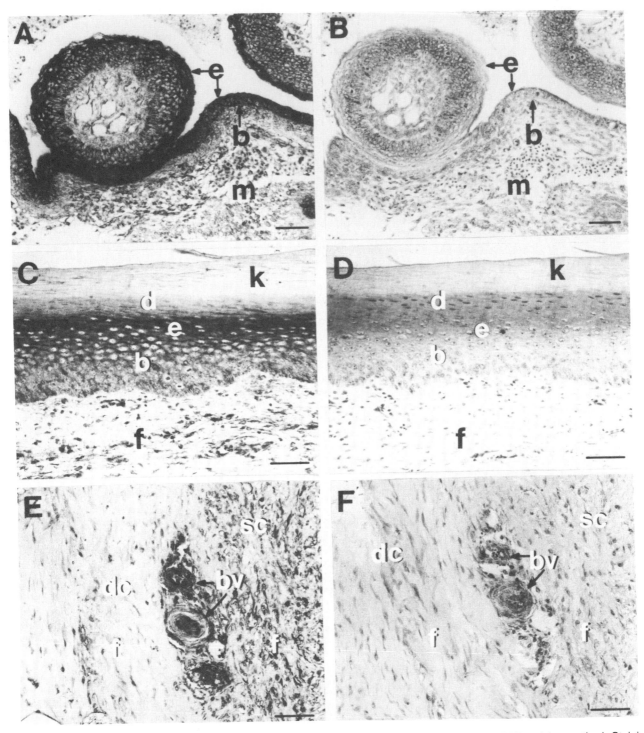

Figure 4 The presence of the 34-kD protein in embryonic and adult chicken skin visualized by the PAP staining method. Staining with rabbit anti-34-kD protein antibody (*A,C,E*); with preimmune antibody (*B,D,F*). Intense staining was seen in the superficial epithelial cell layer (e) of embryonic skin and feather rudiments (*A*). Lower levels of staining were detected in the basal epithelial cell layers (b). Mesenchymal cells (m) were not appreciably stained. Staining of a longitudinal section of adult tongue is shown in *C* and *D*. The basal epithelial layer (b) is lightly stained whereas the more mature epithelial cells (e) are intensely stained. Cells in the later stages of keratinization and nuclear degeneration (d) and the fully keratinized layer (k) are unstained. Significant staining of fibroblasts (f) of connective tissue was observed. Sections through an area of adult chicken comb that reveal variations in the intensity of staining of fibroblasts (f) are shown in *E* and *F*. Fibrocytes present in areas of dense collagen (dc) were frequently unstained, whereas fibroblasts in areas of sparse collagen (sc) or in the vicinity of blood vessels (bv) were intensely stained. In sections stained by the PAP method, positive staining was indicated by the presence of a brown diaminobenzidine reaction product. All sections were counterstained with Gill's hematoxylin. Bars, 50 μm.

tened cells, which are more highly keratinized and are beginning to exhibit nuclear degeneration, are unstained with the anti-34-kD protein antibody as is the outermost layer. A similar distribution for the 34-kD protein was observed in sections of embryonic skin (Fig. 4A). When the sections were incubated with control antibodies, only low levels of staining were detectable by the PAP technique (Fig. 4B,D,F).

Not all fibroblasts present in the dermis expressed detectable amounts of the 34-kD protein. Fibroblasts in the vicinity of blood vessels and in areas of connective tissue where collagen was sparse appeared to contain

significant amounts of the 34-kD protein (Fig. 4E,F), whereas fibrocytes in areas of dense collagen did not express appreciable amounts of this protein (Fig. 4E,F). This variation in the level of the 34-kD protein may reflect differences in the age and/or differentiation state of these cells.

The distribution of the 34-kD protein was also surveyed in several organs that contain well-developed epithelial cell layers. Throughout the respiratory tract, the epithelial cells were intensely stained with the specific antibodies, as shown for trachea in Figure 5A. In the embryonic intestine (Figure 5C), the 34-kD protein was

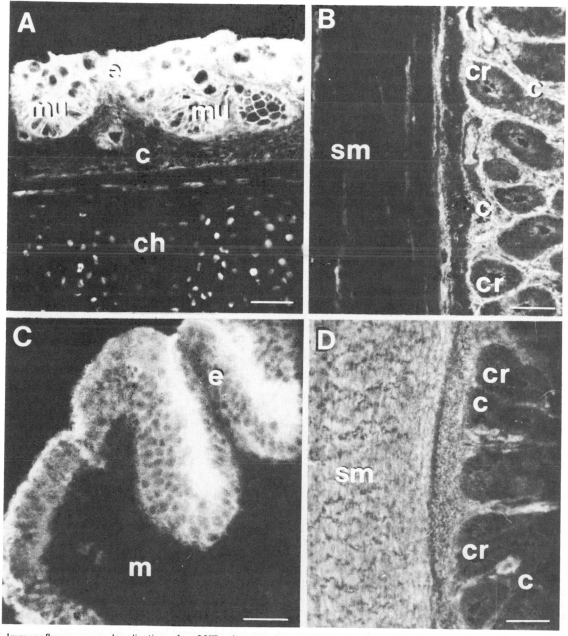

Figure 5 Immunofluorescence localization of pp60^{src} substrates in trachea and intestine. Sections incubated with monoclonal anti-34-kD protein antibody, (A,B,C); with monoclonal anti-vinculin antibody (D). In the adult trachea (A), significant staining of epithelial cells (e) mucous-secreting epithelial cells (mu), connective tissue (c), and chondrocytes (ch) was observed. The localization of the 34-kD protein and vinculin in adult intestine is compared in B and D. (sm) Smooth muscle; (cr) crypts of Lieberkuhn; (c) vascularized connective tissue. A section of embryonic intestine is shown (C). (e) Cuboidal epithelial cells lining intestinal lumen; (m) mesenchymal smooth muscle precursors. Bars, 50 μm.

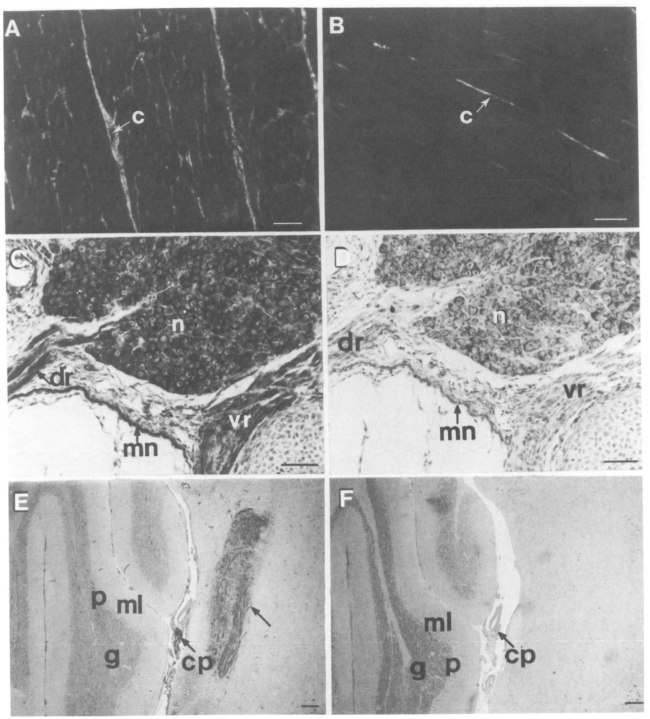

Figure 6 The 34-kD protein content of muscle and nerve tissue determined by immunofluorescence or PAP staining techniques. Frozen sections of adult cardiac muscle (*A*) or breast skeletal muscle (*B*) were incubated with monoclonal antibodies to the 34-kD protein followed by fluorescent rabbit anti-mouse IgG. Paraffin sections of 13-day embryonic dorsal root ganglion (*C,D*) and sagittal sections containing adult cerebellum and brain stem (*E,F*) were incubated with rabbit antibodies to the 34-kD protein (*C, E*), or preimmune antibodies (*D,F*); staining was visualized by the PAP method. The cardiac muscle and skeletal muscle cells were unstained; in both muscle sections, only the vascularized connective tissue (c) was stained. In the embryonic dorsal root ganglion, large ganglion neurons (n) and fibers of the dorsal root (dr) and ventral root (vr) were intensely stained. The membranes that enclose the spinal cord (mn) also showed positive staining. In adult cerebellum, the granule cells (g), Purkinje cells (p), and fibers of the molecular layer (ml) were not stained; however, one region of the brainstem (arrow) was intensely stained. In addition, parts of the choroid plexus (cp) were stained by the anti-34kD protein antibodies. (*A,B*) Bar, 50 μm, 173×; (*C,D*) bar, 50 μm, 216×; (*E,F*) bar, 200 μm, 27×.

concentrated at the edges of the cuboidal epithelial cells lining the lumen. The underlying mesenchyme did not contain the 34-kD protein; however, in adult intestine (Fig. 5B), connective tissue cells that arise from the embryonic mesenchyme contain substantial amounts of the protein. In contrast to the embryonic epithelial cells, the 34-kD protein was not detected in the mature epithelial cells of the crypts of Lieberkuhn except perhaps along the apical surface. The distribution of the 34-kD protein in the intestine was different from that of another potential pp60^{src} substrate, the cytoskeletal-associated protein, vinculin (compare Fig. 5B,D).

The 34-kD protein was not present in most neural cells examined. For example, in cerebellum (Fig. 6E,F), cells of the granular and Purkinje layers and fibers of the molecular layer contained little, if any, 34-kD protein. However, the protein was found in some localized regions of the brainstem (Fig. 6E,F). The 34-kD protein was also present in the large ganglion neurons of the embryonic dorsal root ganglion (Fig. 6C,D). As in other tissues, endothelial cells of blood vessels and fibroblasts in the meninges contained substantial amounts of this protein.

The 34-kD protein was not found in muscle cells of various organs from 13-day embryonic or adult chickens. Immunofluorescence staining of thin sections of cardiac muscle, skeletal muscle of the breast, and intestinal smooth muscle incubated with the anti-34-kD monoclonal antibody are shown in Figure 6, A and B, and Figure 5B, respectively. In these sections, only the connective tissue showed bright staining.

Summary

We have described the preparation of a monoclonal antibody that recognizes the 34-kD pp60^{src} substrate. This antibody was used to localize the 34-kD protein to the inner surface of the plasma membrane. The immunofluorescence staining pattern obtained with the anti-34-kD protein antibody is similar to that of α-spectrin, suggesting that the 34-kD protein may also be associated with the cytoskeleton. Tissue distribution studies established that the 34-kD protein is not expressed in all cells and that its expression is not correlated with the division state of a cell. Significant changes were observed in the level of the 34-kD protein in cells of several tissues during differentiation and maturation. Taken together, the membrane localization and tissue distribution studies raise the possibility that the 34-kD protein may play a role in the transmission of differentiation signals from the cell surface.

Acknowledgments

We thank Dr. Elizabeth Repasky of Roswell Park Memorial Institute for generously providing the antibodies to chicken α-spectrin. We gratefully acknowledge the excellent technical assistance of Ms. Mary Jo Przyborski and thank Mr. Steven Chin for histological services as well as many helpful discussions. This work was supported by U.S. Public Health Service grants AI-11378 and Am-04256. M.E.G. was a Biomedical Fellow of the Revson Foundation.

References

Amini, S. and A. Kaji. 1983. Association of pp36, a phosphorylated form of the presumed target protein for the *src* protein of Rous sarcoma virus, with the membrane of chicken cells transformed by Rous sarcoma virus. *Proc. Natl. Acad. Sci.* **80**: 960.

Bishop, J.M. and H.E. Varmus. 1982. Functions and origins of retroviral transforming genes. In *Molecular biology of tumor viruses*, 2nd edition: *RNA tumor viruses* (ed. R. Weiss et al.), p. 999. Cold Spring Harbor Laboratory, Cold Spring Harbor, New York.

Burridge, K.M. and J. Feramisco. 1980. Microinjection and localization of a 130k protein in living fibroblasts: A relationship to actin and fibronectin. *Cell* **19**: 587.

Burridge, K., T. Kelly, and P. Mangeat. 1982. Nonerythrocyte spectrin: Actin-membrane attachment to proteins occuring in many cell types. *J. Cell Biol.* **95**: 478.

Carpenter, G., L. King, Jr., and S. Cohen. 1979. Rapid enhancement of protein phosphorylation in A-401 cell membrane preparation by epidermal growth factor. *J. Biol. Chem.* **254**: 4884.

Cheng, Y.-S.E. and L.B. Chen. 1981. Detection of phosphotyrosine-containing 34,000 dalton protein in the framework of cells transformed with Rous sarcoma virus. *Proc. Natl. Acad. Sci.* **78**: 2388.

Cooper, J.A. and T. Hunter. 1981a. Changes in protein phosphorylation in Rous sarcoma virus transformed chicken embryo cells. *Mol. Cell. Biol.* **1**: 165.

———. 1981b. Four different classes of retroviruses induce phosphorylation of tyrosines present in similar cellular proteins. *Mol. Cell. Biol.* **1**: 394.

———. 1983. Identification and characterization of cellular targets for tyrosine protein kinases. *J. Biol. Chem.* **258**: 1108.

Cooper, J.A., D.F. Bowen-Pope, E. Raines, R. Ross, and T. Hunter. 1982. Similar effects of platelet-derived growth factor and epidermal growth factor on the phosphorylation of tyrosine in cellular proteins. *Cell* **31**: 263.

Courtneidge, S.A., A.D. Levinson, and J.M. Bishop. 1980. The protein encoded by the transforming gene of avian sarcoma virus (pp60^{src}) and a homologous protein in normal cells (pp60$^{proto-src}$) are associated with the plasma membrane. *Proc. Natl. Acad. Sci.* **77**: 3783.

Courtneidge, S., R. Ralston, K. Alitalo, and J.M. Bishop. 1983. Subcellular location of an abundant substrate (p36) for tyrosine-specific protein kinases. *Mol. Cell. Biol.* **3**: 340.

Decker, S. 1982. Phosphorylation of the Mr = 34,000 protein in normal and Rous sarcoma virus-transformed rat fibroblasts. *Biochem. Biophys. Res. Commun.* **109**: 434.

Edelman, G.M. and I. Yahara. 1976. Temperature sensitive changes in surface modulating assemblies of fibroblasts transformed by mutants of Rous sarcoma virus. *Proc. Natl. Acad. Sci.* **73**: 2047.

Ek, B., B. Westermark, A. Wasteson, and C.-H. Heldin. 1982. Stimulation of tyrosine specific phosphorylation by platelet-derived growth factor. *Nature* **295**: 419.

Erikson, E. and R.L. Erikson. 1980. Identification of a cellular protein substrate phosphorylated by the avian sarcoma virus-transforming gene product. *Cell* **21**: 829.

Erikson, E., D.J. Shealy, and R.L. Erikson. 1981a. Evidence that viral transforming gene products and epidermal growth factor stimulate phosphorylation of the same cellular protein with similar specificity. *J. Biol. Chem.* **256**: 11381.

Erikson, E., R. Cook, G.J. Miller, and R.L. Erikson. 1981b. The same normal cell protein is phosphorylated after transformation by avian sarcoma viruses with unrelated transforming genes. *Mol. Cell. Biol.* **1**: 43.

Geiger, B. 1979. A 130k protein from chicken gizzard: Its location at the termini of microfilament bundles in cultured chicken cells. *Cell* **18**: 193.

Greenberg, M.E. and G.M. Edelman. 1983a. Comparison of the 34,000-Da pp60^{src} substrate and a 38,000-Da phosphoprotein identified by monoclonal antibodies. *J. Biol. Chem.* **258**: 8497.

———. 1983b. The 34kD-pp60^{src} substrate is located at the inner face of the plasma membrane. *Cell* **33**: 767.

Greenberg, M.E., R. Brackenbury, and G.M. Edelman. 1984. Changes in the distribution of the 34kD pp60^{src} substrate during differentiation and maturation of chicken tissues. *J. Cell Biol.* (in press).

Hunter, T. and J.A. Cooper. 1981. Epidermal growth factor induces rapid tyrosine phosphorylation of proteins in A431 human tumor cells. *Cell* **24**: 741.

Hunter, T. and B.M. Sefton. 1982. Protein kinases and viral transformation. In *The molecular actions of toxins and viruses* (ed. P. Cohen and S. Van Heyningen), p. 333. Elsevier Biomedical Press, Amsterdam.

Kasuga, M., Y. Zick, D.L. Blith, F.A. Karlsson, H.U. Häring, and C.R. Kahn. 1982. Insulin stimulation of phosphorylation of the β subunit of the insulin receptor. *J. Biol. Chem.* **257**: 9891.

Krueger, J.G., E. Wang, and A.R. Goldberg. 1980. Evidence that the *src* gene product of Rous sarcoma virus is membrane associated. *Virology* **101**: 25.

Lenk, R. and S. Penman. 1979. The cytoskeletal framework and poliovirus metabolism. *Cell* **16**: 289.

Levine, J. and M. Willard. 1981. Fodrin: Axonally transported polypeptides associated with the internal periphery of many cells. *J. Cell Biol.* **90**: 631.

Nakamura, K.D., R. Martinez, and M.J. Weber. 1983. Tyrosine phosphorylation of specific proteins after mitogen stimulation of chicken embryo fibroblasts. *Mol. Cell. Biol.* **3**: 380.

Nigg, E.A., J.A. Cooper, and T. Hunter. 1983. Immunofluorescent localization of a 39,000-dalton substrate of tyrosine protein kinases to the cytoplasmic surface of the plasma membrane. *J. Cell Biol.* **96**: 1601.

Pawson, T., J. Guyden, T.-H. Kung, K. Radke, T. Gilmore, and G.S. Martin. 1980. A strain of Fujinami sarcoma virus which is temperature-sensitive in protein phosphorylation and cellular transformation. *Cell* **22**: 767.

Petruzzelli, L.M., S. Ganguly, C.J. Smith, M.H. Cobb, C.S. Rubin, and O.M. Rosen. 1982. Insulin activates a tyrosine-specific protein kinase in extracts of 3T3-L1 adipocytes and human placenta. *Proc. Natl. Acad. Sci.* **79**: 6792.

Poirier, F., G. Calothy, R.E. Karess, E. Erikson, and H. Hanafusa. 1982. Role of pp60^{src} kinase activity in the induction of neuroretinal cell proliferation by Rous sarcoma virus. *J. Virol.* **42**: 780.

Radke, K. and G.S. Martin. 1979. Transformation by Rous sarcoma virus: Effects of *src* gene expression on the synthesis and phosphorylation of cellular polypeptides. *Proc. Natl. Acad. Sci.* **76**: 5212.

Radke, K., T. Gilmore, and G.S. Martin. 1980. Transformation by Rous sarcoma virus: A cellular substrate for transformation-specific protein phosphorylation contains phosphotyrosine. *Cell* **21**: 821.

Radke, K., V.C. Carter, P. Moss, P. Dehazya, M. Schliwa, and G.S. Martin. 1983. Membrane association of a 36,000-dalton substrate for tyrosine phosphorylation in chick embryo fibroblasts transformed by avian sarcoma viruses. *J. Cell Biol.* **97**: 1601.

Repasky, E.A., B.L. Granger, and E. Lazarides. 1982. Widespread occurrence of avian spectrin in nonerythroid cells. *Cell* **29**: 821.

Sefton, B.M., T. Hunter, and J.A. Cooper. 1983. Some lymphoid cell lines transformed by Abelson murine leukemia virus lack a major 36,000-dalton tyrosine protein kinase substrate. *Mol. Cell. Biol.* **3**: 56.

Sefton, B.M., T. Hunter, E.H. Ball, and S.J. Singer. 1981. Vinculin: A cytoskeletal target of the transforming protein of Rous sarcoma virus. *Cell* **24**: 165.

Willingham, M.C., G. Jay, and I. Pastan. 1979. Localization of the avian sarcoma virus *src* gene product to the plasma membrane of transformed cells by electron microscopy immunocytochemistry. *Cell* **18**: 125.

Multigenic Control of Tumorigenesis: Three Distinct Oncogenes Are Required for Transformation of Rat Embryo Fibroblasts by Polyoma Virus

F. Cuzin, M. Rassoulzadegan, and L. Lemieux

Centre de Biochimie du CNRS, Université de Nice, 06034 Nice, France

The multistep nature of carcinogenesis is a widely accepted concept. Each step toward the tumorigenic state involves a variety of changes in the structure, metabolism, and regulatory processes of the cell. This evolution, however, can be triggered by many oncogenic viruses as a result of the expression of a single oncogene (for reviews, see this volume). This highly pleiotropic effect of a unique gene may be understood if its product acts on a critical cellular target that, in turn, regulates, either directly or indirectly, a variety of cellular genes, or if it is itself a highly multifunctional protein.

It now appears, however, that the evolution of other tumor viruses, such as polyoma virus (Rassoulzadegan et al. 1980, 1981, 1982a, 1983) or adenoviruses (Houweling et al. 1980; Van den Elsen et al. 1982; Ruley 1983), has developed sets of separate oncogenes whose coordinated expression is necessary for the development of a fully tumorigenic phenotype and which appear to correspond to distinct critical interactions with cellular control systems.

Polyoma virus is a useful model of such multigenic, multistep tumorigenesis. It can now be analyzed in detail, mostly due to the construction by R. Kamen and co-workers (Treisman et al. 1981; Tyndall et al. 1981) of cloned genes that separately encode the various oncogenic proteins. No less than three distinct oncogenes appear to be acting in a coordinated manner in the induction of the virus-induced tumor state in primary rat embryo fibroblast (REF) cells. None of these genes is able to produce by itself a fully transformed state. All three of them, however, separately induce defined alterations of the cell growth controls and cell structure. Their products act on distinct cellular targets: the chromatin (large T protein), the plasma membrane (middle T protein), and possibly the cytoskeleton (small T protein).

The first part of the work described in this article was performed in collaboration with A. Carr and A. Cowie (Imperial Cancer Research Fund Laboratories, London), R. Treisman (Harvard University, Cambridge, Mass.), and R. Kamen (Genetics Institute, Boston, Mass.). A complete description of the experimental procedures can be found in the corresponding papers (Rassoulzadegan et al. 1982a, 1983).

The genetic structure of polyoma early region and the biochemical properties of its protein products

A region of the polyoma genome of ~3 kb in length is continuously expressed in virus-transformed and tumor cells. It corresponds to the part of the genome transcribed during the early phase of the lytic cycle in permissive mouse cells. Three overlapping genes in alternate translational reading frames (Fig. 1) direct the synthesis of distinct proteins via the production of distinct mRNAs by means of different splicing processes operating on a common primary transcript (for review, see Kamen et al. 1980). The three proteins, of respective apparent molecular weights of 105,000 (large T), 56,000 (middle T), and 22,000 (small T), constitute the viral T antigens that are immunoprecipitated by antibodies present in the serum of tumor-bearing animals (for review, see Ito 1980). Large T antigen appears to be located exclusively in the nucleus, middle T antigen in the cytoplasmic membranes, and small T antigen in the cytosol. As its SV40 equivalent (Tjian 1978), the polyoma large T protein binds with very high affinities to defined nucleotide sequences within the region of the promoters and the origin of replication of the viral genome (Gaudray et al. 1981). It exhibits an intrinsic ATPase activity (Gaudray et al. 1980) and carries a nucleotide binding site (Clertant and Cuzin 1982), distinct from the ATPase catalytic site (P. Clertant and F. Cuzin, in prep.). In vivo studies using mutants expressing a thermolabile protein have demonstrated at least two distinct regulatory roles of the large T protein during the lytic cycle of the virus in permissive cells—the initiation of viral DNA synthesis (Francke and Eckhart 1973), and the repression of early mRNA synthesis (Cogen 1978). Middle T antigen by contrast, is a membrane protein (for review, see Ito, 1980). Only a minor fraction of the protein is phosphorylated in vivo on a tyrosine residue, but the protein is tightly associated with a tyrosine kinase activity, which is likely to correspond to the c-src gene product (Courtneidge and Smith 1983). No in vitro activity could be so far associated with the small T protein. In vivo, it is found in the soluble cytoplasmic fraction, and microinjection studies have led Graessmann et al. (1980) to the conclusion that it could be required for the disruption of actin cables characteristic of the transformed cell.

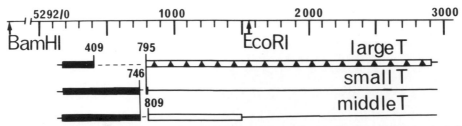

Figure 1 Map of the early region of polyoma virus. (*Top line*) Nucleotide numbers according to Soeda et al. (1979) and cleavage sites of the *Bam*HI and *Eco*RI enzymes. Boxes represent the coding regions for the three indicated proteins, with different symbols according to the reading frame used on the messenger and dashed lines to represent the introns.

More than one polyoma early gene product is required for expression of a fully transformed phenotype

A series of converging results pointed to the middle T protein as an important effector in the maintenance of the tumoral phenotype (for review, see Ito 1980). The absolute defect in transformation of the *hr-t* mutants jamin 1970; Fluck et al. 1977), which lack both middle T and small T proteins but synthesize a normal large T protein, indicated that large T alone is not sufficient for transformation. At the same time, however, results obtained in our laboratory indicated that cell lines derived from FR3T3 rat fibroblast cells by transformation with the *tsa* mutant (Fried 1965), which express a thermolabile large T protein but normal middle T and small T proteins (Trejo-Avila et al. 1981), were temperature dependent for the maintenance of the transformed state (Seif and Cuzin 1977). This observation led us to postulate that, at least in these lines, the large T protein exerts a transformation maintenance function, and, furthermore, we could assign this function to an aminoterminal domain of the protein (Rassoulzadegan et al. 1981). We proposed on this basis a model implying the cooperative action of at least two gene products, middle T and large T, in the maintenance of the transformed state (Rassoulzadegan et al. 1980).

An important breakthrough in the analysis of the respective roles of the viral early proteins in cell transformation resulted from the construction in 1981, by R. Kamen and his colleagues, then at the Imperial Cancer Research Fund Laboratories in London, of modified viral genomes, each encoding only one of these proteins (Treisman et al. 1981). These authors showed that transfer of the DNA of plasmid pPyMT1, encoding only middle T protein, induces transformation of rat fibroblasts of an established line (Rat-1) with an efficiency only slightly lower than that of wild-type polyoma DNA. This observation led them to conclusions that obviously were not consistent with the results of our own studies on the *tsa* mutants. An active collaboration was then started between our laboratories to solve this apparent contradiction.

After confirming the ability of pPyMT1 DNA to transform FR3T3 cells, which had been used previously for transformation experiments with the *tsa* mutant, we investigated the properties of the transformants induced by pPyMT1. All these lines (MTT lines) were found to express in high-serum medium (10% newborn calf serum) a series of transformation characters (ability to grow at high density, grow in soft agar, and produce plasminogen activator), and also to induce tumors in Fischer rats in a manner indistinguishable from wild-type polyoma transformants. However, they all lacked the ability to grow in the presence of low concentrations of serum, which is characteristic of SV40 and polyoma transformants (Smith et al. 1971; Kaplan and Ozanne 1982). When seeded on plastic in the presence of only 0.5% calf serum, MTT transformants grew to confluency and then stopped. When seeded in suspension in agarose medium at the same low serum concentration, they did not divide. The cells recovered the flat morphology characteristic of the original FR3T3 fibroblast. In fact, a complete reversion to the normal phenotype was observed in low-serum medium. This opened the way to identify by complementation analysis the viral protein necessary for the marked changes in the serum factor requirements characteristic of fully transformed cells. Results like those listed in Table 1 demonstrated that only the DNAs encoding the large T protein could efficiently rescue the ability of MTT cells to form colonies in suspension or foci in the presence of limiting concentrations of serum.

After the first clear-cut demonstration by Treisman et al. (1981) that the middle T protein plays a necessary role in the oncogenic process, these data demonstrated that this protein is not sufficient for the expression in vitro of a fully transformed phenotype (Rassoulzadegan et al. 1982a) and therefore probably is not sufficient for the induction in vivo of a complete tumoral development. This was illustrated independently by the observation that the corresponding plasmid DNA, pPyMT1, was unable to transform truly normal rodent cells—embryonic fibroblasts in primary cultures (Rassoulzadegan et al. 1983). In agreement with this conclusion, Asselin and co-workers (1983) observed that injection of pPyMT1 DNA into newborn animals does not lead to tumor formation, as it does in the case of the wild-type DNA.

Immortalization of rodent embryo fibroblasts by the large T protein

In view of the inability of a gene encoding only the middle T protein to transform primary cells, we asked whether an immortalization function might be exerted either by

Table 1 Complementation of MTT Cells for Growth in Agarose Medium at Low Serum Concentration

Plasmid	Viral protein(s) encoded	Colonies per 10^5 cells in agarose medium supplemented with	
		0.5% serum	10% serum
pBR322	none	0	$>10^4$
pPY1	large T, middle T, small T	47	NT[a]
pNG1	large T	38	NT
pPyLT1	large T	22	NT
pPyMT1	middle T	0	NT
pPyST1	small T	0	NT

The indicated DNAs were transferred by the protoplast fusion technique (Rassoulzadegan et al. 1982b) into cells of the MTT4 line, derived from FR3T3 by transfer of plasmid pPyMT1 and focus selection in high-serum medium (Rassoulzadegan et al. 1982a). Cells were seeded (10^5 cells/60-mm plate) 24 hr later in agarose-gelified DMEM containing the indicated amount of newborn calf serum (GIBCO). Colonies were counted after 3 weeks.
[a]NT, not tested.

the large T or by the small T proteins. Immortality, in this context, is defined as the unlimited growth potential in culture exhibited by many tumoral cell lines and by the nontumorigenic 3T3-type lines (Todaro and Green 1963). The pioneer work of Vogt and Dulbecco (1963) had long ago demonstrated that immortality is conferred on primary cells by polyoma transformation. A convenient assay was provided by the observation (Todaro and Green 1963) that rodent embryo fibroblasts, in contrast to cells of established lines, are unable to grow in culture at low cell density. Rat or mouse embryo fibroblasts were thus seeded as very sparse cultures after transfer of the various polyoma genes. We noticed that a fraction of the cells that had received a gene encoding the large T protein were able to form flat colonies under these conditions. Transfer of plasmids encoding either middle T protein only or small T protein only had no effect above the background frequency observed for untreated cells (see Table 2). Colonies were also obtained after transfer of a wild-type polyoma genome, but in this case, they had the dense appearance typical of transformed cells. Cells were picked from several large T-induced colonies and propagated further. Representative lines have been maintained for more than 120 cell generations in culture (40 weekly transfers) without any apparent decrease in cell viability or in growth rate that could indicate the occurrence of a crisis period. As expected from the flat appearance of the colonies, the growth properties of these established cell lines in Dulbecco's modified Eagle's medium (DMEM) containing 10% newborn calf serum were in general similar to those of the "normal" 3T3 lines; in attached cultures, cell division was arrested at a low saturation density corresponding to a complete monolayer and cells did not divide when seeded in suspension in agarose medium. Their flat morphology, indicative of an organized cytoskeleton, was identical to that of primary and 3T3 cells. Unlike these cells, how-

ever, they could grow in DMEM supplemented with only 0.5% calf serum, a property dependent in transformed cells on the expression of the large T protein (see above). A continuous requirement for an activity of the viral protein for cell growth in culture was demonstrated by experiments using a recombinant DNA encoding a *tsa* thermolabile large T protein. Cell lines could be established and maintained at the permissive temperature (33°C) but they stopped growing immediately after transfer to the restrictive temperature (40°C) (Rassoulzadegan et al. 1983).

Aminoterminal localization of the domain of the large T protein involved in transformation

Using the set of assays developed for large T-dependent transformation characters, we could confirm one of our earlier conclusions, namely that, unlike the function(s) of large T protein in viral DNA replication, large T's role in the maintenance of the transformed state can be exerted by truncated forms deleted from the carboxyterminal part of the protein. This hypothesis was supported by the results of experiments using plasmid DNAs that include only the viral sequences between the *Bam*HI and the *Eco*RI sites (promoter region and 5' 40% of the coding region; see Fig. 1) from modified genomes that cannot express middle and small T proteins (*hr-t* mutant NG18, large T-only plasmid pPyLT1). After transfer of these plasmids into rat fibroblasts, a novel T antigen species was observed, phosphorylated in vivo as the full-sized protein, and immunoprecipitated by the same antiserums. Its molecular weight (40 kD) was close to that predicted from the nucleotide sequence (36.7 kD). These plasmid DNAs encoding a truncated large T protein were as efficient as the complete large T-only genes in conferring serum-independent growth ability on MTT cells (Rassoulzadegan et al. 1982a) and unlimited growth potential on primary rat and mouse fibroblasts (Rassoulzadegan et al. 1983).

Maintenance of the transformed phenotype does not require the small T protein

In the course if this work, a large collection of transformed lines was constituted, either from established rat fibroblast lines (Rat-1, FR3T3) or from mouse and rat primary fibroblast cells, which express various combinations of the three early gene products. Although their properties led to the assignment of specific and additive functions in transformation to middle T and large T proteins, no clear conclusion could be drawn on a possible function of the small T protein. As already mentioned, we could detect no difference in the growth patterns in culture or tumorigenic properties between cell lines expressing all three proteins and cell lines that lack a functional small T gene (MTT lines complemented by transfer of a large T or truncated large T gene). We also noticed that cells expressing either only middle T (in high serum medium) or middle T and large T proteins (in both low- and high-serum medium) exhibited the characteristic compact morphology of wild-type transformants. By contrast, cells expressing only the large T protein remained flat and extended like embryonic fibroblasts or 3T3 cells. This observation, more recently confirmed by indirect immunofluorescence visualization of the cytoskeleton (M. Grisoni et al., in prep.), indicates that middle T protein, when properly complemented either by serum factors or by the activity of the large T gene, induces a complete disruption of actin cables. This conclusion is at variance with previous indications that, in the case of SV40, the small-T protein is required for changes in cytoskeletal structures (Graessmann et al. 1980). This discrepancy may only mean that the different systems of oncogenes of polyoma and SV40 cannot be functionally compared at this stage, in spite of the high levels of homology observed locally in amino acid sequences, especially in their small T polypeptides.

The only effect of the small T gene (plasmid pPyST1) that could be observed in cells of an established line was a low efficiency of complementation of the serum requirement of MTT transformants; selection either by growth in suspension or by focus formation in the presence of 0.5% serum after transfer of pPyST1 DNA into MTT cells yielded very small colonies or foci of slow-growing cells, and we did not succeed in further cultivating these cells in low-serum medium (Rassoulzadegan et al. 1982a). This inefficient, but reproducible, complementation is reminiscent of the observations of Asselin et al. (1983) suggesting that small T protein can complement middle T protein in the absence of large T protein for tumor induction in the animal.

A function of the small T protein in the establishment of transformation in primary fibroblast cells

Only two viral functions would appear logically from these results to be required for the establishment of a fully transformed cell line from an embryonic fibroblast: the large T immortalization function and the middle T function inducing the terminal transformation and tumoral properties. In agreement with this scheme, we observed that cell lines established by transfer of large T into primary fibroblasts could be subsequently transformed by transfer of the middle T-only plasmid pPyMT1 (Rassoulzadegan et al. 1983).

A paradoxical result was, however, obtained when we tried to transform REF cells by the simultaneous transfer of large T and middle T genes (Table 2); no stably transformed line could be isolated by focus formation under these conditions. Combinations of middle T and small T or large T and small T genes were similarly inefficient. Transformation could only be achieved by transfer of a wild-type viral genome, or of a combination of modified genomes that would allow the simultaneous synthesis of the three early proteins (M. Rassoulzadegan, et al., in prep.). These results demonstrate a requirement for the small T protein for transformation of the fully normal REF cells.

One possible explanation for this effect might have been in the differences between the immortalization and the transformation assays; immortalization was measured by colony formation on cells actively dividing in low-density cultures, whereas focus formation was monitored after seeding at confluent densities. Immortalization by large T protein might require active growth conditions unless small T would be expressed simultaneously. This hypothesis could be ruled out, because transfer of the large T gene produced established lines with equivalent frequencies in cells maintained at high density and in actively growing cells and because these frequencies were not significantly affected by cotransfer of the small T-only gene (Tables 3 and 4). The results altogether suggest that, during growth in culture of established lines, cellular functions become progressively expressed that render the cell susceptible to a set of oncogenes originally not sufficient to transform. The three early polyoma proteins thus appear to act in a coordinated way for the transformation of embryo fibroblasts into tumor cells.

Expression of small T protein reduces the tightness of cell adhesion to substratum

To try to elucidate the role of small T protein in transformation, we looked for cellular changes induced by transfer of this gene alone into normal rat cells (REF and FR3T3 cells). A first, striking observation was that, during the first days after transfer, a large proportion of the recipient cells were floating in the medium. This phenomenon was never observed using protoplast fusion for the transfer of other genes (Rassoulzadegan et al. 1982b). Remarkably, these floating cells were not dead but maintained an organized structure and an extended flat morphology. Groups of such cells attached to each other could be observed, with occasional mitotic figures. These "floating islands" were indeed growing, but at a reduced rate, and they reattached to the plastic plates after the first 5–10 days. This loss of adhesiveness could be quantitated by measuring the kinetics of cell detachment during exposure to dilute trypsin solutions (Fig. 2).

These observations are likely to correspond to the transitory expression of the gene after transfer. They are

Table 2 Transforming Ability of Various Combinations of Polyoma Virus Early Genes on FR3T3 and REF Cells

Plasmid	Viral protein(s) encoded	Transforming efficiency on	
		REF cells[b]	FR3T3 cells[c]
pBR322	none	0	0
pPy1	LT,MT,ST	74	69
pPyLT1	LT	0	0
pPyMT1	MT	0	58
pPyST1	ST	0	0
pBC1051	MT,ST	0	26
pPyMT1 + pPyLT1	MT,LT	0	62
pMT-TT	MT,TT	0	55
pBC1051 + pPyLT1	LT,MT,ST	9	NT[d]
pMT-TT + pPyST1	TT,MT,ST	3	NT

DNA of the indicated plasmid, or combination of plasmids, was transferred into either FR3T3 or REF cells by the protoplast fusion technique (Rassoulzadegan et al. 1982b). Plasmid pBC1051 includes a complete polyoma genome, but, due to a point mutation of the large T donor splice, expresses only middle T and small T proteins (Nilsson and Magnusson 1983). Plasmid pMT-TT includes in the same DNA molecule the DNA sequences encoding middle T from pPyMT1 and the BamHI–EcoRI fragment of plasmid pPyLT1, encoding the aminoterminal 40% of large T. Cells were seeded 24 hr after fusion at a density of 10^4 cells/60-mm plate in medium supplemented with 10% newborn calf serum (GIBCO). Plates were stained with Giemsa and colonies were counted after 1 month.
[a]LT, large T; MT, middle T; ST, small T; TT, truncated form of large T.
[b]Foci per 6×10^5 cells.
[c]Foci per 7×10^4 cells.
[d]NT, not tested.

now being confirmed and extended by experiments based on the selection of permanent lines by transfer of a plasmid carrying the small T gene linked to a dominant selectable marker, resistance to the drug G418 (Colbère-Garapin et al. 1981). Resistant clones could be selected after transfer of this plasmid, but the cells were loosely attached and did not reattach after trypsinization. Addition of fibronectin allowed attachment and further growth of the resistant cells. Lines are now being established and propagated in this way in the hope that we can analyze this quite specific effect of the viral protein. Whether it is related, and in what manner, to its effect in the establishment of the tumoral state remains entirely to be demonstrated.

Table 3 Cotransfer of the Small T or of the Middle T Gene Does Not Affect the Efficiency of Large T-induced Immortalization

Plasmid	Viral protein(s) encoded[a]	Immortalization efficiency (colonies per 6×10^5 cells)	Morphology of colonies	Growth characteristics of derived cell lines
pBR322	none	0	—	—
pPY1	LT,MT,ST	60	dense	transformed
pPyLT1	LT	35	flat	normal
pPyMT1	MT	0	—	—
pPyST1	ST	0	—	—
pBC1051	MT,ST	0	—	—
pMT-TT	MT,TT	42	flat	normal
pBC1051 + pPyLT1	LT,MT,ST	28	dense	transformed

Transfer of the indicated plasma or combination of plasmids was performed as in the experiment described in Table 2. Immortalized cells were selected by colony formation as previously described (Rassoulzadegan et al, 1983). Cells from three independent colonies were picked in each set and cultures were grown up to saturation: "normal" and "transformed" growth indicate growth arrest at confluency and at higher densities, respectively.
[a]See Table 2 notes for abbreviations.

Table 4 Growth Conditions after Transfer Do Not Affect the Efficiency of Immortalization by the Large T Gene

Plasmid	Viral protein(s) encoded[a]	Immortalization efficiency after 9 days	
		at confluency	of active growth[a]
pBR322	none	0	0
pPY1	LT,MT,ST	15	12
pPyLT1	LT	7	6
pPyMT1	MT	0	0
pPyST1	ST	0	0
pPyLT1 + pPyST1	LT,ST	9	9

Transfer of the indicated plasmid or combination of plasmids was performed as in the experiment described in Table 2. After transfer, parallel cultures were either maintained in active growth below confluency or seeded at confluent growth-inhibiting densities. Nine days later, both sets of cultures were trypsinized and the proportion of cells able to grow as colonies after seeding at very low density (10^3 cells/plate) was measured.

[a]See Table 2 notes for abbreviations.
[b]Colonies per 10^4 cells.

Discussion

Over the past 3 years, several systems of mutigenic determinants of the tumor state have been discovered, first in DNA tumor viruses—adenoviruses (Houweling et al. 1980; Van den Elsen et al. 1982; Ruley 1983) and polyoma virus (Rassoulzadegan et al. 1980, 1981, 1982a, 1983). Of obvious interest is the recent discovery by Land et al. (1983) and by Ruley (1983) that the distinct and additive alterations of the cellular growth control identified in the viral tumorigenesis pathway are likely to correspond to similar steps in the oncogenic process triggered by the known human oncogenic determinants: The polyoma large T protein, the adenovirus E1A, and the *myc* gene functions, on one hand, the polyoma middle T protein and the *ras* gene functions, on the other, complement each other for the transformation of REF cells. The multigenic determination of tumor formation by DNA viruses does not appear (any more) as a specialized mechanism of no general interest.

In this wider perspective, it is interesting to note that polyoma virus has developed not only two but, in fact, three distinct oncogenes; we can now conclude that a function of the small T protein is necessary, in addition to and in conjunction with the functions of the large T and middle T proteins, for REF transformation. These proteins interact with the three obvious cellular targets in oncogenesis, genomic control (large T), membrane structure and function (middle T), and the cell attachment system (small T). One is led immediately to ask whether a small T-like function might be exerted by a still unknown class of cellular oncogenes. Since the requirement for small T is not apparent in the commonly used established lines and since it might be, as the large T functions, complemented by serum factors, such an activity might have been so far not detected, but might be critical under in vivo conditions. One may further speculate that such a function could not only act in the es-

tablishment of the tumoral state, as evidenced by our present results. The only clear effect observed after transfer of the small T gene is at the level of the cell interaction with its substratum. Such a function could be of importance in the pathology of the tumors, possibly in the acquisition of a metastatic potential.

Alternatively, one might ask whether oncogenes that appear to exert functions similar to those of large T, like the adenovirus E1A or the *myc* genes (Land et al. 1983; Ruley 1983), would not also exert the establishment function of the polyoma small T gene. In this case, the polyoma oncogene systems would once more have dissociated, and therefore allow us to identify, critical steps of the tumorigenic process.

Experiments are in progress to expand further our knowledge of the immortalization potential of the large T gene. Results obtained on rodent embryonic fibroblasts clearly indicate that the large T function(s) sufficient for immortalization does not otherwise extensively affect the physiology of rodent fibroblasts. Therefore, one may hope they could lead to the establishment of permanent cell lines from other differentiated tissues, and from other species, that might retain their differentiated properties. Two exploratory series of experiments that have been performed so far have led to encouraging results. Results to be published elsewhere (M. Rassoulzadegan et al., in prep.) indicate that long-term cultures can be obtained from mouse lymphocytes and from human myoblast cells after transfer of pPyLT1 plasmid DNA, under culture conditions that did not allow the survival of the untreated control cultures for more than a limited time. Various clones obtained from the total spleen lymphocyte population expressed in vitro either surface immunoglobulins or the T-lymphocyte-specific antigens.

An independent interest of these systems stems from the fact that the molecular biology of these viruses is by

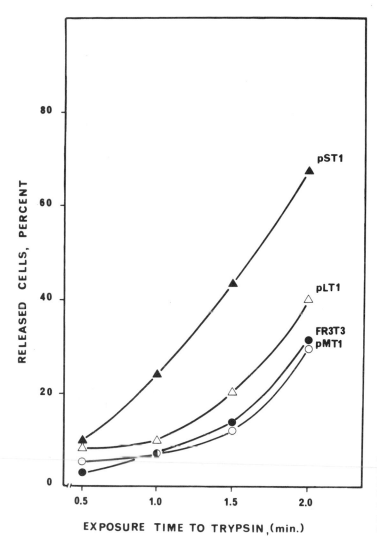

Figure 2 Trypsin sensitivity of FR3T3 cells after transfer of the genes separately encoding the three early viral proteins. FR3T3 cells (10^5 cells/35-mm plate) were fused with bacterial protoplasts (Rassoulzadegan et al. 1982b) carrying the indicated plasmids. Parallel cultures were washed and incubated at 37°C with 2 ml of a 0.2% trypsin solution. At the indicated times, the released cells were counted.

far one of the most advanced in the eukaryotic field. For instance, our knowledge of the regulatory activities exerted by the large T proteins of SV40 and polyoma viruses, although still fragmentary, is far in advance of what we know of the *myc* protein and already suggests possible mechanisms at the molecular level. In light of this, we currently are studying the DNA-binding properties of polyoma large T protein and its possible activity in the control of the expression of cellular genes. As its SV40 counterpart (Tjian 1978; Rio et al. 1980), the polyoma protein binds with high affinities to defined nucleotide sequences in the viral genome (Gaudray et al. 1981), thereby controlling its replication and transcription. We have recently isolated segments of mouse DNA which, in transformed cells, are also recognized with high affinity by the large T protein (Galup et al. 1983 and in prep.). On the other hand, by differential screening of libraries of cDNA representative of the messenger population of cells expressing either only large T or only middle T protein, we could isolate probes corresponding

to cellular genes that appear to be specifically induced in these cells (N. Glaichenhaus et al., in prep.). We hope that such approaches may lead to some insights on the molecular basis of the early step of the tumorigenic process which appears to be induced both by large T protein and by the cellular oncogenes of the *myc* group (Land et al. 1983).

Acknowledgments

In addition to the collaborative work mentioned in the text, we are indebted to R. Kamen for many helpful discussions and generous gifts of materials. We are grateful to S. Nilsson and G. Magnusson for the communication of unpublished results and for the gift of plasmid pBC1051. We thank L. Carbone, F. Tillier, and M.L. Varani for skilled technical assistance. This work was made possible by grants from the Ministère de l'Industrie et de la Recherche and from the Institut National de la Santé et de la Recherche Médicale (France).

References

Asselin, C., C. Gélinas, and M. Bastin. 1983. Role of the three polyoma virus early proteins in tumorigenesis. *Mol. Cell. Biol.* **3**: 1451.

Benjamin, T.L. 1970. Host range mutants of polyoma virus. *Proc. Natl. Acad. Sci.* **67**: 394.

Clertant, P. and F. Cuzin. 1982. Covalent affinity labeling by periodate-oxidized (γ-^{32}P)ATP of the large-T proteins of polyoma and SV40 viruses. *J. Biol. Chem.* **257**: 6300.

Cogen, B. 1978. Virus-specific early RNA in 3T6 cells infected by a tsA mutant of polyoma virus. *Virology* **85**: 222.

Colbère-Garapin, F., F. Horodniceanu, P. Kourilsky, and A.C. Garapin. 1981. A new dominant hybrid selective marker for higher eucaryotic cells. *J. Mol. Biol.* **150**: 1.

Courtneidge, S.A. and A.E. Smith. 1983. Polyoma virus transforming protein associates with the product of the c-*src* cellular gene. *Nature* **303**: 435.

Fluck, M.M., R.J. Staneloni, and T.L. Benjamin. 1977. Hrt and ts-a: Two early gene functions of polyoma virus. *Virology* **77**: 610.

Francke, B. and W. Eckhart. 1973. Polyoma gene function required for viral DNA synthesis. *Virology* **55**: 127.

Fried, M. 1965. Isolation of temperature-sensitive mutants of polyoma virus. *Virology* **25**: 669.

Galup, C., L. Trejo-Avila, E. Mougneau, L. Lemieux, P. Gaudray, M. Rassoulzadegan, and F. Cuzin. 1983. The oncogenic function(s) of the large T protein of polyoma virus. *INSERM* (in press).

Gaudray, P., P. Clertant, and F. Cuzin. 1980. ATP phosphohydrolase (ATPase) activity of a polyoma virus T antigen. *Eur. J. Biochem.* **109**: 553.

Gaudray, P., C. Tyndall, R. Kamen, and F. Cuzin. 1981. The high affinity binding site on polyoma virus DNA for the viral large-T protein. *Nucleic Acids Res.* **9**: 5697.

Graessmann, A., M. Graessmann, R. Tjian, and W.C. Topp. 1980. Simian virus 40 small-t protein is required for loss of actin cable network in rat cells. *J. Virol.* **33**: 1182.

Houweling, A., P.J. van den Elsen, and A.J. van der Eb. 1980. Partial transformation of primary rat cells by the leftmost 4.5% fragment of adenovirus 5 DNA. *Virology* **105**: 537.

Ito, Y. 1980. Organization and expression of the genome of polyoma virus. In *Viral Oncology* (ed. G. Klein), p. 447. Raven Press, New York.

Kamen, R., J. Favaloro, J. Parker, R. Treisman, L. Lania, M. Fried, and A. Mellor. 1980. Comparison of polyoma virus transcription in productively infected mouse cells and transformed rodent cell lines. *Cold Spring Harbor Symp. Quant. Biol.* **44**: 63.

Kaplan, P.L. and B. Ozanne. 1982. Polyoma virus-transformed cells produce transforming growth factor(s) and grow in serum-free medium. *Virology* **123**: 372.

Land, H., L.F. Parada, and R.A. Weinberg. 1983. Tumorigenic conversion of primary embryo fibroblasts requires at least two cooperating oncogenes. *Nature* **304**: 596.

Nilsson, S.V. and G. Magnusson. 1983. T-antigen expression by polyoma mutants with modified RNA-splicing. *EMBO J.* (in press).

Rassoulzadegan, M., B. Binétruy, and F. Cuzin. 1982b. High frequency of gene transfer after fusion between bacteria and eukaryotic cells. *Nature* **295**: 257.

Rassoulzadegan, M., P. Gaudray, M. Canning, L. Trejo-Avila, and F. Cuzin. 1981. Two polyoma gene functions involved in the expression of the transformed phenotype in FR3T3 rat cells. I. Localization of a transformation maintenance function in the proximal half of the large-T coding region. *Virology* **114**: 489.

Rassoulzadegan, M., A. Cowie, A. Carr, N. Glaichenhaus, R. Kamen, and F. Cuzin. 1982a. The roles of individual polyoma virus early proteins in oncogenic transformation. *Nature* **300**: 713.

Rassoulzadegan, M., E. Mougneau, B. Perbal, P. Gaudray, F. Birg, and F. Cuzin. 1980. Host-virus interactions critical for cellular transformation by polyoma virus and simian virus 40. *Cold Spring Harbor Symp. Quant. Biol.* **44**: 333.

Rassoulzadegan, M., Z. Naghashfar, A. Cowie, A. Carr, M. Grisoni, R. Kamen, and F. Cuzin. 1983. Expression of the large T protein of polyoma virus promotes the establishment in culture of "normal" rodent fibroblast cells. *Proc. Natl. Acad. Sci.* **80**: 4354.

Rio, D., A. Robbins, R. Myers, and R. Tjian. 1980. Regulation of simian virus 40 early transcription *in vitro* by a purified tumor antigen. *Proc. Natl. Acad. Sci.* **77**: 5706.

Ruley, H.E. 1983. Adenovirus early region 1A enables viral and cellular transforming genes to transform primary cells in culture. *Nature* **304**: 602.

Seif, R. and F. Cuzin. 1977. Temperature-sensitive growth regulation in one type of transformed rat cells induced by the *tsa* mutant of polyoma virus. *J. Virol.* **24**: 721.

Smith, H., C. Scher, and G.J. Todaro. 1971. Induction of cell division in medium lacking serum growth factor by SV40. *Virology* **44**: 359.

Soeda, E., J.R. Arrand, N. Smolar, J.E. Walsh, and B.E. Griffin. 1979. Coding potential and regulatory signals of the polyoma virus genome. *Nature* **283**: 445.

Tjian, R. 1978. The binding site on SV40 DNA for a T antigen-related protein. *Cell* **13**: 165.

Todaro, G.J. and H. Green. 1963. Quantitative studies on the growth of mouse embryo cells in culture and their development into established lines. *J. Cell Biol.* **17**: 299.

Treisman, R., U. Novak, J. Favaloro, and R. Kamen. 1981. Transformation of rat cells by an altered polyoma virus genome expressing only the middle-T protein. *Nature* **292**: 595.

Trejo-Avila, L., P. Gaudray, and F. Cuzin. 1981. Two polyoma virus gene functions involved in the expression of the transformed phenotype in FR3T3 rat cells. II. The presence of the 56K middle-T protein in the cell membrane is not sufficient for maintenance. *Virology* **114**: 501.

Tyndall, C., G. La Mantia, C.M. Thacker, J. Favaloro, and R. Kamen. 1981. A region of the polyoma virus genome between the replication origin and late protein coding sequences is required in *cis* for both early gene expression and viral DNA replication. *Nucleic Acids Res.* **9**: 6231.

Van den Elsen, P.J., S. de Pater, A. Houweling, J. van der Veer, and A. van der Eb. 1982. The relationship between regions E1A and E1B of human adenoviruses and cell transformation. *Gene* **18**: 175.

Vogt, M. and R. Dulbecco. 1963. Steps in the neoplastic transformation of hamster embryo cells by polyoma virus. *Proc. Natl. Acad. Sci.* **49**: 171.

The Polyoma *hr-t* Gene—
An "Oncogene" with a Purpose

T.L. Benjamin

Department of Pathology, Harvard Medical School, Boston, Massachusetts 02115

The *hr-t* gene of polyoma virus represents a conditional, host-dependent function for virus growth. The block in *hr-t* mutant growth in normal mouse 3T3 cell lines results in virus yields on the order of a few percent of those of a wild-type viral infection. *hr-t* mutants grow nearly as well as the wild type in polyoma-transformed 3T3 cell lines and in certain primary mouse cell cultures. The *hr-t* function is also essential for efficient virus replication in the mouse, polyoma's natural host. The hypothesis put forward to explain the host-range behavior of these mutants proposes the existence of cellular permissive factors under control of the *hr-t* gene. *hr-t* mutants, therefore, replicate well only in those cell types that constitutively express these factors. The fact that *hr-t* mutants replicate poorly in the intact host indicates that permissive factor(s) are not expressed constitutively and must be induced by action of the *hr-t* gene in vivo.

The inability of *hr-t* mutants to induce the expression of cellular permissive factors results in a complete failure to induce cell transformation. Thus, the two aspects of the *hr-t* mutant phenotype—the conditional block in virus growth and the nonconditional block in transformation—are manifestations of the same genetic alteration. *hr-t* mutants encode a normal large T antigen but are defective in both small and middle T antigens; their mutations have been mapped within a segment of the viral DNA encoding an amino acid sequence of 112 residues shared by the small T and middle T proteins. Biological and molecular biological studies of *hr-t* mutants have recently been reviewed (Benjamin 1982).

The work reported here describes recent efforts to understand the roles of the small T and middle T proteins in the biological processes controlled by the *hr-t* viral gene. Experiments have taken two directions. The first concerns structure-function relationships involving the middle T antigen. The approach utilizes site-directed mutagenesis to construct mutants with specific alterations in middle T without affecting small T. The effects of these alterations on the various phosphorylation reactions involving middle T are examined, along with their biological effects in transformation. Studies with two mutants are described. One shows the importance of the carboxyterminal hydrophobic tail of the middle T protein in membrane association, in phosphorylation both in vitro and in vivo, and in cell transformation. The other confirms the importance of retaining Tyr-315, the major site of in vitro phosphorylation, for biological activity in transformation.

The second line of work concerns the natural role of the *hr-t* gene in the virus growth cycle. Results indicate that the *hr-t* function is required for encapsidation of viral minichromosomes, and that modifications of VP-1 may be essential for the process of virion assembly.

Methods of Experimental Procedures

In vitro mutagenesis
Procedures utilizing phage M13 cloning, priming with oligonucleotides, screening, and reconstruction of mutant viral genomes have been described (Carmichael et al. 1982).

Cell transformation
The F111 rat embryo fibroblast cell line has been used for focus and soft agar growth assays as described (Fluck and Benjamin 1979).

Analysis of virus assembly and VP-1 subspecies
Procedures involved in studying encapsidation of viral minichromosomes and two-dimensional gel analysis of VP-1 subspecies are described in Garcea and Benjamin (1983a).

Results

Middle T phosphorylation and the action of the *hr-t* gene in cell transformation
The various phosphorylation reactions involving polyoma middle T antigen are presumed to be important in the biological actions of the virus. Genetic evidence strongly suggests that these activities are crucial to the virus' ability to cause cell transformation (Benjamin 1982). To gain a better understanding of this relationship, we have used site-directed mutagenesis to construct viral mutants with specific alterations in the distal portion of the middle T protein, outside of the region shared with small T. This has been carried out with a subgenomic wild-type viral DNA fragment cloned into bacteriophage M13 as a template and synthetic oligonucleotides containing the desired mutations as primers. Two mutants with single base substitutions have been made and studied (see Fig. 1). Each mutant has been reconstructed along with a wild-type control derived from unmutated sequences in the recombinant phage. The presence of the single base-pair difference has been confirmed in each case by DNA sequencing.

Membrane association mediated by the carboxyterminal portion of middle T is essential for cell transformation as well as for phosphorylation in vivo and in vitro
Py-1387-T contains a C $\rightarrow$ T transition at nucleotide position 1387 (see Fig. 1, top). The consequence of this

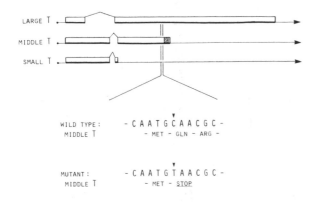

WILD TYPE:
MIDDLE T
- C A A T G C A A C G C -
- MET - GLN - ARG -

MUTANT:
MIDDLE T
- C A A T G T A A C G C -
- MET - STOP

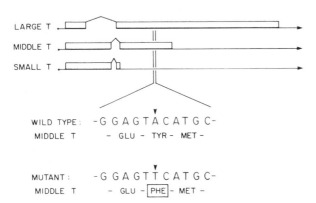

WILD TYPE:
MIDDLE T
- G G A G T A C A T G C -
- GLU - TYR - MET -

MUTANT:
MIDDLE T
- G G A G T T C A T G C -
- GLU - PHE - MET -

Figure 1 Oligonucleotide mutagenesis of middle T antigen. (*Top*) Py-1387-T has a "stop" codon at position 385, upstream from the hydrophobic tail (▨). (*Bottom*) Py-1178-T has tyrosine replaced by phenylalanine at position 315.

mutation is introduction of a TAA "stop" codon in place of a CAA glutamine codon in the middle T protein, 37 amino acids in from the carboxyl terminus (Carmichael et al. 1982). In the overlapping large T frame, there is a change of alanine (GCA) to valine (GTA); this change has no effect on large T function in viral DNA synthesis, since mutant and wild-type viruses grow equally well on a variety of mouse cell lines.

Py-1387-T induces a truncated (51K) middle T protein which is found almost exclusively in the soluble (cytosol) fraction of infected cells, rather than in membrane fractions as first observed for the wild-type middle T (Ito et al. 1977). The carboxyterminal portion of middle T, lacking in the mutant, contains a stretch of 22 uncharged, largely hydrophobic amino acids that presumably mediates membrane attachment. Similar sequences are found in membrane-spanning segments of viral and cellular glycoproteins; however, unlike these proteins, middle T lacks an aminoterminal "signal" sequence and inserts posttranslationally with its aminoterminal portion facing the cytoplasm (Schaffhausen et al. 1982a).

Py-1387-T fails to induce morphological transformation of F111 cells and fails to induce growth of these cells in soft agar. The consequences of the mutation in terms of phosphorylation are equally profound. The 51K middle T protein completely lacks the tyrosine-specific activity measured in immune precipitates, and also fails to be phosphorylated in vivo by the kinase that normally produces the 58K "active" form of middle T. Since both the tyrosine and the serine/threonine sites are present in the mutant protein, the failure of these phosphorylation reactions to occur presumably results from the failure of the protein to become membrane associated. A small amount of incorporation of [^{32}P]orthophosphate into the 51K protein occurs in vivo, and this appears to be exclusively at the site of phosphorylation of the 56K species (Carmichael et al. 1982).

Substitution of Tyr-315 by phenylalanine in middle T drastically weakens the virus in transformation

Py-1178-T contains an A → T transversion, the sole consequence of which is to replace tyrosine at residue 315 by phenylalanine (see Fig. 1, bottom). Tyr-315 is considered to be the major site of phosphorylation of middle T in the immune complex assay based on the following observations. The middle T antigens of a variety of deletion strains were analyzed using a two-dimensional partial proteolysis mapping procedure. The major in vitro phosphorylation, known to be on tyrosine (Eckhart et al. 1979), is contained in an 18K carboxyterminal peptide produced by cleavage with *Staphylococcus aureus* V8 protease (Schaffhausen and Benjamin 1981a,b). This peptide contains two tyrosines, at positions 315 and 322. In mutants dl1013 and dl1014, the tyrosine at 322 is deleted and yet the mutants transform well and show strong in vitro kinase activity (Magnusson and Berg 1979; Schaffhausen and Benjamin 1981a). A second line of evidence comes from use of an antiserum prepared against a nonapeptide with a sequence matching that of the Tyr-315 region of middle T (residues 311–319). Immune precipitates of wild-type middle T made with this antiserum show virtually no kinase activity. Activity is recovered following dissociation of the immune complexes with a soluble nonapeptide (Schaffhausen et al. 1982b).

By constructing Py-1178-T encoding phenylalanine instead of tyrosine at position 315, we hoped to preserve maximally the character of the wild-type middle T protein while preventing phosphorylation at this site (G.G. Carmichael et al., in prep.). The mutant retains a detectable level of middle T-associated kinase activity in vitro, corresponding to roughly 20% that of the wild-type control. Mapping of the in vitro phosphorylated mutant protein by proteolytic and chemical cleavage indicates that the residual activity is primarily on Tyr-322 (G.G. Carmichael et al., in prep). The mutant protein shows normal 56K and 58K in vivo phosphorylation.

Tests for transformation comparing Py-1178-T with its wild-type counterpart, Py-1178-A, show a drastic reduction in the ability of the mutant to transform. Foci appear in mutant-infected cultures, but at significantly later times and at a reduced frequency compared with the wild-type control (see Table 1). The efficiency of

Table 1 Test for Transformation of Rat Cells by Py-1178-A and Py-1178-T

| Virus | Input (pfu) | Foci | | | Agar |
		7 days	10 days	14 days	14 days
Py-1178-A	2×10^6	40	>50	>100	>100
	1×10^5	5	60	80	30
	5×10^3	0	3	4	2
Py-1178-T	6×10^7	0	0	8	0
	6×10^6	0	1	2	0

F111 rat embryo cells were infected with either the wild-type virus Py-1178-A (encoding tyrosine at residue 315) or mutant virus Py-1178-T (encoding phenylalanine) at the indicated input titer (pfu). Cultures were trypsinized 24 hr later and replated both on plastic in Dulbecco's medium with 5% calf serum and in soft agar. Counts of foci were made by microscopic examination at 7, 10, and 14 days after replating, and clones in soft agar were counted at 14 days. Foci induced by the mutant Py-1178-T were small compared with those induced by the wild-type virus. See also Fig. 2.

transformation by the mutant is two to three orders of magnitude less than the wild type in focus assays. Furthermore, the mutant foci are small and qualitatively "weak," and require microscopic examination to detect efficiently (see Fig. 2). Cells within the typical mutant focus grow less densely, are more adherent, and retain a more bipolar shape than their wild-type-transformed counterparts. Py-1178-T is even more defective when compared with Py-1178-A in soft agar growth assays (see Table 1). Rare colonies can be seen, however. Mutant foci grown out and tested in soft agar initially fail to grow, but eventually may give rise to variants that do grow.

VP-1 modification and the action of the *hr-t* gene in productive infection

The conditional host-dependent growth properties of *hr-t* mutants result from a failure of the mutants to induce the appearance of cellular permissive factors essential to the virus growth cycle (Goldman and Benjamin 1975; Staneloni et al. 1977; Benjamin 1982). Only when infecting cells that constitutively express these factors do *hr-t* mutants replicate well. Recent experiments have been directed toward understanding the basis of the poor growth characteristic of *hr-t* mutants in nonpermissive hosts such as 3T3 cells. Results, which are summarized below, indicate that the defect occurs not at the level of synthesis of virion components but rather in assembly of the components into infectious viral particles. Furthermore, the block in assembly is accompanied by a failure to generate modified forms of the major capsid protein VP-1 that are apparently required for encapsidation of the viral minichromosome (Garcea and Benjamin 1983a,b).

hr-t mutants are "early" mutants with a "late" phenotype

hr-t mutants make 30–40% as much viral DNA as wild-type virus and a normal amount of capsid proteins in 3T3 cells, yet they produce only a few percent as many infectious particles as wild type. When analyzed by sedimentation of [³H]thymidine-labeled nucleoprotein complexes, the mutants show accumulation of replicating (95S) and mature (75S) minichromosomes that fail to undergo transition to virion structures (240S). The failure to encapsidate minichromosomes is a defect readily complemented in *trans*, achieved by coinfection with wild-type virus.

The block in encapsidation is accompanied by a failure to generate modified forms of VP-1

VP-1 extracted from wild-type infected 3T3 cells can be resolved into at least four subspecies by conventional two-dimensional gel electrophoresis. In contrast, *hr-t* mutant-infected cells show VP-1 in a predominantly unmodified form. The following observations taken together suggest that VP-1 modifications may be essential for virus assembly: (1) modified forms of VP-1 are present with a fixed stoichiometry in purified virions of both mutant and wild type. (2) *hr-t* mutants by themselves generate only small amounts of the modified VP-1 subspecies and a proportionately small yield of infectious particles. However, upon infection of permissive cells, or upon coinfection of nonpermissive cells along with wild-type virus, normal amounts of modified VP-1 are made and *hr-t* mutant minichromosomes are efficiently assembled into viral particles. (3) Mutants with temperature-sensitive lesions in VP-1 produce modified subspecies in normal amounts and yet fail to assemble (Garcea et al. 1983a). (4) In vitro translation of late polyoma mRNA gives rise to modified forms of VP-1 (Hunter and Gibson 1978). The latter two findings indicate that VP-1 modifications depend on a functional *hr-t* gene and occur before incorporation into virions.

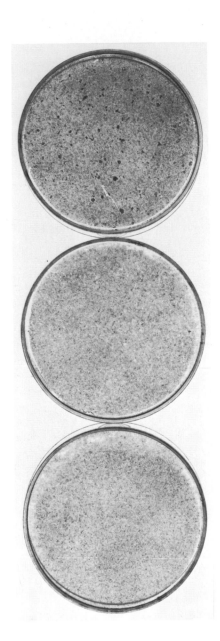

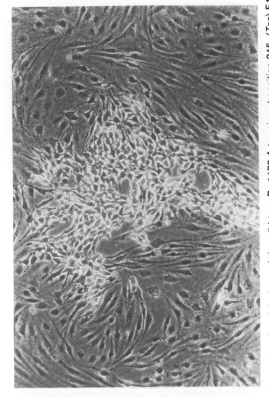

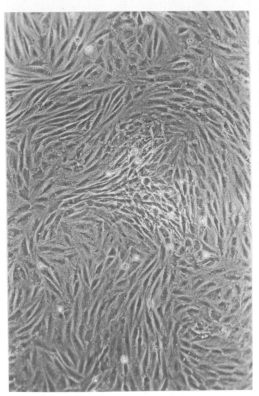

Figure 2 Focus assay for transformation comparing Py-1178-T and Py-1178-A. The mutant PY-1178-T contains phenylalanine and the wild-type Py-1178-A tyrosine at position 315. *(Top)* F111 rat embryo fibroblast cultures. *(Left)* Mock-infected; *(center)* infected with 5 × 10⁶ pfu Py-1178-T; *(right)* infected with 2 × 10⁵ pfu Py-1178-A. *(Bottom)* Microscopic appearance of typical foci induced by Py-1178-T *(left)* and Py-1178-A *(right)*. Magnification, 125×, phase.

Modifications of VP-1 include phosphorylation and acetylation

Two of the VP-1 variants can be labeled with [³²P]orthophosphate. Both phosphoserine and phosphothreonine are found following acid hydrolysis. [¹⁴C]Acetate appears to label primarily one of the four variants that is not labeled by ³²P (R.L. Garcea et al., in prep.).

Small T antigen may suffice for generating modified VP-1 subspecies and for normal growth in 3T3 cells

Py-1387-T encodes normal small T and large T antigens, but is defective for middle T antigen (see Fig. 1). This mutant resembles wild-type virus in its growth on 3T3 cells and in its ability to generate the modified subspecies of VP-1. Similar results have been obtained with RX-3, a defective mutant encoding only a normal small T antigen and replicating in the presence of an *hr-t* mutant helper to provide large T function (R.L. Garcea et al., in prep.). Restoration of small T alone to an *hr-t* mutant lacking both small T and middle T is apparently sufficient to overcome the encapsidation defect in 3T3 cells; it is not clear, however, whether small T suffices for growth in the animal.

Discussion

Protein modification reactions are fundamental to the biological actions of the *hr-t* gene, providing a common theme that unites the seemingly disparate roles of this gene in virus growth and cell transformation. Several manifestations of protein modification have been traced to the *hr-t* gene: phosphorylation of middle T in vivo involving serine and/or threonine at two distinct sites (Schaffhausen and Benjamin 1981a); phosphorylation of middle T on tyrosine in vitro (Eckhart et al. 1979); phosphorylation of VP-1 on serine and threonine, and acetylation of VP-1 (R.L. Garcea et al., in prep.); and hyperacetylation of encapsidated histones H3 and H4 (Schaffhausen and Benjamin 1976). Apart from phosphorylation of the 56K form of middle T antigen in vivo, all of the above modifications either fail to occur or occur at significantly reduced levels with *hr-t* mutants.

Curiously, there is no evidence to suggest that either small T or middle T antigen directly carries out any of these modifications. The middle T protein apparently lacks intrinsic ATP-binding ability (Schaffhausen et al. 1982a), and the middle T gene can be expressed in *Escherichia coli* without associated kinase activity (K. Palme and W. Eckhart, in prep.; B.S. Schaffhausen et al., in prep.). The origins and sequences of action of the various kinases that act on middle T are not fully known. However, based in part on evidence from *hr-t* mutant NG-59, Py-1387-T, and Py-1178-T, the following sequence may be suggested. Some molecules of middle T are phosphorylated on a serine or threonine by a cellular kinase during or soon after synthesis on "free" polysomes. The middle T antigens of all three mutants are phosphorylated at the "56K" site in this manner. This phosphorylation has no recognized function. Following insertion into some membrane component, a small fraction of middle

T molecules is phosphorylated at a different serine or threonine site by the "58K kinase," producing the more active form of middle T in the in vitro kinase assay. Phosphorylation of middle T at the 58K site by this enzyme may promote the association of middle T with one or more cellular tyrosine-specific kinases at the membrane. The recent demonstration of *c-src* in middle T immunoprecipitates makes this protein a likely candidate for the activity seen in the in vitro assay (Courtneidge and Smith 1983). Results with Py-1178-T indicate the importance of an interaction in vivo between the 315–322 region of middle T and a tyrosine kinase. Interaction of activated middle T with *c-src* or other kinase may stimulate the activity of the latter or alter its substrate specificity.

Based on the maturation studies with *hr-t* mutants, polyoma small T antigen may play a role in VP-1 modification and virus assembly. As in the case of middle T antigen, this action is indirect, implying a regulatory rather than an enzymatic function of small T. The enzymes that modify VP-1 are cellular, and most likely correspond to the putative cellular permissive factors through which the *hr-t* gene controls virus growth (Goldman and Benjamin 1975; Staneloni et al. 1977). How the *hr-t* gene products bring about the VP-1 modifications needed for virus assembly remains obscure.

Although current results suggest a distinct separation in the roles of the small T and middle T proteins, the possibility remains that these two related viral proteins cooperate and interact in some manner in the processes of virus growth and persistence in the intact host and tumorigenesis (Benjamin 1982). Neoplastic transformation, unrelated per se to virus growth, may be considered an accidental consequence of the strategy used in polyoma virus assembly which requires the setting into play of a series of protein modification reactions involving host components and leading to VP-1 as a final target. In the "all pentamer" model of the polyoma capsid, three different bonding patterns between VP-1 monomers are evident (Rayment et al. 1982), and the generation of chemically modified forms of VP-1 may be required in the assembly of the particle (Klug 1983).

Acknowledgments

This work has been supported by grants 19567 and 25390 from the National Cancer Institute.

References

Benjamin, T.L. 1982. The hr-t gene of polyoma virus. *Biochim. Biophys. Acta* **695**: 69.

Carmichael, G.G., B.S. Schaffhausen, D.I. Dorsky, D.B. Oliver, and T.L. Benjamin. 1982. Carboxy terminus of polyoma middle-sized tumor antigen is required for attachment to membranes, associated protein kinase activities, and cell transformation. *Proc. Natl. Acad. Sci.* **79**: 3579.

Courtneidge, S. and A. Smith. 1983. Polyoma virus transforming protein associates with the product of the c-src cellular gene. *Nature* **303**: 435.

Eckhart, W., M.A. Hutchinson, and T. Hunter. 1979. An activity phosphorylating tyrosine in polyoma T antigen immunoprecipitates. *Cell* **18**: 925.

Fluck, M. and T.L. Benjamin. 1979. Comparisons of two early

gene functions essential for transformation in polyoma virus and SV40. *Virology* **96**: 205.

Garcea, R.L. and T.L. Benjamin. 1983a. Host range transforming gene of polyoma virus plays a role in virus assembly. *Proc. Natl. Acad. Sci.* **80**: 3613.

Garcea, R.L. and T.L. Benjamin. 1983b. Isolation and characterization of polyoma nucleoprotein complexes. *Virology* **130**: 65.

Goldman, E. and T.L. Benjamin. 1975. Analysis of host range of non-transforming polyoma virus mutants. *Virology* **66**: 372.

Hunter T. and W. Gibson. 1978. Characterization of the mRNAs for the polyoma virus capsid proteins VP-1, VP-2 and VP-3. *J. Virol.* **28**: 240.

Ito, Y., J. Brocklehurst, and R. Dulbecco. 1977. Virus-specific proteins in the plasma membranes of cells lytically infected or transformed by polyoma virus. *Proc. Natl. Acad. Sci.* **74**: 4666.

Klug, A. 1983. Architectural design of spherical viruses. *Nature* **303**: 378.

Magnusson, G. and P. Berg. 1979. Construction and analysis of viable deletion mutants of polyoma virus. *J. Virol.* **32**: 523.

Rayment, I., T. Baker, D. Caspar, and W. Murakami. 1982. Polyoma virus capsid structure at 22.5 Å resolution. *Nature* **295**: 110.

Schaffhausen, B.S. and T.L. Benjamin. 1976. Deficiency in histone acetylation in non-transforming host range mutants of polyoma virus. *Proc. Natl. Acad. Sci.* **73**: 213.

―――. 1981a. Comparison of phosphorylation of two polyoma virus middle T antigens *in vivo* and *in vitro*. *J. Virol.* **40**: 184.

―――. 1981b. Protein kinase activity associated with polyoma virus middle T antigens. *Cold Spring Harbor Conf. Cell Proliferation.* **8**: 1281.

Schaffhausen, B.S., H. Dorai, G. Arakere, and T.L. Benjamin. 1982a. Studies of polyoma virus middle T antigen—Relationship to cell membranes and apparent lack of ATP binding activity. *Mol. Cell. Biol.* **2**: 1187.

Schaffhausen, B.S., T.L. Benjamin, L. Pike, J. Casnellie, and E. Krebs. 1982b. Antibody to the nonapeptide NH_2-glu-glu-glu-glu-tyr-met-pro-met-glu-COOH is specific for polyoma middle T antigen and inhibits *in vitro* kinase activity. *J. Biol. Chem.* **257**: 12467.

Staneloni, R.J., M.M. Fluck, and T.L. Benjamin. 1977. Host range selection of transformation defective "hr-t" mutants of polyoma virus. *Virology* **77**: 598.

Tyrosine Phosphorylation and Polyoma Virus Middle T Protein

S.A. Courtneidge, B. Oostra, and A.E. Smith

Biochemistry Division, National Institute for Medical Research, Mill Hill, London NW7 1AA, England

Shortly after the discovery that $pp60^{v-src}$, the transforming protein of Rous sarcoma virus (RSV), had an associated kinase activity that could be detected in immunoprecipitates (Collett and Erikson 1978; Levinson et al. 1978), a similar activity was shown to be associated with middle T, the transforming protein of polyoma virus (Schaffhausen and Benjamin 1979; Smith et al. 1979). Subsequently, it was found that in both cases the kinase involved was unusual in that it phosphorylated tyrosine residues (Eckhart et al. 1979; Hunter and Sefton 1980). Since that time, overwhelming evidence has accumulated that the tyrosine kinase activity of $pp60^{v-src}$ is an intrinsic property of the protein itself and that the activity plays a crucial role in transformation by RSV (Bishop and Varmus 1982). Several other retroviral transforming proteins have also been shown to have tyrosine kinase activity, and cellular proteins with a similar activity have been identified (Bishop and Varmus 1982). These include the cellular homologs of some of the viral transforming proteins (such as $pp60^{c-src}$) and the cellular receptors for some growth factors (e.g., epidermal growth factor [EGF] and platelet-derived growth factor [PDGF]) and hormones (e.g., insulin) (Courtneidge 1984). Therefore, it seems established that tyrosine kinases play a role in transformation by retroviruses and in cellular regulation. By contrast, the relationship between polyoma virus and its associated kinase activity and the relevance of this association to transformation has proved much more difficult to elucidate.

There have been no reports that middle T protein synthesized in vitro or produced by genetic manipulation in bacterial cells has kinase activity, whereas similar experiments have been possible with $pp60^{v-src}$ (Erikson et al. 1978; Gilmer and Erikson 1981; McGrath and Levinson 1982). Similarly, there is no detectable increase in the abundance of phosphotyrosine in polyoma virus-transformed cells following transformation by polyoma virus (Sefton et al. 1980 and unpubl.). It has likewise proved difficult to detect phosphotyrosine on middle T protein isolated from cells, even though such a modification is readily detected following the in vitro kinase reaction (Smith et al. 1980). Although these findings raise doubts as to the role of tyrosine phosphorylation in transformation by middle T protein, they certainly do not exclude such a possibility. It is conceivable that an early event in the action of middle T does involve tyrosine phosphorylation on a regulatory protein but that, for example, the protein involved is present in such small amounts that the overall level of phosphotyrosine is not measurably altered, or the protein is not fractionated on two-dimensional gel systems and therefore goes undetected. Furthermore, the correlation between the transforming potential of different viral mutants and the kinase activity associated with the middle T protein they encode remains unexplained (Smith and Ely 1983).

We considered that if middle T is not a tyrosine kinase, it must specifically associate with such a cellular enzyme, at least in vitro, and that the identification of the cellular protein involved and its possible role in transformation warranted further investigation. Here we summarize our recent data which showed that middle T protein is associated with the cellular tyrosine kinase $pp60^{c-src}$ (Courtneidge and Smith 1983). We describe other studies below that probe the requirement for phosphorylation of middle T in transformation. By using in vitro mutagenesis to alter an in vitro phosphorylation site (Tyr-315), we found no change in the ability to transform cells. We interpreted these results to show that phosphorylation of middle T protein, at least at Tyr-315, is not essential (Oostra et al. 1983). We propose that transformation by middle T protein may result in part because association with middle T alters the activity or specificity of $pp60^{c-src}$, thus altering processes normally involved in the regulation of cellular proliferation.

Methods of Experimental Procedures

Cells and assays
Growth of the A2 strain of polyoma virus in 3T6 cells, conditions for labeling with [^{35}S]methionine, preparation of extracts, and origin of all antisera except that described below have been described (Smith et al. 1979, 1980; Courtneidge and Smith 1983). Kinase assays were performed as previously (Smith et al. 1979), except when assaying for $pp60^{c-src}$, which used a modified procedure (Courtneidge and Smith 1983). Conditions for partial proteolysis fingerprints and gel electrophoresis have been described in Smith et al. (1980).

Sucrose density analysis
Cells were infected with polyoma virus and approximately 42 hours after infection were labeled with [^{35}S]methionine for a further 4 hours. Preparation of lysates and sucrose density gradient centrifugation was as described (Courtneidge and Smith 1983), except to reduce the background of nonspecifically bound proteins, the immunoprecipitation protocol was made more stringent. Immunoprecipitates were formed as before and collected using *Staphylococcus aureus* that had pre-

viously been suspended in an extract of approximately 10^7 uninfected 3T6 cells and washed three times with RIPA buffer and once with Tris-buffered saline (TBS). Immunocomplexes were eluted from the immunoadsorbent in 4 M $MgCl_2$, 100 mM NaCl, 1 mM EDTA, 10 mM Tris (pH 7.2), and 1% NP-40. After centrifugation to remove the bacteria, the supernatant was adjusted to 0.25 M $MgCl_2$ by dilution; the immunocomplexes were collected by adsorption to a fresh sample of uninfected cell extract-adsorbed bacteria, washed once with RIPA buffer and once with TBS, and then eluted into sample buffer for electrophoresis in polyacrylamide gels.

Purification of middle T protein

3C3 wild-type, middle T-transformed Rat-1 cells (10^6) (B.K. Ely and A.E. Smith, in prep.) were injected intraperitoneally in 4-week old Fischer rats. Soft, *petit pois*-sized tumors developed, particularly on the mesentery, within 2–3 weeks. Tumors were washed, broken in a Waring Blendor, and homogenized in a loose-fitting glass homogenizer using TBS containing 0.5% NP-40, 1 mM EDTA, 1 mM dithiothreitol (DTT), and 1% trasylol. After standing 30 minutes on ice, the homogenate was centrifuged at 30,000 rpm for 30 minutes. The supernatant fraction was pretreated with *S. aureus* bacteria, made up to 0.5 M NaCl, and passed through a 2-ml Sepharose precolumn and a 1-ml column containing 10 mg of antibody to peptide C covalently attached to protein A-Sepharose, as described by Schneider et al. (1982). After extensive washing, the column was eluted with 2 ml of TBS containing 0.2% NP-40 and I mM peptide C. Fractions were made up to 10 mM $MnCl_2$ and after addition of 1 μCi [γ-^{32}P]ATP incubation was continued for 10 minutes at 30°C.

Peptide C corresponds to amino acids 311–329 of polyoma virus middle T protein. It was synthesized using the solid-phase Merrifield procedure, coupled to bovine serum albumin (BSA) via a carboxyterminal lysine, and antibody was raised in rabbits as described (Harvey et al. 1982). Specific antibody was purified by chromatography on peptide C-Sepharose.

Results

Middle T associates with pp60^{c-src}

The middle T-associated kinase activity is usually detected by addition of [^{32}P]ATP to washed immunoprecipitates, followed by analysis of the labeled proteins by polyacrylamide gel electrophoresis. Under those conditions, middle T protein itself becomes phosphorylated (see Fig. 1A, lane 2). We reasoned that if the kinase associated with middle T protein is a cellular protein it should be possible to detect the enzyme in immunoprecipitates of middle T. We tested for the presence of pp60^{c-src}, one of the few identified cellular tyrosine protein kinases. When serum from rabbits bearing RSV-induced tumors (TBR serum) was added to washed immunoprecipitates prior to kinase reaction, the phosphorylation of immunoglobulin (Ig) heavy chains, in addition to middle T, was detected (Fig. 1A, lane 4). Since the TBR serum used is known to have activity against

pp60^{c-src} (Opperman et al. 1979), we interpreted this result to mean that washed immunoprecipitates made using, for example, antiserum raised against polyoma virus-transformed cells (anti-T serum), contain pp60^{c-src}. Such a finding gave support to the notion that the kinase activity measured in vitro results at least in part from the presence of a cellular enzyme. Therefore, we sought further evidence to distinguish whether the activity was present because cross-reacting antibodies present in the antisera immunoprecipitate the two proteins separately, or because middle T protein and pp60^{c-src} form a stable complex, and, consequently, immunoprecipitation of one protein results in coprecipitation of at least a fraction of the other.

Several different antisera have now been tested in the assay to detect pp60^{c-src} described above. Perhaps the most convincing data come from the use of antisera raised against synthetic peptides corresponding to sequences from either middle T protein or pp60^{c-src}. Such experiments showed that, for example, an antibody raised against the carboxyterminal six amino acids of middle T (Walter et al. 1981) and extensively purified by immunoaffinity chromatography on peptide-Sepharose was able to immunoprecipitate the activity that phosphorylates TBR Ig as efficiently as anti-T serum. Such immunoprecipitation was inhibited by prior addition of synthetic peptide, indicating that the determinant recognized was the hexapeptide sequence from middle T protein. Such evidence argues strongly against the possibility that the results obtained reflect an activity in the antiserum against middle T that cross-reacts with pp60^{c-src} and favors the alternative explanation that a complex between middle T and pp60^{c-src} is present in extracts.

If this is the case, it should be possible to detect middle T protein in immunoprecipitates formed using antiserum to pp60^{c-src}. TBR serum was used to immunoprecipitate extracts from polyoma virus-transformed cells, and kinase assays were performed using the washed immunoprecipitates. As expected, pp60^{c-src} present in the immunoprecipitate phosphorylated the Ig heavy chain of the TBR serum but, in addition, middle T was also labeled (Fig. 1B, lane 2). Only the Ig heavy chain was phosphorylated in control cell extracts (Fig. 1B, lane 1), and in separate experiments the TBR serum failed to immunoprecipitate [^{35}S]methionine-labeled middle T synthesized in vitro (data not shown). The latter experiment argues that the TBR serum is not able to recognize middle T directly, again tending to exclude the possibility of a cross-reacting activity in the TBR serum.

Our interpretation of the kinase assays described above is illustrated in diagramatic fashion in Figure 1. In conventional middle T immunoprecipitates, a complex of middle T and pp60^{c-src} is attached to the *S. aureus* via the antibody to middle T. When ATP is added to the immunoprecipitate, the middle T protein is phosphorylated. Addition of TBR prior to kinase assay has the effect of adding another substrate for the pp60^{c-src} kinase, so that now both middle T and TBR Ig are labeled. Similarly, when pp60^{c-src} is immunoprecipitated from polyoma virus-transformed cells using TBR serum, the immunopre

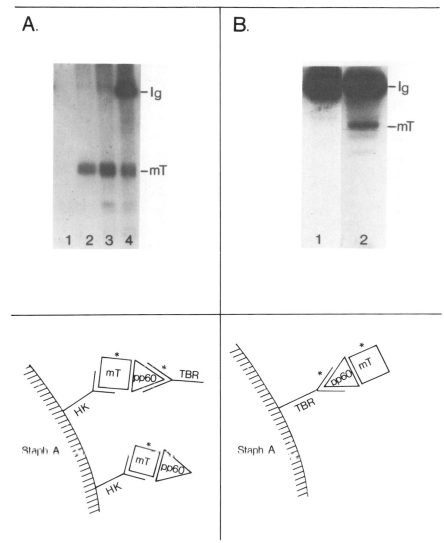

Figure 1 Kinase activities associated with middle T protein and pp60[c-src]. (*A*) (Lane *1*) Polyoma virus-transformed cells immunoprecipitated with normal hamster serum; (lane *2*) polyoma virus-transformed cells immunoprecipitated with hamster anti-T serum (HK
serum); (lane *3*) as lane *2* except normal rabbit serum added before assay; (lane *4*) as lane *2* except antibodies reactive against
pp60[c-src] (TBR serum) added before assay. (*B*) (Lane *1*) Rat-1 cells immunoprecipitated with TBR serum; (lane *2*) polyoma virus-
transformed cells immunoprecipitated with TBR serum. (*Lower half*) Schematic illustration of what we envisage to be happening in
the kinase reactions shown above. (Staph. A) *Staphylococcus aureus*; (HK) hamster anti-T serum; (TBR) tumor-bearing rabbit serum,
i.e. anti-pp60[c-src]; (mT) middle T antigen of polyoma virus; (pp60) pp60[c-src]; (*) radioactive phosphate covalently attached to the
proteins during the kinase assay.

cipitates also contain associated middle T. During the
kinase assay, both the TBR Ig and middle T become
phosphorylated. These results led us to seek further evidence for a complex between middle T and pp60[c-src].

Immunoprecipitation of middle T protein by antiserum
against pp60[c-src] and of pp60[c-src] by antiserum against
middle T can be achieved using extracts from [35]S- and
[32]P-labeled cells, consistent with the idea of a complex
between the two proteins (Courtneidge and Smith 1983).
This is also supported by sucrose density gradient analysis of the metabolically labeled proteins. We already
knew that the pp60[v-src] sedimented as a monomer (Levinson et al. 1980). Similar analysis of pp60[c-src] either
labeled with [35S]methionine (Fig. 2C) or by kinase as-

says (Courtneidge and Smith 1983), showed that it, too,
sedimented with an apparent molecular weight of approximately 60 kD. By contrast, pp60[c-src] from polyoma
virus-transformed cells sedimented over a broad area of
the gradient with fractions with apparent molecular
weights of approximately 60,000 and 220,000 detected
either by metabolic labeling (Fig. 2B) or by associated
kinase activity. Earlier analysis of both the fraction of
middle T able to accept phosphate in the kinase reaction
(Schaffhausen and Benjamin 1981a; Walter et al. 1982)
and the middle T-associated kinase able to phosphorylate rat Ig (Courtneidge and Smith 1983) showed an
apparent molecular weight of approximately 220,000.
Analysis of metabolically labeled extracts from polyoma

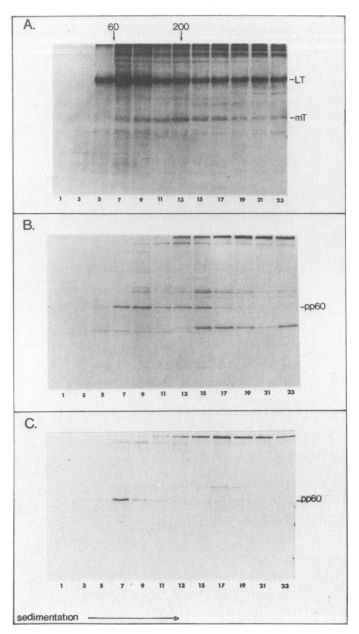

Figure 2 Sedimentation analysis of metabolically labeled middle T protein and pp60$^{c\text{-}src}$. (*A*) Polyoma virus-infected 3T6 cells immunoprecipitated with anti-T serum. (*B*) Polyoma virus-infected 3T6 cells immunoprecipitated with TBR serum. (*C*) Uninfected 3T6 cells immunoprecipitated with TBR serum.

virus-infected cells (Fig. 2A) showed a broad distribution of middle T across the gradient with a proportion of the protein sedimenting in the same region as the heavy fraction of pp60$^{c\text{-}src}$. Thus, transformation by polyoma virus is accompanied by a shift in the apparent molecular weight of a substantial fraction of pp60$^{c\text{-}src}$ to a heavier form that cosediments with the kinase-active fraction of middle T protein.

Purification of middle T protein

To assess the specificity and strength of binding of middle T protein and pp60$^{c\text{-}src}$, as well as to determine whether other proteins can also associate with middle T, we have attempted a purification of middle T protein. To do this,

we have made use of an antibody to a synthetic peptide (corresponding to amino acids 311–329 of middle T) which has the useful property of recognizing middle T in such a way that the bound protein is eluted in the presence of 1 mM peptide in nondenaturing buffers. The antibody was first immunoaffinity purified on peptide-Sepharose and then covalently attached to protein A-Sepharose. As a source of middle T, we used tumors generated in the peritoneal cavity of young rats in response to injected transformed cells. Middle T protein was eluted from the column using peptide and fractions tested for kinase activity in solution by addition of Mn^{++}/ATP. Figure 3A shows the elution profile obtained. Partial proteolysis (Fig. 3B) and two-dimensional finger

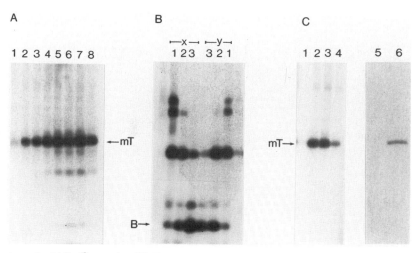

Figure 3 Partial purification of middle T protein. (*A*) Fractions (1–8) eluted from a 1-ml column of peptide antibody-protein A-Sepharose with 1 mM peptide, and assayed for kinase activity by addition of 10 mM Mn^{++} and 1 μCi [γ-^{32}P]ATP. (*B*) Partial proteolysis fingerprint of [^{32}P]middle T labeled in an immunoprecipitate kinase assay using crude extracts (x) and a solution kinase assay using pooled enriched middle T (y). B indicates the characteristic 18-kD carboxyterminal fragment. 1, 2, and 3 indicate addition of 0.01, 0.1, and 1 mg/ml V8 protease per slot. (*C*) [^{32}P]middle T was labeled in the solution kinase assay and immunoprecipitated with normal hamster serum (1), hamster anti-T serum (2), purified antibody raised against the carboxyterminal six amino acids of middle T (3), (4) as 3 but in the presence of 10 μg synthetic peptide, normal rabbit serum (5), TBR serum (6).

printing (data not shown) of the labeled protein showed it to be authentic middle T, bearing phosphate on tyrosine in the usual positions.

It is difficult to estimate the degree of purification. However, solid-phase kinase activity assays in immunoprecipitates of the material added to the column, the flowthrough, wash, and the eluted fractions indicate that the bulk of detectable kinase-active middle T is recovered in the peptide-eluted fraction. Measurements of the amount of protein in the eluted peak are complicated by the presence of the peptide. By separating the protein and peptide fractions on Sepharose G-50 and assuming a 100% recovery, an estimate of the purification as 5000-fold is obtained. Silver staining of polyacrylamide gels of the enriched fraction shows that several proteins are present, including one that is labeled in the kinase reaction and migrates in the position characteristic of middle T protein. Further purification is in progress and should allow us to determine which proteins are specifically bound to middle T.

When the enriched protein is labeled with [^{32}P]ATP and then fractionated on a sucrose gradient, the labeled fraction sediments rapidly with an apparent molecular weight of 220,000 (data not shown; see also Walter et al. 1982). The partially purified middle T protein is precipitated by all the antisera to middle T we have tested. As shown in Figure 3C, the enriched middle T is also precipitated by TBR serum, indicating that it remains associated with pp60$^{c\text{-}src}$. We take these results to mean that the complex between middle T and pp60$^{c\text{-}src}$ is retained throughout the enrichment procedure.

Tyr-315 and transformation

Irrespective of the identity of the kinase involved, we have asked whether the phosphorylation of middle T as

detected in vitro is a necessary step in the transformation process. To do this, we have used site-directed mutagenesis of cloned DNA coding for middle T. Experiments to establish the location of the tyrosine residue(s) in middle T that become phosphorylated rely on the analysis of ^{32}P-labeled middle T by partial proteolysis fingerprinting. Figure 4B shows an example in which wild-type middle T either metabolically labeled with [^{35}S]methionine or ^{32}P-labeled in vitro in the kinase reaction was digested with various amounts of V8 protease. Reproducible degradation patterns are produced and show that of two major, stable methionine-labeled fragments labeled A and B, only one (B) is labeled with [^{32}P]phosphate. Closer examination shows that the labeled fragment B migrates slightly more slowly than its methionine-labeled counterpart, and we return to this point later.

To map fragments A and B, similar analysis was performed with [^{35}S]methionine-labeled middle T species specified by various deletion mutants. Figure 4A shows an example using *dl*8 and *dl*23 (Griffin and Maddock 1979), which indicates that a band of similar mobility to fragment A is shared by wild-type and both mutant species, whereas a band with mobility similar to fragment B is present in wild-type and *dl*8 but lacking in *dl*23. If it is assumed that the V8 cleavage sites are unaltered by the presence of the deletions, then from the known positions of the deletions in the mutants used, we can conclude that fragment A originates from the aminoterminal half of middle T. Consistent with this, analysis of middle T labeled with [^{35}S]cysteine (which by chance is present almost exclusively in the aminoterminal domain) and [^{35}S]fmet-tRNA$_F$ (which labels only the aminoterminal residue) shows that only fragment A is labeled under these conditions (data not shown). Fragment B is probably from the carboxyterminal half of middle T pro-

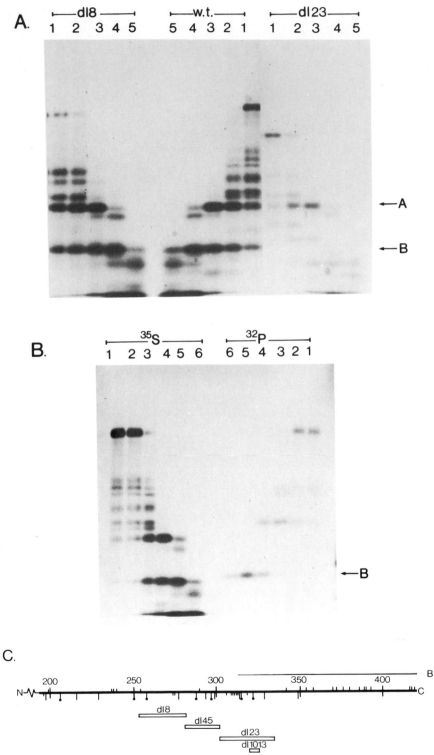

Figure 4 Partial proteolysis fingerprints of different middle T antigens. (*A*) [³⁵S]methionine-labeled middle T from wild-type, *dl*8, and *dl*23 infected cells was treated with increasing amounts of V8 protease; (lanes *1–5*) 5 μl, 0.001, 0.01, 0.1, 1.0, and 10 mg/ml protease per slot. (*B*) Wild-type middle T from infected cells either metabolically labeled with [³⁵S]methionine or labeled with ³²P in immunoprecipitates using [γ-³²P]ATP was treated with (lanes *1–6*) 5 μl, 0, 0.001, 0.01, 0.1, 1.0, and 10 mg/ml V8 protease per slot. (*C*) Schematic representation of the carboxyterminal half of middle T showing regions deleted in mutants mentioned in the text, and the likely origin of V8 protease fragment B. (Knobs) Position of tyrosine residues; (long downward bars) glutamic acid residues likely to be cleavage sites for V8 protease; (short downward bars) glutamic acid residues less likely to be cleavage sites; (upward bars) lysine and arginine residues; the numbers refer to amino acids in middle T.

tein. Since *dl*45 middle T (Bendig et al. 1980) also generates the normal-sized fragment B (data not shown), the cleavage site to produce fragment B is probably downstream of the deletions in *dl*8 and *dl*45 and present within the sequences deleted in *dl*23 (Fig. 4C).

To map the phosphorylation sites within middle T protein, similar analysis of mutant ^{32}P-labeled middle T species has been performed. Making the further assumption that the phosphorylation sites on the mutant middle T species are unaltered, it can be deduced that Tyr-315 is a phosphorylation site, since there are only two tyrosine residues (315 and 322) downstream of the deletion of *dl*45 and mutants (e.g., *dl*1013 and *dl*1014, Magnusson et al. 1981) that lack Tyr-322 still accept phosphate (Fig. 4C). We should emphasize, however, that this conclusion is dependent on the validity of the assumptions mentioned and does not exclude the possibility of phosphorylation at other sites in middle T. Schaffhausen and Benjamin (1981b) also concluded that Tyr-315 is a phosphorylation site in middle T.

In spite of the reservations, Tyr-315 is interesting because it is preceded by a tract of six glutamic acid residues that bears sequence homology to a sequence in pp60^{v-src} preceding a tyrosine that is phosphorylated (Smart et al. 1981) and to a sequence in the polypeptide hormone, gastrin, preceding a tyrosine that is sulfated (Baldwin 1982). Furthermore, all deletion mutants so far reported that lack Tyr-315 and part of the surrounding region are defective in transformation, whereas those that flank the region are transformation competent (Smith and Ely 1983). These considerations led us to probe the sequence requirements in this area in more detail.

A family of mutations (Table 1) around the glutamic acid tract, including one in which Tyr-315 was converted to phenylalanine, were produced using deletion loop mutagenesis and oligonucleotide-directed mutagenesis (Oostra et al. 1983). All the mutants retained the ability to transform cells, as judged by the production of foci overlaying a monolayer of Rat-1 cells following transfection with plasmid DNAs using the calcium phosphate technique. The transformed cells grew in agar with high cloning efficiency and produced tumors in young rats. Control experiments to probe the integrated DNA con-

firmed that cells transformed by the mutant lacking Tyr-315 do indeed contain mutant DNA sequences. We interpret these results to mean that phosphorylation of Tyr-315 is not an essential step in the transformation process, nor in the production of tumors in animals.

Surprisingly, we found that all the middle T species from the mutant transformed cell lines retained the ability to accept phosphate in the kinase reaction (e.g., Fig. 5A). In the case of the mutant lacking Tyr-315, this result must mean that other tyrosines are labeled. Partial proteolysis fingerprints of the mutant middle T showed that a band of mobility similar to fragment B remained labeled (Fig. 5B), suggesting that because Tyr-315 was absent Tyr-322 must be labeled, since it is the only tyrosine residue present. Fragment B produced by the mutant has a slightly increased mobility reminiscent of that seen above when ^{35}S- and ^{32}P-wild-type-labeled fragments B were compared (see also Oostra et al. 1983).

V8 protease is reported to cleave to the carboxyterminal side of glutamic acid residues except those followed by proline or glutamic acid (Houmard and Drapeau 1972). Thus, if the V8 cleavage site to produce fragment B is downstream of the deletion in *dl*45, the most likely site is the bond after Glu-314 (Fig. 4C). If this were the case, wild-type fragment B would have tyrosine at its amino terminus. We suggest that the reduced mobility of wild-type ^{32}P-labeled fragment B is caused by phosphorylation at the amino terminus. If this explanation is correct, with the mutant lacking Tyr-315 (where phosphate can no longer be present at the amino terminus), the mobility of fragment B would be expected to revert to normal, as indeed was found to be the case.

Further evidence that Tyr-322 is phosphorylated comes from two-dimensional tryptic fingerprint analysis of ^{32}P-labeled middle T (R. Harvey et al., in prep., unpubl.) and from cyanogen bromide fragment analysis (B. Schaffhausen, pers. comm.). Recently, we and others (T. Hunter, pers. comm.) have obtained other evidence that Tyr-250 of middle T protein is also phosphorylated in the kinase reaction.

Discussion

We consider that together the evidence presented here and previously established the existence of the complex between middle T and pp60^{c-src}. This finding leads us to doubt whether middle T protein has an intrinsic tyrosine kinase activity, and to suggest as an alternative that the middle T-associated activity measured in vitro reflects the presence of bound pp60^{c-src}.

Many questions remain to be answered about the complex between middle T protein and pp60^{c-src}. From the apparent molecular weight of the complex, it is possible that other proteins are also present. So far, we have no evidence for such proteins. We also do not know whether the complex exists in cells. It is stable in vitro to a wide variety of buffers containing different concentrations of salts, detergents, and chelating agents, but direct evidence for the presence of complex in cells is difficult to obtain.

Table 1 Family of Mutations around Glutamic Acid Tract

pAS101	Glu. Glu. Glu. Glu. Glu. Glu. Tyr. Met. Pro. Met
pAS131	——————————————— Phe —————
pAS132	——————————————— Ile —————
pAS133	——————————— Lys ——— Ile —————
pAS134	———————————Lys. Lys. ———————
pAS135	——————— Lys ———————————
pAS136	Lys ———— Lys. Lys. Lys———————
pAS137	———— Lys ——————— Ile ———

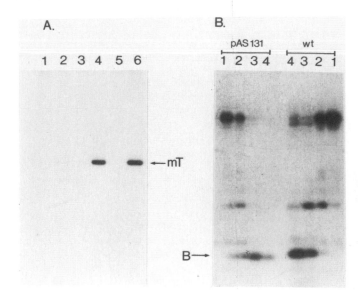

Figure 5 Kinase activity associated with middle T from cells infected with a mutant lacking Tyr-315. (*A*) Kinase reactions were performed on immunoprecipitates of extracts from uninfected (lanes *1* and *2*), wild-type (lanes *3* and *4*), pAS131-transformed cells (lanes *5* and *6*), and the labeled proteins separated by gel electrophoresis. (Lanes *1, 3,* and *5*) Normal hamster serum; (lanes *2, 4,* and *6*) hamster anti-T serum. (*B*) Partial proteolysis fingerprints of the middle T from wild-type and pAS131-transformed cells (lanes *1–4*) produced by addition of 5 μl, 0, 0.01, 0.1, and 1.0 mg/ml V8 protease per slot.

Perhaps the most important question about the complex is its relevance to transformation. The only evidence available at present is the correlation between the presence of associated pp60$^{c\text{-}src}$ and the transforming potential of various mutant middle T species. All mutants tested that have the ability to transform have been found to have associated pp60$^{c\text{-}src}$, whereas several that lack transforming activity (such as the *hr-t* mutant SD15; Carmichael and Benjamin 1980) have no associated pp60$^{c\text{-}src}$ (unpubl. results). Some transformation-defective mutants (such as *dl*23) retain bound pp60$^{c\text{-}src}$. However, we know of no example of a mutant that does transform but does not have associated pp60$^{c\text{-}src}$. If the complex is important in transformation, we would predict this phenotype is impossible. We are currently testing this hypothesis by creating new deletion and point mutations within middle T and testing for the ability to bind and to transform.

The evidence summarized here suggests that phosphorylation of middle T, at least on Tyr-315, is not essential in transformation. Previous deletion mutants have already shown that four of the other five tyrosine residues in the carboxyterminal unique portion of middle T can be removed in one mutant or another without loss of transforming activity (Smith and Ely 1983). Recently, however, we have shown that the remaining tyrosine residue in the carboxyterminal half, at position 250, is phosphorylated in vitro. We have subsequently changed this residue to phenylalanine by oligonucleotide-directed mutagenesis, and the biological properties of the mutant are currently being studied. If the mutant does transform, we will be forced to conclude either that phosphorylation occurs either in the aminoterminal half of middle T or at any of the sites in the carboxyterminal half with no particular specificity. We find the latter suggestions unat-tractive and tentatively conclude that phosphorylation is not important.

Further studies are required to establish whether any properties of middle T or of polyoma virus itself are affected by the alteration of Tyr-315 and surrounding region. Our experiments have only involved calcium phosphate transfection of plasmid DNAs containing middle T-coding sequences into Rat-1 cells, under a limited range of conditions. Although there is no doubt that it is possible to obtain tumors in rats containing middle T that lacks Tyr-315, it is conceivable that when tested as reconstructed virus or using different cell types the Tyr-315 minus mutant may reveal a measurably different phenotype.

Our present working hypothesis, based on the work summarized here, is that the complex between middle T protein and pp60$^{c\text{-}src}$ is directly involved in transformation by polyoma virus. We do not know the function of the complex but we do not believe that phosphorylation of middle T by pp60$^{c\text{-}src}$ plays any role. Because pp60$^{c\text{-}src}$ is conserved, at least from *Drosophila* to man (Shilo and Weinberg 1981; Bishop and Varmus 1982), we assume it is functionally important. Because production of a slightly altered form of the protein, as occurs in cells infected with RSV (which codes for pp60$^{v\text{-}src}$) leads to cellular transformation, we assume that the function of the protein is in some aspect of the regulation of cellular proliferation. We predict, therefore, that by binding to pp60$^{c\text{-}src}$, middle T protein perturbs either the activity or the specificity of pp60$^{c\text{-}src}$, and this somehow results in increased cellular proliferation.

Acknowledgments

We thank Peter Gillett, Yvette Hartley, Rob Harvey, and Ros Smith for technical assistance.

References

Baldwin, G.S. 1982. Gastrin and the transforming protein of polyoma virus have evolved from a common ancestor. *FEBS Lett.* **137**: 1.

Bendig, M., T. Thomas, and W. Folk. 1980. Viable deletion mutant in the medium and large-T antigen coding sequences of the polyoma virus genome. *J. Virol.* **33**: 1215.

Bishop, J.M. and H.E. Varmus. 1982. Functions and origins of retroviral transforming genes. In *Molecular biology of tumor viruses* 2nd edition: *RNA tumor viruses* (ed. R. Weiss et al.). Cold Spring Harbor Laboratory, Cold Spring Harbor, New York.

Carmichael, G.C. and T.L. Benjamin. 1980. Identification of DNA sequence changes leading to loss of transforming ability in polyoma virus. *J. Biol. Chem.* **255**: 230.

Collett, M.S. and R.L. Erikson. 1978. Protein kinase activity associated with the avian sarcoma virus src gene product. *Proc. Natl. Acad. Sci.* **75**: 2021.

Courtneidge, S.A. 1984. The phosphorylation of tyrosyl residues. In *The enzymology of post-translational modification of proteins* (ed. R.B. Freedman and H.C. Hawkins), vol. 2. Academic Press, London. (In press.)

Courtneidge, S.A. and A.E. Smith. 1983. Polyoma virus transforming protein associates with the product of the c-*src* cellular gene. *Nature* **303**: 435.

Eckhart, W., M.A. Hutchinson, and T. Hunter. 1979. An activity phosphorylating tyrosine in polyoma T antigen immunoprecipitates. *Cell* **18**: 925.

Erikson, R., M. Collett, and R.L. Erikson. 1978. *In vitro* synthesis of a functional ASV transforming gene product. *Nature* **274**: 919.

Gilmer, T. and R.L. Erikson. 1981. The Rous sarcoma virus transforming protein pp60*src* expressed in *E. coli* functions as a protein kinase. *Nature* **294**: 771.

Griffin, B.E. and C. Maddock. 1979. New classes of viable deletion mutants in the early region of polyoma virus. *J. Virol.* **31**: 645.

Harvey, R., R. Faulkes, P. Gillett, N. Lindsay, E. Paucha, A. Bradbury, and A.E. Smith. 1982. An antibody to a synthetic peptide that recognises SV40 small-t antigen. *EMBO J.* **1**: 473.

Houmard, J. and G.R. Drapeau. 1972. Staphylococcal protease: A proteolytic enzyme specific for glutamoyl bonds. *Proc. Natl. Acad. Sci.* **69**: 3506.

Hunter, T. and B. Sefton. 1980. Transforming gene product of Rous sarcoma virus phosphorylates tyrosine. *Proc. Natl. Acad. Sci.* **77**: 1311.

Levinson, A.D., H. Oppermann, L. Levintow, H.E. Varmus, and J.M. Bishop. 1978. Evidence that the transforming gene of ASV encodes a protein kinase associated with a phosphoprotein. *Cell* **45**: 561.

Levinson, A.D., H. Oppermann, H.E. Varmus, and J.M. Bishop. 1980. The purified product of the transforming gene of avian sarcoma virus phosphorylates tyrosine. *J. Biol. Chem.* **255**: 11973.

Magnusson, G., M.J. Nilsson, S.M. Dilworth, and N. Smolar. 1981. Characterization of polyoma virus mutants with altered middle and large-T antigens. *J. Virol.* **39**: 673.

McGrath, J.P. and A.D. Levinson. 1982. Bacterial expression of an enzymatically active protein encoded by RSV src gene. *Nature* **295**: 423.

Oostra, B.A., R. Harvey, B.K. Ely, A.F. Markham, and A.E. Smith. 1983. Transforming activity of polyoma virus middle-T antigen probed by site-directed mutagenesis. *Nature* **304**: 456.

Oppermann, H., A.D. Levinson, H.E. Varmus, L. Levintow, and J.M. Bishop. 1979. Uninfected vertebrate cells contain a protein that is closely related to the product of the avian sarcoma virus transforming gene (*src*). *Proc. Natl. Acad. Sci.* **76**: 1804.

Schaffhausen, B.S. and T.L. Benjamin. 1979. Phosphorylation of polyoma T antigens. *Cell* **18**: 935.

⸺. 1981a. Protein kinase activity associated with polyoma virus middle-T antigen (ed. O.M. Rosen and E.G. Krebs). *Cold Spring Harbor Conf. Cell Proliferation* **8**: 1281.

⸺. 1981b. Comparison of phosphorylation of two polyoma virus middle-T antigens *in vivo* and *in vitro*. *J. Virol.* **40**: 184.

Schneider, C., R.A. Newman, D.R. Sutherland, U. Asser, and M.F. Greaves. 1982. A one-step purification of membrane proteins using a high efficiency immunomatrix. *J. Biol. Chem.* **257**: 10766.

Sefton, B.M., T. Hunter, K. Beemon, and W. Eckhart. 1980. Evidence that the phosphorylation of tyrosine is essential for cellular transformation by Rous sarcoma virus. *Cell* **20**: 807.

Shilo, B.-Z. and R.A. Weinberg. 1981. DNA sequences homologous to vertebrate oncogenes are conserved in *Drosophila melanogaster*. *Proc. Natl. Acad. Sci.* **78**: 6789.

Smart, J.E., H. Oppermann, A.P. Czernilofsky, A.F. Purchio, R.L. Erikson, and J.M. Bishop. 1981. Characterisation of sites for tyrosine phosphorylation in the transforming protein of Rous sarcoma virus and its cellular homologue. *Proc. Natl. Acad. Sci.* **78**: 6013.

Smith, A.E. and B.K. Ely. 1983. The biochemical basis of transformation by polyoma virus. *Adv. Viral Oncol.* **3**: 3.

Smith, A.E., R. Smith, B. Griffin, and M. Fried. 1979. Protein kinase activity associated with polyoma virus middle-T antigen *in vitro*. *Cell* **18**: 915.

Smith, A.E., M. Fried, Y. Ito, N. Spurr, and R. Smith. 1980. Is polyoma virus middle-T antigen a protein kinase? *Cold Spring Harbor Symp. Quant. Biol.* **44**: 141.

Walter, G., M.A. Hutchinson, T. Hunter, and W. Eckhart. 1981. Antibodies specific for the polyoma virus middle-T antigen. *Proc. Natl. Acad. Sci.* **78**: 4882.

⸺. 1982. Purification of polyoma virus middle-T tumor antigen by immunoaffinity chromatography. *Proc. Natl. Acad. Sci.* **79**: 4025.

Evaluation of the Importance in Cell Transformation of the Sequence of Polyoma Virus Middle T Antigen around Glu-Glu-Glu-Glu-Tyr-Met-Pro-Met-Glu

Y. Ito

Laboratory of Molecular Oncology, National Cancer Institute, Frederick Cancer Research Facility, Frederick, Maryland 21701

Polyoma virus oncogenes code for three proteins commonly called large, middle, and small T antigens (for review, see Ito 1980). Recent progress in cell transformation experiments using cultured primary murine cells has revealed that all three T antigens are required for the full transforming activity of the virus (Rassoulzadegan et al. 1983). Polyoma virus, therefore, is useful in dissecting the complex biological processes of cell transformation, since various biochemical functions required for cell transformation are carried out by the three different proteins.

Large T antigen is a DNA-binding protein and is localized mainly in the nuclei of transformed cells. Although full-sized, large T antigen is required for viral DNA replication, only the aminoterminal 40% of large T antigen is needed for the role it plays in cell transformation. It has been suggested that the aminoterminal 40% of large T antigen can establish cell lines with unlimited growth potential from primary cells that have only a limited doubling capability (Rassoulzadegan et al. 1983). Cell lines established with the aid of large T antigen are reported to have lower serum requirements than spontaneously established cell lines. Large T antigen-induced cell lines (Rassoulzadegan et al. 1983) and a spontaneously established cell line expressing only large T antigen do not express most of the other properties usually associated with cell transformation, such as anchorage-independent growth. In the latter case, cells are indistinguishable from parental cells by all the criteria tested (Lania et al. 1979). The concept that immortalization of primary cells or establishment of cell lines are prerequisites to oncogenic transformation has also been discussed recently by several other authors (Land et al. 1983; Newbold and Overell 1983; Ruley 1983). Biochemical properties and subcellular localization of small T antigen is not well known. It is believed that small T antigen plays some roles when primary cells are to be transformed (Rassoulzadegan et al. 1983). Cell transformation by polyoma virus does not occur in the absence of middle T antigen. Although primary cells cannot be transformed by a modified viral DNA clone that can express only middle T antigen, established cell lines can be transformed by that modified viral DNA clone (Treisman et al. 1981). Transformed cells expressing only middle T antigen, however, are able to maintain the phenotype of transformed cells only in the medium containing high concentrations of serum (Rassoulzadegan et al. 1982).

A number of mutants have been isolated that have deletions in the region of the genome where parts of both large and middle T antigens are encoded (Griffin and Maddock 1979; Magnusson and Berg 1979; Bendig et al. 1980; Ding et al. 1982; Nilsson et al. 1983). This set of mutants transforms cells, but the phenotype of these transformed cells varies depending upon the positions of the deletions. The most extreme cases are those of the mutants dl8 and dl23 (Griffin and Maddock 1979); cells transformed by dl8 grow faster than wild-type transformed cells as colonies in soft agar or as dense foci on a plastic surface in liquid medium, whereas cells transformed by dl23 grow more slowly than wild-type transformed cells (Ito et al. 1980). The effect on transformation caused by the deletion is generally considered to be due to the alteration of the properties of middle T antigen. From these and other results, we suggested that middle T antigen is primarily responsible for the induction of the phenotype of transformed cells (Ito et al. 1980). From the analysis of dl23 and other mutants that have deletions overlapping with that of dl23 (Fig. 1), it has been suggested that the sequence around Glu-Glu-Glu-Glu-Tyr-Met-Pro-Met-Glu, which spans from the amino acid 311 to 319 of middle T antigen, is important in this function (Ding et al. 1982; Nilsson et al. 1983).

Middle T antigen is a membrane protein (Ito et al. 1977; Ito 1979; Carmichael et al. 1982) and is associated with an activity that phosphorylates middle T antigen on tyrosine in vitro (Eckhart et al. 1979; Schaffhausen and Benjamin 1979; Smith et al. 1979, 1980). The major phosphate acceptor in this reaction is reported to be Tyr-315, which is included in the nonapeptide mentioned above (Schaffhausen and Benjamin 1981). Middle T antigens of mutants dl8 and dl23 are associated with higher or lower middle T antigen phosphorylating activity, respectively (Smith et al. 1979). Middle T antigens of nontransforming mutants, hr-t, and one that lacks the carboxyterminal hydrophobic region are not associated with this enzyme activity (Schaffhausen and Benjamin 1979; Carmichael et al. 1982). From these results, together with those mentioned above, middle T antigen phosphorylating activity appears to be responsible for inducing the phenotype of transformed cells. This en-

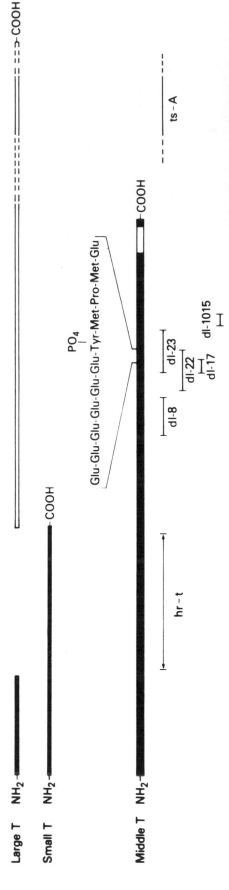

Figure 1 Schematic diagram of the map positions of the mutants of polyoma virus used in the present studies. The data are obtained from Soeda and Griffin (1978) and Hattori et al. (1979) for *hrt*, from Smolar and Griffin (1981) for *dl8* and *dl23*, from Magnusson et al. (1981) for *dl1015*, and from Ding et al. (1982) for *dl22* and *dl17*. The tyrosine residue present in the blown-up sequence is at 315, which has been suggested to be a phosphate acceptor in the in vitro protein kinase reaction mediated by middle T antigen-associated kinase activity (Schaffhausen and Benjamin 1981). The blank area at the carboxyterminal end of middle T antigen indicates the position of the cluster of hydrophobic amino acids (Soeda et al. 1980b).

zyme activity is associated with only a subfraction of middle T antigen (Walter et al. 1982; Segawa and Ito 1982), and the activity is almost exclusively recovered in the plasma membrane fraction (Segawa and Ito 1982). A subfraction of middle T antigen is phosphorylated in vivo. Only a small fraction of the phosphate is on tyrosine residues (Segawa and Ito 1982). A majority of in vivo phosphorylated middle T antigen is also recovered in the plasma membrane fraction, whereas a large fraction of middle T antigen is present in the fractions other than the plasma membrane fraction (Segawa and Ito 1982).

These observations, taken together, suggest that the removal of the region of middle T antigen around the nonapeptide mentioned above does not affect the transformation frequency significantly. Instead it reduces the ability of middle T antigen to induce the transformation phenotype drastically, possibly by reducing the activity that phosphorylates middle T antigen on tyrosine, as measured by the level of middle T antigen phosphorylation in vitro. The middle T antigen phosphorylation reaction appears to occur specifically in the plasma membrane.

My laboratory has been studying the importance of the nonapeptide region of middle T antigen by several different approaches. In this paper, I will summarize the results with respect to (1) the effect of growth factor(s) on tyrosine phosphorylation of middle T antigen, (2) the properties of the antibodies raised against the nonapeptide, and (3) a mouse cell DNA sequence that specifically hybridizes with the segment of viral genome encoding this nonapeptide region of middle T antigen.

Materials and Methods

Mouse DNA library
A Balb/c mouse DNA library prepared in Charon 28 λ phage was obtained from P. Leder (National Institute of Child Health and Development).

Enzymes
Restriction endonucleases and T4 DNA ligase were obtained from Bethesda Research Laboratories and New England Biolabs and were used according to supplier's recommended conditions.

Low-stringency hybridization
Nitrocellulose filters containing immobilized DNA fragments were incubated with approximately 2×10^7 cpm of nick-translated [^{32}P] DNA (2×10^8 cpm/μg) in $6\times$ SSC at 60–63° for 16–20 hours. The nitrocellulose filters were then extensively washed in $6\times$ SSC containing 0.1% SDS at the same temperature as that used for hybridization.

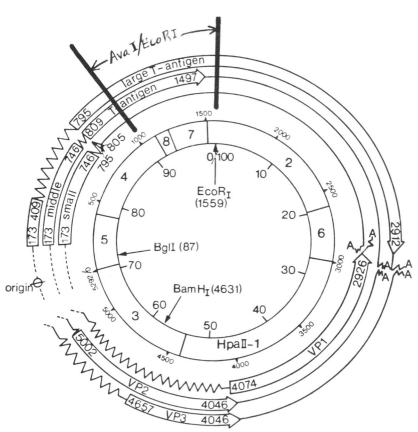

Figure 2 A 544-bp fragment of polyoma virus DNA between the *Ava*I site at nucleotide 1016 and the *Eco*RI site at nucleotide 1560 with respect to the coding regions for three T antigens. The circular map of the polyoma virus genome shown here and in Fig. 6 is from Ito and Griffin (1982).

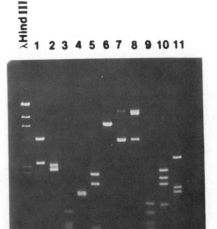

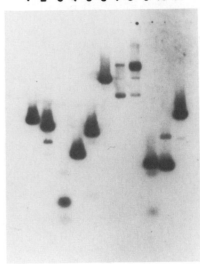

Figure 3 Southern blot analysis of p28H1 DNA using ^{32}P-labeled polyoma virus DNA. p28H1 DNA was digested with restriction endonucleases, separated by electrophoresis in 1% agarose gel, and stained with ethidium bromide. (*Left panel*) The extreme left lane shows λ DNA cut with *Hind*III as a size marker. The DNA fragments in the agarose gel were transferred to nitrocellulose filter by blotting and hybridized with 2 × 10[7] cpm of ^{32}P-labeled polyoma virus DNA at 6 × SSC, 60°C for 18 hr. The filter was extensively washed in 6 × SSC containing 0.1% SDS, dried, and exposed to X-ray film for 16 hr (*right panel*). (Lane *1*) *Hind*III; (lane *2*) *Bgl*I; (lane *3*) *Hae*III; (lane *4*) *Hha*I; (lane *5*) *Hinf*I; (lane *6*) *Hpa*I; (lane *7*) *Kpn*I; (lane *8*) *Mbo*I; (lane *9*) *Msp*I; (lane *10*) *Rsa*I; (lane *11*) *Taq*I.

Results and Discussion

Enhancement of middle T antigen tyrosine phosphorylation by epidermal growth factor

As mentioned above, both a subfraction of middle T antigen associated with an activity that phosphorylates middle T antigen on tyrosine in vitro and a subfraction that is phosphorylated in vivo are recovered in the plasma membrane fraction. Moreover, phosphatase treatment of the immunoprecipitates containing middle T antigen reduces the middle T antigen phosphorylating activity, suggesting that phosphorylation of unspecified protein present in the immunoprecipitates (possibly middle T antigen itself) appears to be essential for this enzyme activity (Segawa and Ito 1982). During the search for cellular protein kinases that would influence middle T antigen phosphorylating activity, it was found that epidermal growth factor (EGF) enhances this activity (Segawa and Ito 1983). When the plasma membrane fraction isolated from polyoma virus-transformed cells is incubated with [γ-32P]ATP, middle T antigen becomes phosphorylated on tyrosine. When the plasma membrane preparation is treated with EGF prior to the incubation with [γ-32P]ATP, tyrosine phosphorylation of middle T antigen is enhanced by about threefold in an EGF receptor-mediated manner. It is interesting to note that middle T antigen appears functionally to be in close association with the EGF receptor which is located in the plasma membrane (Carpenter et al. 1978). This is consistent with the earlier observations mentioned above that the middle T antigen phosphorylation reaction appears to occur specifically in the plasma membrane.

When EGF was added to the culture of intact cells transformed by the virus, it was not clear whether the EGF treatment had any enhancing effect on middle T antigen phosphorylating activity. This might have been due to the fact that polyoma virus-transformed cells were known to secrete some mitogenic factor(s) that would have obscured the effect of added EGF. As mentioned above, the cells expressing only middle T antigen can maintain the full transformation phenotype only when they are kept in the medium containing a high concentration of serum (Rassoulzadegan et al. 1982), suggesting that a function of middle T antigen might be enhanced by externally added growth factor(s). Spontaneously established rat cells, Rat-1, expressing only middle T antigen (Treisman et al. 1981) could not be maintained in good condition for a prolonged period. Three independent clones of such cells were, therefore, starved for serum for 15 hours in the medium containing 0.5% fetal bovine serum (FBS) and treated for 1 hour with 100 ng /ml of EGF, medium containing 20% fresh FBS, or the conditioned medium (serum-free 48-hr supernatant obtained from the culture of polyoma virus-transformed rat cells). Middle T antigen was extracted from the treated cells together with appropriate control cells, and its associated kinase activity was compared. After the treatment with EGF, 20% FBS, or conditioned medium, in vitro tyrosine phosphorylation increased by about 1.7, 1.9, or 1.5 times, respectively. The increment is small but reproducible.

It appears that there is a basal level of an apparent

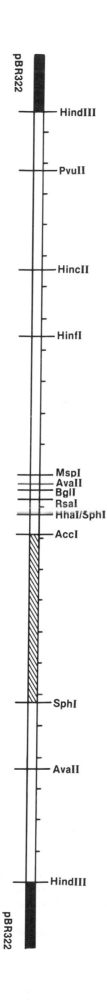

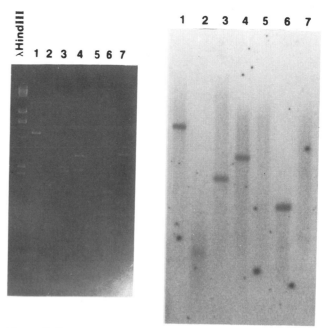

Figure 5 Southern blot analysis of polyoma virus DNA using ^{32}P-labeled p28H1 DNA. Polyoma virus DNA was digested with restriction endonucleases, separated by electrophoresis in 0.8% agarose gel, and stained with ethidium bromide. (*Left panel*) The extreme left lane shows λ DNA cut with *Hind*III as a size marker. The DNA fragments in the gel were transferred to a nitrocellulose filter by blotting and were hybridized with 2×10^7 cpm of ^{32}P-labeled p28H1 DNA at $6 \times$ SSC, 63°C for 18 hr. The filter was extensively washed in $6 \times$ SSC containing 0.1% SDS, dried, and exposed to X-ray film for 16 hr (*right panel*). (Lane *1*) *Ava*I; (lane *2*) *Hae*III; (lane *3*) *Hha*I; (lane *4*) *Hind*III; (lane *5*) *Hpa*II, (lane *6*) *Mbo*I, (lane *7*) *Pvu*II.

EGF-independent tyrosine phosphorylation and that EGF enhances the level of phosphorylation. The basal level could be due to an autophosphorylation or due to a cellular tyrosine kinase tightly associated with middle T antigen, such as pp60^{c-src}, a cellular homolog of a transforming protein of avian sarcoma virus that has been reported recently to be in tight association with a subfraction of middle T antigen (Courtneidge and Smith 1983). Enhancement of middle T antigen tyrosine phosphorylation by EGF could be either a direct phosphorylation by the EGF receptor kinase, a tyrosine kinase, or an indirect one involving one or more cellular kinase(s) whose activity could be enhanced by the EGF receptor kinase. Further studies are necessary to distinguish these various possibilities.

It is interesting to note that the conditioned medium obtained from the supernatant of the culture of polyoma virus-transformed cells also enhances the tyrosine phosphorylation of middle T antigen. It has been shown that similarly obtained conditioned medium contains a transforming growth factor (TGF) (Kaplan and Ozanne 1982).

Figure 4 Restriction enzyme map of p28H1 DNA. The shaded region between the *Acc*I site and *Sph*I site contains the sequence that hybridizes with polyoma virus DNA.

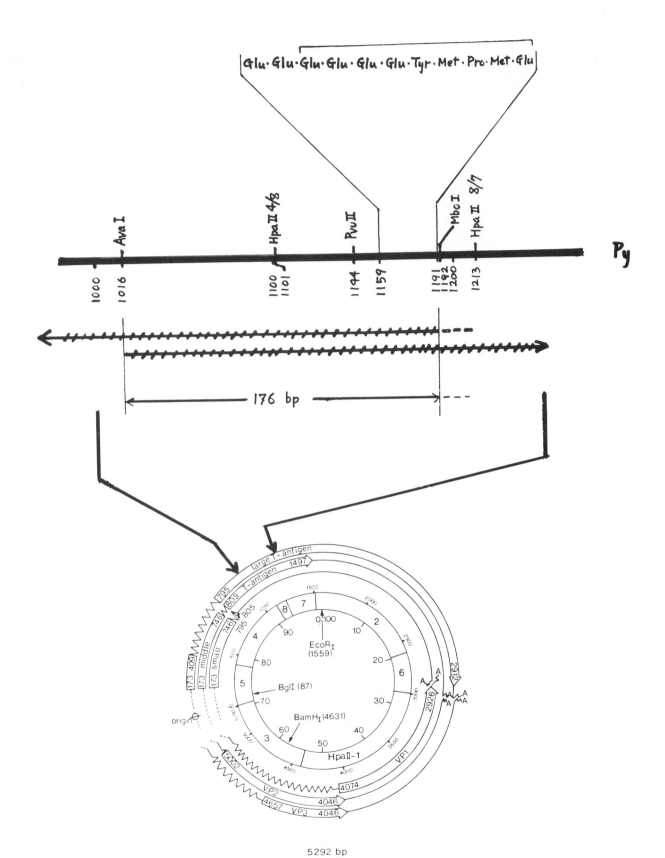

Figure 6 A diagram showing the region of polyoma virus genome where p28H1 DNA hybridizes. A 176-bp segment of polyoma virus DNA between the *Ava*I site at nucleotide 1016 and the *Mbo*I site at nucleotide 1192 contains the sequence that hybridizes with p28H1 DNA. The region encoding the nonapeptide discussed in the text is included in this segment.

Therefore, it is possible that the active component in the conditioned medium is TGF. TGF is defined operationally as polypeptide growth factors that are able to confer the transformed phenotype on normal cells (DeLarco and Todaro 1978). It has been suggested that cells expressing transforming proteins of retroviruses are able to respond to TGF more strongly than untransformed cells (Kaplan et al 1982). The TGF secreted from retrovirus-transformed cells has two components, α and β. TGF α has some sequence homology with EGF and is able to bind to the EGF receptor (Marquardt et al. 1983). TGF β does not bind to the EGF receptor. For the full TGF activity, both components need to bind to their receptors. The TGF α can be substituted with EGF for this function (Roberts et al. 1982).

The TGF secreted by polyoma virus-transformed cells does not bind to the EGF receptor (Todaro et al. 1976; Kaplan and Ozanne 1982). Nevertheless, it has been shown that EGF enhances the effect of TGF secreted from polyoma virus-transformed cells (Kaplan and Ozanne 1982). It is not known whether the polyoma virus-induced TGF corresponds to TGF β. In any event, our results suggest an interesting possibility that some growth factors, including EGF and the TGF from polyoma virus-transformed cells, may induce the transformation phenotype by enhancing the function of middle T antigen.

A cellular protein cross-reactive with the antibodies against the nonapeptide of middle T antigen

Antibodies were raised against the sequence Glu-Glu-Glu-Glu-Tyr-Met-Pro-Met-Glu. The purpose of raising antibodies against this peptide was multifold: to obtain monospecific antibodies against middle T antigen for general use including affinity purification of middle T antigen, to characterize tyrosine phosphorylation of middle T antigen in vitro (Schaffhausen et al. 1982), and to see if there is a cellular protein that reacts with the antibodies. Since the peptide represents the functionally important region of middle T antigen and is considered to include the phosphate acceptor site on the middle T protein, it is particularly interesting to ask the question whether or not there is a cellular protein with such a structure or sequence that could be a cellular homolog of middle T antigen or a cellular target of a phosphorylation reaction mediated by middle T antigen-associated kinase.

The antibodies react well with native as well as denatured middle T antigen. In addition, the antibodies immunoprecipitate a cellular protein with an apparent molecular weight of 130,000 from mouse and rat cells. In some cases, a 33-kD protein is also immunoprecipitated. Immunoprecipitation of middle T antigen as well as 130K and 33-kD proteins is blocked by the peptide. The antibodies label microfilaments of untransformed mouse, rat, human, and chicken cells by immunofluorescence. This labeling is also blocked by the peptide. The labeling pattern and distribution under a variety of conditions is indistinguishable from those of anti-actin antibodies, although the anti-peptide antibodies do not immunoprecipitate actin. The mobility of the 130K pro-

tein in SDS-polyacrylamide gel electrophoresis is very similar to the mobilities of vinculin and myosin light-chain kinase. Neither of these proteins, however, corresponds to the 130K protein. At present, it is not known whether the 130K protein is associated with microfilament. The 33-kD protein does not seem to be tropomyosin (32–40 kD).

In considering the significance of the present observations, it is important to establish whether the same antibodies react with middle T antigen, microfilament protein(s), and the 130-kD and 33-kD proteins. This is because the anti-peptide antibodies are probably not monoclonal and, therefore, there is a possibility that different subpopulations of the antibodies react with different proteins, although the antibodies are directed against a very short peptide. If it is proved that the same antibodies can react both with middle T antigen and cellular protein(s), it would then be worth rigorously studying the possibility that the cross-reaction we observe may have some serious biological meaning (Ito et al. 1980).

Molecular cloning of mouse cell DNA sequences that hybridize with a segment of polyoma virus genome encoding the nonapeptide region

There were two reasons for attempting to isolate mouse cell DNA sequences that would hybridize with a part of the polyoma virus genome encoding the unique region of middle T antigen: It was hoped that one might be able to identify (1) a hypothetical protooncogene corresponding to middle T antigen or (2) a mouse gene(s) encoding a protein that is unrelated to middle T antigen but shares some sequences with middle T antigen. The 130K protein recognized by the anti-peptide antibodies mentioned above could correspond to the gene product of either one of them.

Comparison of the nucleotide sequences of the genomes of polyoma virus and simian virus 40 (SV40) has revealed that a strong homology exists between the genomes of the two viruses to such a degree that one might speculate that they may have evolved from the same ancestor (Soeda et al. 1980a). Although a large part of the coding region is homologous, there is a segment of polyoma virus DNA that does not have a counterpart in the SV40 DNA. That segment of polyoma virus DNA corresponds exactly to the region of the genome where the majority of the unique region of middle T antigen is encoded. In addition, there is a sequence, AATAAA, at nucleotide 1476 where the carboxyterminal end of middle T antigen is encoded. The sequence AATAAA at nucleotide 2915 is mainly used by the viral RNA as a polyadenylation signal and the sequence at nucleotide 1476 does not seem to be used at a significant level as an RNA-processing signal in productive infection of the virus. However, the presence of this sequence and the fact that the majority of the unique region of middle T antigen is encoded in the segment of DNA that is missing in the SV40 genome makes one speculate that the segment might have been picked up by the virus from mouse DNA during the evolution of the virus. This mechanism would be reminiscent of that of oncogene-containing retroviruses by which they acquire protooncogene sequences in host cell DNA into viral genomes. One notable obstacle in accepting this hypothesis is the fact that the segment uses two different reading frames throughout the length of the segment with the coding capacity of some 25-kD polypeptide. If the original mouse DNA segment had only one open reading frame, how could the second reading frame be opened to be a part of large T antigen?

When viral sequences in transformed mouse cells were analyzed, it was noted that there was no detectable hybridization between viral DNA and mouse DNA. If some mouse DNA sequences hybridize with viral DNA, they must hybridize very weakly. The fact that polyoma virus and SV40 DNAs share strong sequence homology in spite of the fact that they do not hybridize even under the low stringency hybridization conditions suggests that the sequence with meaningful homology could not be detected by the nucleic acid hybridization technique. This notion justifies the attempts to identify cellular sequences homologous to viral DNA using very low-stringency hybridization.

To increase the chance of detecting such a hypothetical sequence, approximately 10% of the total viral DNA that is likely to represent the coding sequence for the functionally important part of middle T antigen was preselected. The selected region is a 544-bp segment between the *Ava*I site at nucleotide 1016 and the *Eco*RI site at nucleotide 1560 (Fig. 2). This fragment was purified, labeled with ^{32}P by nick-translation, and used as a probe to screen the mouse DNA library made in λ phage. The hybridization conditions used were 6× SSC at 60° for 16–18 hours. Possible candidate clones were identified and recloned. About 10 clones were isolated from the second screening, and five of them were selected and grown in a large scale. λ phage DNAs from these clones were digested with several restriction endonucleases and were subjected to Southern blot analysis using ^{32}P-labeled polyoma virus DNA as a probe. One of the clones, Cl 28, yielded a 2.4-kb *Hind*-III fragment that contains virtually all the hybridizable fragment. This 2.4-kb *Hind*III fragment was subcloned in pBR322. One of these clones was designated as p28H1 and was further analyzed by Southern blot hybridization using more restriction endonucleases (Fig. 3). From the results shown in Figure 3, and additional results not shown here, a preliminary restriction enzyme map of the clone was obtained and is shown in Figure 4. Most of the hybridizable sequence has been localized to an ~500-bp fragment between *Acc*I and *Sph*I sites shown in Figure 4.

To test exactly which region of the polyoma virus genome hybridizes with this clone p28H1, polyoma virus DNA was digested with several restriction endonucleases and examined by Southern blot analysis using ^{32}P-labeled p28H1 DNA as a probe. As shown in Figure 5, *Ava*I 1, *Hae*III 1, *Hha*I 2, *Hind*III 1, and *Mbo*I 1 fragments hybridize well with p28H1 DNA. However, no hybridization was observed to any fragment generated by

*Hpa*II and *Pvu*II. Figure 6 summarizes the results of this analysis. The region of the genome of polyoma virus that hybridizes with p28H1 lies mostly within nucleotides 1016 and 1192. *Hpa*II 8 fragment is likely to contain a hybridizable sequence, but the fragment (112 bp) may be too small to be immobilized efficiently to a nitrocellulose filter. This may explain the results (shown in Figure 5) that none of the fragments generated by *Hpa*II hybridize with ^{32}P-labeled p28H1 DNA.

The *Pvu*II site at nucleotide 1144 divides the *Pvu*II 2 fragment (1174 bp) on the left side and the *Pvu*II 3 fragment (888 bp) on the right side, as shown in Figure 6. Both of the fragments are large enough to be immobilized to a nitrocellulose filter. Figure 5 shows no hybridization of ^{32}P-labeled p28H1 DNA to any of these two fragments. The result must mean, therefore, that a rather short stretch of viral DNA, including the *Pvu*II site at 1144, can form a relatively stable hybrid with p28H1 DNA and that either of the two fragments generated by digestion with *Pvu*II at nucleotide 1144 can no longer form stable hybrids with p28H1 DNA under the conditions used in the experiments. The *Mbo*I 7 fragment that lies between nucleotides 1192 and 1318 is 126 bp long and it is not likely to be immobilized efficiently to a nitrocellulose filter. Therefore, it is not clear at present whether this 126-bp-long fragment can hybridize to p28H1 DNA. In any event, it is extremely interesting to note in Figure 6 that the region of viral DNA previously identified to encode a functionally important region of middle T antigen is included in the short stretch of the segment that can form a relatively stable hybrid with the mouse cell DNA segment isolated in the present experiment. Nucleotide sequence analysis of cloned mouse DNA segments should answer many questions already mentioned above, notably the question of whether this sequence represents a proto-oncogene corresponding to middle T antigen.

References

Bendig, M.M., T. Thomas, and W.R. Folk. 1980. Viable deletion mutants in the medium and large T-antigen coding sequences of the polyoma virus genome. *J. Virol.* **33:** 1215.

Carmichael, G.G., B.S. Schaffhausen, D.I. Dorsky, D.B. Oliver, and T.L. Benjamin. 1982. Carboxy terminus of polyoma middle-sized tumor antigen is required for attachment to membranes, associated protein kinase activities and cell transformation. *Proc. Natl. Acad. Sci.* **79:** 3579.

Carpenter, G., L. King, Jr., and S. Cohen. 1978. Epidermal growth factor stimulates phosphorylation in membrane preparations *in vitro. Nature* **276:** 409.

Courtneidge, S.A. and A.E. Smith. 1983. Polyoma virus transforming protein associates with the product of the c-*src* cellular gene. *Nature* **303:** 435.

DeLarco, J.E. and G.J. Todaro. 1978. Growth factors from murine sarcoma virus-transformed cells. *Proc. Natl. Acad. Sci.* **75:** 4001.

Ding, D., S.M. Dilworth, and B.E. Griffin. 1982. *Mlt* mutants of polyoma virus. *J. Virol.* **44:** 1080.

Eckhart, W., M-A. Hutchinson, and T. Hunter. 1979. Ac activity phosphorylating tyrosine in polyoma T antigen immunoprecipitates. *Cell* **18:** 925.

Griffin, B.E. and C. Maddock. 1979. New class of viable deletion mutants in the early region of polyoma virus. *J. Virol.* **31:** 645.

Hattori. J., G.G. Carmichael, and T.L. Benjamin. 1979. DNA sequence alterations in Hr-t deletion mutants of polyoma virus. *Cell* **16**: 505.

Ito, Y. 1979. Polyoma virus-specific 55K protein isolated from plasma membrane of productively infected cells is virus coded and important for cell transformation. *Virology* **98**: 261.

———. 1980. Organization and expression of the genome of polyoma virus. In *Viral oncology* (ed. G. Klein), p. 447. Raven Press, New York.

Ito, Y. and B.E. Griffin. 1982. Genetic map of polyoma virus. In *Genetic maps* (ed. S.J. O'Brien), p. 86. National Institutes of Health, Washington, D.C.

Ito, Y., J.R. Brocklehurst, and R. Dulbecco. 1977. Virus-specific proteins in the plasma membrane of cells lytically infected or transformed by polyoma virus. *Proc. Natl. Acad. Sci.* **74**: 4666.

Ito, Y., N. Spurr, and B.E. Griffin. 1980. Middle T antigen as primary inducer of full expression of the phenotype of transformation by polyoma virus. *J. Virol.* **35**: 219.

Ito, Y., Y. Hamagishi, K. Segawa, T. Dalianis, E. Appella, and M. Willingham. 1983. Antibodies against a nonapeptide of polyoma virus middle T antigen: A cross-reaction with a cellular protein(s). *J. Virol.* **48**: 709.

Kaplan, P.L. and B. Ozanne. 1982. Polyoma virus-transformed cells produce transforming growth factor(s) and grow in serum-free medium. *Virology* **123**: 372.

Kaplan, P.I., M. Anderson, and B. Ozanne. 1982. Transforming growth factor production enables cells to grow in the absence of serum: An autocrine system. *Proc. Natl. Acad. Sci.* **79**: 485.

Land, H., L.F. Parada, and R.A. Weinberg. 1983. Tumorigenic conversion of primary embryo fibroblasts requires at least two cooperating oncogenes. *Nature* **304**: 596.

Lania, L., M. Griffiths, B. Cooke, Y. Ito, and M. Fried. 1979. Untransformed rat cells containing free and integrated DNA of a polyoma non-transforming (hr-t) mutant. *Cell* **19**: 793.

Magnusson, G. and P. Berg. 1979. Construction and analysis of viable deletion mutants of polyoma virus. *J. Virol.* **32**: 523.

Magnusson, G., M.-G. Nilsson, S.M. Dilworth, and N. Smolar. 1981. Characterization of polyoma mutants with altered middle and large T antigens. *J. Virol.* **39**: 673.

Marquardt, H., M.W. Hunkapiller, L.E. Hood, D.R. Twardzik, J.E. DeLarco, J.R. Stephenson, and G.J. Todaro. 1983. Transforming growth factors produced by retrovirus-transformed rodent fibroblasts and human melanoma cells: Amino acid sequence homology with epidermal growth factor. *Proc. Natl. Acad. Sci.* **80**: 4684.

Newbold, R.F. and R.W. Overell. 1983. Fibroblast immortality is a prerequisite for transformation by EJc-Ha-*ras* oncogene. *Nature* **304**: 648.

Nilsson, S.V., C. Tyndall, and G. Magnusson. 1983. Deletion mapping of a short polyoma virus middle T antigen segment important for transformation. *J. Virol.* **46**: 284.

Rassoulzadegan, M., A. Cowie, A. Carr, N. Glaichenhaus, R. Kamen, and F. Cuzin. 1982. The role of individual polyoma virus early proteins in oncogenic transformation. *Nature* **300**: 713.

Rassoulzadegan, M., Z. Naghashfar, A. Cowie, A. Carr, M.

Grisoni, R. Kamen, and F. Cuzin. 1983. Expression of the large T protein of polyoma virus promotes the establishment in culture of "normal" rodent fibroblast cell lines. *Proc. Natl. Acad. Sci.* **80**: 4354.

Roberts, A.B., M.A. Anzano, L.C. Lamb, J.M. Smith, C.A. Frolik, H. Marquardt, G.J. Todaro, and M.B. Sporn. 1982. Isolation from murine sarcoma cells of novel transforming growth factors potentiated by EGF. *Nature* **295**: 417.

Ruley, H.E. 1983. Adenovirus early region E1A enables viral and cellular transforming genes to transform primary cells in culture. *Nature* **304**: 602.

Schaffhausen, B.S. and T.L. Benjamin. 1979. Phosphorylation of polyoma T antigen. *Cell* **18**: 935.

———. 1981. Comparison of phosphorylation of two polyoma virus middle T antigens *in vivo* and *in vitro*. *J. Virol.* **40**: 184.

Schaffhausen, B., T.L. Benjamin, L. Pike, J. Casnellie, and E. Krebs. 1982. Antibody to the nonapeptide Glu-Glu-Glu-Glu-Tyr-Met-Pro-Met-Glu is specific for polyoma middle T antigen and inhibits *in vitro* kinase activity. *J. Biol. Chem.* **257**: 12467.

Segawa, K. and Y. Ito. 1982. Differential subcellular localization of *in vivo* phosphorylated and nonphosphorylated middle-sized tumor antigen of polyoma virus and its relationship to a middle sized tumor antigen phosphorylating activity in vitro. *Proc. Natl. Acad. Sci.* **79**: 6812.

———. 1983. Enhancement of polyoma virus middle T antigen tyrosine phosphorylation by epidermal growth factor. *Nature* **304**: 742.

Smith, A.E., R. Smith, B.E. Griffin, and M. Fried. 1979. Protein kinase activity associated with polyoma virus middle T antigen *in vitro*. *Cell* **18**: 915.

Smith, A.E., M. Fried, Y. Ito, N. Spurr, and R. Smith. 1980. Is polyoma virus middle T antigen a protein kinase? *Cold Spring Harbor Symp. Quant. Biol.* **44**: 141.

Smolar, N. and B.E. Griffin. 1981. DNA sequences of polyoma virus early deletion mutants. *J. Virol.* **38**: 958.

Soeda, E. and B.E. Griffin. 1978. Sequences from the genome of a nontransforming mutant of polyoma virus. *Nature* **276**: 294.

Soeda, E., T. Maruyama, J.R. Arrand, and B.E. Griffin. 1980a. Host-dependent evolution of three papova viruses. *Nature* **285**: 165.

Soeda, E., J.R. Arrand, N. Smolar, J.E. Walsh, and B.E. Griffin. 1980b. Coding potential and regulatory signals of the polyoma virus genome. *Nature* **283**: 445.

Todaro, G.J., J.E. DeLarco, and S. Cohen. 1976. Transformation by murine and feline sarcoma viruses specifically blocks binding of epidermal growth factor to cells. *Nature* **264**: 26.

Treisman, R., U. Novak, J. Favaloro, and R. Kamen. 1981. Transformation of rat cells by an altered polyoma virus genome expressing only the middle T protein. *Nature* **292**: 595.

Walter, G., M.A. Hutchinson, T. Hunter, and W. Eckhart. 1982. Purification of polyoma virus medium-size tumor antigen by immunoaffinity chromatography. *Proc. Natl. Acad. Sci.* **79**: 4025.

The Oncogene of Avian Myeloblastosis Virus Is an Altered Proto-oncogene

J.S. Lipsick, W.J. Boyle, M.A. Lampert, and M.A. Baluda

UCLA Jonsson Comprehensive Cancer Center and Department of Pathology, School of Medicine, Los Angeles, California 90024

Acutely transforming retroviruses contain transduced cellular genetic information. These acquired cellular sequences play no essential role in the viral life cycle but are oncogenic for host cells (Bishop and Varmus 1982; Bister and Duesberg 1982). Two distinct, but not necessarily mutually exclusive, models have been proposed for the mechanism of transformation by retroviral oncogenes. The altered proto-oncogene (or qualitative) model ascribes acute retroviral oncogenicity to a structural alteration in the viral oncogene product relative to its normal cellular counterpart, the proto-oncogene (Baluda et al. 1983; Duesberg 1983). The alternative gene dosage (or quantitative) model proposes that such oncogenicity is due to inappropriately increased levels of expression of essentially normal "cellular oncogene" sequences while under control of strong viral transcriptional promoter elements (Bishop 1981; Klein 1981). Recent structural studies of numerous retroviral oncogenes and related cellular proto-oncogenes have tended to support the altered proto-oncogene model (for review, see Duesberg 1983). The oncogene of avian myeloblastosis virus (AMV) represents the most marked alteration of a proto-oncogene examined to date. As we shall discuss, the viral oncogene (*myb*) resulting from the transduced cellular genetic elements (*amv*), differs dramatically from its normal cellular counterpart (*proto-amv*) in gene structure, transcript structure, protein structure, and intracellular protein location.

In addition, it appears that proto-oncogene expression does not occur in the AMV-induced leukemic myeloblasts that we have examined. Since such leukemic cells are polyclonal in chickens and represent multiple transformation events, all target cells for AMV thus seem to be devoid of *proto-amv* expression. *proto-amv* might be turned off by viral transformation, but this is unlikely because it is possible to induce *proto-amv* expression in leukemic myeloblasts that maintain viral oncogene expression (J. Lipsick and M. Dvorak, unpubl.). Also, no other retroviral oncogene products are known to turn off their proto-oncogene counterparts when the latter are normally expressed. The lack of *proto-amv* expression in AMV-induced leukemic myeloblasts argues strongly against models for AMV transformation that require concurrent expression of the proto-oncogene as well as the viral oncogene (Graf and Beug 1978).

Methods of Experimental Procedures

Cells

The BM2 leukemic myeloblast cell line that contains AMV provirus but no integrated helper virus has been described previously (Duesberg et al. 1980). Bursal and thymic lymphocytes were harvested from 17-day-old white leghorn chicken embryos.

Antisera and immunoprecipitation

Preparation of synthetic peptides and anti-peptide antisera, cell labeling, and immunoprecipitation have been described previously (Boyle et al. 1983).

Subcellular fractionation

Nuclei were isolated essentially according to Birckbichler and Prime (1973), using 0.1% Kyro EOB for BM2 cell fractionation and 0.01% digitonin for bursal and thymic lymphocyte fractionation. Postnuclear supernatants were then centrifuged at 100,000g for 1 hour, yielding a "soluble" supernatant fraction (S100) and a "membranous" precipitate fraction (P100). All fractions were then dissolved in the detergent buffer used for immunoprecipitation (Boyle et al. 1983).

Immunofluorescence

Smears of single-cell suspensions on glass slides were air dried and fixed in acetone. Anti-peptide antisera previously absorbed against a chicken liver cellular homogenate were preincubated with or without the appropriate peptide in excess. The cell smears were then incubated with these antisera at 1:20 dilution for 30 minutes at 25°C, washed with phosphate-buffered saline (PBS) (pH 7.4) for 30 minutes, incubated with goat anti-rabbit IgG conjugated to fluorescein isothiocyanate (Sigma) at 1:20 dilution for 30 minutes, and washed again with PBS.

Results and Discussion

Biology and structure of AMV

AMV was originally derived from two chickens with Marek's disease, a herpes virus-induced T-cell lymphomatosis (for review, see Baluda et al. 1983). Standard AMV causes acute myeloblastic leukemia within a few weeks when high-titered viral stocks are injected into chicken embryos or day-old chicks. The virus is also capable of transforming hematopoietic tissues in vitro, giving rise to multiplying cells with morphology similar to the leukemic cells seen in chickens (Baluda and Goetz 1961; Moscovici 1975). However, unlike all other acutely transforming retroviruses studied to date, AMV does not transform fibroblasts in vitro nor does it acutely cause nonmyeloblastic disease in vivo.

AMV itself is replication defective and requires coinfection with a helper virus to generate infectious viral particles. However, cells transformed by AMV but not infected with helper virus produce noninfectious particles that contain viral RNA, *gag*- and *pol*-encoded proteins, but no *env* gene products (Duesberg et al. 1980). Oligonucleotide mapping of viral RNA and restriction and heteroduplex analysis of cloned proviral DNA have shown that AMV contains a near total deletion of the *env* gene relative to its natural helper virus, MAV-1, as seen in Figure 1 (Duesberg et al. 1980; Souza et al. 1980). In the place of deleted *env* sequences, AMV has acquired avian cellular sequences (Roussel et al. 1979; Souza et al. 1980). As has been shown for other proto-oncogenes, these cellular sequences have been highly conserved during vertebrate evolution (Roussel et al. 1979; Bergmann et al. 1981).

The related acutely transforming retrovirus E26 contains at least a portion of the *proto-amv* sequences found in AMV (Roussel et al. 1979; Bister et al. 1982). However, this virus causes predominantly erythroblastosis in vivo and has been reported to transform fibroblasts as well as hematopoietic cells in vitro (Graf et al. 1979). The structure of E26 resembles that of MC29, with the cellular insert abutting a partially deleted *gag* gene and with near total deletion of viral *pol* and *env* sequences (Beug et al. 1982; Bister et al. 1982). In addition, E26 appears to contain additional cellular sequences unrelated to *amv* (LePrince et al. 1983a; Nunn et al. 1983). Whether the differing oncogenic spectra of AMV and E26 are due to these additional cellular sequences or to the differing viral contributions to their oncogene products is at present unknown.

Organization and transcription of the AMV oncogene and proto-oncogene

The region of the cloned AMV provirus containing the 1200-bp cellular insert (*amv*) has been sequenced (Klempnauer et al. 1982; Rushlow et al. 1982). Comparison of the AMV sequence with that of cloned MAV-1 helper virus in the regions of recombination (N. Kan, unpubl.) reveals (1) that the 5' recombination event occurred 111 bp upstream from the termination codon of the MAV-1 *pol* gene precisely at the viral *env* subgenomic mRNA splice site (Schwartz et al. 1983), and (2) that the 3' recombination event occurred 33 bp upstream from the termination codon of the MAV-1 *env* gene. The cellular insert (*amv*) contains a single, long, open reading frame interrupted only once by a single termination codon at nucleotide 84 from the 5' recombination site. This reading frame is continuous with both the 5' *pol* and 3' *env* open reading frames. Therefore, (1) cellular sequences provide an altered 27-amino-acid carboxyl terminus of the AMV *pol* gene product, and (2) viral *env* sequences provide an altered 11-amino-acid carboxyl terminus for the AMV transforming gene product (Fig. 2).

Further examination of the *amv* sequence revealed consensus transcription regulatory sequences within the cellular insert at appropriate distances from the 5' proximal ATG initiation codon within *amv* at nucleotide 439 from the 5' end. This led to the prediction of a 30,000-molecular-weight, AMV-specific transforming protein (Rushlow et al. 1982). However, as will be discussed below, the actual size of the transforming protein is 48,000, requiring translation of nearly the entire cellular insert and presumably initiating in the spliced 5' viral leader of the subgenomic *amv*-specific mRNA. Interestingly, in vitro translation of viral RNA does give rise to a 30,000-molecular-weight protein apparently related to *amv*. Such translation of genomic and/or subgenomic mRNAs may use the "cryptic" cellular initiation site found within the *amv* insert (Anderson and Chen 1981; Bister and Duesberg 1982; Klempnauer et al. 1983).

The RNA for the transforming protein of AMV is a

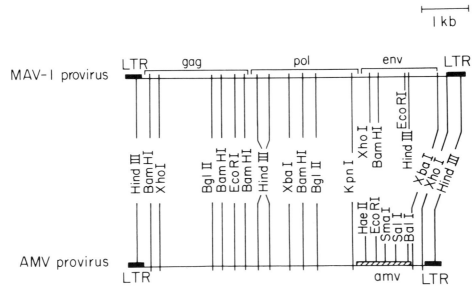

Figure 1 The structure of AMV and its natural helper virus MAV-1. Restriction enzyme sites are from Souza et al. (1980). Viral gene assignments are based on homologous restriction sites in the sequence of RSV (Schwartz et al. 1983).

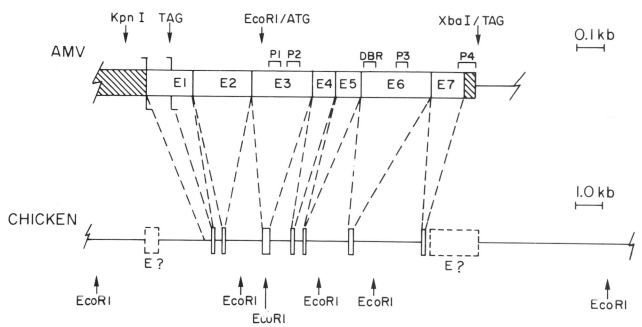

Figure 2 The structure of the AMV cellular insert (*amv*) and of the homologous chicken gene (*proto-amv*). (☐) AMV coding sequences of cellular origin (Rushlow et al. 1982; Klempnauer et al. 1982); (▨) viral coding sequences of Δ *pol* (5′) and Δ *env* (3′); (▢) *proto-amv* coding sequences not present in AMV; (———) non-coding sequences. P1, P2, P3, and P4 are sites of synthetic peptides against which antisera were raised (Boyle et al. 1983). DBR indicates the site of a potential DNA-binding region (see Fig. 6). Two potential splice acceptor sites for generating the *amv*-specific subgenomic message are indicated by large brackets.

spliced subgenomic message similar in structure to the *env*- and *src*-specific messages of Rous sarcoma virus (RSV). The 2-kb *amv*-specific subgenomic mRNA contains U_5-*amv*-U_3 sequences, but no large portions of *gag* or *pol* sequences (Chen et al. 1981; Gonda et al. 1981). Since *gag* sequences are highly conserved in avian retroviruses, the 2-kb mRNA is likely to contain a 5′ viral leader sequence arising from the splice donor site 18 bp within *gag*-encoding sequences that is used to generate subgenomic *env* and *src* mRNAs in RSV (Hackett et al. 1982; Schwartz et al. 1983). The AMV transforming protein would thus have a short *gag* amino terminus as well as a short *env* carboxyl terminus as described above, neither of which would be present in the cellular homolog.

Two potential splice acceptor sites for *amv*-specific subgenomic mRNA are found near the 5′ end of the cellular insert. The first such site occurs at the 5′ viral–cellular junction and is positioned identically to the site presumably used to generate *env* mRNA in RSV and MAV-1 (Schwartz et al. 1983; N. Kan et al. unpubl.). However, such splicing would yield a message continuing in the wrong reading frame relative to the *gag* leader sequence and would terminate prematurely shortly 3′ to this splice site. The second potential splice site occurs within the cellular insert 86 bp downstream from the first site and would precisely splice out the single TAG termination codon at this position (Klempnauer et al. 1982). Elimination of this termination codon would generate a translatable message in the proper reading frame.

By definition, the chicken *proto-amv* gene should con-

tain all of the cellular sequences present in AMV except for mutations. However, as is the case in most eukaryotic genes, including many proto-oncogenes, these coding sequences are separated by noncoding intervening sequences (Breathnach and Chambon 1981). Restriction enzyme analysis and probing with *amv* DNA fragments revealed the presence of an 8–9-kb *proto-amv* domain in chicken genomic DNA containing at least six major *proto-amv* segments separated by five DNA regions lacking homology with *amv* (Perbal et al. 1983). Partial DNA sequencing of the chicken *proto-amv* region has detected an additional sixth intervening sequence (Fig. 2) and has shown that all seven cellular regions of *amv* homology are bounded by consensus splice recognition sequences (Klempnauer et al. 1982). Comparison of *amv* and homologous *proto-amv* sequences reveals 15 base changes that predict 11 differing amino acids in these regions. Restriction enzyme mapping and heteroduplex analysis of cloned human *proto-amv* genomic DNA have revealed a conserved structure for this region in vertebrate DNA (Franchini et al. 1983; LePrince et al. 1983b).

Transcription of *proto-amv* sequences appears to be specific to hematopoietic tissues in the chicken, with the highest levels observed in thymus and embryonic bursa (Chen 1980; Gonda et al. 1982; M. Dvorak, unpubl.). A similar hematopoietic tissue distribution has been observed in the mouse (Mushinski et al. 1983), embryonic cat (Busch et al. 1983), and in a survey of human tumors (Westin et al. 1982). A 4.0-kb *proto-amv* mRNA nearly twice the size of the *amv*-specific viral subgenomic mRNA is seen in avian, murine, feline, and human hematopoietic tissues (Gonda et al. 1982; Westin et al. 1982; Busch et al. 1983; Mushinski et al. 1983). Mapping of this *proto-amv* mRNA using cellular genomic probes has revealed in avian and human genomic DNA the presence of presumed coding sequences both 5′ and 3′ to the region of homology with the viral oncogene that are dispersed over at least 13 kb (Franchini et al. 1983; Gonda and Bishop 1983; M. Dvorak, unpubl.). Thus, the AMV oncogene contains substantial 5′ and 3′ coding region deletions relative to *proto-amv*. Mapping of *proto-amv* mRNA with well-defined probes has also revealed that the cellular message is generated using the second potential AMV splice acceptor site described above (M. Dvorak, unpubl.). The 5′ viral-cellular recombination event has therefore occurred within a cellular intron. This implies that the 5′ recombination must have occurred at the DNA level following genomic insertion of MAV-1, rather than by recombination of viral and cellular mRNAs.

Identification of the AMV transforming protein and its cellular homolog

The identification of the AMV transforming protein proved difficult for several reasons. First, this protein is not fused to a major portion of a viral structural protein. Therefore, the strategy of identifying an altered viral gene product with antisera directed against subviral components was unsuccessful in the case of AMV (Silva and Baluda 1980; Duesberg et al. 1980). Second, AMV causes rapidly and uniformly fatal leukemia only in chickens and transforms no other known cell type, so that production of tumor-bearing animal sera such as that used to identify pp60^{src} (Brugge and Erikson 1977) was not possible. Finally, since AMV is a replication-defective virus, isolation of conditional mutants for the transforming function has been problematic.

To circumvent these difficulties, antisera were raised against several synthetic peptides predicted from the open reading frame of *amv* (Fig. 2). Such a strategy had been used successfully to identify numerous proteins, including transforming proteins of both DNA and RNA tumor viruses (Walter et al. 1980; Lerner 1982). Three such antisera to distinct *amv* peptides specifically identified a protein of 48,000 m.w. in an AMV-transformed cell line and in numerous freshly isolated AMV-induced leukemic buffy coats. This 48,000 m.w. protein was not found in normal chicken hematopoietic tissues, fibroblasts, or fibroblasts infected with the helper virus MAV-1. Thus, it was concluded that this protein, p48^{amv}, is the product of the AMV transforming gene (Boyle et al. 1983). p48^{amv} is not glycosylated and does not appear to act as a protein kinase in vitro in immunoprecipitates, as do many other retroviral transforming proteins (Collett and Erikson 1978). p48^{amv} appears to be phosphorylated to a very small extent in intact cells (W. Boyle et al. unpubl.).

One of the antisera that specifically recognized p48^{amv} also specifically precipitated the 135,000 m.w. putative transforming protein of E26 virus (Boyle et al. 1983).

This further demonstrated the *amv*-specificity of the antiserum. It also proved that the E26 transforming protein does indeed contain *amv* as well as *gag*-encoded sequences, as had been predicted from the genomic structure of this virus (Bister et al. 1982).

The same three distinctly different antipeptide antisera that specifically immunoprecipitated p48^{amv} in leukemic myeloblasts also specifically recognized a 110,000 m.w. protein present in 17-day chicken embryonic thymus which expresses high levels of *proto-amv* mRNA (Boyle et al. 1983). This protein is also specifically immunoprecipitated from chicken 17-day embryonic bursa (a B-lymphoid precursor tissue), 13-day embryonic spleen (a predominantly myeloid organ), adult thymus (a T-lymphoid precursor tissue), and adult bone marrow, all of which contain *proto-amv* mRNA (Chen 1980; Gonda et al. 1982; M. Dvorak, unpubl.). This protein has not been detected in any nonhematopoietic tissues tested to date nor in AMV-transformed leukemic myeloblasts. Thus, it appears that the normal cellular homolog of the viral p48^{amv} is the much larger p110$^{proto-amv}$. This is consistent with the relative sizes of their mRNAs as described above.

Recent experiments show that p110$^{proto-amv}$ is also not glycosylated and does not act as a protein kinase in vitro in immunoprecipitates. However, in contrast to p48^{amv}, p110$^{proto-amv}$ appears to be strongly phosphorylated in intact cells.

Other workers (Klempnauer et al. 1983) who used a different approach, an antiserum against proteins coded by a fused plasmid-growth hormone-*amv* vector, have recently detected a protein presumably identical to p48^{amv} in an AMV-transformed cell line. This same antiserum also detected a putative *proto-amv*-encoded protein of 75,000 m.w. in avian erythroblastosis virus (AEV)-transformed erythroblasts that had previously been shown to express *proto-amv* mRNA (Gonda et al. 1982). It is possible that this 75,000 m.w. protein represents an altered or alternately spliced *proto-amv* gene product. However, no data for normal tissues were presented by these workers.

Subcellular location of p48^{amv} and p110$^{proto-amv}$

If the altered proto-oncogene hypothesis were true for AMV, then the viral *amv* and cellular *proto-amv* gene products should differ in biological properties as well as in structure. As a first approach to understanding the function(s) of these proteins, their location(s) within the cell have been determined. Both subcellular fractionation and immunofluorescence studies using the anti-*amv* peptide antibodies described above have identified the viral p48^{amv} as a nuclear protein in *amv*-transformed myeloblasts (Figs. 3 and 5a,b). In contrast, the p110$^{proto-amv}$ cellular homolog is found exclusively in the cytoplasm of embryonic bursal and thymic lymphocytes (Figs. 4 and 5c,d). This differing subcellular location does not appear to be a property attributable to hematopoietic transformation in general, because MSB-1, a cell line from a chicken T-cell lymphoma induced by Marek's disease virus that expresses *proto-amv* mRNA contains cyto-

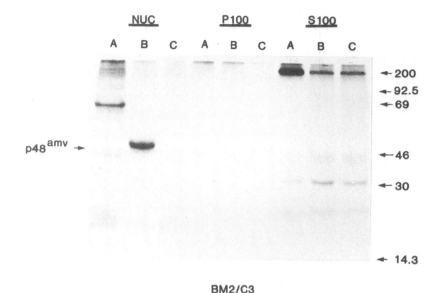

BM2/C3

Figure 3 The AMV transforming protein p48^{amv} is located in the nucleus of BM2 leukemic myeloblasts. Subcellular fractions were immunoprecipitated with normal rabbit serum (lanes *A*), anti-serum to *amv*-peptide 4 (lanes *B*), or anti-serum to *amv*-peptide 4 preincubated with excess peptide 4 (lanoo *C*).

plasmic but not nuclear p110$^{proto-amv}$. Nor is the nuclear location of p48^{amv} likely to be due to viral coding sequences, since many *gag*-fusion retroviral oncogene products are nonnuclear in location and since *env* gene products are not present in cell nuclei. Nuclear localization of proteins appears to be an intrinsic property of their primary structure (Dingwall et al. 1982). Thus, in the case of p48^{amv}, the nucleotropic sequences appear to be cellular in origin.

Among retroviral oncogene products examined so far, only the *myc*- and *fos*-encoded proteins have also been localized in the cell nucleus (Abrams et al. 1982; Donner et al. 1982; T. Curran, pers. comm.). Since p48^{amv} is a candidate DNA-binding protein because of its nuclear location and its possible regulatory function in hematopoiesis, the *amv* protein sequence was compared to that of the known DNA-binding region common to many gene regulatory proteins (Anderson et al. 1982; Sauer et al. 1982). An intriguing similarity is seen between an internal region of *amv* and the helix-turn-helix region common to many phage and bacterial gene regulatory proteins, including λ *cro*, λ *repressor*, and *E. coli lac* repressor products (Fig. 6). Assessment of the significance of this structural similarity must await further elucidation of the function of p48^{amv} in the cell. Since p110$^{proto-amv}$ should contain the same protein sequence, perhaps it or a pro-

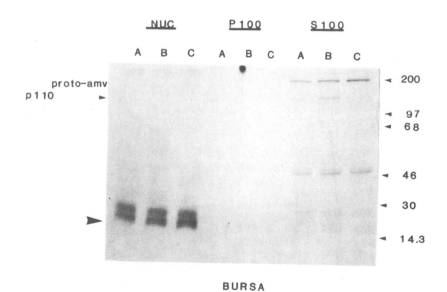

BURSA

Figure 4 The cellular homolog of the AMV transforming protein p110$^{proto-amv}$ is located in the cytoplasm of embryonic bursal lymphocytes. Subcellular fractions were immunoprecipitated as in Fig. 3, using antiserum to *amv*-peptide 1.

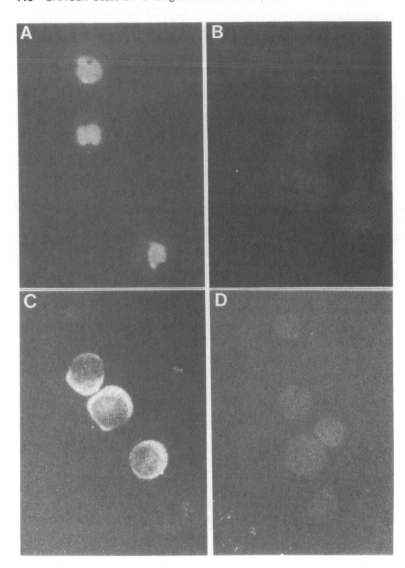

Figure 5 Indirect immunofluorescence confirms the differing subcellular locations of p48^{amv} and p110$^{proto-amv}$. BM2 leukemic myeloblasts stained with antiserum to *amv*-peptide 4 in the absence (*A*) or presence (*B*) of excess *amv*-peptide 4. Embryonic bursal lymphocytes stained with antiserum to *amv*-peptide 1 in the absence (*C*) or presence (*D*) of excess peptide 1.

cessed, as yet unidentified, product also binds specific nucleic acid sequences. Protein interaction with chromosomal DNA need not be restricted to the nucleus, since there is no nuclear membrane during mitosis.

The potential role of *proto-amv* in leukemogenesis

The cellular homolog of the MC29 leukemia virus (*c-myc*) has recently been strongly implicated in the pathogenesis of non-MC29-induced bursal lymphomas in chickens, certain mouse plasmacytomas, and human Burkitt's lymphomas (Hayward et al. 1981; Erickson et al. 1983; Taub et al. 1982; for review, see Klein 1983). Similarly, the cellular homolog of the *erb-B* oncogene of AEV has been implicated in non-AEV-induced erythroblastic leukemias in chickens (Fung et al. 1983). A similar role for *proto-amv* might exist in non-AMV-induced oncogenesis. Three lines of evidence support this possibility.

First, a survey of human neoplasms and cell lines has revealed that *proto-amv* mRNA is expressed only in hematopoietic tissues (Westin et al. 1982). Interestingly,

a promyelocytic human leukemia cell line HL60, which expresses *proto-amv* and can be induced to differentiate in vitro, no longer expresses *proto-amv* mRNA once differentiated. This suggests a role for this gene in maintenance of the transformed phenotype. The *proto-amv* RNA species identified in human neoplasms thus far have been approximately 4 kb in size, suggesting that they are not grossly altered gene products and that an increased gene dosage mechanism may be involved. However, elevated proto-oncogene expression does not necessarily imply transformation. Increased expression of these cellular genes occurs in stem cells and regenerating tissues as well as in neoplasms (Scolnick et al. 1981; Goyette et al. 1983). Recent studies have shown that p110$^{proto-amv}$ is induced in T lymphocytes stimulated to divide by the immunomimetic mitogen concanavalin A (J. Lipsick, unpubl.). Thus, expression of *proto-amv* may be a general property of many rapidly dividing hematopoietic cell lineages, whether transformed or not.

Also, a potential role for *proto-amv* in human carci-

A.

Homology of p48^amv to DNA Binding Regulatory Proteins

p48^amv	GLN-asn-his-thr-ALA-asn-tyr-pro-GLY-trp-his-ser-thr-thr-VAL-ala-asp-asn-thr-arg
lambda repressor	GLN-glu-ser-val-ALA-asp-lys-met-GLY-met-gly-gln-ser-gly-VAL-gly-ala-leu-phe-asn
lambda cro	GLN-thr-lys-thr-ALA-lys-asp-leu-GLY-val-tyr-gln-ser-ala-ILE-asn-lys-ala-ile-his
434 repressor	GLN-ala-glu-leu-ALA-gln-lys-val-GLY-thr-thr-gln-gln-ser-ILE-glu-gln-leu-glu-asn
434 cro	GLN-thr-glu-leu-ALA-thr-lys-ala-GLY-val-lys-gln-gln-ser-ILE-gln-leu-ile-glu-ala
P22 repressor	GLN-ala-ala-leu-GLY-lys-met-val-GLY-val-ser-asn-val-ala-ILE-ser-gln-trp-gln-arg
P22 cro	GLN-arg-ala-val-ALA-lys-ala-leu-GLY-ile-ser-asp-ala-ala-VAL-ser-gln-trp-lys-glu
lac repressor of E. coli	LEU-tyr-asp-val-ALA-glu-tyr-ala-GLY-val-ser-tyr-gln-thr-VAL-ser-arg-val-val-asn

```
                              ***************
          helix      turn          helix
```

B.

Hydropathy of p48^amv and Known DNA Binding Regulatory Proteins

GLN--xxx--xxx--xxx--ALA--xxx--xxx--xxx--xxx--GLY--xxx--xxx--xxx--xxx--xxx--GLY--xxx--xxx--xxx--VAL--xxx--xxx--xxx--xxx--xxx--xxx

	GLN			ALA					GLY					GLY			VAL
p48^amv	−3.5	−3.5	−0.7	+1.8	−3.5	+1.3	−1.6	−0.4	−0.9	3.2	−0.8	−0.7	+0.7	−4.2	+1.8	−3.5	−0.7	−4.5
consensus	−2.5	−1.0	3.2	+1.7	+1.6	3.3	+1.8	3.1	+0.4	1.2	3.2	−0.9	+0.4	4.4	−1.9	+1.9	−0.4	−2.8
	(2.8)	(2.4)	(2.6)	(1.8)	(0.5)	(1.2)	(2.7)	(1.2)	(0)	(1.9)	(1.2)	(0.8)	(3.0)	(1.3)	(0.2)	(1.5)	(3.3)	(2.3)	(4.0)	(2.1)

Figure 6 The AMV oncogene encodes a potential DNA-binding region. (A) Sequences for the known DNA-binding regions of seven proteins are compared with a segment of amv-encoded protein. Boxes indicate highly conserved amino acids. (B) Hydropathy of the amv-encoded protein in this region is compared with that of these seven proteins. Values for each amino acid range from −4.5 to +4.5 in increasing hydrophobicity (Kyte and Doolittle 1982). Standard deviations for the mean consensus values of the seven known DNA-binding proteins are given in parentheses.

nogenesis comes from the recent chromosomal localization of this gene. Human *proto-amv* is located on chromosome 6 at q22–24 (Dalla-Favera et al. 1982; Harper et al. 1983). This locus is near break points seen in consistent chromosomal translocations present in subgroups of human acute lymphocytic leukemia, melanoma, and ovarian carcinoma. Numerous proto-oncogenes have been localized near such break points, suggesting that as for *c-myc*, translocation of these genes may play a role in neoplastic transformation (see Rowley 1983 for review). The *proto-amv* locus should be examined for rearrangement in the neoplasms listed above.

Finally, a recent study of Abelson murine leukemia virus (Ab-MLV)-induced murine B-cell neoplasms has revealed a distinct subclass of such tumors, all of which contain rearranged and transcribed *proto-amv* loci. Interestingly, these neoplasms do not require the continued presence of Ab-MLV for maintenance of transformation (Mushinski et al. 1983). These findings suggest a possible role for the *proto-amv* gene product in the etiology of this non-AMV-induced neoplasm. Thus, further studies on alteration of *proto-amv* may shed light on the oncogenic mechanism of various non-AMV-induced as well as AMV-induced leukemias and lymphomas.

Acknowledgments

We wish to thank S. Aaronson, S. Benedict, R. Doolittle, P. Duesberg, R. Gallo, N. Kan, C. Moscovici, T. Papas, and P. Reddy for scientific collaboration and helpful discussions. This work was supported by grant CA-10197 from the U.S. Public Health Service. J.S.L. is a fellow designate of the Leukemia Society of America.

References

Abrams, H.D., L.R. Rohrschneider, and R.N. Eisenman. 1982. Nuclear location of the putative transforming protein of avian myelocytomatosis virus. *Cell* **29:** 427.

Anderson, S.M. and J.H. Chen. 1981. In vitro translation of avian myeloblastosis virus RNA. *J.Virol.* **40:** 107.

Anderson, W.F., Y. Takeda, O.H. Ohlendorf, and B.W. Matthews. 1982. Proposed α-helical super-secondary structure associated with protein DNA recognition. *J. Mol. Biol.* **159:** 745.

Baluda, M.A. and I.E. Goetz. 1961. Morphological conversion of cell cultures by avian myeloblastosis virus. *Virol.* **15:** 185.

Baluda, M.A., B. Perbal, K.E. Rushlow, and T.S. Papas. 1983. Avian myeloblastosis virus: A model for the generation of viral oncogenes from potentially oncogenic cellular genetic elements. *Folia Biol.* **29:** 18.

Bergmann, D.G., L.M. Souza, and M.A. Baluda. 1981. Vertebrate DNAs contain nucleotide sequences related to the transforming gene of avian myeloblastosis virus. *J. Virol.* **40:** 450.

Beug, H., M.J. Hayman, and T. Graf. 1982. Myeloblasts transformed by the avian acute leukemia virus E26 are hormone-dependent for growth and for the expression of a putative *myb*-containing protein, p135 E26. *EMBO J.* **1:** 1069.

Birckbichler, P.J. and I.F. Pryme. 1973. Fractionation of membrane-bound polysomes, free polysomes and nuclei from tissue cultured cells. *Eur. J. Biochem.* **33:** 368.

Bishop, J.M. 1981. Enemies within: The genesis of retrovirus oncogenes. *Cell* **23:** 5.

Bishop, J.M. and H. Varmus. 1982. Functions and origins of retroviral transforming genes. In *Molecular biology of tumor viruses*, 2nd edition: *RNA tumor viruses* (ed. R. Weiss et al.), p. 999. Cold Spring Harbor Laboratory, Cold Spring Harbor, New York.

Bister, K. and P.H. Duesberg. 1982. Genetic structure and transforming genes of avian retroviruses. *Adv. Viral Oncol.* **1:** 3.

Bister, K., M. Nunn, C. Moscovici, B. Perbal, M.A. Baluda, and P.H. Duesberg. 1982. Acute leukemia viruses E26 and avian myeloblastosis virus have related transformation-specific RNA sequences but different genetic structures, gene products, and oncogenic properties. *Proc. Natl. Acad. Sci.* **79:** 3677.

Boyle, W.J., J.S. Lipsick, E.P. Reddy, and M.A. Baluda. 1983. Identification of the leukemogenic protein of avian myeloblastosis virus and of its normal cellular homologue. *Proc. Natl. Acad. Sci.* **80:** 2834.

Breathnach, R. and P. Chambon. 1981. Organization and expression of split genes coding for proteins. *Annu. Rev. Biochem.* **50:** 349.

Brugge, J.S. and R.L. Erikson. 1977. Identification of a transformation-specific antigen induced by an avian sarcoma virus. *Nature* **269:** 346.

Busch, M.P., B.G. Devi, L.H. Soe, B. Perbal, M.A. Baluda, and P. Roy-Burman. 1983. Characterization of the expression of cellular retrovirus genes and oncogenes in feline cells. *Hematol. Oncol.* **1:** 61.

Chen, J.H. 1980. Expression of endogenous avian myeloblastosis virus information in different chicken cells. *J. Virol.* **36:** 162.

Chen, J.H., W.S. Hayward, and C. Moscovici. 1981. Size and genetic content of virus-specific RNA in myeloblasts transformed by avian myeloblastosis virus (AMV). *Virology.* **110:** 128.

Collett, M.S. and R.L. Erikson. 1978. Protein kinase activity associated with the avian sarcoma virus *src* gene product. *Proc. Natl. Acad. Sci.* **75:** 2021.

Dalla-Favera, R., G. Franchini, S. Martinotti, F. Wong-Staal, R.C. Gallo, and C.M. Croce. 1982. Chromosomal assignment of the human homologues of feline sarcoma virus and avian myeloblastosis virus *onc* genes. *Proc. Natl. Acad. Sci.* **79:** 4714.

Dingwall, C., S.V. Sharnick, and R.A. Laskey. 1982. A polypeptide domain that specifies migration of nucleoplasmin into the nucleus. *Cell* **30:** 449.

Donner, P., I. Greiser-Wilke, and K. Moelling. 1982. Nuclear localization and DNA binding of the transforming gene product of avian myelocytomatosis virus. *Nature* **296:** 262.

Duesberg, P.H. 1983. Retroviral transforming genes in normal cells? *Nature* **304:** 219.

Duesberg, P.H., K. Bister, and C. Moscovici. 1980. Genetic structure of avian myeloblastosis virus, released from transformed myeloblasts as a defective virus particle. *Proc. Natl. Acad. Sci.* **77:** 5120.

Erikson, J., A. Ar-Rushdi, H.L. Drwinga, P.C. Nowell, and C.M. Croce. 1983. Transcriptional activation of the translocated *c-myc* oncogene in Burkitt lymphoma. *Proc. Natl. Acad. Sci.* **80:** 820.

Franchini, G., F. Wong-Staal, M.A. Baluda, C. Lengel, and S.R. Tronick. 1983. Structural organization and expression of human DNA sequences related to the transforming gene of avian myeloblastosis virus. *Proc. Natl. Acad. Sci.* **80:** 7385.

Fung, Y.-K.T., W.G. Lewis, L.B. Crittenden, and H.J. Kung. 1983. Activation of the cellular oncogene *c-erbB* by LTR insertion: Molecular basis for induction of erythroblastosis by avian leukosis virus. *Cell* **33:** 357.

Gonda, T.J. and J.M. Bishop. 1983. Structure and transcription of the cellular homolog (*c-myb*) of the avian myeloblastosis transforming gene (*v-myb*). *J. Virol.* **46:** 212.

Gonda, T.J., D.K. Sheiness, and J.M. Bishop. 1982. Transcripts from the cellular homologs of retroviral oncogenes, distribution among chicken tissues. *Mol. Cell. Biol.* **2:** 617.

Gonda, T.J., D.K. Sheiness, L. Fanisher, J.M. Bishop, C. Moscovici, and M.G. Moscovici. 1981. The genome and intracellular RNAs of avian myeloblastosis virus. *Cell* **23**: 279.

Goyette, M., C.J. Petropoulos, P.R. Shank, and N. Fausto. 1983. Expression of a cellular oncogene during liver regeneration. *Science* **219**: 510.

Graf, T. and H. Beug. 1978. Avian leukemia viruses: Interaction with their target cells *in vivo* and *in vitro*. *Biochem. Biophys. Acta* **516**: 269.

Graf, T., N. Oker-Blom, T.G. Todorov, and H. Beug. 1979. Transforming capacities and defectiveness of avian leukemia viruses OK10 and E26. *Virology.* **99**: 431.

Hackett, P.B., R. Swannstrom, H.E. Varmus, and J.M. Bishop. 1982. The leader sequence of the subgenomic mRNAs of Rous sarcoma virus is approximately 390 nucleotides. *J. Virol.* **41**: 527.

Harper, M.E., G. Franchini, J. Love, M.I. Simon, R.C. Gallo, and F. Wong-Staal. 1983. Chromosomal sublocalization of human c-*myb* and c-*fes* cellular *onc* genes. *Nature* **304**: 169.

Hayward, W.S., B.G. Neel, and S.M. Astrin. 1981. Activation of a cellular *onc* gene by promoter insertion in ALV-induced lymphoid leukosis. *Nature* **290**: 475.

Klein, G. 1981. The role of gene dosage and genetic transpositions in carcinogenesis. *Nature* **294**: 313.

―――. 1983. Specific chromosomal translocations and the genesis of B-cell derived tumors in mice and men. *Cell* **32**: 311.

Klempnauer, K.H., T.J. Gonda, and J.M. Bishop. 1982. Nucleotide sequence of the retroviral leukemia gene v-*myb* and its cellular progenitor c-*myb*: The architecture of a transduced oncogene. *Cell* **31**: 453.

Klempnauer, K.H., G. Ramsay, J.M. Bishop, M.G. Moscovici, C. Moscovici, J.P. McGrath, and A.D. Levinson. 1983. The product of the retroviral transforming gene v-*myb* is a truncated version of the protein encoded by the cellular oncogene c-*myb*. *Cell* **33**: 345.

Kyte, J. and R.F. Doolittle. 1982. A simple method for displaying the hydropathic character of a protein. *J. Mol. Biol.* **157**: 105.

LePrince, D., A. Gegonne, I. Gull, C. deTaisne, A. Schneeberger, C. Lagrou, and D. Stehelin. 1983a. A putative second cell-derived oncogene of the avian leukaemia retrovirus E26. *Nature* **306**: 395.

LePrince, D., S. Saule, C. deTaisne, A. Gegonne, A. Begue, M. Righi, and D. Stehelin. 1983b. The human DNA locus related to the oncogene *myb* of avian myeloblastosis virus. *EMBO J.* **2**: 1073.

Lerner, R.A. 1982. Tapping the immunological repertoire to produce antibodies of predetermined specificity. *Nature* **299**: 592.

Moscovici, C. 1975. Leukemic transformation with avian myeloblastosis virus: Present status. *Curr. Top. Microbiol. Immunol.* **71**: 79.

Mushinski, J.F., M. Potter, S.R. Bauer, and E.P. Reddy. 1983. DNA rearrangement and altered RNA expression of the c-*myb* oncogene in mouse plasmacytoid lymphosarcomas. *Science* **220**: 795.

Nunn, M.F., P.H. Seeburg, C. Moscovici, and P.H. Duesberg. 1983. Tripartite structure of the avian erythroblastosis virus E26 transforming gene. *Nature* **306**: 391.

Perbal, B., J.M. Cline, R.L. Hillyard, and M.A. Baluda. 1983. Organization of chicken DNA sequences homologous to the transforming gene of avian myeloblastosis virus. *J. Virol.* **45**: 925.

Roussel, M., S. Saule, C. Lagrou, C. Rommens, H. Beug, T. Graf, and D. Stehelin. 1979. Three new types of viral oncogene of cellular origin specific for hematopoietic cell transformation. *Nature* **281**: 452.

Rowley, J.D. 1983. Human oncogene locations and chromosome aberrations. *Nature* **301**: 290.

Rushlow, K.E., J.A. Lautenberger, T.S. Papas, M.A. Baluda, B. Perbal, J.G. Chirikjian, and E.P. Reddy. 1982. Nucleotide sequence of the transforming gene of avian myeloblastosis virus. *Science* **216**: 1421.

Sauer, R.T., R.R. Yocum, R.F. Doolittle, M. Lewis, and C.O. Pabo. 1982. Homology among DNA-binding proteins suggests use of a conserved supersecondary structure. *Nature* **298**: 447.

Schwartz, D.E., R. Tizard, and W. Gilbert. 1983. Nucleotide sequence of Rous sarcoma virus. *Cell* **32**: 853.

Scolnick, E.M., M.O. Weeks. T.Y. Shih, S.K. Ruschetti, and T.M. Dexter. 1981. Markedly elevated levels of an endogenous *sarc* protein in a hematopoietic precursor cell line. *Mol. Cell. Biol.* **1**: 66.

Silva, R.R. and M.A. Baluda. 1980. Avian myeloblastosis virus proteins in leukemic chicken myeloblasts. *J. Virol.* **35**: 766.

Souza, L.M., J.N. Strommer, R.L. Hillyard, M.C. Komaromy, and M.A. Baluda. 1980. Cellular sequences are present in the presumptive avian myeloblastosis virus genome. *Proc. Natl. Acad. Sci.* **77**: 5177.

Taub, R., I. Kirsch, C. Morton, G. Lenoir, D. Swan, S. Tronick, S. Aaronson, and P. Leder. 1982. Translocation of the c-*myc* gene into the immunoglobulin heavy chain locus in human Burkitt lymphoma and murine plasmocytoma cells. *Proc. Natl. Acad. Sci.* **79**: 7837.

Walter, G., K.H. Scheidtmann, A. Carbone, A.P. Laudano, and R.F. Doolittle. 1980. Antibodies specific for the carboxy and amino-terminal regions of simian virus 40 large tumor antigen. *Proc. Natl. Acad. Sci.* **77**: 5197.

Westin, E.H., R.C. Gallo, S.K. Arya, L.M. Souza, M.A. Baluda, S.A. Aaronson, and F. Wong-Staal. 1982. Differential expression of the *amv* gene in human hematopoietic cells. *Proc. Natl. Acad. Sci.* **79**: 2194.

myc-related Genes in Viruses and Cells

T.S. Papas, N.K. Kan, D.K. Watson, C.S. Flordellis, M.C. Psallidopoulos,
J. Lautenberger, and K.P. Samuel
Laboratory of Molecular Oncology, National Cancer Institute, Frederick, Maryland 21701

P. Duesberg
Department of Molecular Biology and Virus Laboratory, University of California, Berkeley, California 94720

A 1.6-kb nucleic acid sequence, now termed *myc*, was first identified as part of the transforming (*onc*) gene of avian myelocytomatosis virus MC29 (Duesberg et al. 1977; Mellon et al. 1978). Subsequently, the same sequence was found to be associated with three other avian tumor viruses, namely MH2 (Duesberg and Vogt 1979), CMII (Bister et al. 1979), and OK10 (Bister et al. 1980). The oncogenic spectra of the *myc*-containing avian tumor viruses are the broadest among retroviruses; they cause acute leukemia, carcinomas, and sarcomas and transform fibroblasts as well as hematopoietic cells in tissue culture. Because of their leukemogenic potential, they have been termed acute leukemia viruses (Weiss et al. 1982). Our laboratory was the first to clone (Lautenberger et al. 1981) and determine the nucleotide sequence of the proviral genome of MC29 (Reddy et al. 1983). As yet, *myc* sequences have not been found in nonavian retroviruses.

Sequences very closely related to *myc* have also been found in the DNA of normal avian and mammalian species including man (Sheiness et al. 1980; Robins et al. 1982; Taub et al. 1982; Watson et al. 1983a,b). Moreover, cellular *myc* (*c-myc* or *proto-myc*) sequences are expressed in normal cells (Eva et al. 1982; Gonda et al. 1982; Müller et al. 1982; Vennstrom et al. 1982). To study the relationship between viral and cellular *myc* sequences, we have isolated and sequenced a molecular clone of the chicken (Robins et al. 1982; Watson et al. 1983a) and of the human (Watson et al. 1983b) proto-*myc* locus.

Since *proto-myc* sequences are also expressed and, in some cases, overexpressed or rearranged in certain tumor cells (Hayward et al. 1981; Marcu et al. 1983; Payne et al. 1982; Westin et al. 1982; Erikson et al. 1983), it has been speculated that cellular *myc*-related genes have oncogenic potential like their viral counterparts. Most recently, the viral *myc* sequence has been reported to play a role in converting primary rat cells to cell lines in vitro (Land et al. 1983). However, despite such speculation, there is as yet no direct or consistent

circumstantial evidence that *c-myc* sequences have an oncogenic function like viral *myc* sequences (Duesberg 1983).

In the following, we describe a detailed sequence and product comparison of the *myc*-related *onc* genes of MC29 and MH2 with the *myc*-related genes of normal chicken and human cells. These comparisons provide an initial step toward the understanding of the differential function of the viral and cellular genes, the former being direct-acting transforming entities, the latter mediators of unknown cell functions. We will summarize current and previous data showing that the viral and *myc*-related cellular genes are not isogenic (Reddy et al. 1983; Watson et al. 1983a,b). The *myc*-related genes of MC29, CMII, and OK10 appear to be genetic hybrids consisting of elements derived from (essential) virion structural genes, typically *gag* (and also *pol* in the case of OK10) and a largely conserved 1.6-kb *myc* element (see below). We show that the *myc* gene of MH2 is not linked to Δ*gag*. The cellular *proto-myc* genes share with the viral genes the 3'-terminal 1.6 kb of *myc*, interrupted by a species-specific intron of about 1 kb. However, the 5' regions of the cellular genes are different from viral counterparts although they are as yet incompletely defined. Our results clearly indicate that the 3' 1.6-kb domains of all *v-myc* and *c-myc* isolates are highly conserved, whereas the 5' regions of the respective viral and cellular genes are variable.

Materials and Methods

Molecular cloning and nucleotide sequence analysis

A normal chicken locus homologous to the *myc* sequence of the transforming gene of MC29 (*v-myc*) was further subcloned in the plasmid vector pBR322 and then utilized for sequence analysis. Appropriate endonuclease-resistant DNA fragments were labeled, and all subsequent experiments were carried out as described (Watson et al. 1983a,b). The nucleotide sequence analysis of the human *c-myc* locus was determined in a similar manner.

Figure 1 (*See page 154 for figure.*) Comparison of nucleotide sequences of the chicken c-myc (cc-myc) and human c-myc (hc-myc) and the transforming gene of MC29 (v-myc). The apostrophe indicates identity with the chicken c-myc sequence. Dashes represent nucleotide deletions. Negative numbers represent upstream sequences from the two well-defined downstream exons (Watson et al. 1983a,b). Underlined sequences (−1623 to −2175) represent the third noncoding human upstream exon. Also highlighted are the donor (⌐) and acceptor (⌐) signals, polyadenylation signals, and protein translational termination site. Intervening sequences are represented (I) (Watson et al. 1983a,b).

```
              -3181      -3171      -3161      -3151      -3141      -3131      -3121      -3111      -3101      -3091      -3081
CC-MYC   CTGCAGT TAGTTTCTCT GCATATAATT ATATTGCAGC ACAGGATTAT GATTTTCAAC CCTAGGTGTA CTGGAGTAAT TTTGAAGTAT TTCTGCTGCT TCCAGCTGAA

              -3071      -3061      -3051      -3041      -3031      -3021      -3011      -3001      -2991      -2981      -2971
CC-MYC   TTTCGATGGC TTTTACAGCT CTGAGAGCAT TACTGTGTAT TGGGTCATTC TGATACTGTT CTTAAATGAG TAAAAGAACC ATAGAATGGT TTGAGTTGGA AGGGACCTTC

              -2961      -2951      -2941      -2931      -2921      -2911      -2901      -2891      -2881      -2871      -2861
CC-MYC   AAAGGTCATC TAGTCCAACA TCCCTGCAAT GAGCTGGGAC ATCTACAGCT TGATCAGAGC CCTGTAGAGC CTGGCTTTGA GTGTCTCCAG GGATGGGGCA TCCACCACCT

              -2851      -2841      -2831      -2821      -2811      -2801      -2791      -2781      -2771      -2761      -2751
CC-MYC   CTCTGGGCAA CCCGTTCCAG TGCCTCACTG CCCTTATTTT AAAAAAAACA TCTTCCTAAT ATCCAGTCTA AATCTCCCCT GTCCTACTTT GAAACCATTT CCCCATGTCC

              -2741      -2731      -2721      -2711      -2701      -2691      -2681      -2671      -2661      -2651      -2641
CC-MYC   TATCACAAGA AACCCTCCTA AAGAGTCTGT CTCCTTCTTT CTGGTAGCAT CCCTACGAAC TTTCACACTG GGTCAATTCA GATCCTGCCC CTTTCTGGCA GAATCCTTCA

              -2631      -2621      -2611      -2601      -2591      -2581      -2571      -2561      -2551      -2541      -2531
CC-MYC   GCCACGCTAT TTCCAGTCAC ACCAGCAAAG TCCACTACAG ACACAGCGTT GTAGCATTCA AGAACAGCAC GATGTATTTT AAGCCACCTA GGAGCAAGAG CAAACCCAAT

              -2521      -2511      -2501      -2491      -2481      -2471      -2461      -2451      -2441      -2431      -2421
CC-MYC   GCTTAAAATT GGGCACTGCTC AGCACTCCCC GTTTCTGATC CCCTCTTCTT GTTTTCATGA ATCCGTACC CTTTGCTACC CAACAGCGAC AGAAAGGGCT GCGAAGTGCA
MCV      ----GCTGC 'CT'A'T'CG GCTC'GTGAA 'CCCAGCGGG AG'''GGGAG 'GGAAATC'' TATTTG''AA A'GGAGACGG GCG'G'T'CT GTGGG''GG 'GAC'G'G'

              -2411      -2401      -2391      -2381      -2371      -2361      -2351      -2341      -2331      -2321      -2311
CC-MYC   CTCGGAGCGG AATTTGGCTG CAAACATTCC GCTGCTCAGC GGAAATGGGC GATTTCCACT TAAAAAAAAA AAGGGGGGGG GGGGATTTTT TTTTTTTTTT TTTCATTATT
MCV      'C'''GCT'T 'G'C'TA'AC A'T'ATG'TA TG'AACG'TG AA'C'GCAAT ACAGC'TTA' A'GG'G'G'' 'G''TACC'T 'CATGA'GA' 'GG'GGAAG' AAGGTGGTAC

              -2301      -2291      -2281      -2271      -2261      -2251      -2241      -2231      -2221      -2211      -2201
CC-MYC   TTTTTCGCCG GGAGGGGTTC GTGCAGGTGC CGGGCCGGGG CTGCGCGCTG CATCCCGCGG GCGCTATCGG GCGCCGGGAG AGGGCGCGAT GGCCCCACGG TAGCGTTGGC
MCV      GA'CGT'''T TATTA''AAG ''AACA'ACG G'TCTTACAC GGATTG'AC' ATCTA'TT'A TTC'GCATA' TA'AAAT'TT GTATTTAAG' 'C'TAGCTC'' ''A'AA'AAA
HC-MYC   ---------- ---------- --------C' ''''TTCCCA AA'AGAGG' 'G'GGG'GAA AA'AA'AAA' ATC'TCTCTC GCTAAT'TCC 'C''A'CG'C CCTTTA'AAT

              -2191      -2181      -2171      -2161      -2151      -2141      -2131      -2121      -2111      -2101      -2091
CC-MYC   CGTGGGAAAG CCGGGGCCGCC CCCAGCGCCG GGGAACCGCA ACGGGGGGAT GGATGGGGAG GGGGGTGCGG GGGTCCTCCC GCCCGGCGAT CCGTGTTCCT TTTG'T'ACC
MCV      ''CCATTTTA ''ATC'AC'A 'ATT'GT'T' GGACC'C'GA T' GAT''ACAGA CCG'T'A'TC CCTAAC'ATT AC''CGCC''T 'AAT'AA'CA GAAG'C'T'A TTTG'T'ACC
HC-MYC   GCGA''GTCT GGAC'G'TGA GGACC'C'GA 'CTGTG'TGC T''C''CCGC CACC''CC'G' CCCC'GC''T C'T'CTGCC' 'GAGAAGGGC AGGGCTT''C
                                                                         start non-coding exon

              -2081      -2071      -2061      -2051      -2041      -2031      -2021      -2011      -2001      -1991      -1981
CC-MYC   CTACGCTTAG AAATGATACA AATACTTATA AGTCCGTTTG GTGTGCGTGT GTGTGTGGGG GGAGGGGGGG GGGAGGGGGG GAAAATAAATG CGAAATAAAT
MCV      'CGACG'G'T CGT'AGGGA' T'GTGG'CGG CCA'A'GCGT 'GCGATCCTG 'CATCC'' TCTC'CTTAA C'''CA''A C'AT'ACCCT AGT'G'GGG' GCTGCGGCT'
HC-MYC   AG'G'''G' CGGGA'A'AG ''CGGAGGG' G'GATCGCGC TGAGTATAAA AGCC'GTTTT C''G'CTTTA TCT'ACTC'C T'TA'TAATT CC'GCG'GA' GC'G'GGG'G

              -1971      -1961      -1951      -1941      -1931      -1921      -1911      -1901      -1891      -1881      -1871
CC-MYC   AAGAAATGCA TGAGAAATAG GAATGATATA TATGTATATA TCTTAGCGGG GTGCCCGCAG GTGCGGGTAT TGCAGCGGGA GGGGGCGGAA TAGCGGTCCC GCGGGGCCGG
MCV      'G''GGGCAG AAGCTG'GT' ACG'GGG'GG G'GC'CC'CG G'CGG'G''C AA'GT''GC ACCGG'AAC' CAG''A'TCG TT''AAG'CG GGAA''AAG' C''AC'A'T'
HC-MYC   CGAGCGG''G GCC'GCTAG' 'TGGA'G'GC CGG'CGAGC' GAGCT'''CT 'C'GG''TCC TG'GAA'GGA GATCCG'A'C 'AATA'GG'G CTT''CCT'T 'GCCCAG'CC

              -1861      -1851      -1841      -1831      -1821      -1811      -1801      -1791      -1781      -1771      -1761
CC-MYC   GAAGACGCGA TGCGGAGCGC CCCGTCGGGT CTCGGCTCGG CGCACCTCCG GGGATGGGTA ACGGGGAAGG GGTGACCCCG GGGTGGGGAA GGAGCCGCTG GGTGAGGGGC
MCV      AGCAGTC'AC CC'A'GCGTT GATTCT''TC GC'C'G'GGA TCA'A'AGCAT' 'AAGCC'TC' TAAA''TGAT TTC'T''G'' 'T'AAAACCT ATT''G'AAA AACCTCTCCT
HC-MYC   TCCCG'TGAT CC'CC'''CA G'G''C'CA AC''CTTG''' 'ATC'ACGAA ACTT''CCC' TA'CA'CG'' C'G'CA'TTT 'CACT''A'C TT'CAACACG C'A'CAA''A

              -1751      -1741      -1731      -1721      -1711      -1701      -1691      -1681      -1671      -1661      -1651
CC-MYC   TGCGGAGCGA GCGGGGGGGG GTGCAGAGCC CCCGGGGGTC ACCTTGCAGC CGCTCCCCCC GCAGCCTCCT CCTCCCGTTT AATCCTCCGG GATAACGAAG CAGCGACACG
MCV      'CTAAGAA'G AAATA'''GC CATGTTGT'' 'T'TTACAAA ''GGAA'GGT' GCT'ATGT'T C'CT'AGA' TA'ATTCCCC GGGGTCAT'' '''CC'ATTA 'C''G'''T
HC-MYC   C'''ACT'TC T''AC'C'G' 'A'GCT'TT' TG'CCATT'G GGGACA'TT' 'C'G''G'TG C''GAC''G 'G'T''TGAA 'GG'TCT'GT TGC'G'TGCT T''ACG'TG'

              -1641      -1631      -1621      -1611      -1601      -1591      -1581      -1571      -1561      -1551      -1541
CC-MYC   GGCGGGGGGTG CGCGAGCTAC GGACGCTCCT TTGTGCCGGT AGGGTAGCCG GCAACCGCCC CGCCCGCAGC CGCGTTACGG GTGGACACGG AGCGTGAACC TCCCCTGCCG
MCV      CA'CCA'CG' GCAAT'G'' TTGG'AAATC GG'A'AGTTA 'AAACCG'TC' 'A'AGG'ACA G'TTAC'T'T GAG'AA''AA
HC-MYC   ATTTTTTTC' G'TAGTGG'A AAC'AGGTAA GCACCGAA'' CCAC'T'''T TTT'ATTTAT TTTTTTATCA 'TTTAATGCT 'A'ATG'GTC GAATGCCTAA ATAGGGGTGTC
                          end non-coding exon └ start intron

              -1531      -1521      -1511      -1501      -1491      -1481      -1471      -1461      -1451      -1441      -1431
CC-MYC   CCGTCGGGGG GCAGCGGGAG GAGGGGGAGC GGAGAGCGAG GAGGGAAGGA GGGAGGGGGG AAGGCAGCGA GGAGGGAAGC AGCGAGGGAGC GCCCTTTTCA TCCCCGCTCG
MCV      AGT'TT''TT 'GGATTA'G' 'GA''AG'G TCTCTC'ACA CAG'TCCG'AG T'C'TC'A'A ''CCAGCAAC ''C'GC'A'T 'CA''G 'GGAGGAAGT GGGAGAAA'A
HC-MYC   TTT''TCCCA TTCCT'C'CT ATT'ACACTT TTCTCAGAGT AGTTATG'T' ACTG'''CT' GG'TGG'G'G TA'TCC'GAA CTG''TCG'G 'TAAAG'GAC 'TGT'AAGAT

              -1421      -1411      -1401      -1391      -1381      -1371      -1361      -1351      -1341      -1331      -1321
CC-MYC   TATTTTTTTT TTTTTTTTAC TATGTTTACT CCTTGTAGTA AGAGAAAAAA AACCAACCGC TGCTCCGCAT CGCCTCTCCC CGGCCCCTCT CCCTGCCCTT CGCCGCGCGG
MCV      AC'G'GCAGC GAGA'GCG'A G''GCGC'G GAG''AACTG ''ACACCTA' 'ACCGT'GGC 'CATCCTGCT AT'ATT''GG AA'AG''ATT G'CTGTAAT' 'G'GC'A'AG'
HC-MYC   GGGAGAGGAG AAGGCAGAGG G'AAACGGGA ATG'TTT'TA AGACTACCCT TTC''G'TTT CTG'CTTATG AATATATTCA ''TGACT'' ''''GG''G GA'ATT'CTG

              -1311      -1301      -1291      -1281      -1271      -1261      -1251      -1241      -1231      -1221      -1211
CC-MYC   CTCCCTCCCG CCCGCCCAGC TCCGGCTCGC AGTACTCGG GGGGGGCACG GAGCCCCTCG GCCGCCCCCT CGCGGCGCGC CCTCCCCGCT CACGGAGCCC GCGCGGGAGCG
MCV      ''GGC''T 'TC'T'CTT ATGT'GGGAG T'GTT'GTAT CCTTCC'TG' CG'GGGTGG'A AGA''AG'AG G''AAT'CT'A TCG''G'G'G 'AA'A'CCAA
HC-MYC   ''TTA'TGT' TTAATTGCT' ''T''G'TTT G'GGGG'T'' ''TT''TTT 'C'GTGGG'A 'AAAG'''' T''AT'CT'A G''''TT'GA GTA''GA'G CATATCGC'T

              -1201      -1191      -1181      -1171      -1161      -1151      -1141      -1131      -1121      -1111      -1101
CC-MYC   GGGGCGAGCG GGAGGGAGAT GAAGCGGCGA CGCGCACCGC GAGAGCGCGC ACTCGCGGGG CCCCGCCGTG CCGCTCGTGC TCCCGCCCCC GCTGCATCTC CCGCCCGCCC
MCV      ''CG'''C 'A'G'CAC'CG 'GTCA'''TC 'TG'GC'G'' 'CTGA'TGA' TGGGCAA'' T''GG'GA'GA G'TTG''A'T A'TG'T''G' C'GTGG'GG' 'ATG''TGTA
HC-MYC   'T'TGAGC'A 'ATC'CTCCG 'C'GC''CT' 'TT'TC''CG TCTCCG'GAG GGCATTTAAA TTT''G'TCA ''ATT'CT' GA'A'''''GGA 'AC'G'CACT G''G'GCGT'

              -1091      -1081      -1071      -1061      -1051      -1041      -1031      -1021      -1011      -1001       -991
CC-MYC   CTCGCCGGCG CTTTAAAGAC AGCAAAGCAA CTTAACTTCT ATTGTACCGG ACGGAGCGCG CCGCGCCGCC TTGGACCGTA CAATCTGCCG CACGCCGGGA AGGGCAGCCC
MCV      G'GATTAA'A 'AGAGGGAC' C''CTG'ACC C''CTGGAGC CAAAATTGAT CACA''ACT' G'TGATACGG 'CA'GA'CA' GGGCT'A'GA TC'C'GATT' CTAT'GCAGA
HC-MYC   'CGC'''C'T 'G'CCCCGCGG C''ATTCCA'C 'CGCC''GA' CC'T'TAA'A 'GTTG''ATT TG''TTTTTA AAAAG'AA'' AT'CAATTTA A'AC'T'''T CTCTCAGAGGT

               -981       -971       -961       -951       -941       -931       -921       -911       -901       -891       -881
CC-MYC   TCTCCGCTGT ATTTTTTTTC TCATCGTGGT GGGGAGAAGC GATCTACGTT CTCCCGGCGT TTTGGCTCCC TTTTTTCCCC CGTCTTCTCC GGCGGTTCTT TTTATATTT
MCV      AG'GGAAGCG C''A'G'CCT C'CGGC''C' 'CCGCATGAT 'TCACGAA'T 'TAATGA'A'' 'A'TTTAGGA CC'GCC''AT ATG'C'TATG 'AT''ACGC' 'GGGG'G'CC
HC-MYC   GT'AG'AC'' GG'G''GGGT AGGCGCA''C A''G'A''AG 'GAGGCGAGG A'GTGTC''A ''CTC''GGA A'CG''GA'T T'GAAAAA'' A'G'CGAA'C 'CCGC'CCCA

               -871       -861       -851       -841       -831       -821       -811       -801       -791       -781       -771
CC-MYC   TATCTCCAAT TTCCTGATTT TGTTGTTCCC CGCACCGCCC GCAATTATTG CCTCGCTCCG TCTCGCAGCC GGCGCGTTGG AGGAGCCGGT GAGTGGCGGG GCTCCGCTTT
MCV      A'CTC'AG'C GGTTAT'GCG GCGGCCA'T' GCG'C''G A''CCC'GC' AACG'TCAA' GACG'GG'GA ACG'AC'AAC TT'GAT''C'T T'AA''GCTT AGCTGATGGG
HC-MYC   GCC''GACTC CC'TGCCGCG GCCGCCCT'G G'TGT'CT'G CGCCCG'GAT G'GGAGGAAC 'GCGAGGAG' ''G''TC''' GC'GTT'CAG A'CA'CT'CT A'C'TTGG'G

               -761       -751       -741       -731       -721       -711       -701       -691       -681       -671       -661
CC-MYC   ACCCATCACT CGATCCCGGC CGGTCGGGCT GACAGCGGGG GGCCGCGGGA CCGCGGCTCC CTCCCGGGGG ACGCGGCGCT GCTCCGGGCA CGGCGCCGCCC CATCCTTCTC
MCV      'TGGTGGG'A ACCCA'AGG' TCAGGCC''A TTATTAAGAC C'GG'GAATT GGTTGCTATT ACGG''TC'' CTCTCCA'GC 'T'TA'A'A' GTTGC'CGG' TGG'GGAAC'
HC-MYC   GGGGTGG'T'C G'GGGA'GTA TC'CA'C'GG 'T'TCT'GC' CAGTTGCATC T'CGTAT''A G'G'GAA''' 'G'T'C'C'' AT'ATTATTT GACAC'C''' TTGTA''TAT

               -651       -641       -631       -621       -611       -601       -591       -581       -571       -561       -551
CC-MYC   CGTGCTCCTCG GCTTGGATAT ATAATTCTAT TTTTTGGAGG GGGGGGGGGG GTGGGGAGG GCAAGAAGCA TTTGCTTCTC CGCGTACGCA CGGCAGGTTA TGCTTATTGC
MCV      T'CAGGTC'A TGGGC'GACA TC'CGCAGGG ACCA'CTGA' TCCTTT'TT' A'TTC'CCAA T'GGCTTAT' AAG''GGT'G A'G'GT'AG' 'CT'CC'CCT 'C'GCGCG'G
HC-MYC   G'A'GGG'GT TAAA'CCCGC GGCTGAGCTC GCCACTCCA' CC''C'A'A' AAA'AA''AA AA AGCT'GCAA' AGGAG'GT'G A'GA'T''GGG ''GGG'CG'G

               -541       -531       -521       -511       -501       -491       -481       -471       -461       -451       -441
CC-MYC   ACATATATAC GTATATATAT GTGCGTGTGT GGATATATAT GTATATATGA TAAATTTGGC AAAGTTTGCC CAGCTCCGTG CACGGCCAGG TGGGTGGCTG GGGAGCAGCC
MCV      CTCCGGTG'T CAT'GAC'GC T'TA'GCA'A A'TC'C'GCC AG''''CAG C'GC''ATA GGGCAGCA'' 'TC'A'A'C GC'AA'A'CC GCA'CGG''' G'CCCC'GC' C'''''G'GG
HC-MYC   GGCCG'GG'G G'A'GGG'AGGT 'G'A'GG'A' 'CGGTGCCGG GGGGGTA'G AG'GCGGCTA GGGCGCGAGT GC'AA'C'GC 'T'GAT''GGG ''GGG'CG'G
                                                                                         v-myc/chicken homology

               -431       -421       -411       -401       -391       -381       -371       -361       -351       -341       -331
CC-MYC   CGGCTCTGCG CTGGGAGCTA CCGGCCCTTC TCGCCCGGTT CCCGGTGCCG GAGCTGGGCA CCGGCTGAGC GCGGCGGCTG CGGGAGCTGT GCCCGAGCGG AGCCCCTCCG
MCV      ---------- ---------- ---------- ---------- ---------- ---------- ---------- ---------- ---------- ---------- ----------
HC-MYC   TTCACGCAGC 'GCTAGCGCC 'A'''G'C'' ''''''TTC'C 'TTCAG'TG' CGCAAAACTT TGT''CTT'G ATTTT'''AA ATT'TTT'CC T'A'CGC'AC CT''''GCGGC
```

Figure 1 (*See page 153 for legend.*)

```
                   -321        -311        -301        -291        -281        -271        -261        -251        -241        -231        -221
CC-MYC   GAGAGTCGCG  GGGAGAGCGC  TCCGGGCGTC  CCCGGGCGCT  GACCCCTCGA  TGGACGGGGT  CGCGACTCCC  GGTCGCCCCG  CTGAGCTGGG  GAGGGGGTGA  GGCGGGGGGC
MCV      ----------  ----------  ----------  ----------  ----------  ----------  ----------  ----------  ----------  ----------  ----------
HC-MYC   TTCTTAA'G'  C'CCAG'GC'  GATTTCGA'T  ''TCT''CGC  TG'GGGG'CG  ACTC'C'''C  TTT'CGCT''  ''G'T''G'   GG'''G'''   'CTC''CG'G  CA'CAA'CCG

                   -211        -201        -191        -181        -171        -161        -151        -141        -131        -121        -111
CC-MYC   TCACGAGGGG  TCGTGCTTTT  TATTATTATT  ATTATTTTAT  TATTATTATT  AGTTTATATA  TATATATATA  TATATAAATC  AATCTGACGG  CGCGGGGTGC  CGGGAGGGAG
MCV      ----------  ----------  ----------  ----------  ----------  ----------  ----------  ----------  ----------  ----------  ----------
HC-MYC   CTGGTTCACT  AA'''G'C'   CCGAGA''GC  'GGGGAC'G'  CCAA'GGGGG  T'AAAGGG'G  CTCCC'TAT   'CCCCC'CCA  'GA'CAC'CA  GC''CTT'AG  G''ATA'CTC

                   -101        -91         -81         -71         -61         -51         -41         -31         -21         -11         -1
CC-MYC   CGCTGCGTGC  CGAGGGTCGA  TCTCCCCCGG  CTATAGGGGC  GGGGGGAGCG  GAGCCTCGCG  GCCCCAGGCG  CGGCTCACCG  GGCCCCCCCG  TGTCCCCCTC  CCGCCCGCAG
MCV      ----------  ----------  ----------  ----------  ----------  ----------  ----------  ----------  ----------  ----------  ----------
HC-MYC   T''AAG'G'A  GAG'TTCG'G  A''GTGG'''  GCACT'C''G  CT'C'CCAG'  TTT''G'A'C  AAGA'CCCTT  TAA''''AGA  CTG''T''''  CT'TGTGTG'  ''CG'TC'''
```

```
         start of exon                    30                                  60                                  90
CC-MYC   ┌GCA GCA GCC GCC GCG ATG CCG CTC AGC GCC AGC CTC CCC AGC AAG AAC TAC GAT TAC GAC TAC GAC TCG GTG CAG CCC TAC TTC TAC TTC
V-MYC    │''' ''' ''' ''' ''' ''' ''' ''' ''' ''' ''' ''' ''' ''' ''' ''' ''' ''' ''' ''' ''' ''' ''' ''' ''' ''' ''' ''' ''' '''
HC-MYC   └CAG C'T C'' ''G A' ''' ''C ''' 'A' 'TT ''' T'' A'' 'A' 'G' ''' 'T ''C CT' ''' ''' ''' ''' ''' ''' ''' ''' 'G' 'T ''' ''G'
```

```
                                   120                                 Pst I 150                                 180
CC-MYC   GAG GAG GAG GAG GAG AAC TTC TAC CTG GCG GCG CAG CAG CGG GGC GAG GAG CTG CAG CCT CCC GCC CCG TCC GAG GAC ATC TGG AAG AAG
V-MYC    ''' ''' ''' ''' ''' ''' ''' ''' ''' ''' ''' ''' ''' ''' ''' ''' ''' ''' ''' ''' ''' ''' ''' ''' ''' ''' ''' ''' ''' '''
HC-MYC   --- ''C ''' ''' ''' ''' ''' ''' 'A' --- --- ''' 'A' CAG ''' ''' ''' ''C 'G ''C AG ''' ''T ''' ''' ''' 'A
```

```
                                   210                                 240                                 270
CC-MYC   TTT GAG CTC CTG CCC ACG CCG CCC CTC TCG CCC AGC CGC CGC TCC AGC CTG --- --- --- --- --- --- GCC GCC GCC --- --- TCC ---
V-MYC    ''' ''' ''' ''' ''' ''' 'T' ''' ''' ''' ''' ''' ''' ''' ''' ''' ''' ''' ''' ''' ''' ''' ''' ''' ''' ''' --- --- ''' ---
HC-MYC   ''C ''' 'G ''' ''' ''C ''' ''' 'G ''C ''T ''' ''' 'G'G ''C TGC TCG CCC TCC TAC GTT ''G 'T' A'A CCC TTC ''' CTT
```

```
                                   300                                 330                                 360
CC-MYC   --- --- --- --- --- --- --- --- --- TGC TTC CCT TCC ACC GCC GAC CAG CTG GAG ATG GTG ACG GAG CTG CTC GGG GGG GAC ATG GTC
V-MYC    --- --- --- --- --- --- --- --- --- ''' ''' ''' ''' ''' ''' ''' ''' ''' ''' ''' ''' ''' ''' ''' ''' ''' ''' ''' ''' '''
HC-MYC   CGG GGA GAC AAC GAC GGC GGT GGC GGG A'' ''' --- --- ''G ''' ''' ''' ''' ''C ''' ''' ''G ''A ''A ''' ''G
```

```
                                   390                                 420                                 450
CC-MYC   AAC CAG AGC TTC ATC TGC GAC CCG GAC GAC GAA TCC TTC GTC AAA TCC ATC ATC ATC CAG GAC TGC ATG TGG AGC GGC TTC TCC GCC GCC
V-MYC    ''' ''' ''' ''' ''' ''' ''' ''' ''' ''' ''' ''' ''' ''' ''' ''' ''' ''' ''' ''' ''' ''' ''' ''' ''' ''' ''' ''' ''' '''
HC-MYC   ''' ''' ''T ''' ''' ''' ''' ''' ''' ''' ''' 'G A'' ''' A'' ''' AA' ''' ''' ''' ''T ''' ''' ''' ''' ''' 'G'
```

```
                                   480                                 510                                 540
CC-MYC   GCC AAG CTG GAG AAG GTG GTG TCG AAG CTC GCC ACC TAC CAA GCC TCC CGC CGG GAG GGG GCC CCC GCC GCC GCC TCC CGA CCC GGC
V-MYC    ''' ''' ''' ''' ''' ''' ''' ''' ''' ''' ''' ''' ''' ''' ''' ''' 'A' ''' ''' ''' ''' ''' ''' ''' ''' ''' ''' ''' '''
HC-MYC   ''' ''' ''C --- --- --- ''C 'A ''' ''G ''' T'' ''G ''T G'G ''' AAA ''C A'C ''' AG' C'G AA' C'' G'' ''C --- '''
```

```
                                   570                                 600                                 630
CC-MYC   CCG CCG CCC TCG GGG CCG CCG CCT CCT CCC GCC GGC CCC GCC GCC TCG GCC GGC CTC TAC CTG CAC GAC CTG GGA GCC GCG GCC GAC
V-MYC    ''' ''' ''' ''' ''' ''' ''' ''' ''' ''' ''' ''' ''' ''' ''' ''' ''' ''' ''' ''' ''' ''' ''' ''' ''' ''' ''' ''' '''
HC-MYC   'AC AGC GT' 'GC TCC A'C T'C AGC --- --- --- --- --- --- --- --- --- T'G ''' ''G ''T A'C ''' ''C ''' T'A ''G
```

```
                                   660                                 690                                 720
CC-MYC   TGC ATC GAC CCC TCG GTG GTC TTC CCC TAC CCG CTC AGC GAG CGC GCC --- CCG CGG GCC --- GCC CCG CCC GGC GCC AAC CCC --- ---
V-MYC    ''' ''' ''' ''' ''' ''' ''' ''' ''' ''' ''' ''' ''' ''' ''' ''' ''' ''' ''' ''' ''' ''' ''' ''' ''' ''' ''' ''' ''' '''
HC-MYC   ''' ''' ''' ''' ''' ''' ''' ''' ''T ''A ''C A'' AG' TCG ''C AA' T'' TGC ''' T'' 'AA 'A' T'' 'G' G'' TTC TCT
```

```
                                   750                                 780                                 810
CC-MYC   GCG GCT --- --- --- CTG CTG --- --- --- --- --- --- --- 'GG --- --- --- --- --- --- GTC GAC ACG CCG CCC ACG
V-MYC    ''' ''' ''' ''' ''' ''' ''' --- --- --- --- --- --- --- --- --- ''' ''' ''' ''' --- --- ''' ''' ''' ''' ''' '''
HC-MYC   C'' T'C TCG GAT TCT ''' 'C TCC TCG ACG GAG TCC TCC CCG CAG ''C AGC CCC GAG CCC CTG GTG CTC CAT 'AG ''G ''A ''' ''C
```

```
         end of exon  start of exon      840                                 870                                 900
CC-MYC   ACC AGC AGC GAC TCG GAA│GAA GAA CAA GAA GAA GAT GAG GAA ATC GAT GTC GTT ACA TTA GCT GAA GCG AAC GAG TCT GAA TCC AGC ACA
V-MYC    ''' ''' ''' ''' ''' ''G│''G ''' ''' ''' ''T ''G ''A ''' ''' ''' ''' ''' ''' ''' ''T T'T G'G 'AA A'G AG' C'G 'CT C'' 'GC AAA ''G T''
HC-MYC   ''' ''' ''' ''' ''' ''T│'G ''G ''' ''' ''T ''G ''A ''' ''' ''' ''' ''' ''' ''' ''T T'T G'G 'AA A'G AG' C'G 'CT C'' 'GC AAA ''G T''
```

```
                                   930                                 960                                 990
CC-MYC   GAG TCC AGC ACA GAA GCA TCA GAG GAG CAC TGT AAG CCC CAC CAC AGT CCG CTG GTC CTC AAG CGG TGT CAC GTC AAC ATC CAC CAA CAC
V-MYC    ''' ''' ''' ''' ''' ''' ''' ''' ''' ''' ''' ''' ''' ''' ''' ''' ''' ''' ''' ''' ''' ''' ''' ''' ''' ''' ''' ''' ''' '''
HC-MYC   ''' ''T G'A T'' CCT T'T G'T 'GA 'GC ''' A'C ''A ''T 'CT ''' ''C ''A ''' A'' ''C ''' TC' 'CA ''T ''G ''
```

```
                                   1020                                1050                                1080
CC-MYC   AAC TAC GCT GCT CCT CCC TCC ACC AAG GTG TAC CCA GCC GCC AAG AGG CTA AAG TTG GAC AGT GGC AGG GTC CTC AAA CAG ATC AGC
V-MYC    ''' ''' ''' ''' ''' ''' ''' ''' ''' ''' ''' ''' ''' ''' ''' ''' ''' ''' ''' ''' ''' ''' ''' ''' ''' ''' ''' ''' '''
HC-MYC   ''' ''' ''A ''G ''' ''' ''' ''T CG' AA' ''C ''T ''T ''T ''' ''' G'C ''' ''' 'T' ''A ''' ''G 'G' ''' '''
```

```
                                   1110                                1140                                1170
CC-MYC   AAC AAC CGA AAA TGC TCC AGT CCC ACG TCA GAC TCA GAG GAG AAC GAC AAG AGG ACG CAC AAC GTC TTG GAG CGC CAG CGA AGG
V-MYC    ''' ''' ''' ''' ''' ''' ''' ''' ''' 'T' ''' ''' ''' ''' ''' ''' ''' ''' ''' ''' ''' ''' ''' ''' ''' ''' ''' '''
HC-MYC   A'' ''C A'G T'C ''G A'C ''' ''T T' ''' ''' ''A ''' ''' ''' A'G
```

```
                                   1200                                1230                                1260
CC-MYC   AAT GAG CTG AAG CTG AGT TTC TTT GCC CTG CGT GAC CAG ATA CCC GAG GTG GCC AAC AAC GAG AAG GCG CCC AAG GTT GTC ATC CTG AAA
V-MYC    ''' ''' ''' ''' ''' ''' ''' ''' 'C' ''' ''' ''' ''' ''' ''' ''' ''' ''' ''' ''' ''' ''' ''' ''' ''' ''' ''' ''' ''' '''
HC-MYC   ''C ''' ''A ''G ''C ''T ''' ''' ''' ''' ''C ''G ''' T'' 'AA ''' ''T ''A ''' ''C ''' ''' ''A ''T ''A ''
```

```
                                   1290                                1320                                1350
CC-MYC   AAA GCC ACG GAG TAC GTT CTG TCT ATC CAA TCG GAC GAG CAC AGA CTA ATC GCA GAG AAA GAG CAG TTG AGG CGG AGG AGA GAA CAG TTG
V-MYC    ''' ''' ''' ''' ''' ''' ''' ''' 'C' ''' ''' ''' ''' ''' ''' ''' ''' ''' ''' ''' ''' ''' ''' ''' ''' ''' ''' ''' ''' '''
HC-MYC   ''' ''' ''A 'CA ''A'C ''' ''C G'' ''' G'A ''G ''' ''A 'AG ''C ''T T'T ''A G'G ''C TT ''' C'' AAA C'A C'' ''' '''
```

```
                                   1380                                start non-coding region  1410                       1450
CC-MYC   AAA CAC AAA CTT GAG CAG CTA AGG AAC TCT CGT GCA TAG G AACTCTTGGA CATCACTTAG AATACCCCAA ACTAGAGTGA AACTATGATA AAATATTAGT
V-MYC    ''' ''' ''' ''C ''' ''' ''' ''' ''' ''' ''' ''' ''A ' G'AAAG'AAG G'AA''GATT CC'T'TAAC' GAA'TGTCCT GAGC'ATCAC CT''GAACT
HC-MYC   ''' ''' ''A ''' ''' ''' ''' 'A' ''' ''' C'' ''' T'' ''G ''A
```

```
                                   1500                                              1550
CC-MYC   GTTTCTAATA TCACTCATGA ACTACATCAG TCCATTGAGT ATGGAACTAT TGCAACTGCA TGCTGTGCGA CTTAACTTGA GACTACACAA CCTTGGCCGA ATCTCCGAA
V-MYC    '''''''''' '''''''''' '''''''''' '''''''''' '''''''''' '''''''''' '''''''''' '''''''''' '''''''''' '''''''''' ''''''''''
HC-MYC   ''''''AAA'G CATGATCAA' TGC'ACCTCA CAACC'TG'C TGA'TCT'GA GA'TGAAAG' ''TTA'CCAT' A'GT'AACTG CCTC'A'TTG GAC'TTGG'C ''AAAA'''
```

```
                                   1600                                              1650
CC-MYC   C GGTTTGGCCA GAACCTCAAA ACTGCCTCAT AATTGATACT TTGGGCATAA GGGATGATGG GACATTCTTC ATGCTTGGGG ATGAACTCTT CAACTTTTTT TCTTTTA
V-MYC    ' '''''''''' '''''''''' '''''''''' '''''''''' '''''''''' '''''''''' '''''''''' '''''''''' '''''''''' '''''_'''' ''''''''
HC-MYC   ' TT'''TATGC TTA''ATCTT TT'TTT'TC' TTAAC'G'T' 'GTATTTA'G AATTGTT'TT A'A'AAT''T 'A'A''TACA CAATGT''C' 'TGTAAA'A' 'GCCA'T
```

```
         start Δ env                    1700                                              1750              polyadenylation signal
CC-MYC   AAA TTTTGTATTT AAGGCATTTT TTCTTAGCGA GAATTCCAAA TAGAGTTGTC CCCAGATTGC TGTATATATT TACACATCTT CTTGCCATGT AAATACCTTT AATAA
V-MYC    ''' '''''''''' ''''''''''CC 'GG'GGC'CT
HC-MYC   ''' 'G'AAATAAC TTTAATAAAA CGT'''TA'C AGT'A''CG A'TTTCAA' ''TAGT''ATA GTACCTA
                           polyadenylation signal           poly A addition site
```

```
                                   1800                   poly A addition site          1850                       1880
CC-MYC   AGTCT TTATAGAAAA ATGTGCAACA TTAATACACA GCAGTTGTGG GAACTGGATT TATACTTGTC TTGAACTTGT GTGCCATAAC ATTTCACAGT TTTGTTTTTT ATT
```

Results

Comparing myc nucleotide sequences of the transforming gene of MC29 with those of the chicken and human proto-myc genes

To determine the structural and functional relationship between the chicken and human c-myc locus and the genome of MC29, we have aligned these three sequences on the basis of nucleotide sequence homology (Fig. 1). Several distinct features can be detected, and these are highlighted in Figure 2. Both the chicken and human proto-myc locus contain at least two coding exons interrupted by one noncoding sequence, starting at position 1 and terminating at position 1389 (Fig. 1). They are directly defined as exons by consensus splice donor and acceptor signals and indirectly by the absence of the intron in the viral myc sequence. Protein products of the proto-myc genes with molecular weights of 50,000–60,000 have been identified here (see below). The two exons in both c-myc and v-myc have a common reading frame and a unique conserved translational termination signal TAG (v-myc, chicken c-myc) and TAA (human c-myc) located at position 1387. Beyond this terminator signal, a noncoding stretch of nucleotides is conserved in both v-myc and chicken c-myc. However, in the human c-myc, the corresponding sequences are divergent. Direct comparison of viral and cellular myc genes reveals a stretch of 12 nucleotides (-462 to -473, Fig. 1) shared by MC29 and chicken c-myc but not present in the human c-myc. A perfect splice donor consensus sequence at the 3' border of this 12-bp sequence, e.g., at position -46, indicates a possible upstream exon in chicken c-myc. It would follow that (1) a possible upstream chicken proto-myc exon terminates at position -461 and that (2) the probable recombinational event between a leukemia virus and proto-myc, that generated MC29, occurred in this upstream proto-myc exon at position -474.

To determine how mRNA could be generated from the cellular myc loci, we have looked within these sequences for signals that terminate mRNA. Two consensus signals involved in the termination of mRNA are AATAAA at position 1771 and CACA at position 1807; the corresponding signals for the human homolog are at positions 1685 and 1707.

To identify transcriptional initiation signals in both chicken and human c-myc, sequences 5' to the overlap with v-myc were subjected to sequence analysis. We have extended these sequences 3185 bp upstream in the chicken and 2278 bp in the human. Three approaches have been used to determine the initiation of mRNA from these sequences: (1) examination of the nucleotide sequence for consensus transcriptional signals; (2) utilization of specific [^{32}P]DNA probes from restriction fragments of the genomic c-myc clones (a, b, c, d, e, f, g, h, i, and j for chicken, and a', b', c', and d' for human; see Fig. 2), for hybridization to mature mRNA in the appropriate cells; and (3) direct comparison with sequences generated from cDNA libraries.

To understand how mRNA is initiated in the chicken,

c-myc DNA fragments were isolated from the upstream sequence, as indicated in the legend of Figure 2. Mature 2.5-kb mRNA was detected with probes h, i, and j; weaker signals were obtained with probes a, d, and f; and probes b, c, d, and g gave negative results (not shown). Examination of the chicken c-myc region defined by a, d, and f, identified three possible splice donor signals at positions -2967, -1921, and -1770. If the consensus splice donor signal located at position -2967 were utilized, it is possible that a mRNA could initiate at position -3134 utilizing the "TATA" box at position -3161. This would generate a mRNA that would include both of the cellular coding exons shared with MC29 and MH2 and an uncertain amount of 5', possibly noncoding, sequences. The exact size of the resulting mRNA is uncertain because of uncertainty about the exact 5' end of the mRNA and the question whether other (possibly noncoding) exons exist between the splice donor at -2967 and the acceptors at the 5' ends of the two coding exons shared with the viruses. For example, any mRNA initiating within -1 kb to -3 kb could include an exon, starting at a potential splice acceptor at position -621 up to the splice donor at position -461. The end of this exon would be shared with the 5' end of the myc sequence of MC29 (Fig. 1). Alternatively, a mRNA could initiate in this exon downstream from a potential promoter within this region around position -505 and terminate in an exon downstream from those sequences shared with the viruses to generate a 2.5-kb RNA. The ATG signal at position 16 appears the most likely translation initiation codon for the 2.5-kb proto-myc mRNA. The size of the predicted protein is 47 kD. If the splice donor at -1921 were utilized, a mRNA could again initiate at position -3124, utilizing the same "TATA" box at position -3161. This mRNA would include over 1 kb of 5' sequences and the 1.6 kb of the c-myc-coding exons, for a total of over 2.6 kb. The resulting protein could initiate at the first ATG at -1975 and would have 22 amino acids in addition to the 47-kD protein coded by the downstream exons. If the splice donor site located at -1770 were utilized, a mRNA could be generated from two positions, one at -3134 utilizing the TATA box at -3161, the other at -1923 utilizing the TATA box at -1946. The predicted protein generated from these mRNAs would have 21 amino acids plus those resulting from the two downstream exons. The multiple mRNAs found in chicken cells and predicted from DNA sequence studies could be templates for more than one protein coded by the chicken c-myc locus.

We have identified in human c-myc a stretch of nucleotides 1622 bp upstream from the 5' coding exon (-1623 to -2175, Fig. 1), present in the 2.5-kb mature mRNA in human cells. These experiments were carried out with DNA fragments a', b', c', and d' (Fig. 2): Probes a' and c' detect the 2.5-kb mRNA; probes derived from b' and d' gave negative results (data not shown; methods as for Fig. 8). Careful examination of this region reveals the presence of a mRNA initiation site containing a potential capping site (-2175, Fig. 1) and a TATAAT box (-2203, Fig. 1). This region contains several ter-

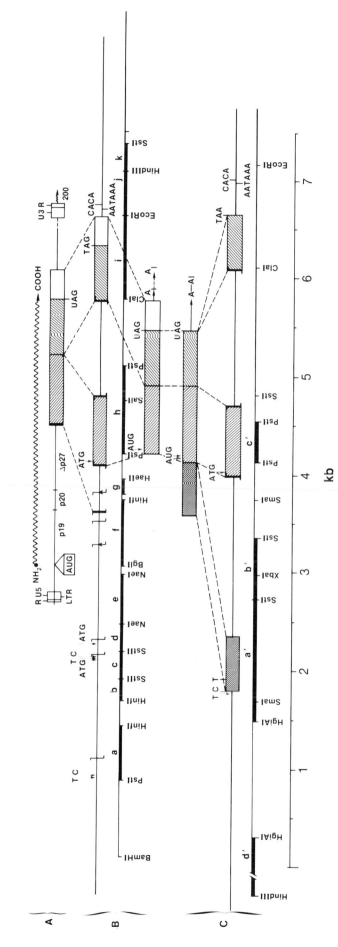

Figure 2 Summary of the major features of the nucleotide sequence analysis of the chicken *c-myc* locus, the human homolog, and the transforming gene of MC29. (A) Proviral genome of MC29 virus; (B) chicken *c-myc* locus and the virus-related region of the *c-myc* mRNA; (C) human *c-myc* locus and the 2.5-kb mRNA. Restriction map and the important features of these genes, including the open reading frames and possible signals for initiation of transcription and translation are illustrated. Hatched areas represent conserved exons shared by these genes. Shaded areas represent human *c-myc*-specific coding regions. Arrows indicate positions (TTATA box) and C (capping site) and ATG; ([ ) and ([ ) represent donor and acceptor signals. Arrows under line B designate positions of LTR insertions in avian leukosis virus-induced lymphomas.

minators with no open reading frame and no translational initiation signal (ATG). We can therefore conclude that this region in the human *proto-myc* gene may represent a noncoding exon. Direct comparison of these sequences with the corresponding sequences derived from a cDNA mouse library (Stanton et al. 1983) revealed that this region is highly conserved between humans and mice. Interestingly, these sequences are not found in the chicken, at least in the corresponding upstream region.

The data generated from these approaches lead to the general conclusion that the human *c-myc* locus is possibly less complex than the chicken homolog.

Protein products predicted from sequence analysis

Comparing the gene products predicted from the nucleotide sequence of the chicken and human *c-myc* loci and the MC29 *onc* gene reveals two distinct domains, the 5' unique domains and the closely related 3' coding domains (Fig. 2). The major difference between the human and chicken *c-myc* genes and the MC29 *onc* gene is in the unique 5' domain. In the MC29 gene, this domain carries 452 amino acids of the retroviral *gag* gene that are not shared with the gene products of the *c-myc* loci. By contrast, the 5' domains of the cellular genes appear to be largely noncoding regions. A schematic comparison of shared and unique amino acids among the proteins encoded by the related 3' domains of MC29, chicken, and human *c-myc* is shown in Figure 3. The p110 MC29 (110 kD) protein encoded by the *myc* domain differs by seven amino acids from the chicken *c-myc* product encoded by the two 3' exons. Much greater variation is found if the human *c-myc* is compared with the viral and chicken *myc*-related genes (Fig. 3), primarily around the coding regions that flank the splicing points. This is consistent with a higher rate of evolutionary change in the exon region nearest the introns. Moreover, the introns of the two cellular genes are completely divergent.

Identification of the chicken *c-myc* gene product(s)

Sequence analysis of the chicken *c-myc* locus revealed an open reading frame shared with the MC29 virus that may generate several putative protein(s). Several models have been discussed above as to how these proteins can be generated from distinct mRNAs. To test these models, we have generated two types of antisera, one raised against synthetic peptides derived from the DNA sequences and the other against a fragment of the MC29

Δ*gag–myc* protein synthesized in *Escherichia coli* (Lautenberger et al. 1983a,b,c). The *myc*-related proteins of Q8 quail cells and chicken embryo fibroblasts transformed by MC29 were labeled with [³⁵S]methionine and then precipitated with both types of antisera. Both antisera immunoprecipitated the p110 *gag–myc* protein from MC29-infected cells (lanes B, C, and D in Fig. 4). The same antisera immunoprecipitated a major and a minor protein from normal cells migrating at 53 kD and 60 kD, respectively (lanes E, G, and H in Fig. 4). These proteins were not detected when preimmune antisera were used (lane F) and both were competed out when synthetic peptide was included in the incubation mixture (lanes I and J). We therefore conclude that the chicken *c-myc* locus generates at least two products—a major 53-kD protein and a minor 60-kD protein. We do not exclude the possibility that other proteins were generated from this locus but were not detected because of technical limitations.

Avian carcinoma virus Mill Hill (MH2) contains a specific sequence, *mht,* and shares a *myc* sequence with MC29, CMII, and OK10 viruses

We have cloned the integrated genome of the MH2 virus from MH2-transformed nonproducer cells. The size of the DNA provirus is 5.2 kb and its complete genetic structure is 5'-Δ*gag*(1.9 kb)-*mht*(1.2 kb)-*myc*(1.3 kb) and a noncoding *c* region (0.2 kb)-3'. Thus, MH2 differs from MC29, CMII, and OK10 in its unique *mht* sequence. A comparison of MH2 and MC29 proviral genomes is shown in Figure 5.

The *gag–myc* junction in molecularly cloned, proviral MC29 DNA is located between the two *Pst*I sites shown in Figure 5b. The restriction pattern of the cloned MH2 proviral DNA indicated that 5' of the left *Pst*I site there exists a high degree of homology between the two viruses. The restriction patterns of the proviral DNAs 3' of the right *Pst*I site were again almost identical up to the rightmost *Hae*II site, suggesting that the MH2 proviral genome contained most of the *myc* sequence found in MC29. These data were consistent with the results from the Southern blot analysis in that the MH2 1.4-kb *Bam–Bam* fragment hybridized only to the 1.1-kb *Bam–Pst gag*-related 5' fragment of MC29 and the MH2 3.2-kb *Bam–Bam* fragment hybridized only to the 1.5-kb *Pst–Bam myc*-related 3' fragment of MC29 (Fig. 5b,c). The *Xho*I site within the *myc* sequence of MH2 is due to a

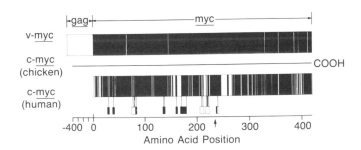

Figure 3 Comparison of predicted amino acid sequence of the chicken *c-myc* to the *myc* sequence of the transforming gene of MC29 and to the human *c-myc*. Solid areas represent identical amino acids. Differences are shown by open areas. Open and solid boxes represent deletions and insertions, respectively. Arrows designate boundary between exons.

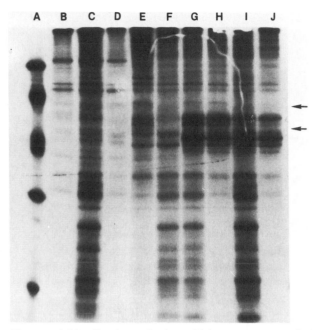

Figure 4 Identification of the chicken *c-myc* product. [^{35}S]methionine-labeled cell lysates from Q8 cells transformed with MC29 (lanes *B,C,D*) and uninfected chicken embryo fibroblasts (lanes *E–J*) were precipitated with two types of antisera—one raised against synthetic peptide derived from DNA sequences (lanes *G,H,I,J*) and the other against a fragment of the *v-myc* protein synthesized in *E. coli* (lanes *B,C,E*). (Lane *F*) Precipitation with preimmune antisera. (Lanes *I,J*) 5 μg of synthetic peptide was included in the incubation mixture.

single-base mutation at position 2900 in MC29 DNA (Kan et al. 1984). However, between the *Pst*I sites in MH2 there was an extra sequence of about 1.2 kb that was not present in the genome of MC29. Furthermore, the restriction pattern of this fragment did not correspond to that of either the *gag* or *pol* sequences of Rous sarcoma virus (RSV) (Schwartz et al. 1983), indicating that the extra sequence in MH2 was unrelated to these viruses. We refer to this MH2-specific sequence as *mht*.

The structure of MH2 provirus and the cellular origin of its *mht* sequence

DNA sequence analysis of the 6.5-kb RI-resistant DNA insert that includes the MH2 provirus (Kan et al. 1984) indicated that the 3′ RI site of this insert was located 1 kb downstream from the 3′ proviral long terminal repeat (LTR). DNA sequences at the junctions of Δ*gag–mht* and *mht–myc* are shown in Figure 6. The nucleotide sequence of MH2 that encompasses the *gag–mht* junction is shown juxtaposed with the corresponding *gag* sequence of RSV in Figure 6. The *gag–mht* junction is near the *Bam*HI site which is 2 kb downstream from the 5′ *Eco*RI site. The overlap between the *gag*-nucleotide sequences of RSV and MH2 stops at sequence position 1923 of RSV (Schwartz et al. 1983). Thus, by comparison with the RSV genome the Δ*gag* region of MH2 contains the complete p27 and p12 minus 63 amino acids at its carboxyterminal end.

Juxtaposition of the *mht–myc* junction sequence with

those of chicken *c-myc* (Watson et al. 1983a) and MC29 (Reddy et al. 1983) showed (Fig. 6B) that there were 25 nucleotides that the *myc* sequence of MH2 shared with the *c-myc* sequence of the chicken that are not present in the sequence of MC29 (Fig. 6B). These *myc* nucleotides map immediately 5′ to the major 5′ chicken *proto-myc* coding exon at positions − 1 to − 25 and probably function as a splice acceptor in *proto-myc* (Fig. 1). A short *mht* nucleotide sequence of MH2 that is related to a possibly homologous *myc* element of MC29 is underlined in Figure 6, A and B. The overlap between the 3′ end of the *gag* region of MC29 with the *gag* gene of RSV at RSV sequence position 1728 (Schwartz et al. 1983) is also shown in Figure 6B.

Data derived from the nucleotide sequence of the MH2 proviral genome indicate that the open reading frame that initiates in the *gag* gene extends into the *mht* region with termination codons present in all three frames approximately 100 nucleotides from the *mht–myc* junction point. The open reading frame within the *myc* portion of MH2 is the same as those of MC29 and chicken *myc*. Single-base mutations are found, however, within the MH2 *myc* that do not alter the open reading frame. The translational termination signal TAG was found to be conserved and at the same position as in the *v-myc* of MC29 and *c-myc* (1387, Fig. 1). The splice acceptor signal at the 5′ end of *myc* that is shared by MH2 and *proto-myc* suggests the presence of a spliced MH2 mRNA with possible donor sequences coming from the 5′ terminal region of the MH2 provirus. Thirty-eight nucleotides of the 3′ noncoding *myc* sequences present in both MC29 and *c-myc* are also found in the *myc* portion of MH2. We have not found envelope-related sequences in MH2. It is therefore concluded that MH2 is a defective virus with a Δ*gag–mht* and a *myc* gene. The *gag* region of MH2 is larger than that of MC29. The *gag* region of MH2 lacks 63 amino acids from p12 and completely lacks p15. MH2 lacks the polymerase and the envelope sequences entirely.

To determine whether *mht* was part of the *c-myc* locus of the chicken or derived from a different chromosomal site, endonuclease-digested chicken DNA was hybridized to *mht* and *myc* DNA after agarose gel electrophoresis. Probes containing only *mht* sequences hybridized to endonuclease restriction fragments of chicken DNA that are different from the fragments of the *c-myc* locus (lanes B, C, E, and F, Fig. 7). Digestion of the same DNA with *Eco*RI (lanes A and D) indicated that both *myc* and *mht* are contained within a 15-kb DNA fragment. Whether this represents physical linkage of these genes or simple comigration of the fragments remains to be resolved. Previous experiments have indicated that *mht* is not located within 5 kb from either side of *myc* sequences (Kan et al. 1983). To determine whether *c-mht* is transcriptionally active, we have assayed normal chicken cells for *mht*-related mRNA. We have identified a single RNA species migrating at 3.8 kb (Fig. 8B) that is larger than the predominant *myc* RNA (Fig. 8A). These results indicate that MH2 contains only a subset of a larger, transcriptionally active cellular gene.

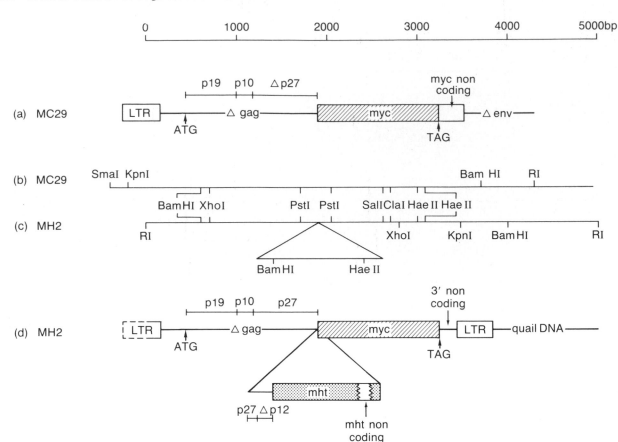

Figure 5 Comparison of the major structural features between MC29 and MH2 proviral genomes. Restriction enzyme maps of MC29 and MH2 proviral genomes are shown in *b* and *c*, respectively. The restriction sites shared by both viruses are listed between the maps, whereas the sites unique to each virus are listed above (*b*) and below (*c*) the maps. MH2 DNA contains an extra sequence of 1.4 kb between the two *Pst*I sites. Genetic maps of MC29 and MH2 are shown in *a* and *d*, respectively; 1.2 kb of the extra sequence in MH2 is designated *mht*. The reading frame of *myc* gene in MH2 is assumed to be the same as that in MC29. The dotted lines in MH2 5′ LTR represent sequences.

Discussion

The Δ*gag–myc* gene of MC29

The Δ*gag–myc* transforming gene of MC29 is a genetic hybrid that consists of 1.5 kb derived from the *gag* gene of avian retroviruses and 1.6 kb from the avian *proto-myc* gene. The 5′ end of the *proto-myc*-derived sequences in MC29 contains a short 13-nucleotide sequence from a *proto-myc* region that maps 474 bp upstream of the major 5′ *proto-myc* exon shared with MC29. The 13-nucleotide sequence obviously functions as an exon in MC29. It is not clear as yet whether it functions as an exon or intron in the *proto-myc* gene. Because a terminator signal is present 5′ to this region at position −500, these 13 nucleotides cannot encode amino acids in *c-myc* protein. However, these nucleotides may be part of an upstream noncoding exon that may start with a splice acceptor at position −622 and terminate with a splice donor at position −461. The bulk of the *myc* sequence of MC29 is derived from the two 3′ *proto-myc* exons, separated by a 1-kb intron. The Δ*gag–myc* gene of MC29 terminates in 0.3 kb of non-coding sequence that is colinear with the 3′ terminus of the *proto-myc* gene.

The *myc*-related gene of MH2

As reported here and elsewhere (Kan et al. 1983, 1984), the genetic structure of MH2 differs fundamentally from that of MC29 in that the *myc* sequence is not directly linked to a truncated *gag* gene. Instead, it appears to be part of or most of a spliced gene that includes a short 5′ virion (possibly *gag*) sequence. Sequence analysis indicates that compared with the *myc* sequence of MC29, the *myc* sequence of MH2 continues to overlap with *proto-myc* upstream of the 5′ boundary of the two exons shared with MH2 for 22 nucleotides into the adjacent *proto-myc* intron. Thus, MH2 shares with chicken *proto-myc* the intron-exon junction at the 5′ border of the two major coding exons of *proto-myc*. It is likely that this region serves in the virus the same splice acceptor function that it is thought to serve in the *proto-myc* gene. The *myc* sequence of MH2 also shares the TAG stop codon with those of MC29 and *proto-myc* and 38 noncoding *myc* nucleotides following this stop codon (Kan et al. 1984).

The *mht* sequence of MH2

In addition to *myc* sequences, MH2 contains a unique 1.3-kb sequence, *mht*, which together with the adjacent

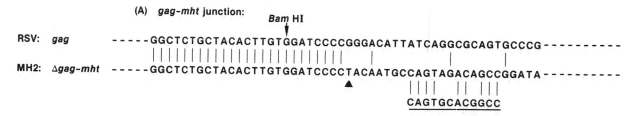

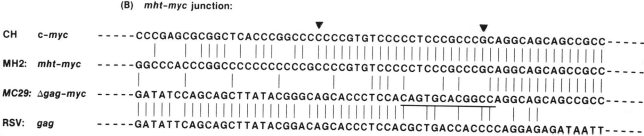

Figure 6 The 5′ and 3′ recombination junction between *gag–mht* (A) and *mht–myc* (B). The vertical lines indicate the area of sequence homology. The RSV *gag* sequences are from Schwartz et al. (1983). Note the presence of 22 bases in *v-mht* are present in *c-myc* but not in the *v-myc*.

5′ 1.9-kb *gag* region of the Δ*gag–mht* hybrid gene encodes the *gag*-related p100 MH2 protein. This protein was thought to be the sole transforming protein of MH2 (Weiss et al. 1982).

However, in view of the two-gene structure of MH2, it remains to be determined what role the *mht*-related and *myc*-related genes play in transformation by MH2. It is conceivable that the Δ*gag–mht* gene is sufficient to transform, however alternative models suggest a possible cooperative function. Preliminary evidence indicates that our MH2 proviral clone is infectious upon transfection onto chicken embryo fibroblasts together with helper virus (MAV-1) DNA. This provides a model for future genetic definition of the roles of Δ*gag–mht* and *myc* genes in the transforming function of MH2.

On the origin of MC29 and MH2 from *proto-myc*
Comparisons of the *myc*-related sequences of MC29, MH2, and chicken *proto-myc* also indicate that the putative recombinational events that generated these viruses from avian *proto-myc* and an avian retrovirus must have been different. In MC29, the 5′ recombination occurred in a region that appears to be an exon or may be an intron in *proto-myc* 474 bp upstream from the two major *proto-myc* exons shared with the virus.

By contrast, the recombination events that generated MH2 would have involved the intron preceding the 5′ boundary of the major coding exons of avian *proto-myc*. Thus, the retroviral transductions of *myc* sequences from avian *proto-myc* that have generated MC29 and MH2 appear to have involved different sites in avian *proto-myc*.

The avian and human *proto-myc* genes and the avian *proto-mht* gene
The exact 5′ boundaries of the avian and human *proto-myc* genes remain to be determined. Nevertheless, the evidence that avian and human *proto-myc* share the two closely related 3′ exons, but differ in introns and in their, as yet, incompletely defined 5′ regions, suggests that the two 3′ exons define conserved structural and functional domains. It is largely these domains that are also shared with the viral *onc* genes. However, the *myc*-related *onc* genes of MC29, CMII, and OK10 are linked to a truncated *gag* gene, whereas the avian and human *proto-myc* genes and the *myc* gene of MH2 are not. Nevertheless, it is likely that at least the chicken *proto-myc* gene contains potential coding sequences that are not part of p110. This is suggested because *myc*-related mRNAs ranging from 2.5 kb to 6.0 kb have been found in normal cells (Sheiness et al. 1980; Gonda et al. 1982) and because preliminary evidence signals the presence of cellular *myc*-related proteins larger than p53 (Fig. 4). The potential coding sequence of the avian *proto-mht* gene must be larger than that of the 1.2-kb *v-mht* sequence, since we have identified a *proto-mht* mRNA of 3.8-kb in normal cells (Fig. 8). Thus, the viral *mht* sequence appears to be a subset of a larger, cellular *proto-mht* gene.

Are *proto-myc* genes functional equivalents of viral *myc*-related genes?
The close structural homology between viral *onc* genes and cellular prototypes suggests that the two types of genes are functionally related. However, it remains to be determined whether the viral genes are functional

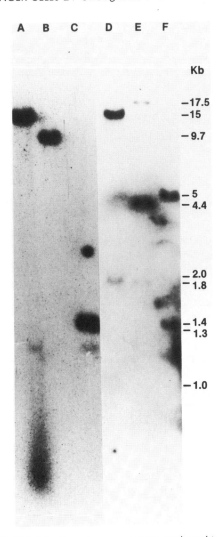

A B C D E F

Kb

—17.5
—15

—9.7

—5
—4.4

—2.0
—1.8

—1.4
—1.3

—1.0

Figure 7 Hybridization of *v-myc*, *c-myc*, and *v-mht* to chicken embryo fibroblast DNA. DNA was digested with *Eco*RI (lanes A and D), *Bam*HI (lanes B and E), and *Hind*III (lanes C and E). Aliquots (20 μg) were fractionated in 0.8% agarose, electrophoresed, transferred to nitrocellulose, and hybridized to nick-translated probes. Lanes A, B, and C hybridized to an 862-bp *Cla*I–*Eco*RI fragment of chicken *c-myc* containing 3′ exon *myc*-specific sequences. Lanes D, E, and F hybridized to an 843-bp *Taq*I–*Taq*I fragment of MH2 proviral DNA containing *mht*-specific sequences.

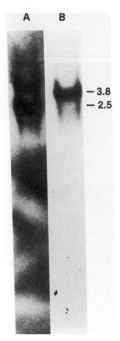

A B

—3.8
—2.5

Figure 8 Expression of *mht* sequence in chicken embryo fibroblasts. Aliquots (5 μg) of poly(A)-selected RNA from normal chicken fibroblasts was fractionated by electrophoresis through a 1% agarose gel containing 2.2 M formaldehyde and 1× MOPS buffer (20 mM MOPS [pH 7.0], 5 mM NaOAC, 1 mM EDTA). RNA was transferred to nitrocellulose and hybridized to nick-translated probes. (Lane A) 862-bp *Cla*I–*Eco*RI *myc* fragment; (lane B) 843-bp *Taq*I–*Taq*I *mht*-specific fragment. (See Kan et al. 1984.)

equivalents or functional variants of cellular genes. If *proto-myc* genes were functional equivalents of viral *onc* genes, they would be potential cancer genes that could play a role in virus-negative cancers (the vast majority of animal cancers). Assuming functional equivalence between viral and cellular *myc* genes, it has been proposed that upstream regulation of *proto-myc* by retroviral promoter insertion (Hayward et al. 1981) or translocation may cause B-cell lymphomas (Taub et al. 1982; Erikson et al. 1983; Marcu et al. 1983) or that gene amplification of *proto-myc* may cause other tumors including myelocytic leukemias (Collins and Groudine 1982; Dalla-Favera et al. 1982). Although there is circumstantial evidence consistent with this view, elevated *proto-myc* expression is not consistently found in the respective

tumors, and such tumors are quite dissimilar from those caused by authentic virus, e.g., lymphomas versus the carcinomas, acute leukemias, and sarcomas caused by viruses of the MC29 subgroup. Furthermore, expression of *proto-myc* in various normal cells argues against a direct role of *proto-myc* genes in carcinogenesis (see above).

Our data provide an alternative explanation for the functional dissimilarities between *proto-myc* and viral *myc* genes. It is likely that both classes of genes share a significant functional domain, encoded in the conserved 1.6 kb of *myc* sequences, but that the qualitative, structural differences that exist between viral and cellular genes represent either specific regulatory or functional domains that determine oncogenicity in the viral genes and normal function in cellular genes.

The major structural differences between viral and cellular *myc*-related genes are the virus-specific *gag* regions of the *onc* genes of MC29, CMII, and OK10. These could alter the topography of the *onc* gene products compared with the cellular *myc* products. The *myc* protein of MC29, for example, is thought to be a nuclear DNA-binding protein (Donner et al. 1982). The cellular *myc* products that lack Δ*gag* may be located at a different site. Alternatively, the viral *gag* and possible cell-specific regions of the cellular *myc* proteins(s) may have regulatory functions affecting a shared functional domain of viral and cellular *myc* proteins acting on identical cellular targets.

It remains to be determined whether the *myc*-related gene of MH2, which appears to lack a *gag* region, is functionally more closely related to the *proto-myc* genes than the hybrid *myc* genes of MC29, CMII, and OK10. An understanding of its role might be an important link between the oncogenic viral hybrid *myc* genes and the cellular genes whose functions are as yet unknown.

Acknowledgments

This work was supported by National Institutes of Health grant CA 11426 to P.D. from the National Cancer Institute. We thank M. Nunn for critical comments on the manuscript.

References

Bister, K., H.-C. Löliger, and P.H. Duesberg. 1979. Oligonucleotide map and protein of CMII: Detection of conserved and nonconserved genetic elements in avian acute leukemia viruses CMII, MC29 and MH2. *J. Virol.* **32**: 208.

Bister, K., G. Ramsay, M.J. Hayman, and P.H. Duesberg. 1980. OK10, an avian leukemia virus of the MC29 subgroup with a unique genetic structure. *Proc. Natl. Acad. Sci.* **77**: 7142.

Collins, S. and M. Groudine. 1982. Amplification of endogenous *myc*-related DNA sequences in a human myeloid leukemia cell line. *Nature* **298**: :679.

Dalla-Favera, R., F. Wong-Staal, and R.C. Gallo. 1982. Onc gene amplification in promyelocytic leukemia cell line HL-60 and primary leukemia cells of the same patient. *Nature* **299**: 61.

Donner, P., I. Greiser-Wilke, and K. Moelling. 1982. Nuclear localization and DNA binding of the transforming gene product of avian myelocytomatosis virus. *Nature* **296**: 262.

Duesberg, P.H. 1983. Retroviral transforming genes in normal cells? *Nature* **304**: 219.

Duesberg, P.H. and P.K. Vogt. 1979. Avian acute leukemia viruses MC29 and MH2 share specific RNA sequences: Evidence for a second class of transforming gene. *Proc. Natl. Acad. Sci.* **76**: 1633.

Duesberg, P.H., K. Bister, and P.K. Vogt. 1977. The RNA of avian acute leukemia virus MC29. *Proc. Natl. Acad. Sci.* **74**: 4320.

Erikson, J., A. Ar-Rushdi, H.L. Drwinga, P.C. Nowell, and C. Croce. 1983. Transcriptional activation of the translocated c-*myc* oncogene in Burkitt lymphoma. *Proc. Natl. Acad. Sci.* **80**: 820.

Eva, A., K.C. Robbins, P.R. Anderson, A. Srinivasen, S.R. Tronick, E.P. Reddy, N.W. Ellmomre, A.T. Galen, J.A. Lautenberger, T.S. Papas, E.H. Westin, and F. Wong-Staal. 1982. Cellular genes analogous to retroviral *myc* genes are transcribed in human tumor cells. *Nature* **295**:116.

Gonda, T.J., D.K. Sheiness, and J.M. Bishop. 1982. Transcripts from the cellular homologs of retroviral oncogenes: Distribution among chicken tissues. *Mol. Cell. Biol.* **2**: 617.

Hayward, W.S., B.J. Neel, and S.M. Astrin. 1981. Activation of a cellular *onc* gene by promoter insertion in ALV-induced lymphoid leukosis. *Nature* **290**: 475.

Kan, N., C. Flordellis, C. Garon, P.H. Duesberg, and T. Papas. 1983. Avian carcinoma virus MH2 contains a specific sequence, *mht*, and shares the *myc* sequence with MC29, CMII and OK10 viruses. *Proc. Natl. Acad. Sci.* **80**: 6566.

Kan, N., C. Flordellis, G. Mark, P. Duesberg, and T. Papas. 1984. Nucleotide sequence of avian carcinoma virus MH2: Two potential *onc* genes, one related to avian virus MC29, the other to murine sarcoma virus 3611. *Proc. Natl. Acad. Sci.* (in press).

Land, H., L.F. Parada, and R.A. Weinberg. 1983. Tumorigenic conversion of primary embryo fibroblasts requires at least two cooperating oncogenes. *Nature* **304**: 596.

Lautenberger, J.A., D. Court, and T.S. Papas. 1983a. High-level expression in *Escherichia coli* of the carboxy-terminal sequences of the avian myeloblastosis virus (MC29) v-*myc* protein. *Gene* **23**: 75.

Lautenberger, J.A., L. Ulsh, T.Y. Shih, and T.S. Papas. 1983b. High-level expression of *Escherichia coli* of enzymatically active Harvey murine sarcoma virus p21 *ras* protein. *Science* **221**: 858.

Lautenberger, J.A., R.A. Schulz, C.F. Garon, P.N. Tsichlis, and T.S. Papas. 1981. Molecular cloning of avian myelocytomatosis virus (MC29) transforming sequences. *Proc. Natl. Acad. Sci.* **78**: 1518.

Lautenberger, J.A., N.C. Kan, D. Court, T. Pry, S. Showalter, and T.S. Papas. 1983c. High-level expression of oncogenes in *Escherichia coli*. In *Gene analysis techniques* (ed. T.S. Papas et al.), vol. 3, p. 147. North Holland/Elsevier. (In press.)

Marcu, K.B., L.J. Harris, L.W. Stanton, J. Erikson, R. Watt, and C.M. Croce. 1983. Transcriptionally active c-*myc* oncogene is contained within NIARD, a DNA sequence associated with chromosome translocations in B-cell neoplasia. *Proc. Natl. Acad. Sci.* **80**: 519.

Mellon, P., A. Pawson, K. Bister, G.S. Martin, and P.H. Duesberg. 1978. Specific RNA sequences and gene products of MC29 avian acute leukemia virus. *Proc. Natl. Acad. Sci.* **75**: 5874.

Müller, R., D.J. Harmon, J.M. Tremblay, M.J. Cline, and I.M. Verma. 1982. Differential expression of cellular oncogenes during pre- and postnatal development of the mouse. *Nature* **299**: 640.

Neel, B.F., G.P. Gregory, C.E. Rogler, A.M. Skalka, G. Ju, F. Hishinuma, T. Papas, S. Astrin, and W. Hayward. 1982. Molecular analysis of the c-*myc* locus in normal tissue and in avian leukosis virus-induced lymphomas. *J. Virol.* **44**: 158.

Payno, G.S., J.M. Dishop, and H.E. Varmus. 1982. Multiple arrangements of viral DNA and activated host oncogene in bursal lymphomas. *Nature* **295**: 209.

Reddy, E.P., R.K. Reynolds, D.K. Watson, R.A. Shulz, J. Lautenberger, and T.S. Papas. 1983. Nucleotide sequence analysis of the proviral genome of avian myelocytomatosis virus (MC29). *Proc. Natl. Acad Sci.* **80**: 2500.

Robins, T., K. Bister, C. Garon, T, Papas, and P. Duesberg. 1982. Structural relationship between a normal chicken DNA locus and the acute transforming gene of the avian acute leukemia virus MC29. *J. Virol.* **41**: 635.

Schwartz, D.E., R. Tizard, and W. Gilbert. 1983. Nucleotide sequence of Rous sarcoma virus. *Cell* **32**: 853.

Sheiness, D.K., S.H. Hughes, H.E. Varmus, E. Stubblefield, and J.M. Bishop. 1980. The vertebrate homologue of the putative transforming gene of avian myelocytomatosis virus: Characteristics of the DNA locus and its RNA transcript. *Virology* **105**: 415.

Stanton, L.W., R. Watt, and K.B. Marcu. 1983. Translocation breakage are truncated transcripts of c-*myc* oncogene in murine plasmacytomas. 1983. *Nature* **303**: 401.

Taub, R., R. Kirsch, C. Morton, G. Levin, D. Swan, S. Tronick, S. Aaronson, and P. Leder. 1982. Translocation of the c-*myc* gene into the immunoglobulin chain locus in human Burkitt's lymphoma and murine plasmacytoma cells. *Proc. Natl. Acad. Sci.* **79**: 7837.

Vennstrom, B., D. Sheiness, J. Zabielski, and J.M. Bishop. 1982. Isolation and characterization of c-*myc*, a cellular homolog of the oncogene (v-*myc*) of avian myelocytomatosis virus strain 29. *J. Virol.* **42**: 773.

Watson, D.K., E.P. Reddy, P.H. Duesberg, and T.S. Papas. 1983a. Nucleotide sequence analysis of the chicken c-myc gene reveals homologous and unique coding regions by comparison with the transforming gene of avian myelocytomatosis virus MC29, gag-myc. *Proc. Natl. Acad. Sci.* **80**: 2146.

Watson, D.K., M.C. Psallidopoulos, K.P. Samuel, R. Dalla-Favera, and T.S. Papas. 1983b. Nucleotide sequence analysis of human c-*myc* locus, chicken homologue, and myelocytomatosis virus MC29 transforming gene reveals a highly conserved gene product. *Proc. Natl. Acad. Sci.* **80**: 3642.

Weiss, R.A., N.M. Teich, H. Varmus, and J.M. Coffin, eds. 1982. *The molecular biology of tumor viruses*, 2nd edition: *RNA tumor viruses*. Cold Spring Harbor Laboratory, Cold Spring Harbor, New York.

Westin, E.H., F. Wong-Staal, E.P. Gelman, R. Dalla-Favera, T.S. Papas, J.A. Lautenberger, A. Eva, E.P. Reddy, S.R. Tronick, S.A. Aaronson, and R.C. Gallo. 1982. Expression of cellular homologues of retroviral *onc* genes in human haematopoietic cells. *Proc. Natl. Acad. Sci.* **79**: 2494.

Evolutionary Relationships among Oncogenes of DNA and RNA Tumor Viruses: *myc, myb*, and Adenovirus E1A

R. Ralston and J.M. Bishop

George W. Hooper Foundation and Department of Microbiology and Immunology, School of Medicine, University of California, San Francisco, California 94143

Structural and functional homologies have been found among proteins encoded by several retroviral oncogenes, demonstrating the existence of families of these genes (Bishop and Varmus 1982). Because the retroviral oncogenes have cellular homologs, the existence of similar families among these "cellular oncogenes" is also implied (for review, see Bishop 1983). Cellular genes belonging to these families have been found in such evolutionarily distant species as humans (Spector et al. 1978; Dalla-Favera et al. 1982), fruit flies (Shilo and Weinberg 1981; Simon et al. 1983), nematodes (Shilo and Weinberg 1981), and brewer's yeast (E. Scolnick and S. Reed, pers. comm.), consistent with the hypothesis that these genes have evolved from a small number of ancestral sequences (Bishop 1983). The role of the cellular oncogenes in normal cells is not known, but it is generally presumed that they act in controlling growth and development.

We now describe evidence for a new family of oncogenes, with the retroviral oncogenes *v-myc* and *v-myb* as prototypes. Proteins encoded by these two genes are found in the nuclei of infected cells (Abrams et al. 1981; Donner et al. 1982; K.-H. Klempnauer, pers. comm.). Unexpectedly, this family also includes the E1A region of adenoviruses, whose products are required for viral oncogenesis (for review, see Flint 1980) and are located in the nucleus (Jochemsen et al. 1982; Feldman and Nevins 1983; Yee et al. 1983). Our findings suggest that the oncogenes of RNA and DNA tumor viruses may at least in some instances share evolutionary origins and function according to common principles.

Results

Having obtained the nucleotide and deduced amino acid sequences of the retroviral oncogenes *v-myc* (Alitalo et al. 1983) and *v-myb* (Klempnauer et al. 1982), we undertook a computer search for related proteins among the current entries in the Protein Sequence Database of Dayhoff (Dayhoff et al. 1983). The search revealed that the proteins encoded by *v-myc* and *v-myb* each contained several short strings of amino acids that were either identical or very similar to strings of amino acids in the proteins encoded by the E1A region of adenovirus type 12 (Ad12) (Perricaudet et al. 1980). Manual inspection of these sequences revealed several distinctive features. In particular, *v-myc* and Ad12 E1A shared two strings of amino acids that were either identical or conservative substitutions, one of which was unusually acidic:

v-myc	...AASAGLY...	...SDSEEEQEED...
Ad 12 E1A	...AASEGLFL...	...SDSEDEQDEN...

Other examples included the sequence: serine, (aromatic), Z, X, X, X, aspartic acid (where X tends to be acidic), near the aminotermini, and a sequence of two/three basic residues followed by a cysteine, near the carboxyl termini:

v-myc	...S F I CDPD...	..NRKCS...
Ad12	...S Y QEAED...	...RRRCA...
v-myb	...SWTEEED...	...HHHCT...

These sequences were found by manually searching for uncommon amino acids (e.g., tryptophan) and amino acids that tend to be conserved during evolution (e.g., cysteine). These and other structural similarities, together with the similarity in subcellular localization of the proteins encoded by *v-myc* and E1A (the subcellular localization of the *v-myb* protein was not known at this point in our comparisons) and the role of E1A in oncogenesis, suggested that further investigation of potential relationships might prove fruitful.

It was apparent from the initial homology search and manual inspection of the sequences that structural relationships between these proteins, if they existed, would not involve extensive strings of identical residues. Analysis of several well-established protein families has demonstrated that proteins can have very similar tertiary structures and closely related functions even though their primary structures are only distantly related (Rossman and Argos 1977, 1981). In the present case, however, the tertiary structures of these proteins have not been determined nor are their biochemical functions known. These difficulties have been overcome in other cases because knowledge of many sequences belonging to a protein family (or "superfamily") has allowed identification of regions of sequence conservation and variability as well as favored amino acid substitutions within these regions (Dayhoff 1978). This information could then be used to evaluate the relatedness of other proteins whose amino acid sequences contained few identities when compared with any single member of the family, but showed clear consistencies when compared with the family as a whole. The approach is analogous

165

to the establishment of taxonomic characters that permit phylogenetic classifications among distantly related species. Similarly, our approach in investigating potential relationships among the proteins encoded by *v-myc*, *v-myb*, and E1A was aimed at identifying consistent characteristics of their primary structures and, where possible, correlating these with biochemical or biological information.

Evaluating the significance of the relationships

Our initial results indicated only that similarities of uncertain significance might exist among the proteins encoded by *v-myc*, *v-myb*, and Ad12 E1A. To evaluate further the relationships among these proteins, we turned to the matrix comparison devised by McLachlan (McLachlan 1971). This method of sequence comparison has several advantages for analyzing distantly related proteins: (1) it calculates all possible comparisons between short strings of amino acids from two proteins by construction of a matrix, (2) it takes into account the probability of amino acid substitutions, and (3) it gives an estimate of the statistical significance of the relationship using a rigorously defined set of assumptions that are based on structural considerations. We were also able to enhance the strength of the comparisons by using the sequences for the related but nonidentical E1A regions of adenoviruses type 5 (Ad5) (Perricaudet et al. 1979), type 7 (Ad7) (Dijkema et al. 1980), and type 12 (Ad12) (Perricaudet et al. 1980), and the sequences for *v-myc* (Alitalo et al. 1983) and human *c-myc* (Colby et al. 1983).

The sequences were compared by using the data for both adenovirus 12 E1A and *v-myc* as reference standards (Fig. 1). The results indicated appreciable homology among the E1A proteins of Ad5, Ad7, and Ad12, as anticipated; intermediate homologies between the *myc* and E1A proteins; and weak but detectable homology between *myb* and both *myc* and E1A. The homology between *myc* and *myb* is slightly more extensive than that between *myc* and the E1A proteins of Ad5 and Ad7.

Aligning the homologies among viral transforming proteins

Having found evidence of significant relationships among these oncogene products, we arranged the sequences to obtain maximum alignment of their homologous regions (Fig. 2). It was apparent from the matrix comparisons that we would be looking for distant relationships, presumably sufficient to conserve tertiary structure and homologous functions of proteins, but not involving extensive strings of identical amino acids. Therefore, we employed a multistep strategy that first aligned the proteins already known to be related (the E1A proteins as one example, the viral and cellular *myc* proteins as another), then used the homologies between the most closely related members of the two groups to align both sets of sequences. This method had the advantage of emphasizing consistencies within each group: making conserved sequences more apparent and providing information about allowable substitutions and regions of variability. Finally, *v-myb* was aligned with the *myc* and E1A sequences.

In each case, the alignments were accomplished as follows. First, occasional regions where the proteins to be compared shared identical strings of amino acids were found and used to define fixed positions in the alignments (examples include residues 14–20, 61–63, 97–100, 117–119, 172–180, 243–247, and 271–288). Regions between the strings of identities were then aligned by inspection, using the string-matching data from the matrix comparisons to identify regions of similar sequence. Judgments of similarity are based on statistical analysis of substitution frequencies for pairs of amino acids in 16 protein families (McLachlan 1971). As the alignment proceeded, we were aided by the use of closely related sequences (the family of E1A proteins on the one hand, the *myc* proteins on the other) to locate areas where variation in sequence length (i.e., insertions or deletions of sequence) is tolerated, and to evaluate the significance of individual amino acid substitutions. For example, in areas where it was difficult to match type-12 E1A and *v-myc*, the other related sequences often provided guides to alignment. After the initial alignment of all seven available sequences was completed, it was rechecked several times to maximize the alignments among all of the sequences.

The final alignments of the various amino acid sequences revealed regions of homology distributed along the entire lengths of the proteins. The homologies involve conservative substitutions of amino acids more frequently than identical residues. Relationships are most apparent between *myc* and Ad12 E1A, and between *myc* and *myb*. There are nevertheless regions where E1A is more closely related to *myb* than to *myc*. The utility of our strategy is illustrated by the relationships we were able to perceive between *myc* and *myb*. These became apparent through the recognition of sequences conserved in both the E1A proteins and the *myc* proteins. Thus, the regions in which E1A and *myc* are most closely related are generally related to *myb* as well. Once perceived, the relationships between *myc* and *myb* proved to be as great as those between *myc* and Ad5 or Ad7 E1A.

While performing the alignments, we discovered a previously unappreciated duplication of sequence in the aminoterminal domain of *v-myb* (Fig. 2C). The rightward unit of the repeat is included in the alignments illustrated by Figure 2A, the leftward unit is not. Analogous repetitions are not apparent in any of the other proteins studied here.

Justifying gaps in the sequence alignments

To achieve the alignments illustrated by Figure 2, it was necessary to place gaps at various positions in the amino acid sequences. Insertions and deletions of amino acid sequence occur frequently in evolutionarily related proteins and are observed as gaps in protein sequence alignments (Dayhoff 1978). For example, numerous gaps are needed to align the amino acid sequences of the serine proteases (Fig. 3A). In general, the gaps occur at similar locations in the various proteins, thereby indicating regions where variations in sequence length can

Comparisons to:

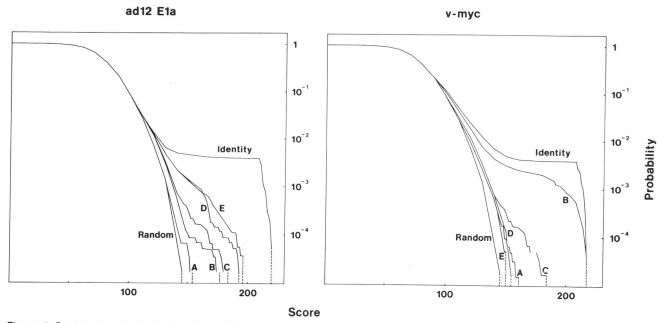

Figure 1 Statistical analysis of relatedness. The sequences of proteins encoded by E1A, *myc*, and *myb* were compared using the matrix procedure of McLachlan (McLachlan 1971) and a VAX 11/780 computer. The sequences encoded by 12S mRNAs were used for the E1A proteins. Two reference sequences were used for the comparisons, the sequence of Ad12 E1A (*left panel*) and the sequence of *v-myc* from MC29 virus (*right panel*). Standards for unrelated sequences with identical amino acid compositions were obtained by comparing the sequences to randomly scrambled versions of themselves. The results of this comparison give the leftward-most curves in the plots. The complete identity obtained when a sequence is compared against itself is defined by the rightward-most curves. Curves describing proteins related by nonidentical sequences fall between the two extremes. The sequences used in the comparisons were *v-myb* (A), *c-myc* (B), Ad5 E1A (D), and Ad7 E1A (E). Curve C (*v-myc* compared with Ad12 E1A or Ad12 E1A compared with *v-myc*) is the same in both panels. Probability is plotted as a function of score. The actual sequences used for the matrix comparison are shown in Fig. 2A.

be tolerated (Lesk and Chothia 1980, 1982; Greer 1981). In this example, the positions of variation arise from the tertiary structure of the proteins, since they represent loops on the surfaces of the native molecules (Delbaere et al. 1975; Greer 1981).

Figure 3B illustrates the placement of gaps in the aligned sequences of the E1A, *myc*, and *myb* proteins. It is apparent that there is a general (but not inevitable) concurrence between the positions of gaps in the related E1A proteins and the proteins encoded by the two retroviral oncogenes. The frequency of gaps is comparable to that observed among distantly related members of the serine protease family. The manner in which gaps in the alignments reflect regions of permissible structural variation is dramatized by the need to use two relatively large gaps to align satisfactorily the very closely related sequences of *v-myc* and *c-myc* and the need to use 17 gaps to align the E1A sequences (see Figs. 2A and 3B).

We conclude that the consistent disposition of gaps along the aligned sequences of E1A, *myc*, and *myb* adds to the credibility of the alignments and suggests that the proteins have related structures. Related observations have been made previously in detailed studies of the serine proteases. These studies demonstrated that distinctions between structurally conserved and structurally

variable regions of related proteins can be used to minimize erroneous alignments of sequence (Greer 1981).

The disposition and number of gaps in the sequence alignments is also consistent with other features of these proteins. Hydrophobicity calculations (Chou and Fasman 1978) indicated that all of the proteins analyzed here are predominantly hydrophilic (data not shown). In addition, the amino acid sequences are uncommonly rich in proline, glycine, and serine, residues that tend to disrupt regular secondary structure. These observations suggest that the tertiary structures of these proteins probably contain many solvent-accessible loops. In other protein families, such structures tend to be hotspots for insertions and deletions (Lesk and Chothia 1980, 1982).

Recent work has indicated that splice junctions within amino acid sequences are generally located on the surfaces of native proteins, frequently within or near regions of length variation in related proteins (Craik et al. 1983). The splice junctions for E1A, *myc*, and *myb* are located in rough accord with this principle (see Fig. 3B).

How did the homologies among E1A, *myc*, and *myb* arise?

The unexpected structural homology between proteins encoded by oncogenes of RNA tumor viruses and DNA tumor viruses raises the question of the origin of this relationship. The issue of convergence versus divergence as the basis of structural relationships between proteins is usually not resolvable unless the number of identical amino acids is commandingly large (Doolittle 1981). However, the current tendency in such arguments seems to favor divergence. Indeed, the premise that it is easier to duplicate and then modify genetic components rather than to assemble new genes de novo from random beginnings has led Doolittle to propose that all proteins have evolved from a small number of ancestral sequences (Doolittle 1981). In the case of *myc* and *myb*, the small number of identities and lack of information about higher-order structure or function make any decision between convergence and divergence necessarily subjective. For *v-myc* and Ad12 E1A, however, we can show that the relationship is unlikely to be due solely to convergence.

Because convergence is defined as structural similarity resulting from functional requirements, its effect must be due to selection at the protein level. Figure 4 shows the nucleotide sequences of Ad12 E1A and *v-myc* in two widely separated regions of amino acid sequence homology. The nucleotide sequences show many identities in these regions, indeed, more than would be expected on the basis of amino acid similarities. For example, the two pairs of aligned serine codons in the upper panel are identical, even though there are 72 possible combinations. In addition, there are strings of identities in the nucleotide sequences that are apparent when two gaps are introduced (lower panel). These identities are not in the reading frame and would not be expected to occur through convergence. However, such identities could be accounted for by two frameshift mutations during evolution of one of the sequences. The unexpected similarities in the nucleotide sequences of Ad12 E1A and *myc* suggest the existence of a common ancestral sequence. The origin of such a sequence could be either common ancestry of adenoviruses and eukaryotic cells

or recombination between ancestral viral sequences and cellular *myc* sequences.

Discussion

We have sought to identify distant relationships among proteins with potentially similar functions by using families of closely related proteins to define structurally conserved and variable regions that should persist even in divergent relatives (Rossman and Argos 1977, 1981). Thus, by first aligning independently the proteins encoded by several E1A genes and the proteins encoded by *v-myc* and *c-myc*, we were able to perceive relationships between the E1A and *myc* proteins. It may be significant that the E1A sequences of Ad12 are most closely related to *myc*, since Ad12 is the most highly oncogenic of the three strains of adenoviruses we have used in our comparisons. In a more refined application of our strategy, we uncovered homologies between *myc* and *myb* only by first comparing the proteins encoded by these genes to the E1A proteins.

The placement of gaps to achieve sequence alignments might be viewed as unduly arbitrary. Our use of gaps was strongly constrained, however, by the requirement that we be able to align seven different sequences derived from three different families of proteins (E1A, *myc*, and *myb*). We prefer this form of constraint to arbitrary assignments of "penalties" for the introductions of gaps in alignments (McLachlan 1971; Doolittle 1981).

The number of identical amino acids in pairwise comparisons between proteins from different families (*myc*, *myb*, and E1A) ranges from 15% to 21%. Although the overall number of identities is not high, it is significant that they tend to occur in similar positions among all of these proteins. The number of identities compares favorably with data for distantly related members of well-established families such as the globins (Dayhoff 1978), cytochromes (Dayhoff 1978), dehydrogenases (Rossman and Argos 1977; Wierenga and Hol 1983), repressors (Sauer et al. 1983), and serine proteases (Delbaere

Figure 2 Alignment of related sequences. The deduced amino acid sequences for E1A, *myc*, and *myb* were arranged to achieve maximum alignment of homologous regions (*A*). Shown are the complete sequences of the smaller E1A proteins (Perricaudet et al. 1979, 1980; Dijkema et al. 1980), residues 97–372 of *v-myc* (Alitalo et al. 1983), residues 102–386 of human *c-myc* (Colby et al. 1983), residues 63–334 of *v-myb* (Klempnauer et al. 1982), and residues 63–334 of chicken *c-myb* (Klempnauer et al. 1982). The residues deleted in the Ad5 mutant *dl*311 (Carlock and Jones 1981) are indicated by the bar above the Ad5 E1A sequence (residues 206–226). *B* aligns the additional domain in the larger E1A proteins with homologous regions from the other proteins. Capital letters denote the amino acids found in the larger but not the smaller E1A proteins. For Ad5 E1A, the sequence unique to the protein encoded by the 13S mRNA follows the Gly at alignment position 180. A 20-residue gap must be inserted between this Gly and the first Glu of the unique sequence to align it with the homologous sequence of Ad12 E1A. Also shown are the amino acid sequences from the larger E1A proteins of the Ad5 host-range mutants H5*hr*440 (Solnick and Anderson 1982), H5*in*500 (Carlock and Jones 1981), and H5*hr*1 (Riccardi et al. 1981). H5*hr*440 terminates at the Glu shown in the lower panel. H5*in*500 is an insertion-frameshift mutant that alters the sequence of the unique region and terminates at the Ile shown. H5*hr*1 is a deletion-frameshift mutant that terminates at the Ile shown. The mutations in H5*in*500 and H5*hr*1 affect only the products of the 13S mRNAs. H5*hr*440 also contains a mutation that prevents splicing of the 12S mRNA, so that only the mutant protein is made. In all of the alignments, asterisks denote identities between amino acid residues or substitutions occur with greater-than-average frequency among related proteins as established by McLachlan (McLachlan 1971); boxes are used to emphasize regions where comparison of both Ad12 E1A to *v-myc* and *v-myc* to *v-myb* reveal strings of homology whose likelihood exceeds average expectation, again according to the scores assigned by McLachlan. The direct repeat in the amino terminus of *myb* is shown in *C*. The sequence begins with the first amino acid of the *myb*-specific region of AMV. This duplication is also present in the amino terminus of *c-myb* (Klempnauer et al. 1982). The amino acid differences in *c-myb* are indicated above and below the *v-myb* sequences. The positions of the splice junctions in *c-myb* are shown by arrowheads.

A Alignment of Sequences

```
                    10          20          30          40          50          60
ad5 E1a    MR HIICHGGV I--TEEMAAS LL DQL IEEVL ADNLPPP-SH FEPPTLHELY DL-- DVTAP
ad7 E1a    MR HLRFLPQE IISSFETGIE ILEFV VNTLM GDDPEPPVQP FDPPTLHDLY DL-- EVDGP
ad12 E1a   MR TEMT-PLV L--SYQEADD ILEHL VDNFF -NEVPSDDDL Y-VPSLYELY DL-- DVESA G
                *  **            ***         *  *              **        **  ***

v-myc      -V TELLGGDM VNQSFICDPD DE SFVKSIII QDCM WSGFS A A-AKLEKVVS EKLA TYQAS
c-myc      -V TELLGGDM VNQSFICDPD DE TFIKNIII QDCM WSGFS A A-AKL---VS EKLA SYQAA
             *  **  ** **** ****   *     *  *  *    ****  *  ***         ** *****

v-myb      -WHNHLNPEV KKTSWTEEED RI IYQ AHKRL GNR-WAEIA K L-LPGRTDNA VK-N HWNSTM
c-myb      -WHNHLNPEV KKTSWTEEED RI IYQ AHKRL GNR-WAEIA K L-LPGRTDNA IK-N HWNSTM
```

```
                    70          80          90         100         110         120
ad5 E1a    --E DPNEE AV SQI----FPD S--VML AVQE GIDLLTFFPA --PG SPEPPH LSRQP EQ QPEQ
ad7 E1a    --E DPNEG AV NGF----FTD S--MLL AADE GLDINPPPET SVTPGVVVES GRGGKK LPDS
ad12 E1a   --E DNNEQ AV NEF----FPE S--LIL AASE GL-FLPEPPV -LSPVC---E PIGGEC MPQL
              * *        *        **     **** ** ***        **   *     ** *

v-myc      RREGGPAAAS RPGPPPSGPP PPPAGP AASA GL-YLHDLGA -AAADCI--D PSVV--FPYP
c-myc      RKD SGSPNPA RGHS------ S------VCSTS SL-YLQDLSA -AASECI--D PSVV--FPYP
           ***  **  **       +     *            **   * * **      *   * *** **  ***

v-myb      RRK VEQEGY P QESSKAGPPS ATTGFQ KSSH IMAFAHNPPA --GPLPGAGQ APLG SDYPYY
c-myb      RRK VEQEGY L QESSKAGL PS ATTGFQ KSSH IMAFAHNPPA --GPLPGAGQ APLG SDYPYY
```

```
                   130         140         150         160         170         180
ad5 E1a    RALGPVSMPN LV-------- ---------- --- PEVIDL TCH -EA-GF PPSDDEDEEG
ad7 E1a    ---------- ---------- ---------- --- GAAEMDL RCY -EE-GF PPSDDEDGET
ad12 E1a   H--------- ---------- ---------- --- PEDMDL LCY -EM-GF PCSDSEDEQD
                                                       **         *******

v-myc      LDERAPRAAP ---------- ---------- --- PGANPAAL LGV -DTPPT TSSDSEEEQE
c-myc      LNDSSSPKSC ASQDSSAFSP SSDSLLSSTE SP PQGSPEPL VLHE EETPPT TSSDSEEEQE
            ***_+                               **  * **   ++       **

v-myb      HIAEPQNV-- ---------- ---------- --- PGQIPYPV ALHI -NIINV PQPAAAAIQR
c-myb      HIAEPQNV-- ---------- ---------- --- PGQIPYPV ALHV -NIVNV PQPAAAAIQR
```

```
                   190         200         210         220         230         240
ad5 E1a    ------PVS- EPEPEPEPE PEPARP TRRP -KMAPAILRR PTSPVSRECN SSTDSC-DSG
ad7 E1a    EQ------ST -----HTAVN EGVKA ASDVF -KLDCPELPG HGCPVSDDES PSPDSTT---
ad12 E1a   EN-GMAHVS- -----ASAAA AAADRE REEF -QLDHPELPG HNCPVSDNE- PEPNSTLDGD
            **  *         ****  ****    *****               *  *

v-myc      EDEEIDVVTL AEANESESST ESSTE ASEEH CKPHHSPLVL KRCHV----- ----------
c-myc      DEEEIDVVSV EKRQAPGKRS ESGSP SAGGH SKPPHSPLVL KRCHV----- ----------
            + * ** *  **  +     **   *       ***           * *

v-myb      HYTDED-PEK EKR---IKEL ELLLM STENE LKGQQA-LPT ---------- ----------
c-myb      HYNDED-PEK EKR---IKEL ELLLM STENE LKGQQA-LPT ---------- ----------
```

```
                   250         260         270         280         290         300
ad5 E1a    PSNTPPE--- ---------I HPVVPLCPIK PVAVRVGGRR Q-AVECIEDL L--NEPGQ--
ad7 E1a    ---SPPEIHA PAPAN-VCKP IPVKPKPGKR PAVDKLEDLL EGG-DGPLDL STRKLPRQ
ad12 E1a   ERPSPPKLGS AVP------- -----EGVIK PVPQRVTGRR RCAVESILDL IQEEEREQTV
               *                     *      * **** **  *** ***     *****  *

v-myc      NIHQHNY--A APPSTKVEYP AAKRLKLDSG RVLKQISNNR KCSSPRTLDS EENDKRRTHN
c-myc      STHQHNY--A APPSTRKDYP AAKRVKLDSV RVLRQISNNR KCTSPRSSDT EENVKRRTHN
               *      **  *   *         *   ** *      *  + * ***  ***    **+   *  *

v-myb      QNHTANY--- -PGWHSTTVA DNTRTSGDNA PV-SCLGEHH HCTPSPPVDH GCLPEESA-S
c-myb      QNHTANY--- -PGWHSTTVA DNTRTSGDNA PV-SCLGEHH HCTPSPPVDH GCLPEESA-S
```

```
                   310         320         330
ad5 E1a    PLD-LSCK-R P-RP
ad7 E1a
ad12 E1a   PVD-LSVK-R P-RCN
              *   *  *   *

v-myc      ------VLER Q-RRNELKLR FFA-LRDQIP EVAN-
c-myc      ------VLER Q-RRNELKRS FFA-LRDQIP ELEN-
                  * *** *  *       **  ****  *

v-myb      PARCMIVHQS NILDNVKNLL EFAETLQLID SFLN-
c-myb      PARCMIVHQS NILDNVKNLL EFAETLQLID SFLN-
```

B Alignment of Sequences Unique to Large E1a Proteins

```
H5hr440 E1a    ---E
H5in500 E1a    ---EEF VLDYVEHPG IPGTVAGLVI ITGGIRGTQI LCVRFAI
H5hr1 E1a      ---EEF VLDYVEHPG HGCR SCHYHR RNTGTQILCV RFAI
ad5 E1a        ---EEF VLDYVEHPG HGCR SCHYHR RNTGDPDIMC SLCYMRTCGM FVYS-
ad7 E1a        -asdvf -kldcpelpg hgcK SCEFHR NNTGMKELLC SLCYMRMHCH FTYS-
ad12 E1a       -ereef -qldhpelpg hncK SCEHHR NSTGNTDLMC SLCYLRAYNM FIYS-
                *****    *  ** **       *  **

v-myc          -aseeh ckphhsplvl krchv----- ---------- ---------- -----
c-myc          -saggh skpphsplvl krchv----- ---------- ---------- -----
                ****     *  **** *

v-myb          -stene lkgqqa-lpt ---------- ---------- ---------- -----
c-myb          -stene lkgqqa-lpt ---------- ---------- ---------- -----
```

C Direct Repeat in the N-terminus of *myb*

```
      1        10          20          30          40          50
                            I                    L         V
      NRTDVQCQHR WQKVLNPELN KGPWTKEEDQ RVIEHVQKYG PKRWSDIAKH LKGRIG
      ***  *  *** ***** *  ****** **  *** ** * *  ******* **  * *  *
      KQCRER WHNHLNPEVK KTSWTEEED- RIIYQAHKRL GNRWAEIAKL LPGRTDNAVK
                                                                  I
      60        70          80          90         100        110
```

Figure 2 (*See facing page for legend.*)

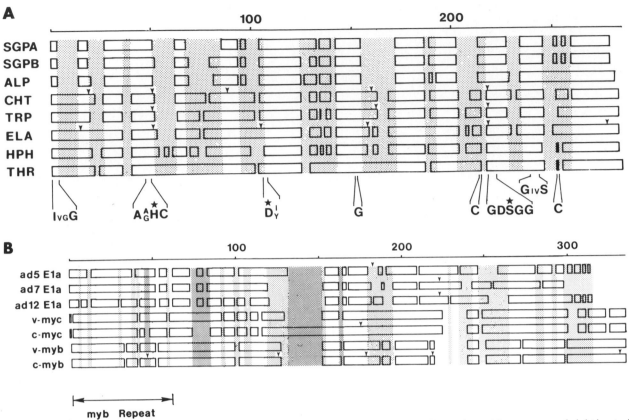

Figure 3 Topographical homologies. (*A*) Gap positions in alignments of serine proteases. The amino acid sequences of eight bacterial and eukaryotic serine proteases and haptoglobin (Craik et al. 1983) have been redrawn to represent contiguous residues in the alignments as blocks. The sequences shown are chymotrypsin (CHT), trypsin (TRP), elastase (ELA), haptoglobin (HPH), thrombin (THR), *S. griseus* proteases A and B (SGPA, SGPB), and α-lytic protease (ALP). The consensus regions of length variation are emphasized by shading. The positions of splice junctions in the mRNAs are mapped onto the amino acid sequences (indicated by arrowheads). Amino acids that are invariant in these proteases are shown in bold type below the block alignments. The number of invariant residues, though small, is larger that the number of invariant residues in the globin superfamily (3/170) (Dayhoff 1978). The active-site residues are indicated with stars as a guide to topography. Haptoglobin (HPH) differs from the consensus residues in having TAKN instead of AAH*C and GDAGS instead of GDS*GG. All of the proteases shown in the block alignments have related tertiary structures (Delbaere et al. 1975). The gaps shown in the alignment map to loops in the tertiary structures (Delbaere et al. 1975; Greer 1981). Note that the conserved residues are widely distributed along the sequences. (*B*) Gap positions in alignments of the *myc*, *myb*, and E1A proteins. The sequence alignments in Fig. 2A have been redrawn to represent contiguous residues by blocks. The 17 gaps that occur in the alignment of the E1A proteins as a group, and that are not due to alignment with *myc* or *myb* are shown by the lightly shaded areas. The three gaps that occur in the alignment of the *myc* sequences are indicated by darkly shaded areas. These shaded areas reflect regions of polypeptide length variation (i.e., insertions or deletions of sequence) within the *myc* or E1A families. The positions of splice junctions are indicated by arrowheads. The position of the direct repeat in the *myb* sequences (Fig. 2C) is also indicated.

et al. 1975; Craik et al. 1983), in which homologous regions were defined much as we have done here.

Several features of the oncogenes we have compared sustain our conclusion that these genes are all relatives of one another. First, the proteins encoded by *myc* (Abrams et al. 1981; Donner et al. 1982) *myb* (K.-H. Klempnauer, pers. comm.), and E1A (Jochemsen et al. 1982; Feldman and Nevins 1983; Yee et al. 1983) are all located in the nucleus of transformed cells. Second, it has recently been shown that E1A and *v-myc* serve similar establishment functions in transformation of cells in culture (Land et al. 1983; Ruley 1983). We learned of these results only after presenting our arguments for a structural relationship between *myc*, *myb*, and E1A. Third, genetic analyses have shown that for Ad5, the larger E1A protein encoded by the 13S mRNA is essential for the function of E1A in cellular transformation (Riccardi et al. 1981). By contrast, there is evidence that the smaller of the two E1A proteins may be sufficient for transformation by Ad12 (Jochemsen et al. 1982). In accord with this contrast, a string of homologous sequence shared by *v-myc* (residues 208–225 in the upper portion of Fig. 2) and the smaller E1A protein of Ad7 and Ad12 is contained instead in the larger E1A protein of Ad5 (Fig. 2B). Ad5 mutants whose lesions are within this region of homology, such H5*hr*440 (Solnick and Anderson 1982) or H5*in*500 (Carlock and Jones 1981) (Fig. 2B), are transformation defective. In contrast, the E1A mutants H5*hr*1 (Riccardi et al. 1981) (Fig. 2B) and *dl*311 (Jones and Shenk 1979) (Fig. 2A) retain transformation

```
ad12    ProCysSerAspSerGluAspGluGlnAspGluAsn
        CCCTGTAGCGATTCGGAAGACGAGCAAGACGAGAAC
        ** * ***** ******** ** ***** ** *
        ACCAGCAGCGACTCGGAAGAAGAACAAGAAGAAGAT
v-myc   ThrSerSerAspSerGluGluGluGlnGluGluAsp


ad12    ProValProGl-nArgValThrGlyArgArgArgCys
        CCTGTGCCTCA-GCGGGTGACTGGGAGGCGTAGATGT
        ** ***** * * * ** * ***
        AGCGT-CCTCAAACAGATCAGCAACAACCGAAAATGC
v-myc   ArgVa-lLeuLysGlnIleSerAsnAsnArgLysCys
```

Figure 4 Nucleotide sequence homologies between *myc* and Ad12 E1A. The nucleotide sequences of *v-myc* and Ad12 E1A corresponding to positions 171–192 and 271–282 in Fig. 2 are shown. Asterisks indicate identical nucleotides. The nucleotide sequence of chicken *c-myc* is identical to *v-myc* in these regions (Watson et al. 1983).

ability, although the phenotype is cold-sensitive in cells transformed by H5*hr*1 (Ho et al. 1982; Babiss et al. 1983).

There are nevertheless significant differences in the biological effects of these oncogenes. For example, *v-myc* is capable of transforming avian fibroblasts and macrophages, whereas *v-myb* can transform avian macrophages but not fibroblasts (see Bishop and Varmus 1982). The E1A proteins by themselves do not cause transformation, but can extend the growth potential of ("immortalize") primary newborn rat kidney cells (NRK) (see Flint 1980). Also, *v-myc* is apparently unable to transform mammalian cells, although its effect on primary NRKs is similar to E1A (Ruley et al., this volume). Although we have identified significant similarities in the sequences of the proteins encoded by these oncogenes, the differences are also clearly important and may relate to corresponding differences in their biological effects.

From previous analyses of proteins related to the tyrosine-specific protein kinases (Bishop and Varmus 1982; Bishop 1983), and from our present demonstration of distant relationships among E1A, *myc*, and *myb*, it appears increasingly likely that retroviral oncogenes and their cellular progenitors have evolved from a small number of ancestral genes, and that the E1A genes of adenovirus share evolutionary origins with *myc* and *myb*. The preservation of structurally conserved sequences in homologous positions raises the possibility that the proteins all have similar structural features that in turn underlie related functions.

Acknowledgments

We thank Robert J. Fletterick and Stephen Sprang for helpful discussions and for assistance with computations, Hugo Martinez for assistance in screening the Protein Sequence Database, Karl-Heinz Klempnauer, Kari Alitalo, Arthur D. Levinson, R. Weinberg, and E. Ruley for communicating their results prior to publication, and Gary Ramsay for critical reading of the manuscript. R.R. was supported by a fellowship from the National Institutes of Health. This work was supported by grants from the National Cancer Institute and the American Cancer Society.

References

Abrams, H.D., L.R. Rohrschneider, and R.N. Eisenman. 1981. Nuclear location of putative transforming protein of avian myelocytomatosis virus. *Cell* **29:** 427.

Alitalo, K., J.M. Bishop, D.H. Smith, E.Y. Chen, W.W. Colby, and A.D. Levinson. 1983. Nucleotide sequence of the *v-myc* oncogene of avian retrovirus MC-29. *Proc. Natl. Acad. Sci.* **80:** 100.

Babiss, L.E., H.S. Ginsberg, and P.B. Fisher. 1983. Cold-sensitive expression of transformation by a host range mutant of type 5 adenovirus. *Proc. Natl. Acad. Sci.* **80:** 1352.

Bishop, J.M. 1983. Cellular oncogenes and retroviruses. *Annu. Rev. Biochem.* **52:** 301.

Bishop, J.M. and H.E. Varmus. 1982. Functions and origins of retroviral transforming genes. In *Molecular biology of tumor viruses*, 2nd edition: *RNA tumor viruses* (ed. R. Weiss et al.), p. 999. Cold Spring Harbor Laboratory, Cold Spring Harbor, New York.

Carlock, L.R. and N.C. Jones. 1981. Transformation-defective mutant of type 5 containing a single altered E1a mRNA species. *J. Virol.* **40:** 657.

Chou, P. and Q. Fasman. 1970. Empirical predictions of protein conformation. *Annu. Rev. Biochem.* **47:** 251.

Colby, W.W., E.Y. Chen, D.H. Smith, and A.D. Levinson. 1983. Identification and nucleotide sequence of a human locus homologous to the v-myc oncogene of avian myelocytomatosis virus MC29. *Nature* **302:** 722.

Craik, C.S., W.J. Rutter, and R.J. Fletterick. 1983. Splice junctions: Association with variation in protein structure. *Science* **220:** 1125.

Dalla-Favera, R., E.R. Gelmann, S. Martinotti, G. Franchini, T.S. Papas, R.C. Gallo, and F. Wong-Staal. 1982. Cloning and characterization of different human sequences related to the onc gene (v myc) of avian myeloblastosis virus (MC29). *Proc. Natl. Acad. Sci* **79:** 6497.

Dayhoff, M.O. 1978. *Atlas of protein sequence and structure*, vol. 5, suppl. 3. National Biomedical Research Foundation, Washington, D.C.

Dayhoff, M.O., L.T. Hunt, W.C. Barker, B.C. Orcutt, L.S. Yeh, H.R. Chen, D.G. George, M.C. Blomquist, and G.C. Johnson. 1983. *Protein sequence computer data base*. National Biomedical Research Foundation, Washington, D.C.

Delbaere, L.T.J., W.L.B. Hutcheon, M.N.G. James, and W.E. Theissen. 1975. Tertiary structural differences between microbial serine proteases and pancreatic serine enzymes. *Nature* **257:** 758.

Dijkema, R., B.M.M. Dekker, and H. van Ormondt. 1980. The nucleotide sequence of the transforming *Bgl*II-H fragment of adenovirus type 7 DNA. *Gene* **9:** 141.

Donner, P., I. Greiser-Wilke, and K. Moelling. 1982. Nuclear localization and DNA binding of the transforming gene product of avian myelocytomatosis virus. *Nature* **296:** 262.

Doolittle, R.F. 1981. Similar amino acid sequences: Chance or common ancestry? *Science* **214:** 149.

Feldman, L.T. and J.R. Nevins. 1983. Localizations of the adenovirus E1Aa protein, a positive-acting transcriptional factor, in infected cells. *Mol. Cell. Biol.* **3:** 829.

Flint, S.J. 1980. Transformation by adenoviruses. In *Molecular biology of tumor viruses*, 2nd edition: *DNA tumor viruses* (ed. J. Tooze), p. 547. Cold Spring Harbor Laboratory, Cold Spring Harbor, New York.

Greer, J. 1981. Comparative model-building of the mammalian serine proteases. *J. Mol. Biol.* **153:** 1027.

Ho, Y.-S., R. Galos, and J. Williams. 1982. Isolation of type 5 adenovirus mutants with a cold-sensitive host range phenotype. *J. Virol.* **122:** 109.

Jochemsen, H., G.S.G. Daniels, J.J.L. Hertoghs, P.I. Schrier, P.J. van den Elsen, and A.J. van der Eb. 1982. Identification of adenovirus-type 12 gene products involved in transformation and oncogenesis. Genetic evidence of adenovirus transformation maintenance function. *Virology* **122:** 15.

Jones, N. and T. Shenk. 1979. Isolation of adenovirus type 5 host range deletion mutants defective for transformation in rat embryo cells. *Cell* **17:** 683.

Klempnauer, K.-H., T.J. Gonda, and J.M. Bishop. 1982. Nucleotide sequence of the retroviral leukemia gene v-*myb* and its cellular progenitor c-*myb*: The architecture of a transduced oncogene. *Cell* **31:** 453.

Land, H., L.F. Parada, and R.A. Weinberg. 1983. Tumorigenic conversion of primary embryo fibroblasts requires at least two cooperating oncogenes. *Nature* **304:** 596.

Lesk, A. and C. Chothia. 1980. How different amino acid sequences determine similar protein structures: The structure and evolutionary dynamics of the globins. *J. Mol. Biol.* **136:** 225.

―――. 1982. Evolution of proteins formed by β-sheets. II. The core of the immunoglobulin domains. *J. Mol. Biol.* **160:** 325.

McLachlan, A.D. 1971. Tests for comparing related amino-acid sequences. Cytochrome *c* and cytochrome c_{551}. *J. Mol. Biol.* **61:** 409.

Perricaudet, M., J.M. le Moullec, and P. Tiollais. 1980. Structure of two adenovirus type 12 transforming polypeptides and their evolutionary implications. *Nature* **288:** 174.

Perricaudet, M., G. Akusjarvi, A. Virtanen, and U. Pettersen. 1979. Structure of two spliced mRNAs from the transforming region of human subgroup C adenoviruses. *Nature* **281:** 694.

Riccardi, R.P., R.L. Jones, C.L. Cepko, P.A. Sharp, and B.E. Roberts. 1981. Expression of early adenovirus genes requires a viral encoded acidic polypeptide. *Proc. Natl. Acad. Sci.* **78:** 6121.

Rossman, M.G. and P. Argos. 1977. The taxonomy of protein structure. *J. Mol. Biol.* **109:** 99.

―――. 1981. Protein folding. *Annu. Rev. Biochem.* **50:** 497.

Ruley, H.E. 1983. Adenovirus early region 1A enables viral and cellular transforming genes to transform primary cells in culture. *Nature* **304:** 602.

Sauer, R.T., R.R. Yocum, R.F. Doolittle, M. Lewis, and C.O. Pabo. 1983. Homology among DNA-binding proteins suggests use of a conserved super-secondary structure. *Nature* **298:** 447.

Shilo, B.-Z. and R.A. Weinberg. 1981. DNA sequences homologous to vertebrate oncogenes are conserved in *Drosophila melanogaster*. *Proc. Natl. Acad. Sci.* **78:** 6789.

Simon, M.A., T.B. Kornberg, and J.M. Bishop. 1983. Three loci related to the *src* oncogene and tyrosine-specific protein kinase activity in *Drosophila*. *Nature* **302:** 837.

Solnick, D. and M.A. Anderson. 1982. Transformation-deficient adenovirus mutant in expression of region 1A but not region 1B. *J. Virol.* **42:** 106.

Spector, D., H.E. Varmus, and J.M. Bishop. 1978. Nucleotide sequences related to the transforming gene of avian sarcoma virus are present in DNA of uninfected vertebrates. *Proc. Natl. Acad. Sci.* **75:** 4102.

Watson, D.K., E.P. Reddy, P.H. Duesberg, and T.S. Papas. 1983. Nucleotide sequence analysis of the chicken c-*myc* gene reveals homologous and unique coding regions by comparison with the transforming gene of avian myelocytomatosis virus MC29, *gag-myc*. *Proc. Natl. Acad. Sci.* **80:** 2146.

Wierenga, R.K. and W.G.J. Hol. 1983. Predicted nucleotide-binding properties of p21 protein and its cancer-associated variant. *Nature* **302:** 842.

Yee, S.-P., D.T. Rowe, M.K. Tremblay, M. McDermott, and P.E. Branton. 1983. Identification of human adenovirus early region 1 products by using antisera against synthetic peptides corresponding to the predicted carboxy termini. *J. Virol.* **46:** 1003.

Properties of the Avian Viral Transforming Proteins *gag-myc, myc,* and *gag-mil*

K. Moelling, T. Bunte, I. Greiser-Wilke, and P. Donner

Max-Planck-Institut für Molekulare Genetik, Ihnestrasse 63, D-1000 Berlin 33, Federal Republic of Germany

E. Pfaff

Institut für Mikrobiologie der Universität, Im Neuenheimer Feld 220, D-69 Heidelberg, Federal Republic of Germany

The acute avian leukemia viruses (ALV) can be classified into three groups by their oncogenic spectra as well as by homologies of their oncogenes (for reviews, see Bishop 1982; Graf and Stehelin 1982). One of these groups comprises the avian myelocytomatosis viruses MC29, the oncogene of which has been designated *myc*. *myc*-related sequences have been identified in three MC29-related viral isolates, the Mill Hill No. 2 (MH2), the myelocytomatosis virus CMII, and Oker Blom's isolate OK10. Another group is represented by the avian erythroblastosis virus (AEV), which codes for two oncogenes, *erb-A*, which is linked to the structural protein *gag*, and *erb-B* (Vennström and Bishop 1982), both of which are unrelated to *myc* (Roussell et al. 1979). The avian myeloblastosis viruses (AMV) and E26 belong to the third group.

The viruses of the MC29 family induce myelocytomatosis and liver, as well as kidney, carcinomas in vivo and transform fibroblasts and macrophages in vitro (Graf and Beug 1978). The sequences responsible for the oncogenicity of these viruses are encoded by the transformation-specific *myc* sequence. Deletions within this region result in transformation-defective mutants, three of which have been described—Q10A, Q10C, and Q10H. These mutants spontaneously arose in an MC29-transformed quail cell line Q10. The mutants are not tumorigenic in animals and show an altered ability to transform bone marrow cells, yet they transform fibroblasts as efficiently as the wild type (Ramsay et al. 1980, 1982a). One of these mutants, Q10H, was passaged through chicken fibroblasts in tissue culture and regained deleted *myc* sequences. This recovered virus, HB-1, does not cause the typical MC29 tumor spectrum in animals but gives rise to rapid lymphomas (Ramsay et al. 1982b). The extent of restoration of wild-type *myc* sequences is still unknown.

Although the *myc* sequences in the case of MC29, CMII, and OK10 are highly related, less homology has been reported between MC29 and MH2 (Roussell et al. 1979; Sheiness et al. 1980). Recently, MH2 was found to be much more oncogenic than MC29 in vivo and it exhibits a higher efficiency of transformation in quail fibroblasts in vitro (Linial 1982), suggesting some more distant relationship between the two.

Most of the viral *myc* sequences are expressed as *gag-myc* polyproteins with the known exception of OK10, which codes for a *myc*-containing polyprotein but also expresses a subgenomic *myc*-specific message (Pfeifer et al. 1981; Saule et al. 1982). We have characterized the avian *gag-myc* polyproteins by using monoclonal antibodies against the viral structural protein p19, which represents the amino terminus of the *gag* portion (Greiser-Wilke et al. 1981). Using these antibodies, we were able to purify the *gag myc* proteins and demonstrate that they bind to double-stranded DNA in vitro (Donner et al. 1982).

Here we report on properties of transforming proteins of OK10 and MH2. Whereas the *gag*-containing polyprotein from OK10 closely resembles other *gag-myc* polyproteins, MH2 does not code for a typical *gag-myc* polyprotein. Rather, this protein exhibits novel properties; it binds to RNA in vitro and was designated here as *gag-mil*. Both OK10 and MH2, furthermore, code for a 55,000-m.w. *myc*-specific protein, p55^{myc}, which is a phosphoprotein located in the nucleus. We identified this protein by *myc*-specific antibodies prepared against a carboxyterminal peptide.

Methods of Experimental Procedures

Cells and viruses

The MC29-transformed fibroblasts used are an established quail fibroblast cell line, designated MC29-Q8-NP, which does not produce any virus (Bister et al. 1977). MH2 is a cell line of MH2-transformed quail nonproducer fibroblasts that was kindly supplied to us by C. Moscovici (University of Florida and Veterans Administration Hospital, Gainesville, Fla.). CMII cells were established as a quail fibroblastic cell line in this laboratory. The OK10-transformed quail cell line OK10-QDP9C, a defective producer line, was established by S. Pfeifer-Ohlsson and was kindly supplied to us by Dr. A. Vaheri (University of Helsinki, Helsinki, Finland). AEV-cl23 is a nonproducer, AEV-transformed, established chicken fibroblast cell line kindly supplied to us by S. Martin (University of California, Berkeley, Ca.). Three transformation-defective deletion mutant-transformed quail fibroblast lines, Q10A, Q10C, and Q10H, were kindly supplied to us by M. Hayman (Imperial Cancer Research Fund, London, England). HB-1 transformed quail fibroblasts originated from T. Graf and H. Beug (EMBL, Heidelberg, West Germany). Cells were grown in Dulbecco's modified Eagle's medium in the presence of 8% calf or 20% chicken serum.

Radioactive labeling of cells, immunofluorescence, indirect immunoprecipitation procedure, immune affinity column chromatography, DNA filter-binding assay, and RNA filter-binding assay have been described before (Bunte et al. 1982,1983; Donner et al. 1982,1983).

Anti-*myc* antibodies

A synthetic peptide representing nine amino acids of the carboxyl terminus of the avian viral *myc* protein was synthesized by Bachem Co. (Bubendorf, Switzerland) and

was used for immunization of rabbits. The rabbits were boosted twice before the serum was used.

Immunoblotting technique

The procedure was performed essentially as described by Towbin et al. (1979). Bacterial lysates containing 50 μg of protein in total were transferred electrophoretically onto nitrocellulose sheets. One strip was stained with amido black for protein and the other one was saturated with binding buffer (3% bovine serum albumin, 10 mM Tris-HCl [pH 7.4], 140 mM NaCl) and then incubated with 1:10 dilution of rabbit-anti-*myc* serum. As second

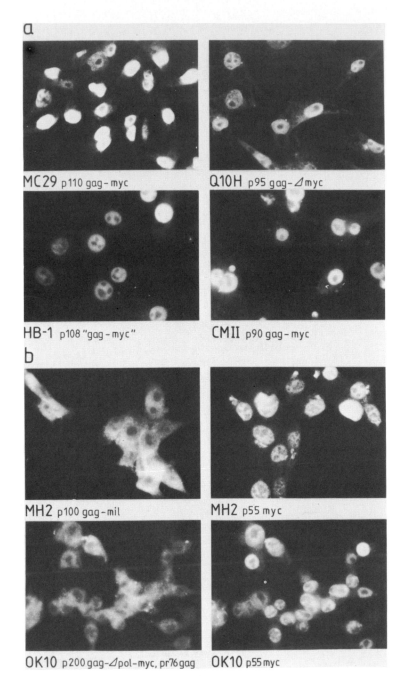

Figure 1 Indirect immunofluorescence analysis of transformed fibroblasts. (*a*) IgG of monoclonal antibodies against p19 and fluorescein-labeled second antibody was used to analyze quail cell lines transformed with MC29 wild-type, Q10H mutant, HB-1 recovered virus, and CMII virus. (*b*) MH22- and OK 10-transformed cells were analyzed with anti-p19 monoclonal IgG (*left*) and anti-*myc* serum (*right*).

antibody, goat anti-rabbit serum labeled with rhodamine was used to allow identification of the immunocomplex by fluorescence.

"McKay assay"

Cells were lysed with 50 mM Tris-HCl (pH 7.5), 0.1% Triton X-100, and 200 mM NaCl, and nuclei were isolated and treated by ultrasonification. The clarified supernatant was treated with immune affinity column material containing anti-p19 IgG. Radioactively labeled DNA fragments were mixed with the immobilized protein as described (McKay 1981). The precipitate was washed with the same buffer used for lysis. Buffers with increasing salt concentrations were applied and the residual precipitate analyzed for DNA.

Results

Cellular localization of *gag-myc, myc,* and *gag-mil,* proteins

Established nonproducer fibroblast cell lines transformed by MC29, MH2, CMII, OK10 and the three deletion mutants Q10A, Q10C, and Q10H, and the recovered virus HB-1, which express virus-specific transforming proteins but do not produce virus, were analyzed. The cellular localization of their *gag*-related polyproteins was analyzed by monoclonal antibodies against p19, the amino terminus of *gag*. The *gag*-unrelated *myc*-specific proteins were tested using antibodies against a *myc*-specific carboxyterminal synthetic peptide. Using these two types of antibodies, indirect immunofluorescence analysis was performed. Figure 1a shows that the wild-type protein p110$^{gag-myc}$ of MC29, the p95$^{gag-\Delta myc}$ of one of its three deletion mutants Q10H, the p108 "*gag-myc*" protein of HB-1, and the p90$^{gag-myc}$ protein of CMII all reside in the nucleus of transformed fibroblasts using monoclonal antibody against p19 for these experiments. Control experiments demonstrating the specificities of all the reactions shown have been published (Bunte et al. 1982,1983; Donner et al. 1982,1983). Figure 1b shows cytoplasmic fluorescence with anti-p19 monoclonal antibodies in the case of OK10 as well as MH2 (Fig. 1b, left part). Since the OK10 cell line used codes also for pr76^{gag}, the protein precursor of the structural *gag* proteins, cytoplasmic fluorescence also arises through the contribution of this polyprotein (Donner et al. 1982). However, the p100^{gag}-related polyprotein of MH2 was considered to be of *gag-myc* type (Hu et al. 1978; Hu and Vogt 1979). Such a molecule would be expected to be a nuclear protein by analogy to *gag-myc* proteins and not cytoplasmic as is shown in Figure 1b. Using *myc*-specific antibodies with MH2 cells, nuclear fluorescence is indeed observed. The same result is obtained with OK10 cells. The type of nuclear fluorescence detected with anti-p19 and anti-*myc* antibodies is indistinguishable; nucleoli are always excluded.

Cell fractionation analyses have confirmed that at least 60% of the *gag-myc* proteins are located in detergent-stripped nuclei and that the MH2 polyprotein is cytoplasmic (Donner et al. 1982; Bunte et al. 1983). Twenty percent of the wild-type and mutant *gag-myc* proteins were detected in a chromatin preparation (Bunte et al. 1982). Furthermore, pulse-chase experiments indicated that most of the p110$^{gag-myc}$ protein migrates to the nucleus within 30–60 minutes (Bunte et al. 1982).

The *myc* protein is a phosphoprotein of 55K

Since no *myc*-specific antibodies were available, a *myc* protein without a *gag*-portion has not yet been described. We prepared antibodies against a synthetic peptide representing nine amino acids of the carboxyl terminus of the avian viral *myc* protein and used them in an indirect immunoprecipitation of metabolically labeled transformed fibroblasts. The precipitated *myc*-specific proteins are the p110$^{gag-myc}$ of MC29 superinfected with RAV-60 helper virus, and a p55 *myc* protein from OK10 and MH2 cellular lysates. In addition to the *myc* protein expressed from a subgenomic message, OK10 also codes for a large polyprotein p200$^{gag-\Delta pol-myc}$ (Saule et al. 1982), which is also recognized by anti-*myc* as well as by anti-p19 antibodies (Fig. 2a). The p100 of MH2 is not recognized by anti-*myc* sera in agreement with its absence from the nucleus. P100 is not of *gag-myc* type, and is designated p100$^{gag-mil}$ in these studies.

The *gag-myc* wild-type proteins are known to be phosphorylated (Ramsay et al. 1982a); p100$^{gag-mil}$ is phosphorylated as well (Fig. 2b). Furthermore, p55^{myc} in OK10 and MH2 cells is also phosphorylated (Fig. 2b). The specificity of the *myc* antibody is demonstrated by competition with excess of synthetic peptide. Furthermore, it does not precipitate an analogous protein from control cells (Fig. 2a,b).

Purification of *gag*-related polyproteins

To characterize the in vitro properties of *gag*-related transforming proteins, transformed nonproducer cells of all the MC29 family members as well as mutant and recovered viruses were metabolically labeled, lysed, and applied to immune affinity columns consisting of monoclonal IgG against p19. The purification achieved by this method is about 3000- to 4000-fold. The amount of protein recovered from 5×10^8 cells (10–20 mg cell protein) is about 2 μg of the respective polyprotein with a specific activity of 2×10^5 cpm/μg. About 20,000 molecules of p110$^{gag-myc}$ are present in one MC29 cell. The various purified proteins are shown in Figure 3 (top). To control the effect of the *gag* precursor itself, virus-producing cells were also extracted by immune affinity column. In addition to pr76^{gag}, other p19-related intermediates can be detected in these cells (see slot indicated by SR-D). Also, for comparison, Fujinami sarcoma virus-transformed rat embryo fibroblasts were analyzed by immune affinity column chromatography. The purified p130$^{gag-fps}$ protein is an active protein kinase that phosphorylates itself as well as other substrates spe-

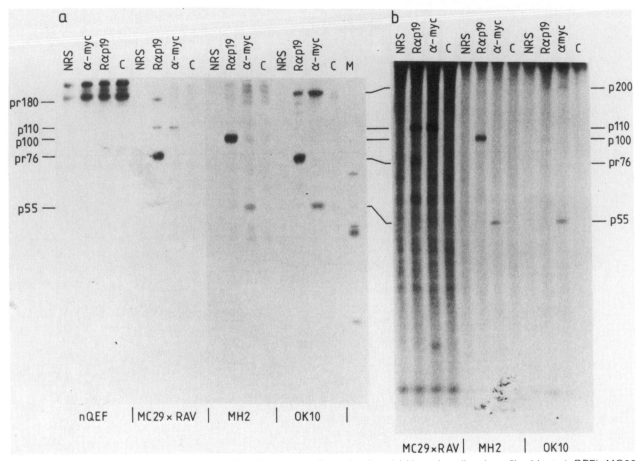

Figure 2 Immunoprecipitation of transformed cells with *myc*-specific antibodies. (*a*) Normal quail embryo fibroblasts (nQEF), MC29 cells superinfected with RAV-60 helper virus (MC29 × RAV), OK10, and MH2 nonproducer cells were labeled with [³⁵S]methionine, lysed, and used for indirect immunoprecipitation with normal rabbit serum (NRS), rabbit anti-p19 serum (Rαp19), anti-*myc* serum (α-*myc*), and anti-*myc* serum mixed with 5 μg of synthetic peptide for competition (C). (*b*) MC29-, OK10-, and MH2-transformed cells were labeled with ³²P in vitro, lysed, and used for immunoprecipitation as described in *a*. M indicates marker proteins.

cifically in the amino acid tyrosine (P. Donner et al., in prep.). Purification of the OK10^{gag}-related proteins shows predominantly pr76^{gag} present in this cell line, as well as the p200$^{gag-\Delta pol-myc}$ polyprotein. Some minor bands of unknown specificity show up in addition (Fig. 3, top).

The purified *gag*-related polyproteins were subsequently analyzed for their abilities to bind to DNA in vitro in a filter-binding assay. Double-stranded metabolically ([³H]thymidine)-labeled cellular DNA (100,000 cpm/μg) was sheared to about 20 kb in size; about 200,000 cpm were used per assay. In the presence of 70 mM NaCl, 0.1 μg of p110$^{gag-myc}$ protein retained about 1 μg of DNA on the filter (Fig. 3a). DNA binding was sensitive to salt ions. At 180 mM, NaCl binding was reduced to 50% (Donner et al. 1983).

Binding of the wild-type protein p110$^{gag-myc}$ to DNA in vitro was compared with that of the three mutant proteins with deletions in their *myc* portions. All three deletion mutants exhibit a 10- to 20-fold reduced DNA-binding ability in vitro (Donner et al. 1983). These data indicate a correlation between DNA-binding ability of *myc*-spe-

cific proteins and transforming ability in the animal. The polyprotein of HB-1 is presently under investigation.

Since the actual target cells in the animal are bone marrow cells, and not fibroblasts as analyzed here, MC29-transformed nonproducer bone marrow cells were isolated and the p110$^{gag-myc}$ protein purified. It also binds to DNA indistinguishably from the p110$^{gag-myc}$ of fibroblastic origin (Fig. 3b) (Donner et al. 1983).

The ability to bind to DNA in vitro was also observed with the p90$^{gag-myc}$ protein of CMII and the mixture of the two proteins p200$^{gag-\Delta pol-myc}$ and pr76^{gag} from OK10 (Fig. 3b). Since pr76^{gag} itself does not bind to DNA in vitro (Fig. 3b) (Donner et al. 1982), this ability can be attributed to the p200^{myc}-containing polyprotein. Preliminary evidence indicates that also the purified p55^{myc} protein binds to DNA in vitro.

The p100$^{gag-mil}$ of MH2 interacted with DNA in spite of its cytoplasmic localization. However, it exhibited another unique property; it binds to poly(A)-containing cytoplasmic RNA in vitro in a filter-binding assay (Fig. 3c) (Bunte et al. 1983). Its role in the cytoplasm therefore may involve interaction with RNA. Another cytoplasmic

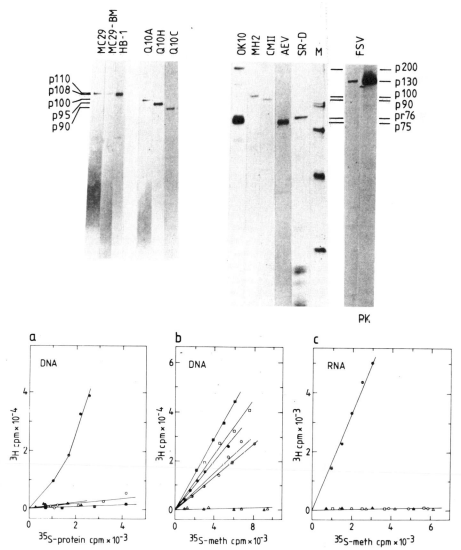

Figure 3 Filter-binding assay with purified *gag*-related transforming proteins. At the top, autoradiograms of *gag*-polyproteins are shown after purification by anti-p19 immune affinity column. The purified p130$^{gag-fps}$ protein of FuSV is also known after autophosphorylation (PK). The purified proteins were analyzed for protein–nucleic acid interaction in filter-binding assays (*bottom*). Either ^{3}H-labeled, sheared, double-stranded cellular DNA or poly(A)-containing cytoplasmic RNA was mixed with the purified proteins in vitro and then analyzed by filter binding. (*a*) (●) MC29 wild-type; (o, ▲, ■) Q10A, Q10C, and Q10H deletion mutants. (*b*) (o) MC29 from fibroblasts; (■) MC29 from bone marrow; (◑) OK10; (●) MH2; (□) CMII; (▲) AEV; (△) SR-D. (*c*) Same nomenclature as *b*.

protein is the *gag-erb-A* protein of AEV (Donner et al. 1983). This protein, however, binds neither to DNA nor to RNA in vitro (Fig. 3c). Its properties are still unknown.

Specificity of DNA-protein interaction in vitro

Binding of the p110$^{gag-myc}$ protein to DNA in vitro raised the question about the nature of the DNA–protein interaction. The p110$^{gag-myc}$ protein does not bind to single-stranded DNA in vitro (P. Donner and K. Moelling, unpubl.). It was also shown that binding to double-stranded DNA can be more readily displaced by homopolymeres such as poly(dG)-poly(dC) rather than by poly(dA)-poly(dT), with the first one being 1000-fold more efficient (Donner et al. 1983).

Another transforming protein, the T antigen of SV40, which is also a DNA-binding protein, has been shown to interact specifically with its own origin of replication, a region that harbors a specific 72-bp repeat (McKay 1981). In analogy to T antigen, a DNA–protein interaction was assayed with the p110$^{gag-myc}$ protein. Restricted DNA fragments of SV40 double-stranded DNA, of cloned MC29 DNA provirus into a pBR322 vector, and cloned SR-D provirus in pBR322 were radioactively labeled in vitro and treated with p110$^{gag-myc}$ coupled to immune affinity material to perform an immunoprecipitation. The p110 protein was not treated by denaturing buffers (SDS or extreme pH values) to preserve a potential sequence specificity. The immune complex was washed and subsequently treated with increasing concentrations of salt ions (NaCl). No specific DNA fragment was resistant to salt elution. All fragments were released simultaneously at about 200–500 mM salt (Fig.

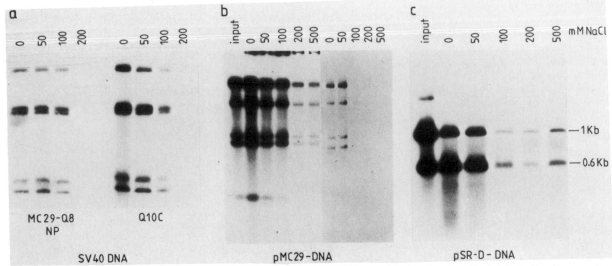

Figure 4 Precipitation of DNA fragments by *gag-myc* protein. (*a*) SV40 DNA, restricted and radioactively labeled in vitro, was treated with p110$^{gag-myc}$ and p90$^{gag-\Delta myc}$ of MC29 and Q10C, respectively, immobilized by anti-p19 IgG to immune affinity beads for immunoprecipitation as described (McKay 1981). The precipitates were treated with indicated concentrations of salt. The remaining complex was analyzed by SDS-gel electrophoresis and autoradiography. (*b*) ^{32}P-labeled MC29 cloned DNA restricted with *Bam*HI was used instead of SV40 DNA. A control was performed using the beads without protein for precipitation (*right part*). (*c*) Two DNA fragments of cloned SR-D DNA were used for precipitation. The 0.6-kb fragment contained LTR and the 1-kb fragment contained no LTR sequences.

4). Precipitation of the DNA fragments was not due to interaction between DNA and immunobeads (see control, Fig. 4). The binding of p110 was furthermore analyzed with a 0.6-kb DNA fragment containing the avian viral long terminal repeat (LTR) of SR-D. Another 1-kb viral DNA fragment without an LTR was used for comparison. Even though slightly more of the 0.6-kb fragment still bound at 500 mM salt than of the 1-kb fragment,

further studies with these DNA fragments have to be performed to allow conclusions.

Discussion

We have described properties of the transformation-specific protein *myc* coded for by MC29 viruses. The protein is expressed as a *gag-myc* polyprotein in some of the MC29 strains such as MC29 itself, CMII, and

Table 1 Avian Retroviral Transforming Proteins

	Virus	Protein	N[a]	C[b]	DNA b.p.[c]	RNA b.p.	PK[d]
I	FSV	p130$^{gag-fps}$		+	−	−	+
	MC29	p110$^{gag-myc}$	+		+		−
	mutants	p90–p100$^{gag-\Delta myc}$	+		(±)		−
	revertant	p108$^{"gag-myc"}$	+				
IIA							
	CM II	p90$^{gag-myc}$	+		+		
	MH 2	p100$^{gag-mil}$	−	+	+	+	
		p55^{myc}	+		+		
	OK10	p200$^{gag-\Delta pol-myc}$	+		+		
		p55^{myc}	+		+		
IIB	AEV	p75$^{gag-erb-A}$		+	−	−	−
		(p68^{erb-B})					
	AMV	(p48^{amv})					
IIC							
	E26	p135$^{gag-amv-ets}$			+		
	RAV-0						
III		pr76^{gag}		+	−	−	−
	RPV						

This table summarizes all the viruses and their polyproteins analyzed. The molecular weights are indicated by kilodaltons.
[a]N, stripped nuclei.
[b]C, cytoplasmic fraction.
[c]b.p., binding protein.
[d]PK, protein kinase.

OK10, whereas a *myc*-specific protein without a viral *gag* portion was detected in MH2- and OK10-transformed cells. The molecular weight of the *myc*-protein was determined as 55 kD in both cases (Fig. 2). Detection of this protein became possible by synthesis of a peptide against the carboxyl terminus of the avian viral *myc* protein, the sequence of which was published recently (Alitalo et al. 1983). Antibodies against the peptide precipitate the p110*gag-myc* polyprotein without recognizing *gag*-related proteins such as pr76*gag*, indicating its *myc*-specificity.

Whereas a p55*myc* protein was anticipated to exist in OK10-transformed cells in addition to a *gag*-linked *myc* polyprotein from the existence of a subgenomic *myc*-specific message (Saule et al. 1982), existence of p55*myc* in MH2-transformed cells was unexpected. Its p100*gag*-related polyprotein had been considered as *gag-myc*, mainly on the basis of analogy to other MC29 viruses (Hu et al. 1978; Hu and Vogt 1979). Only recently, a very oncogenic MH2-transformed cell line has been described lacking p100, which expressed a subgenomic *myc*-specific message (Pachl et al. 1983).

The results reported here indicate that p100 does not exhibit any *gag-myc* type properties; rather it appears to be a unique polyprotein in its ability to interact with RNA in vitro (Fig. 3) (Bunte et al. 1983). p100 was designated *gag-mil* since this protein appears MH2 specific and may be involved in the rather unusual properties of this virus to cause a high incidence of hepatocarcinomas (Alexander et al. 1979). In addition, a p55*myc* protein was identified in MH2-transformed cells. MH2 therefore resembles in its genetic composition AEV, which codes for two oncogenes, *gag-erb-A* and *erb-B*. Even though transformation properties of AEV reside predominantly in *erb-B*, *gag-erb-A* plays a role during cellular differentiation and exerts an enhancing effect on transformation (Frykberg et al. 1983). A concerted action between *gag-mil* and *myc* may occur in MH2 transformation as well and result in different oncogenicity than is caused by *myc* alone.

The properties of p55*myc* do not seem to exhibit any differences compared with *gag-myc* polyproteins in terms of their cellular localizations in transformed fibroblasts. Their in vitro DNA-binding properties also appear to be similar (unpubl.).

The purified *gag-myc* polyproteins bind to DNA in vitro (Donner et al. 1982). This in vitro property correlates with transformation, since the purified polyproteins from three transformation-defective deletion mutants exhibit a 10- to 20-fold reduced DNA-binding ability (Fig. 3) (Donner et al. 1983). The in vitro properties of the recovered virus HB-1 still remain unclear.

To analyze the function of DNA–protein interaction and the molecular mechanism resulting in malignant transformation, the nature of the DNA binding was further investigated. By analogy to the SV40-coded T antigen, a DNA–protein interaction was analyzed (McKay 1981), which, however, did not reveal a preferential binding of p110*gag-myc* to certain SV40 DNA fragments or the oncornaviral LTR region (Fig. 4). These results may either indicate that the action of *myc* protein does not function through recognition of specific sequences or alternatively that the assay conditions need to be improved. All in vitro studies performed with p110*gag-myc* such as DNA footprinting, effect on DNA synthesis, or RNA transcription suffer from lack of material.

A summary of all properties of the various transformation-specific proteins determined in these studies appears as Table 1. Binding of p55*myc* and p135*gag-amv-ets*, the polyprotein of E26, to DNA in vitro are still preliminary observations.

Acknowledgments

We are indebted to G. Czerny and S. Richter for expert technical assistance. We thank Dr. H. Schuster for encouragement and support of this study. The work was supported by the Deutsche Forschungsgemeinschaft, Stiftung Volkswagenwerk, Stiftung Unterberg, and Fonds der Chemischen Industrie.

References

Alexander, R.W., C. Moscovici, and P.K. Vogt. 1979. Avian oncovirus Mill Hill no. 2: Pathogenicity in chickens. *J. Natl. Cancer Inst.* **62:** 359.

Alitalo, K., J.M. Bishop, D.H. Smith, E.Y. Chen, W.W. Colby, and A.D. Levinson. 1983. Nucleotide sequence of the v-myc oncogene of avian retroviruses MC29. *Proc. Natl. Acad. Sci.* **80:** 100.

Bishop, J.M. 1982. Retroviruses and cancer genes. *Adv. Cancer Res.* **37:** 1.

Bister, K., M.J. Hayman, and P.K. Vogt. 1977. Defectiveness of avian myelocytomatosis virus MC29: Isolation of long-term nonproducer cultures and analysis of virus-specific polypeptide synthesis. *Virology* **82:** 431.

Bunte, T., I. Greiser-Wilke, and K. Moelling. 1983. The transforming protein of the MC29-related virus CMII is a nuclear DNA-binding protein whereas MH2 codes for a cytoplasmic RNA-DNA binding polyprotein. *EMBO J.* **2:** 1087.

Bunte, T., I. Greiser-Wilke, P. Donner, and K. Moelling. 1982. Association of gag-myc proteins from avian myelocytomatosis virus wild-type and mutants with chromatin. *EMBO J.* **1:** 919.

Donner, P., I. Greiser-Wilke, and K. Moelling. 1982. Nuclear localization and DNA-binding of the transforming gene product of avian myelocytomatosis virus. *Nature* **296:** 262.

Donner, P., T. Bunte, I. Greiser-Wilke, and K. Moelling. 1983. Reduced DNA-binding ability of purified transformation-specific proteins from deletion mutants of the acute avian leukemia virus MC29. *Proc. Natl. Acad. Sci.* **80:** 2861.

Frykberg, L., S. Palmieri, H. Beug, T. Graf, M.J. Hayman, and B. Vennström. 1983. Transforming capacities of avian erythroblastosis virus mutants deleted in the erbA or erbB oncogenes. *Cell* **32:** 227.

Graf, T. and H. Beug. 1978. Avian leukemia viruses: Interaction with their target cells in vivo and in vitro. *Biochim. Biophys. Acta* **516:** 269.

Graf, T. and D. Stehelin. 1982. Avian leukemia viruses: Oncogenes and genome structure. *Biochim. Biophys. Acta* **651:** 245.

Greiser-Wilke, I., M.K. Owada, and K. Moelling. 1981. Isolation of monoclonal antibodies against the avian oncornaviral protein p19. *J. Virol.* **39:** 325.

Hu, S.S.F. and P.K. Vogt. 1979. Avian oncovirus MH2 is defective in *gag, pol,* and *env. Virology* **92:** 278.

Hu, S.S.F., C. Moscovici, and P.K. Vogt. 1978. The defectiveness of Mill Hill 2, a carcinoma-inducing avian oncovirus. *Virology* **89:** 162.

Linial, M. 1982. Two retroviruses with similar transforming genes exhibit differences in transforming potential. *Virology* **119:** 382.

McKay, R.D.G. 1981. Binding of a simian virus 40 T antigen-related protein to DNA. *J. Mol. Biol.* **145:** 471.

Pachl, C., B. Biegalke, and M. Linial. 1983. RNA and protein encoded by MH2 virus: Evidence for subgenomic expression of v-myc. *J. Virol.* **45:** 133.

Pfeifer, S., R.F. Pettersson, A. Kallio, N. Oker-Blom, and A. Vaheri. 1981. Avian acute leukemia virus OK10 has an 8.2 kb genome and modified glycoprotein gp78. *J. Virol.* **40:** 533.

Ramsay, G., T. Graf, and M.J. Hayman. 1980. Mutants of avian myelocytomatosis virus with smaller gag gene-related proteins have an altered transforming ability. *Nature* **288:** 170.

Ramsay, G., M.J. Hayman, and K. Bister. 1982a. Phosphorylation of specific sites in the gag-myc polyproteins encoded by MC29-type viruses correlates with their transforming ability. *EMBO J.* **1:** 1111.

Ramsay, G.M., P.J. Enrietto, T. Graf, and M.J. Hayman. 1982b. Recovery of myc-specific sequences by a partially transformation-defective mutant of avian myelocytomatosis virus, MC29, correlates with the restoration of transforming activity. *Proc. Natl. Acad. Sci.* **79:** 6885.

Roussel, M., S. Saule, C. Lagrou, C. Rommens, H. Beug, T. Graf, and D. Stehelin. 1979. Three new types of viral oncogene of cellular origin specific for haematopoietic cell transformation. *Nature* **281:** 452.

Saule, S., A. Sergeant, G. Torpier, M.B. Raes, S. Pfeifer, and D. Stehelin. 1982. Subgenomic mRNA in OK10 defective leukemia virus-transformed cells. *J. Virol.* **42:** 71.

Sheiness, D., K. Bister, C. Moscovici, L. Fanshier, T. Gonda, and J.M. Bishop. 1980. Avian retroviruses that cause carcinoma and leukemia: Identification of nucleotide sequences associated with pathogenicity. *J. Virol.* **33:** 962.

Towbin, H., T. Staehelin, and J. Gordon. 1979. Electrophoretic transfer of proteins from polyacrylamide gels to nitrocellulose sheets: Procedure and some applications. *Proc. Natl. Acad. Sci.* **76:** 4350.

Vennström, B. and J.M. Bishop. 1982. Isolation and characterization of chicken DNA homologous to the two putative oncogenes of avian erythroblastosis virus. *Cell* **28:** 135.

Analysis and Purification of *v-myc* Proteins Using Anti-peptide Antibodies

S.R. Hann, M.A. Bender,* and R.N. Eisenman

Hutchinson Cancer Research Center, Seattle, Washington 98104
*Department of Pathology, School of Medicine, University of Washington, Seattle, Washington 98105

The proteins encoded by the various forms of the *myc* oncogene have proven to be rather elusive. This stems from the lack of a suitable antiserum reactive with *myc*-related proteins. In the absence of such sera, most studies on *myc* proteins concentrated on the *gag-myc* fusion protein (P110$^{gag-myc}$) synthesized by the defective avian leukemia virus MC29. Because this protein also contained polypeptide regions derived from the *gag* gene, it could easily be identified by readily available anti-*gag* sera (Bister et al. 1977). Anti-*gag* sera were also used to identify lower-molecular-weight forms of the MC29 P110$^{gag-myc}$ produced by mutants of MC29 that contained deletions in *myc* (Ramsay and Hayman 1982) and failed to transform hematopoietic cells (Ramsay et al. 1980). Furthermore, anti-*gag* sera were essential in establishing the nuclear localization of MC29 P110$^{gag-myc}$ (Abrams et al. 1982; Donner et al. 1982).

The availability of nucleotide sequencing data on avian and mammalian *myc* genes (Alitalo et al. 1983; Colby et al. 1983; Reddy et al. 1983; Watson et al. 1983) has made it possible to synthesize peptides corresponding to defined regions of the protein. Such peptides can then be used to raise antisera that one hopes will react with the complete protein. We have recently been able to show that an antiserum prepared against a peptide corresponding to the carboxyterminal 12 amino acids of MC29 *v-myc* (anti-*v-myc* 12C) specifically precipitates the known *gag-myc* fusion proteins produced by the defective leukemia viruses MC29, CMII, and OK10. In addition, proteins of 62 kD and 61/63 kD were precipitated by anti-*v-myc* 12C from OK10- and MH2-transformed cells, respectively (Hann et al. 1983). These two viruses synthesize their *myc* proteins from subgenomic mRNAs which lack *gag* sequences (Chiswell et al. 1981; Pachl et al. 1983) and thus could not be identified without sera specifically reactive with *myc* proteins. The anti-*v-myc* 12C serum also recognizes comigrating 62-kD proteins from several avian bursal lymphoma cell lines in which the *c-myc* gene has been activated, presumably by insertion of a retroviral promoter region. All of these proteins were shown to be phosphoproteins, and all were found, by both immunofluoresence and cell fractionation techniques, to be localized in nuclei of their respective transformed cells (Hann et al. 1983).

In this paper, we describe some technical studies carried out with anti-*v-myc* 12C as well as with several other antisera prepared against peptides corresponding to different regions of *v-myc*. These regions were chosen because they were especially hydrophilic and therefore more likely to lie at the exposed surface of the native protein (Hopp and Woods 1981). In addition, we show by tryptic peptide mapping techniques that the proteins precipitated by anti-*v-myc* 12C from MH2- and OK10-infected cells are related. Finally, we present data indicating that the anti-carboxyterminal peptide sera can be used for purification of native *myc*-related proteins.

Methods of Experimental Procedures

Preparation of anti-peptide sera

Peptide synthesis was carried out by the solid-phase method of Merrifield (Barany and Merrifield 1980) using a Vega Biochemicals Automated Peptide Synthesizer. Synthesis, cleavage from the resin, and extraction and purification of peptides were as described (Hann et al. 1983). A tyrosine residue was coupled to the amino terminus of each *myc* peptide to facilitate the cross-linking of the peptide to bovine serum albumin (BSA) by the *bis*-diazotized benzidine procedure of Bassiri et al. (1979). The peptide-BSA conjugates were injected into New Zealand White rabbits with repeated injections at monthly intervals. Bleedings followed injections by 10 days. IgG fractions were obtained from the rabbit sera by precipitation in 50% ammonium sulfate and affinity chromatography on protein A-Sepharose. The set of IgG subclasses thus obtained was passed first through a column of BSA linked to Sepharose and then through a column consisting of the immunizing peptide linked to Sepharose. The bound antibody was eluted with 5 M NaI and 1 mM sodium thiosulfate at 4°C and immediately dialyzed against phosphate-buffered saline (Gentry et al. 1983). The concentration of antibody was determined by absorbance at 280 nm. The affinity-purified antibody preparation was stored frozen at −80°C until first use and was thereafter stored at 4°C (for details, see Hann et al. 1983.) Anti-*gag* serum was prepared from disrupted avian myeloblastosis virus (AMV) virions as described previously (Eisenman et al. 1980).

Immune assays

Radioimmunoprecipitations were carried out exactly as previously described using rabbit antiserum and Formalin-fixed *Staphylococcus aureus*. Final washed pellets were dissolved in SDS-electrophoresis sample buffer and boiled 3 minutes, and the supernatant was analyzed by SDS-PAGE (Hann et al. 1983). For competitive inhibition of antibody precipitation (blocking) experiments, 20 μg of peptide per 10 μg of affinity-purified antiserum were mixed and incubated for 30 minutes at 4°C and used directly in the precipitation assay.

Immunoblot analysis utilized the method of Towbin et al. (1979) with some modifications. Crude nuclei were prepared from subconfluent cells by lysis in hypotonic buffer with 0.5% NP-40 followed by centrifugation at 2000 rpm for 10 minutes. The pellet was resuspended in RIPA buffer, sonicated, and made 1× in electrophoresis sample buffer containing 5% SDS and 4% β-mercaptoethanol. Samples containing equivalent amounts of material as determined by absorbance at 280 nm were electrophoresed on SDS discontinuous polyacrylamide gels (SDS-PAGE). Each well of the slab gel contained material derived from approximately 3×10^6 to 4×10^6 cells. Following electrophoresis, the gel was overlaid with a nitrocellulose sheet (BA85, S&S) and proteins electrophoretically transferred from the gel to the sheet in a Trans-Blot Cell (Bio-Rad). The transfer buffer consisted of 0.25 M Tris (pH 8.3), 192 M glycine, and 20% v/v methanol. Transfer was usually for 18 hours at 6 v/cm² at 4°C. After transfer, the nitrocellulose sheet was washed for 1 hour in Buffer A (0.15 M NaCl, 0.05 M Tris-Cl [pH 7.4], 0.005 M EDTA, 0.25% gelatin, and 0.05% NP-40). The blot is then incubated in Buffer A containing 10 μg/ml of antibody for 2 hours at 4°C. After three 10-minute rinses in Buffer A, the sheet is incubated for 20 minutes in Buffer A containing 2×10^5 cpm of iodinated (^{125}I) protein A. The sheet is then rinsed for three 10-minute intervals in Buffer A made up to 1 M NaCl and 0.4% sarcosyl and finally washed rapidly in distilled water before being covered with Saran Wrap and exposed to X-ray film in a cassette containing two intensifying screens.

Tryptic peptide mapping

For tryptic peptide mapping, proteins were eluted from the gel slices in the presence of L-1-tosylamido-2-phenylethyl chloromethyl ketone (TPCK)-trypsin, oxidized in performic acid, and prepared for chromatography as described previously (Eisenman et al. 1980). The lyophilized peptide pellet was dissolved in 20 μl 90% formic acid and then brought to 100 μl with distilled water. The sample was then injected onto a reverse-phase HPLC column (MCH-10, Varian) using a Varian 5000 liquid chromatography system. The sample was washed into the column with 4.5% formic acid. Peptides were eluted with a gradient of 65% ethanol in 4.5% formic acid. The column was maintained at 40°C and the flow rate was 0.5 ml/minute. Fractions (0.5 ml) were collected and the radioactivity determined in a liquid scintillation counter.

Affinity purification of *myc* proteins

We followed the method of Walter et al. (1982). For preparation of immunoabsorbent beads, 3.5 mg of affinity-purified anti-v-*myc* 18C was cross-linked to 1 g of cyanogen bromide-activated Sepharose 4B (Pharmacia) according to the procedure recommended by the manufacturer. For affinity chromatography, approximately 300 μl of labeled cell lysate (corresponding to 2×10^6 to 4×10^6 cells) were incubated with 50 μl of immunoabsorbent beads (corresponding to 50 μg of anti-v-

myc 18C); incubation was for 2.5 hours at 4°C. The beads were then washed four times in 500 μl RIPA buffer (0.15 M NaCl, 10 mM Tris-Cl [pH 7.4], 1% NP-40, 1% deoxycholate, 0.1% SDS, and 0.5% aprotinin) containing 1 mM dithiothreitol (DTT). Specific protein was then eluted from the beads by washing in RIPA buffer containing 10 mM MgCl₂, 1 mM DTT, and the indicated amount of peptide. For electrophoretic analysis of the labeled released protein, the final wash supernatant was made 1× in SDS-electrophoresis sample buffer, boiled 3 minutes, and fractionated by SDS-PAGE using a slab gel.

Results and Discussion

Use of anti-peptide antibodies in precipitation and immunoblot assays

Affinity-purified antisera (see Methods) were prepared to four peptides corresponding to different regions of the MC29 v-*myc* protein as deduced from the nucleotide sequence (Alitalo et al. 1983; Watson et al. 1983):

1. Peptide v-*myc* 12C, consisting of the 12 carboxy-terminal amino acids of MC29 v-*myc*. The affinity-purified antiserum has been designated anti-v-*myc* 12C and was described in detail in Hann et al. (1983).
2. Peptide v-*myc* 18C, consisting of the 18 carboxy-terminal amino acids of MC29 v-*myc*. The affinity-purified antiserum is referred to as anti-v-*myc*-18C.
3. Peptide v-*myc* N231/243 consisting of residues 231–243 from the *gag-myc* boundary of MC29 (using the numbering system of Alitalo et al. 1983). The antiserum is designated anti-v-*myc* N231/243.
4. Peptide v-*myc* N113/122 consisting of residues 113–122 from the MC29 *gag-myc* boundary. The affinity-purified antiserum is referred to as anti-v-*myc* N113/122.

A more complex antiserum was prepared by immunizing with a mixture of BSA cross-linked peptides v-*myc* 18C, v-*myc* N231/243, and v-*myc* N113/122. Because the resulting antiserum reacted predominantly with the carboxy-terminal peptide region, it was affinity-purified using peptide v-*myc* 18C. Most of its activity could be blocked, however, by peptide v-*myc* 12C. It is designated anti-v-*myc* 18C'.

Figure 1 shows an analysis of immunoprecipitates from a detergent extract of [^{35}S]methionine-labeled MC29-transformed quail cells (Q8 line) using three different anti-peptide antibodies. The P110$^{gag-myc}$ protein is precipitated quite effectively by both the anti-v-*myc* 12C and the anti-v-*myc* 18C' preparations (Fig. 1, lanes 1 and 2). However, competitive inhibition of precipitation of both these antibodies was found to occur with peptide v-*myc* 12C. Inhibition with anti-v-*myc* 12C was complete, whereas, inhibition with anti-v-*myc* 18C' was only about 90% complete (data not shown, but see Figs. 2 and 3). This suggests that anti-v-*myc* 18C' is reacting primarily with the 12 carboxyterminal amino acids of v-*myc*. When antibodies directed against a peptide close to the amino terminus of v-*myc* (peptide v-*myc* N113/122) are used,

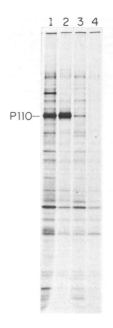

Figure 1 Radioimmunoprecipitations using anti-*v-myc* peptide antibodies with regional specificity. A 100-mm plate of Q8 cells was labeled for 90 min with 500 μCi [³⁵S]methionine, extracted in RIPA buffer, and the cleared lysate divided into four aliquots. Each sample was treated with the indicated affinity-purified anti-peptide antibody and fixed *S. aureus*. The resulting immuno-precipitate was analyzed by SDS-PAGE on a 10% gel. A radioautograph of the dried gel is shown. (Lane *1*) Anti-*v-myc* 12C; (lane *2*) anti-*v-myc* 18C′; (lane *3*) anti-*v-myc* N113/122; (lane *4*) anti-*v-myc* N113/122 preincubated with 10 μg of peptide N113/122.

In the experiment shown in Figure 2, nuclei were prepared from Q8 cells as well as from cells infected with MC29 mutants deleted at a region around the *Cla*I site within *myc*. These mutant-infected cells were derived and characterized by Hayman and co-workers (Ramsay and Hayman 1982) and have been shown to produce *gag-myc* fusion proteins smaller than the P110*ᵍᵃᵍ⁻ᵐʸᶜ* of wild-type MC29. For each sample, duplicate aliquots of nuclei were electrophoresed and transferred to nitrocellulose in parallel. One nitrocellulose sheet was then probed with anti-*v-myc* 18C′ and the duplicate sheet probed with an anti-*v-myc* 18C′ preparation that had been preincubated with peptide *v-myc* 12C. The data in Figure 2 show that the anti-peptide serum effectively recognizes the MC29 and mutant *myc* proteins. In the blot using anti-*v-myc* 18C′ that had been preincubated with peptide 12C, we observe an almost total loss of the relevant bands. The incomplete inhibition may be due to low amounts of antibody reactive with residues 13–18 which are not contained in the competing peptide. The bands observed in Figure 2 correspond to what was previously observed for the *myc*-deletion mutants using anti-*gag* sera (Ramsay and Hayman 1982). The fact that a carboxyterminal anti-peptide serum recognizes proteins from all these mutants indicates that the deletions are internal to the *myc*-coding region.

The anti-*v-myc* 18C′ also recognizes proteins at 62 kD and a doublet at 61 kD and 63 kD in nuclear extracts from OK10- and MH2-transformed cells, respectively

we detect a relatively low level of precipitation of MC29 P110*ᵍᵃᵍ⁻ᵐʸᶜ* (Fig. 1, lane 3). Precipitation of P110*ᵍᵃᵍ⁻ᵐʸᶜ* by anti-*v-myc* N113/122 is specific, because it is blocked by addition of the corresponding peptide (Fig. 1, lanes 3 and 4). Another antiserum, anti-*v-myc* N231/243, raised against a more central region of *v-myc*, failed to precipitate detectable levels of P110*ᵍᵃᵍ⁻ᵐʸᶜ* (data not shown). Because essentially equivalent amounts of affinity-purified antibodies were used in all these precipitation assays, it would seem likely that the poor efficiencies exhibited by anti-*v-myc* N231/243 and anti-*v-myc* N113/122 result from masking of determinants due to protein conformation. However, boiling of labeled lysates in SDS did not increase the efficiencies of precipitation with anti-*v-myc* N113/122 (data not shown). In any event, it is clear that the carboxyterminal antibodies are the most effective in terms of their reactivity with both native and denatured *myc* proteins.

It was of interest to determine whether the anti-peptide sera would recognize *myc*-related proteins in an immunoblot assay. This method involves probing a nitrocellulose sheet, onto which SDS-PAGE-fractionated proteins have been electrophoretically transferred, with antisera and ¹²⁵I-labeled protein A. This is a sensitive procedure that allows the analysis of relatively small amounts of cells or tissue samples which are difficult or impossible to label metabolically (Towbin et al. 1979).

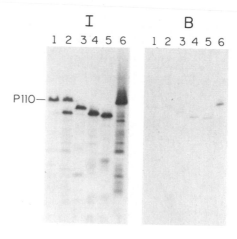

Figure 2 Immunoblots of nuclear extracts using anti-*v-myc* peptide antibodies: analysis of MC29 and deletion mutant proteins. Nuclei were pelleted from detergent extracts of the indicated cells, dissolved in SDS-electrophoresis sample buffer, and duplicate samples fractionated by SDS-PAGE on two 10% gels. The proteins were then electrophoretically transferred to nitrocellulose sheets as described in Methods. Blot *I* (Immune) was treated with 10 μg/ml anti-*v-myc* 18C′; blot *B* (Block) was treated with anti-*v-myc* 18C′ that had been preincubated with 0.25 mg/ml peptide 12C. Both sheets were then treated with ¹²⁵I-labeled Protein A. (Lanes *1*) MC29-transformed quail cell nuclei (Q8 line); (lanes *2*) MC29-transformed quail cell nuclei (Q10.1 line); (lanes *3*) deletion mutant QF4A nuclei; (lanes *4*) deletion mutant Q10C nuclei; (lanes *5*) deletion mutant Q10H nuclei; (lanes *6*) MC29 revertant-transformed quail cell nuclei (HB1C13).

(Fig. 3). These would appear to be the same proteins as detected in extracts of labeled cells after immunoprecipitation with a similar antiserum (anti-*v-myc* 12C; Hann et al. 1983). Although anti-*v-myc* 12C precipitated essentially equal amounts of MC29 P110$^{gag-myc}$ and the MH2 and OK10 proteins from labeled extracts, the 18C′ serum appears to be less efficient at detecting the latter two proteins compared with P110$^{gag-myc}$ in the immunoblot assay. We tentatively attribute this to some difference in the carboxyterminal regions of these proteins, which results in less efficient antibody binding in the immunoblot assay. We note that recognition of the MH2 and OK10 proteins by anti-*v-myc* is blocked by preincubation of the antisera with peptide *v-myc* 12C, indicating that the recognition is specific for these *myc*-related sequences (Fig. 3). Another anti-peptide serum, anti-*v-myc* N231/243, failed to recognize *myc*-related proteins in either radioimmunoprecipitation or immunoblot assays (data not shown).

Tryptic mapping of MH2 p61/63 and OK10 p62
As a first step towards comparative structural analysis of *myc*-encoded proteins, we have prepared tryptic maps of the *myc*-related proteins of MH2 and OK10. Although both the OK10 and MH2 proteins are specifically precipitated with anti-*v-myc* 12C and both are phosphorylated, the MH2 p61/63 appears as a doublet and OK10 p62 as a single band in radioimmunoprecipitation assay (Hann et al. 1983) and in immunoblots (Fig. 3). To prepare peptide maps of these proteins, transformed cells were labeled with [^{35}S]methionine and the *myc*-related proteins precipitated with anti-*v-myc* 12C and analyzed on SDS-PAGE. The MH2 p61/63 doublet and OK10 p62 bands were eluted from their gel slices in the presence of TPCK-trypsin, oxidized in performic acid, and fractionated by liquid chromatography on a reverse-phase

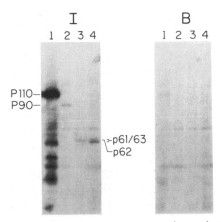

Figure 3 Immunoblots of nuclear extracts using anti-*v-myc* peptide antibodies: analysis of MC29, CMII, OK10, and MH2 proteins. Nuclei were analyzed on immunoblots as described in the legend to Fig. 2. (Blot *I*) Anti-*v-myc* 18C′; (blot *B*) anti-*v-myc* 18C′ preincubated with peptide 12C. (Lanes *1*) MC29-transformed quail cell nuclei (Q8 line); (lanes *2*) CMII-transformed quail cell nuclei; (lanes *3*) OK10-transformed quail cell nuclei; (lanes *4*) MH2-transformed quail cell nuclei. Each well contained nuclei from approximately 3 × 10^6 cells.

column using a gradient of ethanol in formic acid. Figure 4 shows the pattern of [^{35}S]methionine-containing peptides eluted from the column for MH2 p61/63 and for OK10 p62.

Comparison of the two peptide profiles shows three groups of peaks (peaks 1, 2, and 4 in Fig. 4) that apparently coeluted within the gradients for the two proteins as well as a major peak eluting at the same point in the postgradient methanol wash. A fifth heterogeneous peak elutes at markedly different positions in the MH2 profile compared with the OK10 profile (peak 3). The picture that emerges is that these two *v-myc*-encoded proteins have overall a similar pattern of methionine tryptic peptides with at least one major difference. At this point, we cannot say whether the peptide differences or the heterogeneity of some of the peaks are due to posttranslational modifications such as phosphorylation, acetylation, or glycosylation or to amino acid changes in the *v-myc*-coding regions. Another problem concerns the number of peptides detected here. The MC29 *v-myc* and chicken *c-myc* amino acid sequences that were derived from the nucleotide sequences (Alitalo et al. 1983; Colby et al. 1983; Reddy et al. 1983) predict four methionine tryptic peptides clustered in the aminoterminal portion of the proteins. Our finding of five or more methionine tryptic peptides in the MH2 and OK10 proteins may indicate the presence of either additional coding sequences or posttranslational modification of only a portion of these *v-myc*-encoded proteins. A more trivial explanation could be that one of the peaks (most likely the flowthrough) represents undigested material and, thus, is not a real peptide. More detailed analysis will be required to determine the origin of the observed differences in peptide pattern and number.

Affinity purification of MC29 P110$^{gag-myc}$ and OK10 p62^{v-myc} using anti-peptide antibodies
Purification of *myc*-encoded proteins in a biologically active form will probably be important in assaying *myc* activity and function. Donner et al. (1982) had previously used a monoclonal antibody against a *gag* protein to bind MC29 P110$^{gag-myc}$ to an immune-affinity column. However, elution from the column required 50% ethylene glycol at pH 2.0, probably leading to denaturation of the protein. Here we use a method described by Walter et al. (1982) with which specific proteins from cell extracts are bound to anti-peptide antibody linked to Sepharose beads. The antigen is released by using an excess of peptide in isotonic buffer containing mixed detergents at neutral pH. Using this procedure, a 2500-fold purification of polyoma virus middle T antigen was achieved, and the kinase associated with middle T was found to retain activity (Walter et al. 1982).

To purify the *v-myc* proteins encoded by MC29 and OK10, lysates were prepared from [^{35}S]methionine-labeled virally transformed quail cells. Aliquots of lysate corresponding to protein from approximately 2 × 10^6 to 4 × 10^6 cells were incubated with Sepharose beads to which 40–50 µg of affinity-purified anti-*v-myc* 18C had been covalently cross-linked. Following extensive wash-

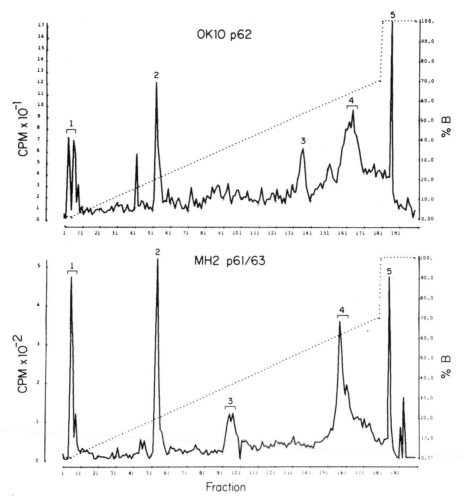

Figure 4 Methionine tryptic peptide maps of OK10 p62 and MH2 p61/63. OK10 and MH2-transformed cells were labeled with [³⁵S]methionine, lysed in RIPA buffer, and immunoprecipitates formed using anti-*v-myc* 12C. The relevant bands were excised from the gel and the proteins eluted with TPCK-trypsin and oxidized in performic acid. The peptides were dissolved in formic acid and subjected to chromatography on a reverse-phase HPLC column, as described in Methods. Peptides were eluted from the column with a gradient of Buffer B (65% ethanol and 4.5% formic acid) indicated by the dotted line. Fractions 180–200 were eluted in 100% methanol.

ing of the beads with RIPA buffer, they were finally washed in buffer containing different concentrations of peptide *v-myc* 18C. The supernatant remaining from this wash was then analyzed on SDS-PAGE for presence of labeled protein. The position of P110$^{gag-myc}$ is demonstrated by radioimmunoprecipitations with anti-*gag* (Fig. 5A, lane 1) and anti-*v-myc* 18C (Fig. 5A, lane 2). Figure 5A, lanes 3–6, also shows the effect of increasing concentrations of peptide *v-myc* 18C on the elution of MC29 P110 from the anti-*v-myc* 18C-linked Sepharose beads. When the beads are washed with buffer lacking peptide, we fail to observe release of P110$^{gag-myc}$ (Fig. 5A, lane 3). However, when 5–25 μg of peptide are added to the wash buffer, we detect substantial release of P110$^{gag-myc}$ (Fig. 5A, lanes 4–6). No release of IgG from the beads following the peptide elution was observed as determined by Coomassie blue staining of the gels. Relatively low amounts of presumably contaminating cellular proteins are observed on the gels (Fig. 5). Recently, we

have been able to reduce such contamination by more extensive washing prior to elution (cf. Figs. 5, A and B).

Not all the P110$^{gag-myc}$ is released from the beads, even when high levels of peptide are used for elution. This was shown by treating extract-incubated beads with SDS at 100°C for 3 minutes (Fig. 5A, lane 7). The existence of material that cannot be released with saturating amounts of peptide suggests the presence of a population of antibodies with relatively high affinity for the carboxyl terminus of *v-myc* proteins. Although this places a limit on the amount of *v-myc* protein that can be recovered by peptide elution, it also raises the possibility of obtaining a population of antibodies of high uniform affinity for *myc* proteins.

Figure 5B demonstrates that the peptide elution method can also be used to isolate the OK10 p62^{v-myc} protein. In this experiment, we varied the temperature of the buffer used for bead washing and peptide elution in an attempt to increase the efficiency of elution of bound

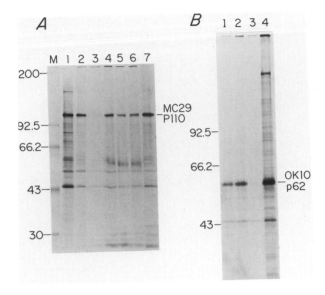

Figure 5 Immunoaffinity purification of *myc* proteins. A detergent extract corresponding to 2×10^6 to 4×10^6 cells was incubated with Sepharose beads to which approximately 50 μg anti-*v-myc* 18C had been coupled covalently. Following extensive washing, the beads were treated with RIPA buffer containing the indicated amount of peptide *v-myc* 18C and the beads pelleted. The remaining supernatant was made 1× in SDS-electrophoresis sample buffer, boiled, and fractionated by SDS-PAGE on a 10% gel. Equal amounts of extract were used for each lane. Radioautographs of dried gels are shown. (*A*) Extract from MC29-transformed quail cells (Q8). (Lane *M*) Molecular-weight markers (molecular weights in kilodaltons). (Lane *1*) Anti-*gag* radio-immunoprecipitate; (lane *2*) anti-*v-myc* 18C radioimmunoprecipitate; (lanes *3–6*) extracts incubated with immunoabsorbent beads and the beads washed with 0 μg peptide (lane *3*), 5 μg peptide (lane *4*), 15 μg peptide (lane *5*), and 25 μg peptide (lane *6*). (Lane *7*) Beads treated with SDS-electrophoresis sample buffer following incubation with extract. (*B*) Extract from OK10-transformed quail cells. Beads were eluted with 5 μg of peptide. Beads were washed and eluted at 4°C (lane *1*); ambient temperature (lane *2*); 37°C (lane *3*). (Lane *4*) Beads treated with SDS-electrophoresis sample buffer following incubation with extract.

protein. We found that increasing the temperature from 4°C to ambient temperature results in an approximately twofold increase in p62$^{v\text{-}myc}$ elution (Fig. 5B, lanes 1 and 2). Increasing the wash and elution temperature to 37°C, however, resulted in failure to detect p62$^{v\text{-}myc}$ after the treatment with peptide (Fig. 5B, lane 3). The higher temperature may have led to loss of the protein in the initial RIPA washes. Comparison of the amount of p62$^{v\text{-}myc}$ released with peptide (Fig. 5B, lane 2) to that of a parallel sample released by boiling in SDS (Fig. 5B, lane 4) indicates that a substantial fraction of p62$^{v\text{-}myc}$ was not eluted in excess peptide, as was also observed for MC29 P110$^{gag\text{-}myc}$ above.

Once a specific protein is eluted from antibody-linked beads with excess peptide, it can be separated from detergent and peptide by precipitation or by column chromatography. In a preliminary study, we eluted MC29 P110$^{gag\text{-}myc}$ as described above and precipitated the

eluate in cold acetone. Protein recovered from the precipitate was then microinjected into the cytoplasm of uninfected quail fibroblast cells. The cells were fixed and stained by indirect immunofluorescence with rabbit anti-*gag* antibodies. Our initial experiment showed weak perinuclear and nuclear fluorescence at 6 hours after cytoplasmic injection (M. Bender and J. Izant, unpubl.). These studies suggest that immunoaffinity chromatography using anti-peptide sera may provide a simple procedure for purification of biologically active *myc*-encoded protein.

Acknowledgments

We are grateful to H. Abrams, L. Rohrschneider, L. Gentry, and C. Tachibana for helpful discussions, and to Pei-Feng Cheng for a gift of iodinated protein A. This work was supported by grant CA20525 to R.N.E. from the National Cancer Institute. R.N.E. is a Scholar of the Leukemia Society of America. M.A.B. is supported by National Institutes of Health-NIGMS NRSA GMO7266.

References

Abrams, H.D., L.R. Rohrschneider, and R.N. Eisenman. 1982. Nuclear localization and DNA binding of the putative transforming gene product of avian myelocytomatosis virus. *Cell* **29:** 427.

Alitalo, K., J.M. Bishop, D.H. Smith, E.Y. Chen, W.W. Colby, and A.D. Levinson. 1983. Nucleotide sequence of the v-*myc* oncogene of avian retrovirus MC29. *Proc. Natl. Acad. Sci.* **80:** 100.

Barany, G. and R.B. Merrifield. 1980. Solid-phase peptide synthesis. In *The peptides: Analysis, synthesis, and biology* (ed. E. Gross and J. Meienhofer), vol. 2, p.1. Academic Press, New York.

Bassiri, R., J. Dvorak, and R.D. Utiger. 1979. Thyrotropin-releasing hormone. In *Methods in hormone radioimmunoassay* (ed. B.M. Jaffe and H.R. Behrman), p. 45. Academic Press, New York.

Bister, K., M. Hayman, and P.K. Vogt. 1977. Defectiveness of MC29: Isolation of long-term non-producer cultures and analysis of viral polypeptide synthesis. *Virology* **82:** 431.

Chiswell, D.J., G. Ramsay, and M.J. Hayman. 1981. Two virus-specific RNA species are present in cells transformed by defective leukemia viruses OK10. *J. Virol.* **40:** 301.

Colby, W.W., E.Y. Chen, D.H. Smith, and D.A. Levinson. 1983. Identification and nucleotide sequence of a human locus homologous to the v-*myc* oncogene of avian myelocytomatosis virus MC29. *Nature* **301:** 723.

Donner, P., I. Greiser-Wilke, and K. Moelling. 1982. Nuclear localization and DNA binding of the transforming gene product of avian myelocytomatosis virus. *Nature* **296:** 262.

Eisenman, R., W.S. Mason, and M. Linial. 1980. Synthesis and processing of polymerase proteins of wild-type and mutant avian retroviruses. *J. Virol.* **36:** 62.

Gentry, L.E., L.R. Rohrschneider, J.E. Casnellie, and E.G. Krebs. 1983. Antibodies to a defined region of pp60^{src} neutralize the tyrosine specific kinase activity. *J. Biol. Chem.* **258:** 11219.

Hann, S.R., H.D. Abrams, L.R. Rohrschneider, and R.N. Eisenman. 1983. Proteins encoded by the v-myc and c-myc oncogenes: Identification and localization in acute leukemia virus transformants and bursal lymphoma cells lines. *Cell* **34:** 789.

Hopp, T.P. and K.R. Woods. 1981. Prediction of protein antigenic determinants from amino acid sequences. *Proc. Natl. Acad. Sci.* **78:** 3824.

Pachl, C., B. Biegalke, and M. Linial. 1983. RNA and protein encoded by MH2 virus: Evidence for subgenomic expression of v-myc. *J. Virol.* **45:** 133.

Ramsay, G. and M.J. Hayman. 1982. Isolation and biochemical characterisation of partially transformation-defective mutants of avian myelocytomatosis virus strain MC29: Localization of the mutation to the *myc* domain of the 110,000 dalton polyprotein. *J. Virol.* **41:** 745.

Ramsay, G., T. Graf, and M.J. Hayman. 1980. Mutants of avian myelocytomatosis virus with smaller *gag*-gene related proteins have an altered transforming ability. *Nature* **288:** 170.

Reddy, E.P., R.K. Reynolds. D.K. Watson, R.A. Schultz, J. Lautenberger, and T.S. Papas. 1983. Nucleotide sequence analysis of the avian myelocytomatosis virus (MC29). *Proc. Natl. Acad. Sci.* **80:** 2500.

Towbin, H., T. Staehelin, and J. Gordon. 1979. Electrophoretic transfer of proteins from polyacrylamide gels to nitrocellulose sheets: Procedure and some applications. *Proc. Natl. Acad. Sci.* **76:**4350.

Walter, G., M.A. Hutchinson, T. Hunter, and W. Eckhart. 1982. Purification of polyoma virus medium-size tumor antigen by immunoaffinity chromatography. *Proc. Natl. Acad. Sci.* **79:** 4025.

Watson, D.K., M.C. Psallidopoulos, K.P. Samuel, R. Dalla-Favera, and T.S. Papas. 1983. Nucleotide sequence analysis of human c-myc locus, chicken homologue, and myelocytomatosis virus MC29 transforming gene reveals a highly conserved gene product. *Proc. Natl. Acad. Sci.* **80:** 3642.

Activation of the *c-myc* Gene in Avian and Human B-cell Lymphomas

K.G. Wiman,* C.K. Shih,* M.M. Goodenow,* A.C. Hayday,† H. Saito,†
S. Tonegawa,† and W.S. Hayward*

*Memorial Sloan-Kettering Cancer Center, New York, New York 10021
†Massachusetts Institute of Technology, Cambridge, Massachusetts 02139

In recent years it has become clear that the genomes of possibly all eukaryotic cells contain a set of genes with oncogenic potential. Most of these genes, which are called cellular oncogenes or proto-oncogenes, are homologous to the transforming genes of avian and mammalian retroviruses. The cellular oncogenes are highly conserved throughout evolution, and are thought to perform functions essential to the normal cell in the control of cell growth and development (Bishop 1981; Teich et al. 1982). Mutational events that lead to abnormal regulation of a proto-oncogene, or to alterations in the properties of the gene product of a proto-oncogene, can induce neoplastic transformation. The concept of activation of a cellular gene being responsible for induction of neoplasia emerged from studies showing that proviral integration adjacent to the host *c-myc* gene leads to enhanced expression of that gene and neoplastic growth (Hayward et al. 1981; Payne et al. 1982). Recent investigations indicate that the same gene may be activated by chromosomal translocation in nonvirally induced tumors. We shall discuss here mechanisms for activation of the *c-myc* gene by proviral integration, and present data from our laboratory suggesting how chromosomal translocation involving the *c-myc* gene might lead to neoplastic disease. We will point out similarities and differences between activation of the *c-myc* gene by proviral integration and chromosomal translocation.

Activation of *c-myc* by Avian Leukosis Virus

The slowly transforming retroviruses are the most abundant retroviruses in nature and are probably responsible for a majority of naturally occurring, virally induced neoplasms. In contrast to the rapidly transforming, or acute retroviruses, the slowly transforming retroviruses do not have a transforming gene and they induce neoplasia only after a prolonged latent period. Furthermore, unlike the acute retroviruses, they do not transform cells in tissue culture (Hanafusa 1977). For a long time, the mechanisms by which the slowly transforming retroviruses induce neoplastic transformation was not understood. However, analyses of chicken B-cell lymphomas induced by avian leukosis virus (ALV) have provided strong evidence that induction of tumor formation occurs as a result of insertion of proviral sequences adjacent to the host *c-myc* gene in more than 80% of the ALV-induced lymphomas. Moreover, levels of *c-myc* mRNA were elevated 30–100-fold compared with normal tissue, and

in most of the tumors the *c-myc* mRNA was found to contain viral sequences derived from the long terminal repeat (LTR) of the integrated provirus. Thus, initiation of transcription from the transcriptional promoter in the LTR, and readthrough into the adjacent host *c-myc* gene would lead to enhanced expression of this gene, and neoplastic transformation.

Further studies have demonstrated that in most ALV-induced B-cell lymphomas, proviral integration occurs upstream of the two coding exons of the *c-myc* gene, but downstream of a putative 5′ noncoding exon, and *c-myc* promoters (Shih et al. 1984). Consequently, proviral integration results in displacement of normal cellular regulatory sequences and placement of the *c-myc* gene under viral transcriptional control. Since proviral integration displaces the 5′ noncoding exon of *c-myc*, the *c-myc* mRNA synthesized from such a truncated *c-myc* gene will be devoid of sequences derived from the first, noncoding exon of *c-myc*. As will be discussed in more detail below, a role has been proposed for the 5′ noncoding sequences of the *c-myc* mRNA in translational control (Saito et al. 1983). According to the model, removal of these sequences results in enhanced translational efficiency of the *c-myc* mRNA. If correct, this model would imply that the *c-myc* gene is activated at the translational level as well as at the transcriptional level in most ALV-induced lymphomas.

In a minority of the cases of ALV-induced lymphomas that have been analyzed, proviral integration was found to be upstream of the *c-myc* gene, but in the opposite transcriptional orientation, and in one case downstream of *c-myc* (Payne et al. 1982). In these lymphomas, the transcriptional promoter in the proviral LTR cannot serve as initiation site for transcription of the *c-myc* gene. Instead, the transcription of the *c-myc* gene is likely to be increased by proviral enhancer sequences acting on a cellular promoter. The fact that such orientations of the integrated provirus relative to *c-myc* occur only in a small proportion of ALV-induced lymphomas indicates that proviral integration in the same transcriptional orientation, upstream of the coding sequence, is the most efficient means of activating the *c-myc* gene.

Although altered control of *c-myc* expression is a general feature of ALV-induced lymphomas, mutations within the coding sequence of *c-myc* leading to structural changes of the *c-myc* gene product might also play some role in activating the oncogenic potential of *c-myc*. Indeed, point mutations have been found within the *c-myc*-coding sequences in one ALV-induced lymphoma (D. Westaway and H. Varmus, pers. comm.). A final answer to this question must await nucleotide sequence analysis of the *c-myc* gene in a number of ALV-induced lymphomas.

Activation of *c-myc* by Chromosomal Translocation

Many types of human neoplasias are consistently associated with certain chromosomal defects (Rowley 1982; Yunis 1983). This information, and the demonstration of *c-myc* activation by ALV integration, led to the proposal that proto-oncogenes might be activated by a translocation event joining the coding sequences of a proto-oncogene with positive control elements belonging to another gene (Hayward et al. 1981; Klein 1981). This notion has recently received substantial support from studies of murine plasmacytomas and human Burkitt's lymphomas. Virtually all Burkitt's lymphomas and a number of non-Burkitt's lymphomas, carry a reciprocal translocation involving chromosome 8, and chromosomes 2, 14, or 22 (Zech et al. 1976; Bernheim et al. 1981). The 8,14 translocation occurs in about 90% of the cases. Quite recently, the immunoglobulin heavy-chain locus was localized to chromosome 14, band q32, by in situ hybridization (Kirsch et al. 1982). This is exactly the site involved in the common 8,14 translocation in Burkitt's lymphomas. An analogous pattern of reciprocal chromosomal translocations has been found in mouse plasmacytomas. These findings led to the suggestion that an oncogene on the donor chromosome is activated by translocation to the transcriptionally active immunoglobulin gene regions (Klein 1981). Recent work in several laboratories has indeed shown that the human *c-myc* gene is localized on chromosome 8, band q24, which is precisely the chromosomal segment involved in the typical Burkitt's lymphoma translocations (Dalla-Favera et al. 1982b; Neel et al. 1982; Taub et al. 1982). The genes for the immunoglobulin κ and λ chains have been localized to chromosomes 2 and 22, respectively; again, these are the sites involved in variant Burkitt's lymphoma translocations (Malcolm et al. 1982; Taub et al. 1982). Thus, these observations seem to suggest that the translocation leads to constitutively high levels of expression of the *c-myc* gene, and consequently to neoplasia, by bringing *c-myc* under the control of an immunoglobulin transcriptional element.

In attempts to elucidate possible mechanisms by which *c-myc* might be activated by rearrangement with an immunoglobulin locus, we have analyzed the translocated *c-myc* gene in two B-cell lymphoma cell lines of the Burkitt's type, Manca and AW-Ramos. Both cell lines are IgM producers, carry the 8,14 translocation, and form tumors in nude mice (Klein et al. 1975; Nishikori et al. 1984). Southern blot analyses indicated that the *c-myc* gene is rearranged in both cell lines. We have isolated clones containing *c-myc* and adjacent immunoglobulin sequences from genomic libraries constructed from each of these cell lines. Figure 1 shows a restriction map of part of the human IgM locus. The

position of a recently identified enhancer element (Hayday et al. 1984) is indicated. This transcriptional enhancer element augments the transcription of an adjacent gene in a transfection assay by several orders of magnitude. The normal human *c-myc* gene, which is also shown in Figure 1, has been sequenced by a number of groups (Battey et al. 1983; Bernard et al. 1983; Colby et al. 1983). It has three exons, the second and third of which contain the coding information for the *c-myc* gene product. The initiation methionine codon is located close to the 5' boundary of the second exon. The first exon has been localized approximately 1.5 kb upstream of the second exon in both mice and humans (Battey et al. 1983; Saito et al. 1983; Stanton et al. 1983). This exon is not translated, since no initiation codon is present, and a number of termination codons exist in all three reading frames. As can be seen in the figure, the *c-myc* gene has recombined with the IgM locus in both Manca and AW-Ramos. This is consistent with data obtained by other investigators, demonstrating that *c-myc* is frequently translocated to the IgM locus in Burkitt's lymphomas (Taub et al. 1982; Bernard et al. 1983). The precise points of chromosomal recombination were mapped in Manca and AW-Ramos by determining the nucleotide sequence of the relevant portion of the rearranged *c-myc* gene, and by comparing with the nucleotide sequence of the normal *c-myc* gene. In Manca, the point of recombination is 292 nucleotides 3' of the first exon. Thus, the translocation has resulted in a truncated *c-myc* gene, which is devoid of the first, noncoding exon and associated transcriptional promoters. The recombination point with respect to the IgM locus is immediately downstream of the J segments, but 5' to the enhancer element. As a result, the transcriptional enhancer element is located approximately 2 kb upstream of the *c-myc* gene in Manca, and should exert its enhancing activity on *c-myc*. That this is indeed the case has been demonstrated in a transcription assay (Hayday et al. 1984). In contrast, the recombination point in AW-Ramos is located 340 nucleotides upstream from a cap site at the 5' boundary of the 5' exon. Thus, all three *c-myc* exons remain intact. The recombination point with respect to the IgM locus is within the μ switch segment, less than 2 kb 5' to the exons encoding the constant heavy-chain domains. As a consequence, the known immunoglobulin transcriptional enhancer element is not joined to the *c-myc* gene in AW-Ramos.

The two rearranged *c-myc* genes described here represent two different examples of *c-myc* rearrangements as regards position of the recombination point relative to the first exon. In murine plasmacytomas, the majority of the chromosomal recombination points seem to occur within, or downstream of the first exon (Cory et al. 1983; Stanton et al. 1983). In human Burkitt's lymphomas, however, a considerable proportion of the cases have recombination points upstream of the first exon of *c-myc*, like AW-Ramos (Battey et al. 1983; Bernard et al. 1983; Hamlyn and Rabbitts 1983). The recombination point in the Ig locus usually occurs within the μ switch segment. The arrangement of the two genes in Manca, on the other

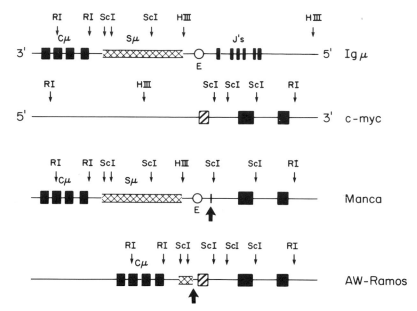

Figure 1 Restriction maps of part of the IgM locus, the normal *c-myc* gene, and the translocated *c-myc* genes in the Manca and AW-Ramos cell lines. The IgM locus is shown with the 3' end to the left and the 5' end to the right. The constant-region exons (C$_\mu$), the switch region (S$_\mu$), and the six functional J segments are indicated. A recently identified immunoglobulin enhancer sequence (see text) is represented by E. Coding *c-myc* exons are denoted by black boxes, and the noncoding *c-myc* exon is indicated by the hatched box. Fat arrows indicate the point of chromosomal recombination in Manca and AW-Ramos, and thin arrows indicate cleavage sites for *Eco*RI (RI), *Hind*III (HIII), and *Sac*I (ScI).

hand, is unusual in that the immunoglobulin transcriptional enhancer element located between the J segments and the C$_\mu$ exons is brought into close contact with the *c-myc* gene. This is the only case observed so far, in which the known immunoglobulin enhancer element has been shown to act directly on the translocated *c-myc* gene.

The normal *c-myc* gene is expressed as (at least) two mRNA species of approximately 2.3 kb and 2.4 kb, respectively. This is probably due to the presence of two alternative transcription initiation sites, 170 bp apart (Battey et al. 1983; Saito et al. 1983). Northern analysis has demonstrated elevated levels of expression of *c-myc* in Manca cells compared with a control cell line derived from Epstein-Barr virus (EBV)-infected peripheral blood lymphocytes. Two major *c-myc* mRNA species of 2.2 kb and 2.6 kb are expressed at levels comparable to the *c-myc* mRNA levels in HL-60, a promyelocytic leukemia cell line that exhibits an 8–32-fold amplification of the *c-myc* gene (Collins and Groudine 1982; Dalla-Favera et al. 1982a). The high levels of *c-myc* mRNA in Manca cells have been shown to result from the immunoglobulin transcriptional enhancer element acting on cryptic promoters in the first *c-myc* intron (Hayday et al. 1984). The *c-myc* gene appears to be expressed at slightly elevated levels also in AW-Ramos cells. As expected, two *c-myc* mRNA species of normal size are detected, although the increment of expression is more obvious for the larger (2.4 kb) mRNA species. It is not clear whether or not the observed level of expression of *c-myc* in AW-Ramos cells has any significance in activating the oncogenic potential of *c-myc*. One problem with this type of analysis

is the choice of control cell. Should the level of *c-myc* mRNA in the EBV-transformed cells be considered "control level," or is *c-myc* expression somehow increased, perhaps as a consequence of EBV infection? Moreover, it is conceivable that activation of the *c-myc* gene does not require high levels of *c-myc* mRNA, but occurs through disruption of a temporal control mechanism, leading to inappropriate expression of *c-myc* (Hayward et al. 1982). Thus, *c-myc* expression at a time when this gene would normally be inactive is likely to be the important factor in transformation. The idea that the *c-myc* gene is controlled in a timed fashion has received support from analyses of the effects of various mitogens on *c-myc* expression (Kelly et al. 1983). If the *c-myc* gene in AW-Ramos is, in fact, activated at the transcriptional level, resulting in increased or constitutive *c-myc* expression, the question arises as to how such activation is brought about. An attractive hypothesis is that the IgM locus harbors other as yet unidentified transcriptional enhancer elements that would influence the expression of the *c-myc* gene in AW-Ramos. Alternatively, the translocation may displace important control sequences normally located upstream of the *c-myc* gene, leading to an altered regulation of *c-myc* expression.

We recently proposed a model for activation of the translocated *c-myc* gene at the translational level (Saito et al. 1983). This model is based on the observation that sequences within the first and second exons in the *c-myc* gene are complementary to each other, allowing a stem-loop structure in the *c-myc* mRNA to form. Such an mRNA would be translated with a considerably reduced efficiency. However, removal of the complementary sequences in the first exon, e.g., by proviral integration or chromosomal translocation, would result in enhanced translational efficiency of the mRNA. Since the translocated *c-myc* gene in Manca cells is devoid of the first, noncoding exon, the truncated mRNA synthesized from this gene should be translated at high efficiency if the translational control hypothesis is valid. Even if this hypothesis turns out to be wrong, the possibility exists that the unusually long 5' noncoding sequence of the *c-myc* mRNA is significant in the regulation of the *c-myc* gene by other mechanisms.

Unlike the Manca *c-myc* gene, the *c-myc* gene in AW-Ramos cells is apparently not truncated. Therefore, activation of this *c-myc* gene at the translational level according to the model described here, does not seem probable. Nucleotide sequence analysis of the AW-Ramos *c-myc* gene has, in fact, shown that the sequence complementarity regions in the first and second exons are identical to the corresponding sequences in the normal *c-myc* gene (K.G. Wiman et al., in prep.). Thus, it appears that whereas the Manca *c-myc* gene is activated at the transcriptional level by an immunoglobulin enhancer element, and possibly also at the translational level, by displacement of the first exon, neither of these mechanisms is applicable to the translocated *c-myc* gene in AW-Ramos.

The translocation of *c-myc* to the immunoglobulin locus brings this gene into a genetically unstable region, characterized by an unusually high frequency of somatic mutations (Tonegawa 1983). During normal B-cell differentiation somatic mutations accumulate in a rearranged V_H segment upon VDJ joining, and are subsequently selected by antigen stimulation. In a large proportion of Burkitt's lymphomas, the *c-myc* gene is translocated to approximately the same position relative to the C_μ exons and the S_μ segment as is normally occupied by a rearranged V_H gene. An intriguing possibility is that this gene arrangement results in the introduction of somatic mutations in the *c-myc* gene by an enzymatic system that has evolved as a means of increasing antibody diversity. Somatic mutations in the *c-myc* gene could in principle affect regulatory sequences or coding sequences. Multiple mutations in the coding sequence of a translocated *c-myc* gene have recently been demonstrated in Raji, a Burkitt's lymphoma cell line (Rabbitts et al. 1983). The mutations were confined to the 5' part of *c-myc*, up to a point in the intron between the second and third exon, giving rise to 16 amino acid changes in the *c-myc* protein. It is too early to tell whether mutations have occurred also in regulatory sequences. At any rate, this information together with the fact that mutations have been found in the coding sequence of the chicken *c-myc* gene in an ALV-induced lymphoma, seems to suggest that certain alterations of the structure of the *c-myc* protein might in some cases contribute in expressing the full oncogenic potential of the *c-myc* gene.

We have carried out nucleotide sequencing of the AW-Ramos *c-myc* gene to determine whether this gene has acquired somatic mutations affecting regulatory sequences or coding sequences. No nucleotide changes were found when the sequence of the two coding exons of the AW-Ramos *c-myc* gene was compared with the sequence of the two coding exons of the normal *c-myc* gene (Colby et al. 1983; K.G. Wiman et al., in prep.). Thus, the translocated *c-myc* gene in AW-Ramos encodes a *c-myc* protein that is identical to the normal *c-myc* protein. This information is in agreement with data obtained by Battey et al. (1983). These authors were not able to find any nucleotide changes in the coding region of a translocated *c-myc* gene from Burkitt's lymphoma BL22. Therefore, it seems clear that mutations in *c-myc* coding sequences giving rise to an altered *c-myc* protein are not an essential feature of *c-myc* activation in human B-cell lymphomas.

In conclusion, it seems clear that transcriptional activation of *c-myc* is an important factor in induction of neoplasia by this gene. In ALV-induced lymphomas, transcriptional activation occurs as a result of integration of a proviral LTR adjacent to the *c-myc* gene. Transcriptional activation of the translocated *c-myc* gene in human B-cell lymphomas has, in one case, been shown to result from the effect of an immunoglobulin enhancer element. It remains to be seen whether enhancer-like sequences in the immunoglobulin locus play a role in *c-myc* activation in other human B-cell lymphomas. Translational activation of the *c-myc* gene in at least a proportion of ALV-induced lymphomas and human B-cell lymphomas might possibly occur by removal of sequences necessary for translational control. Alterations in the structure of the *c-myc* protein as a result of mutations in *c-myc*-coding sequences may in some cases be yet another mechanism contributing in expressing the oncogenic potential of *c-myc*. The ultimate answer to the question of *c-myc* activation will undoubtedly come from analyses of rearranged and normal *c-myc* genes in a functional assay. Such an assay for the activated *c-myc* gene is currently being developed in a number of laboratories, including our own, and should soon shed some light on the enigma of *c-myc* activation and neoplastic transformation.

Acknowledgments

A. Manwell is gratefully acknowledged for expert technical assistance. This work was supported by grants from the National Institutes of Health (grant CA34502), Bristol Meyers, and The Kleberg Foundation (W.S.H.). K.G.W. is a recipient of a European Molecular Biology Organization long-term fellowship. M.M.G. is the recipient of a postdoctoral fellowship from the Damon Runyon/Walter Winchell Cancer Fund.

References

Battey, J., C. Moulding, R. Taub, W. Murphy, T. Stewart, H. Potter, G. Lenoir, and P. Leder. 1983. The human *c-myc* oncogene: Structural consequences of translocation into the IgH locus in Burkitt lymphoma. *Cell* **34:** 779.

Bernard, O., S. Cory, S. Gerondakis, E. Webb, and J.M. Adams. 1983. Sequence of the murine and human cellular *myc* oncogenes and two modes of *myc* transcription in B lymphoid tumors. *EMBO J.* **2:** 2375.

Bernheim, A., R. Berger, and G. Lenoir. 1981. Cytogenetic studies on African Burkitt's lymphoma cell lines: t(8;14);

t(2;8) and t(8;22) translocations. *Cancer Genet. Cytogenet.* **3:** 307.

Bishop, J.M. 1981. Enemies within: The genesis of retrovirus oncogenes. *Cell* **23:** 5.

Colby, W.W., E.Y. Chen, D.H. Smith, and A.D. Levinson. 1983. Identification and nucleotide sequence of a human locus homologous to the v-*myc* oncogene of avian myelocytomatosis virus MC29. *Nature* **301:** 722.

Collins, S. and M. Groudine. 1982. Amplification of endogenous *myc*-related DNA sequences in a human myeloid leukemia cell line. *Nature* **298:** 679.

Cory, S., S. Gerondakis, and J.M. Adams. 1983. Interchromosomal recombination of the cellular oncogene c-*myc* with the immunoglobulin heavy chain locus in murine plasmacytomas in a reciprocal exchange. *EMBO J.* **2:** 697.

Dalla-Favera, R., F. Wong-Staal, and R.C. Gallo. 1982a. *onc* gene amplification in promyelocytic leukemia cell line HL-60 and primary leukemic cells of the same patient. *Nature* **299:** 61.

Dalla-Favera, R., M. Bregni, J. Erikson, D. Patterson, R.C. Gallo, and C.M. Croce. 1982b. Human c-*myc onc* gene is located on the region of chromosome 8 that is translocated in Burkitt lymphoma cells. *Proc. Natl. Acad. Sci.* **79:** 7824.

Hamlyn, P.H. and T.H. Rabbitts. 1983. Translocation joins c-*myc* and immunoglobulin 1 genes in a Burkitt lymphoma revealing a third exon in the c-*myc* oncogene. *Nature* **304:** 135.

Hanafusa, H. 1977. Cell transformation by RNA tumor viruses. In *Comprehensive virology* (ed. H. Frankel-Conrat and R.R. Wagner), vol. 10, p. 401. Academic Press, New York.

Hayday, A.C., S.D. Gillies, H. Saito, C. Wood, K. Wiman, W.S. Hayward, and S. Tonegawa. 1984. Activation of a translocated human c-*myc* gene by an enhancer in the immunoglobulin heavy-chain locus. *Nature* **307:** 334.

Hayward, W.S., B.G. Neel, and S.M. Astrin. 1981. Activation of a cellular *onc* gene by promoter insertion in ALV-induced lymphoid leukosis. *Nature* **290:** 475.

————. 1982. Avian leukosis viruses: Activation of cellular "oncogenes." *Adv. Viral Oncol.* **1:** 207.

Kelly, K., B.H. Cochran, C.D. Stiles, and P. Leder. 1983. Cell-specific regulation of the c-*myc* gene by lymphocyte mitogens and platelet-derived growth factor. *Cell* **35:** 603.

Kirsch, I.R., C.C. Morton, K. Nakahara, and P. Leder. 1982. Human immunoglobulin heavy chain genes map to a region of translocations in malignant B lymphocytes. *Science* **216:** 301.

Klein, G. 1981. The role of gene dosage and genetic transpositions in carcinogenesis. *Nature* **294:** 313.

Klein, G., B. Giovanella, A. Westman, J.S. Stehlin, and D. Mumford. 1975. An EBV-genome-negative cell line established from an American Burkitt lymphoma; receptor characteristics, EBV infectibility and permanent conversion into EBV-positive sublines by *in vitro* infection. *Intervirology* **5:** 319.

Malcolm, S., P. Barton, C. Murphy, M.A. Ferguson-Smith, D.L. Bently, and T.H. Rabbitts. 1982. Localization of human immunoglobulin K light chain variable region genes to the short arm of chromosome 2 by *in situ* hybridization. *Proc. Natl. Acad. Sci.* **79:** 4957.

Neel, B.G., S.C. Jhanward, R.S.K. Chaganti, and W.S. Hayward. 1982. Two human c-*onc* genes are located on the long arm of chromosome 8. *Proc. Natl. Acad. Sci.* **79:** 7842.

Nishikori, M., H. Hansen, S.C. Jhanward, J. Fried, P. Sordillo, B. Koziner, K. Llyod, and B. Clarkson. 1984. Establishment of a near tetraploid B-cell lymphoma cell line with duplication of the 8,14 translocation. *Cancer Genet. Cytogenet.* (in press).

Payne, G.S., J.M. Bishop, and H.E. Varmus. 1982. Multiple arrangements of viral DNA and an activated host oncogene (c-*myc*) in bursal lymphomas. *Nature* **295:** 209.

Rabbitts, T.H., P.H. Hamlyn, and R. Baer. 1983. Altered nucleotide sequences of a translocated c-*myc* gene in Burkitt lymphoma. *Nature* **306:** 760.

Rowley, J.D. 1982. Identification of the constant chromosome regions involved in human hematologic malignant disease. *Science* **216:** 749.

Saito, H., A.C. Hayday, K. Wiman, W.S. Hayward, and S. Tonegawa. 1983. Activation of the c-*myc* gene by translocation: A model for translational control. *Proc. Natl. Acad. Sci.* **80:** 7476.

Shih, C.-K., M.M. Goodenow, M. Linial, and W.S. Hayward. 1984. Nucleotide sequence 5′ of the chicken c-*myc* coding region: Localization of a non-coding exon that is absent from *myc* transcripts in most ALV-induced lymphomas. *Proc. Natl. Acad. Sci.* (in press).

Stanton, L.W., R. Wait, and K.B. Marcu. 1983. Translocation, breakage and truncated transcripts of c-*myc* oncogene in murine plasmacytomas. *Nature* **303:** 401.

Taub, R., I. Kirsch, C. Morton, G. Lenoir, D. Swan, S. Tronick, S. Aaronson, and P. Leder. 1982. Translocation of the c-*myc* gene into the immunoglobulin heavy chain locus in human Burkitt lymphoma and murine plasmacytoma cells. *Proc. Natl. Acad. Sci.* **79:** 7837.

Teich, N., J. Wyke, T. Mak, A. Bernstein, and W. Hardy. 1982. Pathogenesis of retrovirus-induced disease. In *Molecular biology of tumor viruses*, 2nd edition: *RNA tumor viruses* (ed. R. Weiss et al.), p. 785. Cold Spring Harbor Laboratory, Cold Spring Harbor, New York.

Tonegawa, S. 1983. Somatic generation of antibody diversity. *Nature* **302:** 227.

Yunis, J.J. 1983. The chromosomal basis of human neoplasia. *Science* **221:** 227.

Zech, L., U. Haglund, K. Nilsson, and G. Klein. 1976. Characteristic chromosomal abnormalities in biopsies and lymphoid cell lines from patients with Burkitt and non-Burkitt lymphomas. *Int. J. Cancer* **17:** 47.

Tumorigenesis by Mouse Mammary Tumor Virus May Involve Provirus Integration in a Specific Region of the Mouse Chromosome and Activation of a Cellular Gene

C. Dickson, G. Peters, R. Smith, and S. Brookes

Laboratory of Viral Carcinogenesis, Imperial Cancer Research Fund Laboratories, London, WC2A 3PX, England

Mouse mammary tumor virus (MMTV) is a congenitally transmitted B-type retrovirus, known to be the major causative agent of mammary carcinomas in strains of mice that suffer a high incidence of this disease (Moore et al. 1979; Cardiff and Young 1980). The available biological and biochemical evidence suggests that the MMTV genome comprises a single, replication-competent component, carrying the three replicative genes, *gag, pol,* and *env,* characteristic of the Retroviridae. However, MMTV is unusual in having the potential for an additional gene, given the acronym *orf,* since a substantial open reading frame is present near the 3' end of the genome, distal to and partially overlapping with *env* (Dickson and Peters 1981; Sen et al. 1981; Redmond and Dickson 1983). Curiously these *orf* sequences occur within a portion of the genome that becomes duplicated during the formation of the long terminal repeat (LTR) segments at each end of the integrated DNA provirus (Dickson et al. 1981; Donehower et al. 1981; Fasel et al. 1982; Kennedy et al. 1982). Although it is possible that this extra gene, or indeed other viral genes, may contribute to tumorigenesis, it is clear that *orf* does not constitute a "typical" viral oncogene as found in many other oncogenic retroviruses. In the first place, no cellular homolog to *orf* can be detected other than as the LTR components of endogenous MMTV proviruses. Second, MMTV does not induce morphological transformation of cells in tissue culture. In view of the unusual tissue tropism of MMTV and its generally poor infectivity in culture systems, it could be argued that this latter feature simply reflects our inability to propagate appropriate target cells. However, in vivo, up to 80% of the mammary epithelium may become productively infected with virus and yet maintain an apparently normal phenotype (Cohen et al. 1979b; Cardiff and Young 1980). Thus, while almost all viremic female mice eventually succumb to the disease, in terms of the total number of MMTV-infected cells, a tumor is a relatively rare event. This, and the long interval between infection and the appearance of tumors, suggests that tumorigenesis is most likely a result of some stochastic event rather than expression of a viral oncogene.

One obvious possibility for such a mechanism is insertional mutagenesis, in that integration of a provirus into chromosomal DNA may perturb the expression of adjacent cellular genes (Varmus 1982). Since the vast majority of such integrative events would presumably be either harmless or lethal to the cell, they would not be phenotypically discernible among a mass population of infected cells. A tumor would therefore represent the rare instance in which the perturbation conferred a selective growth advantage on an individual cell, causing it to proliferate into a clonal, neoplastic colony. Consistent with such a notion, MMTV-induced tumors are known to be clonal and to contain one or more integrated proviruses in addition to the endogenous units present in all normal tissues (Cohen et al. 1979b; Cohen and Varmus 1980; Fanning et al. 1980; Groner et al. 1980; Morris et al. 1980; Nusse and Varmus 1982; Peters et al. 1983). A prediction of the model would be that in each tumor, one such acquired provirus should reside in a defined chromosomal domain. By cloning fragments of DNA spanning the junctions between proviral and cellular sequences, we and others have obtained evidence that this is indeed the case in MMTV-induced carcinomas (Nusse and Varmus 1982; Peters et al. 1983). Interestingly, two quite independent provirus integration regions have been identified in this way, designated *int-1* and *int-2,* each spanning about 25 kb of cellular DNA. Here we describe the identification and characterization of *int-2* and present evidence that sequences within the *int-2* region are expressed in poly (A)$^+$ RNA in specific mammary tumors.

Methods of Experimental Procedures

Preparation and analysis of tissue DNA

The mammary tumors from which molecular clones were derived were obtained by injecting purified virus released from the Mm5MT/C1 mammary carcinoma cell line into newborn BALB/c mice (Dickson and Peters 1981). The tumors subsequently used for mass screening with molecularly cloned probes were either hormone-dependent or -independent tumors arising in the BR6 strain of mice. BR6 mice, developed as an inbred line from an original C57BL × R111 cross (Foulds 1949), suffer a high incidence of spontaneous mammary carcinomas, presumably as a result of milk-borne MMTV characteristic of the R111 parent. These BR6 tumors and other tissues were generously provided by Dr. Audrey Lee of this institute.

Freshly dissected tissues, normally tumor and spleen, were disrupted by Dounce homogenization and deproteinized by treatment with Pronase (1 mg/ml) and SDS (1%) as previously described (Peters et al. 1983). After extractions with phenol and chloroform, the high-molecular-weight DNA was recovered by spooling from ethanol, redissolved in 10 mM Tris-HCl (pH 7.8), 1 mM EDTA, and dialyzed exhaustively against this buffer at room temperature (Peters et al. 1983). The nucleic acid concentration was calculated from the absorbance at 260 nm.

DNA samples (10–15 μg) were digested to completion with an excess of the appropriate restriction enzymes in a standard buffer containing 20 mM Tris-HCl (pH 7.6), 50 mM NaCl, 10 mM magnesium acetate, 5 mM 2-mercaptoethanol, and 100 μg/ml bovine serum albumin (BSA). The resultant DNA fragments were then fractionated by electrophoresis in 0.8% agarose gels and transferred onto nitrocellulose filters according to standard procedures (Maniatis et al. 1982; Peters et al. 1983). Fragments of λ DNA generated with the enzyme *Hind*III were used as size markers.

Preparation and analysis of tissue RNA

Either freshly dissected or frozen tissues were homogenized in a mixture of 4 M guanidinium thiocyanate, 0.1 M 2-mercaptoethanol, 0.5% Sarcosyl, and 25 mM HEPES (pH 7.0) using a Sorvall Omnimix. RNA was then recovered from the homogenate by centrifugation through a cushion of 5.7 M CsCl in 25 mM HEPES (pH 7.0) at 100,000g for 16–20 hours (Chirgwin et al. 1979). The pellet of RNA was dissolved in 10 mM Tris-HCl (pH 7.8), 1 mM EDTA, and 0.1% SDS and reprecipitated by addition of sodium acetate (0.2 M) and ethanol (2 vol). The polyadenylated RNA fraction was then prepared by binding to poly(rU)-Sepharose in a buffer containing 0.5 M NaCl, 10 mM Tris-HCl (pH 7.8), 1 mM EDTA, and 0.1% SDS. The bound material amounting to between 5% and 10% of the applied RNA was subsequently eluted with sterile distilled water and precipitated with ethanol.

Samples of poly(A)$^+$ RNA (5 μg) were denatured by incubation in RNA electrophoresis buffer (20 mM MOPS [pH 7.0], 1 mM EDTA, and 5 mM sodium acetate) containing 2.2 M formaldehyde and 50% formamide at 60°C for 10 minutes. The RNAs were then fractionated in 1.2% agarose gels containing RNA electrophoresis buffer and 2.2 M formaldehyde, and transferred to nitrocellulose by blotting in 20× SSC (Thomas 1980). The filters were baked at 80°C for 2 hours to immobilize the RNA and prepared for hybridization as described below.

Radioactive probes and molecular hybridization

Molecularly cloned fragments of MMTV or cellular DNA were generally excised from the respective plasmids by digestion with appropriate restriction enzymes and recovered by electroelution. Samples of DNA (0.5 μg) were labeled by nick-translation in the presence of [α-^{32}P]dCTP (2000–3000 Ci/mmole from Amersham International) as described elsewhere (Peters et al. 1983).

The specific activity of the resultant probes was between 5 × 10^7 and 1 × 10^8 cpm/μg of DNA. Nick-translated probes were denatured at 100°C for 2 minutes, quenched in ice, and diluted to a final concentration of approximately 5 × 10^5 cpm/ml in hybridization buffer containing 50% formamide. Hybridizations were performed at 42°C for 24–48 hours and the nitrocellulose filters were then washed in 0.1× SSC and 0.1% SDS at 65°C for 1 hour prior to autoradiography (Peters et al. 1983).

Molecular cloning procedures and analysis of clones

The majority of techniques employed in the isolation of molecular clones followed standard protocols or have been described in previous reports (Maniatis et al. 1982; Peters et al. 1983). Briefly, high-molecular-weight tumor DNA was digested to completion with *Eco*RI and ligated into the separated arms of the bacteriophage vectors λgtWES.λB or λL47.1. After packaging in vitro, the recombinant plaques were plated on *E. coli* LE392 and screened using MMTV-specific probes. Phage containing the host-virus junction fragments were plaque-purified and propagated in small-scale cultures for isolation of DNA. The required DNA inserts were then transferred into the plasmid vector pAT153 for larger-scale purification and characterization.

Results

Analysis of acquired proviruses in MMTV-induced tumors

We set out initially to test the hypothesis that all MMTV-induced mammary tumors should have a provirus integrated into a limited region of chromosomal DNA. The approach was therefore to isolate and compare recombinant DNA clones containing the cellular DNA sequences around the sites of provirus integration in a number of independent tumors. To begin with, we chose to examine tumors induced in the BALB/c strain of mice since this particular strain has a relatively simple and well-characterized pattern of endogenous MMTV sequences (Cohen et al. 1979a; Morris et al. 1980; Traina et al 1981). Tumors were induced by injecting newborn mice with virus produced in tissue culture from a mammary tumor cell line of C3H mouse origin. High-molecular-weight DNA was prepared from each tumor, digested with the restriction enzyme *Eco*RI, and analyzed by agarose gel electrophoresis and Southern blotting procedures. The enzyme *Eco*RI cleaves the MMTV provirus at a single site close to the midpoint so that each complete proviral unit should yield two characteristic fragments representing the junctions between viral and cellular DNA (Cohen et al. 1979b). The two junction fragments can be distinguished from one another by using cloned MMTV DNA probes specific for either the 5′ or 3′ side of the *Eco*RI site (Peters et al. 1983). As an example, Figure 1 shows the results of an analysis of two BALB/c tumors using a 3′-specific probe such that each provirus is represented by a single band on the autoradiograph. A normal tissue control is also included

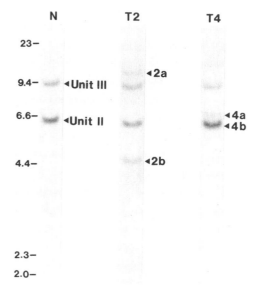

Figure 1 Analysis of acquired MMTV proviruses in mammary tumors induced in BALB/c mice. DNA from virally induced tumors (T2 and T4) and from normal tissue (N) was digested with *Eco*RI, fractionated on a 0.8% agarose gel, and analyzed by blot hybridization procedures, using a probe specific for the 3′ end of the MMTV provirus. Unit II and unit III refer to the two endogenous MMTV units (*Mtv-8* and *Mtv-9*) present in the germline of BALB/c mice that yield 3′ virus–cell junction fragments of 6.2 kb and 9.2 kb, respectively. 2a, 2b, 4a, and 4b identify new 3′ junctions created by integration of the infecting MMTV proviruses. The approximate size of each fragment was estimated relative to a series of molecular-weight markers (indicated in kb) derived from *Hind*III digestion of λ DNA.

to illustrate the pattern derived from the endogenous units present in the BALB/c germline, namely 3′ *Eco*RI fragments of 6.2 kb and 9.2 kb from unit II (*Mtv-8*) and unit III (*Mtv-9*), respectively (Traina et al. 1981). From this analysis, it was apparent that both tumors contained two additional 3′-junction fragments as compared with normal tissue, although one of the novel bands in tumor T4 was obscured by the endogenous unit of the same size (Fig. 1). The fact that such new junctions can be detected by this technique indicates that these tumors are probably clonal growths derived from individual infected cells. Moreover, the variable sizes of these new fragments, 11.4 kb and 4.7 kb in tumor T2 and 7.0 kb and 6.2 kb in tumor T4, confirm that provirus integration can take place at multiple, possibly random sites in the host DNA.

Cloning of virus–cell junction fragments

Ideally, we hoped to find a tumor with only one newly acquired provirus, but the majority of tumors that we have examined contain between two and six. The tumors shown in Figure 1 were among the simplest examples found and were therefore used to prepare recombinant DNA libraries. *Eco*RI-digested DNA was ligated into the bacteriophage vectors λgtWES.λB or λL47.1 and recombinant plaques were screened using MMTV-specific probes. In this way, clones representing all four of the new 3′-junction fragments from tumors T2 and T4 were

isolated and characterized by restriction enzyme digestion. The restriction maps of the respective clones 2a, 2b, 4a, and 4b are shown in Figure 2.

A number of conclusions can be drawn from these maps. In the first place, no rearrangement or deletion of viral sequences has been detected in these and other cloned junctions, although occasional restriction-site polymorphism has been observed. Second, all four fragments shown represent newly acquired proviruses derived from the input virus and are readily distinguishable from the endogenous units. In screening the tumor DNA libraries, clones containing the 3′ ends of endogenous units II and III were also isolated and characterized in detail (data not shown). Finally, no obvious similarities exist between the cellular DNA flanking the four proviral elements.

Despite this latter finding, it was still possible that these flanking cellular sequences constituted part of a more extensive common integration region. To make the comparison more rigorous, specific probes were prepared for the cellular DNA adjacent to each of the four integrated proviruses as depicted in Figure 2. The selected restriction fragments were first tested for the absence of repetitive sequence elements by hybridization to total cellular DNA, and subsequently were cloned into appropriate pAT153-based plasmid vectors. Each of these probes was shown to recognize a unique *Eco*RI fragment in normal cellular DNA (Fig. 3). However, the sizes of the so-called "unoccupied sites" were different for all four integration events. As expected, each probe also recognized two *Eco*RI fragments in the respective tumor DNA, one derived from the normal allele on the uninterrupted chromosome, the second being the new virus–cell junction on the other chromosome. In a truly monoclonal tumor, the intensities of these two bands would be expected to be equal, but such a situation can be readily upset by the presence of any normal tissue, such as stroma, in the initial tumor biopsy.

Having prepared these probes, the important question was obviously whether they detected any analogous interruptions in cellular DNA from other mammary tumors. To examine this issue, DNA was prepared from 40 independent tumors arising in the BR6 strain of mice. DNA from each tumor was digested with *Eco*RI blotted onto nitrocellulose and hybridized with each of the four specific cellular DNA probes. With the 2a probe, the 9.7-kb *Eco*RI fragment present in normal DNA was interrupted by viral sequences in one additional tumor (data not shown). The fact that two independent tumors must therefore have an MMTV provirus in the same, small region of cellular DNA is highly significant and unlikely to have arisen by chance. However, a much more dramatic result was obtained with the 4a probe in that the 10.0-kb *Eco*RI site was disrupted in 12 additional tumors. No such interruption was detected with either of the 2b and 4b probes.

Examples of these analyses with the 4a probe are presented in Figure 4. As shown in Figure 4A, all of these positive tumors contained the expected 10.0-kb *Eco*RI fragment plus at least one novel fragment recognized by

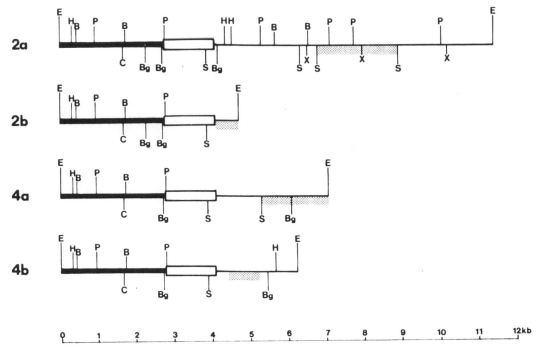

Figure 2 Characterization of cloned virus–cell junction fragments. The four new 3′ junction fragments from tumors T2 and T4, designated 2a, 2b, 4a, and 4b (Fig. 1) were obtained as recombinant DNA clones in suitable phage vectors. The respective *Eco*RI fragments were then transferred into the plasmid vector pAT153, propagated in bulk, and characterized by digestion with various combinations of the following restriction enzymes: *Eco*RI (E), *Hin*dIII (H), *Bam*HI (B), *Pst*I (P), *Sac*I (S), *Cla*I (C), and *Bgl*II (Bg). The sizes of the various digestion products were computed relative to a series of plasmid-derived standards of known nucleotide sequence and viral specific fragments were identified by blot hybridization with appropriate probes. Unique viral sequences are represented by the heavy lines, the viral LTR by open-boxed segments, and cellular DNA by the thin lines. Fragments of cellular DNA that were selected as unique sequence probes are depicted as stipled segments underlying each restriction map.

the 4a probe. The presence of the normal chromosomal allele makes it unlikely that these novel fragments reflected restriction site polymorphism in this region of DNA, and since the new fragments varied in size, being generally less than 10.0 kb, they could not have resulted from incomplete digestion of the DNA. More importantly, similar novel fragments were also recognized by a 3′-specific viral probe, as indicated in Figure 4B, suggesting that they were generated by the insertion of viral DNA. The exceptional case (track e) in which two new fragments were detected by the 4a probe, presumably resulted from provirus integration within the 1.75 kb of cellular DNA represented by the probe. One further conclusion that can be drawn from these results is that since

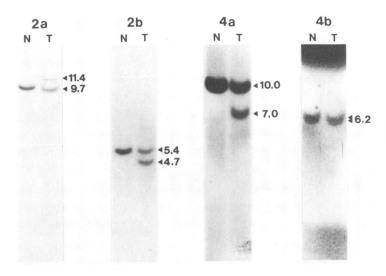

Figure 3 Detection of MMTV proviral integration sites using specific cellular probes. The unique-sequence cellular probes 2a, 2b, 4a, and 4b, derived from the four virus–cell junction fragments shown in Fig. 2, were used to probe Southern blots of *Eco*RI-digested DNA from either normal tissue (N) or the corresponding tumor (T). As indicated, each probe recognized a single *Eco*RI fragment in normal tissue representing the uninterrupted allele present on both chromosomes. In contrast, with the appropriate tumor DNA, the probes recognized both the unoccupied site on one chromosome and the respective novel junction fragment generated by provirus integration on the other. The size of each fragment was calculated relative to known standards and by detailed restriction mapping.

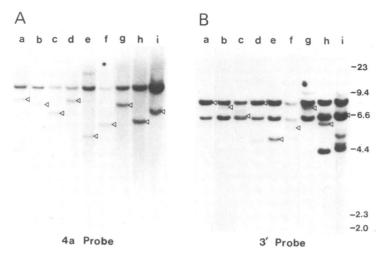

Figure 4 Analysis of tumors containing an MMTV provirus within the site recognized by probe 4a. DNA from nine selected mammary tumors, from BR6 mice, was digested with *Eco*RI, fractionated by electrophoresis in a 0.8% agarose gel, and transferred to a nitrocellulose filter. The filter was then hybridized successively to the 4a cellular DNA probe (*A*) and a 3′-specific viral probe (*B*). In addition to the expected 10.0-kb *Eco*RI fragment, the 4a probe detected at least one novel fragment (▷) in each tumor. A corresponding fragment was also recognized by 3′-specific viral sequences, suggesting that each novel band resulted from MMTV provirus insertion. The sizes of the *Hin*dIII-digested λ DNA markers are indicated in kilobases. (Data reprinted, with permission, from Peters et al. 1983.)

all the new junction fragments recognized by the 4a probe also included the 3′ end of the virus, these proviruses must be in the same orientation as the original 4a junction. Similarly, the two 2a-positive tumors contained proviruses in the same orientation (not shown).

Characterization of the unoccupied integration sites
From the foregoing data, it is clear that the *Eco*RI fragments recognized by the 2a and 4a probes constituted common integration regions in MMTV-induced tumors. To characterize these regions in more detail, the original recombinant phage libraries were rescreened with these cellular DNA probes and additional clones were isolated that contained the respective unoccupied 9.7-kb and 10.0-kb *Eco*RI fragments. The detailed restriction maps of these fragments indicated that they were quite clearly distinct from one another and, by comparison with the junction fragments mapped in Figure 2, that no gross rearrangements had occurred as a result of provirus integration.

The 10.0-kb fragment recognized by 4a was also found to be essentially free of repetitive sequence elements when used as a hybridization probe at high stringency. Thus, with this entire unoccupied site as the probe, both the 5′- and 3′-junction fragments generated by provirus integration could be detected on the same Southern blot. From the combined sizes of these fragments (19.8 ± 0.5 kb), we concluded that, within the limits of this type of analysis, the proviruses integrated within this region had not suffered major deletions (Peters et al. 1983). These measurements also permitted more accurate mapping of the provirus integration sites and indicated that although the precise sites varied from tumor to tumor, they were not randomly distributed throughout the 10.0-kb region (see below).

The exclusive use of the enzyme *Eco*RI in these experiments, although convenient, restricted the range of the analyses to 9.7 kb and 10.0 kb, respectively, with the 2a and 4a probes. Therefore, two approaches were taken to extend the scope of these studies. In the first

instance, Southern blots were prepared using alternative restriction enzymes in an attempt to find larger fragments detectable with these probes. For example, the enzyme *Xba*I generates a unique 24-kb fragment from normal mouse DNA that encompasses the 4a probe, and five additional tumors were identified in which a provirus had integrated within this fragment. However, the availability of only the two *Eco*RI clones from which to prepare probes placed severe limitations on this type of analysis and it was considered essential to isolate further molecular clones containing DNA adjacent to each of the 9.7-kb and 10.0-kb *Eco*RI fragments. This was achieved by screening a phage library prepared from BALB/c DNA partially digested with *Hae*III and *Alu*I such that the average size of the DNA inserts was approximately 15–20 kb (originally constructed in the laboratory of L. Hood). Two positive phage clones were identified by screening with the 10.0-kb *Eco*RI fragment as probe. Surprisingly, when duplicate filters from the library were screened with the 2a probe, the same two plaques (plus one other) were identified as positive. Thus, the two probes 2a and 4a derived from independent tumors must be very closely linked in mouse cellular DNA and identify sections of the same provirus integration region.

DNA was isolated from each of these clones and characterized by restriction enzyme mapping. The deduced maps overlapped with one another and were in perfect agreement with the previous analyses of the 9.7-kb and 10.0-kb *Eco*RI fragments. This permitted construction of the extended map of the integration region (Fig. 5) and indicated that the two *Eco*RI fragments identified by the 2a and 4a probes were separated by only 1.6 kb of cellular DNA. The data also revealed an important conclusion concerning the relative orientations of the proviruses within the 9.7-kb and 10.0-kb regions. By comparing the deduced cellular map with those of the original junction fragments in Figure 2, it is clear that these two proviruses, and consequently all other examples detected by the respective probes, must be in opposite transcriptional orientations. Thus, within this

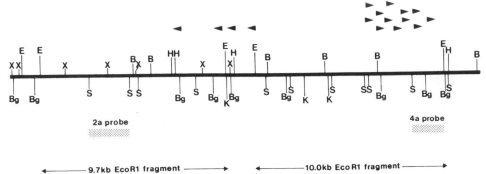

Figure 5 Restriction map and location of proviruses within the common integration region (*int-2*). Recombinant phage clones containing overlapping fragments of BALB/c DNA were detected by hybridization to the 2a and 4a probes, as described in the text, and characterized by digestion with various combinations of the restriction enzymes *Eco*RI(E), *Hind*III (H), *Bam*HI (B), *Sac*I (S), *Kpn*I (K), *Xba*I (X), and *Bgl*II (Bg). The position of the 2a and 4a probes and the corresponding 9.7-kb and 10.0-kb *Eco*RI fragments are indicated. The arrowhead symbols represent the approximate location and transcriptional orientation of MMTV proviruses in 16 independent tumors.

extended region, two clusters of provirus integration sites have been mapped such that viral transcription is directed away from a central section in which no insertions have yet been detected. The extent of this central section remains uncertain as additional examples of proviral integrations are still being mapped, using the more extensive repertoire of probes now available.

Expression of RNA from the integration region

The distribution and orientation of proviruses integrated within this defined chromosomal domain are clearly not random. Therefore, we considered that the pattern of integration sites may be reflecting the location of a cellular gene within this region of cellular DNA. The most attractive possibility was that the two clusters of integration sites may be symmetrically disposed around a cellular transcription unit. Poly(A) RNA was therefore prepared from selected tumors, fractionated under denaturing conditions, and blots were probed using DNA fragments specific for the internal section of the integration region. As shown in Figure 6, RNA transcripts were detected specifically in those tumors in which a provirus was integrated in this region. The major transcript was approximately 3.2 kb in size with possible minor species at around 3.7 kb and 2.5 kb, the significance of which is presently unclear. However, even in the positive tumors, the level of this RNA is very low. Relative to the viral 35S and 24S mRNAs detected on the same blots, we estimated that transcripts derived from this integration region amounted to only tens of copies per cell. Other mammary tumors, normal mammary gland, and selected adult mouse tissues did not show evidence of transcription from this region, suggesting that provirus integration may be activating RNA synthesis from an otherwise silent gene.

Discussion

The starting hypothesis for these studies was the assertion that tumorigenesis by MMTV is mediated by proviral activation of a cellular gene. Such a notion would predict that in all MMTV-induced mammary tumors, at least one newly acquired provirus should be present and in a limited region of chromosomal DNA. To test this prediction, we have examined and prepared probes specific for the sites of provirus integration in two independent tumors. The cellular sequences detected by these probes showed no obvious homology or similarity, confirming the general belief that retrovirus integration can take place at essentially random sites in the host DNA. However, DNA fragments recognized by two of these probes, 2a and 4a, derived from different tumors, were found to be very closely linked in mouse chromosomal DNA. Moreover, the characteristic fragments identified by these probes were also found to be interrupted by insertion of viral sequences in a significant proportion of other mammary tumors, suggesting that a defined integration locus does indeed exist (Figs. 4 and 5; Peters et al. 1983).

Provirus integration within this chromosomal domain has now been detected in a total of 22 independent mammary tumors. However, as this only represents around 50% of the total number of tumors examined, the question remains as to the situation in the other 50%. One explanation would be that we have not identified the limits of the integration region and that the range of the probes must be extended beyond the present 30 kb to detect further proviral integration events. Alternatively, other integration regions may exist that harbor proviruses in the tumors that score negative with our probes. During the course of our studies, Nusse and Varmus (1982) reported the results of an analogous series of experiments describing a 25–30-kb region of mouse DNA, designated MMTV *int-1*, in which they could detect an integrated provirus in 70% of the C3H mammary tumors they examined. However, on the basis of restriction enzyme mapping and cross-hybridization of probes, the *int-1* locus and the region we have described here, which we have termed *int-2*, appear quite different. Moreover, they have recently been mapped to different mouse chromosomes, *int-1* being on chromosome 15 and *int-2* on

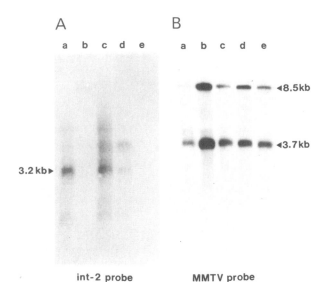

A B

a b c d e   a b c d e

◄8.5kb

◄3.7kb

3.2kb►

int-2 probe   MMTV probe

Figure 6 Expression of RNA from the MMTV integration region. Total poly(A)⁺ RNA (5 μg) from five independent BR6 mammary tumors was fractionated under denaturing conditions and transferred onto nitrocellulose filters by standard blotting procedures. The filters were then hybridized to either (A) a 1.8-kb SacI DNA fragment from the central portion of the common integration region (see Fig. 5) or (B) MMTV LTR sequences. Those tumors that showed evidence for provirus integration in this defined region (lanes a, c, and d; C. Dickson et al., unpubl.) express specific RNA transcripts detectable with cellular DNA probes from the region, whereas other tumors (lanes b and e) do not. The size of the major transcript was estimated to be 3.2 kb as indicated. All five tumors expressed comparable amounts of the expected 35S (8.5 kb) and 24S (3.7 kb) viral RNA transcripts (B). The level of expression of the cellular transcripts can be assessed from the exposure time for the autoradiographs shown in A (6 days) and B (6 hr).

chromosome 7, which confirms that they represent discrete loci (Peters et al. 1984; R. Nusse and D. Cox, pers. comm.).

The conclusion that two distinct provirus integration regions may be implicated in the same neoplastic disease raises the issue of whether other such regions might exist. As discussed above, the full extents of int-1 and int-2 may be larger than the regions presently characterized, but a substantial number of mammary tumors show no evidence of provirus integration in either int-1 or int-2. For example, approximately 25% of the BR6 tumors we have examined presently fall into this category (C. Dickson et al., unpubl.). It is, therefore, possible that the approach we have described here has the potential of identifying further cellular loci which may contribute to mammary carcinogenesis.

Several arguments support the conclusion that provirus integration in the int-2 region is significant for mammary carcinogenesis rather than fortuitous. For example, although both of the original tumors, T2 and T4, contained other proviruses in different regions of cellular DNA, the probes specific for these alternative integration sites, 2b and 4b, did not detect proviral insertions in any of 40 independent BR6 tumors examined. Thus, it would seem unlikely that 2a and 4a should coincidentally rep-

resent integration in a preferred region whereas 2b and 4b do not. Moreover, within int-2, the sites of integration are variable and distributed over a range of about 20 kb, suggesting that the proviruses were unlikely to be targeted to this region by localized DNA sequence homology. The distribution of proviruses is also clearly nonrandom, raising the possibility that the precise location and orientation of the integrating provirus may be constrained by its subsequent influence on the proliferative capacity of the cell. However, the most compelling evidence that integration within int-2 may be causal rather than a fortuitous event during carcinogenesis is the presence in tumors of RNA transcripts derived from this region of DNA. The fact that such RNAs have only been detected in tumors that have sustained a provirus integration in int-2 (Fig. 6) argues strongly in favor of a mechanistic link between the two observations.

The exact location and extent of the int-2 transcription unit is currently under investigation, but preliminary indications are that the RNA is homologous to the segment of int-2 DNA that lies between the two groups of mapped integration sites. Thus, whatever the transcriptional orientation of the int-2 gene, the MMTV proviruses that appear to influence its expression are directed away from the gene. An exactly analogous situation apparently applies to the int-1 region (R. Nusse, pers. comm.). It is clear then that the MMTV proviruses do not activate the cellular gene by simple promoter insertion as commonly found in the lymphomas and erythroleukemias induced by avian leukosis virus (ALV) (Fung et al. 1981, 1983; Hayward et al. 1981; Neel et al. 1981; Payne et al. 1982). The situation does however resemble the less common cases of lymphomas in which the ALV-provirus is directed away from the cellular gene (Payne et al. 1982). Other parallels between ALV- and MMTV-induced disease are apparent. For example, tumorigenesis by ALV and MMTV is frequently preceded by the appearance of nodules of hyperplastic cells in the bursa and mammary gland, respectively (De Ome et al. 1959; Neiman et al. 1980). These preneoplastic lesions are believed to be precursors of the clonal populations of tumor cells that eventually develop. In the case of ALV, the cellular genes implicated in the tumorigenic process have been identified as progenitors of known viral oncogenes, such as myc and erb (Fung et al. 1981, 1983; Hayward et al. 1981; Neel et al. 1981; Payne et al. 1982). With MMTV, on the other hand, there is too little information regarding the nature and expression of the int-2 gene to decide whether it constitutes a true oncogene. If it does, then it may well prove to be a novel example since we have so far detected no homology between int-2 and a selection of known viral oncogenes (Peters et al. 1983), nor with the dominant transforming gene detected by transfection of mammary carcinoma DNA (Lane et al. 1981; M.A. Lane and C. Dickson et al., unpubl.).

If int-2 does constitute a cellular oncogene, it is perhaps significant that it does not appear to be expressed in any of the adult mouse tissues tested, including midpregnancy mammary gland (C. Dickson et al., unpubl.). Thus, the provirus seems to turn on an otherwise silent gene as opposed to increasing a basal level of expression. Whether structural alterations are also involved, as is the case for some other cellular oncogenes, remains to be determined, but this appears less likely in view of the distances over which MMTV proviruses are distributed within the *int-2* region. The mechanism by which the MMTV provirus exerts its effect is therefore unclear. Considerable attention is currently being paid to the presence of so-called enhancer elements in the genomes of papovaviruses, in some retroviral LTRs, and as components of cellular transcription units (Khoury and Gruss 1983). Such elements are *cis*-acting and operate irrespective of orientation and position relative to the gene in question. There is also evidence that they may display inherent species or tissue specificity (de Villiers et al. 1982; Banerji et al. 1983; Gillies et al. 1983; Queen and Baltimore 1983; Spandidos and Wilkie 1983). Thus, although standard assays for enhancer activity have not detected such a function in the MMTV LTR (Lee et al. 1981), it is conceivable that an analogous element with a strict tissue specificity for mammary epithelial cells may indeed exist. Since enhancer activity may be blocked by the introduction of a strong transcription promoter between the element and the assayed gene (de Villiers et al. 1982; Wasylyk et al. 1983), this situation would also offer a rationalization for the orientation of proviruses relative to the *int-2* gene. However, until more is known about the structure and function of *int-2*, such considerations must remain speculative.

References

Banerji, J., L. Olson, and W. Schaffner. 1983. A lymphocyte-specific cellular enhancer is located downstream of the joining region in immunoglobulin heavy chain genes. *Cell* **33**: 729.

Cardiff, R.D. and L.J.T. Young. 1980. Mouse mammary tumor biology: A new synthesis. *Cold Spring Harbor Conf. Cell Proliferation* **7**: 1105.

Chirgwin, J.M., A.E. Przybyla, R.J. MacDonald, and W.J. Rutter. 1979. Isolation of biologically active ribonucleic acid from sources enriched in ribonuclease. *Biochemistry* **18**: 5294.

Cohen, J.C. and H.E. Varmus. 1980. Proviruses of mouse mammary tumor virus in normal and neoplastic tissues from GR and C3Hf mouse strains *J. Virol.* **35**: 298.

Cohen, J.C., J.E. Majors, and H.E. Varmus. 1979a. Organization of mouse mammary tumor virus-specific DNA endogenous to BALB/c mice. *J. Virol.* **32**: 483.

Cohen, J.C., P.R. Shank, V.L. Morris, R. Cardiff, and H.E. Varmus. 1979b. Integration of the DNA of mouse mammary tumor virus in virus-infected normal and neoplastic tissue of the mouse. *Cell* **16**: 333.

De Ome, K.B., L.J. Faulkin, Jr., H.A. Bern, and P.B. Blair. 1959. Development of mammary tumors from hyperplastic alveolar nodules transplanted into gland-free mammary fat pads of female C3H mice. *Cancer Res.* **19**: 515.

de Villiers, J., L. Olson, J. Banerji, and W. Schaffner. 1982. Analysis of the transcriptional enhancer effect. *Cold Spring Harbor Symp. Quant. Biol.* **46**: 911.

Dickson, C. and G. Peters. 1981. Protein-coding potential of mouse mammary tumor virus genome RNA as examined by in vitro translation. *J. Virol.* **37**: 36.

Dickson, C., R. Smith, and G. Peters. 1981. In vitro synthesis of polypeptides encoded by the long terminal repeat region of mouse mammary tumour virus DNA. *Nature* **291**: 511.

Donehower, L.A., A.L. Huang, and G.L. Hager. 1981. Regu-

latory and coding potential of the mouse mammary tumor virus long terminal redundancy. *J. Virol.* **37**: 226.

Fanning, T.G., J.P. Puma, and R.D. Cardiff. 1980. Selective amplification of mouse mammary tumor virus in mammary tumors of GR mice. *J. Virol.* **36**: 109.

Fasel, N., K. Pearson, E. Buetti, and H. Diggelmann. 1982. The region of mouse mammary tumor virus DNA containing the long terminal repeat includes a long coding sequence and signals for hormonally regulated transcription. *EMBO J.* **1**: 3.

Foulds, L. 1949. Mammary tumours in hybrid mice: The presence and transmission of the mammary tumour agent. *Br. J. Cancer* **3**: 230.

Fung, Y.-K.T., A.M. Fadly, L.B. Crittenden, and H.-J. Kung. 1981. On the mechanism of retrovirus-induced avian lymphoid leukosis: Deletion and integration of the proviruses. *Proc. Natl. Acad. Sci.* **78**: 3418.

Fung, Y.-K.T., W.G. Lewis, L.B. Crittenden, and H.-J. Kung. 1983. Activation of the cellular oncogene c-erbB by LTR insertion: Molecular basis for induction of erythroblastosis by avian leukosis virus. *Cell* **33**: 357.

Gillies, S.D., S.L. Morrison, V.T. Oi, and S. Tonegawa. 1983. A tissue-specific transcription enhancer element is located in the major intron of a rearranged immunoglobulin heavy chain gene. *Cell* **33**: 717.

Groner, B., E. Buetti, H. Diggelmann, and N.E. Hynes. 1980. Characterization of endogenous and exogenous mouse mammary tumor virus proviral DNA with site-specific molecular clones. *J. Virol.* **36**: 734.

Hayward, W.S., B.G. Neel, and S.M. Astrin. 1981. Activation of a cellular oncogene by promoter insertion in ALV induced lymphoid leukosis. *Nature* **290**: 475.

Kennedy, N., G. Knedlitschek, B. Groner, N.E. Hynes, P. Herrlich, R. Michalides, and A.J.J. van Ooyen. 1982. Long terminal repeats of endogenous mouse mammary tumour virus contain a long open reading frame which extends into adjacent sequences. *Nature* **295**: 622.

Khoury, G. and P. Gruss. 1983. Enhancer elements. *Cell* **33**: 313.

Lane, M.-A., A. Sainten, and G.M. Cooper. 1981. Activation of related transforming genes in mouse and human mammary carcinomas. *Proc. Natl. Acad. Sci.* **78**: 5185.

Lee, F., R. Mulligan, P. Berg, and G. Ringold. 1981. Glucocorticoids regulate expression of dihydrofolate reductase cDNA in mouse mammary tumor chimaeric plasmids. *Nature* **294**: 228.

Maniatis, T., E.F. Fritsch, and J. Sambrook, eds. 1982. *Molecular cloning. A laboratory manual.* Cold Spring Harbor Laboratory, Cold Spring Harbor, New York.

Moore, D.H., C.A. Long, A.B. Vaidya, J.B. Sheffield, A.S. Dion, and E.Y. Lasfargues. 1979. Mammary tumor viruses. *Adv. Cancer Res.* **29**: 347.

Morris, V.L., J.E. Vlasschaert, C.L. Beard, M.F. Milazzo, and W.C. Bradbury. 1980. Mammary tumors from BALB/c mice with a reported high mammary tumor incidence have acquired new mammary tumor virus DNA sequences. *Virology* **100**: 101.

Neel, B.G., W.S. Hayward, H.L. Robinson, J. Fang, and S.M. Astrin. 1981. Avian leukosis virus-induced tumors have common proviral integration sites and synthesize discrete new RNAs: Oncogenesis by promoter insertion. *Cell* **23**: 323.

Neiman, P.E., L. Jordan, R.A. Weiss, and L.N. Payne. 1980. Malignant lymphoma of the bursa of Fabricius: Analysis of early transformation. *Cold Spring Harbor Conf. Cell Proliferation* **8**: 519.

Nusse, R. and H.E. Varmus. 1982. Many tumors induced by the mouse mammary tumor virus contain a provirus integrated in the same region of the host genome. *Cell* **31**: 99.

Payne, G.S., J.M. Bishop, and H.E. Varmus. 1982. Multiple arrangements of viral DNA and an activated host oncogene in bursal lymphomas. *Nature* **295**: 209.

Peters, G., C. Kozak, and C. Dickson. 1984. Mouse mammary tumor virus integration regions *int-1* and *int-2* map on different mouse chromosomes. *Mol. Cell Biol.* **4**: 375.

Peters, G., S. Brookes, R. Smith, and C. Dickson. 1983. Tumorigenesis by mouse mammary tumor virus: Evidence for a common region for provirus integration in mammary tumors. *Cell* **33**: 369.

Queen, C. and D. Baltimore. 1983. Immunoglobulin gene transcription is activated by downstream sequence elements. *Cell* **33**: 741.

Redmond, S.M.S. and C. Dickson. 1983. Sequence and expression of the mouse mammary tumour virus *env* gene. *EMBO J.* **2**: 125.

Sen, G.C., J. Racevskis, and N.H. Sarkar. 1981. Synthesis of murine mammary tumor viral proteins in vitro. *J. Virol.* **37**: 963.

Spandidos, D.A. and N.M. Wilkie. 1983. Host-specificities of papillomavirus, Moloney murine sarcoma virus and Simian virus 40 enhancer sequences. *EMBO J.* **2**: 1193.

Thomas, P.S. 1980. Hybridization of denatured RNA and small DNA fragments transferred to nitrocellulose. *Proc. Natl. Acad. Sci.* **77**: 5201.

Traina, V.L., B.A. Taylor, and J.C. Cohen. 1981. Genetic mapping of endogenous mouse mammary tumor viruses: Locus characterization, segregation, and chromosomal distribution. *J. Virol.* **40**: 735.

Varmus, H.E. 1982. Recent evidence for oncogenesis by insertion mutagenesis and gene activation. *Cancer Surveys* **1**: 309.

Wasylyk, B., C. Wasylyk, P. Augereau, and P. Chambon. 1983. The SV40 72bp repeat preferentially potentiates transcription starting from proximal natural or substitute promoter elements. *Cell* **32**: 503.

Oncogene Activation by Proviral Insertion

R. Nusse and A. Van Ooyen

Department of Virology, Antoni van Leeuwenhoekhuis, Netherlands Cancer Institute, 1066 CX Amsterdam, The Netherlands

D. Westaway, Y.K. Fung, and H.E. Varmus

Department of Microbiology and Immunology, University of California Medical Center, San Francisco, California 94143

C. Moscovici

Department of Pathology, University of Florida and Veteran's Administration Medical Center, Gainesville, Florida 32602

Certain cellular genes are deployed diversely during oncogenesis, and a correspondingly diverse arsenal of techniques is now available for discovering those genes. Experimental convergence over the past several years has revealed that largely overlapping sets of cellular genes may be (1) transduced by retroviruses to form highly oncogenic viruses; (2) expressed more efficiently as a consequence of adjacent proviral insertions; (3) mutated by single-base substitutions, acquiring the ability to transform heterologous cells; (4) grossly amplified in number to generate heightened levels of expression; or (5) translocated from normal chromosomal contexts to novel ones (for reviews, see Cooper 1982; Bishop 1983; Klein 1983).

In this brief paper, we review recent efforts in our laboratories to pursue evidence that some retroviruses lacking their own oncogenes can induce tumors by serving as insertional mutagens (Varmus 1982). This phenomenon is experimentally attractive because it can lead us to new cellular oncogenes, illustrate features of eukaryotic gene regulation, serve as a model for other types of chromosomal rearrangements, and assist in more precise definition of the multiple stages in oncogenesis long predicted from clinical observations. The insertion mutation hypothesis, in its simplest form, supposes that proviral DNA can be integrated at virtually any site in the chromosomes of an infected host cell; in one or a few cells, proviral DNA is integrated near a cellular oncogene capable of initiating tumor formation in that cell type. The level of expression (or the structure of the product) of the oncogene is altered by the insertion, most commonly because a retroviral promoter or enhancer augments transcriptional activity. The insertion mutation then favors outgrowth of the mutant cell, and additional mutations, at varied sites and by varied mechanisms, may contribute further to tumor progression.

The "activation" of c-*myc* in avian bursal lymphomas may itself be a multistep phenomenon

The idea that retroviral insertion mutations of cellular oncogenes might be a crucial factor in tumorigenesis first took strong hold upon the scientific imagination with the identification of a known proto-oncogene, c-*myc*, as the integration site for avian leukosis virus (ALV) proviruses in a large number of chicken bursal lymphomas (Hayward et al. 1981). Proviruses in the c-*myc* locus are associated with intracellular levels of c-*myc* RNA 20–100-fold higher than in convenient control cells, with the provirus either providing a promoter for c-*myc* (when positioned upstream from c-*myc* in the same transcriptional orientation) or contributing an enhancer element to c-*myc* (when positioned upstream in the opposite transcriptional orientation or downstream from c-*myc*) (Hayward et al. 1981; Neel et al. 1981; Payne et al. 1981, 1982). These findings suggested that the first step in lymphomagenesis is the insertion of an ALV provirus in a suitable site for augmentation of c-*myc* expression, with selection for the rare cell in which it occurred. The prediction that additional uncommon events contribute to tumor development was supported by the observation that a presumed mutant form of another gene, now called *Blym* (Goubin et al. 1983), gives lymphoma DNA competence to transform mouse NIH-3T3 cells (Cooper and Neiman 1980, 1981).

More detailed study of mutant c-*myc* loci molecularly cloned from bursal lymphomas suggests that multiple uncommon events may be required to achieve full neoplastic potential at the site of the insertion mutations. This possibility was foreshadowed by the frequent description of truncated ALV proviruses within c-*myc* domains (Fung et al. 1981; Hayward et al. 1981; Payne et al. 1981, 1982), and it has been strengthened by our recent analysis of mutant c-*myc* loci from the lymphoid leukosis tumors, LL3 and LL4. The proviruses in these loci have suffered deletions likely to have occurred subsequent to integration; in addition, adjacent to one insertion mutation, we have found evidence for somatic mutations that affect the coding potential of c-*myc* and may thereby also contribute to tumor progression (D. Westaway et al., in prep.).

A summary of the central findings is illustrated in Figure 1. The narrow open boxes in both sections of the figure show the two c-*myc* exons (flanked by splice donor and acceptor sites) that encompass virtually all of the v-*myc* sequences found in the genome of MC29, an avian retrovirus that encodes a 100-kD *gag-myc* fusion protein

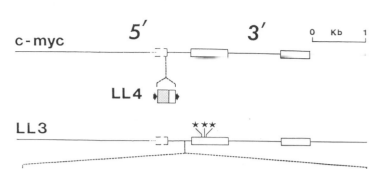

Figure 1 Secondary mutations at provirally mutated *c-myc* loci in bursal lymphomas LL3 and LL4. For explanation, see text.

(Alitalo et al. 1983; Reddy et al. 1983; Watson et al. 1983). The dashed box represents a region of uncertain size that contains at least 12 bp also found in *v-myc*; this sequence is followed by a splice donor consensus sequence (and therefore may constitute another exon), positioned about 450 bp upstream from the first of the known large exons (W. Hayward and M. Linial, pers. comm.). Additional exons further upstream from the illustrated exons are likely to supply the remainder of the sequences found in the normal *c-myc* mRNA of 2.5 kb.

The proviral insert in tumor LL4 lies within the "hypothetical" exon, about 470 bp to the 5′ side of the first large exon, in the same transcriptional orientation. Restriction mapping of tumor DNA and relevant cloned restriction fragments indicates that the entire proviral insert is small, about the size of a single long terminal repeat (LTR). Nucleotide sequencing reveals a solitary LTR that appears to be derived from an integrated provirus: Two bp are absent from each end of the LTR and 6 bp of host sequence are duplicated to flank the LTR (Varmus 1983). In tumor LL3, the provirus is oriented in the transcriptional sense opposite to that of *c-myc* and resides approximately 125 bp to the 5′ side of the first large *c-myc* exon. The provirus has suffered a large internal deletion extending from a site within the nontranslated leader, near the 3′ end of the tRNA primer binding site, to the p27 coding region of the *gag* gene. The sequences of the host–viral junctions indicate that this provirus was also inserted by a normal mechanism, without subsequent rearrangements of adjacent cellular DNA, since 2 bp have been lost from each LTR, 6 bp have been duplicated at the insertion site, and the *c-myc* sequence on the 3′ side of the provirus confirms the assignment of transcriptional orientations.

Since both of these mutant proviruses lack the packaging signal for viral RNA (Shank and Linial 1980) and some or all of the tRNA primer binding site, they cannot have been directly transcribed from mutant viruses present in the infecting stock; instead they must have arisen de novo either during reverse transcription or (more likely) after proviral integration. The "solo" LTR in LL4 appears to be the residue of homologous recombination between 5′ and 3′ LTRs, whereas the internal deletion in the LL3 provirus reveals no more than two homologous

base pairs at the recombination sites. There are numerous precedents for both types of events involving proviruses and similarly structured transposable elements (Varmus 1983); their frequency, measured for proviruses in cultured somatic cells, is low, $\sim 10^{-6}$ events per cell generation (Varmus et al. 1981). Thus, there would appear to be a requirement for selection of the deletion mutations. The selective factor(s) could be the attenuation of viral gene expression or augmented expression of *c-myc*. Both deletions probably eliminate the possibility of expressing viral structural genes in these tumors: No other acquired proviruses are present in either tumor (Payne et al. 1981), the LL4 provirus has lost all known coding domains, and the LL3 provirus lacks the initiation codon for *gag* and *gag-pol* and the splice donor site for *env* mRNA. Cells bearing the deleted proviruses might therefore escape a host immune response directed against viral antigens present in the original tumor cell. The proviral deletions might also have positive effects upon the enhanced expression of *c-myc*. For example, homologous recombination between the LTRs in tumor LL4 might have removed an inhibiting effect of the 5′ LTR upon the promoter for *c-myc* transcription in the 3′ LTR; an effect of this type has been observed in another experimental context by Cullen et al. (1984).

During our studies of these two mutant *c-myc* loci, we noted that a *Sac*I site normally present in the first large coding exon is absent in the LL3 allele (Payne et al. 1981). Since the site is present in both alleles in normal tissue from the animal in which LL3 arose, the alteration that eliminated the site must have been a somatic mutation (D. Westaway et al., in prep.). Nucleotide sequencing of 180 bp at the 5′ end of the implicated exon reveals three nucleotide substitutions represented by stars above the LL3 *c-myc* exon in Figure 1: a silent G → A transition in codon 57 that destroys the *Sac*I recognition site, a silent C → A transversion in codon 46, and another C → A substitution in codon 63, converting it from a proline to a threonine codon. Although we cannot be certain that the latter two differences from the reported sequence of *c-myc* are truly somatic mutations rather than genetic polymorphisms, it seems likely that the three changes occurred in one concerted event and were selected for as a result of the amino acid alterations introduced by codon 63 (and perhaps by other mutations in the unsequenced part of c-myc). Thus, these results extend the conclusions drawn from the proviral deletion mutations by suggesting that other kinds of secondary mutations may alter the nature (e.g., the oncogenicity) of the c-myc gene product. Of course, more direct genetic tests of such ideas are now required, but it appears that multiple steps toward full neoplasia can occur by proviral insertions, deletions, and base substitutions within a single locus.

Discovery of a novel cellular oncogene at the site of proviral insertion mutations in mouse mammary tumors

Mammary carcinomas are induced after long latency in laboratory mice by the mouse mammary tumor virus (MMTV), a retrovirus that appears to lack a host-derived oncogene; the tumors are clonal growths bearing from one to several new MMTV proviruses (Cohen et al. 1979). In the hopes of finding cellular oncogenes implicated in mammary tumorigenesis, we have asked whether any cellular loci can be identified as targets for insertion mutation by MMTV proviruses in tumor cells. By screening over 25 primary tumors in C3H mice, we encountered one tumor bearing a single new provirus; molecular cloning of a large portion of this provirus, its flanking DNA, and normal mouse DNA representing the uninterrupted insertion site was then exploited to generate several probes for the cellular locus (Nusse and Varmus 1982). Examination of DNA from several other tumors showed that 19 of 26 tumors carried MMTV proviruses within a 20-kb domain that we have called int-1 (Fig. 2). The proviruses appear to be arranged about equally on either side of a central region that is transcribed in tumors but not in tumor-free, MMTV-infected mammary glands.

Tests for homology between the int-1 domain and 16 viral retroviral oncogenes have failed to reveal any similarity, suggesting that the transcribed region represents a novel mammary oncogene. (In addition, int-1 clones do not anneal to DNA enriched for the NIH-3T3 cell transforming gene described in mammary tumor DNA by Lane et al. [1981] [G. Cooper and M.A. Lane, unpubl.].) Like other cellular oncogenes, int-1 is highly conserved among metazoan organisms, with sequences homologous to the transcribed region detectable in Drosophila, fish, birds, and several mammals, including man. However, unlike most oncogenes, except c-mos (Muller et al. 1982; Bishop 1983), int-1 is not usually expressed; no int-1 RNA has been detected in a variety of mouse cell lines and tissues, save mammary tumors, most of which have documented int-1 insertion mutations. int-1 has been assigned to chromosome 15 in the mouse (Nusse et al. 1984) and to chromosome 12 in man (R. Nusse and A. Geurts van Kessel, unpubl.); however, no rearrangements (other than the MMTV insertion mutations) have yet been shown to involve these chromosomes in mammary tumors. Mapping of int-1 RNA with the S1 nuclease technique and incomplete nucleotide sequencing of int-1 genomic and cDNA clones indicate that at least four exons are present in the gene. However, the protein product of int-1 has not yet been identified.

Activation of expression of int-1 commonly occurs by an indirect mechanism

One of the most curious features of the insertion mutations in the int-1 locus is the orientation of the MMTV proviruses: Virtually all of the proviruses are either on the 5′ side of the int-1 gene in the opposite transcriptional orientation or on the 3′ side of the gene in the same orientation (Nusse et al. 1984; see Fig. 2). These conclusions are based upon restriction mapping of genomic DNA bearing the mutant alleles and determination of the direction of transcription of int-1 (from left to right on the map as we have drawn it). In view of results with ALV mutations in the c-myc locus, it is surprising to find that none of the 19 C3H tumors in our original collection exhibit MMTV proviruses positioned appropriately to provide an LTR promoter for int-1. (Furthermore, none of the proviruses appear to have sustained deletion mu-

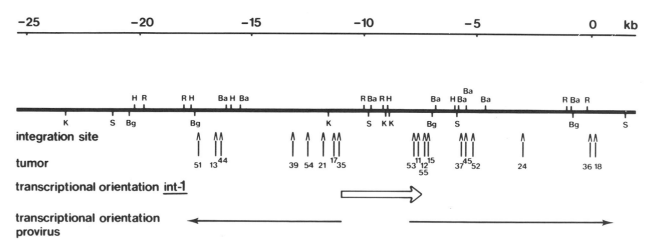

Figure 2 Physical and transcriptional map of the mouse int-1 locus showing the positions of inserted proviruses in tumors with the indicated numbers, the direction of transcription of the proviruses and of int-1, and recognition sites for EcoRI (R), BamHI (Ba), HindIII (H), BglII (Bg), SstI (S), and KpnI (K).

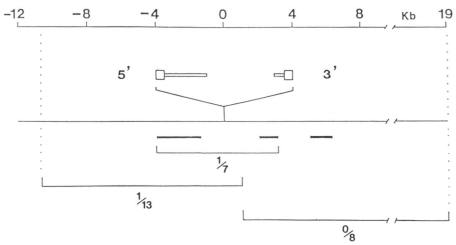

Figure 3 An attempt to identify a common proviral domain in MAV-induced nephroblastomas. (Open boxes) The cloned regions of MAV proviral DNA from the initial tumor; (solid bars) derivation of molecular probes for the flanking cellular sequences; (brackets) the domains tested in 15 tumors (including the initial tumor) for rearrangements.

tations detectable by restriction mapping of uncloned DNA.) Some tumors, however, contain hybrid transcripts, with *int-1* sequences linked to MMTV sequences. In these cases (tumors 11, 12, 15, 53, and 55 in Fig. 2), the proviral insertions have been mapped to a region a few hundred bp to the 5' side of the polyadenylation site for *int-1* RNA. In most tumors, *int-1* RNA measures approximately 2.6 kb in length; in the tumors with insertions near the polyadenylation site, *int-1* RNA is appreciably longer, generally 3.2–3.8 kb. We have used the "sandwich hybridization" method to show that these transcripts are longer because they include sequences from the MMTV LTR (Nusse et al. 1984). In these instances, transcription of *int-1* appears to proceed into the U_3 region of the 5' LTR of MMTV proviruses so that polyadenylation occurs at the site provided by the LTR. We have described a similar situation in a bursal lymphoma with a truncated provirus on the 3' side of *c-myc* (Payne et al. 1982).

Our results favor the notion that MMTV proviral DNA provides a transcriptional enhancer to the *int-1* domain. This interpretation might seem to be at odds with evidence that the MMTV promoter is comparatively weak, often requiring enhancers derived from other viral genomes for efficient expression (Huang et al. 1981; Lee et al. 1981) and that most viral enhancer elements are derived from what are considered to be strong promoters. However, it should be noted that (1) the proviral insertions convert a normally silent gene to one expressed rather inefficiently, with less than 10 copies of *int-1* RNA per cell; (2) enhancers may demonstrate decided preference for certain cellular environments (Banerji et al. 1983; Gillies et al. 1983) and (perhaps) for certain target genes; and (3) glucocorticoids stimulate transcription from the MMTV LTR (Huang et al. 1981; Lee et al. 1981), perhaps by a mechanism that is akin to enhancement (Chandler et al. 1983; Hynes et al. 1983; Majors and Varmus 1983), suggesting that the enhancement of *int-*

1 transcription may also be abetted by hormonal effects. The disposition of MMTV proviruses around the *int-1* gene may be relevant to the mechanism of enhancement: If the enhancer is located in the U_3 region of the LTR and active upon proximal promoters (deVilliers et al. 1983; Waslyk et al. 1983), the orientation of proviruses away from *int-1* would avoid the interposition of an MMTV promoter between the enhancer and the *int-1* promoter.

Are genetic targets for insertion mutations specific for certain cell lineages and predictive of chromosomal rearrangements?

The pursuit of retroviral insertion mutations in a number of contexts has unveiled some tantalizing correlations between the cellular genes that are mutated and the type of tumor cells in which those mutations are found. Thus proviruses of four readily distinguishable viruses—ALV, chicken syncytial virus (a reticuloendotheliosis virus), ring-necked pheasant virus, and myeloblastosis-associated virus—have been regularly found in the *c-myc* locus of avian bursal lymphomas (see above; Noori-Daloii et al. 1981; G. Simon and W. Hayward, pers. comm.; D. Westaway and C. Moscovici, unpubl.). Conversely, DNA of one virus—Rous associated virus-1 of the ALV group—can be found either in the *c-myc* locus in bursal lymphomas or in the *c-erb-B* locus in erythroblastosis (Fung et al. 1983).

On the other hand, at least two loci, the *int-1* locus described above and the *int-2* locus identified by Peters et al. (1983), appear to be independent targets for insertion mutations conducive to mammary tumors; moreover, not all tumors have insertions in one of these two domains, suggesting that other loci may yet be implicated. These latter findings could be interpreted to mean that there exist several mammary-specific oncogenes; alternatively, *int-1*, *int-2*, and other unidentified loci might be specific for tumor induction in certain types of cells within the mammary gland (Dulbecco et al. 1983). Recent attempts to define insertion mutations in MLV-induced thymic lymphomas indicate that the situation may be yet more complex, with some tumors bearing proviruses in or near c-myc and some bearing proviruses in commonly interrupted but uncharacterized loci (Tsichlis et al. 1983; D. Steffen, A. Hayday, P. Tsichlis, and J. Adams, pers. comm.). In any case, the determinants of the suggested specificities remain obscure; the influences of preferred integration sites, cell-specific enhancer activities, and gene products that meddle in differentiating processes have yet to be assessed satisfactorily.

The recent evidence for chromosomal translocations involving c-myc in B-cell tumors of mice and man (Klein 1983) provokes speculation that insertion mutations may be harbingers of other kinds of rearrangements affecting the same gene, particularly in tumors of the same type. A wider screening of tumors—e.g., of erythroleukemias for aberrations of c-erb-B or of mammary carcinomas for aberrations of int-1 or int-2—will be required to address this issue.

How general is the role of insertion mutation in tumorigenesis by viruses without oncogenes?

Results from several laboratories, summarized in the preceding section, support the idea that insertion mutations of cellular genes may be a common initiating step in tumorigenesis by certain retroviruses, particularly those that lack oncogenes derived from cellular genes. However, there appear to be exceptions. Considerable evidence links the oncogenic activity of the spleen focus-forming virus of the Friend virus complex to its unusual env gene, a recombinant gene that encodes a glycosylated fusion protein of about 45 kD (Troxler et al. 1980). Second, efforts to identify genetic targets for insertion mutations in B-cell tumors induced by the bovine leukemia virus have been unavailing (Kettmann et al. 1983); if insertion mutations do occur, either many sites are at risk or the proviruses can act over vast distances.

We have encountered similar difficulties in attempts to identify a target for insertion mutations during the induction of nephroblastomas in chickens by the myeloblastosis-associated virus (MAV). Most of these large tumors are clonal growths bearing multiple MAV proviruses. Although MAV proviruses are found in c-myc in bursal lymphomas, our examination of over 10 nephroblastomas has failed to reveal rearrangements of the c-myc locus (D. Westaway, unpubl.). Therefore, we have attempted to isolate an afflicted cellular gene by the "transposon tagging" procedure used to find int-1. Both ends of a MAV provirus with flanking cellular DNA were cloned from one tumor that carries a single detectable provirus (Fig. 3). Molecular probes derived from host sequences surrounding the integration site were used to survey about 30 kb of cellular DNA for interrupting proviruses in 14 tumors. Only DNA from the original tumor showed evidence of insertions in this region (Fig. 3); hence, further work in required to determine whether insertion mutations are instrumental in renal tumorigenesis by MAV.

Acknowledgments

Work in our laboratories is supported by grants CA 19287, CA 12705, AI 18782, and CA 09043 from the National Institutes of Health and MV48J from the American Cancer Society to H.E.V. and J.M.B.; and from the Netherlands Cancer Society Queen Wilhemina Fonds to R.N. and A.v.O.

References

Alitalo, K., J.M. Bishop, D.H. Smith, E.Y. Chen, W.W. Colby, and A.D. Levinson. 1983. Nucleotide sequence of the v-myc oncogene of avian retrovirus MC-29. *Proc. Natl. Acad. Sci.* **80:** 100.

Banerji, J., L. Olson, and W. Schaffner. 1983. A lymphocyte specific enhancer element is located downstream of the joining region in immunoglobulin heavy chain genes. *Cell* **33:** 729.

Bishop, J.M. 1983. Cellular oncogenes and retroviruses. *Annu. Rev. Biochem.* **52:** 301.

Chandler, V.L., B.A. Maler, and K.R. Yamamoto. 1983. DNA sequences bound specifically by glucocorticoid receptor in vitro render a heterologous promoter hormone responsive in vivo. *Cell* **33:** 489.

Cohen, J.C., P.R. Shank, V.L. Morris, R. Cardiff, and H.E. Varmus. 1979. Integration of the DNA of mouse mammary tumor virus in virus-infected normal and neoplastic tissues of the mouse. *Cell* **16:** 33.

Cooper, G.M. 1982. Cellular transforming genes. *Science* **217:** 801.

Cooper, G.M. and P.E. Neiman. 1980. Transforming genes of neoplasms induced by avian lymphoid leukosis viruses. *Nature* **287:** 659.

———. 1981. Two distinct candidate transforming genes of lymphoid leukosis virus-induced neoplasms. *Nature* **292:** 857.

Cullen, B.R., P.T. Lomedico, and G. Ju. 1984. Transcriptional interference in avian retroviruses—Implications for the promoter insertion model of leukemogenesis. *Nature* **307:** 241.

de Villiers, J., L. Olson, J. Banerji, and W. Schaffner. 1983. Analysis of the transcriptional "enhancer" effect. *Cold Spring Harbor Symp. Quant. Biol.* **47:** 911.

Dulbecco, R., M. Unger, B. Armstrong, M. Bowman, and P. Syka. 1983. Epithelial cell types and their evolution in the rat mammary gland determined by immunological markers. *Proc. Natl. Acad. Sci.* **80:** 1033.

Fung, Y.K.T., A.M. Fadly, L.B. Crittenden, and H.J. Kung. 1981. On the mechanism of retrovirus-induced avian lymphoid leukosis: Deletion and integration of the proviruses. *Proc. Natl. Acad. Sci.* **78:** 3418.

Fung, Y.K., W.G. Lewis, L.B. Crittenden, and H.-J. Kung. 1983. Activation of the cellular oncogene c-erbB by LTR insertion: Molecular basis for induction of erythroblastosis by avian leukosis virus. *Cell* **33:** 357.

Gillies, S.D., S.L. Morrison, V.T. Oi, and S. Tonegawa. 1983. A tissue-specific transcription enhancer element is located in the major intron of a rearranged immunoglobulin heavy chain gene. *Cell* **33:** 717.

Goubin, G., D.S. Goldman, J. Luce, P.E. Neiman, and G.M. Cooper. 1983. Molecular cloning and nucleotide sequence of a transforming gene detected by transfection of chicken B-cell lymphomas DNA. *Nature* **302:** 114.

Hayward, W.S., B.G. Neel, and S.M. Astrin. 1981. Activation of a cellular onc gene by promoter insertion in ALV-induced lymphoid leukosis. *Nature* **290:** 475.

Huang, A.L., M. Ostrowski, D. Berard, and G.L. Hager. 1981. Glucocorticoid regulation of the Ha-MuSV p21 gene conferred by sequences from the mouse mammary tumor virus. *Cell* **27:** 245.

Hynes, N., A.J.J. v. Ooyen, N. Kennedy, P. Herrlich, H. Ponta, and B. Groner. 1983. Subfragments of large terminal repeat cause glucocorticoid responsive expression of mouse mammary tumor virus and of an adjacent gene. *Proc. Natl. Acad. Sci.* **80:** 3637.

Kettmann, R., J. Deschamps, D. Couez, J.J. Claustriaux, R. Palm, and A. Burny. 1983. Chromosome integration domain for bovine leukemia provirus in tumors. *J. Virol.* **47:** 146.

Klein, G. 1983. Specific chromosomal translocations and the genesis of B cell derived tumors in mice and men. *Cell* **32:** 311.

Lane, M.A., A. Sainten, and G.M. Cooper. 1981. Activation of related transforming genes in mouse and human mammary carcinomas. *Proc. Natl. Acad. Sci.* **78:** 5185.

Lee, F., R. Mulligan, P. Berg, and G.M. Ringold. 1981. Glucocorticoids regulate expression of dihydrofolate reductase cDNA in mouse mammary tumor virus chimaeric plasmids. *Nature* **294:** 228.

Majors, J.E. and H.E. Varmus. 1983. A small region of the mouse mammary tumor virus long terminal repeat confers glucocorticoid hormone regulation on a linked heterologous gene. *Proc. Natl. Acad. Sci.* **80:** 5866.

Muller, R., D.J. Slamon, J.M. Tremblay, M.J. Cline, and I.M. Verma. 1982. Differential expression of cellular oncogenes during pre- and postnatal development of the mouse. *Nature* **299:** 640.

Neel, B.G., W.S. Hayward, H.L. Robinson, J. Fang, and S.M. Astrin. 1981. Avian leukosis virus-induced tumors have common proviral integration sites and synthesize discrete viral RNAs: Oncogenesis by promoter insertion. *Cell* **23:** 323.

Noori-Daloii, M.R., R.A. Swift, H.I. Kung, L.B. Crittenden, and R.L. Witter. 1981. Specific integration of REV proviruses in avian bursal lymphomas. *Nature* **294:** 574.

Nusse, R. and H.E. Varmus. 1982. Many tumors induced by the mouse mammary tumor virus contain a provirus integrated in the same region of the host genome. *Cell* **31:** 99.

Nusse, R., A. van Ooyen, D. Cox, Y.W. Fung, and H.E. Varmus. 1984. Mode of proviral activation of a putative mammary oncogene (int-1) on mouse chromosome 15. *Nature* **307:** 131.

Payne, G.S., J.M. Bishop, and H.E. Varmus. 1982. Multiple arrangements of viral DNA and an activated host oncogene in bursal lymphomas. *Nature* **295:** 209.

Payne, G.S., S.A. Courtneidge, L.B. Crittenden, A.M. Fadly, J.M. Bishop, and H.E. Varmus. 1981. Analysis of avian leukosis virus DNA and RNA in bursal tumors: Viral gene expression is not required for maintenance of the tumor state. *Cell* **23:** 311.

Peters, G., S. Brookes, R. Smith, and C. Dickson. 1983. Tumorigenesis by mouse mammary tumor virus: Evidence for a common region for provirus integration in mammary tumors. *Cell* **33:** 369.

Reddy, E.P., R.K. Reynolds, D.K. Watson, R.A. Schultz, J. Lautenberger, and T.S. Papas. 1983. Nucleotide sequence analysis of the proviral genome of avian myelocytomatosis virus (MC29). *Proc. Natl. Acad. Sci.* **80:** 2500.

Shank, P.R. and M. Linial. 1980. Avian oncovirus mutant (SE21Q1b) deficient in genomic RNA: Characterization of a deletion in the provirus. *J. Virol.* **36:** 450.

Troxler, D.H., S.K. Ruscetti, and E.M. Scolnick. 1980. The molecular biology of Friend virus. *Biochim. Biophys. Acta* **605:** 305.

Tsichlis, P.N., P. Gunter Strauss, and L.R. Hu. 1983. A common region for proviral DNA integration in Mol MuLV-induced rat thymic lymphomas. *Nature* **302:** 445.

Varmus, H.E. 1982. Recent evidence for oncogenesis by insertion mutagenesis and gene activation. *Cancer Surveys* **1:** 309.

———. 1983. Retroviruses. In *Mobile genetics elements* (ed. J.A. Shapiro), p. 411. Academic Press, New York.

Varmus, H.E., N. Quintrell, and S. Ortiz. 1981. Retroviruses as mutagens: Insertion and excision of a nontransforming provirus alter expression of a resident transforming provirus. *Cell* **25:** 23.

Waslyk, B., C. Waslyk, P. Augereau, and P. Chambon. 1983. The SV40 72 bp repeat preferentially potentiates transcription starting from proximal natural or substitute promoter elements. *Cell* **32:** 503.

Watson, D.K., E.P. Reddy, P.H. Duesberg, and T.S. Papas. 1983. Nucleotides sequence analysis of the chicken c-myc gene reveals homologous and unique coding regions by comparison with the transforming gene of avian myelocytomatosis virus MC29, delta-gag-myc. *Proc. Natl. Acad. Sci.* **80:** 2146.

The *Blym-1* Transforming Gene in Chicken and Human B-cell Lymphomas

A. Diamond,* J. Devine,* M.A. Lane,† and G.M. Cooper*

*Laboratory of Molecular Carcinogenesis and †Laboratory of Molecular Immunobiology, Dana-Farber Cancer Institute and Departments of Pathology, Harvard Medical School, Boston, Massachusetts 02115

Cellular transforming genes in lymphoid neoplasms

The phenotypic changes that accompany neoplastic development are generally believed to be a result of genetic alterations. Support for this concept has come from the demonstration that the DNAs of a variety of neoplastic cells can induce the morphological transformation of mouse NIH-3T3 cells by transfection with high efficiency whereas the DNA of normal cells cannot. In addition, the DNAs of NIH-3T3 cells that have been transformed by cellular DNA acquire the capacity to transform other mouse cells in secondary transfection experiments. In numerous examples, the exogenous transforming DNA has been shown by blot hybridization techniques to be transferred to the recipient mouse cells and similarly transferred in subsequent rounds of transfections. These results provide direct evidence that at least in some cases dominant genetic alterations have occurred during carcinogenesis and these transforming genes can be efficiently detected by transfection.

Activated transforming genes have been detected in the DNA of carcinomas, sarcomas, a neuroblastoma, lymphomas, and leukemias (for review, see Cooper 1982). Over 90% of the DNAs of lymphoid neoplasms have been shown to be capable of efficiently transforming mouse cells by transfection, implicating these transforming sequences in the disease process (Cooper and Neiman 1980; Lane et al. 1982a,b). Lane et al. (1982 a,b) have examined the transforming genes of various B- and T-lymphocyte neoplasms of mouse and human origin by restriction endonuclease sensitivity studies. These experiments have revealed that in multiple isolates of B- and T-lymphocyte neoplasms representing the same stage of differentiation the same transforming gene is activated. In contrast, the transforming genes of B- and T-lymphocyte neoplasms representing different stages of differentiation are different, indicating that there are stage-specific transforming genes activated in neoplasms of this type, and that these genes are well-conserved between mouse and man. These results also imply that these genes may be involved in the normal development of these cells.

The activated transforming gene of chicken B-cell lymphomas

Infection of susceptible chickens with lymphoid leukosis virus (LLV) results in the appearance of a variety of neoplasms, including bursal lymphomas, after a long latency period. LLVs are retroviruses that do not appear to contain oncogeneic sequences, in contrast to the acutely transforming retroviruses that contain specific viral transforming genes and induce tumors with a short latency period. The long latency periods required for LLVs to induce tumors is thought to be a consequence of the necessity for a number of steps to occur prior to tumor development. These steps may be correlated to early events in pathogenesis such as the appearance of pre-neoplastic follicles in the bursa of infected birds approximately 40 days after infection. Although most of these follicles eventually regress, approximately 1% are thought to progress further to metastatic lymphomas (Neiman et al. 1980).

The mechanism with which LLVs induce bursal lymphomas has been well studied. Hayward et al. (1981) have reported that in 80–90% of bursal lymphomas induced by LLVs viral long terminal repeat (LTR) sequences were present in the vicinity of the chicken *c-myc* gene, the cellular gene homologous to the transforming sequences of the avian myelocytomatosis virus strain MC29. Integration of either the entire LLV genome or LTR sequences near *c-myc* results in the activation of *c-myc* transcription by 20–100-fold. In most cases, the LLV sequences integrate downstream from the *c-myc* gene, and it has been proposed that promotion from viral regulatory signals into the *c-myc* gene results in increased mRNA levels. Additional work by Payne et al. (1982) has shown that transcriptional activation of *c-myc* can also occur when LLV sequences are integrated in either orientation downstream or upstream from *c-myc*, indicating that other viral regulatory elements, such as enhancer elements, are involved. Such enhancer elements have been found in a number of viral LTR sequences (Laimons et al. 1982; Jolly et al. 1983; Luciw et al. 1983). These results clearly implicate the *c-myc* gene in the pathogenesis of bursal lymphomas.

Transfection studies with bursal lymphoma DNAs have shown that this DNA can induce the transformation of mouse NIH-3T3 cells with an efficiency of approximately 0.1 transformant per μg of DNA (Cooper and Neiman 1980). Analysis of mouse transformant DNAs by Southern blot hybridization has indicated that the *c-myc* gene was not transferred to the mouse cells, providing evidence for a second transforming gene in bursal lymphomas (Cooper and Neiman 1981). Thus, there appear to be at least two genes involved in lymphomagenesis, the *c-myc* gene directly influenced by the LLV genome and a transforming gene detected by transfection.

The activated transforming gene of the RP9 bursal lymphoma cell line has recently been isolated (Goubin

211

et al. 1983). A recombinant phage library was made from the DNA of NIH-3T3 cells transformed by RP9 DNA and screened by sib selection using the biological assay of transfection. A single clone positive in the transfection was isolated and designated *ChBlym-1*. This clone had an insert of cellular DNA of 4.5 kb and a transforming activity of 1×10^3 to 5×10^3 transformants per μg of DNA. This activity is similar to that observed for other cloned transforming genes. Hybridization experiments indicated that *ChBlym-1* was not homologous to any previously isolated retroviral genes (Goubin et al. 1983).

Sequence analysis of *ChBlym-1* predicted a small protein of 65 amino acids that is rich in arginine (9.2%) and lysine (12.3%) (Goubin et al. 1983). In addition, the predicted amino acid sequence is hydrophilic at the ends and contains a central sequence of 14 amino acids that is hydrophobic. The nucleotide sequence of *ChBlym-1* was shown by a computer-assisted homology search to be 36% homologous to the aminoterminal regions of the transferrin family of proteins. Transferrins are a class of high-molecular-weight, iron-binding proteins that are essential growth factors for cells grown in serum-free media. The involvement of transferrins in the control of cell growth has been implicated because expression of both transferrin-related molecules (Brown et al. 1982) and transferrin receptors (Judd et al. 1980; Omary et al. 1980; Reinherz et al. 1980; Goding et al. 1981; Haynes et al. 1981; Sutherland et al. 1981) has been correlated with cell proliferation. In addition, transferrin has been shown to be a lymphocyte mitogen (Dillner-Centerlind 1979). It is intriguing that a transforming gene product is homologous to a family of growth control-related proteins. Recently, the product of the simian sarcoma virus transforming gene, *v-sis*, has been shown to be homologous to platelet-derived growth factor (Doolittle et al. 1983; Waterfield et al. 1983). It remains to be seen if more transforming genes will be related to other growth factors.

It has also been shown by blot hybridization that *ChBlym-1* is homologous to a small family of chicken genes present in both lymphoma and normal cells of the same birds (Goubin et al. 1983). In addition, *ChBlym-1* has also been shown to be homologous to a small gene family present in human DNA, indicating that these sequences are well conserved throughout vertebrate evolution. With this in mind, we hypothesized that sequences related to *ChBlym-1* may be activated in human neoplasms. We chose to look at Burkitt's lymphoma because it represents a B-cell neoplasm at an intermediate stage of development, as does chicken bursal lymphoma.

Transforming activity of Burkitt's lymphoma DNAs

Six Burkitt's lymphoma cell lines were analyzed for transforming activity. They were the Raji and Namalwa Epstein Barr virus (EBV)-positive African cell lines; BJAB, an African EBV-negative cell line; and CW678, EW36, and MC116, EBV-negative American Burkitt's lymphoma cell lines (Diamond et al. 1983). The DNAs of all these cell lines transformed NIH-3T3 cells with efficiencies be-

tween 0.1 and 1.0 transformant per μg of DNA in both primary and secondary rounds of transfections. In contrast, the DNA of three EBV-immortalized lymphocyte cell lines failed to induce transformation of mouse cells. EBV-immortalized cells differ from Burkitt's lymphoma cells because they are karyotypically normal, polyclonal, and cannot induce tumors in nude mice (Nilsson 1979). These results indicated that the transforming activity detected in the DNA of six Burkitt's lymphoma cell lines is specific for the lymphomas.

To determine if the transforming activity observed was due to the acquisition of the same gene by mouse cells, restriction endonuclease sensitivity studies were performed (Diamond et al. 1983). The DNAs of six Burkitt's lymphoma cell lines were inactivated by digestion with *Bam*HI but not by digestion with *Hin*dIII, *Eco*RI, or *Xho*I, indicating that in each case the same transforming gene was activated.

The activated transforming gene in Burkitt's lymphoma DNA

The activated transforming gene detected in Burkitt's lymphoma DNA by transfection has been cloned by virtue of its homology to *ChBlym-1* (Diamond et al. 1983). DNA from the CW678 Burkitt's lymphoma cell line was partially digested with *Mbo*I, and DNA of approximately 15–25 kb was inserted into the *Bam*HI site of the L47.1 λ vector, packaged in vitro, and screened by plaque hybridization using *ChBlym-1* as a hybridization probe. Then 15 positively hybridizing clones were selected, amplified, and tested by transfection for transforming activity. One of these clones efficiently transformed mouse cells (2×10^4 to 3×10^4 transformants per pmole of DNA) and was designated *HuBlym-1*. Hybridization experiments revealed that *HuBlym-1*, like *ChBlym-1*, was not homologous to any of the viral transforming genes *myc*, Ha-*ras*, Ki-*vas*, *fms*, *erb*, *abl*, *src*, *sis*, *fes*, *mos*, and *rel*. The restriction enzyme map of *HuBlym-1* indicated it was not homologous to a new member of the *ras* family, N-*ras*. N-*ras* has recently been shown to be activated in the AW Ramos Burkitt's lymphoma cell line (Murray et al. 1983). In addition, *HuBlym-1* is also not homologous to *Tlym-I*, a transforming gene isolated from a T-cell lymphoma (M.-A. Lane et al., in prep.).

To confirm that the activated gene cloned from a Burkitt's lymphoma cell line was the same gene detected by transfection of total genomic DNA, restriction endonuclease sensitivity studies were performed (Diamond et al. 1983). The cloned DNA was inactivated by digestion with *Bam*HI and not by *Xho*I, *Eco*RI, or *Hin*dIII. This pattern of enzyme sensitivity exactly matches that observed for total Burkitt's lymphoma DNA. Direct evidence that *HuBlym-1* is the activated transforming gene detected by transfection with cellular DNA has come from hybridization experiments which demonstrated that a 5-kb *Hin*dIII fragment present in the DNA of normal fibroblasts and six Burkitt's lymphoma cell lines that hybridized to a *HuBlym-1* probe was also present in the DNA of NIH-3T3 cells transformed by Burkitt's lymphoma DNA but not in the DNA of mouse cells. These same experiments revealed that whatever the mode of activation of *HuBlym-1*, it does not appear to include gene amplification or gross genetic rearrangements since the 5-kb *Hind*III band containing *HuBlym-1* sequences is present in similar amounts in both the DNAs of normal human fibroblasts and Burkitt's lymphoma cells. In addition, activation also appears not to be a consequence of increased *HuBlym-1* transcriptional activity because there is not a higher level of *HuBlym-1* mRNA in Burkitt's lymphoma cells as compared with that of immortalized lymphocytes (J. Devine, unpubl.). It therefore appears that activation of *HuBlym-1* probably involves a small structural alteration. Single-base mutations have been shown to be responsible for the activation of members of the *ras* family of transforming genes (Reddy et al. 1982; Tabin et al. 1982; Taparowsky et al. 1982; Capon et al. 1983; Shimizu et al. 1983; Yuasa et al. 1983), and it is possible that similar types of mutations result in activation of *HuBlym-1*.

Neoplastic development of B-cell lymphomas

The pathogenesis of Burkitt's lymphoma resembles that of avian B-cell lymphomas. LLV integration near the chicken *c-myc* gene results in *c-myc* transcriptional activation. Chicken *c-myc* is not, however, the gene responsible for the transforming activity of bursal lymphoma DNA. The transforming gene has been shown to be *ChBlym-1*. In Burkitt's lymphoma, EBV has been shown to be a contributing factor in the occurrence of the disease, although the role that EBV plays has yet to be determined (Epstein and Achong 1979). Burkitt's lymphoma cells typically exhibit a chromosomal translocation between chromosomes 8 and either 14, 2, or 22 (Klein 1981; Rowley 1982). A number of investigators have placed the human *c-myc* gene precisely at the breakpoint on chromosome 8 and have shown that it translocates to the recipient chromosome (Dalla-Favera et al. 1982; Neel et al. 1982; Taub et al. 1982; Marcu et al. 1983). These results clearly implicate *c-myc* in the disease process. As in chicken B-cell lymphomas, *c-myc* is not the gene detected by transfection. This was *HuBlym-1*. Thus, both chicken B-cell lymphomas and Burkitt's lymphoma have early viral involvements—*c-myc* activation and activation of a *Blym* transforming gene detectable by transfection. The similarities between these two systems imply that these events are significant in the development of tumors. Furthermore, since both these lymphomas include neoplastic and preneoplastic stages, it is conceivable that these events can be correlated to the various stages resulting in neoplasia.

Acknowledgments

These studies were supported by a fellowship to A.D. from the Damon Runyon-Walter Winchell Cancer Fund, a travel fellowship to J.D. from the Imperial Cancer Research Fund, London, and a faculty research award to G.M.C. from the American Cancer Society.

References

Brown, J.P., R.M. Hewick, I. Hellström, K.E. Hellström, R.F. Doolittle, and W.J. Dreyer. 1982. Human melanoma-associated antigen is structurally and functionally related to transferrin. *Nature* **296:** 171.

Capon, D.J., E.Y. Chen, A.D. Levinson, P.H. Seeburg, and D.V. Goeddel. 1983. Complete nucleotide sequence of the T24 human bladder carcinoma oncogene and its normal homologue. *Nature* **302:** 33.

Cooper, G.M. 1982. Cellular tranforming genes. *Science* **217:** 801.

Cooper, G.M. and P.E. Neiman. 1980. Transforming genes of neoplasms induced by avian lymphoid leukosis viruses. *Nature* **287:** 656.

———. 1981. Two distinct candidate transforming genes of lymphoid leukosis virus induced neoplasms. *Nature* **292:** 857.

Dalla-Favera, R., M. Gregni, J. Erikson, D. Patterson, R.C. Gallo, and C.M. Croce. 1982. Human c-myc onc gene is located on the region of chromosome 8 that is translocated in Burkitt lymphoma cells. *Proc. Natl. Acad. Sci.* **79:** 7824.

Diamond, A., G.M. Cooper, J. Ritz, and M.-A. Lane. 1983. Identification and molecular cloning of the human *Blym* transforming gene activated in Burkitt's lymphomas. *Nature* **305:** 112.

Dillner Centorlind, M.-L. S. Hammarström, and P. Perlman. 1979. Transferrin can replace serum for *in vitro* growth of mitogen-stimulated T lymphocytes. *Eur. J. Immunol.* **9:** 942.

Doolittle, R.F., M.W. Hunkapiller, L.E. Hood, S.G. Devare, K.C. Robbins, S.A. Aaronson, and H.N. Antoniades. 1983. Simian sarcoma virus onc gene, v-sis, is derived from the gene (or genes) encoding a platelet-derived growth factor. *Science* **221:** 275.

Epstein, M.A. and B.G. Achong. 1979. In *The Epstein-Barr virus* (ed. M.A. Epstein and B.G. Achong), p. 321. Springer-Verlag, New York.

Goding, J.W. and G.F. Burns. 1981. Monoclonal antibody OKT-9 recognizes the receptor for transferrin on human acute lymphocytic leukemia cells. *J. Immunol.* **127:** 1256.

Goubin, G., D.S. Goldman, J. Luce, P.E. Neiman, and G.M. Cooper. 1983. Molecular cloning and nucleotide sequence of a transforming gene detected by transfection of chicken B-cell lymphoma DNA. *Nature* **302:** 114.

Haynes, B.F., M. Hemler, T. Cotner, D.L. Mann, G.S. Eisenbarth, J. Strominger, and A.S. Fauci. 1981. Characterization of a monoclonal antibody (5E9) that defines a human cell surface antigen of cell activation. *J. Immunol.* **127:** 347.

Hayward, W.S., B.G. Neel, and S.M. Astrin. 1981. Activation of a cellular onc gene by promoter insertion in ALV-induced lymphoid leukosis. *Nature* **290:** 475.

Jolly, D.J., A.C. Esty, S. Subramani, T. Friedmann, and I.M. Verma. 1983. Elements in the long terminal repeat of murine retroviruses enhance stable transformation by thymidine kinase gene. *Nucleic Acids Res.* **11:** 1855.

Judd, W., C.A. Poodry, and J.L. Strominger. 1980. Novel surface antigens expressed on dividing cells but absent from non-dividing cells. *J. Exp. Med.* **152:** 1430.

Klein, G. 1981. The role of gene dosage and genetic transpositions in carcinogenesis. *Nature* **294:** 313.

Laimons, L.A., G. Khoury, C. Gorman, B. Howard, and P. Gruss. 1982. Host-specific activation of transcription by tandem repeats from simian virus 40 and Moloney murine sarcoma virus. *Proc. Natl. Acad. Sci.* **79:** 6453.

Lane, M.-A., D. Neary, and G.M. Cooper. 1982a. Activation of a cellular transforming gene in tumors induced by Abelson murine leukemia virus. *Nature* **300:** 659.

Lane, M.-A., A. Sainten, and G.M. Cooper. 1982b. Stage-specific transforming genes of human and mouse B- and T-lymphocyte neoplasms. *Cell* **28:** 873.

Luciw, P.A., J.M. Bishop, H.E. Varmus, and M.R. Capecchi. 1983. Location and function of retroviral and SV40 sequences that enhance biochemical transformation after microinjection of DNA. *Cell* **33:** 705.

Marcu, K.B., L.J. Harris, L.W. Stanton, J. Erikson, R. Watt, and C.M. Croce. 1983. Transcriptionally active c-*myc* oncogene is contained within NIARD, a DNA sequence associated with chromosome translocations in B-cell neoplasia. *Proc. Natl. Acad. Sci.* **80:** 519.

Murray, M.J., J.M. Cunningham, L.F. Parada, F. Dautry, P. Lebowitz, and R.A. Weinberg. 1983. The HL-60 transforming sequence: A ras oncogene coexisting with altered myc genes in hematopoietic tumors. *Cell* **33:** 749.

Neel, B.G., S.C. Jhanwar, R.S.K. Chaganti, and W.S. Hayward. 1982. Two human c-onc genes are located on the long arm of chromosome 8. *Proc. Natl. Acad. Sci.* **79:** 7842.

Neiman, P.S., L. Jordan, and R. Weiss. 1980. Malignant lymphoma of the bursa of fabricius: Analysis of early transformation. *Cold Spring Harbor Conf. Cell Proliferation* **7:** 519.

Nilson, D.K. 1979. The nature of lymphoid cell lines and their relationship to the virus. In *The Epstein-Barr virus* (ed. M.A. Epstein and B.G. Achong), p. 225. Springer-Verlag, New York.

Omary, M.B., I.S. Trowbridge, and J. Minowada. 1980. Human cell-surface glycoprotein with unusual properties. *Nature* **286:** 888.

Payne, G.S., J.M. Bishop, and H.E. Varmus. 1982. Multiple arrangements of viral DNA and an activated host oncogene in bursal lymphomas. *Nature* **295:** 209.

Reddy, E.P., R.K. Reynolds, E. Santos, and M. Barbacid. 1982. A point mutation is responsible for the acquisiton of transforming properties by the T24 human bladder carcinoma oncogene. *Nature* **300:** 149.

Reinherz, E.L., P.C. Kung, G. Goldstein, R.H. Levey, and S.F. Scholssman. 1980. Discrete stages of human intrathymic differentiation: Analysis of normal thymocytes and leukemic lymphoblasts of T-cell lineage. *Proc. Natl. Acad. Sci.* **77:** 1588.

Rowley, J. 1982. Identification of constant chromosome regions involved in human hematologic malignant disease. *Science* **216:** 749.

Shimizu, K., M. Goldfarb, Y. Suard, M. Perucho, Y. Li, T. Kamata, J. Feramisco, E. Stavnezer, J. Fogh, and M.H. Wigler. 1983. Three human transforming genes are related to the viral ras oncogenes. *Proc. Natl. Acad. Sci.* **80:** 2112.

Sutherland, R., D. Dlia, C. Schneider, R. Newman. J. Kemshead, and M. Greaves. 1981. Ubiquitous cell-surface glycoprotein on tumor cells is proliferation-associated receptor for transferrin. *Proc. Natl. Acad. Sci.* **78:** 4515.

Tabin, C.J., S.M. Bradley, C.I. Bargmann, R.A. Weinberg, A.G. Papageorge, E.M. Scolnick, R. Dhar, D.R. Lowy, and E.H. Chang. 1982. Mechanism of activation of a human oncogene. *Nature* **300:** 143.

Taparowsky, E., Y. Suard, O. Fasano, K. Shimizu, M. Goldfarb, and M. Wigler. 1982. Activation of the T24 bladder carcinoma transforming gene is linked to a single amino acid change. *Nature* **300:** 762.

Taub, R., I. Kirsch, C. Morton, G. Lenoir, D. Swan, S. Tronick, S. Aaronson, and P. Leder. 1982. Translocation of the c-myc gene into the immunoglobulin heavy chain locus in human Burkitt lymphoma and murine plasmacytoma cells. *Proc. Natl. Acad. Sci.* **79:** 7837.

Waterfield, M.D., G.T. Scrace, N. Whittle, P. Stroobant, A. Johnsson, A. Wasteson, B. Westermark, C.-H. Heldin, J.S. Huang, and T. Deuel. 1983. Platelet derived growth factor is structurally related to the putative transforming protein p28[sis] of simian sarcoma virus. *Nature* **204:** 305.

Yuasa, Y., S.K. Srivastava, C.Y. Dunn, J.S. Rhim, E.P. Reddy, and S.A. Aaronson. 1983. Acquisition of transforming properties by alternative point mutations with c-bas/has human proto-oncogene. *Nature* **303:** 775.

Amplification of Cellular Oncogenes in Tumor Cells

M. Schwab, K. Alitalo, H.E. Varmus, and J.M. Bishop

George W. Hooper Foundation and Department of Microbiology and Immunology, School of Medicine, University of California, San Francisco, California 94143

The oncogenes of retroviruses arose by transduction and modification of normal vertebrate genes now known as "cellular oncogenes" (Bishop 1982). Although cellular oncogenes first came to light as the apparent progenitors of viral oncogenes, a variety of circumstantial evidence presently suggests that the cellular genes themselves may contribute to tumorigenesis initiated by diverse causes. The contribution of cellular oncogenes to tumorigenesis could take either of two forms: (1) inappropriately enhanced expression that overburdens cells with a normal protein encoded by a cellular oncogene or (2) mutational damage that changes the functions of the gene product. Evidence for both scenarios has surfaced and been reviewed elsewhere (Bishop 1982). This paper has a more limited purview: We summarize the evidence that expression of cellular oncogenes can be enhanced by gene amplification and treat the possibility that these events might figure in tumorigenesis.

There are at least three means by which the expression of a cellular oncogene could be augmented. First, mutations within regulatory elements could unleash the gene from its usual constraints. Ironically, this most obvious of mechanisms has yet to be encountered in the study of either experimental or naturally arising tumors. Second, rearrangements of DNA could bring the gene under the sway of foreign regulatory influences. Two examples of this possibility are now known: insertion of retroviral DNA in the vicinity of cellular oncogenes (Nusse et al., this volume) and chromosomal translocations that alter the context within which a cellular oncogene resides (Klein 1983). Third, spontaneous or evoked amplification of chromosomal DNA could increase the "dose" of a cellular oncogene and, hence, the amount of its protein product. Amplification of cellular oncogenes in tumor cells has come into view only recently, but as the search for its occurrence has broadened, so has the frequency with which it has been found and the diversity of the oncogenes affected.

Tumor cells may contain either of two karyotypic manifestations of gene amplification—double minute chromosomes (DMs) and homogeneously staining regions (HSRs) within macrochromosomes. Once considered to be relatively rare features of human tumors, improved scrutiny is now revealing these abnormalities in as many as 20% of all solid tumors examined (J. Trent, pers. comm.). The molecular nature of DMs and HSRs was first worked out in a specialized setting—the emergence of tumor cells resistant to cytoxic drugs during the course of chemotherapy or of experimental selection in cell culture (Schimke et al. 1978). But it is also clear that DMs and HSRs can be present in tumor cells prior to the initiation of any form of therapy (for examples, see Schimke 1982) and it is in this setting that we chose to explore the possible amplification of cellular oncogenes.

Methods of Experimental Procedures

Cell lines and tumors

COLO 201, 205, and 320 were obtained from the American Type Culture Collection (Semple et al. 1978; Quinn et al. 1979), Y1 cells from D. George (George and Powers 1981), established lines of human neuroblastoma cells from F. Gilbert (New York University, N.Y.), G. Brodeur (Washington University, St. Louis, Mo.), and J. Trent (University of Arizona, Tucson), samples of primary neuroblastomas at the time of resection with the assistance of Drs. J. Kushner, M.R. Harrison, and V. Levin (University of California, San Francisco), and viable cell suspensions of primary neuroblastomas after karyotyping from J. Trent and from J. Casper.

Procedures for molecular hybridization

We have described previously our procedures for analysis of DNA by Southern blotting, for screening cellular RNA for expression of cellular oncogenes, and for analysis of poly(A)$^+$ cellular RNA by Northern blotting (Schwab et al. 1983a).

Analyzing cellular proteins for the products of cellular oncogenes

Antisera against the products of cellular ras genes were kindly provided by M. Furth and E. Scolnick (Furth et al. 1982). Antisera against the product of cellular myc were prepared in our laboratory (Alitalo et al. 1983b). Immunoprecipitations and analysis by immunofluorescence were performed as described previously.

Analysis of chromosomes

Karyotypes were analyzed after either trypsin-Giemsa or quinacrine staining. DMs were isolated according to published procedures (George and Powers 1981). Hybridization to chromosomes in situ was performed with tritium-labeled DNA from molecular clones as described previously (Harper and Saunders 1981; Alitalo et al. 1983a; Schwab et al. 1983a).

Results

Amplification of cellular oncogenes in human and mouse tumors

Table 1 summarizes the amplifications of cellular oncogenes reported to date in human and mouse tumor cells, chosen for examination because they bear either DMs or HSRs. Although the sampling of tumors is for the moment still small, the prevalence of known cellular oncogenes in the amplified DNA is remarkable. Cell lines derived from seven different types of tumors and bearing either DMs or HSRs have been examined; each line displays amplification of a recognizable cellular oncogene. The amplified genes identified to date include *c-myc*, *c-myb*, *c*-Ki-*ras*, and a newly described potential oncogene tentatively denoted N-*myc* in recognition of its amplification in the cells of human neuroblastomas (Schwab et al. 1983b). The extent of gene amplification varies from five- to many hundredfold over the single copy found in the haploid genome in normal cells.

Although none of the amplified genes has been examined in full detail, mapping with restriction endonucleases indicates that the structure of most of the genes has not been greatly disturbed by the process of amplification. We have found only one exception to this statement. COLO 320 cells contain two forms of amplified *c-myc*, one whose general topography appears normal and one which has suffered a rearrangement (probably a translocation or insertion of foreign DNA) upstream of its coding region (Alitalo et al. 1983a; M. Schwab, unpubl.). COLO 320 cells are available as clones containing only DMs and clones containing only HSRs (Semple et al. 1978; Alitalo et al. 1983a). The normal and rearranged versions of *c-myc* are of roughly equal abundance in the cells containing DMs, whereas the normal version of the amplified gene predominates

in the cells containing HSRs (Alitalo et al. 1983a); the rearranged version is present only in what appears to be a single copy.

Amplification of N-*myc* in human neuroblastoma

The exceptional frequency with which DMs and HSRs occur in cells derived from human neuroblastomas prompted an extensive survey of these cells for amplification of known cellular oncogenes. In our initial survey, we recognized that DNA related to *c-myc* was amplified in numerous lines of neuroblastoma cells (Table 2). Further study revealed, however, that the amplified gene was not the previously isolated, prototypic version of human *c-myc*, but rather a very distant kin that we have provisionally denoted N-*myc* (Schwab et al. 1983b). The principal homology between prototypic human *c-myc* and N-*myc* is limited to two blocks of 74 and 59 nucleotide pairs within the leftward of the two exons that contain the open reading frame encoding the *c-myc* protein (Schwab et al. 1983b). Other investigators have cloned at least three loci from human DNA that share some homology with a 5′ domain of human *c-myc* (Dalla Favera et al. 1982b). The published restriction maps of these loci are different from the map that we have obtained for N-*myc*, so it is likely that N-*myc* is a previously unrecognized gene.

We have found amplification of N-*myc* in all but one of the cell lines derived from human neuroblastomas that we have examined (Table 2), and this line (SK-N-SH) contains neither DMs nor HSRs (Brodeur et al. 1981). In addition, five out of nine samples from primary tumors resected prior to institution of chemotherapy displayed amplification of N-*myc* (Schwab et al. 1983b; M. Schwab et al.; J. Trent; both unpubl.). Results with other malignant tumors derived from the neurectoderm have varied; we have found N-*myc* amplified in only one (Y79) of several cell lines derived from retinoblastomas, and no amplification of the gene in lines from melanomas (Table 2; M. Schwab et al., unpubl.).

Table 1 Amplification of Cellular Oncogenes in Tumor Cells

Tumor	Oncogene	Amplification	Expression enhanced
HL60 (APML)	*c-myc*	20 ×	yes
COLO 320 (carcinoma)	*c-myc*	50 ×	yes
Y1 (adrenocortical)	*c*-Ki-*ras*	50 ×	yes
COLO 201/205 (colon carcinoma)	*c-myb*	10 ×	yes
K562 (CML)	*c-abl*	10 ×	yes
Neuroblastoma	"N-*myc*"	5–200 ×	yes
SCLC → LCV (carcinoma of lung)	*c-myc*	5–30 ×	yes

The table summarizes all available reports of amplified cellular oncogenes. References are given in the text. Data on COLO 320, Y1, COLO 201/205, and neuroblastoma represent the authors' own work. Abbreviations: (APML) acute promyelocytic leukemia; (COLO) Colorado; (SCLC) small-cell lung carcinoma; (LCV) large-cell variant (a more malignant form of SCLC).

Table 2 The Amplification of N-*myc*

Origin of DNA	Nature of specimen	HSR on chromosome	Presence of DMs	Extent of amplification of N-*myc*
MCN-1	Nb/c	—	+	8–10
Kelly	Nb/c	13p, markers	−	100–120
NGP	Nb/c	4p16,12q13	−	120–140
NLF	Nb/c	9q13	−	20–25
CHP-134	Nb/c	6q,7p		20–25
CHP-126	Nb/c	5q33	+	100–120
IMR-32	Nb/c	1p34	−	15–20
NMB	Nb/c	13p11	+	100–120
SK-N-SH	Nb/c	—	−	0
AR	Nb/T	?	?	80–100
SH	Nb/T	?	?	8–10
LG	Nb/T	?	?	5
GK	Nb/T	?	?	5
Y79	Rb/c	1p34	−	20
HL60	APML	—	+	0
K562	CML	—	−	0
HA-A	melanoma	7p	−	0
HA-L	melanoma	7p	−	0
COLO 320	carcinoma	X	+	0
Human epidermal fibroblasts	normal	—	−	0

Amplification of N-*myc* was estimated by molecular hybridization, using a molecular clone representing a portion of N-*myc* and Southern blots of DNAs from cell lines and tumors (for details, see Schwab et al. 1983b). Specimens are denoted as follows: (Nb/c) neuroblastoma cell line; (Nb/T) neuroblastoma, resected prior to chemotherapy; (Rb/c) retinoblastoma cell line; (APML) acute promyelocytic leukemia; (CML) chronic myelogenous leukemia.

Normal human cells contain a single haploid copy of N-*myc* located on the short arm of chromosome 2 (M. Schwab et al.; A. Sakaguchi; both unpubl.). By contrast, amplified N-*myc* is situated in HSRs on chromosomes other than number 2 in the various cell lines analyzed to date (Table 2).

Cytological locations of amplified cellular oncogenes

Neither DMs nor HSRs were apparent in the earliest reported instances of amplified cellular oncogenes (Collins and Groudine 1982, 1983; Dalla Favera et al. 1982a). Therefore, we exploited the existence of both karyotypic abnormalities in our materials to test the expectation that the amplified cellular oncogenes were located within these abnormalities. DMs isolated from the COLO 320, Y1, and neuroblastoma cell lines contained the appropriate amplified oncogenes (M. Schwab et al.; D. George; both unpubl.). Similarly, hybridization in situ revealed that amplified c-*myc*, c-Ki-*ras*, and N-*myc* were located on the HSRs in COLO 320, Y1, and neuroblastoma cell lines, respectively (Alitalo et al. 1983a; Schwab et al. 1983a,b). None of the HSRs were located at the chromosomal position occupied by the corresponding unamplified cellular oncogene, so it appears that in each instance the chromosomal domain bearing the cellular oncogene has been both amplified and translocated. This conclusion was immediately apparent from the banding patterns of chromosomes in the case of Y1 and neuroblastoma cells. For COLO 320 cells, however, it was necessary to use hybridization in situ with a molecular probe specific for the X chromosome to prove the location of the very large HSRs that occupy the bulk of both arms of the marker chromosome (K. Alitalo et al.; C.C. Lin; both unpubl.).

Expression of amplified cellular oncogenes

Gene amplification increases the amount of template available for production of RNA and, in most cases, augments expression of the amplified gene (Schimke et al. 1978; Schimke 1982). Amplification of cellular oncogenes conforms to this rule: Expression of the amplified genes listed in Table 1 is enhanced to levels that are in rough accord with the extent of gene amplification (Dalla Favera et al. 1982a; Alitalo et al. 1983a; Schwab et al. 1983a,b; M. Schwab et al., unpubl.). The enhancement is not limited to synthesis of RNA. Y1 cells contain exceptionally large amounts of the protein encoded by c-Ki-*ras* situated on the plasma membrane (Schwab et al. 1983a), and COLO 320 cells contain an abundant protein that is likely to be the as yet poorly characterized product of human c-*myc* (M. Schwab et al.; G. Evan and

G. Ramsay; both unpubl.). Analysis of RNA by Northern blotting has demonstrated that amplification of the cellular oncogenes has no gross effect on the structure of the RNA transcribed from the amplified genes (Schwab et al. 1983a; M. Schwab et al., unpubl.). It appears likely, however, that the damaged version of amplified c-myc in COLO 320 cells gives rise to a shortened form of c-myc RNA that predominates over the normal c-myc transcript in COLO 320 cells containing DMs (M. Schwab et al., unpubl.). We cannot presently say whether this anomaly has any functional consequence.

Discussion

The role of gene amplification in tumorigenesis

It is easy to suggest, but difficult to prove, that amplification and enhanced expression of cellular oncogenes has contributed to the genesis of the tumors studied in this report. One point raises the argument above pure conjecture. DMs are unstable elements that are generally lost from growing cells unless the enhanced expression of a gene within the DMs confers a selective advantage upon the cells (Schimke 1982). Since DMs were present at the time several of the tumors studied here were explanted into culture, and since DMs have survived innumerable generations of cell growth thereafter, we cannot avoid the suspicion that gene amplification has helped sustain the growth of the tumor cells. We cannot be certain that the identified cellular oncogenes are responsible for the impact of gene amplification, but it seems more than coincidence that, in every instance studied to date, karyotypic evidence of gene amplification in tumor cells not subjected to chemotherapy has been accompanied by amplification of either a previously identified cellular oncogene or a gene that can be recognized by its kinship to a known oncogene (i.e., N-myc). myc).

At what point in tumorigenesis might gene amplification come into play? We do not know, and we are confronted by two apparently contrasting clues. On the one hand, insertional mutagenesis is an early event (perhaps the first event) in the genesis of tumors by retroviruses without oncogenes of their own (Nusse et al., this volume); the consequence of insertional mutagenesis is enhanced expression of a cellular oncogene along the lines described here for gene amplification (although it is possible that mutations are also sustained by the coding element of the induced oncogene) (Westaway et al. 1984). On the other hand, amplification and enhanced expression of c-myc apparently occurs in concert with the conversion of human carcinoma of the lung cells to a more malignant phenotype—an advanced stage in the evolution of these tumor cells (J. Minna, pers. comm.). Of course, there may be no mandatory sequence of events for the genesis of any particular tumor, merely the requirement for a concerted set of genetic (and perhaps epigenetic) abnormalities before the full malignant phenotype is achieved. In such a scheme, enhanced expression of an oncogene could play its part whenever amplification happened to occur.

Reconstructing the evolution of karyotypic abnormalities in tumor cells

The sequence in which DMs and HSRs might arise has been controversial (Schimke 1982). At least three different scenarios have been suggested: (1) an amplified domain of DNA might depart a chromosome to engender DMs, which at some subsequent time reinsert by homologous recombination at their chromosomal site of origin to produce an HSR; (2) DMs might serve as vehicles for translocation of amplified DNA to new chromosomal locations; or (3) HSRs may arise in situ by amplification of DNA that never leaves its original position in a chromosome. Our findings add to previous indications that DMs can precede HSRs in the lives of tumor cells and that the creation of HSRs can be a form of translocation.

DMs apparently appeared prior to HSRs in many of the neuroblastoma cell lines we have examined and in COLO 320. In the neuroblastomas, amplified DNA (traced as N-myc) has been translocated from the normal position of N-myc on the short arm of chromosome 2 to new positions on at least eight other chromosomes. We have yet to find an instance where the amplified DNA resides at the normal chromosomal location of N-myc. Similarly, amplified c-myc in COLO 320 has been translocated from the normal location of human c-myc (8q24) to an X chromosome.

The current karyotype of COLO 320 must have arisen from an elaborate sequence of events which, to a first approximation, we can reconstruct as follows. (1) At some point during the genesis of the tumor, a domain of DNA that included c-myc began to amplify. A rearrangement also affected c-myc early in the course of events; the normal and rearranged versions of the gene then amplified in concert, eventually generating DMs that carry roughly equal portions of normal and rearranged c-myc. (2) COLO 320 cells now contain only one copy of chromosome 8 (C.C. Lin, pers. comm.). It is conceivable that the missing copy of chromosome 8 represents the original source of amplified DNA. (3) In cells containing translocations between autosomal and X chromosomes, the remaining normal X chromosome is usually inactive (late replicating) (Van Dyke et al. 1981). We were therefore surprised to find that both the normal X chromosome and the HSR chromosome in COLO 320 cells are active (early replicating) (M. Schwab et al.; C.C. Lin; both unpubl.). We presume that one copy of the X chromosome was lost early in the history of the tumor and that, as is often the case in leukemias of females (Levan and Mitelman 1978), it was the inactive X chromosome that was lost (COLO 320 cells originated from a female). The active X chromosome might then have duplicated by nondisjunction. (4) At some subsequent time, possibly after the cells had been established in culture, amplified DNA from the DMs inserted into the long arm of one of the two copies of active X chromosome to produce the HSR first described in the karyotype of COLO 320 cells (Semple et al. 1978). Further rearrangements, either additional insertions of amplified DNA from DMs or translocations from the long arm, extended the HSR to occupy virtually the entire long arm and produced in addition an HSR bearing c-myc on the short arm of the same X chromosome (Alitalo et al. 1983a). The HSRs appear to have been built mainly of the normal rather than the rearranged version of c-myc, suggesting that only portions of the amplified DNA in DMs recombine with chromosomes to engender HSRs.

N-myc: A new oncogene?

The homology with c-myc that permitted the recognition of N-myc, and the consistency with which N-myc is amplified and its expression enhanced in neuroblastoma cells, raise the possibility that N-myc is an authentic cellular oncogene. The family of human myc genes appears to be quite large: There are at least three genes in addition to N-myc that share partial homology with the prototypic c-myc (Dalla Favera et al. 1982b), and by using a molecular clone of v-myc as a hybridization probe, we have detected even further genetic loci that probably belong in the myc family (M. Schwab et al., unpubl.).

The evidence that cellular myc genes can contribute to tumorigenesis is for the moment circumstantial: The prototypic c-myc is affected by the characteristic chromosomal translocations found in Burkitt's lymphoma and mouse plasmacytomas (Klein 1983); c-myc has been found to be amplified in several forms of human tumors (see Table 1); N-myc is amplified with great consistency in human neuroblastomas (Table 2); insertion of retroviral DNA in the vicinity of chicken c-myc may be the initial event in the genesis of bursal lymphomas (Nusse et al., this volume); and c-myc can collaborate with other oncogenes in the tumorigenic transformation of primary embryonic cells (Land et al. 1983). The effects of chromosomal translocations on the expression of c-myc are presently in dispute. By contrast, insertion of retroviral DNA in the vicinity of chicken c-myc and the amplification of either c-myc or N-myc almost certainly enhance the expression of these genes. For example, N-myc is not amplified in the neuroblastoma cell line SK-N-SH and expression of the gene in these cells is negligible (M. Schwab et al., unpubl.), whereas expression of N-myc in other neuroblastoma cell lines and in tumors is enhanced roughly in accord with the extent of gene amplification.

A gene termed N-ras that is capable of transforming established lines of rodent cells in culture has been identified in the SK-N-SH line of neuroblastoma cells (Shimizu et al. 1983). Therefore, it is reasonable to wonder whether the activity of N-ras and the enhanced expression of N-myc might represent two collaborating genetic events in the genesis of neuroblastomas. At the moment, however, these two events have not been found in the same tumor or cell line: N-myc is not amplified in the SK-N-SH line, and N-ras activity has not been reported in any other sample of neuroblastoma.

The domain of amplified DNA in neuroblastoma cells is predictably large (Kanda et al. 1983) and may therefore contain genes other than N-myc that are important to tumorigenesis. But we see no reason for the moment to exclude the possibility that amplification of N-myc represents both a molecular marker for neuroblastoma and an important factor in the genesis of this tumor.

Acknowledgments

We are indebted to Drs. D. George, J. Trent, G. Brodeur, F. Gilbert, and C.C. Lin for collaborative work included in this summary, and to J. Marinos and J. LaBaer for assistance. This work was supported by grants from the National Cancer Institute and the American Cancer Society. M.S. is a Heisenberg fellow of Deutsche Forschungsgemeinschaft; K.A. was a fellow of the NIH Fogarty International Center.

References

Alitalo, K., M. Schwab, C.C. Lin, H.E. Varmus, and J.M. Bishop. 1983a. Homogeneously staining chromosomal regions contain amplified copies of an abundantly expressed cellular oncogene (c-myc) in malignant neuroendocrine cells from a human colon carcinoma. Proc. Natl. Acad. Sci. **80**: 1707.

Alitalo, K., G. Ramsay, J.M. Bishop, S. Ohlsson, W.W. Colby, J.P. McGrath, and A.D. Levinson. 1983b. Identification of nuclear proteins encoded by viral and cellular myc oncogenes. Nature **306**: 274.

Bishop, J.M. 1982. Retroviruses and cancer genes. Adv. Cancer Res. **37**: 1.

Brodeur, G.M., A.A. Green, F.A. Hayes, K.J. Williams, D.L. Williams, and A.A. Tsiatis. 1981. Cytogenetic features of human neuroblastomas and cell lines. Cancer Res. **41**: 4678.

Collins, S. and M. Groudine. 1982. Amplification of endogenous myc-related DNA sequences in a human myeloid leukaemia cell line. Nature **298**: 679.

———. 1983. Rearrangement and amplification of c-abl sequences in the human chronic myelogenous leukemia cell line K-562. Proc Natl. Acad. Sci. **80**: 4813.

Dalla Favera, R., F. Wong-Staal, and R.C. Gallo. 1982a. onc gene amplification in promyelocytic leukaemic cell lines HL-60 and primary leukaemic cells of the same patient. Nature **299**: 61.

Dalla Favera, R., E.P. Gelmann, S. Martinotti, G. Franchini, T.S. Papas, R.C. Gallo, and F. Wong-Staal. 1982b. Cloning and characterization of different human sequences related to the onc gene (v-myc) of avian myelocytomatosis virus (MC29). Proc. Natl. Acad. Sci. **79**: 6497.

Furth, M.E., L.J. Davis, B. Fleurdelys, and E.M. Scolnick. 1982. Monoclonal antibodies to the p21 products of the transforming gene of Harvey murine sarcoma virus and of the cellular ras gene family. J. Virol. **43**: 294.

George, D.L. and V.E. Powers. 1981. Cloning of DNA from double minutes of Y1 mouse adrenocortical tumor cells: Evidence for gene amplification. Cell **24**: 117.

Harper, M.E. and G.F. Saunders. 1981. Localization of single copy DNA sequences on G-banded human chromosomes by in situ hybridization. Chromosoma **83**: 431.

Kanda, N., R. Schreck, F. Alt, G. Bruns, D. Baltimore, and S. Latt. 1983. Isolation of amplified DNA sequences from IMR-32 human neuroblastoma cells: Facilitation by fluorescence-activated flow sorting of metaphase chromosomes. Proc. Natl. Acad. Sci. **80**: 4069.

Klein, G. 1983. Specific chromosomal translocations and the genesis of B-cell-derived tumors in mice and men. Cell **32**: 311.

Land, H., L.F. Parada, and R.A. Weinberg. 1983. Tumorigenic conversion of primary embryo fibroblasts requires at least two cooperating oncogenes. Nature **304**: 596.

Levan, G. and F. Mitelman. 1978. Absence of late-replicating X-chromosome in a female patient with acute myeloid leukemia and the 8;21 translocation. J. Natl. Cancer Inst. **62**: 273.

Quinn, L.A., G.E. Moore, R.T. Morgan, and L.K. Woods. 1979. Cell lines from human colon carcinoma with unusual cell products, double minutes, and homogeneously staining regions. *Cancer Res.* **39**: 4914.

Schimke, R.T., ed. 1982. *Gene amplification.* Cold Spring Harbor Laboratory, Cold Spring Harbor, New York.

Schimke, R.T., R.J. Kaufman, F.W. Alt, and R.F. Kellems. 1978. Gene amplification and drug resistance in cultured mammalian cells. *Science* **202**: 1051.

Schwab, M., K. Alitalo, H.E. Varmus, J.M. Bishop, and D. George. 1983a. A cellular oncogene (c-Ki-*ras*) is amplified, overexpressed, and located within karyotypic abnormalities in mouse adrenocortical tumour cells. *Nature* **303**: 497.

Schwab, M., K. Alitalo, K.-H. Klempnauer, H.E. Varmus, J.M. Bishop, F. Gilbert, G. Brodeur, M. Goldstein, and J. Trent. 1983b. Amplified DNA with limited homology to the *myc* cellular oncogene is shared by human neuroblastoma cell lines and a neuroblastoma tumor. *Nature* **305**: 245.

Oemple, T.V., L.A. Quinn, L.K. Woods, and G.E. Moore. 1978. Tumor and lymphoid cell lines from a patient with carcinoma of the colon for a cytotoxicity model. *Cancer Res.* **38**: 1345.

Shimizu, K., M. Goldfarb, M. Perucho, and M. Wigler. 1983. Isolation and preliminary characterization of the transforming gene of a human neuroblastoma cell line. *Proc. Natl. Acad. Sci.* **80**: 383.

Van Dyke, D.L., J.P. Abraham, K. Maeda, L. Weiss, and M. Poel. 1981. Multiple active X chromosomes in myelofibrosis with myeloid metaplasia. *Cancer Genet. Cytogenet.* **3**: 137.

Westaway, D., G. Payne, and H.E. Varmus. 1984. Deletions and base substitutions in provirally mutated c-*myc* alleles may contribute to the progression of B-cell tumors. *Proc. Natl. Acad. Sci.* (in press).

Consistent Chromosomal Rearrangements in Human Malignant Disease and Oncogene Location

J.D. Rowley

Department of Medicine, University of Chicago, Chicago, Illinois 60637

Consistent chromosomal abnormalities, particularly translocations, inversions, or deletions, are frequently observed in the malignant cells of a number of human cancers and leukemias. The most data relating particular chromosomal aberrations with specific types of leukemia are available for the myeloid leukemias.

In chronic myeloid leukemia (CML), a translocation involving chromosomes 9 and 22 (t[9;22][q34;q11]) is seen in over 90% of patients who have a Philadelphia (Ph^1 or 22q−) chromosome. About 4% of patients have a simple variant translocation that appears to involve chromosome 22 and some chromosome other than chromosome 9; an equal number have a more complex translocation that involves three or more chromosomes including 9, 22, and some other chromosome.

For the acute myeloid leukemias, certain structural aberrations are specifically (or relatively specifically) associated with particular morphologic subtypes. Thus, in the differentiation of the granulocytic lineage, a t(8;21)(q22;q22) is associated with myeloblastic leukemia in which some of the cells show minimal further maturation, whereas a t(15;17)(q22;q21) is seen only in promyelocytic leukemia. Monoblastic leukemia is associated with translocations or deletions of the long arm of chromosome 11. A recent observation is that in leukemia with some differentiation of both granulocytes and monocytes, and in which the marrow eosinophils have abnormal basophilic granules, an inversion of chromosome 16 (inv[16][p13q22]) or a deletion of chromosome 16 at q22 is a regular feature. We have now studied four patients with a t(6;9)(p23;q34) who show an excess of basophils in the bone marrow. This is of interest because an increase in basophils is a feature of CML, and the break in chromosome 9 appears to involve the same band in both types of leukemia.

Among the recent exciting developments in cancer research, none has been more remarkable than the cloning of the breakpoints in the t(8;14) in Burkitt's lymphoma and the t(9;22) in CML. The fact that proto-oncogenes are found at the breakpoints, e.g., c-myc in Burkitt's and c-abl in CML, only serves to emphasize the significance of chromosomal rearrangements in malignant cells. At present, 14 proto-oncogenes or transforming DNA sequences have been localized to human chromosomes and at least one-half have been located at chromosomal bands that are involved in translocations or deletions.

The study of the chromosomal pattern in the affected cells of a number of human tumors has been one of the most rapidly advancing areas in cancer research over the last 20 years. Major advances in our understanding of the specificity of some of the abnormalities have occurred in the last 13 years with the application of new chromosome-banding techniques. These techniques allow the identification of each human chromosome and of parts of chromosomes as well. The most significant early observation was the identification of the Philadelphia (Ph^1) chromosome in chronic myelogenous leukemia by Nowell and Hungerford (1960). The abnormality appeared to be a deletion of about one-half of the long arm of one G-group chromosome. Changes in modal chromosome number or morphology were detected in only 50% of patients with acute leukemia and there seemed to be little pattern to the observed aberrations. With the advent of chromosome-banding techniques in 1970, however, we could identify each chromosome, and an examination of leukemic cells now revealed a pattern of recurring abnormalities that could be associated with particular morphologic subtypes of acute leukemia. We have just entered the third and most exciting period, which will be devoted to an understanding of the consistent changes at the molecular level. This period has had an auspicious beginning with the observation that many of the chromosomal aberrations seen in leukemia and lymphoma involve structural aberrations of chromosomal segments that contain cellular proto-oncogenes.

Chromosomal Patterns in Acute Nonlymphocytic Leukemia (ANLL)

An analysis of chromosomal patterns, to be relevant to a malignant disease, must be based on a study of the karyotype of the tumor cells themselves. In the case of leukemia, the specimen is usually a bone marrow aspirate that is processed immediately or is cultured for 24–48 hours (Testa and Rowley 1981). The presence of at least two "pseudodiploid" or hyperdiploid cells or three hypodiploid cells, each showing the same abnormality, is considered evidence of an abnormal clone. All abnormalities discussed in this paper are clonal. In most instances, cells from unaffected tissues will have a normal karyotype, so the chromosomal abnormalities observed in the malignant cells represent somatic mutations in an otherwise normal individual.

In the following discussion, the chromosomes are

identified according accepted nomenclature (ISCN 1978). The total chromosomal number is indicated first, followed by the sex chromosomes, and then by the gains, losses, or rearrangements of the autosomes. A + sign or − sign before a number indicates a gain or loss, respectively, of a whole chromosome; a + or − after a number indicates a gain or loss of part of a chromosome. The letters "p" and "q" refer to the short and long arms of the chromosome, respectively. Translocations are identified by "t" followed by the chromosomes involved in the first set of brackets; the chromosome bands in which the breaks occurred are indicated in the second brackets. Uncertainty about the chromosome or band involved is signified by "?".

Common chromosomal gains and losses in ANLL

The most common chromosomal abnormalities seen in a variety of leukemias are summarized in Table 1. With regard to gains and losses of chromosomes, the most frequent extra chromosome is chromosome 8 and the one most frequently missing is 7. Moreover, each of these chromosomal changes occurs as the only change in at least one-half of the patients whose cells show this aberration. Many of the other changes are only seen in patients with more complex karyotypes, which suggests that they are secondary events.

Consistent structural aberrations in ANLL

One of the major advances in cytogenetics has been the correlation of particular chromosomal structural rearrangements, usually translocations, with specific subtypes of acute leukemia, four of which will be discussed in this section.

The 8;21 translocation in acute myeloblastic leukemia (AML-M2)

Kamada et al. (1968) recognized that a subgroup of ANLL patients may be characterized by an abnormality most likely representing a translocation between a C- and a G-group chromosome. The exact nature of this abnormality was resolved by Rowley (1973), who used the Q-banding technique to determine that it is a balanced translocation between chromosomes 8 and 21 (t[8;21][q22;q22]). The frequency with which this translocation occurs seems to vary from one laboratory to another, but it accounted for 10% (25/249) of the abnormal cases recently reviewed by Rowley and Testa (1982). In this review, the t(8;21) was found to be the most frequent abnormality in children with ANLL, being reported in 17% (10/60) of karyotypically abnormal cases. The abnormality appeared to be restricted patients with a diagnosis of M2 (acute myeloblastic leukemia with maturation) according to the French-American-British (FAB) classification (Bennett et al. 1976). At the 2nd International Workshop on Chromosomes in Leukemia (1980), all 43 cases with a t(8;21) and adequate bone marrow material available for cytological review had a diagnosis of M2. However in the 4th Workshop (1984), 3 of 44 t(8;21) patients appeared to have acute myelomonocytic leukemia (M4).

The 15;17 translocation and acute promyelocytic leukemia (APL)

A structural rearrangement involving chromosomes 15 and 17 in APL was first recognized by Rowley et al. (1977). Of the 80 patients with APL who were reviewed at the 2nd International Workshop on Chromosomes in Leukemia (1980), 33 (41%) had a t(15;17) alone (23 cases) or with other abnormalities, 7 had other types of chromosomal changes, and 40 had a normal karyotype. The data from our series at the University of Chicago is somewhat different in that every one of the 27 patients with APL de novo whom we have studied has had a t(15;17) (Larson et al. 1984). Various technical factors involved in processing samples are clearly an important factor leading to these apparent discrepancies. The rearrangement was not found in patients with any other type of leukemia or other solid tumor; moreover, it has not been reported as a constitutional abnormality. There is controversy over the exact breakpoints in both chromosomes 15 and 17. We recently have been successful in obtaining longer chromosomes, and the breakpoints appear to be 15q22 and 17q21.1 (Larson et al. 1984).

Table 1 Common Chromosome Changes in Leukemia

Type	Gains	Losses	Rearrangements
CML			
chronic phase	—	—	t(9;22)
blast crisis	+8, +Ph[1]	rare; −7	t(9;22), i(17q)
ANLL			
AML-M2	+8	−7; less −5	t(8;21)
APL	—	—	t(15;17)
AMMoL	+8	−7	inv(16) or del(16q)
AMoL	—	—	t(11q) or del(11q)
ALL			
Null	+21; +6	rare; −9	t(9;22)
B cell	—	—	t(8;14), t(2;8), t(8;22)
T cell	—	—	—

Structural alterations of 11q in acute monocytic leukemia (M5)

In addition to the consistent translocations just discussed, Berger et al. (1980) recently presented 10 cases of acute monocytic leukemia (AMoL-M5) that had an unexpectedly high incidence of rearrangements of the long arm of chromosome 11. More recently, they reported on 34 patients, 24 of whom had type-a or poorly differentiated and 10 of whom had type-b or well-differentiated monocytic leukemia (Berger et al. 1982). Thirteen of the 34 appeared to have a normal karyotype, nine had various abnormalities, and twelve had aberrations involving 11q, thus confirming their initial observation. Abnormalities of 11q occurred most frequently in children with monoblastic leukemia (type a) (6/8); adults with monoblastic leukemia had the next highest incidence (5/16); the incidence in monocytic (type b) leukemia was low, namely one of three children and zero of seven adults.

Aberrations of 11q differ from the t(8;21) and t(15;17) in three ways. First, the breakpoint in 11q usually involves band 11q23–24 but can also occur in 11q13–14; in Berger's series, 11q23–24 was affected in nine patients and 11q13–14 in three others. Second, the other chromosome involved in the translocation is variable, although 9p and 19 appear to be affected more often than others. Finally, 11q aberrations have been reported in patients with acute leukemia other than AMoL-M5. In a series of children reported by Kaneko et al. (1982), a translocation involving 11q was seen in a patient with AML-M2, although the cytochemical reaction of the leukemic cells was of the monocytic type. On review of these cases, they may be reclassified as M5. On the other hand, it may be that the chromosomal analyses have revealed a spectrum of morphologic features in AMoL not heretofore suspected.

Inv(16) in acute myelomonocytic leukemia (M4)

We have recently identified a new chromosomal abnormality that appears to be restricted to one subtype of ANLL. The abnormality is an inversion of chromosome 16 that has been identified only in acute myelomonocytic leukemia (AMMoL) (Le Beau et al. 1983). The patient population from which we have identified those with an abnormal chromosome 16 is summarized in Table 2. It is remarkable that approximately 20% of our patients with M4 leukemia have this aberration, which is just being identified. This situation has occurred, in large part, because the aberration is subtle and it is easily overlooked in contracted chromosomes with indistinct bands. It is our interpretation that a break has occurred in the short arm of chromosome 16 (band p13) and in the long arm (band q22) with inversion of the intervening segment. This results in a very metacentric chromosome.

The chromosomal abnormality is associated with unusual morphology of the eosinophils that appear to be immature with a mixture of eosinophilic and basophilic-staining granules in their cytoplasm. The basophilic granules are larger, more irregular, and more numerous than those occasionally seen in immature eosinophils. Among the first 11 patients with this syndrome, the eosinophil granules were periodic acid Schiff-positive in eight who were tested and the naphthol-ASD-chloracetate esterase was positive in all seven who were tested. In our experience, these reactions are negative in normal eosinophil granules. An earlier report also noted abnormalities of chromosome 16 that were associated with an excess of marrow eosinophils (Arthur and Bloomfield 1983).

Translocations in Lymphoid Neoplasms

The data presented here were selected from a large amount of information available on the chromosomal pattern in a number of lymphoid neoplasms (Rowley and Fukuhara 1980). They were selected because they provide the background for illustrating the next step in our understanding of the role of consistent chromosomal changes in malignant transformation. This section will review the consistent translocations seen in Burkitt's lymphoma and in some patients with B-cell ALL.

Consistent translocations in Burkitt's lymphoma and B-cell acute lymphoblastic leukemia (ALL)

Manolov and Manolova (1972) identified a consistent abnormality in the cells of five of six fresh Burkitt's lymphomas and in seven of nine cultured cell lines. They observed an additional band at the end of the long arm of one chromosome 14 (14q+). Zech et al. (1976) first observed that in all metaphase cells of adequate quality, the end of one chromosome 8 was consistently absent. They suggested that the missing part of chromosome 8 was translocated to chromosome 14, t(8;14)(q24;q32). The t(8;14) has also been observed in nonendemic Burkitt's tumors from America, Europe, and Japan (for review, see Mitelman 1981). Thus, there is no doubt that the t(8;14) is a highly characteristic chromosomal anomaly

Table 2 Incidence of Inv(16)—University of Chicago

Condition	Number
Patients, ANLL de novo	174
Patients, AMMoL-M4	60
M4 patients, inv(16)	14 (23%)[a]
typical abnormal eosinophils	11
very low percentage of abnormal eosinophils	1
questionably abnormal eosinophils	2

[a]Two also have del(16q).

in Burkitt's tumors; it has also been observed in some other lymphoid malignant diseases. The t(8;14) was identified in Burkitt's tumors that lacked any markers positive for Epstein-Barr virus (EBV) as well as in EBV-positive tumors.

As additional Burkitt's tumors were examined, it became apparent that there were at least two other related translocations that could occur. All three translocations involved chromosome 8 with a break in the same band, 8q24. One variant translocation involved chromosome 2 with a break in the short arm(t[2;8][p13;q24]) and one involved chromosome 22 with a break in the long arm in the same band affected in CML (t[8;22][q24;q11]). These same translocations have been seen in some patients with B-cell ALL, indicating the relatedness of Burkitt's lymphoma and B-cell ALL (Mitelman 1981). Complex, three-way translocations have also been observed affecting the t(8;14). We recently studied a patient with B-cell ALL who had a complex translocation (Kaneko et al. 1982). In the leukemic cells, most of the long arm of chromosome 5 was translocated to chromosome 8 and the end of chromosome 8 was translocated to chromosome 14, producing the typical 14q+ marker chromosome; presumably the end of chromosome 14 was translocated to chromosome 5.

Defining the critical recombinant chromosome

It is now apparent that the sites of consistent translocations pinpoint chromosomal segments that contain genes critically involved in malignant transformation. Isolation and analysis of these segments of DNA have high scientific priority. The evidence for Burkitt's lymphoma is exciting and clearly points the way to future research in this area. The loci for the immunoglobulin genes are on the three chromosomes other than chromosome 8, involved in translocations in Burkitt's lymphoma. Thus, the locus for the heavy-chain complex is on chromosome 14, that for κ is on chromosome 2, and that for λ is on chromosome 22. Moreover, with the use of chromosomal hybridization in situ, the κ light-chain genes have been mapped to the short arm of chromosome 2 (band 2p12–13), the heavy-chain gene has been mapped to 14q32, and the λ light-chain gene has been mapped to 22q11 (for review, see Rowley 1982).

An even more direct association between translocation types and gene function has been reported by Lenoir et al. (1982). They analyzed the type of immunoglobulin produced in either Burkitt's tumor cell lines or in fresh tumor cells and correlated this information with the karyotype of the tumors. All three lines with a t(2;8) expressed κ light chains and all five cell lines with a t(8;22) expressed λ light chains. For 17 cell lines with t(8;14), 9 were κ and 8 were λ producers.

There are two recombinant chromosomes in each translocation, and it would appear useful to determine which is the critical recombinant (Rowley 1982). Each of the three common translocations in myeloid leukemia—9;22, 8;21, and 15;17—also occurs in a variant form in a limited number of patients, and one can use these to determine whether one recombinant chromo-

some is constant in these variant forms. Based on these data, the critical event leading to malignant transformation in these types of myeloid leukemia is related to the juxtaposition of 9q to 22q in CML, that of 21q to 8q in AML, and that of the end of 17q to 15q in APL.

Chromosomal Location of Proto-oncogenes

One of the most exciting revelations in the past year has involved the cellular oncogenes and their chromosomal location. Much of the excitement derives from the observation that many oncogenes are located in the bands that are involved in consistent translocations (Fig. 1). The specific rearrangement of the *c-myc* gene and the immunoglobulin loci is discussed by others in this volume and will not be covered in this review. The *c-mos* gene is located on band 8q22 (Neel et al. 1982); what its relationship is to the t(8;21) in AML is currently unknown. The Abelson oncogene has been shown to translocate to the Ph¹ chromosome in the t(9;22) in CML (De Klein et al. 1982). This is an important observation from the genetic viewpoint because this is the first gene known to be on chromosome 9 that has been shown to translocate to chromosome 22. This establishes the fact that the translocation is reciprocal.

Some known oncogenes have not been implicated in structural rearrangements. Thus, it was assumed for some time that *c-fes*, known to be on chromosome 15, would be involved in the t(15;17) in APL. Such is not the case; first, from work of Sheer et al. (1983), we know that *c-fes* is not on the 15q+ chromosome. Moreover, *c-fes* has been localized to the end of chromosome 15 (Harper et al. 1983) and thus is some distance from the breakpoint.

Of particular interest is *c-Ha-ras*, which is on 11p13 (Jhanwar et al. 1983); a deletion of this region as a constitutional abnormality is associated with aniridia and a predisposition to Wilms' tumor (Riccardi et al. 1978). Moreover, we have described a patient with a normal karyotype whose Wilms' tumor cells had a deletion of 11p13 (Kaneko et al. 1981). On the other hand, several patients with Wilms' tumor and a constitutional deletion of 11p are heterozygous for restriction enzyme sites for the *c-Ha-ras*. This indicates that the gene is outside of the deleted segment of 11p. Thus, in a number of leukemias, lymphomas, or cancers, chromosomal regions previously defined by cytogeneticists as sites of consistent rearrangements are found to be the sites of proto-oncogenes.

The challenge for the future in the myeloid leukemias is first to find a way to isolate the DNA from the breakpoints, then to identify the genes involved, and finally to determine the alterations in gene function that are related to the translocations or deletions. Unless we are very lucky, this task will be more difficult in the myeloid leukemias than in Burkitt's lymphoma for two reasons. We do not have suitable cell lines available to provide a continuing source of cells for DNA analysis. There are, for example, no cell lines with a t(15;17) or a t(8;21). Those from patients with CML generally have a very rearranged

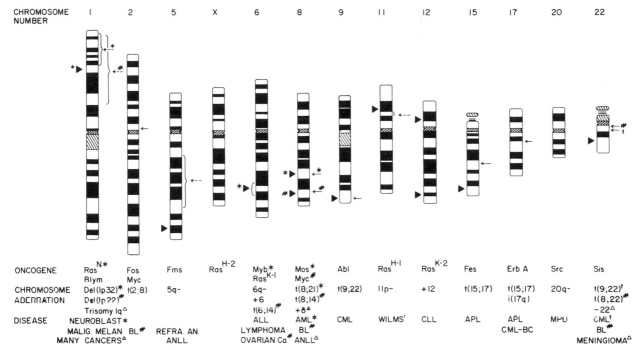

Figure 1 Diagram of chromosomes containing known cellular oncogenes; the number is above each chromosome, and the oncogenes, karyotypic aberrations, and neoplastic diseases associated with these aberrations are indicated below the chromosomes. The arrowhead (▶) to the left of each chromosome indicates the band carrying the cellular oncogene; the arrow to the right of a chromosome identifies specific bands involved in consistent translocations (←) or deletions (⟵) observed in patients having the disorders listed. Under chromosome 1, *Blym* has been localized to 1p32 (*▶); the deletions distal to 1p32 and 1p22 are associated with neuroblastoma or malignant melanoma, respectively. For chromosome 6, *c-myb* has been localized to 6q22-24 (*▶). The t(6;14) is found in ovarian cancer. Under chromosome 8, * indicates the *c-mos* and the t(8;21) in AML-M2 and # indicates *c-myc* and t(2;8), t(8;14), or t(8;22) in Burkitt lymphoma (BL). In chromosome 12, the *c-ras*$^{K-2}$ shows two regions of homology with in situ hybridization. (Refra. an.) Refractory anemia; (CLL) chronic lymphocytic leukemia; (MPD) myeloproliferative disorders; (p) short arm of the chromosome; (q) long arm of the chromosome.

karyotype. The second problem is the lack of information regarding which genes in myeloid cells will be analogous to the immunoglobulin genes in B-cell tumors. It may be that the *c-onc*, such as *c-mos* or *c-abl* will be at the breakpoint, and cloned DNA from these genes can be used to isolate the breakpoint. If this is not the case, then the search for the DNA from each breakpoint may be a very tedious one. As is clear from the harvest of information regarding *c-myc* in B-cell tumors, the reward is worth the search.

Acknowledgments

This work was supported in part by Public Health Service grants CA 16910, CA 19266, and CA 25568, awarded by the National Cancer Institute, Department of Health and Human Services, and by the Department of Energy, contract number DE-AC02-80EV10360.

References

Arthur, D.C. and C.D. Bloomfield. 1983. Partial deletion of the long arm of chromosome 16 and bone marrow eosinophilia in acute nonlymphocytic leukemia: A new association. *Blood* **61**: 994.

Bennett, J.M., D. Catovsky, M.-T. Daniel, G. Flandrin, D.A.G. Galton, H.R. Gralnick, and C. Sultan. 1976. Proposals for the classification of the acute leukemias. French-American-British (FAB) co-operative group. *Br. J. Haematol.* **33**: 451.

Berger, R., A. Bernheim, H.J. Weh, M.-T. Daniel, and G. Flandrin. 1980. Cytogenetic studies on acute monocytic leukemia. *Leuk. Res.* **4**: 119.

Berger, R., A. Bernheim, F. Sigaux, M.-T. Daniel, F. Valensi, and G. Flandrin. 1982. Acute monocytic leukemia chromosome studies. *Leuk. Res.* **6**: 17.

De Klein, A., A.G. van Kessel, G. Grosveld, C.R. Bartram, A. Hagemeijer, D. Bootsma, N.K. Spurr, N. Heisterkamp, J. Groffen, and J.R. Stephenson. 1982. A cellular oncogene is translocated to the Philadelphia chromosome in chronic myelocytic leukemia. *Nature* **300**: 765.

Fourth International Workshop on Chromosomes in Leukemia. 1984. *Cancer Genet. Cytogenet.* **11**: 249.

Harper, M.E., G. Franchini, J. Love, M.I. Simon, R.C. Gallo, and F. Wong-Staal. 1983. Chromosomal sublocalization of human c-myb and c-fes cellular *onc* genes. *Nature* **304**: 169.

International System for Human Cytogenetic Nomenclature. 1978. *Cytogenet. Cell Genet.* **21**: 309.

Jhanwar, S.C., B.G. Neel, W.S. Hayward, and R.S.K. Chaganti. 1983. Localization of c-ras oncogene family on human germline chromosomes. *Proc. Natl. Acad. Sci.* **80**: 4794.

Kamada, N., K. Okada, T. Ito, T. Nakatsui, and H. Uchino. 1968. Chromosome 21-22 and neutrophil alkaline phosphatase in leukemia. *Lancet* I: 364.

Kaneko, Y., M.C. Egues, and J.D. Rowley. 1981. Interstitial

deletion of 11p limited to Wilms' tumor cells in a patient without aniridia. *Cancer Res.* **41:** 4577.

Kaneko, Y., J.D. Rowley, H.S. Maurer, D. Variakojio, and J.W. Moohr. 1982. Chromosome pattern in childhood acute non-lymphocytic leukemia (ANLL). *Blood* **60:** 389.

Kaneko, Y., J.D. Rowley, D. Variakojis, R.R. Chilcote, I. Check, and M. Sakurai. 1982. Correlation of karyotype with clinical features in acute lymphoblastic leukemia (ALL). *Cancer Res.* **42:** 2918.

Larson, R.A., K. Kondo, J.W. Vardiman, A.E. Butler, H.M. Golomb, and J.D. Rowley. 1984. Every patient with acute pro-myelocytic leukemia may have 15;17 translocation. *Am. J. Med.* (in press).

Le Beau, M.M., R.A. Larson, M.A. Bitter, J.W. Vardiman, H.M. Golomb, and J.D. Rowley. 1983. Association of an inversion of chromosome 16 with abnormal marrow eosinophils in acute myelomonocytic leukemia: A unique cytogenetic-clinicopathological association. *New Engl. J. Med.* **309:** 630.

Lenoir, G.M., J.L. Preud'homme, A. Bernheim, and R. Berger. 1982. Correlation between immunoglobulin light chain expression and variant translocation in Burkitt's lymphoma. *Nature* **298:** 474.

Manolov, G. and Y. Manolova. 1972. Marker band in one chromosome 14 from Burkitt lymphomas. *Nature* **237:** 33.

Mitelman, F. 1981. Marker chromosome 14q + in human cancer and leukemia. *Adv. Cancer Res.* **34:** 141.

Neel, B.G., S.C. Jhanwar, R.S.K. Chaganti, and W.S. Haywood. 1982. Two human c-onc genes are located on the long arm of chromosome 8. *Proc. Natl. Acad. Sci.* **79:** 7842.

Nowell, P.C. and D.A. Hungerford. 1960. A minute chromosome in human granulocytic leukemia. *Science* **132:** 1497.

Riccardi, V.M., E. Sujansky, A.C. Smith, and U. Francke. 1978.

Chromosomal imbalance in the aniridia-Wilms' tumor association: 11p interstitial deletion. *Pediatrics* **61:** 604,

Rowley, J.D. 1973. Identification of a translocation with quin-acrine fluorescence in a patient with acute leukemia. *Ann. Genet.* **16:** 109.

———. 1982. Identification of the chromosome regions involved in human hematologic malignant disease. *Science* **216:** 749.

Rowley, J.D. and S. Fukuhara. 1980. Chromosome studies in non-Hodgkin lymphomas. *Semin. Oncol.* **7:** 255.

Rowley, J.D. and J.R. Testa. 1982. Chromosome abnormalities in malignant hematologic diseases. *Adv. Cancer Res.* **36:** 103.

Rowley, J.D., H.M. Golomb, J. Vardiman, S. Fukuhara, C. Dougherty, and D. Potter. 1977. Further evidence for a non-random chromosomal abnormality in acute promyelocytic leukemia. *Int. J. Cancer* **20:** 869.

Second International Workshop on Chromosomes in Leukemia. 1980. *Cancer Genet. Cytogenet.* **2:** 89.

Sheer, D., L.R. Hiorns, K.F. Stanley, P.N. Goodfellow, D.M. Swallow, S. Povey, N. Heisterkamp, J. Groffen, J.R. Stephenson, and E. Solomon. 1983. Genetic analysis of the 15;17 chromosome translocation associated with acute pro-myelocytic leukemia. *Proc. Natl. Acad. Sci.* **80:** 5007.

Testa, J.R. and J.D. Rowley. 1981. Chromosomes in leukemia and lymphoma with special emphasis on methodology. In *The leukemic cell* (ed. D. Catovsky), p. 184. Churchill-Livingstone, Edinburgh.

Zech, L., U. Haglund, K. Nilsson, and G. Klein. 1976. Characteristic chromosomal abnormalities in biopsies and lymphoid-cell lines from patients with Burkitt and non-Burkitt lymphomas. *Int. J. Cancer* **17:** 47.

myc Oncogene Activation by Chromosomal Translocation

M.D. Cole, S.P. Piccoli, E.J. Keath, P. Caimi, and A. Kelekar
E.A. Doisy Department of Biochemistry, Saint Louis University School of Medicine, St. Louis, Missouri 63104

Specific chromosomal translocations are a consistent feature of many malignant cells, especially cells of hematopoietic origin (Rowley 1982). One common feature of several well-characterized translocations is that they involve the chromosomes that contain the immunoglobulin genes. This is particularly striking for mouse plasmacytomas (Ohno et al. 1979) and human Burkitt's lymphomas (Manolov and Manolova 1972). In both cases, there is a common breakpoint in one chromosome (chromosome 15 in the mouse and chromosome 8 in humans) and a segment is translocated to one of the immunoglobulin gene-containing chromosomes, 12 (heavy) and 6 (κ) in the mouse and 14 (heavy) and 2 (κ) or 22 (λ) in humans (for review, see Klein 1983). It was suggested that these chromosomal aberrations may involve a cellular transformation-related gene (Klein 1981).

Many recent studies have shown that the breakpoint for the chromosomal translocations in both plasmacytomas and Burkitt's lymphomas occurs at a cellular oncogene termed c-myc (Adams et al. 1982; Crews et al. 1982; Shen-Ong et al. 1982; Taub et al. 1982; Erikson et al. 1983; Marcu et al. 1983). The myc oncogene was first identified as the transforming sequence from the acute oncogenic retrovirus MC29 (Roussel et al. 1979). The viral oncogene was subsequently found to have a cellular counterpart (Robins et al. 1982; Vennstron et al. 1982) that is highly conserved in evolution (Sheiness and Bishop 1979) and actively expressed in many normal cells (Gonda et al. 1982). The first suggestion that the cellular myc gene could be involved in oncogenesis came from studies of avian leukosis virus-induced B-cell lymphomas where viral integration apparently enhances the expression of the c-myc gene 10–20-fold (Hayward et al. 1981). Amplified c-myc genes and enhanced c-myc expression have also been found in a human promyelocytic leukemia (Collins and Groudine 1982; Dalla-Favera et al. 1982) and an endocrine-derived carcinoma (Alitalo et al. 1983).

We have characterized the structure of the chromosomal translocation breakpoint at c-myc in several plasmacytomas. Figure 1 shows a summary diagram of the most common configuration of genes found in mouse plasmacytomas, which will be discussed in more detail below. It is important to understand how the chromosomal translocation affects expression of the c-myc gene, especially what influence the Ig gene has on transcription of the shorter c-myc RNA found in tumors (Shen-Ong et al. 1982). Furthermore, it is essential to compare the level of c-myc expression in normal versus transformed cells.

Materials and Methods

DNA and RNA isolation, gel electrophoresis, and Southern and Northern blot analysis were described previously (Shen-Ong et al. 1982). DNA sequencing was performed according to Maxam and Gilbert (1980) using either 5' or 3' end-labeled fragments. Cytoplasmic dot blots were prepared according to White and Bancroft (1982).

Results and Discussion

Structure of the translocation breakpoint

Analysis of the c-myc oncogene locus in mouse plasmacytomas shows a consistent pattern of DNA rearrangements in nearly all tumor lines. Restriction enzyme mapping, Southern blot analysis, and molecular cloning have been used to show that the rearrangements are due to a chromosomal translocation that joins the immunoglobulin heavy-chain locus (chromosome 12) to the c-myc gene (chromosome 15) in most tumor lines that have been characterized (Fig. 1) (Adams et al. 1982; Crews et al. 1982; Shen-Ong et al. 1982; Marcu et al. 1983). A specific immunoglobulin gene (C_α) is involved in the majority of BALB/c plasmacytomas, whereas in NZB tumors the sequences joined to myc have not been defined (Harris et al. 1982).

Figure 1 illustrates that c-myc and C_α are always in opposite transcriptional orientation, but the distance between the two genes can be quite variable, from 1.5 kb in MOPC-46B to 4 kb in MOPC-315. Conversely, the breakpoint within c-myc is almost always within a segment of approximately 1 kb between HindIII and BamHI sites. In one tumor line, TEPC-15, the breakpoint within c-myc falls less than 0.3 kb to the right of the BamHI site.

The chromosomal breakpoint near the C_α gene is almost invariably within a region on the 5' side of the gene that is involved in "switching" between different heavy-chain isotypes (Shen-Ong et al. 1982). This region (S_α) contains a tandem array of small DNA sequences that apparently are recognized by the enzymes involved in the switch (Davis et al. 1980). Presumably the c-myc translocation occurs as the result of an "abortive" switching event, and it was of great interest to determine if some sequence within the c-myc gene shared homology with the "switch" region or if some other common sequence was recognized. Therefore, we have determined the DNA sequence at the translocation breakpoint in two different plasmacytoma lines (MOPC-315 and

227

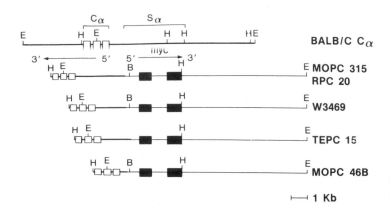

BALB/C C$_\alpha$

MOPC 315
RPC 20

W3469

TEPC 15

MOPC 46B

├──┤ 1 Kb

Figure 1 Summary diagram of the organization of the *c-myc* and C$_\alpha$ genes after chromosomal translocation in the five different plasmacytoma lines. (Reprinted, with permission, from Shen-Ong et al. 1982.)

MOPC-104E) and compared the sequences with other breakpoints that have been determined.

The DNA sequences within the *c-myc* gene that occur in six different plasmacytomas are shown in Figure 2, along with the consensus sequence for the C$_\alpha$ switch region (Davis et al. 1980). Examination of the sequences clearly shows that there is no homology between any of the breakpoints and the S$_\alpha$ sequence. Furthermore, there is no sequence homology among the various *c-myc* breakpoints. Thus, we can conclude that there is no specific DNA sequence within *c-myc* that is recognized as a target for the abortive switching events. Presumably, DNA rearrangements that involve the joining of non-immunoglobulin sequences to the switch region occur at random at unknown frequency in immunoglobulin-producing cells and those that occur near *c-myc* promote neoplastic transformation and hence appear in the resultant tumor.

Although the sequences at the translocation breakpoint share no apparent homology, they are localized within a very small region of the *c-myc* gene. This initially was evident from restriction enzyme digests of many plasmacytoma DNAs in which the DNA rearrangements were found almost invariably to occur within a 1.4-kb *Hind*III–*Bam*HI segment. This region recently has been

shown to encompass the first exon and the first intron of the *c-myc* gene (Stanton et al. 1983).

Figure 3 shows the location of seven breakpoints within the *c-myc* sequence. All of the breakpoints fall within a 0.7-kb region and four are clustered within 250 bp. Clearly there is a preferred region of the *c-myc* gene that is involved in the majority of chromosomal translocations in mouse plasmacytomas. Furthermore, the first *c-myc* intron is also involved in several Burkitt's lymphoma translocations (Dalla-Favera et al. 1983). The fact that the first exon is displaced or disrupted in all plasmacytomas and many Burkitt's lymphomas suggests that there is some selection for breakpoints in this region. One possibility is that the configuration of the chromatin in the first intron makes it prone to chromosomal breaks, such as the presence of a DNase I hypersensitive site. A second possibility is that removal of the first exon alters *myc* expression in a way that promotes tumor transformation, although the first exon does not code for any of the *myc* protein (Stanton et al. 1983). Many additional studies will be required to resolve these questions.

Altered *c-myc* transcripts in plasmacytomas

Chromosomal translocation induces the synthesis of an altered *c-myc* RNA that is 0.4 kb shorter than the normal

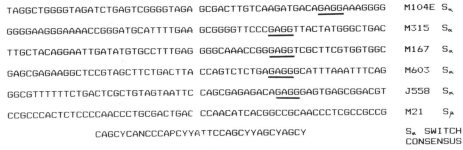

TAGGCTGGGGTAGATCTGAGTCGGGGTAGA GCGACTTGTCAAGATGACAGAGGAAAGGGG   M104E S$_\alpha$

GGGGAAGGGAAAACCGGGATGCATTTTGAA GCGGGGTTCCCGAGGTTACTATGGGCTGAC   M315 S$_\alpha$

TTGCTACAGGAATTGATATGTGCCTTTGAG GGGCAAACCGGGAGGTCGCTTCGTGGTGGC   M167 S$_\alpha$

GAGCGAGAAGGCTCCGTAGCTTCTGACTTA CCAGTCTCTGAGAGGGCATTTAAATTTCAG   M603 S$_\alpha$

GGCGTTTTTTCTGACTCGCTGTAGTAATTC CAGCGAGAGACAGAGGGAGTGAGCGGACGT   J558 S$_\alpha$

CCGCCCACTCTCCCCAACCCTGCGACTGAC CCAACATCACGGCCGCAACCCTCGCCGCCG   M21 S$_\mu$

CAGCYCANCCCAPCYYATTCCAGCYYAGCYAGCY   S$_\alpha$ SWITCH CONSENSUS

Figure 2 Translocation breakpoints from six plasmacytoma lines. The sequence shown is from *c-myc* in each case with the gap at the position where C$_\alpha$ sequences become joined to *c-myc*. The sequences to the right of the gap remain with the *c-myc* gene whereas those to the left are displaced by C$_\alpha$. The breakpoint for MOPC-104E was determined from the sequence of the translocation reciprocal (S.P. Piccoli et al., in prep.). A tetranucleotide (GAGG) that is conserved in all C$_\alpha$-*c-myc* translocations is underlined. The breakpoints other than those from MOPC-315 and MOPC-104E were taken from Calame et al. (1982), Adams et al. (1983), and Dunnick et al. (1983).

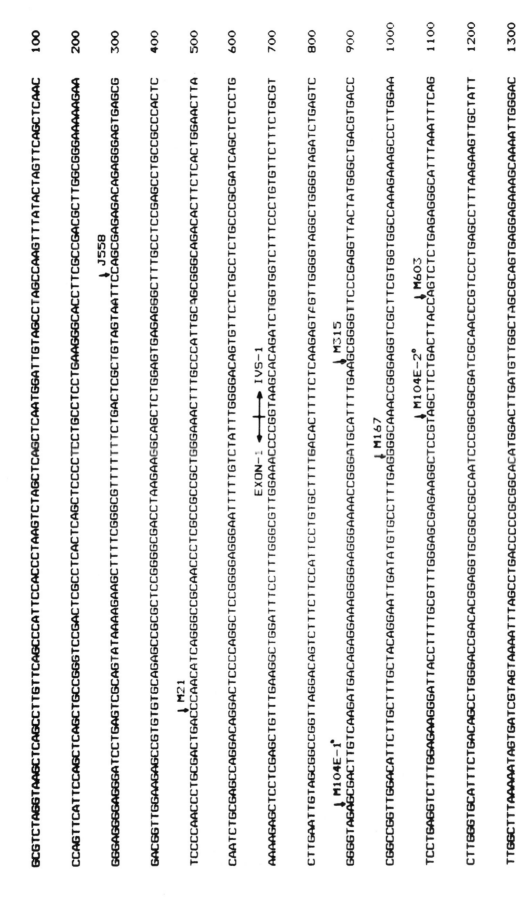

Figure 3 Sequence of the first *c-myc* exon and first intron showing the positions of several breakpoints. The exon 1–intron 1 boundary was taken from Stanton et al. (1983). The breakpoint for the initial C_α-*c-myc* translocation in MOPC-104E is labeled M104E-1°. The breakpoint for the secondary deletion described in Fig. 6 is labeled M104E-2°.

transcript (Shen-Ong et al. 1982). The size of the tumor-specific RNA (2.0–2.1 kb) is the same for all tumor lines, regardless of the distance between C_α and *c-myc*. This suggests that the S_α sequences to the left of the breakpoint do not provide the promoter for the tumor-specific RNA but that the RNA initiates to the right of the breakpoint in *c-myc* sequences that are conserved in all translocated genes. The shorter RNA is the result of displacement of an exon from the *c-myc* gene by the chromosomal translocation (Adams et al. 1983; Stanton et al. 1983), and the tumor-specific RNA initiates in what is presumably the first *myc* intron. We have been interested in determining what sequences within the *c-myc* intron provide the promoter for the tumor-specific RNA and what influence, if any, the C_α gene has on transcription of the *c-myc* oncogene.

RNA transcripts from the *c-myc* intron

Northern blots of normal and tumor RNAs were probed with different segments of the *c-myc* intron to determine which sequences were present in the tumor-specific RNA. Figure 4 shows the pattern of hybridization with two probes that are near the *Bam*HI site. The *Xba*I–*Sst*I fragment hybridizes consistently to two species of RNA of 2.0 kb and 2.4 kb that comigrate with the *c-myc* RNAs detected with probes from the gene coding regions (Shen-Ong et al. 1982). These RNAs were not detected in MOPC-460, which has no break in the *myc* gene, nor in the TEPC-15 where the breakpoint occurs to the right of the *Bam*HI site. The same two species of RNA were evident in MOPC-46B with shorter exposures, although they are obscured in Figure 4 by a broad smear of hybridization that will be discussed in more detail below. A second probe from this region (*Bam*HI–*Sst*I) hybridizes to the same two species of RNA, plus additional

RNAs of both higher and lower molecular weight. These results suggest that the tumor-specific RNAs initiate between *Xba*I and *Sst*I, since this region is common to all of the tumor lines that contain the 2.0-kb and 2.4-kb *c-myc* RNAs.

Previous studies have shown that both 2.0-kb and 2.4-kb *myc* RNAs are produced in plasmacytomas (Adams et al. 1982; Shen-Ong et al. 1982; Marcu et al. 1983). The 2.4-kb species comigrates with the 2.4-kb normal *myc* mRNA but is apparently not the same. As demonstrated above, the 2.4-kb plasmacytoma RNA hybridizes to the *myc* intron whereas the normal *myc* RNA does not. Furthermore, probes specific for the *myc* exon that is displaced by translocation do not detect normal *myc* RNA in most tumor lines (Stanton et al. 1983). Thus, although plasmacytomas contain both normal and translocated *myc* alleles, the normal gene is not expressed at a detectable level. This observation may indicate that expression of the normal *c-myc* gene is shut off in plasma cells or the target cells from which plasmacytomas arise.

Levels of *myc* expression

Several studies have suggested that chromosomal translocation leads to a 10–20-fold increase in the level of *myc* RNA in the cell (Erikson et al. 1983; Marcu et al. 1983; Mushinski et al. 1983). In murine plasmacytomas, nearly all tumor lines have been found to have similar amounts of *myc* RNA, but how this relates to the level in normal cells is still unknown. Earlier studies with total cellular poly(A)-containing RNA suggested that there was no difference in *c-myc* RNA levels in normal and tumor cells (Shen-Ong et al. 1982). However, there was no attempt to quantitate *myc* expression with respect to the number of transcripts per cell. To compare *myc* RNA levels in equivalent number of cells, the cytoplasmic dot

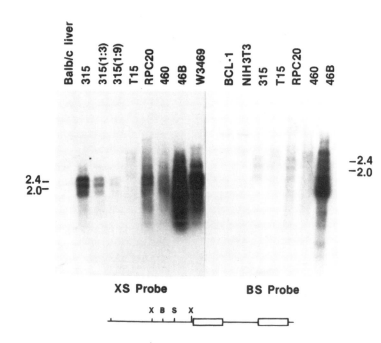

Figure 4 Northern blot hybridization of RNAs transcribed from the *c-myc* intron. Poly(A)-containing RNAs (7 µg, except for the MOPC-315 dilutions) from each cell type were electrophoresed on formaldehyde-agarose gels and transferred to nitrocellulose. The fragments indicated were isolated from pM104H (Shen-Ong et al. 1982), nick-translated, and hybridized to the filters.

blot technique was used. Dot blots from both plasmacytoma and normal splenic B cells were hybridized with a *c-myc* probe. Approximately 25-fold more *myc* RNA was found in plasmacytoma cells than in B cells (Fig. 5). This difference may reflect enhanced transcription of *c-myc* due to the chromosomal translocation. However, it is important to point out that plasmacytomas are rapidly growing and pseudotetraploid, whereas B cells are basically nondividing and diploid. It will be of interest to compare the RNA levels in mitogen-stimulated B cells, especially if the samples can be enriched for actively dividing cells.

Is there an Ig-associated enhancer of *c-myc*?

It has been suggested that an oncogene may be transcriptionally activated by transposition into a functionally active Ig gene region (Klein 1981). This is not the case in plasmacytomas since the translocation involves the nonfunctional Ig allele. Another possibility is that the Ig constant region may have an enhancing activity for any adjacent promoter, as suggested by studies of the C_k locus (Perry et al. 1980). However, analysis of the translocation of MOPC-104E suggests that neither C_α nor S_α are required for expression of the shorter plasmacytoma *myc* RNA.

Initial characterization of the cloned *myc* gene from MOPC-104E demonstrated that the DNA rearrangement was different from that in other BALB/c tumors in which C_α was joined to *myc* by an abortive switching event. A probe from the DNA joined to the *myc* gene in MOPC-104E hybridized to 4.5-kb *Eco*RI and 2.9-kb *Hin*dIII fragments that were not rearranged in tumor cells (Shen-Ong et al. 1982). This sequence has now been identified as the DNA segment flanking the 3' end of the C_α gene (Fig. 6) by both hybridization studies and electron microscopy of heteroduplex molecules (data not shown). Furthermore, the final gene rearrangement was apparently achieved by two steps, the first of which was an abortive C_α switching event similar to that found in other tumor lines. Evidence for the initial switching event comes from the continued presence of the reciprocal of the translocation in the tumor DNA. A single reciprocal fragment can be detected with probes from both S_α and

the displaced 5'-flanking sequence from the *myc* gene (Cory et al. 1983; M. Cole, unpubl.) but not with the C_α coding sequence (Shen-Ong et al. 1982). Subsequent to the abortive switching event, both C_α and all of S_α were apparently deleted joining *myc* to the 3'-flanking sequences from C_α. The DNA sequence at the junction does not appear to contain any residual S_α sequences (S.P. Piccoli and M.D. Cole, in prep.). Thus, the synthesis of the tumor-specific *myc* RNA from the latent promoter in the *myc* intron is not dependent on sequences within either C_α or S_α. This observation raises the possibility that there is a distinct enhancing element on the 3' side of C_α that can act at a distance. An alternative possibility is that the effect of the translocation on *myc* expression is the result of a change in chromatin structure that extends a distance on either side of the IgH locus. Studies of additional tumor lines in which *myc* is not joined to C_α may provide further insight into this question.

The C_α sequence may induce transcripts from the *c-myc* intron other than those that hybridize to the *c-myc* exons. The Northern blot in Figure 4 shows that in addition to the *myc* RNAs of 2.0 kb and 2.4 kb, there is a smear of hybridization that is especially prominent in MOPC-46B. Shorter exposures of the filter hybridized to the *Xba*I–*Sst*I probe appear the same as the filter hybridized to the *Bam*HI–*Sst*I probe, where a band at 1.4 kb is evident over the broad smear. These RNAs do not hybridize to a *c-myc* exon probe (Shen-Ong et al. 1982). A possible explanation for the additional RNAs transcribed from the *myc* intron comes from consideration of the gene organization shown in Figure 1. The C_α and *myc* genes were found to be significantly closer in MOPC-46B than in any other tumor line so any enhancing activity from C_α or its 3'-flanking sequences would be greater. It is not known if the *myc* intron RNAs in MOPC-46B are transcribed from the same or the opposite strand as *c-myc*.

Conclusion

DNA rearrangements induced by chromosomal translocation have been found at the *c-myc* oncogene in 80–90% of mouse plasmacytomas. Most of the rearrangements that have been characterized are the result of abortive immunoglobulin switching events that join C_α to the 5' end of the *myc* gene. The most likely consequence for the translocation appears to be the transcription of elevated levels of *myc* RNA. However, since many tumor cell lines without translocations have equally high levels of *myc* RNA, it is not yet clear that the RNA level found in plasmacytomas is a direct consequence of the translocation. An important feature of murine plasmacytomas is that the translocation breakpoints always occur within the *c-myc* gene. Therefore, in addition to the loss of an untranslated leader sequence, the normal *c-myc* gene control region would also be displaced. This could lead to deregulation of the *c-myc* gene as well as to enhanced transcription. Further studies of the regulation of *c-myc* expression in both normal and tumor cells should provide

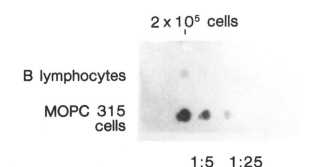

Figure 5 Cytoplasmic dot blots of plasmacytoma and normal B cells after hybridization to a mouse *c-myc* probe (*Bam*HI–*Hin*dIII; Shen-Ong et al. 1982). The 1:5 and 1:25 samples were prepared by diluting an aliquot of the original sample with 15× SSC. The hybridization was eliminated by preincubation of the filters with RNase.

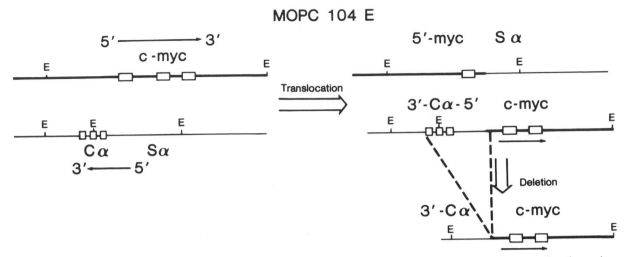

Figure 6 Diagram of the *c-myc* DNA rearrangements in the MOPC-104E tumor line. The DNA fragment representing the reciprocal of the translocation (5′ *c-myc* joined to S_α) has been observed in Southern blots of tumor DNA (see text). The organization of the *c-myc* gene cloned from MOPC-104E was established by hybridization studies and electron microscopy of heteroduplex molecules.

additional insight into the activation of oncogenes by chromosomal translocation.

Acknowledgments

This work was supported by grants from the American Cancer Society, the Sklarow Memorial Trust, and the National Cancer Institute.

References

Adams, J.M., S. Gerondakis, E. Webb, L.M. Corcoran, and S. Cory. 1983. Cellular *myc* oncogene is altered by chromosome translocation to the immunoglobulin locus in murine plasmacytomas and is rearranged similarly in human Burkitt lymphomas. *Proc. Natl. Acad. Sci.* **80:** 1982.

Adams, J.M., S. Gerondakis, E. Webb, J. Mitchell, O. Bernard, and S. Cory. 1982. Transcriptionally active DNA region that rearranges frequently in murine lymphoid tumors. *Proc. Natl. Acad. Sci.* **79:** 6966.

Alitalo, K., M. Schwab, C.C. Lin, H.E. Varmus, and J.M. Bishop. 1983. Homogeneously staining chromosomal regions contain amplified copies of an abundantly expressed cellular oncogene (c-*myc*) in malignant neuroendocrine cells from a human colon carcinoma. *Proc. Natl. Acad. Sci.* **80:** 1707.

Calame, K., S. Kim, P. Lalley, R. Hill, M. Davis, and L. Hood. 1982. Molecular cloning of translocations involving chromosome 15 and the immunoglobulin C_α gene from chromosome 12 in two murine plasmacytomas. *Proc. Natl. Acad. Sci.* **79:** 6994.

Collins, S. and M. Groudine. 1982. Amplification of endogenous *myc*-related DNA sequences in a human myeloid leukaemia cell line. *Nature* **298:** 679.

Cory, S., S. Gerondakis, and J.M. Adams. 1983. Interchromosomal recombination of the cellular oncogene c-*myc* with the immunoglobulin heavy chain locus in murine plasmacytomas is a reciprocal exchange. *EMBO J.* **2:** 697.

Crews, S., R. Barth, L. Hood, J. Prehn, and K. Calame. 1982. Mouse c-*myc* oncogene is located on chromosome 15 and translocated to chromosome 12 in plasmacytomas. *Science* **218:** 1319.

Dalla-Favera, R., F. Wong-Staal, and R.C. Gallo. 1982. *onc* gene amplification in promyelocytic leukaemia cell line HL-60 and primary leukaemic cells of the same patient. *Nature* **299:** 61.

Dalla-Favera, R., S. Martinotti, R. Gallo, J. Erikson, and C.M. Croce. 1983. Translocations and rearrangements of the c-*myc* oncogene locus in human undifferentiated B-cell lymphomas. *Science* **219:** 963.

Davis, M.M., S.K. Kim, and L. Hood. 1980. DNA sequences mediating class switching in α-immunoglobulins. *Science* **209:** 1360.

Dunnick, W., B.E. Shell, and C. Dery. 1983. DNA sequences near the site of reciprocal recombination between a c-*myc* oncogene and an immunoglobulin switch region. *Proc. Natl. Acad. Sci.* **80:** 7269.

Erikson, J., A. ar-Rushdi, H.L. Drwinga, P.C. Nowell, and C.M. Croce. 1983. Transcriptional activation of the translocated c-*myc* oncogene in Burkitt lymphoma. *Proc. Natl. Acad. Sci.* **80:** 820.

Gonda, T.J., D. Sheiness, and J.M. Bishop. 1982. Transcripts from the cellular homologs of retroviral oncogenes: Distribution among chicken tissues. *Mol. Cell. Biol.* **3:** 617.

Harris, L.J., R.B. Lang, and K.B. Marcu. 1982. Non-immunoglobulin-associated DNA rearrangements in mouse plasmacytomas. *Proc. Natl. Acad. Sci.* **79:** 4175.

Hayward, W.S., B.G. Neel, and S.M. Astrin. 1981. Activation of a cellular *onc* gene by promotor insertion in ALV-induced lymphoid leukosis. *Nature* **290:** 475.

Klein, G. 1981. The role of gene dosage and genetic transpositions in carcinogenesis. *Nature* **294:** 313.

———. 1983. Specific chromosomal translocations and the genesis of B-cell-derived tumors in mice and man. *Cell* **32:** 311.

Manolov, G. and Y. Manolova. 1972. Marker band in one chromosome 14 from Burkitt lymphomas. *Nature* **237:** 33.

Marcu, K.B., L.J. Harris, C.W. Stanton, J. Erikson, R. Watt, and C.M. Croce. 1983. Transcriptionally active c-*myc* oncogene is contained within NIARD, a DNA sequence associated with chromosome translocations in B cell neoplasia. *Proc. Natl. Acad. Sci.* **80:** 519.

Maxam, A.M. and W. Gilbert. 1980. Sequencing of labeled DNA with base-specific chemical cleavages. *Methods Enzymol.* **65:** 499.

Mushinski, J.F., S.R. Bauer, M. Potter, and E.P. Reddy. 1983. Increased expression of *myc*-related oncogene mRNA characterizes most Balb/c plasmacytomas induced by pristane or Abelson murine leukemia virus. *Proc. Natl. Acad. Sci.* **80:** 1073.

Ohno, S., M. Babonits, F. Wiener, J. Spira, and G. Klein. 1979. Nonrandom chromosome changes involving the Ig gene-carrying chromosomes 12 and 6 in pristane-induced mouse plasmacytomas. *Cell* **18**: 1001.

Perry, R.P., D.E. Kelley, C. Coleclough, J.G. Seidman, P. Leder, S. Tonegawa, G. Matthyssens, and M. Weigert. 1980. Transcription of mouse K chain genes: Implications for allelic exclusion. *Proc. Natl. Acad. Sci.* **77**: 1937.

Robins, T., K. Bister, C. Garon, T. Papas, and P. Duesberg. 1982. Structural relationship between a normal chicken DNA locus and the transforming gene of the avian acute leukemia virus MC29. *J. Virol.* **41**: 635.

Roussel, M., S. Saule, C. Lagrou, C. Rommens, H. Beug, T. Graf, and D. Stehelin. 1979. Three new types of viral oncogene of cellular origin specific for haematopoietic cell transformation. *Nature* **281**: 452.

Rowley, J.D. 1982. Identification of the constant chromosome regions involved in human hematologic malignant disease. *Science* **216**: 749.

Sheiness, P. and J.M. Bishop. 1979. DNA and RNA from uninfected vertebrate cells contain nucleotide sequences related to the putative transforming genes of avian myelocytomatosis virus. *J. Virol.* **31**: 514.

Shen-Ong, G.L.C., E.J. Keath, S.P. Piccoli, and M.D. Cole. 1982. Novel *myc* oncogene RNA from abortive immunoglobulin-gene recombination in mouse plasmacytomas. *Cell* **31**: 443.

Stanton, L.W., R. Watt, and K.B. Marcu. 1983. Translocation, breakage and truncated transcripts of *c-myc* oncogene in murine plasmacytomas. *Nature* **303**: 401.

Taub, R., I. Kirsh, C. Morton, G. Lenoir, D. Swan, S. Tronick, S. Aaronson, and P. Leder. 1982. Translocation of the *c-myc* gene into the immunoglobulin heavy chain locus in human Burkitt lymphoma and murine plasmacytoma cells. *Proc. Natl. Acad. Sci.* **79**: 7837.

Vennstrom, B., D. Sheiness, J. Zabielski, and J.M. Bishop. 1982. Isolation and characterization of *c-myc*, a cellular homolog of the oncogene (*v-myc*) of avian myelocytomatosis virus strain 29. *J. Virol.* **42**: 773.

White, B.A. and F.C. Bancroft. 1982. Cytoplasmic dot hybridization. *J. Biol. Chem.* **257**: 8569.

Chromosomal Translocations and *c-myc* Activation in Burkitt's Lymphoma

C.M. Croce, J. Erikson, K. Nishikura, A. ar-Rushdi, A. Giallongo, and G. Rovera

The Wistar Institute of Anatomy and Biology, Philadelphia, Pennsylvania 19104

J. Finan and P.C. Nowell

Department of Pathology and Laboratory Medicine, University of Pennsylvania School of Medicine, Philadelphia, Pennsylvania 19104

Since the discovery of the 9;22 translocation in patients with chronic myelogenous leukemia (CML) (Nowell and Hungerford 1960; Rowley 1973, 1983), a variety of specific chromosomal translocations have been observed in malignancies of the hematopoietic system, such as acute promyelocytic leukemia (Rowley 1983), Burkitt's lymphoma (Manolov and Manolova 1972; Zech et al. 1976), and adult B-cell lymphoma (Yunis 1983), and, more recently, in solid tumors (Aurias et al. 1983; Turc-Carel et al. 1983).

Manolov and Manolova (1972) observed an abnormally long chromosome 14 in Burkitt's lymphoma, subsequently shown to be the result of a reciprocal translocation between chromosomes 8 and 14 (Zech et al. 1976). Two variant chromosomal translocations have been observed in a minority (25%) of Burkitt's lymphomas (Van den Berghe et al. 1979; Lenoir et al. 1982); one involves a reciprocal translocation between chromosomes 8 and 22 and the other involves a reciprocal translocation between chromosomes 2 and 8. In all cases, the breakpoint on chromosome 8 is located consistently at band q24 (Van den Berghe et al. 1979; Lenoir et al. 1982). Since the use of somatic cell genetics techniques has allowed the mapping of the genes for human immunoglobulin heavy chains to chromosome 14 (Croce et al. 1979), of λ light-chain genes to chromosome 22 (Erikson et al. 1981), and of κ light-chain genes to chromosome 2 (Malcolm et al. 1982; McBride et al. 1982), it became clear that the immunoglobulin chain genes might be involved in the chromosomal exchanges observed in Burkitt's lymphoma (Erikson et al. 1981).

The involvement of the heavy-chain locus in Burkitt's lymphomas with the t(8;14) chromosomal translocation was shown by using somatic cell hybrids between mouse myeloma cells and Burkitt's lymphoma cells (Erikson et al. 1982). The analysis of the hybrids indicated that the genes for the variable regions of heavy chains translocated to the involved chromosome 8, and the genes for the constant regions remained on chromosome 14 (Erikson et al. 1982). Thus, the heavy-chain locus is split by the chromosomal break occurring in Burkitt's lymphomas with the t(8;14) translocation (Erikson et al. 1982).

Analysis of rodent–human hybrids for the presence of the human homologs of known retroviral oncogenes has allowed the chromosomal localization of several human oncogenes (Dalla Favera et al. 1982b,c,d). One of these, the so-called *c-myc* oncogene that is homologous to the avian virus oncogene, *v-myc*, which can induce B-cell lymphoma in chickens, was found to be located on that small segment of chromosome 8 that translocates to chromosome 14 in Burkitt's lymphoma (Fig. 1) (Dalla Favera et al. 1982c). This finding implies a possible role for the *c-myc* oncogene in the development of the Burkitt's tumor. By using restriction enzyme analysis and probes for the *myc* oncogene and for human immunoglobulin genes, several laboratories have found rearrangements of the *c-myc* oncogene and head-to-head rearrangements between the *c-myc* and the C_μ gene in some Burkitt's lymphomas with the t(8;14) translocation (Dalla Favera et al. 1982c, 1983; Taub et al. 1982). These findings were confirmed by analysis of recombinant DNA clones containing the chromosomal breakpoint (Hamlin and Rabbitts 1983).

Thus, in Burkitt's lymphomas with the t(8;14) chromosomal translocation, the *c-myc* gene moves into close proximity of the heavy-chain locus (Fig. 1). In some cases, the oncogene is rearranged, and in others it is intact within a large *Bam*HI restriction fragment (Dalla Favera et al. 1982c, 1983; Taub et al. 1982; Hamlin and Rabbitts 1983).

Extending these initial observations, we have now ex-

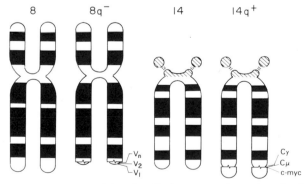

Figure 1 Diagram of the t(8;14) chromosomal translocation in Burkitt's lymphoma. The V_H gene translocates from chromosome 14 to the involved 8 (8q−), whereas the *c-myc* oncogene translocates to the heavy-chain locus.

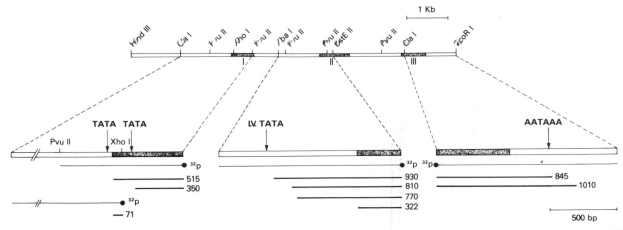

Figure 2 Schematic representation of DNA probes used for S1 nuclease analysis. The structure of the human *c-myc* genomic DNA is schematicaly shown according to Watt et al. (1983a,b) and Colby et al. (1983). A pBR322 subclone, pMyc 41·HE carrying the 8.3-kb HindIII–EcoRI DNA fragment shown in this figure, was used to prepare various S1 probes. A double-stranded 1.3-kb ClaI–XhoI fragment, 5′ ³²P-labeled at the XhoI site within the first exon, and PvuII 0.8-kb fragment were used to analyze the initiation site. The probe used for S1 mapping analysis to detect the novel initiation sites or cryptic splicing sites within the intervening sequences between the first and second exons was a double-stranded 1.4-kb XbaI–BstEII fragment 5′ ³²P-labeled at the BstEII site within the second exon. The probe used for S1 nuclease analysis of the 3′ end of the *c-myc* messages was a DNA fragment ClaI–EcoRI 1.4-kb that was 3′ ³²P-labeled. The location and size of S1 nuclease-resistant DNA products are shown together by the solid bars in the diagram. The approximate locations of the authentic TATA box found by us (Watt et al. 1983a) and another TATA boxlike sequence (I.V. TATA) found within the first intron (Colby et al. 1983) are indicated. The location of the recognition signal sequence (AA TAA) for polyadenylation found by Colby et al. (1983) is also indicated.

amined further the structure and function of the *c-myc* oncogene in Burkitt's tumor cell lines with the usual 8;14 chromosomal translocation and also with the variant 8;22 and 2;8 rearrangements. Our findings and conclusions to date are summarized in the following paragraphs.

Structure of the *c-myc* oncogene

DNA sequence analysis of a genomic *c-myc* clone (Watt et al. 1983) and of *c-myc* DNA clones (Watt et al. 1983b) indicates that the *c-myc* gene is formed by three exons separated by two introns (Fig. 2) (Watt et al. 1983a). The first exon codes for an untranslated leader that has termination codons on all three reading frames (Watt et al. 1983b). The *c-myc* gene has two promoters (TATA boxes) and two transcription initiation sites, one of

which, 160 nucleotides downstream from the first initiation site, is within the first exon (Watt et al. 1983b) (Fig. 2). Both initiation sites are utilized at variable ratios in human B-cell lines (ar-Rushdi et al. 1983). When a chromosomal break occurs within the first exon or in the first intervening sequence, as observed in the JD38 and ST486 lymphoma cell lines with an 8;14 translocation, novel transcripts initiating in the first intervening sequence are expressed (Fig. 2) (ar-Rushdi et al. 1983). The putative promoter site (I.V. TATA) described by Colby et al. (1983) is in the first intervening sequence and is shown in Figure 2.

The *c-myc* oncogene also contains two termination signals as determined by S1 nuclease protection experiments (ar-Rushdi et al. 1983) (Fig. 2). The nucleotide sequence of *c-myc* cDNA indicates that the oncogene

Table 1 Human Lymphoma Cell Lines Used in This Study

Cell line	Diagnosis[a]	Presence of EBV genome	Translocation	Origin
Daudi	BL	+	t(8;14)(q24; q32)	Africa
P3HR-1	BL	+	t(8;14)(q4; q32)	Africa
CA46	BL	–	t(8;14)(q24; q32)	South America
JD38	NBL	–	t(8;14)(q24; q32)	North America
JI	BL	+	t(2;8)(p12; q32)	Europe
LY91	BL	+	t(2;8)(p12; q32)	Africa
LY67	BL	+	t(8;22)(q24; q11)	Africa

[a]Histologic diagnosis: (BL) Burkitt's lymphoma; (NBL) non-Burkitt's lymphoma.

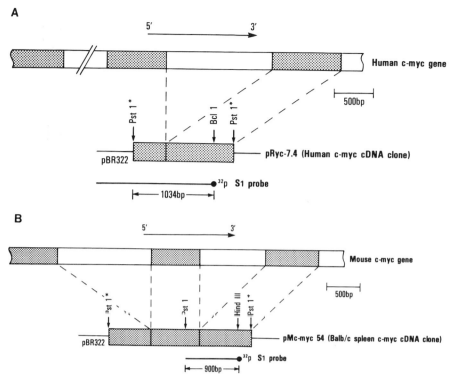

Figure 3 Schematic representation of DNA probes used for S1 nuclease analysis. (A) The structures of the human c-myc cDNA clone pRyc-7.4 which carries a human c-myc cDNA 1.2-kb insert in pBR322 and a part of human c-myc gene are schematically shown according to Nishikura et al. (1983). pRyc-7.4 plasmid DNA was digested by Bcll, 5'-end ^{32}P-labeled, and used as a probe (human c-myc probe). The expected fragment protected by human c-myc mRNA (1034 nucleotides) encompasses most of the protein-coding sequences (Watt et al. 1983b). (B) The structures of the mouse c-myc cDNA clone pMC-myc 54 (Nishikura et al. 1983), which carries a mouse c myc cDNA 2.2-kb insert in pBR322, and a part of mouse c-myc gene are schematically presented according to Nishikura et al. (1983). pMC-myc 54 plasmid was digested by HindIII, labeled with ^{32}P at the 5' end, and cleaved with Pstl. The resulting Pstl–HindIII 900-bp fragment was isolated and used as probe (mouse c-myc S1 probe). The fragment encompasses most of the protein-coding sequences.

can code for a protein of 439 amino acids (48,812 m.w.) (Watt et al. 1983b).

Activation of the translocated c-myc oncogene in Burkitt's lymphomas with the t(8;14) chromosomal translocation

We have previously shown high levels of c-myc transcripts in a number of Burkitt's lymphoma cell lines (Erikson et al. 1983a). These findings have now been extended to additional Burkitt's (and non-Burkitt's B cell) lymphomas with the t(8;14), t(8;22), and t(2;8) chromosomal translocations (Table 1) which had either a normal or a rearranged c-myc oncogene as determined by the S1 nuclease protection procedure using a cDNA probe (Ryc 7.4) specific for the second and the third exon of the c-myc oncogene (Fig. 3) (Nishikura et al. 1983). As shown in Figure 4, the levels of c-myc transcripts were consistently high in all Burkitt's lymphoma cell lines examined, regardless of whether the gene appeared to be rearranged. In Burkitt's lymphoma cell lines with the t(8;14) translocation, the levels of myc transcripts were similar to or higher than those expressed in the HL60 cell line derived from human promyelocytic leukemia cells that contain an amplified c-myc gene and

express levels of c-myc transcripts 20–40-fold higher than normal cells (Dalla Favera et al. 1982a).

To determine whether the high levels of c-myc transcripts observed in Burkitt's lymphoma cells were due to the characteristic translocation involving chromosome 8, we have examined somatic cell hybrids between Burkitt's lymphoma cells and mouse plasmacytoma cells for the expression of human c-myc transcripts by the S1 nuclease protection procedure (Nishikura et al. 1983). We have previously shown that since the mouse and human c-myc genes are not identical, the S1 nuclease protection method can be used to determine the levels of the human and of the mouse c-myc transcripts in hybrid cells, utilizing either a human or a mouse myc cDNA probe, respectively (Fig. 3) (Nishikura et al. 1983). As shown in Table 2, in studies of cell lines with the 8;14 translocation, only the hybrids containing the 14q+ chromosome expressed high levels of human c-myc transcripts. Hybrids containing the untranslocated c-myc gene on the normal chromosome 8 did not express such transcripts. No difference in the levels of mouse c-myc transcripts were detectable in the hybrid clones (Nishikura et al. 1983). Thus, we can conclude that the translocated c-myc gene and the untranslocated c-myc gene that remains on the normal chromosome 8

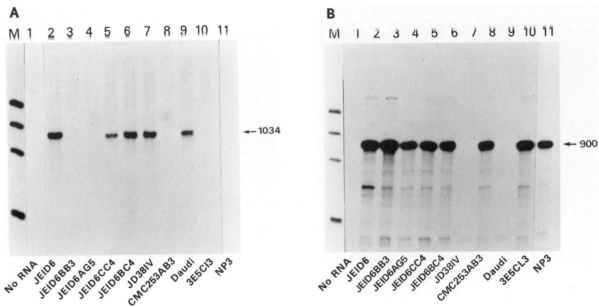

Figure 4 S1 nuclease analysis of *c-myc* RNAs in the hybrid cells between NP3 and Burkitt's lymphoma cell lines with the t(8;14) chromosomal translocation. (*A*) Cytoplasmic RNA (20 μg) was hybridized with human *c-myc* probe or (*B*) mouse *c-myc* S1 probe described in Fig. 3. The parental NP3 used for hybrid preparation is a nonproducer mouse myeloma.

are under different transcriptional control. The *c-myc* gene that is in close proximity to the heavy-chain locus on the 14q+ chromosome is activated while the normal *c-myc* gene is repressed (Table 2) (Nishikura et al. 1983).

We have also examined the levels of *c-myc* transcripts in somatic cell hybrids between NP3 mouse plasmacytoma cells and Epstein-Barr virus-transformed GM 1056 human lymphoblastoid cells. As shown in Table 2, hybrid cells containing the normal chromosome 8 from GM 1056 did not express human *c-myc* transcripts, whereas the parental GM 1056 cells do. Thus, we can conclude that the normal human *c-myc* oncogene is shut off in a mouse plasmacytoma background, whereas the translocated oncogene in the same circumstances, is expressed at high levels.

We have also investigated the levels of human *c-myc* transcripts in hybrid cells between mouse fibroblasts (LM-tk⁻) and P3HR-1 Burkitt's lymphoma cells (Table 2). As shown in Table 2, a dramatic reduction of the levels of human *myc* transcripts occurs in these hybrids (Nishikura et al. 1983). Thus, we can conclude that the level of transcripts of the translocated *c-myc* oncogene is significantly influenced by the differentiated state of the cells harboring the translocated chromosome.

We have also investigated the expression of the untranslocated and of the translocated *c-myc* gene in Burkitt's lymphomas with the t(8;14) chromosomal translocation in which the *c-myc* gene is rearranged head-to-head with the immunoglobulin C_μ gene as determined by Northern blotting analysis using DNA probes specific for the first and for the second and third exon of the *c-myc* oncogene. The probe specific for the second and third exon (Ryc 7.4) detected 2.2–2.4-kb *myc* transcripts

in all Burkitt's lymphomas examined, including Daudi Burkitt's lymphoma cells that carry a normal but translocated *c-myc* gene, and JD38 and ST486 lymphoma cells which carry a rearranged *c-myc* gene that has had the first exon decapitated by the chromosomal translocation (Dalla Favera et al. 1983; ar-Rushdi et al. 1983). On the contrary, we did not detect 2.2–2.4-kb *myc* transcripts in ST486 and JD38 cells using a probe specific for the first exon (ar-Rushdi et al. 1983). Therefore, we conclude that only the translocated *c-myc* gene is expressed in the two lymphoma cell lines that have a rearranged *c-myc* gene. Since we observed short (~0.9 kb) transcripts that hybridized with the *c-myc* first exon in ST486 and JD38 cells, and since we have shown that these transcripts derive from the first exon presumably left behind on the 8q⁻ chromosome because of the translocation, we can also conclude that the enhancers that are capable of increasing *c-myc* transcription must be on both sides of the breakpoint on chromosome 14 (ar-Rushdi et al. 1983).

Somatic cell genetics of the t(8;22) chromosomal translocation in variant Burkitt's lymphomas

A Burkitt's cell line with the variant t(8;22) chromosomal translocation has also been studied by the somatic cell genetics approach to define the mechanisms resulting in *c-myc* activation in these circumstances. Somatic cell hybrids between mouse plasmacytoma cells and BL2 Burkitt's lymphoma cells carrying a t(8;22) chromosomal translocation were examined for the presence and expression of human λ chains and the *c-myc* oncogene. As shown in Table 3, our data indicate that the *c-myc* oncogene remains on the 8q+ chromosome in BL2 cells, and the excluded and rearranged immunoglobulin

Table 2 Transcription of the Mouse and Human c-myc Genes in Mouse × Human Hybrids

Parental cells and hybrid clones	Human isozymes		Human chromosomes						Human oncogenes		Levels of c-myc transcripts	
	GSR	NP	8	8q −	14	14q +	2q −	8q +	c-mos[a]	c-myc	mouse	human
P3HR-1 (BL)	+	+	+	+	+	+	−	−	+	+	−	+ + +
JE1D6 (NP3 × P3HR-1 hybrid)	+	+	+	−	−	+	−	−	+	+	+ + +	+ + +
BB3 (NP3 × P3HR-1 hybrid)	+	−	+	−	−	−	−	−	+	+	+ + +	−
AG5 (NP3 × P3HR-1 hybrid)	+	−	+	−	−	−	−	−	+	+	+ + +	−
CC4 (NP3 × P3HR-1 hybrid)	−	+	−	−	−	+	−	−	−	+	+ + +	+ + +
BC4 (NP3 × P3HR-1 hybrid)	−	+	−	−	−	+	−	−	−	+	+ + +	+ + +
NP3 (mouse plasmacytoma)	−	−	−	−	−	−	−	−	−	−	+ + +	−
JD38 (NBL)	+	+	+	+	+	+	−	−	+	+	−	+ + +
253 A-B3 (NP3 × JD38 hybrid)	+	−	+	−	+	−	−	−	+	+	+ + +	−
Daudi (BL)	+	+	+	+	+	+	−	−	+	+	−	+ + +
3E5 CL3 (NP3 × Daudi hybrid)	+	+	+	+	+	+	−	−	+	+	+ + +	−
JI (BL)	+	+	+	−	+	−	+	+	+	+	−	+ + +
JI 5-3 (NP3 × JI hybrid)	+	+	+	−	+	−	−	−	+	+	+ + +	−
JI 4-2 (NP3 × JI hybrid)	+	+	+	−	+	−	+	+	+	+	+ + +	+ +
GM1056 (EBV transformed)	+	+	+	−	+	−	−	−	+	+	−	+ +
DSK 1B 2A5 (NP3 × GM1056 hybrid)	+	+	+	−	+	−	−	−	+	+	+ + +	−
LM-tk⁻ (mouse fibroblast)	−	−	−	−	−	−	−	−	−	−	+ + +	−
M44 CL2S5 (LM-tk⁻ × P3RH1 hybrid)	−	+	−	−	−	+	−	−	−	+	+ + +	±

[a]The c-mos oncogene resides on band q22 of chromosome 8.

C_λ allele translocates from chromosome 22 to this chromosome 8 (Croce et al. 1983). As a result of the translocation, transcriptional activation of the c-myc oncogene on the rearranged chromosome 8 (8q +) occurs, whereas the c-myc oncogene on the normal chromosome 8 is transcriptionally silent (Table 3). These findings suggest that the translocation of a rearranged immunoglobulin locus to the 3′ side of an unrearranged c-myc oncogene may enhance its transcription and contribute to malignant transformation (Fig. 5).

We have also examined the chromosomes of BL2 cells by the in situ hybridization procedure using a C_λ DNA probe. These analyses indicate that all the C_λ genes translocate from chromosome 22 to chromosome 8 in these BL2 Burkitt's lymphoma cells (Emanuel et al. 1984). On the contrary, we have observed that all the C_λ genes remain on the Philadelphia chromosome (22q −) in chronic myelogenous leukemia (CML) cells with the t(9;22) translocation (Emanuel et al. 1984). Thus, we can conclude that the chromosomal break-

Table 3 Ig Genes and Oncogenes in BL2 Hybrids

Cell line	Human chromosomes[a]				Human Cλ genes			Expression of human λ chains	Human oncogenes		Transcripts of human c-myc
	8	8q +	22	22q −	17 kb (upper band)	12 kb (middle band)	6.8 kb (lower band)		c-myc	c-mos	
BL2	+	+	+	+	+	+	+	+	+	+	+ + +
NP3	−	−	−	−	−	−	−	−	−	−	−
1-9	+ +	−	+ +	+	+	−	+	+	+	+	n.d.[b]
1-15	±	+ +	−	+	+	+	−	−	+	+	+ + +
1-23	+ +	+ +	−	+ +	+	+	−	−	+	−	n.d.
3-1	+ +	−	+ +	+	+	−	+	−	+	+	−
3-2	±	−	+ +	+ +	+	−	+	+	+	+	−
4-35	−	+	+	+	+	+	+	+	+	+	n.d.
17-6	−	+ +	+ +	+	+	+	+	+	+	+	+ + +

[a]Frequency of metaphases with relevant chromosome: (−) none; (±) <10%; (+) 10–30%; (+ +) >30%.
[b](n.d.) Not done.

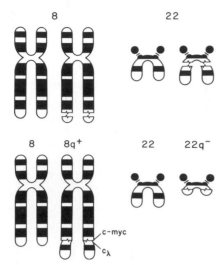

Figure 5 Diagram of the t(8;22) translocation observed in BL2 Burkitt's lymphoma cells. The activated *c-myc* oncogene remains on chromosome 8, whereas the C_λ locus translocates to a region distal to the *c-myc* oncogene.

points in the q11 region of chromosome 22 are different in Burkitt's lymphoma and CML, suggesting different mechanisms of oncogene activation (Emanuel et al. 1984).

Somatic cell genetics of the t(2;8) translocation in variant Burkitt's lymphomas

We have also studied somatic cell hybrids between a mouse plasmacytoma and JI Burkitt's lyphoma cells carrying the t(2;8) chromosomal translocation for the expression of human κ chains and for the presence and rearrangement of the human *c-myc* oncogene and κ-chain genes. Our results indicate that the *c-myc* oncogene is unrearranged and remains on the 8q+ chromosome of JI cells (Table 4) (Erikson et al. 1983b). Two rearranged immunoglobulin C_κ genes were detected: the expressed allele on the normal chromosome 2 and the excluded allele translocated from chromosome 2 to the involved chromosome 8 (8q+) (Table 4) (Erikson et al. 1983a). The distribution of human V_κ and C_κ genes in hybrid clones retaining different human chromosomes indicated that C_κ is distal to V_κ on 2p (Fig. 6), and that the chromosomal breakpoint in this Burkitt's lymphoma is within the V_κ region (Table 4). High levels of transcripts of the *c-myc* gene were found when it resided on the 8q+ chromosome but not on the normal chromosome 8, demonstrating that, as in the 8;22 rearrangement, translocation of a light-chain gene locus to a region distal to the *c-myc* oncogene can enhance *c-myc* transcription.

The *c-myc* proteins

We have synthesized a synthetic peptide specific for the carboxyl terminus of the *c-myc* protein on the basis of the nucleotide sequences of *myc* cDNA (Watt et al. 1983b). Table 5 shows the amino acid sequence of the synthetic peptide used for immunization of rabbits. Antiserum against this synthetic peptide was able to im-

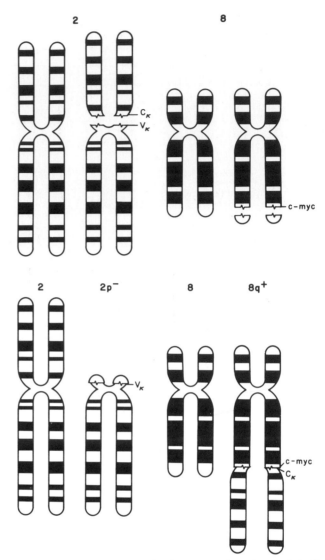

Figure 6 Diagram of the t(2;8) translocation observed in JI Burkitt's lymphoma cells. The activated *c-myc* oncogene remains on chromosome 8, whereas the C_κ gene translocates to a region distal to the *c-myc* oncogene. Since we observe the presence of human V_κ genes in hybrids with either the 2p− or the 8q+ chromosome, we also conclude that the C_κ gene is distal to the V_κ genes on 2p and that the breakpoint occurred in the chromosomal segment carrying V_κ genes.

munoprecipitate a 48-kD protein from [35S]methionine-labeled lysates of different Burkitt's lymphoma cells, HL60 human promyelocytic cells that contain an amplified *c-myc* gene (Dalla Favera et al. 1982a), HeLa cells, human lymphoblastoid cell lines, and COLO 320 colon carcinoma cells that contain an amplified *c-myc* gene (Giallongo et al. 1983). The immunoprecipitation of the 48K protein was inhibited by the carboxyterminal peptide.

We have also immunoprecipitated the *c-myc* protein from mouse plasmacytoma cells and from mouse × human hybrid cells that express high levels of both mouse and human *c-myc* transcripts. These hybrids were de-

Table 4 Human κ Genes and Oncogenes in JI × NP 3 Hybrids

Cells	Human chromosomes[a]				Human isozymes[b]		Human κ chains expression	Human genes			Human oncogenes		Human c-myc transcripts
								C_κ					
	8	8q +	2	2p −	MDH	IDH		15 kb	7.5 kb	V_κ	c-mos	c-myc	
JI	+ +	+ +	+ +	+ +	+	+	+	+	+	+	+	+	+ + +
JI 4-5	−	+ +	−	−	+	−	−	+	−	+	+	+	+ + +
JI 4-5B7	−	+	−	−	+	−	−	+	−	+	+	+	+ +
JI 4-5H11	−	−	−	−	−	−	−	−	−	−	−	−	−
JI 5-4	+	−	−	+ +	−	+	−	−	−	+	+	+	−
JI 6-5	−	−	+ +	−	+	+	+	−	+	+	−	−	−
JI 4-2L	−	+ +	−	−	+	−	−	+	−	+	+	+	+ + +
NP3	−	−	−	−	−	−	−	−	−	+	−	−	−

[a]Frequency of metaphases with relevant chromosomes: (−) none; (+) 10–30%; (+ +) >30%.
[b](MDH) Malate dehydrogenase; (IDH) isocitrate dehydrogenase.

rived from NP3 mouse plasmacytoma and P3HR-1 Burkitt's lymphoma cells. The anti-carboxyterminal antiserum immunoprecipitated the same 48-kD protein from mouse myeloma, Burkitt's lymphoma, and these hybrid cells, but not from a lysate of SK BR5 human breast cancer cells that do not produce c-myc transcripts (Giallongo et al. 1983). The same 48-kD protein was detected in lipopolysaccharide (LPS)-stimulated mouse spleen cells and also in pokeweed mitogen (PWM)-stimulated human B cells (data not shown). Thus, the size of this putative myc protein is consistent with the potential coding region predicted from the c-myc nucleotide sequence, and it is the same for normal and malignant B cells, carrying either a rearranged or an unrearranged c-myc oncogene (Giallongo et al. 1983). Formal proof whether this protein is indeed myc or a protein with homology to the carboxyl terminal of the myc gene product awaits amino acid sequencing.

Conclusions

The result summarized in the preceding sections indicate that the translocation of the c-myc gene to the immu-

noglobulin heavy-chain gene cluster, or the translocation of either the λ-chain locus or the κ-chain locus to a region distal (3′) to the c-myc oncogene, results in the transcriptional activation of the c-myc gene involved in the translocation, whereas the c-myc oncogene on the normal chromosome 8 is transcriptionally silent. In all cases examined thus far, it appears that the critical association in Burkitt's lymphoma cells is between the oncogene and the 5′ side of the immunoglobulin constant-region genes, even though they remain separated to some degree by intervening variable regions and other sequences.

Since no differences in the c-myc gene product have been detected in Burkitt's lymphoma or mouse myeloma cells, with or without c-myc rearrangements, it appears that the expression of high levels of a structurally normal myc product is the significant result of the translocation. Thus, it is reasonable to speculate that when a c-myc gene is located in close proximity to an immunoglobulin locus in a differentiated B lymphocyte, its transcription is enhanced and cannot be shut off, resulting in high constitutive levels of c-myc expression. This could result in a continuous and irreversible proliferative stimulus for the affected B cells, ultimately leading to neoplasia.

Table 5 Carboxyterminal Sequence of the c-myc Gene Product and Synthetic Peptide Used for Immunization

A
NH_2 ..... Gln−Leu−Lys−His−Lys−Leu−Glu−Gln−Leu−Arg−Asn - Ser−Cys−Ala

B
NH_2−Tyr$\overset{*}{}$−Lys−His−Lys−Leu−Glu−Gln−Leu−Arg−Asn−Ser−Cys−Ala

The peptide was produced using a Vega 250 peptide synthesizer. The crude product was purified by gel filtration and reverse-phase chromatography. The major fraction obtained was judged pure by amino acid composition and sequence. The tyrosine residue was added for coupling purposes.
[a]c-myc gene product carboxyterminal sequence.
[b]Sequence of synthetic peptide used for immunization.

References

ar-Rushdi, A., K. Nishikura, J. Erikson, R. Watt, G. Rovera, and C.M. Croce. 1983. Differential expression of the translocated and of the untranslocated c-*myc* Burkitt lymphoma. *Science* **222**: 390.

Aurias, A., C. Rimbaut, D. Buffe, J. Dubousset, and A. Mazabraud. 1983. Chromosomal translocations in Ewing's sarcoma. *N. Engl. J. Med.* **309**: 496.

Colby, W.W., E.Y. Chen, D.H. Smith, and A.D. Levinson. 1983. Identification and nucleotide sequence of a human locus homologous to the v-*myc* oncogene of avian myelocytomatosis virus MC29. *Nature* **301**: 722.

Croce, C.M., M. Shander, J. Martinis, L. Cicurel, G.G. D'Ancona, T.W. Dolby, and H. Koprowski. 1979. Chromosomal location of the human immunoglobulin heavy chain genes. *Proc. Natl. Acad. Sci.* **76**: 3416.

Croce, C.M., W. Thierfelder, J. Erikson, K. Nishikura, J. Finan, G. Lenoir, and P.C. Nowell. 1983. Transcriptional activation of an unrearranged and untranslocated c-*myc* oncogene by translocation of a Cλ locus in Burkitt lymphoma. *Proc. Natl. Acad. Sci.* **80**: 6922.

Dalla Favera, R., F. Wong-Staal, and R.C. Gallo. 1982a. *onc* gene amplification in promyelocytic leukaemia cell line HL-60 and primary leukaemic cells of the same patient. *Nature* **290**: 61.

Dalla Favera, R., R.C. Gallo, A. Giallongo, and C.M. Croce. 1982b. Chromosomal localization of the human homolog (c-sis) of the Simian sarcoma virus onc gene. *Science* **218**: 686.

Dalla Favera, R., S. Martinotti, R.C. Gallo, J. Erikson, and C.M. Croce. 1983. Translocation and rearrangements of the c-myc onc-gene in human undifferentiated B-cell lymphomas. *Science* **219**: 963.

Dalla Favera, R., M. Bregni, J. Erikson, D. Patterson, R.C. Gallo, and C.M. Croce. 1982c. Assignment of the human c-myc onc-gene to the region of chromosome 8 which is translocated in Burkitt lymphoma cells. *Proc. Natl. Acad. Sci.* **79**: 7824.

Dalla Favera, R., G. Franchini, S. Martinotti, F. Wong-Staal, R.C. Gallo, and C.M. Croce. 1982d. Chromosomal assignment of the human homologues of feline sarcoma virus and avian myeloblastosis virus onc-genes. *Proc. Natl. Acad. Sci.* **79**: 4714.

Emanuel, B., E. Wang, P.C. Nowell, J. Selden, and C.M. Croce. 1984. Non-identical 22q11 breakpoint for the t(9:22) of CML and the t(8:22) of Burkitt's lymphoma. *Cytogenet. Cell Genet.* (in press).

Erikson, J., J. Martinis, and C.M. Croce. 1981. Assignment of the human genes for immunoglobulin chains to chromosome 22. *Nature* **294**: 173.

Erikson, J., J. Finan, P.C. Nowell, and C.M. Croce. 1982. Translocation of immunoglobulin V$_H$ genes in Burkitt lymphoma. *Proc. Natl. Acad. Sci.* **179**: 5611.

Erikson, J., A. ar-Rushdi, H.L. Drwinga, P.C. Nowell, and C.M. Croce. 1983a. Transcriptional activation of the c-myc oncogene in Burkitt lymphoma. *Proc. Natl. Acad. Sci.* **80**: 820.

Erikson, J., K. Nishikura, A. ar-Rushdi, J. Finan, B. Emanuel, G. Lenoir, P.C. Nowell, and C.M. Croce. 1983b. Translocation of an immunoglobulin κ locus to a region 3′ of an unrearranged c-*myc* oncogene enhances c-*myc* transcription. *Proc. Natl. Acad. Sci.* **80**: 7581.

Giallongo, A., E. Appella, R. Ricciardi, G. Rovera, and C.M. Croce. 1983. Identification of the c-*myc* oncogene product in normal and malignant B cells. *Science* **222**: 430.

Hamlin, P.H. and T.H. Rabbitts. 1983. Translocation joins c-*myc* and immunoglobulin γ1 genes in a Burkitt lymphoma revealing a third exon in the c-*myc* oncogene. *Nature* **304**: 135.

Lenoir, G.M., J.L. Preud'homme, A. Bernheim, and R. Berger. 1982. Correlation between immunoglobulin light chain expression and variant translocation in Burkitt's lymphoma. *Nature* **298**: 474.

Malcolm, S., P. Barton, C. Murphy, M.A. Ferguson-Smith, D.L. Bentley, and T.H. Rabbitts. 1982. Localization of human immunoglobulin light chain variable region genes to the short arm of chromosome 2 by *in situ* hybridization. *Proc. Natl. Acad. Sci.* **79**: 4957.

Manolov, G. and Y. Manolova. 1972. Marker band in one chromosome 14 from Burkitt lymphoma. *Nature* **237**: 33.

McBride, O.W., P.A. Heiter, G.F. Hollis, D. Swan, M.C. Otey, and P. Leder. 1982. Chromosomal location of human kappa and lambda immunoglobulin light chain constant region genes. *J. Exp. Med.* **155**: 1480.

Nishikura, K., A. ar-Rushdi, J. Erikson, R. Watt, G. Rovera, and C.M. Croce. 1983. Differential expression of the normal and of the translocated human c-myc oncogenes in B cells. *Proc. Natl. Acad. Sci.* **80**: 4822.

Nowell, P.C. and D.A. Hungerford. 1960. Chromosomes of normal and leukemic human leukocytes. *Science* **132**: 1497.

Rowley, J.D. 1973. A new consistent chromosomal abnormality in chronic myelogenous leukaemia identified by quinacrine fluorescence and Giemsa staining. *Nature* **243**: 290.

———. 1983. Identification of the constant chromosome regions. *Science* **216**: 749.

Taub, R., I. Kirsch, C. Morton, G. Lenoir, D. Swan, S. Tronick, S. Aaronson, and P. Leder. 1982. Translocation of the c-*myc* gene into the immunoglobulin heavy chain locus in human Burkitt lymphoma and murine plasmacytoma cells. *Proc. Natl. Acad. Sci.* **79**: 7837.

Turc-Carel, C., I. Philip, M.P. Berger, T. Philip, and G.M. Lenoir. 1983. Letter to the editor. *N. Engl. J. Med.* **309**: 497.

Van den Berghe, H., C. Parloir, S. Gosseye, V. Eglebienne, G. Cornu, and G. Sokal. 1979. Variant translocation in Burkitt lymphoma. *Cancer Genet. Cytogenet.* **1**: 9.

Watt, R., K. Nishikura, J. Sorrentino, A. ar-Rushdi, C.M. Croce, and G. Rovera. 1983a. The structure and nucleotide sequence of the 5′ end of the human c-*myc* gene. *Proc. Natl. Acad. Sci.* **80**: 6307.

Watt, R., L.W. Stanton, K.B. Marcu, R.C. Gallo, C.M. Croce, and G. Rovera. 1983b. Nucleotide sequence of cloned cDNA of the human c-*myc* oncogene. *Nature* **303**: 725.

Yunis, J. 1983. The chromosomal basis of human neoplasia. *Science* **221**: 227.

Zech, L., V. Haglund, N. Nilsson, and G. Klein. 1976. Characteristic chromosomal abnormalities in biopsies and lymphoid-cell lines from patients with Burkitt and non-Burkitt lymphomas. *Int. J. Cancer* **17**: 47.

Activation of *c-myc* Gene by Translocation in a Human Non-Hodgkin's Lymphoma: Transcriptional and Translational Mechanisms

A.C. Hayday, H. Saito, C. Wood, S.D. Gillies, and S. Tonegawa
Center for Cancer Research and Department of Biology, Massachusetts Institute of Technology, Cambridge, Massachusetts 02139

K. Wiman and W.S. Hayward
Memorial Sloan-Kettering Cancer Center, New York, New York 10021

Avian myelocytomatosis virus MC29 induces a broad range of tumors in chickens and will transform chicken fibroblasts and macrophages in vitro. The viral oncogene apparently responsible is *v-myc*. The *v-myc* protein is a fusion product of part of the major viral structural protein (*gag*) sequences and sequences transduced from the chicken genome (Bister et al. 1977; Alitalo et al. 1983b). The transduced sequences are derived from a cellular gene that is termed *c-myc* (Neel et al. 1982b; Robins et al. 1982; Vennstrom et al. 1982).

Activation of chicken *c-myc* has been suggested as the means by which the chronic avian leukosis virus (ALV) induces neoplastic disease. By integrating close to the *c-myc* gene, the ALV provirus can lead to enhanced levels of *c-myc* transcription (Hayward et al. 1981; Payne et al. 1982). In addition, in a human cell line (HL60) derived from an acute promyelocytic leukemia the human *c-myc* gene is amplified approximately 20-fold and there is a concomitant amplification of *c-myc* mRNA (Collins and Groudine 1982; Dalla-Favera et al. 1982a). Amplification of the *c-myc* gene has also been observed in a human colon carcinoma cell line (Alitalo et al. 1983a).

Nonrandom chromosomal translocations have been observed in a wide variety of vertebrate neoplasms (Nowell and Hungerford 1960; Klein 1981). These observations, together with the demonstration of *c-myc* activation by ALV integration, have led to the suggestion that *c-onc* genes might be activated by specific translocation events (Hayward et al. 1981; Klein 1981; Rowley 1982). In support of this notion, recent studies have shown that *c-myc* is translocated in certain lymphoid neoplasms of both mice and man. In particular, murine *c-myc* on chromosome 15 is recombined into the heavy-chain locus of mouse immunoglobulin (Ig) genes (on chromosome 12) in BALB/c plasmacytomas characterized by t(12:15) translocations (Adams et al. 1982; Calame et al. 1982; Sheng-Ong et al. 1982, Taub et al. 1982). The human *c-myc* gene has been mapped to a site on chromosome 8(q24) (Neel et al. 1982a; Taub et al. 1982) that corresponds to the breakpoint associated with translocations in Burkitt's and other non-Hodgkin's lymphomas. In a majority of Burkitt's lymphomas characterized by t(8:14)(q24;q32) translocations, the *c-myc* gene on chromosome 8 is recombined into the Ig heavy-chain (Igh) locus on chromosome 14 (Dalla-Favera et al. 1982b; Taub et al. 1982; Adams et al. 1983). Other Burkitt's lymphomas, featuring translocations t(8,22)(q24;q11) and t(2,8)(p12;q24), possibly recombine the *c-myc* gene close to the Ig λ and κ loci, respectively. Do these translocations directly activate the oncogenic potential of the *c-myc* gene? If so, what is the mechanism for the activation?

To address the above questions, we compared the structure and expression of a normal and translocated human *c-myc* gene. This comparison revealed that the translocated *c-myc* gene is transcribed from cryptic promoters that lie, ordinarily, within intron I of germline *c-myc*. Furthermore, activity at these promoters is dependent upon sequences at a distance upstream from them, in a manner analogous to the dependence of promoter activity upon enhancers. The sequences upstream do contain a potent, tissue-specific transcriptional enhancer, ordinarily associated with the human Igh genes. In addition, these studies led us to hypothesize that the expression of the *c-myc* gene product is ordinarily suppressed at the level of translation, and that this suppression may be removed as a result of *c-myc* translocation.

Results

Human *c-myc* gene consists of three exons

A two-exon structure for both the chicken (Neel et al. 1982b; Robins et al. 1982; Vennstrom et al. 1982) and human (Dalla-Favera et al. 1982c; Colby et al. 1983) *c-myc* genes has been deduced by comparing restriction maps and nucleotide sequences with those of the *v-myc* gene of MC29 virus. However, more recent sequencing analysis of a human *c-myc* cDNA clone (Watt et al. 1983) suggests the presence of a third exon upstream of these two exons. To establish the exon-intron structure of the human *c-myc* gene, a series of DNA fragments were dissected from a cloned genomic *c-myc* gene clone cAIDS4 (Fig. 1) and used as hybridization probes for

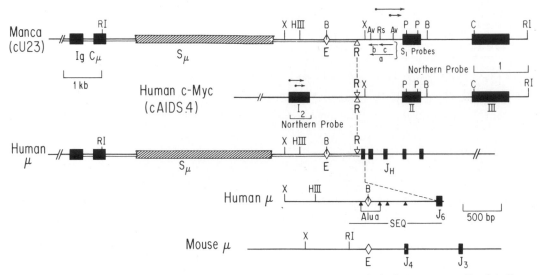

Figure 1 Three cloned segments of DNA are compared: human germline *c-myc* (cAIDS.4), human germline Igh-Cμ, and a human translocated *c-myc* gene (cU.2.3). The derivation of cosmid clones cAIDS.4 and cU.2.3 is described elsewhere (Saito et al. 1983; K. Wiman et al., in prep.). (■) Exons; (double line) chromosome 14 sequences; (single line) chromosome 8 sequences; (R) recombination point between the two; (horizontal arrows) transcription. Restriction sites: (RI) *Eco*RI; (X) *Xba*I; (HIII) *Hind*III; (Av) *Ava*I; (Rs) *Rsa*I; (P), *Pst*I; (B) *Bgl*II; (C) *Cla*I; (Alu) *Alu*I. The complete map for only the first three of these is presented. Sμ and Jₕ refer to switch and joining segments, respectively. The definition of the Jₕ segments is derived from Ravetch et al. (1981), and from our sequencing (-SEQ-) by chemical degradation (Maxam and Gilbert 1980). (E) A transcriptional enhancer element, determined initially for the mouse (Gillies et al. 1983; Neuberger and Calabi 1983) and now for the human (Hayday et al. 1984; this paper).

Northern blotting analysis of *c-myc* mRNA from HeLa cells. The results obtained by these experiments confirmed the existence of a single additional exon at 1.5 kb upstream (data not shown). Hereafter, these exons will be referred to as exons I, II, and III from 5′ to 3′ (see Fig. 1 for the exon-intron structure). The exact 3′ boundary of exon I was determined by comparing the DNA sequence of the genomic clone with that of the published cDNA. As shown in Figure 2, this boundary was assigned to nucleotide 657.

Two major transcription initiation sites in the *c-myc* gene

To localize accurately the 5′ end of exon I on the genomic DNA sequence, we carried out S1 nuclease protection experiments (Berk and Sharp 1977; Weaver and Weissmann 1979) using probes comprised of the two genomic DNA fragments thought to span the 5′ boundary of exon I. The results reported elsewhere (Saito et al. 1983) indicated that two alternative sites define the 5′ boundaries of exon I, one at nucleotide position 104 and the other 279 (see Fig. 2). TATA sequences occur upstream from each of these sites, characteristic of many eukaryotic promoters (Goldberg 1979). No sequence characteristic of splice acceptor sites (Mount 1981) precedes either of the two boundaries (note that the conserved AG dinucleotide alone is not a sufficient condition). The sizes of the *c-myc* mRNAs (2200 bp and 2030 bp plus poly[A]) predicted by summing the sizes of the three exons match well with the sizes (2.3 kb) of the mRNA detected by Northern blotting of HeLa cell RNA. In fact, a close inspection of the Northern data

(Fig. 3) indicated that the 2.3-kb band is a doublet. We conclude that the *c-myc* gene is transcribed from at least two start sites in HeLa cells. The sequences covered by the two probes used in the S1 nuclease protection experiment overlap with the 5′ end of the cDNA sequence reported by Watt et al. (1983). All the above results indicate that no additional introns split the *c-myc* gene in the 5′ region, confirming that this gene is composed of three exons.

Exon 1 constitutes a large untranslated leader segment

We determined the complete DNA sequence of exon I of the human *c-myc* gene by sequencing up to the *Xba*I site in intron I. From this point, the sequence of the remainder of the gene was available from the data of Colby et al. (1983). Within this latter area, however, certain regions, e.g., around pseudopromoters (see below) were resequenced.

One notable feature of exon I is that it is untranslatable: It contains no initiator methionine codon. In addition, it contains numerous translational stop codons in all three frames. As a consequence, the first initiator AUG remains that proposed by Colby et al. (1983), just within exon II.

A second notable feature of exon I is that a 68-nucleotide stretch of it is almost exactly complementary to a 70-bp stretch of exon II (see Figs. 2 and 4). This complementarity allows a stem-loop structure (Fig. 4) to be proposed for *c-myc* RNA. The free energy for such a structure would be about −90 kcal/mole (Tinoco et al. 1973), which is sufficient to maintain it under physiological conditions should it be able to form. This structure would sequester the initiator AUG in the loop and, according to the ''bind and scan'' model for eukaryotic translation (Kozak 1980), would render it inaccessible to efficient translation. There is ample evidence for the bind and scan model (Kozak 1978, 1980), and, in addition, it has been demonstrated that, in prokaryotes, base-pairing in mRNA can reduce its translational efficacy (Kozak and Nathans 1972; Saito and Richardson 1981).

```
SmaI                                                          TATA box              100
CCCGGGTTCC CAAAGCAGAG GGCGTGGGGG AAAAGAAAAA AGATCCTCTC TCGCTAATCT CCGCCCACCG GCCCTTTATA ATGCGAGGGT CTGGACGGCT

  ↓CAP site 1                                                       TaqI               200
GAGGACCCCC GAGCTGTGCT GCTCGCGGCC GCCACCGCCG GGCCCCGGCC GTCCCTGGCT CCCCTCCTGC CTCGAGAAGG GCAGGGCTTC TCAGAGGCTT

                           TATA box                              ↓CAP site 2          300
GGCGGGAAAA AGAACGGAGG GAGGGATCGC GCTGAGTATA AAAGCCGGTT TTCGGGGCTT TATCTAACTC GCTGTAGTAA TTCCAGCGAG AGGCAGAGGG

                                                                                      400
AGCGAGCGGG CGGCCGGCTA GGGTGGAAGA GCCGGGCGAG CAGAGCTGCG CTGCGGGCGT CCTGGGAAGG GAGATCCGGA GCGAATAGGG GGCTTCGCCT

                                                                                      500
CTGGCCCAGC CCTCCCGCTG ATCCCCCAGC CAGCGGTCCG CAACCCTTGC CGCATCCACG AAACTTTGCC CATAGCAGCG GGCGGGCACT TTGCACTGGA

                                                                                      600
ACTTACAACA CCCGAGCAAG GACGGGACTC TCCCGACGCG GGGAGGCTAT TCTGCCCATT TGGGGACACT TCCCCGCCGC TGCCAGGACC CGCTTCTCTG

                PvuII                                   ↓Splice site                  700
AAAGGCTCTC CTTGCAGCTG CTTAGACGCT GGATTTTTTT CGGGTAGTGG AAAACCAGGT AAGCACCGAA GTCCACTTGC CTTTTAATTT ATTTTTTTAT

           TaqI                                                                       800
CACTTTAATG CTGAGATGAG TCGAATGCCT AAATAGGGTG TCTTTTCTCC CATTCCTGCG CTATTGACAC TTTTCTCAGA GTAGTTATGG TAACTGGGGC

                                                                                      900
TGGGGTGGGG GGTAATCCAG AACTGGATCG GGGTAAAGTG ACTTGTCAAG ATGGGAGAGG AGAAGGCAGA GGGAAAACGG GAATGGTTTT TAAGACTACC
                                     Rearrangement point
   TaqI                              in "Manca"                                        1000
CTTTCGAGAT TTCTGCCTTA TGAATATATT CACGCTGACT CCCGGCCGGT CGGACATTCC TGCTTTATTG TGTTAATTGC TCTCTGGGTT TTGGGGGGCT
                                              ▲
              SstI                                                                     1100
GGGGGTTGCT TTGCGGTGGG CAGAAAGCCC CTTGCATCCT GAGCTCCTTG GAGTAGGGAC CGCATATCGC CTGTGTGAGC CAGATCGCTC CGCAGTCGCT

                                                                                      1200
GACTTGTCCC CGTCTCCGGG AGGGCATTTA AATTTCGGCT CACCGCATTT CTGACAGCCG GAGACGGACA CTGCGGCGCG TCCCGCCCGC CTGTCCCCGC

                                                             XbaI                     1300
GGCGATTCCA ACCCGCCCTG ATCCTTTTAA GAAGTTGGCA TTTGGCTTTT TAAAAAGCCA TAATACAAGT TAAAACCTGG GTCTCTAGAG GTGTTAGGAC

                                                                                      1400
GTGGTGTTGG GTAGGCGCAG GCAGGGGAAA AGGGAGGCGA GGATGTGTCC GATTCTCCTG GAATCGTTGA CTTGGAAAAA CCAGGGCGAA TCTCCGCACC

                                                                                      2200
CAGCCCTGAC TCCCCTGCCG CGGCCGCCCT CGGG..............................TAGC TCTGCAAGGG GAGAGGTTCG GGACTGTGGC

                                                             ↓Splice site   2297
GCGCACTGCG CGCTGCGCCA GGTTTCCGCA CCAAGACCCC TTTAACTCAA GACTGCCTCC CGCTTTGTGT GCCCCGCTCC AGCAGCCTCC CGCGACG

                                          TaqI                                 2378
ATG CCC CTC AAC GTT AGC TTC ACC AAC AGG AAC TAT GAC CTC GAC TAC GAC TCG GTG CAG CCG TAT TTC TAC TGC GAC GAG
Met Pro Leu Asn Val Ser Phe Thr Asn Arg Asn Tyr Asp Leu Asp Tyr Asp Ser Val Gln Pro Tyr Phe Tyr Cys Asp Glu

                                             PstI                                      2459
GAG GAG AAC TTC TAC CAG CAG CAG CAG CAG AGC GAG CTG CAG CCC CCG GCG CCC AGC GAG GAT ATC TGG AAG AAA TTC GAG
Glu Glu Asn Phe Tyr Gln Gln Gln Gln Gln Ser Glu Leu Gln Pro Pro Ala Pro Ser Glu Asp Ile Trp Lys Lys Phe Glu

                                                                                      2540
CTG CTG CCC ACC CCG CCC CTG TCC CCT AGC CGC CGC TCC GGG CTC TGC TCG CCC TCC TAC GTT GCG GTC ACA CCC TTC TCC
Leu Leu Pro Thr Pro Pro Leu Ser Pro Ser Arg Arg Ser Gly Leu Cys Ser Pro Ser Tyr Val Ala Val Thr Pro Phe Ser

                                                                                      2615
CTT CGG GGA GAC AAC GAC GGC GGT GGC GGG AGC TTC TCC ACG GCC GAC CAG CTG GAG ATG GTG ACC GAG CTG CTG ........
Leu Arg Gly Asp Asn Asp Gly Gly Gly Gly Ser Phe Ser Thr Ala Asp Gln Leu Glu Met Val Thr Glu Leu Lue ........
```

Figure 2 Nucleotide sequence of exon I of the human *c-myc* gene and the flanking region. Also included is the 5′ end of exon II whose sequence was determined by Colby et al. (1983). Intron and 5′ untranscribed regions are indicated by italics. Predicted amino acid sequence is shown under the nucleotide sequence. The upward arrow indicates the breakage point of the translocation in Manca; downward arrows indicate the transcription initiation sites or splice sites. The two sequences in exon I and exon II that are complementary to each other are underlined.

In a non-Hodgkin's lymphoma, Manca, an active *c-myc* gene is translocated to a site between Ig-J$_H$ and Ig C$_\mu$

The non-Hodgkin's lymphoma Manca (Nishikori et al. 1984) shows a chromosomal translocation (t(8,14)(q24; q32) that is characteristic of many Burkitt's lymphomas (Klein 1981). In situ hybridization of a *v-myc* probe prepared from the chicken acute leukemia virus MC29 (Lautenberger et al. 1981) to Manca chromosomes indicated that the human *c-myc* locus is on that portion of chromosome 8 (Neel et al. 1982a) that is translocated (data not shown).

We constructed a cosmid library from Manca DNA, screened it with the *v-myc* probe, and isolated a genomic DNA clone (clone cU.2.3) spanning the translocation breakpoint. A detailed map of clone cU.2.3 in the region of *c-myc*-Ig linkage was derived by restriction analysis and partial DNA sequencing. It was compared with maps, derived in the same way, of human germline Igh C$_\mu$ and human germline *c-myc*, contained on plasmid pH18-C1-10 and cosmid cAIDS4, respectively (Fig. 1). It can be deduced that in Manca DNA, the human *c-myc* gene on chromosome 8 is fused head-to-head with DNA sequences on chromosome 14, about 6.5 kb 5′ to the first exon of Igh C$_\mu$. The junction on chromosome 14 lies between S$_\mu$ and J$_H$6, at a point that is not normally used for the productive rearrangement of an Igh gene. The junction on chromosome 8 occurs between exons I and II of the *c-myc* gene. As a result, the Manca DNA cloned in cU.2.3 contains neither exon I nor the normal transcriptional start sites for the human *c-myc*. It does, however, retain the initiator AUG and downstream sequences of exons II and III. The *c-myc* exons II and III are fused to sequences from Igh C$_\mu$ that include a region E (see Fig. 1). Region E is a stretch of DNA, between C$_\mu$ and J$_H$, that is in an analogous location to sequences in the mouse genome that have been shown to have tissue-specific transcriptional enhancing activity (Gillies et al. 1983).

The translocated *c-myc* gene is transcribed from multiple sites within the intron I of its normal counterpart

Northern analysis of RNA from Manca cells indicated a high level of *c-myc* transcription (Fig. 3). It is clear that there are multiple transcripts hybridizing to the *c-myc* Northern probe (see Fig. 1). Probes indicated in Figure 1 were used in S1 nuclease protection experiments (Berk and Sharp 1977; Weaver and Weissmann 1979) to map precisely the transcription initiation points of the translocated *c-myc* gene (Hayday et al. 1984). In summary, the major initiation site for the translocated *c-myc* gene is at around nucleotide 364. As shown in Figure 3, sequences 30 bp and 70 bp upstream of this site suggest that this site may be a very efficient promoter. By primer extension of all S1 probes shown in Figure 1, we judge this to be the 5′-most start site for the translocated gene. There are additional start sites that lie closer to exon II, notably at around nucleotide 870. This site is preceded at 28 bp distance by TTTATT. Between these sites there are further S1-sensitive sites, but their designation as initiation sites is uncertain, either because of lack of confirmation by primer extension or because there is faint S1 sensitivity at these sites merely in the presence of yeast carrier RNA.

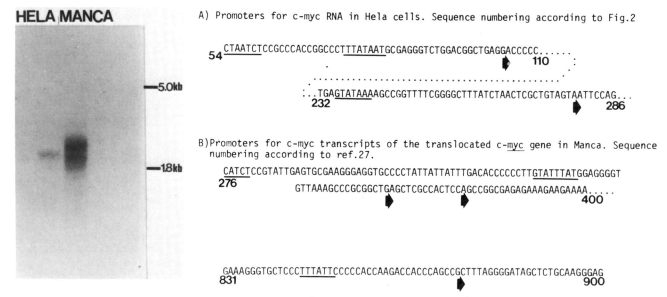

Figure 3 Northern analyses of mRNA from HeLa (1 μg) and Manca (0.3 μg) cells. mRNA was analyzed after the protocols of Thomas (1980) using Northern probe 1 (see Fig. 1) as probe. Ribosomal RNA species were used as size markers. Use of Northern probe 2 (see Fig. 1) continued to detect RNA in the HeLa cell sample, but not in the Manca cell sample (not shown). At right are indicated the DNA sequences about the promoters that we propose generate the transcripts shown. Sequence data in B derives from Colby et al. (1983), but in many places was reconfirmed by chemical degradation (Maxam and Gilbert 1980). Underlined are sequences similar to those consistently found at analogous positions in RNA polymerase II promoters (Breathnach and Chambon 1981).

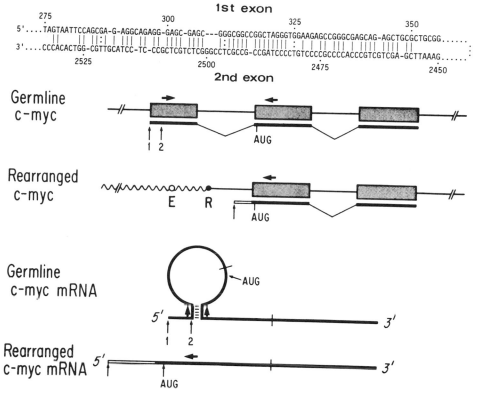

Figure 4 (*A*) Internal sequence complementarity seen in exon I and exon II of the germ line (untranslocated) *c-myc* gene. The nucleotide numbers are the same as those in Fig. 2. The hydrogen bond-forming bases are connected by bars. G-T pairs (which as G-U pairs in RNA are allowed to make weak hydrogen bonds) are indicated by dots. Deletions indicated by dashes are included to maximize the complementarity. (*B*) Schematic representations of the transcription and splicing of the germline (untranslocated) and translocated *c-myc* genes. The germline *c-myc* gene is transcribed from one of the two initiation sites 5′ of exon I, whereas the translocated *c-myc* gene is transcribed from initiation sites within the intron. Only one of the initiation sites in intron I is shown. (*C*) Possible secondary structures of *c-myc* RNA. The germline *c-myc* RNA can form a stem-loop structure, with the initiation AUG codon within the loop: The *c-myc* mRNA from the translocated *c-myc* gene cannot.

If there are no splices between these varied initiation points and exon II, the result would be a series of transcripts ranging in size from 1660 bp to 2300 bp, not including the poly(A) tail (Proudfoot and Brownlee 1976). That this is the case is suggested both by the coincidence of the S1 and primer extension analyses (not shown) and by cDNA cloning. The latter reveals a contiguous transcript extending upstream from exon II at least until position 660. Beyond this point, the S1 nuclease-sensitive sites have been confirmed as initiation (as opposed to splice) points by primer extension (data not shown).

A human tissue-specific transcriptional enhancer element is located between J_H and C_μ

It has previously been shown that sequences derived from the J_H-C_μ region of the murine Igh locus contain a DNA element that enhances the transcription of the associated gene in a manner independent of both position and orientation (Banerji et al. 1983; Gillies et al. 1983). Since (in Manca DNA) the *c-myc* gene is translocated just 300 bp downstream of the human J_H cluster (Fig. 1), we suspected that the high level of *c-myc* transcription in Manca cells (Fig. 3) might be due to a human

enhancer element, which may be located in an analogous region (referred to as E in Fig. 1).

To test this hypothesis, we first attempted to identify the putative human enhancer element. For this purpose, the 2.2-kb *Xba*I fragment (see Fig. 1) containing most of the sequence between the J_H cluster and S_μ, plus about 330 bp derived from the 5′-flanking region of the translocated, truncated *c-myc* gene, was inserted into the *Eco*RI site of pSER (Gillies et al. 1983). This plasmid was derived from pSV2-*gpt* (Mulligan and Berg 1980) by deletion from the latter of the SV40 enhancer sequences. As a result, pSER transforms cells to mycophenolic acid resistance (gpt[+] phenotype) at a frequency greatly reduced by comparison to that of pSV2-*gpt* (5×10^{-6} vs. 10^{-4} in J558L cells). The original level of transformation can be restored by the insertion, into the *Eco*RI site of pSER, of the murine Igh gene-associated enhancer element (Gillies et al. 1983). This was interpreted to mean that the inserted mouse DNA enhanced *Eco*gpt transcription (Gillies et al. 1983). The insertion, in either orientation, of the human 2.2-kb *Xba*I fragment into the *Eco*RI site of pSER (2.3 kb upstream of the *Eco*gpt gene) restored the gpt(+) transformation efficiency of J558L cells to a level exceeding even that of pSV2-*gpt*. The transformation efficiency of pSV2-*gpt* was itself increased 5–10-fold by insertion of the *Xba*I fragment into the *Eco*RI site of that plasmid. By contrast, insertion into the *Eco*RI site (of either pSER of pSV2-*gpt*) of other DNA fragments from either the murine or human Igh locus, did not significantly affect transformation frequencies. In addition, as for the murine Igh enhancer, the potent effect of the human *Xba*I fragment on transformation was specific to lymphoid cells. By comparison with pSV2-*gpt*, pSER molecules containing the *Xba*I fragment, in either orientation, were over 100 times reduced in their ability to transform rodent fibroblasts. In a further experiment, the 2.2-kb *Xba*I fragment was dissected by cleavage with *Alu*I, and the resulting fragments also were tested in the pSER assay. Most, if not all, the enhancing activity could be attributed to the 279-bp fragment, *Alu* a (see Fig. 1).

These transformation experiments strongly suggest that the 2.2-kb human *Xba*I fragment carries within it a tissue-specific transcriptional enhancer element. To prove this point more directly, we examined the effect of this DNA fragment on the transcription of a mouse Igγ2b gene. In short, it was found that in transfected cells, insertion of the *Xba*I fragment could restore Igγ2b transcription to a murine construct that lacked the murine Igh-associated enhancer element (Hayday et al. 1984). The direction and site of insertion was largely irrelevant.

Finally, the nucleotide sequence of a portion of the human *Xba*I fragment (shown to have enhancing activity) was compared with that previously obtained for the analogous area of mouse DNA. There was extensive homology over several hundred nucleotides. Like the mouse sequence, the human sequence contains "corelike" elements (Weiher et al. 1983): The rest of the homology presumably relates to the tissue-specific nature of both enhancers.

Promoters for the translocated *c-myc* gene in Manca are activated by upstream sequences

To investigate whether the high level of *c-myc* transcription in Manca cells was due to the proximity of an enhancer-type element, the transcription of the translocated *c-myc* gene was studied in mouse myeloma cells. J558L cells were transformed by spheroplast fusion (Sandri-Goldin et al. 1983), with either of two plasmids, pSV2.26 or pSV2Δ4. The former contains the 11.7-kb *Eco*RI fragment from cU.2.3 (see Fig. 1) cloned into the *Eco*RI site of pSV2-*gpt* (Mulligan and Berg 1980). The 11.7-kb *Eco*RI fragment contains the translocated and truncated *c-myc* gene, plus about 8 kb of 5′-flanking sequence that includes the Igh enhancer. Plasmid pSV2Δ4 contains a 9.5-kb *Eco*RI fragment cloned into the *Eco*RI site of pSV2-*gpt*. This 9.5-kb fragment is the 11.7-kb *Eco*RI fragment of cU.2.3 from which the central 2.2-kb *Xba*I fragment has been removed. This deletion removes sequences that we identify as having transcriptional enhancing activity (see above).

After transformation with these plasmids, gpt(+) transformants of J558L cells were isolated and assessed for the presence of exogenous DNA. In most cases in which the transforming DNA was pSV2.26, there are single copies of the exogenous DNA (Fig. 5). In most cases, the integration is within the 11.7-kb *Eco*RI fragment, frequently disrupting the *c-myc* gene itself and leading to detectable *Eco*RI fragments smaller than 11.7 kb. By contrast, cells transfected with pSV2Δ4 contain multiple, intact copies of the transfecting species. In addition, the disruption of the *c-myc* sequences after transformation by pSV2.26 was specific to lymphoid cells. As shown in Figure 5, fibroblasts transformed with pSV2.26-assimilated, tandem, intact copies of transfecting DNA. The reasons for this difference in copy number can only be speculated upon (Hayday et al. 1984).

Fortunately, several clones (26.1, 26.2, 26.4, 26.7, 26.8) did contain, intact, the transfected *c-myc* gene and sequences 5′ to it that included the Igh enhancer. These clones were assessed for their transcription of the transfected DNA. As shown in Figure 6, use of S1 probe a (Fig. 1) detected transcription of *c-myc* RNA from the same site as in Manca. By contrast, the clones Δ4.1 and Δ4.2 (data not shown for Δ4.2) contained almost no RNA that would form an S1-resistant hybrid with probe a. In addition, Northern analysis of Δ4.1 and Δ4.2 RNA showed no detectable *c-myc* expression over and above that endogenous to J558L cells (Stanton et al. 1983). Since all transformed cells are maintained under continual selection for *Ecogpt* gene activity, the transfected DNA in Δ4.1 and Δ4.2 cannot be sequestered in a transcriptionally silent area. Rather, it is the removal of sequences beginning 350 bp 5′ to the most upstream detectable start that appears to have dramatically reduced transcription of the translocated *c-myc* gene. Such deletions are characteristic of enhancer mutations (Benoist and Chambon 1981).

The product of the translocated *c-myc* gene may be overexpressed at the translational level

In addition to coming under the influence of the Igh enhancer element, the translocated *c-myc* gene in Manca cells is truncated by loss of exon I. Since the initiator AUG is in exon II, transcripts initiating from the "pseudopromoters," described above, can presumably encode the same *myc* protein as is encoded by germline *c-myc*. (There are no AUG codons between the pseudopromoters and exon II.) However, because exon I is absent from these transcripts, the initiator AUG is no longer sequestered in an inaccessible loop (Fig. 4). Therefore, we would predict that transcripts of the translocated *c-myc* gene will be translated much more efficiently than those of the germline gene.

Discussion

To date, precise sites of *c-myc* rearrangements have been mapped for only a few Burkitt's and non-Hodgkin's lymphomas (Adams et al. 1983; Neuberger and Calabi 1983; K. Wiman et al., in prep; this study). Among these, at least three (Lou, W1, and Manca) have rearrangement sites within exon I or intron I. Similarly, in the three murine plasmacytomas (J558, M167, and M603) for which *myc*

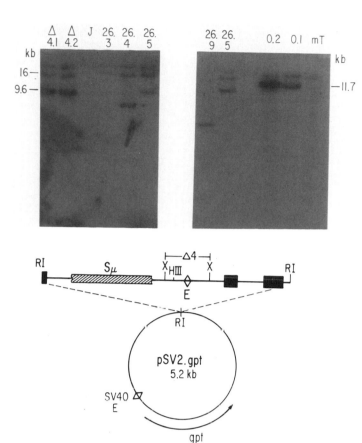

Figure 5 Southern analysis of human *c-myc*-reactive DNA sequences in J558 transformants. DNA from the clones indicated was cleaved with *Eco*RI and, after electrophoresis and transfer, was probed with Northern probe 1 (see Fig. 1). The transfecting DNA species, pSV2.26, is shown below, as well as the deletion that gave rise to pSV2.Δ4. (J) J558L; (mT) parental rat fibroblasts; (0.1, 0.2) sisters of these transformed with pSV2.26. The upper two bands in J and its transformed sister cells are endogenous to J558L cells (Stanton et al. 1983), and the upper band in the mT-derived clones, endogenous to mT cells. mT cells were a kind gift of F. Cuzin. Sizes of fragments were estimated from coelectrophoresis of λDNA cleavage products.

rearrangements have been documented at the nucleotide level, either a complete exon I or the normal transcriptional promoter is lost (Calame et al. 1982; Adams et al. 1983). In addition, Southern gel blotting experiments indicate that the translocation breakpoint is either within exon I or intron I in several other murine plasmacytomas. In short, the loss of exon I may be a feature common to many human Burkitt's lymphomas and most BALB/c plasmacytomas in which *c-myc* is rearranged. Therefore, the overproduction of the *myc* gene product via a translational mechanism of the sort suggested here may be a common feature for cells harboring these translocations.

The above mechanism may also play a role in ALV-induced B-cell lymphomas. The vast majority of proviral integrations in these tumors are located within a region that would correspond to intron I of human *c-myc* (i.e., 0–1 kb upstream from exon II of chicken *c-myc* [Neel et al. 1982b; Payne et al. 1982; M. Goodenow and W. Hayward, unpubl.]). Although the precise boundaries of exon I in the chicken *c-myc* gene have not been defined, sequencing data have revealed a region within the putative exon I that would form a stable stem-loop structure with sequence in exon II (C.-K. Shih et al., unpubl.) in a manner analogous to that described here for human *c-myc* gene.

There are cases where *c-myc* rearrangements occur either downstream (e.g., Payne et al. 1982) at some distance from the *c-myc* gene (e.g., Sheng-Ong et al. 1982) and where it is therefore not easy to apply the translational model for the activation of the *c-myc* gene. In these cases, an overproduction of *c-myc* may be due to transcriptional effects. In fact, a number of studies showed that the level of *c-myc* RNA is generally higher in Burkitt's lymphomas and mouse myelomas than in nontumorigenic human lymphoblastoid lines or normal B cells (Adams et al. 1982; Erikson et al. 1983; Marcu et al. 1983; Mushinski et al. 1983), although the degree of augmentation varies widely, from only marginal (two- to threefold) to substantial (over 10-fold). In Manca, the case described here, the level of the *c-myc* RNA is particularly high. We demonstrate in the present study that in Manca cells the structural *c-myc* gene is translocated to the Ig heavy-chain genetic locus, where it is transcribed from previously cryptic promoters located in what is ordinarily intron I of the *c-myc* gene. The activity of these promoters is dependent upon sequences over 350 bp upstream from them, in a fashion reminiscent of the dependence of promoter activity upon enhancers. Furthermore, we demonstrate that sequences in this region include a potent, lymphoid-specific transcriptional enhancer element, ordinarily involved in the activation of human immunoglobulin, heavy-chain gene transcription. This element is highly homologous to the enhancer element in analogous location in the mouse genome. It may be this element that, in Manca, is responsible for *c-myc*

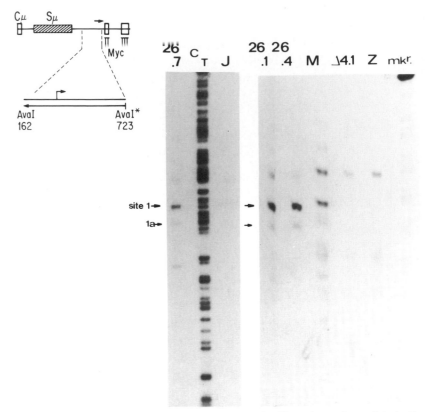

Figure 6 S1 analysis of human *c-myc* mRNA in Manca cells (M), J558L cells, (J), and transformed derivatives of J558L cells, 26.1, 26.4, 26.7 and Δ4.1. The probe was strand-separated S1 probe a (see Fig. 1) as indicated. C/T is a pyrimidine analysis of the sense strand of this fragment. Strand separation and sequencing were by Maxam and Gilbert (1980) with a modification to the former suggested by P. Jat. (Z) Probe alone plus yeast RNA; (arrows) fragments specific to the addition of lymphoid cell RNA. Electrophoresis was on a 6% urea-acrylamide gel for approximately 7 hr.

activation. In the majority of cases of Burkitt's lymphomas and murine plasmacytomas studied to date, the *c-myc* gene is translocated to one of the switch recombination (S) regions and is present on the chromosome that does not carry the defined Igh-associated enhancer. This suggests that either additional enhancer elements associated with Ig genes are yet to be identified, or one or more entirely different mechanism(s) operate(s) for the activation of *c-myc* transcription. One such mechanism has recently been suggested by Croce and his collegues (Nishikura et al. 1983). According to this model, the normal *c-myc* gene is under a negative control, possibly by autorepression, and the translocation releases the *c-myc* gene from this repression. Whether such a mechanism indeed operates or not remains to be tested.

In summary, there clearly exist multiple mechanisms by which the *c-myc* gene can be activated in cancerous cells. These include its amplification in promyelocytic leukemia, and its transcriptional activation by nearby viral elements in ALV-induced lymphomas. On the basis of the present study, we wish to add to this list two additional mechanisms, namely an activation by a translational mechanism that occurs as the result of the gene's disruption during translocation and a transcriptional ac-

tivation of previously cryptic promoters in the *c-myc* gene by, most likely, an enhancer-dependent mechanism.

Acknowledgments

We are indebted to Lena Angman, John McMaster, and Anne Maxwell for excellent technical support, and to Eleanor Basel for painstaking preparation of the manuscript. A.C.H. thanks the Imperial Cancer Research Fund, London, and K. Wiman, the European Molecular Biology Organization for travel and long-term fellowships, respectively. This work was supported by grants AI-17879 (S.T.), CA-14051 (a core grant to S. Luria), and CA-34502 (W.H.) from the National Institutes of Health. Finally, we thank C.M. Croce (Wistar Institute) for a previous gift of pH18-CL-10.

References

Adams, J.M., S. Gerondakis, E. Webb, L.M. Corcoran, and S. Cory. 1983. Cellular *myc* gene is altered by chromosome translocation to an immunoglobulin locus in murine plasmacytomas, and is rearranged similarly in human Burkitt lymphomas. *Proc. Natl. Acad. Sci.* **80**: 1982.

Adams, J.M., S. Gerondakis, E. Webb, J. Mitchell, O. Bernard, and S. Cory 1982. Transcriptionally active DNA region that rearranges frequently in murine lymphoid tumors. *Proc. Natl. Acad. Sci.* **79**: 6966.

Alitalo, K., M. Schwab, C.C. Lin, H.E. Varmus, and J.M. Bishop. 1983. Homogeneously staining chromosomal regions contain amplified copies of an abundantly expressed cellular oncogene (c-myc) in malignant neuroendocrine cells from a human colon carcinoma. *Proc. Natl. Acad. Sci.* **80:** 1707.

Alitalo, K., J.M. Bishop, D.H. Smith, E.Y. Chen, W.W. Colby, and A.D. Levinson. 1983b. Nucleotide sequence of the v-myc oncogene of avian retrovirus, MC29. *Proc. Natl. Acad. Sci.* **80:** 100.

Banerji, J., L. Olson, and W. Schaffner. 1983. A lymphocyte-specific cellular enhancer is located downstream of the joining region in immunoglobulin heavy chain genes. *Cell* **33:** 729.

Benoist, C. and P. Chambon. 1981. *In vivo* sequence requirements of the SV40 early promoter region. *Nature* **290:** 304.

Berk, A.J. and P.A. Sharp. 1977. Sizing and mapping of early adenovirus mRNAs by gel electrophoresis of S1 endonuclease-digested hybrids. *Cell* **12:** 721.

Bister, K., M.J. Hayman, and P.K. Vogt 1977. Defectiveness of avian myelocytomatosis virus MC29: Isolation of long-term non-producer cultures and analysis of virus specific polypeptide synthesis. *Virology* **82:** 431.

Breathnach, R. and P. Chambon. 1981. Organization and expression of eukaryotic split genes, coding for protein. *Annu. Rev. Biochem.* **50:** 349.

Calame, K., S. Kim, P. Lalley, R. Hill, M. Davis and L. Hood. 1982. Molecular cloning of translocations involving chromosome 15 and the immunoglobulin Cα gene from chromosome 12 in two murine plasmacytomas. *Proc. Natl. Acad. Sci.* **79:** 6994.

Colby, W.W., E.Y. Chen, D.H. Smith, and A.D. Levinson. 1983. Identification and nucleotide sequence of a human locus homologous to the v-myc oncogene of avian myelomacytomatosis virus MC29. *Nature* **301:** 722.

Collins, S. and M. Groudine. 1982. Amplification of endogenous myc-related DNA sequences in a human myeloid leukemia cell line. *Nature* **296:** 679.

Dalla-Favera, R., F. Wong-Staal, and R.C. Gallo. 1982a. onc gene amplification in promyelocytic leukemia cell line, HL-60, and primary leukemic cells of the same patient. *Nature* **299:** 61.

Dalla-Favera, R., M. Bregni, J. Erikson, D. Patterson, R. Gallo, and C.M. Croce. 1982b. Human c-myc oncogene is located on the region of chromosome 8 that is translocated in Burkitt lymphoma cells. *Proc. Natl. Acad. Sci.* **79:** 7824.

Dalla-Favera, R., E.P. Gelmann, S. Martinotti, G. Franchini, T.S. Papas, R.C. Gallo, and F. Wong-Staal. 1982c. Cloning and characterization of different human sequences related to the onc gene (v-myc) of avian myelaytomatosis virus (MC29). *Proc. Natl. Acad. Sci.* **79:** 6497.

Erikson, J., A. Ar-Rushdi, H.L. Drwinga, P.C. Nowell, and C.M. Croce. 1983. Transcriptional activation of the translocated c-myc oncogene in Burkitt lymphoma. *Proc. Natl. Acad. Sci.* **80:** 820.

Gillies, S.D., S.L. Morrison, V.T. Oi, and S. Tonegawa. 1983. A tissue-specific transcriptional enhancer element is located in the major intron of a rearranged immunoglobulin heavy chain gene. *Cell* **33:** 717.

Goldberg, M. 1979. "Sequence analysis of *Drosophila* histone genes." Ph.D. thesis, Stanford University, Stanford, California.

Hayday, A.C., S.D. Gillies, H. Saito, C. Wood, K. Wiman, W.S. Hayward, and S. Tonegawa. 1984. Activation of translocated human c-myc gene by an enhancer in the immunoglobulin heavy chain locus. *Nature* **307:** 334.

Hayward, W.S., B.G. Neel, and S.M. Astrin. 1981. Activation of a cellular onc gene by promoter insertion in ALV-induced lymphoid leukosis. *Nature* **290:** 475.

Klein, G. 1981. The role of gene dosage and genetic transpositions in carcinogenesis. *Nature* **294:** 313.

Kozak, M. 1978. How do eukaryotic ribosomes select initiation regions in messenger RNA? *Cell:* **25:** 1109.

————. 1980. Evaluation of the "scanning model" for initiation of protein synthesis in eucaryotes. *Cell* **22:** 7.

Kozak, M. and D. Nathans. 1972. Translation of the genome of a ribonucleic acid bacteriophage. *Bacteriol. Rev.* **36:** 109.

Lautenberger, J.A., R.A. Shultz, C.F. Garon, P.N. Tsichlis, and T.S. Papas. 1981. Molecular cloning of avian myelocytomatosis virus (MC29) transforming sequences. *Proc. Natl. Acad. Sci.* **78:** 1518.

Marcu, K.B., L.J. Harris, L.W. Stanton, J. Erikson, R. Watt, and C.M. Croce. 1983. Transcriptionally active c-myc oncogene is contained within NIARD, a DNA sequence associated with chromosome translocation in B-cell neoplasia. *Proc. Natl. Acad. Sci.* **80:** 519.

Maxam, A. and W. Gilbert. 1980. Sequencing of end labeled DNA with base specific chemical cleavages. *Methods Enzymol.* **65:** 499.

Mount, S.M. 1981. A catalogue of splice junction sequences. *Nucleic Acids Res.* **10:** 459.

Mulligan, R.G. and P. Berg. 1980. Expression of a bacterial gene in mammalian cells. *Science* **209:** 1422.

Mushinski, I.F., S.R. Bauer, M. Potter, and E.P. Reddy. 1983. Increased expression of myc-related oncogene mRNA characterizes most BALB/c plastocytomas induced by pristane or Ableson murine leukemia virus. *Proc. Natl. Acad. Sci.* **80:** 1073.

Neel, B.G., S.C. Jhanwar, R.S.K. Chaganti, and W.S. Hayward. 1982a. Two human c-onc genes are located in the long arm of chromosome 8. *Proc. Natl. Acad. Sci.* **79:** 7842.

Neel, B.G., G.P. Gasic, C.E. Rogler, A.M. Skalka, G. Ju, F. Hishinuma, T. Papas, S.M. Astrin, and W.S. Hayward. 1982b. Molecular analysis of the c-myc locus in normal tissue and in avian leukosis virus-induced lymphomas. *J. Virol.* **44:** 158.

Neuberger, M. and F. Calabi. 1983. Reciprocal chromosome translocation between c-myc and immunoglobulin γ2b genes. *Nature* **305:** 240.

Nishikori, M., H. Hansen, S. Jhanwar, J. Fried, P. Sordillo, B. Koziner, K. Lloyd, and B. Clarkson 1984. Establishment of a near-tetraploid B-cell lymphoma line with duplication of the 8;14 translocation. *Cancer Genet. Cytogenet.* **12:** 39.

Nishikura, K., A. Ar-Rushdi, J. Erikson, R. Watt, G. Rovera, and C.M. Croce. 1983. Differential expression of the normal and of the translocated human c-myc oncogenes in B cells. *Proc. Natl. Acad. Sci.* **80:** 4822.

Nowell, P.C. and D.A. Hungerford. 1960. A minute chromosome in human chronic granulocytic leukemia. *Science* **132:** 1497.

Payne, G.S., J.M. Bishop, and H.E. Varmus. 1982. Multiple arrangements of viral DNA and an activated host oncogene in bursal lymphomas. *Nature* **295:** 209.

Proudfoot, N.J. and G.G. Brownlee. 1976. 3′ Non-coding region sequences in eukaryotic messenger RNA. *Nature* **263:** 211.

Ravetch, J.V., U. Siebenlist, S. Korsmeyer, T. Waldman, and P. Leder. 1981. Structure of the human immunoglobulin μ locus: Characterisation of embryonic and rearranged J and D genes. *Cell* **27:** 583.

Robins, T., K. Bister, C. Garon, T. Papas, and P. Duesberg. 1982. Structural relationship between a normal chicken DNA locus and the transforming gene of the avian acute leukemia virus MC29. *J. Virol.* **41:** 635.

Rowley, J.D. 1982. Identification of the constant chromosome regions involved in human haematologic malignant disease. *Science* **216:** 749.

Saito, H. and C.C. Richardson. 1981. Processing of mRNA by ribonuclease III regulates expression of gene 1.2 of bacteriophage, T7. *Cell* **27:** 533.

Saito, H., A.C. Hayday, K. Wiman, W.S. Hayward, and S. Tonegawa. 1983. Activation of the c-myc gene by translocation: A model for translational control. *Proc. Natl. Acad. Sci.* **80:** 7476.

Sandri-Goldin, R.M., A.L. Goldin, M. Levine, and J.C. Glorioso.

1981. High-frequency transfer of cloned Herpes simplex virus type 1 sequences to mammalian cells by protoplast fusion. *Mol. Cell. Biol.* **1:** 743.

Shen-Ong, G.L.C., E.J. Keath, S.P. Piccoli, and M.D. Cole. 1982. Novel *myc* oncogene RNA from abortive immunoglobulin-gene recombination in mouse plasmacytomas. *Cell* **31:** 443.

Stanton, L.W., R. Watt, and K.B. Marcu. (1983). Translocation, breakage, and truncated transcripts of c-*myc* oncogene in murine plasmacytomas. *Nature* **303:** 401.

Taub, R., I. Kirsch, C. Morton, G. Lenoir, D. Swan, S. Tronicle, S. Aaronson, and P. Leder. 1982. Translocation of the c-*myc* gene into the immunoglobulin heavy chain locus in human Burkitt lymphoma and murine plasmacytoma cells. *Proc. Natl. Acad. Sci.* **79:** 7837.

Thomas, P.S. 1980. Hybridization of denatured RNA and small DNA fragments transferred to nitrocellulose. *Proc. Natl. Acad. Sci.* **77:** 5201.

Tinoco, I., Jr., P.N. Borer, B. Dangler, M.D. Levine, O.C. Uhlenbeck, D.M. Crothers, and J. Gralla. 1973. Improved estimation of secondary structure in ribonucleic acids. *Nat. New Biol.* **246:** 40.

Vennstrom, B., D. Sheiness, J. Zabielski, and J. Bishop. 1982. Isolation and characterization of c-*myc*, a cellular homologue of the oncogene (v-*myc*) of avian myelocytomatosis virus, strain 29. *J. Virol.* **42:** 773.

Watt, R., L.W. Stanton, K.B. Marcu, R.C. Gallo, C.M. Croce, and G. Rovera. 1983. Nucleotide sequence of cloned cDNA of human c-*myc* oncogene. *Nature* **303:** 725.

Weaver, R.F. and C. Weissmann. 1979. Mapping of RNA by a modification of the Berk-Sharp procedure: The 5′ termini of 15S β globin mRNA precursor and mature 10S β globin mRNA have identical map coordinates. *Nucleic Acids Res.* **7:** 1175.

Weiher, H., M. Konig, and P. Gruss. 1983. Multiple point mutations affecting the SV40 enhancer. *Science* **219:** 626.

The Role of Specific Chromosomal Translocations and Trisomies in the Genesis of Certain Plasmacytomas and Lymphomas in Mice, Rats, and Humans

Z. Wirschubsky, F. Wiener, J. Spira, J. Sümegi, C. Perlmann, and G. Klein

Department of Tumor Biology, Karolinska Institutet, S-104 01 Stockholm, Sweden

Specific chromosomal translocations are regularly associated with B-cell-derived tumors in mice, rats, and humans. It has been suggested that these translocations may act in oncogenesis by transposing cellular oncogenes to highly active chromosomal regions (Klein 1981). Recent molecular studies in several laboratories have shown that the translocations associated with mouse plasmacytoma and Burkitt's lymphoma frequently involve quantitatively altered *c-myc* expression.

We were interested in analyzing the relationship between oncogene activation and specific chromosomal aberrations in certain B- and T-cell-derived tumors. A new approach has been developed for the study of gene transpositions in tumors with chromosomal aberrations, based on flow cytometry and chromosome sorting.

Murine Plasmacytomas

Primary murine plasmacytomads (MPC) induced in BALB/c mice have two characteristic chromosomal translocations—rcpt(12;15) or rcpt(6;15) (Ohno et al. 1979).

Immunoglobulin expression

Both translocations affect immunoglobulin (Ig) gene-carrying chromosomes. The Ig heavy-chain genes and κ light-chain genes of the mouse have been localized to chromosomes 12 and 6, respectively (Hengartner et al. 1978; Swan et al. 1979; Meo et al. 1980).

The typical 12;15 translocation was found in both κ- and λ-producing tumors. The variant 6;15 translocation was restricted to a minority of the κ producers, suggesting a functional correlation between the chromosome affected and the type of light chain produced. Seven analyzed λ-producing plasmacytomas all contained the typical 12;15 translocation (Wiener et al. 1980a).

Diploidy and polyploidy

In diploid plasmacytomas, the translocation has affected one of the two homologous chromosomes. In the more frequent tetraploid tumors, two chromosomes were normal and two carried the translocation. This was interpreted to mean that the translocation must have occurred before the polyploidization. Since the majority of primary (0 generation) plasmacytomas were already tetraploid, it can be implied that the translocation occurs at an early

stage, and most probably at the time when the tumor originates.

Oncogene involvement

Klein (1981) has suggested that the plasmacytoma-associated translocations may act by transposing a cellular oncogene on chromosome 15 to active Ig-gene regions where the oncogene is activated to a constitutive and/or abnormal expression. Recent molecular studies (for review, see Klein 1983) have confirmed this hypothesis in showing that a cellular oncogene, *c-myc*, is in the immediate vicinity of the translocation breakpoint on chromosome 15.

In the majority of the plasmacytomas carrying the typical 12;15 translocation studied, *c-myc* breaks off at the first exon and transposes to the S_α region of the unexpressed IgH gene. This leads to a rearrangement of the *c-myc* gene.

A minority of the typical and a majority of the variant translocation-carrying plasmacytomas only contain germ line *c-myc* sequences indicating that the transcriptional unit and its flanking sequences have not been altered. In all likelihood, the entire *c-myc* gene has been displaced, together with its flanking sequences, including the nearest restriction sites to the Ig gene-carrying chromosome.

A minor proportion of the MPCs do not carry either the typical or the variant translocation. In a recent study that involved high-resolution banding analysis, translocation-negative plasmacytomas were found to carry an interstitial deletion, affecting band D3 in one of the two chromosome 15 homologs, i.e., the region corresponding to the breakpoint involved in the typical and the variant translocations (F. Wiener et al., in prep.). The *c-myc* gene was rearranged in one of three such plasmacytomas, whereas the other two contained only germ line sequences (F. Wiener et al., in prep.). The *c-myc* gene was highly transcribed in all three tumors, however (F. Wiener et al., in prep.).

Conceivably, the deletion may have joined the *c-myc* transcriptional unit to an active gene region on the same chromosome and/or has led to the loss of some important regulatory sequences.

Susceptibility to plasmacytomagenesis

BALB/c mice are extraordinarily susceptible to plasmacytoma induction (for review, see M. Potter et al.

1983). To assess whether this susceptibility was determined by some gene carried on chromosome 15, plasmacytomas were induced in AKR(6;15) × BALB/c backcross mice. Since both the BALB/c-derived chromosome 15 and the AKR-derived 6;15 chromosome could serve as the translocation donor, we have concluded that the variation in the susceptibility of these strains to PC induction was probably outside chromosome 15. Another interesting observation was made in the course of these studies. Although seven of ten PCs carried a 12;15 translocation, the remaining three had a variant 6;15 translocation. Interestingly, the exchange involved the distal segments of the same Robertsonian chromosome; in other words, a pericentric inversion had occurred within the AKR-derived 6;15 marker. The occurrence of this extraordinary cytogenetic phenomenon in three different tumors, and with the same breakpoints as in the variant 6;15 translocation where the two chromosomes are separate, underlines the significance of the translocation as an important change, probably directly involved with the genesis of the tumor itself.

Orientation of the IgH locus and *c-myc* activation

Both the 12;15 and the 6;15 translocations arise by reciprocal exchanges (Ohno et al. 1979; F. Wiener et al., in prep.). For the rcpt(12;15), this was also confirmed at the molecular level (Cory et al. 1983) and it was further shown that the 5′ end of the *c-myc* gene is joined to VDJ sequences while the body of the *c-myc* gene has joined to $S_\mu C_\mu$ sequences. The relationship between the chromosomal and molecular exchange is still open to a number of questions, however.

Two alternatives exist: The main part of the transposed *c-myc* gene may be either on the 12q+ or on the 15q− chromosome marker. Cory et al. (1983) suggest the 15q− marker, based upon the suggested orientation of the IgH locus in the mouse as V_H-centromere proximal (Meo et al. 1980; Owen et al. 1981). However, this was only tentatively suggested, and on the basis of data derived from a single recombinant mouse. Even for that mouse, the orientation was only valid on the unproven assumption that a double crossover could be excluded.

This question can be definitely solved, isolating the two reciprocally exchanged chromosomal markers by flow cytometry and analyzing the extracted DNA with *c-myc* and IgH probes, as discussed in the following section.

Chromosome sorting

The typical mouse flow karyotype contains five major peaks, as a rule (Fig. 1a). Figure 1b shows the flow karyotype of a mouse leukemia line homozygous for the Robertsonian 6;15 translocation. The position of the missing normal chromosome 15 pair can be deduced from a comparison of Figure 1, a and b.

In the leukemia line analyzed in Figure 1b (MCF-AKR Rb[6;15]), the Rb(6;15) marker is the only metacentric among the normal acrocentric mouse chromosomes. We have sorted the Rb(6;15)-containing peak and the chromosome 15-depleted peak into slides and stained the chromosomes by Giemsa stain. The Rb(6;15)-containing fraction showed predominantly metacentric chromosomes, whereas the chromosome 15-depleted fraction did not contain any metacentric chromosomes (Z. Wirschubsky, unpubl.).

We have also explored the feasibility of sorting chromosomes from the typical 12;15 translocation-carrying mouse plasmacytoma. Due to the relative homogeneity of mouse chromosomes, the 12q+ and the 15q− markers are within peaks that also contain other chromosomes (Fig. 2). Due to shifts in size and DNA content, the translocation chromosomes could be assigned to the positions indicated in Figure 2. We are presently sorting out these peaks in order to confirm the tentative assignment by appropriate DNA probes.

Burkitt's Lymphoma

Both the EBV-carrying and the EBV-negative varieties of Burkitt's lymphoma were found to carry one of three characteristic chromosomal translocations, t(8;14), t(2;8), and t(8;22). The typical 8;14 translocation was seen in approximately 90% of the cases, whereas the variant 2;8 and 8;22 translocations occurred in about 5% each.

All three translocations affect the same *c-myc*-carrying region (band 8q24). One of the three Ig gene-carrying chromosomes serves as the recipient, with breakpoints in the region corresponding to the Ig locus (for review, see Klein 1983).

Translocations and *c-myc* rearrangement

Somatic hybrid segregation analysis of the Burkitt's lymphoma line Daudi has shown that *c-myc* is displaced from its normal position on chromosome 8q24 to the 14q+ marker (Erikson et al. 1982). In other Burkitt's lymphoma lines, *c-myc* has rearranged to $S_\mu C_\mu$ sequences as shown by the comigration of *c-myc* and μ-hybridizing DNA fragments (Taub et al. 1982; Hamlyn and Rabbitts 1983; see also review by Perry 1983). A substantial part of the typical t(8;14)-carrying Burkitt's lymphoma lines did not show any *myc* rearrangement in DNA hybridization assays, however. Moreover, the same technology failed to reveal any rearrangement in lines carrying the variant translocations. It is possible that the *c-myc* transposition affects the whole *c-myc* locus, with its flanking sequences. Alternatively, *c-myc* may have stayed in its original position in these lines and parts of the Ig genes and/or their flanking sequences may have become transposed to its vicinity. This problem is also suitable for analysis by chromosome sorting.

Variant translocations

Lenoir et al. (1982) found a tight functional correlation between the light-chain product and the chromosome affected by the variant translocations. This could mean that the variant translocations affect the functionally rearranged chromosome, or it may be due to some coupling between the κ and λ rearrangements, respectively, and the occurrence of the corresponding translocation.

a

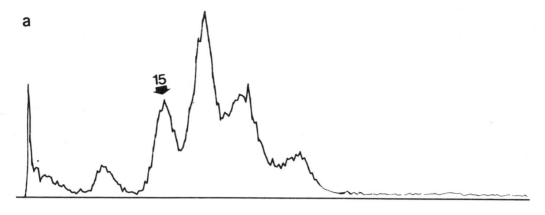

b

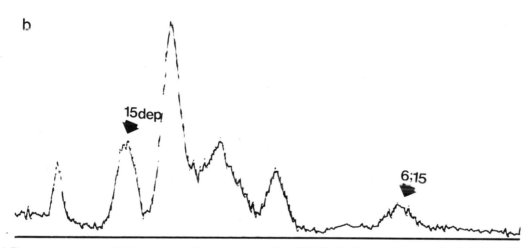

Figure 1 (*a*) Flow karyotype of a 15-trisomic, T-cell leukemia cell line TIKAUT. (*b*) Flow karyotype of a diploid MCF virus-induced T-cell leukemia cell line in AKR Rb6;15 mouse. Peak containing the Rb6;15 chromosome and the 15 chromosome-depleted peak is indicated.

Applications of chromosome sorting

By separating the reciprocally translocated t(2;8), t(8;22), and t(8;14) chromosomes, it will be possible to study the relationship between each chromosomal marker and the *c-myc* oncogene.

Sorting will also permit the localization of the re-arranged, highly transcribed *c-myc* sequences in comparison with their relatively inactive germ line counterparts. It will also clarify the question whether the translocation always affects the nonfunctionally rear-ranged chromosome or may also involve the functionally active Ig locus. The molecular methods that have been used so far can only pick up *c-myc* sequences within or in the immediate vicinity of the probed Ig sequences and introduce therefore, *ipso facto*, a bias for the identifi-cation of rearrangements that affect the nonfunctionally rearranged Ig locus. Separation of the translocated chromosomes and subsequent molecular analysis is free of such bias.

Chromosome sorting

Using the preparation method of Sillar and Young (1982), we have obtained interpretable flow karyotypes from all three types of translocation-carrying Burkitt's lymphoma lines (Wirschubsky et al. 1983).

The translocation chromosomes could be assigned to extra peaks that arose due to the shifts in their DNA content (Fig. 3 a–c). These assignments were facilitated by the fact that the Burkitt's lymphoma lines analyzed did not carry other chromosomes in the regions corre-sponding to the translocated elements, as indicated by conventional chromosome banding analysis and partic-ularly by the detection of the same extra peaks in several independent lines that carried the same translocation.

To assess the purity of the separated chromosomes, we have sorted the 22q − marker from a t(8;22)-carrying Burkitt's lymphoma line MAKU (Zech et al. 1976). Upon reanalysis of the sorted chromosomal fractions, a peak was obtained corresponding to the position of the orig-

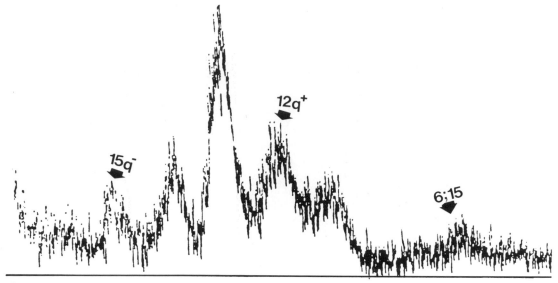

Figure 2 Flow karyotype from a plasmacytoma (CAK TEPC 2003) induced in an AKR Rb6;15 × BALB/c mouse. Peaks containing the Rb6;15 chromosome and the 12q+ and the 15q− markers are indicated.

inal 22q− marker, to the exclusion of other peaks (Wirschubsky et al. 1983).

It has been estimated (Lebo 1982) that a flow rate of 2200 chromosomes/second for about 16 hours would provide chromosomal DNA enriched from about 12 μg of total DNA. This corresponds to approximately 2.5×10^6 to 3×10^6 sorted chromosomes of a single type. Provided that the separated fraction has the required purity, specific sequences would be sufficiently enriched for restriction enzyme analysis and molecular cloning.

Rat Immunocytomas

The LOU/Esl rat strain develops a high frequency of spontaneous immunocytomas (Bazin et al. 1972). Six out of seven investigated rat immunocytomas were found to carry a reciprocal 6;7 translocation (Wiener et al. 1982). Banding homologies were found between this translocation and the chromosomes involved in the typical 12;15 translocations in mouse plasmacytomas (Wiener et al. 1982). The question arises whether the rat 6;7 translocation is really homologous to the MPC- and Burkitt's lymphoma-associated translocations, i.e., involves the *c-myc* and the Ig genes?

Using rat-mouse somatic hybrids that segregated rat chromosomes, we could localize the rat *c-myc* locus to chromosome 7, as postulated (Sümegi et al. 1983). Moreover the *c-myc* locus was rearranged in four of five rat immunocytomas carrying the 6;7 translocation (Sümegi et al. 1983). This suggests that *c-myc* may be involved in the generation of B-cell-derived tumors in a third species.

Mouse T-cell Leukemia

Trisomy of chromosome 15 is a highly specific and regular feature of T-cell leukemias in mice, irrespective of

the inducing agent (Dofuku et al. 1975; Wiener et al. 1978a,b,c; Spira et al. 1979, 1980). The critical segment of chromosome 15 required for duplication is located in the distal part of the chromosome (Wiener et al. 1978b; Spira et al. 1980).

"Duplication hierarchy" of chromosome 15

Different F_1 hybrid combinations were derived from the crossing of two mouse strains with cytogenetically distinguishable chromosomes 15, to analyze the duplication pattern of chromosome 15 in chemically and virally induced leukemias (Fig. 4) (Wiener et al. 1979, 1980b, 1982). The leukemias of F_1 hybrids derived from crosses between cytogenetically different but genetically identical strains (for example, CBA × CBAT6T6 or AKR × AKR Rb 6;15) showed random duplication (Fig. 4). This was also the case when the cross involved genetically closely related strains, such as the CBAT6T6 × C3H F_1 hybrid. This proves that translocated or nontranslocated status of chromosome 15 did not skew the likelihood of the two complementary nondisjunctions. In the CBAT6T6 × AKR combination, all 15-trisomic T-cell leukemias showed exclusive duplication of the AKR-derived chromosome 15. In the CBAT6T6 × C57BL cross, the opposite preference was seen, with the exclusive duplication of the CBAT6T6-derived chromosome. All 15-trisomic leukemias induced in crosses between genetically different strains showed a similar asymmetry, i.e., duplication of one type of chromosome 15 only to the complete exclusion of the other. Crosses involving all genetically unrelated strains are summarized in Figure 4. Since nondisjunction of the homologous chromosomes 15 occurs with equal frequency, the duplication preference observed can only mean that the duplication of one parental strain-derived chromosome 15 is more likely to be associated with the development of leukemia than the

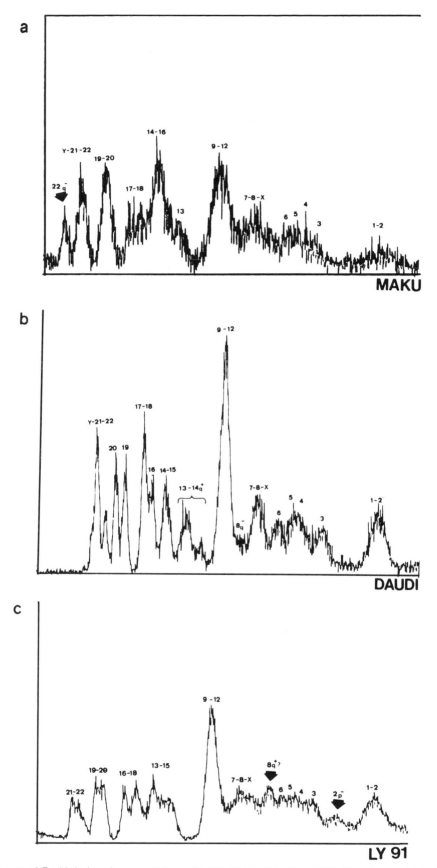

Figure 3 Flow karyotypes of Burkitt's lymphoma cell lines. (*a*) MAKU t(8;22); (*b*) DAUDI t(8;14); and (*c*) LY91 t(2;8). The peaks corresponding to the chromosomal markers are indicated.

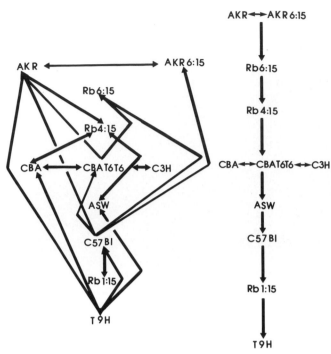

Figure 4 Asymmetrical chromosome 15 duplication. Scale indicates position in duplication hierarchy. F_1 hybrid crosses are indicated with straight lines between the strains.

duplication of the other. This can be interpreted as differences in the likelihood of some regulatory mutation or some other variation in chromosome 15-associated gene(s).

AKR-derived chromosome 15

In leukemias induced in different F_1 hybrids where AKR was one parental partner, the AKR-derived chromosome always showed preferential duplication. This extraordinary dominance may be a result of the selection of the AKR strain for high leukemia incidence. This selection, combined with inbreeding, is known to have fixed several genes that contribute to high leukemia incidence at different levels (for review, see Lilly and Pincus 1973).

Three leukemia-associated viruses have been demonstrated in AKR mice:

1. Gross virus, localized as a provirus at two sites in the genome, AKv-1 and AKv-2 (Rowe 1972).
2. Recombinant MCF virus (Hartley et al. 1977).
3. SL3-3 virus (Nowinsky and Hays 1978; Pedersen et al. 1981).

Although the preferential duplication of the AKR-derived chromosome 15 was observed in chemically induced leukemias as well, we have asked the question whether it could be related to the extraordinary susceptibility of the AKR strain to virus-induced leukemogenesis.

To answer this question, we have induced leukemias in AKR 6;15 × B6Fv-1^n hybrid mice with recombinant N-tropic MCF virus. In this F_1 hybrid, both parental genomes carry the permissive *Fv-1^n* allele, and the chro-

mosomes 15 of the two parents are cytogenetically distinguishable from each other. In four 15-trisomic leukemias analyzed, the AKR-derived chromosome 15 was preferentially duplicated (Z. Wirschubsky et al., in prep.). Thus, it must be concluded that the AKR-derived chromosome 15 duplicates preferentially, even in a viremic mouse where the virus may be presumed to have an equal chance to reintegrate on the chromosome 15 of either parent. Moreover, recent results (Z. Wirschubsky et al., in prep.) show that neither a total replacement of the genetic background nor the induction of a viremic state can change the preferred duplication status of the AKR-derived 15 chromosome. It appears that the reasons for this preference are to be sought in the genetic content of the AKR chromosome itself.

Chromosome 15 and the tumorigenic phenotype: Somatic hybrid studies

Somatic hybrids studied lend support to the involvement of oncogene(s) localized on chromosome 15 in the genesis of T-cell leukemias (Spira et al. 1981). A 15-trisomic, AKR-derived, T-cell lymphoma line TIKAUT was fused with diploid CBAT6T6 fibroblasts. High and low tumorigenic hybrids were analyzed comparatively for their chromosome complement.

High tumorigenic hybrids differed from low tumorigenic hybrids with regard to the number of tumor versus normal parent-derived chromosome 15. In the high tumorigenic group, the leukemia-derived chromosome 15 was amplified (from 3 to 5–6) with a concomitant reduction (from 2 to 1) in the number of normal parent-derived chromosomes 15. In contrast, low tumorigenic hybrids retained their original chromosome complement. It was concluded that amplification of a changed gene on chromosome 15 favored tumorigenic behavior, probably because it helped to overcome some *trans*-acting, restricting influence of its normal homolog.

c-myc rearrangement in TIKAUT

In TIKAUT, the leukemic parent line of these hybrids, Adams et al. (1982) found only a single 33-kb rearranged *Eco*RI *c-myc* fragment. This was in contrast to the majority of the T-cell leukemias tested where only a 21.5-kb *Eco*RI germ line *c-myc* fragment was found. Since TIKAUT has a chromosome-15 trisomy, this also meant that a single chromosome 15 with the rearranged *c-myc* fragment has duplicated twice in two nondisjunction events whereas the normal chromosome 15 was lost. TIKAUT is a serially passaged, mutagenized, universal fuser line derived from a spontaneous AKR leukemia, TKA. We have now tested TKA and found that it contained both a rearranged 33-kb and a germ line 22-kb *Eco*RI *c-myc* fragment (Wirschubsky et al. 1984).

TIKAUT thus provides an interesting case history in tumor progression, with sequential cytogenetic and molecular events that take place during progressive growth. It also emphasizes the importance of the balance between the leukemia-derived chromosome and its normal counterpart for the expression of the tumorigenic phenotype.

Some applications of chromosome sorting to the analysis of mouse leukemias

Some of the changes associated with chromosome 15 of mouse leukemias can be approached by chromosome sorting. This is exemplified by Figure 5a, which shows the flow karyotype of a DMBA-induced T-cell leukemia in SJL mice. This cell line had a cryptical translocation, where the distal part of chromosome 15 was translocated onto the X chromosome (Spira et al. 1980). This is paralleled by the appearance of a sixth peak. Since this line did not have any other translocations in the regions of the large chromosomes 1 and 2, we assigned the X;15 translocation to the extra peak, as indicated in Figure 5a.

The T9H mouse strain has a reciprocal 7;15 translocation. The breakpoint on chromosome 15 corresponds to the 15D2/D3 band, corresponding to the translocation breakpoint in the plasmacytomas. We have analyzed an an Abelson virus-induced T9H leukemic line by flow cytometry. By calculating the relative chromosome content under each peak and by correlating the extra peaks to the translocation chromosomes, a tentative assignment could be worked out, as shown in Figure 5b.

Sorting of the chromosome 15-containing fractions from these lines will permit molecular analysis, including the study of possible retroviral insertions or other DNA rearrangements in the neighborhood of relevant oncogenes.

Acknowledgments

This investigation was supported by the Swedish Cancer Society and by Grant No. 2 R01 CA 14054-10, awarded by the National Cancer Institute.

References

Adams, J.M., S. Gerondakis, E. Webb, J. Mitchell, O. Bernard, and S. Cory. 1982. Transcriptionally active DNA region that rearranges frequently in murine lymphoid tumors. *Proc. Natl. Acad. Sci.* **79**: 6966.

Bazin, H., C. Deckers, A. Becker, and J.F. Hermemans. 1972. Transplantable immunoglobulin secreting tumours in rats. I. General features of LOU/Ws1 strain rat immunocytomas and their monoclonal proteins. *Int. J. Cancer* **10**: 568.

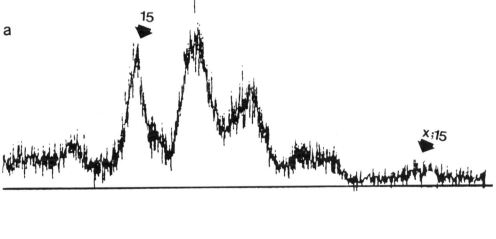

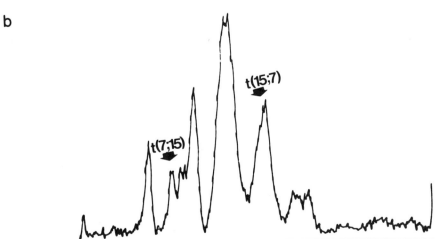

Figure 5 Flow karyotypes of mouse cell lines with translocations affecting chromosome 15. (*a*) SJL-VDJ 6998 line with a X:15 tumor-associated translocation. (*b*) T(7;15)9H cell line induced by Abelson virus. Peaks corresponding to the translocation chromosomes are indicated.

Cory, S., S. Gerondakis, and J.M. Adams. 1983. Interchromosomal recombination of cellular oncogene *c-myc* with the immunoglobulin heavy chain locus in murine plasmacytomas in a reciprocal exchange. *EMBO J.* **2**: 697.

Dofuku, R., J.L. Biedler, B.A. Spengler, and L.J. Old. 1975. Trisomy of chromosome 15 in spontaneous leukemia of AKR mice. *Proc. Natl. Acad. Sci.* **72**: 1515.

Erikson, J., J. Finan, P. Nowell, and C.M. Croce. 1982. Translocation of immunoglobulin Ch genes in Burkitt lymphoma. *Proc. Natl. Acad. Sci.* **79**: 5611.

Hamlyn, P.H. and T.H. Rabbitts. 1983. Translocation joins *c-myc* and immunoglobulin γ 1 genes in a Burkitt lymphoma revealing a third exon in the *c-myc* oncogene. *Nature* **304**: 135.

Hartley, J.W., N.K. Wolford, L.J. Old, and W.P. Rowe. 1977. A new class of murine leukemia virus associated with the development of spontaneous leukemia. *Proc. Natl. Acad. Sci.* **74**: 789.

Hengartner, H., T. Meo, and E. Muller. 1978. Assignment of genes for immunoglobulin kappa and heavy chains to chromosomes 6 and 12 in mouse. *Proc. Natl. Acad. Sci.* **75**: 4494.

Klein, G. 1981. The role of gene dosage and genetic transposition in carcinogenesis. *Nature* **294**: 313.

———. 1983. Specific chromosomal translocations and the genesis of B-cell derived tumors in mice and men. *Cell* **32**: 311.

Lebo, R.V. 1982. Chromosome sorting and DNA sequence localization. *Cytometry* **3**: 145.

Lenoir, G.N., J.L. Preud'homme, A. Bernheim, and R. Berger. 1982. Correlation between immunoglobulin light chain expression and variant translocation in Burkitt's lymphoma. *Nature* **298**: 474.

Lilly, F. and T. Pincus. 1973. Genetic control of murine viral leukemogenesis. *Adv. Cancer Res.* **117**: 231.

Meo, T., J. Johnson, C.V. Beeckey, S.J. Andrews, J. Peters, and A.G. Searle. 1980. Linkage analysis of murine immunoglobulin heavy chain and serum prealbumin genes establish their location on chromosome 12 proximal to the T(5:12)31 H breakpoint in band 12F₁. *Proc. Natl. Acad. Sci.* **77**: 550.

Nowinski, R.C. and F. Hayse. 1978. Oncogenicity of AKR endogenous leukemia viruses. *J. Virol.* **27**: 13.

Ohno, S., M. Babonits, F. Wiener, J. Spira, G. Klein, and M. Potter. 1979. Non-random chromosome changes involving Ig-gene chromosomes (Nos. 12 and 6) in pristane induced mouse plasmacytomas. *Cell* **18**: 1001.

Owen, F.L., R. Riblet, and B.A. Taylor. 1981. The T suppressor cell alloantigen Gsv maps near immunoglobulin allotype genes and may be a heavy chain constant-region marker on a T cell receptor. *J. Exp. Med.* **153**: 801.

Pedersen, F.S., R.L. Crowther, D.Y. Tenney, A.M. Reimold, and W.A. Haseltine. 1981. Novel leukaemogenic retroviruses isolated from cell line derived from spontaneous AKR tumour. *Nature* **292**: 167.

Perry, R.P. 1983. Consequences of myc invasion of immunoglobulin loci: Facts and speculation. *Cell* **33**: 647.

Potter, M., F. Mushinsky, and F. Wiener. 1983. Recent developments in plasmacytoma genesis. *Adv. Viral Oncol.* (in press).

Rowe, W.P. 1972. Studies of genetic transmission of murine leukemia virus by AKR mice. *J. Exp. Med.* **136**: 1271.

Sillar, R. and B.C. Young. 1982. A new method for the preparation of metaphase chromosomes for flow analysis. *J. Histochem. Cytochem.* **29**: 74.

Spira, J., F. Wiener, S. Ohno, and G. Klein. 1979. Is trisomy cause or consequence of murine T cell leukemia development? Studies on Robertsonian translocation mice. *Proc. Natl. Acad. Sci.* **70**: 6619.

Spira, J., F. Wiener, M. Babonits, J. Gamble, J. Miller, and G. Klein. 1981. The role of chromosome 15 in murine leukemogenesis. I. Contrasting behavior of the tumor vs. normal parent-derived chromosomes no. 15 in somatic hybrids of varying tumorigenicity. *Int. J. Cancer* **28**: 785.

Spira, J., M. Babonits, F. Wiener, S. Ohno, Z. Wirschubski, N. Haran-Ghera, and G. Klein. 1980. Non-random chromosomal changes in Thy-1 positive and Thy-1 negative lymphomas induced by 7,12-dimethylbenzanthracene (DMBA) in SJL mice. *Cancer Res.* **40**: 2609.

Sumegi, J., J. Spira, H. Bazin, J. Szpirer, G. Levan, and G. Klein. 1983. Rat c-myc oncogene is located on chromosome 7 and rearranges in immunocytomas with t (6:7) chromosomal translocation. *Nature* **306**: 497.

Swan, D., P. D'Eustachio, L. Leinwand, J. Siedman, D. Keithely, and F.H. Ruddle. 1979. Chromosomal assignment of mouse kappa light chain genes. *Proc. Natl. Acad. Sci.* **76**: 2735.

Taub, R., I. Kirch, C. Morton, G. Lenoir, D. Swan, S. Tronich, S. Aaronson, and P. Leder. 1982. Translocation of the *c-myc* gene into the immunoglobulin heavy chain locus in human Burkitt lymphoma and murine plasmacytoma cells. *Proc. Natl. Acad. Sci.* **79**: 7837.

Wiener, F., M. Babonits, J. Spira, G. Klein, and H. Bazin. 1982. Non-random chromosomal changes involving chromosomes 6 and 7 in spontaneous rat immunocytomas. *Int. J. Cancer* **29**: 431.

Wiener, F., M. Babonits, J. Spira, G. Klein, and M. Potter. 1980a. Cytogenetic studies on the IgA/lambda producing murine plasmacytomas: Regular occurrence of a t(12;15) translocation. *Somatic Cell Genet.* **6**: 731.

Wiener, F., S. Ohno, J. Spira, N. Haran-Ghera, and G. Klein. 1978a. Chromosomal changes (trisomy 15 and 17) associated with tumor progression in leukemias induced by radiation leukemia virus (RadLV). *J. Natl. Cancer Inst.* **61**: 227.

———. 1978b. Cytogenetic mapping of the trisomic segment of chromosome 15 in murine T-cell leukemia. *Nature* **275**: 658.

Wiener, F., J. Spira, M. Babonits, N. Haran-Ghera, and G. Klein. 1980b. Non-random duplication of chromosome 15 in murine T-cell leukemias: Further studies on translocation heterozygotes. *Int. J. Cancer* **26**: 661.

Wiener, F., J. Spira, S. Ohno, N. Haran-Ghera, and G. Klein. 1978c. Chromosome changes (trisomy 15) in murine T-cell leukemia induced by 7,12-dimethylbenz(a)anthracene (DMBA). *Int. J. Cancer* **22**: 447.

———. 1979. Non-random duplication of chromosome 15 in murine T-cell leukemias induced in mice heterozygous for translocation t(14;15)6. *Int. J. Cancer* **23**: 504.

Wirschubsky, Z., C. Perlmann, J. Lindsten, and G. Klein. 1983. Flow karyotype analysis and fluorescence-activated sorting of Burkitt-lymphoma-associated translocation chromosomes. *Int. J. Cancer* **32**: 147.

Wirschubsky, Z., F. Wiener, J. Spira, J. Sümegi, and G. Klein. 1984. Triplication of chromosome no. 15 with an altered c-myc containing EcoRI fragment and elimination of the normal homologue in a T-cell lymphoma line of AKR origin (TIKAUT). *Int. J. Cancer* (in press).

Zech, L., U. Haglund, K. Nilsson, and G. Klein. 1976. Characteristic chromosomal abnormalities in biopsies and lymphoid cell lines from patients with Burkitt and non-Burkitt lymphomas. *Int. J. Cancer* **17**: 47.

Involvement of c-abl in the Philadelphia Translocation

J. Groffen,* N. Heisterkamp, and J.R. Stephenson

Laboratory of Viral Carcinogenesis, National Cancer Institute-FCRF, Frederick Cancer Research Facility, Frederick, Maryland 21701

G. Grosveld and A. de Klein

Department of Cell Biology and Genetics, Erasmus University, 3000 DR Rotterdam, The Netherlands

A series of human cellular sequences designated "oncogenes" has been identified on the basis of sequence homology with retroviral transforming genes (Bishop 1982; Varmus 1982). Evidence for the potential involvement of oncogenes in human cancer is rapidly accumulating. One line of evidence for this possibility is the demonstration that human tumor-derived DNA sequences, isolated on the basis of their ability to transform mouse cells phenotypically in tissue culture, correspond to particular classes of cellular oncogenes (Der et al. 1982; Pulciana et al. 1982; Tabin et al. 1982; Taparowsky et al. 1982; Shimizu et al. 1983). More recently, other human oncogenes have been shown to be involved in highly specific chromosomal translocations characteristic of particular classes of human neoplasia (de Klein et al. 1982; Taub et al. 1982; Adams et al. 1983; Dalla-Favera et al. 1983; Sheer et al. 1983) and amplification of specific cellular oncogenes in tumor cells has been demonstrated (Collins and Groudine 1982; Dalla-Favera et al. 1982; Alitalo et al. 1983). The present studies were undertaken to identify and clone molecularly the human c-abl oncogene, to determine its relationship to other classes of human oncogenes, and, to examine the potential involvement of c-abl in chronic myelogenous leukemia (CML).

Methods

Cell lines and tissues
The parental mouse, human, and Chinese hamster cell lines and the mouse × human and Chinese hamster × human somatic cell hybrids used in the present study are as described in the footnotes to Tables 1–3. Tumor cells from control individuals and patients with CML were obtained through the National Institutes of Health Resource and Logistics Program.

Gel electrophoresis and hybridization
Restriction enzymes were purchased from either New England BioLabs or Bethesda Research Laboratories (BRL) and were used according to the suppliers' specifications. DNAs were digested with restriction enzymes, subjected to electrophoresis through 0.75% agarose gels, and transferred to nitrocellulose (Schleicher and

Schuell, pH 79) essentially as described by Southern (1975). Nick-translation of probes and filter hybridization were as previously described (Groffen et al. 1982). Specific activity of the probes was 2×10^8 to 5×10^8 cpm/μg. Following hybridization, filters were exposed to XAR-2 film (Kodak) for up to 5 days at $-70°C$ with Dupont Lightning Plus intensifying screens.

Preparation of DNA probes
DNA probes were prepared by digesting 150 μg of DNA with appropriate restriction enzymes, followed by electrophoresis through low-melting-point agarose (BRL). Desired bands were excised from gels and brought into solution by heating at 65°C for 30 minutes. Agarose was removed by two extractions with phenol equilibrated with 0.3 M NaOAc (pH 5.0) and one extraction with phenol:chloroform:isoamylalcohol (25:24:1). DNA was precipitated with ethanol and 0.2 M NaOAc (pH 4.8) in the presence of 20 μg/ml Dextran T-500 as carrier.

Nucleic acid sequencing
DNA restriction fragments were prepared, labeled with $[\gamma\text{-}^{32}P]$ATP, and sequenced according to the method of Maxam and Gilbert (1980).

In situ hybridization
Chromosome preparations from peripheral blood of CML patients and control individuals were prepared according to standard techniques. Following RNase treatment, chromosomes were denatured in 70% formamide/$2 \times$ SSC at 70°C for 2 minutes, rinsed three times in $2 \times$ SSC, and dehydrated in ethanol. DNA probes were labeled as described above, denatured for 5 minutes at 70°C at a concentration of 0.2 μg/ml in 50% (v/v) formamide/$2 \times$ SSCP (0.3 M NaCl/0.03 M trisodium-citrate/0.04 M NaPO4 [pH 6])/10% dextran sulfate, combined with a 1000-fold excess of alkali-denatured salmon sperm rDNA carrier, added to the chromosomes, and hybridized for 10 hours at 37°C. Slides were rinsed in three changes of 50% formamide $12 \times$ SSC at 39°C for 15 minutes each, followed by five changes in $2 \times$ SSC at 39°C, and 5 hours washing in $2 \times$ SSC at 4°C. After dehydration in ethanol, slides were exposed to Kodak NTB2 emulsion for 18 days at 4°C, developed, stained with Giemsa, and grains counted.

*Present address: Oncogene Science Inc., Mineola, New York 11501.

Table 1 Localization of *c-abl* on Human Chromosome 9

Hybrids	1	2	3	4	5	6	7	8	9	10	11	12	13	14	15	16	17	18	19	20	21	22	X	*c-abl*
MOG-2	+	+	+	+	+	+	+	+	+	+	+	+	+	+	+	+	+	+	+	+	+	+	+	+
MOG-2 E5	+	−	+	+	+	+	+	+	+	+	−	+	+	+	+	+	+	+	+	+	+	+	+	+
F4SC13C1112	+	−	−	−()	−	−	−	−	+	−	−	−	−	+	−	−	−	−	−	−	−	−	+	+
MOG-2G1	+	−	+	+	+	+	+	+	−	+	−	+	+	+	+	+	+	+	+	+	−	+	+	−
SIR-7A2	+	+	−	−	+	−	+	−	−	+	+	+	−	+	+	+	+	+	+	+	−	+	+	−
SIR-7D1	+	+	−	+	−	−	+	−	−	−	−	+	+	+	+	−	+	+	+	+	−	+	+	−
SIR-7G1	+	−	−	+	−	−	+	−	−	+	+	−	+	+	−	+	+	+	+	+	−	+	+	−
HOR19D2	−	−	−	−	−	−	−	−	−	−	+	−	−	+	−	+	−	−	−	−	−	−	+	−
F4SC13C19	+	−	−	−	−	−	−	−	−	−	−	−	−	+	−	−	−	−	−	−	−	−	+	−
MOG-13/22	+	−	−	−	−	−	−	−	−	−	−	−	−	−	−	−	−	−	−	+	+	+	+	−
FIR 5R3	−	−	−	−	−	−	−	−	−	−	−	−	+	−	−	+	−	−	−	−	−	−	−	−
DUR 4.3	−	−	+	−	+	NT	−	−	−	+	+	+	+	+	+	−	+	+	−	+	+	+	+	−

The derivation of mouse and human somatic cell hybrids, determination of their complements of human chromosome, and identification of human *c-abl*-specific oncogene sequences was as previously described (Heisterkamp et al. 1983b).

Results and Discussion

Isolation of *v-abl* homologous sequences from a cosmid library of human cellular DNA

For use as a molecular probe, a 3.5-kb *Bam*HI restriction fragment encompassing all but a short region of the Abelson murine leukemia virus proviral DNA, was excised λ-AM-1, kindly provided by E.P. Reddy and S.A. Aaronson, and subcloned into pHEP (Heisterkamp et al. 1983a). A *v-abl* DNA probe was prepared from pHEP-Ab by digestion with *Bst*EII and *Bam*HI. For identification of *v-abl* homologous human sequences, high-molecular-weight mouse and human cellular DNAs were digested with *Eco*RI, electrophoresed, transferred to nitrocellulose filters, and hybridized to the the *v-abl Bam*HI–*Bst*EII probe. *v-abl* homologous human DNA restriction fragments of 11, 7.2, 5, 4.0, 3.4, 2.9, and 2.5 kb were clearly resolved. The demonstration of numerous human DNA *Eco*RI restriction fragments hybridizing to *v-abl*, which itself encompasses a region of only 3.0 kb, provided an initial indication that the human *v-abl* homolog must contain extensive intervening sequences. It was also apparent that although strength of homology of human and mouse cellular DNAs with *v-abl* were comparable, the restriction patterns were quite distinct, a finding consistent with previous reports by Goff et al. (1980) and Srinivasan et al. (1981).

To facilitate further characterization of *v-abl* homologous human DNA sequences, a previously described (Groffen et al. 1982) cosmid library of human carcinoma DNA was utilized. Upon screening with the *v-abl Bam*HI–*Bst*EII probe, nine positive cosmid clones were identified. For further characterization of these clones, a series of probes with specificity for subgenomic regions of *v-abl* were prepared. These included *v-abl* $P_{1.7}$ which, in addition to 5′ *v-abl* sequences, contains around 0.6 kb of Moloney murine leukemia virus sequences, two probes corresponding to the central portion of *v-abl* ($P_{0.25}$ and $P_{0.7}$), and a fourth probe specific for the 3′ region (*v-abl* $P_{0.85}$). Of the nine *v-abl* homologous cosmid clones

isolated, three, cos 8, 15, and 18, hybridized to at least two of the specific *v-abl* subgenomic probes. cos 15 contained *Eco*RI fragments of 7.2, 3.4, 2.9, and 2.5 kb, each of which hybridized to the *v-abl* $P_{1.7}$. cos 18 contained *Eco*RI fragments of 4.0 kb and 3.1 kb homologous to *v-abl* $P_{1.7}$, one of which—the 4.0-kb fragment—also hybridized to *v-abl* $P_{0.25}$ and a fragment of 5.0 kb homologous to *v-abl* $P_{0.25}$, $P_{0.7}$, and $P_{0.85}$. The third clone, cos 8, contained *v-abl* homologous *Eco*RI fragments of 7.2, 5.0, 4.0, 3.4, and 2.5 kb.

Restriction maps of *v-abl* homologous sequences within cos 8, 15, and 18, were generated using various combinations of *Eco*RI, *Kpn*I, *Bam*HI, *Hind*III, and *Bgl*II. As summarized in Figure 1, the three cosmid clones contain overlapping cellular sequences corresponding to a single contiguous region of human cellular DNA of around 64 kb. Based upon hybridization with the four individual subgenomic *v-abl* probes, seven distinct regions of *v-abl* homology (exons), interspersed by six nonhomologous regions representing probable intervening sequences (introns), were identified. In addition, colinearity of sequences within the human *v-abl* homolog and the viral *v-abl* gene was established.

Identification of three overlapping cosmid inserts representing the complete *v-abl* homolog

To establish whether the complete human *v-abl* homolog was represented within cos 8, 15, and 18, and whether rearrangements may have occurred during cloning, the composite restriction map of the cloned sequences was compared with that of *v-abl* homologous sequences in human cellular DNA. The latter were identified on the basis of hybridization to individual *v-abl* subgenomic probes. Upon digestion of human cellular DNA, together with a small amount of DNA from cos 15 and 18, and hybridization to *v-abl* $P_{1.7}$, all *v-abl* homologous fragments in cos 15 and 18 comigrated with those in human genomic DNA. *Kpn*I digestion of cellular DNA generated restriction fragments of 18.6, 14.2, 5.6, and 2.8 kb hy-

Table 2 Translocation of *c-abl* from Chromosome 9 to Chromosome 22 in CML

Cell line	Human chromosomes					
	AK1	9	22	9q+	22q−	*c-abl*
Mouse						
NIH-3T3	NT	−	−	−	−	−
Human						
A673	NT	+	+	+	+	+
Mouse × human hybrid						
PgMe-25NU	−	−	+	−	−	−
WESP-2A	−	−	+	+	−	+
Chinese hamster × human hybrid						
10CB-23B	+	+	−	−	−	+
14CB-21A	+	−	−	+	+	−
1CB-17a NU	−	−	+	+	−	+

Cell lines were derived and their human chromosomal complements determined as previously described (de Klein et al. 1982). *c-abl* human oncogene sequences were identified by Southern blot molecular hybridization analysis using human specific probes (de Klein et al. 1982).

Table 3 Translocation of *c-abl* to Chromosome 22 in t(1,9,22)

Hybrids	Human chromosomes																											
	1	2	3	4	5	6	7	8	9	10	11	12	13	14	15	16	17	18	19	20	21	22	X	Y	1p−	1q+	22q−	*c-abl*
8CB-7B	−	−	−	+	+	+	−	−	−	−	−	−	−	+	−	+	+	+	+	−	−	+	−	−	+	+	−	−
8CB-8A	+	−	+	+	+	+	+	+	−	+	+	+	+	+	+	+	+	+	+	+	+	+	+	−	+	+	−	−
12CB-17B	−	−	+	+	+	−	+	+	−	+	+	−	+	−	+	+	+	+	+	+	−	+	+	−	+	−	−	−
WEDY-7	+	+	+	+	+	+	+	+	−	+	−	+	+	+	−	−	+	+	+	+	−	+	−	−	−	+	−	−
WEDY-9	+	+	−	+	+	+	+	+	−	−	+	+	+	+	+	+	+	+	+	+	−	−	−	−	−	+	+	+
17CB-3B	−	+	−	+	+	−	−	−	+	+	−	+	+	+	−	+	+	+	+	+	+	−	−	−	NA	NA	NA	NA
17CB-21C	−	−	−	+	+	−	−	−	+	+	−	−	−	+	+	+	+	−	−	+	−	+	−	−	NA	NA	NA	+

Somatic cell hybrids were derived by fusion of mouse (WEHI-30) or Chinese hamster (a3 or a23) cells with either Ph[1]-positive (8CB-7B, 8CB-8A, 12CB-17B, WEDY-7, WEDY-9) or PH[1]-negative CML leukocytes. Analysis of human chromosomal content and *c-abl* oncogene sequences was as previously described (Bartram et al. 1983b).

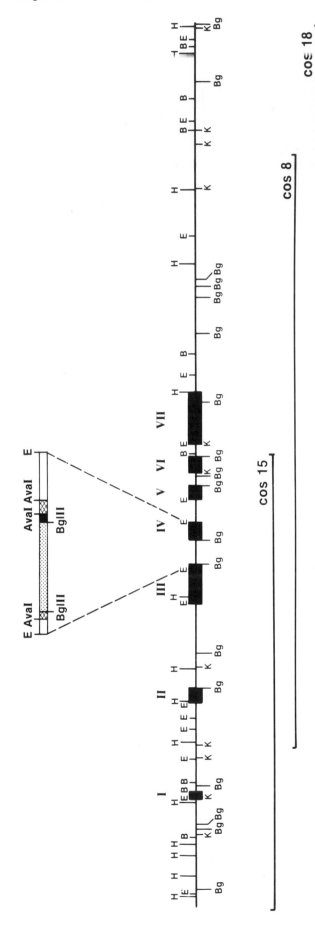

Figure 1 Restriction map of the human *c-abl* oncogene. Regions of homology to *v-abl*-specific probes (■) are designated I through VII. The *c-abl* tyrosine acceptor site region is indicated at an expanded scale in the upper portion of the figure. Cellular DNA inserts within cos 8, cos 15, and cos 18 are shown at the bottom of the figure. Restriction endonucleases include: *BglI* (Bg); *BamHI* (B); *HindIII* (H); *EcoRI* (E); and *Kpn* (K).

bridizing to *v-abl* P$_{1.7}$ whereas *Bam*HI digestion yielded 24.0-kb and 3.4-kb fragments hybridizing with *v-abl* P$_{1.7}$ and a 7.3-kb *v-abl* P$_{0.7}$ homologous fragment. These results are in concordance with the mapping and hybridization data on the cloned DNA shown in Figure 1, arguing against the introduction of major rearrangements of the *c-abl* locus during cloning. It should be noted that the 4.1-kb and 11-kb *Eco*RI fragments, identified upon digestion of total human DNA and hybridization with *v-abl* P$_{1.7}$, are missing from the cloned human *c-abl* sequence represented in cosmids 8, 15, and 18. As discussed in detail elsewhere, these restriction fragments apparently correspond to independent loci of *v-abl* homologous human sequence (Heisterkamp et al. 1983).

c-abl phosphotyrosine acceptor site

The region of *c-abl* containing the phosphotyrosine acceptor site is shown at expanded scale in the upper portion of Figure 1. To map precisely the position of the acceptor tyrosine residue, the 0.14-kb *Bgl*II–*Ava*I restriction fragment was subjected to nucleic acid sequences analysis (Groffen et al. 1983a). Of the three possible reading frames, the first contained six termination codons, the second contained a single TGA stop codon near the middle of the sequence, not followed by any obvious splice acceptor site, whereas the third lacked any termination codons and thus appeared to represent the authentic coding sequence for the *c-abl* gene product. To extend this analysis, we subsequently sequenced the coding region of an adjacent downstream *Ava*I–*Ava*I *c-abl* restriction fragment, and by an analogous approach, the corresponding region of *v-abl*. The amino acid sequences corresponding to each of these regions of nucleic acid sequence are shown in Figure 2. The predicted amino acid sequences of the internal 61 residues were identical, based on either the *v-abl* or *c-abl* nucleic acid sequence. Sixteen additional aminoterminal and 18 carboxyterminal residues correspond to regions for which only *v-abl* sequence was determined.

To determine whether the deduced *c-abl/v-abl* amino acid sequence corresponds to phosphotyrosine acceptor site regions common to the *v-src*-, *v-yes*-, and *v-fes/fps*-encoded transforming proteins, relevant sequences were compared. As shown in Figure 2, the *c-abl/v-abl* sequence contains a total of 38/96 residues in common with all four of the viral acceptor site regions examined. Additional relatedness with individual viral sequences appears somewhat random; some *c-abl/v-abl* residues are in common either with *v-yes* or *v-src* whereas others are shared only with the *v-fes* and *v-fps* gene products. The *c-abl/v-abl*-encoded proteins also contain a tyrosine residue (*) at the position corresponding to the previously identified tyrosine acceptor sites of each of the other oncogene-encoded products examined. Additionally, there is considerable homology (28/96 residues) between *c-abl* and the catalytic subunit of the mammalian ATP-dependent protein kinase (BOV-PK), although the tyrosine acceptor residue of *c-abl/v-abl* is replaced by a tryptophan residue in BOV-PK. Of interest, this substi-

tution is directly adjacent to a threonine residue known to represent one of two phosphorylation sites previously identified in BOV-PK (Shoji et al. 1981).

Localization of *c-abl* to the long (q) arm of chromosome 9

As discussed above, by use of appropriate *v-abl*-specific probes, we were able to discriminate several human *Eco*RI *c-abl* restriction fragments from mouse *c-abl* homologous sequences. This observation made possible the use of somatic cell hybrids as a means of determining the chromosomal localization of the human *c-abl* oncogene (Heisterkamp et al. 1982). As summarized in Table 1, upon analysis of a panel of mouse × human somatic cell hybrids, complete concordance was observed between the presence of human DNA-specific *v-abl* cross-reactive *Eco*RI restriction fragments in the 2.5–5.0 kb size range and human chromosome 9 (Table 1). Each of the other human chromosomes could be excluded by one or more examples of discordance. In a second experiment, four hamster × human somatic cell hybrids, containing only limited complements of human chromosomes, were analyzed for human *c-abl* sequences. Only one clone, C10bCit29, contained human *c-abl*-specific sequences. Of interest, this particular hybrid was positive for each of three isoenzyme markers for human chromosome 9, cytoplasmic soluble *cis*-aconitase (ACONs), AK3 and AKA1. A subclone of C10b, designated C10b2BU, lacked detectable human *c-abl* sequences and by isoenzyme analysis contained only ACONs and AK3, both of which are localized on the short arm of chromosome 9 (Fig. 3). The third marker, AK1, which was not detected in this hybrid, maps on the long arm of chromosome 9. The remaining two hybrids were nonreactive in assays for all three markers for chromosome 9 and lacked detectable sequences hybridizing to the human *c-abl* B$_{0.6}$ probe. These findings localize *c-abl* to the distal portion of the long arm of chromosome 9.

Translocation of *c-abl* to chromosome 22 (Ph[1] chromosome) in CML

The above findings are of interest because of the involvement of the long arm of chromosome 22 (band 22q11) in a specific translocation with the long arm of chromosome 9 (band 9q34), the Philadelphia translocation (Ph[1]), occurring in human CML. The abnormal chromosomes are designated 9q+ and 22q−; of these the 22q− chromosome is observed in 92% of CML cases. We investigated the chromosomal location of the human *c-abl* gene in cases of CML where the Philadelphia translocation is present. Southern blot analyses with *c-abl* and *v-abl* probes were performed on *Eco*RI-digested DNAs from somatic cell hybrids segregating the 9q+ and 22q− chromosomes (de Klein et al. 1982).

The cell hybrids used each contain a full complement of mouse or Chinese hamster chromosomes and a limited number of human chromosomes. The hybrid cell lines were obtained by fusion of cells from mouse (Pg 19 and WEHI-3B) or Chinese hamster (E36 and a3) origin with leukocytes from different CML patients and

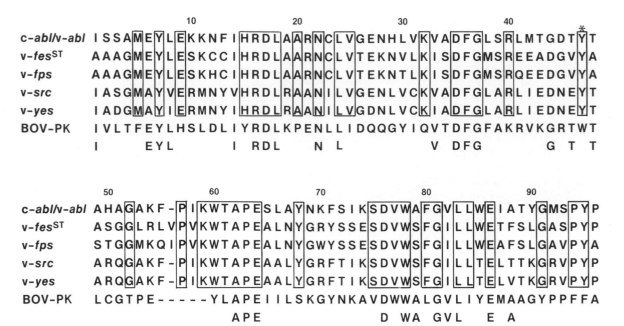

Figure 2 Comparison of the deduced amino acid sequence of the *v-abl* and human *c-abl* phosphotyrosine acceptor sites to analogous regions of the *v-fes*[ST]- (Hampe et al. 1982), *v-fps*- (Shibuya and Hanafusa 1982), *v-src*- (Czernilofsky et al. 1980; Kitamura et al. 1982), and *v-yes*- (Kitamura et al. 1982) encoded transforming proteins and to the catalytic subunit of the mammalian AMP-dependent protein kinase (Shoji et al. 1981). Amino acids common to each of the oncogene-encoded acceptor domains are shown in open boxes, whereas those residues shared by the *c-abl*-encoded sequence and BOV-PK are indicated in the lower portion of the figure. The position of the putative phosphotyrosine acceptor residue (*) is also shown. (A) alanine; (G) glycine; (T) threonine; (C) cysteine; (P) proline; (M) methionine; (V) valine; (I) isoleucine; (L) leucine; (Y) tyrosine; (F) phenylalanine; (W) tryptophan; (D) aspartic acid; (E) glutamic acid; (R) arginine; (K) lysine; (H) histidine; (S) serine; (N) asparagine; (Q) glutamine.

from a normal donor. The human chromosome content of these cells is summarized in Table 2. To maximize specificity for *c-abl* detection, two human *v-abl* restriction fragments with homology to the presumptive 5′ and 3′ proximal *Eco*RI fragments of *c-abl* were isolated. After hybridization and washing to high stringency (0.1 × SSC), the 5′-terminal 0.6-kb *Bam*HI probe and the 3′-terminal 1.1-kb *Hin*dIII–*Eco*RI probe cross-hybridized to only a minimal extent with mouse or hamster *c-abl* sequences. Using these probes, *Eco*RI-restricted DNAs of hybrid cell lines containing chromosomes 22, 9, 9q+, or 22q− were analyzed for human *c-abl* sequences (Table 2). As controls, DNAs from human placenta and from the mouse and Chinese hamster fusion partners were analyzed. Human *c-abl*-specific restriction fragments detected in human placenta DNA were present in DNA from the hybrid cell lines 10 CB-23B (chromosome 9), 1CB-17a NU, and WESP-2A (both containing chromosome 22q−). These bands were not detected in DNA from PgMe-25Nu (chromosome 22), 14CB-21A (chromosome 9q+), Pg19, and WEHI-3B (mouse controls) or E36 and a3 (Chinese hamster controls). Because all other *c-abl* *Eco*RI fragments that hybridize to *v-abl* sequences, are flanked by the 2.9-kb and 5.0-kb *Eco*RI fragments, it seems highly probable that these fragments are also included in the translocation to the Philadelphia chromosome. To test this possibility directly, hybridization was performed using the *v-abl* $P_{1.7}$ probe. Because of the problems with *v-abl* probes in-

dicated above, only WESP-2A, the hybrid containing the most 22q− sequences (50% of the molar amount), was tested. This probe detects human *Eco*RI *c-abl* fragments of 11, 7.2, 4.0, 3.4, 2.9, and 2.5 kb. Of these fragments, the 11-kb band has been shown to map outside the main human *c-abl* locus and will not be considered here. The human 2.9-, 3.4-, 4.0- and 7.2-kb *c-abl* fragments were readily detected in the WESP 2A DNA. The 2.5-kb *Eco*RI human *c-abl* fragment comigrates with a mouse fragment of similar size and thus could not be identified in this analysis.

The hybrid cell lines containing the 9q+ and 22q− chromosomes examined in the present study were obtained from fusion experiments with CML cells from three different individuals. Therefore, we conclude that in the Philadelphia translocation a fragment of chromosome 9 is translocated to chromosome 22q− and that this fragment includes the human *c-abl* sequences. This finding establishes that the translocation is reciprocal, a general assumption which is demonstrated unequivocally by these results. Moreover, the data raise the possibility of involvement of the human *c-abl* gene in the generation of CML.

Search for the t(9;22) junction site

To investigate the possibility that the chromosome 9 breakpoint in the t(9;22) may be localized either within or in close proximity to the human *c-abl* oncogene, high-molecular-weight DNA was isolated from biopsy sam-

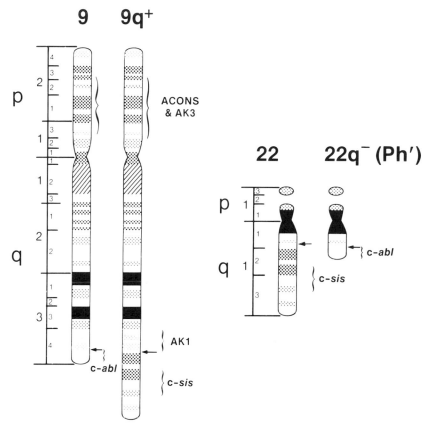

Figure 3 Diagramatic representation of the involvement of *c-abl* and *c-sis* in the Ph¹ translocation. Chromosome banding patterns are as previously shown by Yunis (1982); map positions of ACONS, AK3, and AK1 are as previously reported (Carritt and Povey 1979). Localization of *c-abl* within the terminal portion of chromosome 9(q34), which is translocated to chromosome 22 in CML, is as described in the text. Mapping of *c-sis* to the region of chromosome 22 (q11 to qter) translocated to chromosome 9 is as previously described (Groffen et al. 1983b; Bartram et al. 1983a).

ples of the spleens of three CML patients and from an erythroleukemic cell line K562 established from a CML patient in blast crisis (Heisterkamp et al. 1983b). Each DNA was digested with *Bam*HI and subjected to Southern blot analysis. The restriction enzyme patterns of each of the four CML DNAs were indistinguishable from those of control DNA, when hybridized either to the above described *v-abl* probe, *v-abl* $P_{1.7}$, or probes isolated from different regions of the human *c-abl* locus (data not shown).

Chromosomal walking

As no rearrangements could be detected in the *v-abl* homologous cellular DNA region encompassed by the cosmid clones shown in Figure 1, a probe was prepared corresponding to an 0.4-kb *Hind*III–*Eco*RI fragment (0.4 HE) mapping within the 5′ domain of the human *c-abl* locus (Fig. 4) and was used to screen the original human cosmid library (Heisterkamp et al. 1983b). Although recombinants representative of approximately 10 times the complete human genome were analyzed, no positive clones were obtained. Upon analysis of total human DNA, a *Bam*HI fragment of approximately 14.5 kb was found to hybridize to the 0.4 HE probe. To characterize

this restriction fragment further, a library of size-fractionated *Bam*HI-digested total human DNA was constructed in Charon 30. Upon screening of the library with the 0.4 HE probe, seven positive recombinant phage clones were identified. The insert of one of these positives was subcloned into pBR328 (p5′-*c-abl*) and subjected to detailed restriction enzyme analysis as shown in Figure 4B. No sequences in the 14.5-kb fragment hybridized to any of the *v-abl*-specific probes.

As indicated in Figure 4B, an 0.2-kb probe was prepared from the 5′ terminus of p5′-*c-abl* by digestion with *Bam*HI and *Eco*RI. This probe hybridized to a *Hind*III fragment of around 9.5 kb in all DNAs examined, suggesting that sequences immediately 5′ to the newly cloned region are nonrearranged. As expected, a fragment of 14.5 kb was detected in *Bam*HI-digested normal human DNA, whereas in DNA of CML patient 0319129, an additional *Bam*HI restriction fragment of around 3.1 kb was identified. Similarly, the 0.4-kb HE probe isolated from the 5′ region of *c-abl* hybridized with a 14.5-kb *Bam*HI fragment in the other two CML DNAs. In DNA from CML patient 0319129, however, an extra *Bam*HI fragment of around 30 kb was visible. The most likely explanation for these findings is that one allelic copy of DNA sequences 5′ to *c-abl* in CML patient 0319129 DNA

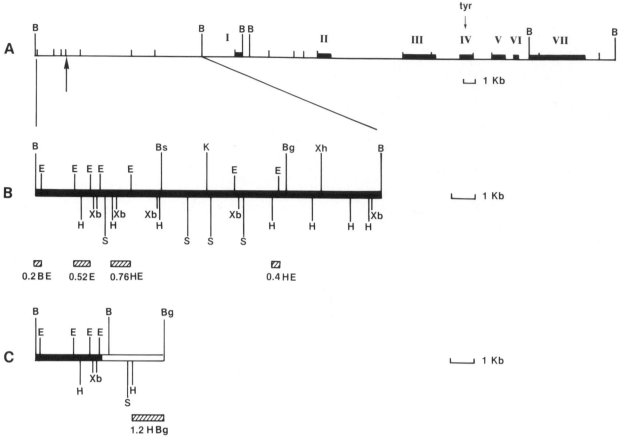

Figure 4 Restriction enzyme analysis of p5′-c-abl and a part of pBglII 9q + . The position of p5′-c-abl in relation to the v-abl homologous regions in the human c-abl locus is indicated in A. Individual exons are designated I through VII. EcoRI sites are marked by small vertical lines; v-abl homologous sequences are indicated by solid bars. The vertical arrow points to the breakpoint in the DNA of CML 0319129. A restriction map of p5′-c-abl is shown in B; probes used in this study, indicated as hatched boxes, are shown beneath the map. The pBglII-9q + fragment in C is a subclone of a 6.0-kb BglII fragment isolated from CML patient 0319129; in B and C the BglII site within 200 bp of the 5′ BamHI site and a HpaI site in between these two restriction sites are not shown. The solid bar indicates sequences from chromosome 9 whereas the open bar represents sequences from chromosome 22. Cloning and subcloning of the p5′-c-abl and BglII-9q + sequences was according to previously described methods (Heisterkamp et al. 1983b). Restriction enzyme maps are based on hybridization data and on results of double digestions of individual fragments isolated from low-melting-point agarose gels. Restriction enzymes include: BamHI (B); BglII (Bg); BstEII (Bs); HindIII (H); SstI (S); XbaI (xb); XhoI (Xh); EcoRI (E); and KpnI (K).

is normal whereas the second is rearranged; these appear to be present in about a 1 : 1 molar ratio.

To define more accurately the region where DNA of patient 0319129 differs from the normal region, probes including an 0.52-kb EcoRI fragment (0.52 E) and an 0.76-kb EcoRI–HindIII fragment (0.76 HE) (see Fig. 4B), were prepared from p5′-c-abl, corresponding to the approximate region of rearranged sequences in the DNA of patient 0319129. Extra DNA fragments were found with these probes upon restriction enzyme digestion of DNA 0319129 with BglII, XbaI, SstI, and HindIII (Fig. 5). The 9.5-kb 5′ HindIII fragment, which hybridized to the 0.52-kb EcoRI probe, seemed to be present in a normal quantative level, as did the 2.0-kb fragment hybridizing to the 0.76-kb HE probe. A rearrangement thus appeared to have taken place within the 1.25-kb HindIII fragment, since, in addition to the normal 1.25-kb HindIII fragment, a fragment of 2.2 kb could be identified.

Molecular cloning of a chromosomal junction fragment

Since human c-abl is translocated to the Philadelphia chromosome (22q −) in CML, we reasoned that the transposed sequences in DNA of CML patient 0319129 should include most of the 14.5-kb BamHI fragment; the 5′ sequences of this fragment would presumably remain on chromosome 9, linked to sequences from chromosome 22, thus accounting for the 3.1-kb BamHI fragment. The 9.5-kb BglII fragment would thus represent the chromosome 22/9 chimeric fragment localized at the Ph¹ translocation breakpoint; the 6.0-kb BglII fragment would contain sequences from chromosomes 9 and 22, on the 9q + chromosome.

To test this model, DNA from CML patient 0319129 was digested with BglII and size-fractionated in the 6–7-kb range, and a library was constructed in BamHI-digested Charon 30 phage arms. Three positive clones

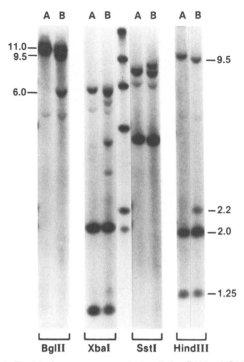

Figure 5 Restriction enzyme analysis of the DNA of CML patient 0319129. Restriction enzymes used and the molecular weights of the fragments in the *Bg*lI and *Hin*dIII digestions are as indicated. γ-^{32}P-labeled *Hin*dIII digestion fragments of DNA in the center of the figure serve as a molecular-weight marker for the *Xba*I and *Sst*I digestions. Southern blots were hybridized with a mixture of the 0.52 E and 0.76 HE probes (see Fig. 4B). (Lanes *A*) DNA of cell line A673; (lanes *B*) DNA of CML 0319129.

were identified upon screening with the 0.2-kb BE probe. Because each of the positive clones contained an additional inserted *Bg*lI fragment, some *Bg*lI sites had remained intact, enabling the subcloning of most of the 6.0-kb *Bg*lI fragment by *Bg*lI–*Hpa*I digestion into plasmid ORF (Weinstock et al. 1983). As shown in the restriction enzyme map of this fragment, the 3′ *Eco*RI site of the 0.52-kb *Eco*RI fragment is still present. In contrast, an *Sst*I site immediately 3′ of it and all other restriction enzyme sites to the 3′ are either missing or different from those found in the same region in p5′-*c-abl* between the *Eco*RI and *Sst*I sites. Sequences 5′ of this point in the 6.0-kb *Bg*lI fragment hybridize to p5′-*c-abl*; sequences 3′ of it do not (results not shown).

To determine the origin of the 6.0-kb *Bg*lI fragment, a 1.2-kb *Hin*dIII–*Bg*lI probe (1.2 HBg) was prepared. Using stringent washing conditions, this probe hybridized to a 5.0-kb *Bg*lI fragment in DNA of the human cell lines A204, but not to sequences in mouse DNA or in rodent-human somatic cell hybrids containing human chromosome 9. A 5.0-kb *Bg*lI fragment was detected in an independent hybrid (PgMe-25Nu) containing chromosome 22 as its only human component. Moreover, using the same probe, both 5.0-kb and 6.0-kb *Bg*lI fragments were identified in the DNA of patient 0319129. The 1.2 HBg probe did not hybridize to sequences in

the human-mouse somatic cell hybrid WESP-2A, which contains the Ph¹ chromosome in the absence of 9,9q + or 22. Thus, the 6.0-kb *Bg*lI fragment cloned from patient 0319129 DNA must contain, in addition to sequences from chromosome 9, sequences originating from the translocated region of chromosome 22. These results are summarized diagramatically in Figure 6.

Amplification of *c-abl* in K562 DNA

Although the K562 cell line has been shown to lack a cytogenetically identifiable Ph¹ chromosome, it was reported to contain a small ring chromosome, probably derived from a Ph¹ chromosome (Klein et al. 1976). As shown in Figure 7D, using the 1.2 HBg probe, a non-amplified 5.0-kb *Bg*lI fragment was detected in K562 DNA. In contrast, human *c-abl* sequences were found to be amplified at least fourfold in K562 DNA, as were sequences up to 17 kb upstream of the most 5′ *v-abl* homologous *Eco*RI region. The 11.0-kb *Eco*RI fragment (Fig. 7A) that hybridized to the *v-abl* P$_{1.7}$ probe but had no linkage with the main human *c-abl* locus was non-amplified and thus served as an internal control. The immunoglobulin light-chain constant region (C$_λ$) (Hieter et al. 1981) is also amplified at least fourfold (Fig. 7B). This latter observation is consistent with the localization of human *c-abl* and C$_λ$ sequences on the same amplifi-

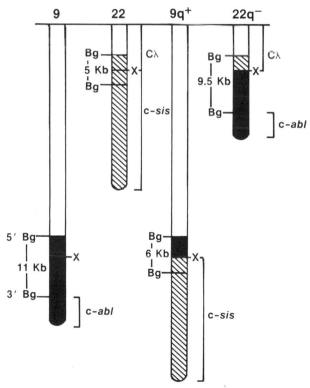

Figure 6 Schematic representation of the t9;22 in CML patient 0319129. The sizes of the *Bg*lI fragments detected with probes from chromosomes 9 and 22 are indicated. Regions in black originate from chromosome 9; hatched regions are from chromosome 22. An X indicates the t(9;22) chromosomal breakpoint. The human *c-sis* oncogene and the C$_λ$ region on chromosome 22 are shown for purpose of orientation.

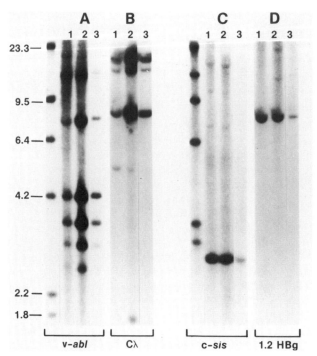

Figure 7 Amplification of *c-abl* in the erythroleukemic cell line K562. Control human DNA (10 μg, lanes *1* in each panel) was run next to 10 μg (lanes *2*) and 2.5 μg (lanes *3*) K562 DNA. ³²P-labeled *Hind*III-digested DNA is included as a molecular-weight standard for panels *A* + *B* (0.6% agarose gels) and for panels *C* + *D* (0.75% agarose gels). (*A*) DNAs were digested with *Eco*RI, and hybridized to *v-abl* P₁.₇. (*B*) *Eco*RI-digested DNAs were hybridized to a *Bgl*II–*Hind*III probe, isolated from a human Cλ clone, Hu λ5 (Hieter et al. 1981). (*C*) *Bam*HI-digested DNA hybridized to a previously described (Groffen et al. 1983b) 1.7-kb *Bam*HI probe prepared from a human *c-sis* cosmid clone. (*D*) *Bgl*II-digested DNAs hybridized to the 1.2 HBg probe described in Fig. 4C.

cation unit, presumably a part of the Ph¹ chromosome. In concordance with this conclusion is the finding that Cλ remains on the Ph¹ chromosome in the t9:22 (C.R. Bartram, unpubl. observ.). In contrast, *c-sis*, which is located on chromosome 22 and transferred to chromosome 9 in the Ph¹ translocation (Groffen et al. 1982; Bartram et al. 1983a), is nonamplified (Fig. 7C). Finally, the fact that the 5.0-kb *Bgl*II fragment normally localized on chromosome 22 is nonamplified in K562 supports the assumption that it is translocated to chromosome 9 in this cell line.

Translocation of *c-abl* to 22q − in t(9;11;22) and t(1;9;22)

To investigate if the *c-abl* gene is involved in the variant forms of CML, chromosomes from a patient with complex Philadelphia translocation, t(9;11;22), a Ph¹-negative patient, and two healthy individuals, respectively, were examined by in situ hybridization (Bartram et al. 1983b). The results of these experiments are summarized in Figure 8. The *c-abl* probe hybridized to the distal part of 9q34 in normal controls. In the CML patient with the complex translocation, the probe hybridized to the normal chromosome 9 and to the Ph¹ chromosome. In

contrast, a strong hybridization signal could be detected only on chromosome 9 at band q34 from the Ph¹-negative patient.

Confirmation of these results was obtained by Southern blot analysis of panels of somatic cell hybrids derived from cells of a second CML patient with the complex translocation t(1;9;22) and a second Ph¹-negative CML patient (Table 3). Hybrid cell lines were obtained by fusion of cells from mouse (WEHI-3B) or Chinese hamster (a3 or a23) origin with the patients's leukocytes. The 3′ *c-abl* probe hybridized to DNA from cell line WEDY-9 (Ph¹) but not to DNA from 8CB-7B, 8CB-8A, or WEDY-7 (chromosome 9q +). Again, the recipient chromosome for the distal part of chromosome 22, 1p −, lacked human *c-abl* sequences (12CB-17B).

Using a panel of hybrid cell lines containing chromosomes 9 or 22 obtained from a patient with Ph¹-negative CML, the human *c-abl* probe consistently hybridized to DNA from cell lines containing chromosome 9 (17CB-3B, 17CB-21C, 16CB-16A, 16CB-20) and not to cell lines containing chromosome 22 in the absence of chromosome 9 (16CB-15A, 16CB-17, 16CB-12, 16CB-1). With respect to the Ph¹-negative CML patient, these results can be explained on the assumption that either nonleukemic cells had been involved in the cell fusion or that only the "normal" chromosomes 22 and 9 had been retained in the hybrids. In the absence of genetic markers to distinguish the respective homologs of chromosomes 9 and 22, these possibilities cannot be resolved. However, since the peripheral leukocytes from the patient contained 98% myeloid cells, and assuming random chromosome segregation in hybrids, it is unlikely that the "normal" chromosomes 22 or 9 are individually segregated.

Conclusions

The present findings localize *c-abl* to human chromosome 9 and demonstrate its translocation to chromosome 22q − (the Ph¹ chromosome) in CML. In one of three CML patient DNAs examined, the Ph¹ chromosomal breakpoint has been localized within 14 kb of the most 5′ *v-abl* homologous region. The possibility that the t(9,22) breakpoint may even map within the 5′ coding region of the human *c-abl* locus cannot be excluded, since at present the position of the most 5′ exon in human *c-abl* has not been determined. Although, as yet, we have not localized the breakpoints in the DNAs of the two other CML patients or in DNA of the cell line WESP-2A, containing the 22q − chromosome, the results of cytogenetic analysis suggest that variability in Ph¹ translocation breakpoints must be very minor. Our findings establish that the site of the Ph¹ translocation breakpoint is not identical in each patient and suggests that breakpoints of other CML DNAs may be located 5′ of the approximately 80 kb of cloned DNA encompassing the human *c-abl* locus. Similarly, the t(8;14) translocation breakpoint in Burkitt's lymphoma involving the human *c-myc* oncogene has been shown to be variable in position (Dalla-Favera et al. 1982; Taub et al. 1982; Adams et

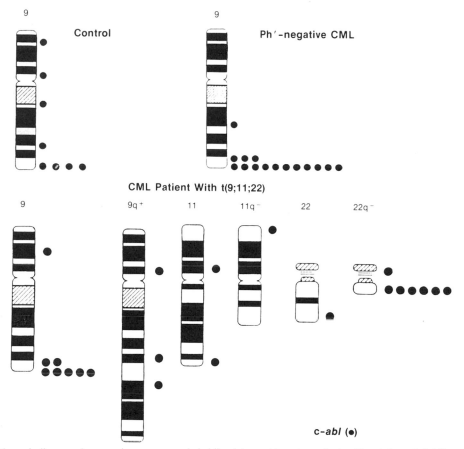

Figure 8 Distribution of silver grains on chromosomes hybridized to *c abl* probes. A significant ($p > 0.001$) grain accumulation is noted over band q34 of chromosome 9 in a healthy control. In a CML patient with a t(9;11;22), the hybridization signal ($p < 0.001$) is found both on the normal chromosome 9 and 22q−, whereas in the Ph[1]-negative CML a grain accumulation is only found on chromosome 9q34 ($p < 0.01$).

al. 1983; Stanton et al. 1983). The orientation of human *c-abl* on chromosome 9, with its 5′ region toward the centromere of the chromosome (Fig. 6), is established by the fact that the breakpoint has been found 5′ to the human *c-abl* locus. The possible involvement of *c-abl* in CML is further indicated by its translocation to the Ph[1] chromosome in the t(9;11;22) and t(1;9;22) complex translocations associated with CML and the specific amplification of *c-abl* and C$_\lambda$ sequence in the K562 cell line. In view of recent evidence implicating immunoglobulin sequences in the activation or alteration of *c-myc* in Burkitt's lymphoma, the localization of the λ immunoglobulin locus (Erikson et al. 1981) and *c-abl* oncogene in close proximity to the Ph[1] breakpoint in CML seems unlikely to be coincidental. Although a number of questions remain to be resolved, these findings strongly implicate *c-abl* in CML and suggest that the mechanism of *c-abl* activation may be analogous to the activation of *c-myc* in Burkitt's lymphoma.

Acknowledgments

We thank A. Geurts van Kessel and N.K. Spurr for providing somatic cell lines; A. Hagemeijer and F.H. Reynolds, Jr., for valuable discussion; P. Leder for the generous gift of the recombinant Huλ5; Gail Blennerhassett and Pamela Hansen for technical assistance; and Beverly Bales for help with the preparation of the manuscript. The work was supported under National Cancer Institute-Public Health Service contract NOI-CP-75380 and by the Netherlands Cancer Society (Koningin Wilhelmina Fonds).

References

Adams, J.M., S. Gerondakis, E. Webb, L.M. Corcoran, and S. Cary. 1983. Cellular *myc* is altered by chromosome translocation to an immunoglobulin locus in murine plasmacytomas and is rearranged similarly in human Burkitt lymphomas. *Proc. Natl. Acad. Sci.* **80:** 1982.

Alitalo, K., M. Schwab, C. Lin, H.E. Varmus, and J.M. Bishop. 1983. Homogenously staining chromosomal regions contain amplified copies of an abundantly expressed cellular oncogene (c-*myc*) in malignant neuroendocrine cells from a human colon carcinoma. *Proc. Natl. Acad. Sci.* **80:** 1707.

Bartram, C.R., A. de Klein, A. Hagemeijer, G. Grosveld, N. Heisterkamp, and J. Groffen. 1983a. Localization of the human c-*sis* oncogene in Ph[1]-positive and Ph[1]-negative chronic myelocytic leukemia by *in situ* hybridization. *Blood* **63:** 223.

Bartram, C.R., A. de Klein, A. Hagemeijer, T. van Agthoven, A. van Kessel, D. Bootsma, G. Grosveld, M. Ferguson-Smith,

T. Davies, M. Stone, N. Heisterkamp, J.R. Stephenson, and J. Groffen. 1983b. Translocation of the human c-*abl* oncogene occurs in variant Ph'-positive but not Ph'-negative chronic myelocytic leukemia. *Nature* **306**: 277.

Bishop, J.M. 1982. Oncogenes. *Sci. Am.* **247**: 81.

Carritt, B. and S. Povey. 1979. Regional assignments of the loci AK₃, ACONS and ASS on human chromosome 9. *Cytogenet. Cell Genet.* **23**: 171.

Collins, S. and M. Groudine. 1982. Amplification of endogenous *myc* related DNA sequences in a human myeloid leukaemia cell line. *Nature* **298**: 679.

Czernilofsky, A.P., A.D. Levinson, H.E. Varmus, J.M. Bishop, E. Fischer, and H.M. Goodman. 1980. Nucleotide sequence of an avian sarcoma virus oncogene (*src*) and proposed amino acid sequence for gene product. *Nature* **287**: 198.

Dalla-Favera, R., S. Martinotti, and R. Gallo. 1983. Translocation and rearrangement of the c-*myc* oncogene locus in human undifferentiated B-cell lymphomas. *Science* **219**: 963.

Dalla-Favera, R., F. Wong-Staal, and R. Gallo. 1982. *onc* gene amplification in promyelocytic leukemia cell line HL-60 and primary leukaemia cells of the same patient. *Nature* **299**: 61.

de Klein, A., A. Guerts van Kessel, G. Grosveld, C.R. Bartram, A. Hagemeijer, D. Bootsma, N.K. Spurr, N. Heisterkamp, J. Groffen, and J.R. Stephenson. 1982. A cellular oncogene is translocated to the Philadelphia chromosome in chronic myelocytic leukaemia. *Nature* **300**: 765.

Der, C.J., T.G. Krontiris, and G.M. Cooper. 1982. Transforming genes of human bladder and lung carcinoma cell lines are homologous to the *ras* genes of Harvey and Kristen sarcoma viruses. *Proc. Natl. Acad. Sci.* **79**: 3637.

Erikson, J., J. Martinis, and C.M. Croce. 1981. Assignment of the genes for human immunoglobulin chains to chromosome 22. *Nature* **22**: 173.

Goff, S.P., E. Gilboa, O.N. Witte, and D. Baltimore. 1980. Structure of the Abelson murine leukemia virus genome and the homologous cellular gene: Studies with cloned viral DNA. *Cell* **22**: 777.

Groffen, J., N. Heisterkamp, F. Reynolds, Jr., and J.R. Stephenson. 1983a. Human c-*abl* phosphotyrosine acceptor site. *Nature* **304**: 57.

Groffen, J., N. Heisterkamp, G. Grosveld, W. van de Ven, and J.R. Stephenson. 1982. Isolation of human oncogene sequences (v-*fes* homolog) from a cosmid library. *Science* **216**: 1136.

Groffen, J., N. Heisterkamp, J.R. Stephenson, A. van Kessel, A. de Klein, G. Grosveld, and D. Bootsma. 1983b. c-*sis* is translocated from chromosome 22 to chromosome 9 in chronic myelocytic leukemia. *J. Exp. Med.* **158**: 9.

Hampe, A., I. Laprevotte, F. Galibert, L.A. Fedele, and C.J. Sherr. 1982. Nucleotide sequences of feline retroviral oncogenes (v-*fes*) provide evidence for a family of tyrosine-specific protein kinase genes. *Cell* **30**: 775.

Heisterkamp, N., J. Groffen, and J.R. Stephenson. 1983a. The human v-*abl* cellular homologue. *J. Mol. Appl. Genet.* **2**: 57.

Heisterkamp, N., J.R. Stephenson, J. Groffen, P.F. Hansen, A. de Klein, C.R. Bartram, and J. Grosveld. 1983b. Localization of the c-*abl* oncogene adjacent to a translocation breakpoint in chronic myelocytic leukemia. *Nature* **306**: 239.

Heisterkamp, N., J. Groffen, J.R. Stephenson, N.K. Spurr, P.N. Goodfellow, B. Solomon, B. Garritt, and W.F. Bodmer. 1982. Chromosomal localization of human cellular homologues of two viral oncogenes. *Nature* **299**: 747.

Hieter, P.A., G.F. Hollis, S.J. Korsmeyer, T.A. Waldmann, and P. Leder. 1981. Clustered arrangement of immunoglobulin lambda constant region genes in man. *Nature* **294**: 536.

Kitamura, N., A. Kitamura, K. Toyoshima, Y. Hirayama, and M. Yoshida. 1982. Avian sarcoma virus Y73 genome sequence and structural similarity of its transforming gene product to that of Rous sarcoma virus. *Nature* **297**: 205.

Klein, E., H. Ben-Bassat, H. Neumann, P. Ralph, J. Zeuthen, A. Polliack, and F. Vánky. 1976. Properties of the K562 cell line derived from a patient with chronic myeloid leukemia. *Int. J. Cancer* **18**: 421.

Maxam, A.M. and W. Gilbert. 1980. Sequencing end-labeled DNA with base-specific chemical cleavages. *Methods Enzymol.* **65**: 499.

Pulciani, S., E. Santos, A. Lauver, L. Long, S. Aaronson, and M. Barbacid. 1982. Oncogenes in solid human tumours. *Nature* **300**: 539.

Sheer, D., L.R. Hiorns, P.N. Goodfellow, J. Trowsdale, E. Solomon, D.M. Swallow, S. Povey, N. Heisterkamp, J. Groffen, and J.R. Stephenson. 1983. Genetic analysis of the 15;17 chromosome translocation associated with acute promyelocytic leukemia. *Proc. Natl. Acad. Sci.* **80**: 5007.

Shibuya, M. and H. Hanafusa. 1982. Nucleotide sequence of Fujinami sarcoma virus: Evolutionary relationship of its transforming gene with transforming genes of other sarcoma viruses. *Cell* **30**: 787.

Shimizu, K., M. Goldfarb, Y. Suard, M. Perucho, Y. Li, T. Kamata, J. Feramisco, E. Stavnezer, J. Fogh, and M. Wigler. 1983. Three human transforming genes are related to the viral *ras* oncogenes. *Proc. Natl. Acad. Sci.* **80**: 2112.

Shoji, S., D.C. Parmelee, R.D. Wade, S. Kumar, L.H. Ericsson, K.A. Walsh, H. Neurath, G.L. Long, J.G. Demaille, E.H. Fischer, and K. Titani. 1981. Complete amino acid sequence of the catalytic subunit of bovine cardiac muscle cyclic AMP-dependent protein kinase. *Proc. Natl. Acad. Sci.* **78**: 848.

Southern, E.M. 1975. Detection of specific sequences among DNA fragments separated by gel electrophoresis. *J. Mol. Biol.* **98**: 503.

Srinivasan, A., E.P. Reddy, and S.A. Aaronson. 1981. Abelson murine leukemia virus. Molecular cloning of infectious integrated proviral DNA. *Proc. Natl. Acad. Sci.* **78**: 2077.

Stanton, L.W., R. Watt, and K.B. Marcu. 1983. Translocation breakage and truncated transcripts of c-*myc* oncogene in murine plasmacytomas. *Nature* **303**: 401.

Tabin, C.J., S.M. Bradley, C.I. Bargmann, and R.A. Weinberg. 1982. Mechanism of activation of a human oncogene. *Nature* **300**: 143.

Taparowsky, E., Y. Suard, O. Fasano, K. Shimizu, M. Goldfarb, and M. Wigler. 1982. Activation of the T24 bladder carcinoma transforming gene is linked to a single amino acid change. *Nature* **300**: 762.

Taub, R., I. Kirsch, C. Morton, and G. Lenoir. 1982. Translocation of the c-*myc* gene into the immunoglobulin heavy chain locus in human Burkitt lymphoma murine plasmacytoma cells. *Proc. Natl. Acad. Sci.* **79**: 7837.

Varmus, H.E. 1982. Form and function of retroviral proviruses. *Science* **216**: 812.

Weinstock, G.M., C. ap Rhys, M.L. Berman, B. Hampar, D. Jackson, T.J. Silhavy, J. Weisemann, and M. Zweig. 1983. Open reading frame expression vectors: A general method for antigen production in *Escherichia coli* using protein fusions to β-galactosidase. *Proc. Natl. Acad. Sci.* **80**: 4432.

Yunis, J.J. 1982. Most cancers may have a chromosomal defect. In *Gene amplification* (ed. R.T. Schimke), p. 297. Cold Spring Harbor Laboratory, Cold Spring Harbor, New York.

Intracisternal A-particle Genes: A Family of *copia*-like Transposable Elements in *Mus musculus*

R.G. Hawley*†, M.J. Shulman†‡, and N. Hozumi*†

*Ontario Cancer Institute and †Department of Medical Biophysics, University of Toronto, Toronto, Ontario, Canada, M4X 1K9 ‡Rheumatic Disease Unit, Wellesley Hospital, Toronto, Ontario, Canada, M4Y 1J3

Intracisternal A particles (IAPs) are retroviruslike entities that are found in many embryonic and transformed cells of *Mus musculus* (Dalton et al. 1961; Wivel and Smith 1971; Kuff et al. 1972; Biczysko et al. 1973; Calarco and Szöllösi 1973; Chase and Pikó 1973; Yotsuyanagi and Szöllösi 1981). These particles, which form by budding at the endoplasmic reticulum, reside in the cisternae. Although they share several properties with B- and C-type retroviruses, such as an intrinsic reverse transcriptase activity (Wilson and Kuff 1972; Wilson et al. 1974; Yang and Wivel 1974; Wong-Staal et al. 1975) and an RNA genome that codes for the A-particle structural protein (Yang and Wivel 1973; Lueders et al. 1977; Paterson et al. 1978), IAPs differ from these retroviruses in that they are not found extracellularly (Dalton et al. 1961; Minna et al. 1974). Furthermore, as purified IAPs have not been found to be infectious (Kuff et al. 1968, 1972), the significance of their presence has remained obscure.

DNA sequences homologous to IAP-associated RNA (IAP genes) are present in about 1000 copies distributed throughout the genome of *M. musculus* (Lueders and Kuff 1977, 1980). The majority of IAP genes are 7 kbp long (Kuff et al. 1981), although variants with internal deletions and substitutions have also been described (Ono et al. 1980). IAP genes contain long terminally redundant sequences (LTRs), similar to those found in the *copia*-like transposable elements of yeast and *Drosophila*, and in the integrated forms of retroviruses (Cole et al. 1981; Kuff et al. 1981; Roeder and Fink 1983; Rubin 1983; Varmus 1983). Like the LTRs of these elements, IAP LTRs end in short inverted repeats that include the terminal dinucleotides 5′TG . . . CA3′ (Kuff et al. 1983b). As well, a 7-kbp IAP gene was found to be flanked by a direct repeat of 6 bp (Kuff et al. 1983b) that, by analogy to other transposable genetic elements, was probably generated during insertion (Kleckner 1981; Roeder and Fink 1983; Rubin 1983).

In this paper, we summarize the data that, taken together, demonstrate the ability of IAP genes to move within the mouse genome. As is the case with other transposable elements (Kleckner 1981; Roeder and Fink 1983; Rubin 1983), IAP genes can influence the expression of the cellular genes at the various loci where they insert. Examples are given demonstrating the inactivation of cellular genes by physical disruption, and the enhancement of cellular gene transcription, presumably by a process akin to promoter insertion (Neel et al. 1981; Payne et al. 1981).

Materials and Methods

Cell lines

X63Ag8 was originally derived from the plasmacytoma MOPC21 and synthesizes IgG1(κ) of unknown specificity (Köhler and Milstein 1975). Sp6 is an IgM(κ)-producing hybridoma cell line derived by fusing X63Ag8 cells with spleen cells from a BALB/c mouse previously immunized with the hapten trinitrophenyl (TNP) (Köhler and Milstein 1976). It originally produced the gamma (γ_1) heavy and kappa (κ_{M21}) light chains of X63Ag8 as well as TNP-specific mu (μ_{TNP}) heavy and kappa (κ_{TNP}) light chains. From Sp6, a subclone (Sp6-A1-14) was isolated that does not produce the γ_1 heavy chain. Sp602 and Sp603 are subclones of Sp6-A1-14. The mutant cell lines igk-1 and igk-20, derived from Sp602, are defective in κ_{TNP} chain synthesis (Köhler and Shulman 1980).

DNA isolation and analysis

Cell and plasmid DNAs were isolated by standard techniques as described in Hozumi et al. (1981b). Nitrocellulose blotting was done according to the method of Southern (1975) as described in Hozumi et al. (1981a). Hybridization was carried out using DNA restriction fragments isolated by preparative acrylamide gel electrophoresis and radiolabeled by nick-translation (Rigby et al. 1977) as described in Hozumi et al. (1981a). The plasmid pHT10 (Blair et al. 1980), used to prepare a *mos*-specific probe, was provided by G. Vande Woude (National Cancer Institute, Bethesda, Md.). The plasmid pα25RH1.6 (R. Greenberg and K. Marcu, unpubl.), which contains the 3′ end of the J558α25 c-*myc* gene (Harris et al. 1982), was supplied by K. Marcu (State University at Stony Brook, New York).

RNA isolation and analysis

RNA was isolated from membrane-bound polyribosomes as described by Marcu et al. (1978). RNA blotting to nitrocellulose was performed as described by Thomas (1980).

Results

Mutant immunoglobulin genes

We have been interested in the molecular mechanisms controlling the expression of the immunoglobulin (Ig) genes of the mouse. One approach that we have taken employs the methods of somatic cell genetics to generate mutant cell lines defective in Ig gene expression. Thus, several mutant mouse hybridomas were derived from a hybridoma (Sp6) which synthesizes IgM(κ) specific for the hapten TNP (Köhler and Shulman 1980). Two of these mutants, igk-1 and igk-20, which are defective in the production of the TNP-specific κ chain (κ_{TNP}), were found to contain rearranged κ_{TNP} genes (Hawley et al. 1982). Molecular cloning of these mutant genes indicated that the rearrangement event in each case was due to the insertion of an IAP gene into one of the introns of the wild-type κ_{TNP} gene (Hawley et al. 1982).

In the case of the mutant κ_{TNP} gene in igk-1, what appears to be a deleted form of an IAP gene (~5 kbp) has inserted into the large intron that separates the κ_{TNP}-variable (V_{TNP}) gene segment from the κ-constant (C_κ) gene segment (Fig. 1). The transcriptional orientation of this IAP gene is in the same direction as κ_{TNP} gene transcription. A low amount of κ_{TNP}-specific mRNA is produced by this cell line (Hawley et al. 1982), roughly in agreement with previous estimates of the amount of κ_{TNP} synthesized (Köhler and Shulman 1980). At this time, the manner in which the IAP gene affects the expression of the igk-1 κ_{TNP} gene remains unknown.

The igk-20 κ_{TNP} gene contains a full-length IAP gene (~7 kbp) that has inserted into the small intron that separates the exon encoding a hydrophobic leader peptide (L_{TNP}) from the V_{TNP} gene segment (Fig. 1). In this case, the transcriptional orientation of the IAP gene is opposite that of the κ_{TNP} gene. A κ_{TNP}-specific mRNA species, which contains both L_{TNP} and V_{TNP} homologous sequences but is slightly larger than the normal κ_{TNP} mRNA, has been identified by RNA blot analysis (Hawley et al. 1982; R. Hawley et al., in prep.). As no κ_{TNP} chain is produced by igk-20, this κ_{TNP}-related mRNA must be defective. We speculate that aberrant splicing to a "cryptic" splice site within the L_{TNP}-V_{TNP} intron could be the cause of this defect. A potential donor splice site (AAA/GTAATT) can be found 34 bp 3' of the normal L_{TNP} donor splice site and 22 bp 5' of the IAP gene insertion site (Hawley et al. 1982; R. Hawley et al., unpubl.). This potential donor splice site shares homology with the donor splice site consensus sequence at seven out of nine positions (Mount 1982). Utilization of this "cryptic" site would render the κ_{TNP} mRNA out of phase in the V_{TNP} coding region. Aberrant splicing from "cryptic" splice sites has been reported for several natural and in vitro-

constructed mutant genes (Nevins 1983). In particular, D. Kelley and R. Perry (pers. comm.) have found that a mutant κ-chain gene from the NZB plasmacytoma PC6684 (Perry et al. 1981) utilizes a "cryptic" splice site at a similar position as that proposed for the igk-20 κ_{TNP} gene. In their example, aberrant splicing from the "cryptic" position is probably the result of mutations in the normal donor splice site that have rendered it nonfunctional (D. Kelley and R. Perry, pers. comm.). In contrast to this, the normally used L_{TNP} donor splice site of the igk-20 κ_{TNP} gene is identical to the wild-type sequence (R. Hawley et al., unpubl.).

IAP gene transcription

By analogy to retroviruses, it might be expected that movement of IAP genes occurs through an RNA intermediate (Varmus 1983). In support of this hypothesis, all examples of IAP gene insertion have been found in particle-producing cells (Hawley et al. 1982; Rechavi et al. 1982; see below). Furthermore, Shen-Ong and Cole (1982) have reported amplification of IAP genes in two plasmacytomas. In each of the cases they examined, the amplified IAP genes were colinear with the IAP-associated RNA. As shown in Figure 2, hybridization of membrane-associated RNA, purified from the mutant hybridomas igk-1 and igk-20, as well as the wild-type hybridoma Sp603 and the X63Ag8 plasmacytoma fuser cell line, with an IAP-specific probe reveals several predominant IAP RNAs superimposed on a background smear. In addition to some low-molecular-weight molecules (~2 kb), each cell line produces IAP RNAs of 7.1 kb and 4.7 kb. We expect that the 7.1-kb IAP RNA corresponds to the transcriptional product of a full-length IAP gene, analogous to the one inserted in the igk-20 κ_{TNP} gene, whereas the 4.7-kb IAP RNA corresponds to transcripts originating from a deleted form of an IAP gene, analogous to the one found in the igk-1 κ_{TNP} gene. Confirmation of these speculations, however, must await direct structural comparisons of these IAP RNAs with the cloned IAP genes.

Association of IAP genes with activated cellular proto-oncogenes

Exogenous retroviruses have occasionally been found to activate cellular proto-oncogenes upon insertion (Hay-

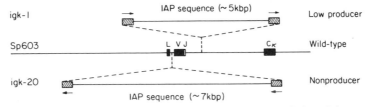

Figure 1 Schematic diagram of wild-type and mutant κ_{TNP} genes. The direction of transcription of the κ_{TNP} genes is from left to right. Ig gene-coding sequences are indicated by open and solid boxes. IAP sequences which are present in the κ_{TNP} genes isolated from igk-1 and igk-20 DNA are represented by lines flanked by hatched boxes above and below the wild-type κ_{TNP} gene, respectively. The approximate positions where the IAP genes have inserted into the wild-type κ_{TNP} gene are indicated. The hatched boxes represent homologous regions (LTRs), which are present at each end of the IAP sequences. Arrows indicate the normal direction of IAP gene transcription. Therefore, IAP gene transcription would be in the same direction as κ_{TNP} gene transcription in igk-1 and in the opposite direction to κ_{TNP} gene transcription in igk-20. Restriction enzyme maps of the cloned wild-type κ_{TNP} gene and the portions of the mutant κ_{TNP} genes that have been cloned can be found in Hawley et al. (1982). The cloning and characterization of the remaining portions of the mutant κ_{TNP} genes will be reported elsewhere (R. Hawley et al., in prep.). Abbreviations: (L) leader sequence; (V) variable region; (J) joining segment; (C_κ) k-chain constant region.

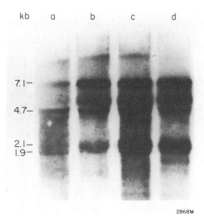

Figure 2 Characterization of IAP sequences in plasmacytoma and hybridoma RNA. RNA (10 μg) from X63Ag8 (lane *a*), Sp603 (lane *b*), igk-1 (lane *c*), and igk-20 (lane *d*) was denatured with glyoxal, electrophoresed through a horizontal 1% agarose gel in 10 mM sodium phosphate buffer at pH 6.9, transferred to nitrocellulose as described by Thomas (1980), and hybridized to a 750-bp *Hin*dIII fragment that was isolated from the 3′ end of an IAP gene and contains IAP internal and LTR sequences (Kuff et al. 1981; R. Hawley et al., unpubl.). Sizes were estimated by comparison with mouse 28S and 18S rRNAs (4.7 kb and 1.8 kb, respectively) and *E. coli* 23S and 16S rRNAs (2.90 kb and 1.54 kb, respectively) (Nelson et al. 1983).

ward et al. 1981; Fung et al. 1983) and the same appears to be true of IAP genes. Recently, Rechavi et al. (1982) reported that the cellular homolog of the Moloney murine sarcoma viral oncogene (*c-mos*) was activated in a mouse plasmacytoma (XRPC24) as a result of a recombination with a repetitive DNA element. Analysis of the sequence of this repetitive element revealed a 90% homology with the sequence of an IAP LTR that was fused to the *c-mos* gene in a head-to-head manner (Kuff et al. 1983a; Newmark 1983). RNA sequences have been found in IAP-producing cells that correspond to transcription of the IAP gene in the direction opposite to that of normal IAP gene transcription (Georgiev et al. 1983).

The presence of these "anti-sense" IAP sequences suggests that the IAP LTR may contain a bidirectional promoter, and it may be the "anti-sense" capability of this promoter that is responsible for *c-mos* gene transcription.

In light of the XRPC24 *c-mos* gene result, we were prompted to examine the structural integrity of the *c-mos* gene in our hybridoma cell lines and in the X63Ag8 plasmacytoma fuser cell line. To this end, *Eco*RI-digested genomic DNA was fractionated on agarose gels, transferred to nitrocellulose, and hybridized to a ³²P-labeled probe containing *mos*-specific sequences. In addition to a 15-kpb band that corresponds to the normal *c-mos* allele, all lanes containing DNA from either the X63Ag8 plasmacytoma, the Sp603 hybridoma, or the igk-1 and igk-20 mutants exhibited an additional band that migrated at 12.5 kbp (Fig. 3A). Digestion of these same DNAs with *Xba*I also revealed an additional band (Fig. 3B). In this case, the extra band was larger (3.3 kbp) than the normal 2.8-kbp *c-mos* band. These results indicate that the X63Ag8 plasmacytoma also contains a rearranged *c-mos* gene and this rearranged gene has been retained in the Sp6 hybridoma and its subclones. Furthermore, the size of the *Eco*RI band (12.5 kbp) is the same size as that of the rearranged *c-mos* gene in the XRPC24 plasmacytoma. Thus, the rearranged *c-mos* gene in X63Ag8 may also be due to an IAP gene insertion. In addition to the rearrangement, the extra band appears to be more intense in X63Ag8 than the band that corresponds to the normal *c-mos* allele (Fig. 3, lanes b). However, both *c-mos* alleles have a similar copy number in all of the hybridomas (Fig. 3).

This is only the second instance of a *c-mos* gene rearrangement in a mouse plasmacytoma. In contrast to this, almost all mouse plasmacytomas contain a rearranged form of the cellular homolog of the avian myelocytomatosis viral oncogene (*c-myc*) (Perry 1983). In some cases, rearrangement of the *c-myc* gene has been shown to be the result of a 15;12 chromosomal trans-

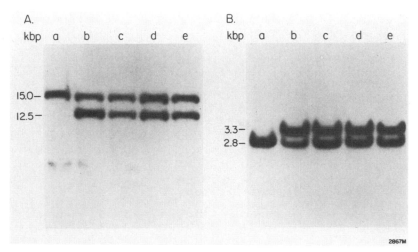

Figure 3 Analysis of the *c-mos* gene in plasmacytoma and hybridoma DNAs. Genomic DNA from BALB/c kidney (lanes *a*), X63Ag8 (lanes *b*), Sp603 (lanes *c*), igk-1 (lanes *d*), and igk-20 (lanes *e*) was digested with *Eco*RI (*A*) or *Xba*I (*B*). Aliquots (20 μg) were electrophoresed through 1% agarose gels, transferred to nitrocellulose, and hybridized with a ³²P-labeled probe prepared from an *Xba*I–*Hin*dIII *v-mos*-specific fragment contained in the plasmid pHT10 (Blair et al. 1980). Fragment sizes were determined by comparison with *Hin*dIII-digested λ phage DNA.

location that links the *c-myc* gene to the Igα heavy-chain constant region (Klein 1983). In addition to this translocational event, which involves the 5' end of the *c-myc* gene, Marcu and his colleagues (Harris et al. 1982) have identified several *c-myc* genes that have also undergone rearrangement at their 3' ends. One such *c-myc* gene (J558α25) has been cloned (Harris et al. 1982). Analysis of the novel DNA sequence at the 3' end of this *c-myc* gene indicated that it is moderately repeated in the mouse genome (R. Greenberg and K. Marcu, pers. comm.). To investigate whether this novel repetitive DNA sequence might be a member of the IAP gene family, a subclone (pα25RH1.6, Fig. 4B) containing the repetitive sequence and the 3' end of the *c-myc* gene from J558α25 (R. Greenberg and K. Marcu, unpubl.) was hybridized to a ³²P-labeled probe containing IAP LTR sequences (see Fig. 2). The IAP LTR sequences contained in this probe are homologous to the LTR sequences of the IAP genes identified by Kuff et al. (1983b). But these LTRs differ from the LTRs of the IAP genes studied by Cole et al. (1981) in the region of the IAP LTR that corresponds to the U5 region of a retroviral LTR (Varmus 1983). Nevertheless, LTRs from both types of IAP genes are about 340 bp and contain a highly conserved *Pst*I site about 150 bp from the 5' end (Cole et al. 1981; Kuff et al. 1981). Other characteristic features of IAP genes are one or two polymorphic *Eco*RI sites located in the body of the IAP gene about 300–800 bp from the *Pst*I site in the 5' LTR (Kuff et al. 1981; Shen-Ong and Cole 1982). Digestion of a plasmid (pg[Tκ2]⁷, Fig. 4B) containing IAP LTR sequences with *Pst*I and *Eco*RI, and hybridization with the IAP LTR probe yielded two reactive fragments (0.90 kbp and 0.33 kbp) as expected (Fig. 4A, right lane a). Digestion of pα25RH1.6 with *Pst*I and *Eco*RI yielded fragments of 4.85 kbp, 0.75 kbp, and 0.36 kbp (Fig. 4A, left lane b).

The 0.75-kbp fragment is common to both plasmids (Fig. 4A) and contains the β-lactamase gene from pBR322 (Sutcliffe 1979). The 4.85-kbp fragment was detected by the IAP LTR probe (Fig. 4A, right lane b). If the IAP-related sequences in the J558α25 *c-myc* clone correspond to a representative IAP gene of the type described by Cole et al. (1981), the lack of homology between the 0.36-kbp fragment and the IAP LTR probe can be explained. Thus, taken together, these results suggest that an IAP gene has inserted at the 3' end of the J558α25 *c-myc* gene and it is oriented in the same transcriptional direction as the *c-myc* gene (Fig. 4B).

Discussion

From these results, it is apparent that movement of IAP genes can occur within the mouse genome during experimental time. That the plasmacytomas and hybridomas in which the IAP gene insertions were found also produce IAPs is consistent with a mechanism of transposition involving an RNA intermediate. In this regard, it is interesting that RNA sequences homologous to the *copia* transposable element in *Drosophila* have been found within viruslike particles (VLPs) as well (Shiba and Saigo 1983). Similar to mouse IAPs, *Drosophila* VLPs contain a reverse transcriptase activity, and apparently the VLP structural protein is encoded by *copia* RNA (Shiba and Saigo 1983). Although it is not known whether *copia* RNA contains direct repeats, analogous to those found at the ends of IAP RNA (Cole et al. 1982) and necessary for the synthesis of a provirallike intermediate (Varmus 1983), the RNA from the *copia*-like transposable element Ty1 of yeast does contain direct repeats (Elder et al. 1983). It would seem, therefore, that reverse transcription of an RNA intermediate might be a widespread mechanism of movement of cellular

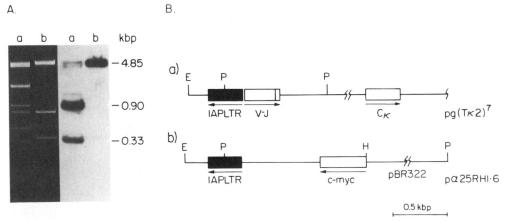

Figure 4 Detection of IAP sequences in a rearranged *c-myc* gene. (*A*) Aliquots (1 μg) of the plasmids pg(Tκ2)' (lanes *a*) and pα25RH1.6 (lanes *b*) were digested with *Pst*I and *Eco*RI, electrophoresed through a 2% agarose gel, transferred to nitrocellulose, and hybridized to a ³²P-labeled probe containing IAP LTR sequences (see Fig. 2). The ethidium bromide-stained gel is shown on the left and the autoradiogram is shown on the right. Fragment sizes were determined by comparison with *Hinf*I-digested pBR322 DNA. (*B*) Schematic diagrams of the plasmids used in A. (*a*) pg(Tκ2)⁷ contains a 9.0-kbp *Bam*HI fragment of the igk-20 κ_TNP gene (Tκ2) (Hawley et al. 1982) that was inserted into the *Bam*HI site of the plasmid pSV2-*gpt* (Mulligan and Berg 1980). (□) Ig gene-coding sequences; (■) an IAP LTR. (*b*) pα25RH1.6 contains a 1.6-kbp *Eco*RI–*Hind*III fragment of the 3' end of the J558α25 *c-myc* gene (Harris et al. 1982) which was inserted into pBR322 (R. Greenberg and K. Marcu, unpubl.). (□) *c-myc*-coding sequences; (■) a presumed IAP LTR. The directions of transcription are indicated by arrows. Restriction enzyme abbreviations: (E) *Eco*RI; (H) *Hind*III; (P) *Pst*I.

DNA sequences in eukaryotes. The recent discovery of dispersed "processed" genes (Sharp 1983) provides support for this hypothesis.

From comparisons of the sizes of restriction fragments detected by blot analysis of genomic DNA, we suspect that independent insertions of IAP genes have occurred at the same chromosomal loci in different cells. For example, the size of the *Eco*RI fragment containing the altered *c-mos* gene in the X63Ag8 plasmacytoma is the same size as the *Eco*RI fragment containing the IAP-*c-mos* fusion gene in the XRPC24 plasmacytoma (Rechavi et al. 1982). Thus, it is possible that the altered X63Ag8 *c-mos* gene arose in the same manner. (This prediction has been confirmed by Canaani et al., this volume.) Similarly, by this criterion, the other 3' rearranged *c-myc* genes observed by Harris et al. (1982) might also correspond to IAP gene insertions like the one identified in the J558α25 *c-myc* gene. In addition, we have recently identified another mutant hybridoma that has lost the expression of its κ-chain gene due to a rearrangement event (Ochi et al. 1983). Interestingly, the size of the *Bam*HI fragment containing the C_κ gene segment is the same size as that observed for the igk-1 κ_{TNP} gene (Hawley et al. 1982), suggesting that the rearrangement in this κ-chain gene might be due to the insertion of an IAP gene as well. Should these other rearrangements correspond to insertions of IAP genes, one interpretation of these results would be that IAP genes exhibit a preference for certain chromosomal loci. However, an alternative possibility would be that insertions of IAP genes occur at random throughout the mouse genome, usually going unnoticed, and occasionally an IAP gene inserts at the same site in different cells, resulting in a selective advantage for the variant cells and the subsequent detection of the mutagenic event. Regardless of which explanation is correct, the finding of IAP genes in similar positions within these loci might reflect a specificity of IAP genes for a particular target sequence in the DNA. In this regard, it is interesting that a 5-bp sequence (AATAA) near the end of the IAP LTR (Kuff et al. 1983b) is also present just downstream from both of the κ_{TNP} gene insertion sites (R. Hawley et al., unpubl.). Short sequences of homology have been reported to exist between the ends of some prokaryotic transposable elements and their target sequences (Kleckner 1981). Whether this 5-bp sequence is a common target sequence that serves to align an incoming IAP gene remains to be determined.

Like other transposable elements, IAP genes can either inactivate cellular genes (e.g., the κ_{TNP} gene) or increase the transcription of cellular genes (e.g., the *c-mos* gene) upon insertion. It is not clear, however, what effect the IAP gene insertion has on the J558α25 *c-myc* gene. The majority of the plasmacytoma *c-myc* genes are presumably activated by a 5' rearrangement event (Kirsch et al. 1981; Adams et al. 1982; Calame et al. 1982; Harris et al. 1982; Shen-Ong et al. 1982). Rearrangement of the 3' end of the *c-myc* gene is not necessary for its activation because only a small portion of plasmacytomas contain transcriptionally active *c-myc* genes with rearranged 3' ends. In the ones that do, the

5' end of the *c-myc* gene is also rearranged (Harris et al. 1982). In addition, these plasmacytomas usually contain another copy of the *c-myc* gene which is only rearranged at the 5' end (Harris et al. 1982). The J558α25 *c-myc* gene is apparently not essential for growth of plasmacytoma cells in tissue culture, as an in vitro derivative of the J558 plasmacytoma does not contain the J558α25 *c-myc* gene (Adams et al. 1982). However, the fact that several *c-myc* genes do have rearranged 3' ends suggests that the 3' rearrangement might contribute in some manner to continued growth of the plasmacytomas in vivo. It is conceivable that the IAP LTR is providing a transcriptional enhancer sequence that allows the one *c-myc* gene to be transcribed at an increased rate (Khoury and Gruss 1983). If so, this situation would be somewhat analogous to that of a chicken bursal lymphoma that was induced by avian leukosis virus (ALV). In this particular tumor, increased expression of the chicken *c-myc* gene was correlated with the presence of an ALV LTR situated at the 3' end of the *c-myc* gene in the same transcriptional orientation as that predicted for the IAP LTR in J558α25 (Payne et al. 1982).

IAP LTRs contain DNA sequences that are presumably involved in the initiation of transcription and polyadenylation (Kuff et al. 1983b). However, the mechanisms controlling IAP gene expression are not known. For example, it is not understood why different IAP genes are activated in different plasmacytomas. IAP gene expression does not appear to be directly linked to Ig gene expression because IAPs are found rarely in normal Ig-producing cells (Dalton et al. 1961; Wivel and Smith 1971). Moreover, there does not appear to be a relationship between the subset of IAP genes activated and the type of Ig produced because similar subsets of IAP genes have been found to be expressed in plasmacytomas producing entirely different types of Ig (Shen-Ong and Cole 1982). With the availability of cloned IAP genes and the advent of high-efficiency gene-transfer techniques, it should be possible to examine the mechanisms controlling the expression of IAP genes by introducing them into cells of different types.

Recently, Rubin and Spradling (1982) described an efficient gene transfer system into *Drosophila* embryos that utilizes transposable element vectors. In their experiments, the genes of interest were inserted into a transposable element and microinjected into the *Drosophilia* embryo along with an intact transposable element. The intact element provided the "transposase" which facilitated the integration of the injected DNA into the *Drosophila* genome. In this way, the sequences within the element were found to be transferred into the recipient DNA in a nontandem and nonpermuted manner whereas the sequences outside the element were not transferred. By analogy, construction and utilization of IAP gene vectors may facilitate the introduction of foreign genes into the mouse germ line.

Acknowledgments

We thank N. Govindji for expert technical assistance, W. Trimble for comments on the manuscript, and R.

Perry and K. Marcu for permission to cite unpublished results. This work was supported by grants from the Medical Research Council, the National Cancer Institute, the Arthritis Society, and the Allstate Foundation. R.G.H. was supported by a Studentship of the Medical Research Council.

References

Adams, J.M., S. Gerondakis, E. Webb, J. Mitchell, O. Bernard, and S. Cory. 1982. Transcriptionally active DNA region that rearranges frequently in murine lymphoid tumors. *Proc. Natl. Acad. Sci.* **79:** 6966.

Biczysko, W., M. Pienkowski, D. Solter, and H. Koprowski. 1973. Virus particles in early mouse embryos. *J. Natl. Cancer Inst.* **51:** 1041.

Blair, D.G., W.L. McClements, M.K. Oskarsson, P.J. Fischinger, and G.F. Vande Woude. 1980. Biological activity of cloned Moloney sarcoma virus DNA: Terminally redundant sequences may enhance transformation efficiency. *Proc. Natl. Acad. Sci.* **77:** 3504.

Calame, K., S. Kim, P. Lalley, R. Hill, M. Davis, and L. Hood. 1982. Molecular cloning of translocations involving chromosome 15 and the immunoglobulin C_α gene from chromosome 12 in two murine plasmacytomas. *Proc. Natl. Acad. Sci.* **79:** 6994.

Calarco, P.G. and D. Szöllösi. 1973. Intracisternal A particles in ova and preimplantation stages of the mouse. *Nat. New Biol.* **243:** 91.

Chase, D.G. and L. Pikó. 1973. Expression of A- and C-type particles in early mouse embryos. *J. Natl. Cancer Inst.* **51:** 1971.

Cole, M.D., M. Ono, and R.C.C. Huang. 1981. Terminally redundant sequences in cellular intracisternal A-particle genes. *J. Virol.* **38:** 680.

———. 1982. Intracisternal A-particle genes: Structure of adjacent genes and mapping of the boundaries of the transcriptional unit. *J. Virol.* **42:** 123.

Dalton, A.J., M. Potter, and R.M. Merwin. 1961. Some ultrastructural characteristics of a series of primary and transplanted plasma cell tumors of the mouse. *J. Natl. Cancer Inst.* **26:** 1221.

Elder, R.T., E.Y. Loh, and R. Davis. 1983. RNA from the yeast transposable element Ty1 has both ends in the direct repeats, a structure similar to retrovirus RNA. *Proc. Natl. Acad. Sci.* **80:** 2432.

Fung, Y.-K.T., W.G. Lewis, L.B. Crittenden, and H.-J. Kung. 1983. Activation of the cellular oncogene c-*erbB* by LTR insertion: Molecular basis for induction of erythroblastosis by avian leukosis virus. *Cell* **33:** 357.

Georgiev, G.P., D.A. Kramerov, A.P. Ryskov, K.G. Skryabin, and E.M. Lukanidin. 1983. Dispersed repetitive sequences in eukaryotic genomes and their possible biological significance. *Cold Spring Harbor Symp. Quant. Biol.* **47:** 1109.

Harris, L.J., R.B. Lang, and K.B. Marcu. 1982. Non-immunoglobulin-associated DNA rearrangements in mouse plasmacytomas. *Proc. Natl. Acad. Sci.* **79:** 4175.

Hawley, R.G., M.J. Shulman, H. Murialdo, D.M. Gibson, and N. Hozumi. 1982. Mutant immunoglobulin genes have repetitive DNA elements inserted into their intervening sequences. *Proc. Natl. Acad. Sci.* **79:** 7425.

Hayward, W.S., B.G. Neel, and S.M. Astrin. 1981. Activation of a cellular *onc* gene by promoter insertion in ALV-induced lymphoid leukosis. *Nature* **290:** 475.

Hozumi, N., R. Hawley, and H. Murialdo. 1981a. Molecular cloning of an immunoglobulin kappa constant gene from NZB mouse. *Gene* **13:** 163.

Hozumi, N., G.E. Wu, H. Murialdo, L. Roberts, D. Vetter, W.L. Fife, M. Whiteley, and P. Sadowski. 1981b. RNA splicing mutation in an aberrantly rearranged immunoglobulin λ I gene. *Proc. Natl. Acad. Sci.* **78:** 7019.

Khoury, G. and P. Gruss. 1983. Enhancer elements. *Cell* **33:** 313.

Kirsch, I.R., J.V. Ravetch, S.-P. Kwan, E.E. Max, R.L. Ney, and P. Leder. 1981. Multiple immunoglobulin switch region homologies outside the heavy chain constant region locus. *Nature* **293:** 585.

Kleckner, N. 1981. Transposable elements in prokaryotes. *Annu. Rev. Genet.* **15:** 341.

Klein, G. 1983. Specific chromosomal translocations and the genesis of B-cell-derived tumors in mice and men. *Cell* **32:** 311.

Köhler, G. and C. Milstein. 1975. Continuous cultures of fused cells secreting antibody of predefined specificity. *Nature* **256:** 495.

———. 1976. Derivation of specific antibody-producing tissue culture and tumor lines by cell fusion. *Eur. J. Immunol.* **6:** 511.

Köhler, G. and M.J. Shulman. 1980. Immunoglobulin M mutants. *Eur. J. Immunol.* **10:** 467.

Kuff, E.L., L.A. Smith, and K.K. Lueders. 1981. Intracisternal A-particle genes in *Mus musculus*: A conserved family of retrovirus-like elements. *Mol. Cell. Biol.* **1:** 216.

Kuff, E.L., N.A. Wivel, and K.K. Lueders. 1968. The extraction of intracisternal A-particles from a mouse plasma-cell tumor. *Cancer Res.* **28:** 2137.

Kuff, E.L., K.K. Lueders, H.L. Ozer, and N.A. Wivel. 1972. Some structural and antigenic properties of intracisternal A particles occurring in mouse tumors. *Proc. Natl. Acad. Sci.* **69:** 218.

Kuff, E.L., A. Feenstra, K. Lueders, G. Rechavi, D. Givol, and E. Canaani. 1983a. Homology between an endogenous viral LTR and sequences inserted in an activated cellular oncogene. *Nature* **302:** 547.

Kuff, E.L., A. Feenstra, K. Lueders, L. Smith, R. Hawley, N. Hozumi, and M. Shulman. 1983b. Intracisternal A-particle genes as movable elements in the mouse genome. *Proc. Natl. Acad. Sci.* **80:** 1992.

Lueders, K.K. and E.L. Kuff. 1977. Sequences associated with intracisternal A particles are reiterated in the mouse genome. *Cell* **12:** 963.

———. 1980. Intracisternal A-particle genes: Identification in the genome of *Mus musculus* and comparison of multiple isolates from a mouse gene library. *Proc. Natl. Acad. Sci.* **77:** 3571.

Lueders, K.K., S. Segal, and E.L. Kuff. 1977. RNA sequences specifically associated with mouse intracisternal A particles. *Cell* **11:** 83.

Marcu, K.B., O. Valabuena, and R.P. Perry. 1978. Isolation, purification, and properties of mouse heavy-chain immunoglobulin mRNAs. *Biochemistry* **17:** 1723.

Minna, J.D., K.K. Lueders, and E.L. Kuff. 1974. Expression of genes for intracisternal A particle antigen in somatic cell hybrids. *J. Natl. Cancer Inst.* **52:** 1211.

Mount, S.M. 1982. A catalogue of splice junction sequences. *Nucleic Acids Res.* **10:** 459.

Mulligan, R.C. and P. Berg. 1980. Expression of a bacterial gene in mammalian cells. *Science* **209:** 1422.

Neel, B.G., W.S. Hayward, H.L. Robinson, J. Fang, and S.M. Astrin. 1981. Avian leukosis virus-induced tumors have common proviral integration sites and synthesize discrete new RNAs: Oncogenesis by promoter insertion. *Cell* **23:** 323.

Nelson, K.J., J. Haimovich, and R.P. Perry. 1983. Characterization of productive and sterile transcripts from the immunoglobulin heavy-chain locus: Processing of μ_m and μ_s mRNA. *Mol. Cell. Biol.* **3:** 1317.

Nevins, J.R. 1983. The pathway of eukaryotic mRNA formation. *Annu. Rev. Biochem.* **52:** 441.

Newmark, P. 1983. What has moved into c-*mos*? *Nature* **301:** 196.

Ochi, A., R.G. Hawley, T. Hawley, M.J. Shulman, A. Traunecker, G. Köhler, and N. Hozumi. 1983. Functional immunoglobulin M production after transfection of cloned immunoglobulin heavy and light chain genes into lymphoid cells. *Proc. Natl. Acad. Sci.* **80:** 6351.

Ono, M., M.D. Cole, A.T. White, and R.C.C. Huang. 1980. Sequence organization of cloned intracisternal A particle genes. *Cell* **21:** 465.

Paterson, B.M., S.S. Segal, K.K. Lueders, and E.L. Kuff. 1978. RNA associated with murine intracisternal type A particle codes for the main particle protein. *J. Virol.* **27:** 118.

Payne, G.S., J.M. Bishop, and H.E. Varmus. 1982. Multiple arrangements of viral DNA and an activated host oncogene in bursal lymphomas. *Nature* **295:** 209.

Payne, G.S., S.A. Courtneidge, L.B. Crittenden, A.M. Fadly, J.M. Bishop, and H.E. Varmus. 1981. Analysis of avian leukosis virus DNA and RNA in bursal tumors: Viral gene expression is not required for maintenance of the tumor state. *Cell* **23:** 311.

Perry, R.P. 1983. Consequences of *myc* invasion of immunoglobulin loci: Facts and speculation. *Cell* **33:** 647.

Perry, R.P., C. Coleclough, and M. Weigert. 1981. Reorganization and expression of immunoglobulin genes: Status of allelic elements. *Cold Spring Harbor Symp. Quant. Biol.* **45:** 925.

Rechavi, G., D. Givol, and E. Canaani. 1982. Activation of a cellular oncogene by DNA rearrangement: Possible involvement of an IS-like element. *Nature* **300:** 607.

Rigby, P.W.J., M. Dieckmann, C. Rhodes, and P. Berg. 1977. Labeling deoxyribonucleic acid to high specific activity *in vitro* by nick translation with DNA polymerase I. *J. Mol. Biol.* **113:** 237.

Roeder, G.S. and G.R. Fink. 1980. Transposable elements in yeast. In *Mobile genetic elements* (ed. J.A. Shapiro), p. 300. Academic Press, New York.

Rubin, G.M. 1983. Dispersed repetitive DNAs in *Drosophila*. In *Mobile genetic elements* (ed. J.A. Shapiro), p. 329. Academic Press, New York.

Rubin, G.M. and A.C. Spradling. 1982. Genetic transformation of *Drosophila* with transposable element vectors. *Science* **218:** 348.

Sharp, P.A. 1983. Conversion of RNA to DNA in mammals: Alu-like elements and pseudogenes. *Nature* **301:** 471.

Shen-Ong, G.L.C. and M.D. Cole 1982. Differing populations of intracisternal A-particle genes in myeloma tumors and mouse subspecies. *J. Virol.* **42:** 411.

Shen-Ong, G.L.C., E.J. Keath, S.P. Piccoli, and M.D. Cole. 1982. Novel *myc* oncogene RNA from abortive immunoglobulin-gene recombination in mouse plasmacytomas. *Cell* **31:** 443.

Shiba, T. and K. Saigo. 1983. Retrovirus-like particles containing RNA homologous to the transposable element *copia* in *Drosophila melanogaster. Nature* **302:** 119.

Southern, E.M. 1975. Detection of specific sequences among DNA fragments separated by gel electrophoresis. *J. Mol. Biol.* **98:** 503.

Sutcliffe, J.G. 1979. Complete nucleotide sequence of the *Escherichia coli* plasmid pBR322. *Cold Spring Harbor Symp. Quant. Biol.* **43:** 77.

Thomas, P.S. 1980. Hybridization of denatured RNA and small DNA fragments transferred to nitrocellulose. *Proc. Natl. Acad. Sci.* **77:** 5201.

Varmus, H.E. 1983. Retroviruses. In *Mobile genetic elements* (ed. J.A. Shapiro), p. 411. Academic Press, New York.

Wilson, S.H. and E.L. Kuff. 1972. A novel DNA polymerase activity found in association with intracisternal A-type particles. *Proc. Natl. Acad. Sci.* **69:** 1531.

Wilson, S.H., E.W. Bohn, A. Matsukage, K.K. Lueders, and E.L. Kuff. 1974. Studies on the relationship between deoxyribonucleic acid polymerase activity and intracisternal A-type particles in mouse myeloma. *Biochemistry* **13:** 1087.

Wivel, N.A. and G.H. Smith. 1971. Distribution of intracisternal A-particles in a variety of normal and neoplastic mouse tissues. *Int. J. Cancer.* **7:** 167.

Wong-Staal, F., M.S. Reitz, Jr., C.D. Trainor, and R.C. Gallo. 1975. Murine intracisternal type A particles: A biochemical characterization. *J. Virol.* **16:** 887.

Yang, S.S. and N.A. Wivel. 1973. Analysis of high-molecular-weight ribonucleic acid associated with intracisternal A particles. *J. Virol.* **11:** 287.

———. 1974. Characterization of an endogenous RNA-dependent DNA polymerase associated with murine intracisternal A particles. *J. Virol.* **13:** 712.

Yotsuyanagi, Y. and D. Szöllösi. 1981. Early mouse embryo intracisternal particle: Fourth type of retrovirus-like particle associated with the mouse. *J. Natl. Cancer Inst.* **67:** 677.

Properties of the Mouse and Human *mos* Oncogene Loci

D.G. Blair, T.G. Wood, A.M. Woodworth, M.L. McGeady, M.K. Oskarsson,
F. Propst, M.A. Tainsky, C.S. Cooper, R. Watson, B.M. Baroudy, and
G.F. Vande Woude

Laboratory of Molecular Oncology, National Cancer Institute, Frederick Cancer Research Facility,
Frederick, Maryland 21701

The acute transforming retroviruses have been useful in demonstrating the role of specific cellular genes in malignant transformation (Bishop 1978, 1981, 1983). A portion of the genome of these viruses is homologous to host chromosomal DNA sequences that represent the cellular progenitors (*c-onc*) to the virus-encoded oncogenes (*v-onc*). The cellular oncogenes are apparently limited in number, present in low or single copy per haploid genome, and are evolutionarily conserved. Although the normal biological functions of these oncogenes have yet to be deciphered, when these genes are acquired by retroviruses their expression is regulated by the retroviral transcriptional control elements. One such acute transforming retrovirus, Moloney sarcoma virus (Mo-MSV), was isolated from a rhabdomyosarcoma that arose in a BALB/c mouse injected with Moloney murine leukemia virus (Mo-MLV) (Moloney 1966). The mouse cellular sequence acquired by Mo-MSV has been designated *v-mos*.

We have previously isolated biologically active recombinant DNA clones containing the entire Mo-MSV proviral genomes of the m1 and HT1 (Vande Woude 1980) strains and used the cloned *v-mos* sequence to identify and isolate the *v-mos* cellular homolog *c-mos*^Mo from normal mouse DNA (Oskarsson et al. 1980) (Fig. 1). We have also cloned a DNA fragment from human placental DNA, *c-mos*^Hu, containing a sequence homologous to *c-mos*^Mo (Watson 1982) (Fig. 1). Using a combination of

Southern blot hybridization (Southern 1975) and nucleotide sequence determinations (Maxam and Gilbert 1980; Reddy et al. 1980), the proviral *v-mos* and cellular mouse and human *c-mos* clones have been compared (Oskarsson et al. 1980; Reddy et al. 1980; Van Beveren et al. 1981). The transduced *v-mos* gene has been inserted into the *env*-coding region of Mo-MLV and codes for a protein of 374 amino acids (Van Beveren et al. 1981). The five aminoterminal codons of the *v-mos* open reading frame are derived from the Mo-MLV *env* gene. A direct comparison of the nucleotide sequences of *v-mos* and *c-mos*^Mo revealed 25 single-base differences in the sequence of 1157 nucleotides (Van Beveren et al. 1981).

Structural elements of *v-mos*, and the cellular *c-mos*^Mo and *c-mos*^Hu loci

The general structural features of the *v-mos*, *c-mos*^Mo, and *c-mos*^Hu are shown in Figure 1. The *v-mos* locus is presented as part of the integrated HT1 MSV provirus locus cloned from transformed mink cells (Vande Woude 1980). The *c-mos*^Mo locus molecularly cloned from the normal BALB/c mouse genome DNA has been previously described (Oskarsson et al. 1980). It contains three repetitive DNA sequences 3' to *mos* that represent members of the mouse B1 (Krayev et al. 1980) repetitive DNA family. An additional B1 repetitive DNA sequence is found 10 kbp upstream from the 5' end of *c-mos*^Mo.

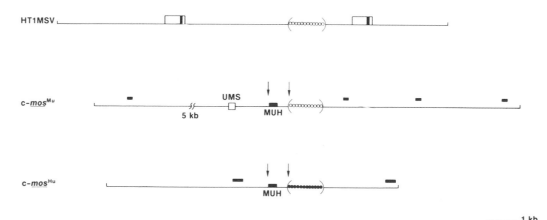

Figure 1 Structural elements of *v-mos* and the cellular *c-mos*^Mo and *c-mos*^Hu loci. A detailed restriction map of the HT1 MSV proviral DNA (McClements et al. 1981) and the cellular *c-mos*^Mo (Oskarsson et al. 1980) and *c-mos*^Hu (Watson et al. 1982) recombinant DNA clones have previously been described. (ooooooo) DNA sequences representing the *v-mos/c-mos*^Mo homology; (●●●●●●●) *c-mos*^Hu homology; (MUH) the *mos* upstream homology; (UMS) the upstream mouse sequence; (■) DNA sequences representing the mouse B1 repetitive DNA family in *c-mos*^Mo and the human *Alu*-repetitive DNA family.

The *c-mos*[Hu] locus has also been described (Watson et al. 1982) and contains two regions that hybridize to probes representing the human *Alu*-repetitive DNA family (Jelinek et al. 1980). The positioning and abundance of the B1 and *Alu* family members in the mouse and human cellular loci does not appear to be conserved.

Southern blot hybridization analysis demonstrates that the only region of shared homology between the Mo-MSV provirus and the *c-mos*[Mo] locus is the acquired *v-mos* gene (Oskarsson et al. 1980). A similar comparison of the *c-mos*[Mo] and *c-mos*[Hu] loci reveals that in addition to the shared homology in *mos*, a second region of homology is also detected 5' to both *c-mos* sequences and is referred to as the *mos* upstream homologous region (MUH) (F. Propst et al., in prep.) (Fig. 1). No other regions of homology were detected in the 5-kb DNA segments 5' to the *c-mos* loci. Mouse MUH is a 217-bp sequence that is 75% homologous to the human MUH, a 212-bp sequence located 353 bp upstream from the first ATG in the *c-mos*[Hu] gene (Fig. 2).

We have sequenced 2000 bp upstream (5') to *c-mos*[Mo] and find that both human and mouse *mos* open reading frames begin at a common conserved ATG that we have designated 1 (Fig. 2). We have determined that the mouse cellular sequence at positions −97 to −95 is ATG and not ATTG as reported (Van Beveren et al. 1981). This difference results in the following changes in the open reading frame of the *c-mos*[Mo] sequence: (1)

the open reading frame beginning at the ATG in position −143 (Fig. 2) now terminates after 36 codons (position −35, Fig. 2); (2) the ATG present in our sequence at position −79 (Fig. 2) initiates an open reading frame that also terminates at position −35 (Fig. 2); (3) open reading frames of *c-mos*[Mo] and *c-mos*[Hu] initiate at a common ATG, when the sequences are aligned by introducing two gaps of 15 and 3 bases into *c-mos*[Mo] and a single gap of 9 bases into *c-mos*[Hu]. The aligned sequences that initiate at equivalent ATGs (position 1, Fig. 2) are 77% homologous and terminate at equivalent opal codons. This yields open reading frames of 343 codons for *c-mos*[Mo] and 346 codons for *c-mos*[Hu].

We have previously identified consensus splice acceptor signals (position −33 in *c-mos*[Mo] and position −29 in *c-mos*[Hu]; Fig. 1) upstream from the position 1 ATG (Fig. 2) (Watson et al. 1981). *mos* expression has not been detected in normal tissues, but the presence of the conserved MUH region, together with the longer *mos* homology, is suggestive of a functional locus.

Identification of the upstream mouse sequence

The molecular elements of the Mo-MSV proviral genome responsible for cell transformation are the acquired *v-mos* sequence and the proviral long terminal repeat (LTR) (Blair et al. 1980; McClements 1981). Although transfection of recombinant DNA containing only the *v-mos* sequence induces a low level of cell transformation,

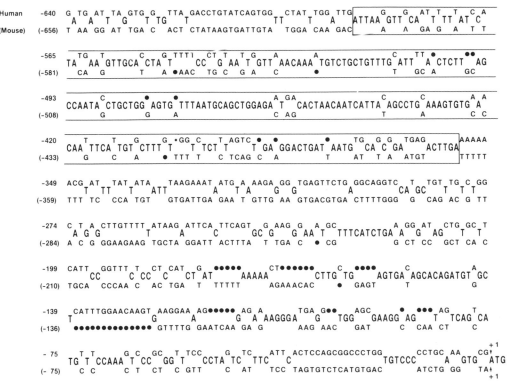

Figure 2 Comparison of the nucleotide sequence of the cellular DNA preceding the *c-mos*[Mo] and *c-mos*[Hu] open reading frame. DNA sequence analysis was performed by the method of Maxam and Gilbert (1980). The *c-mos*[Mo] and *c-mos*[Hu] DNA sequences (see arrows in Fig. 1) are aligned starting from the initiator ATG of the cellular *mos* open reading frames. Sequence homology between the two DNAs is indicated by a single upper-case letter, whereas nonhomology between the two DNA sequences is represented by the respective nucleotide designations for each of the cellular DNAs. The DNA sequence representing the *mos* upstream homology (MUH) is enclosed. Spaces inserted in the nucleotide sequence to maximize the sequence alignment are represented as dots (●).

the transforming activity of *v-mos* is enhanced with equivalent efficiency by introducing an LTR in either a 5′ or 3′ position relative to *v-mos* (Blair et al. 1980; Wood et al. 1983) (Fig. 3A). In contrast to its viral counterpart, *c-mos*[Mo] does not induce morphological transformation in DNA transfection assays (Oskarsson et al. 1980) and RNA transcripts containing *c-mos* have not been detected in normal cells (Frankel and Fischinger 1976; Gattoni et al. 1982). The transforming potential of *c-mos* can be activated by introducing an LTR 5′ to *c-mos* (Blair et al. 1981) (Fig. 3; LS2). However, unlike *v-mos*, insertion of an LTR 3′ to *c-mos*, as in LS1 (Fig. 3), does not result in an equivalent level of activation (Oskarsson et al. 1980; Blair et al. 1981). This difference in activity apparently is not due to differences in the nucleotide sequence of *c-mos* and *v-mos*, since the transforming potential of *c-mos* is efficiently activated by a 5′ LTR.

To explain the low transforming activity observed with an LTR introduced 3′ to *c-mos*, we have examined the RNA transcripts expressed in one of the LS1 transfectants (Fig. 3). A *mos*-specific probe detected a single 3.8-kb RNA transcript in these cells (data not shown),

whereas a probe representing the 3 kb of normal mouse DNA sequences preceding *c-mos* did not hybridize to this RNA transcript. These results suggested that the loss of mouse sequences preceding *c-mos* may be necessary for its activation.

To determine the effect of the upstream mouse sequences (UMS) on activation of the transforming potential of *c-mos*, a series of recombinant DNA clones were constructed, each containing an LTR 3′ to *c-mos* but with varying regions of the mouse DNA sequences upstream (Fig. 4A). Transfection of pLS1, a recombinant clone in which the normal mouse DNA sequences 5′ to the *Sac*I site were removed, induce, like LS1 (Fig. 4A), a low level of cell transformation (Fig. 4B). The transforming efficiency of recombinant DNA clones containing

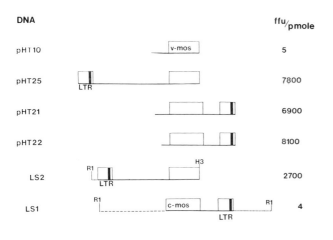

Figure 3 Effect of mouse cellular DNA sequences on the biological activity of *c-mos*[Mo] and *v-mos*. (*A*) The deletion of mouse DNA sequences from pMS1 by digestion with BAL 31 endonuclease has been described (Blair et al. 1981). Two of the resulting clones, pMST7 and pMST30, represent deletions (note arrows) of 1.1 kb and 1.3 kb, respectively. pMSTX was derived from an *Xba*I–*Hin*dIII digest of pmS1. A DNA fragment derived from the HT1 MSV proviral DNA clone containing the 3′ LTR was introduced at the *c-mos*[Mo] *Hin*dIII site in each construct. (*B*) The *Sac*I–*Xba*I DNA fragment was isolated from pmS1 and introduced into the viral sequences preceding *v-mos*: at the *Xba*I site 27 bp 5′ to *v-mos* (pHTMS23); at the *Xba*I site 400 bp 5′ to *v-mos* (pHTMS22); and using *Sac*I linkers, at the *Sma*I site 5′ to *v-mos* (pHTSM23). pHTSM22 was constructed using a *Bgl*II–*Xba*I DNA fragment isolated from pmS1 and inserted at the *Bgl*II site in the viral sequences preceding *v-mos*. All cloned DNAs were linearized by digestion with *Eco*RI prior to transfection (Blair et al. 1980). Restriction enzymes: (Bg 2) *Bgl*II; (H3) *Hin*dIII; (R1) *Eco*RI; (S) *Sac*I; (X) *Xba*I.

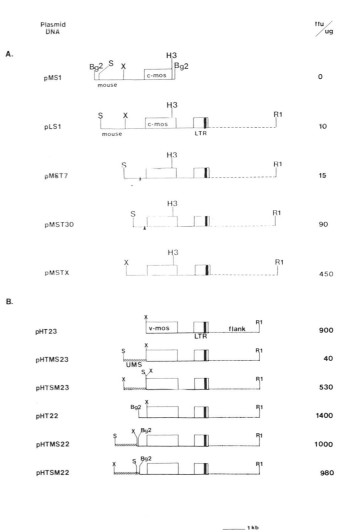

Figure 4 Comparison of the biological activity of cloned *v-mos* and *c-mos* recombinant DNAs. Descriptions of the *v-mos*[Mo] (Blair et al. 1980) and *c-mos*[Mo] (Oskarsson et al. 1980) have previously been published. DNA transfection-transformation assays were performed, as described (Blair et al. 1980). Restriction endonucleases: (H3) *Hin*dIII; (R1) *Eco*RI.

deletions of up to 1.3 kb of mouse DNA sequence (pMST7 and pMST30; Fig. 4A) were also low. However, deletion of all the sequences between the SacI and XbaI sites results in an increased activation of the transforming potential of c-mos (pMSTX, Fig. 4A), suggesting that mouse sequences retained in pMST30 and pMST7 are responsible for the inefficient activation of c-mos. We have determined the entire nucleotide sequence of a 2-kb region upstream from c-mos^{Mo} and show in Figure 5 the regions where the deletions occur in both pMST7 and pMST30. Collectively, this identifies a 184-bp sequence (UMS), position −1835 to −1651 (Fig. 5) from the initiating ATG in c-mos^{Mo}, which functions in a *cis*-acting fashion in preventing activation of the transforming potential of c-mos^{Mo}.

To determine if the UMS can prevent enhancement of the transforming activity of v-mos, we isolated the 1.0-kb SacI–XbaI DNA fragment and inserted this sequence, in both possible orientations, into the viral sequences preceding v-mos (Fig. 4B). The transforming efficiency of pHT23 is reduced 95% by introducing the UMS immediately 5′ to v-mos in the same orientation as it occurs upstream from c-mos^{Mo} (Fig. 4B, pHTMS23), whereas in the reverse polarity UMS reduces the transforming activity approximately 50%. The reduction in transforming efficiency is dependent upon the position UMS is inserted in the viral sequences 5′ to v-mos (Fig. 4B).

When UMS is introduced, in either orientation, into viral sequences 500 bp upstream from v-mos (pHTMS23, pHTMS22; Fig. 3), we observe no significant differences in transforming activity when compared with pHT22. Analysis of the RNA transcripts expressed in cells transformed by pHTMS22 containing UMS 500 bp upstream from v-mos reveals only a 2.9-kb v-mos RNA transcript (data not shown). This RNA is of a size that is compatible with the initiation of this transcript having occurred within the viral sequences preceding v-mos and is similar to the size RNA we have detected in some v-mos 3′ LTR transfectants (Wood et al. 1983). Although the mechanism involved in UMS preventing the activation of c-mos is at present unclear, these results suggest that UMS may prevent readthrough by RNA polymerase and may represent an obligatory termination signal for RNA transcription.

The transforming potential of *c-mos*^{Hu}

The DNA sequences of the human and mouse homologs converge at a common ATG (Watson et al. 1982) in the conserved mos open reading frames. The open reading frames are 75% homologous (Fig. 6) and suggest that c-mos^{Hu}, like c-mos^{Mo} (Blair et al. 1981), may have transforming potential.

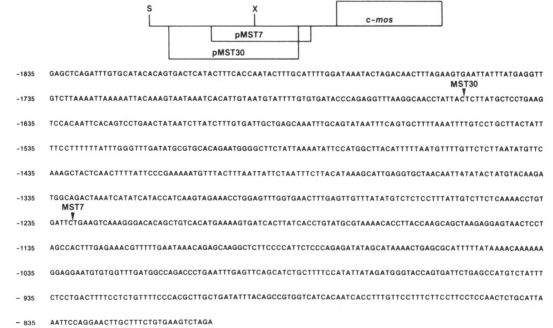

Figure 5 Nucleotide sequence of the *c-mos*^{Mo} UMS. A schematic diagram of the *c-mos*^{Mo} and upstream cellular DNA sequence is shown. The complete nucleotide sequence of the SacI (S)–XbaI (X) DNA fragment is presented and is numbered based upon the first nucleotide in the initiator codon ATG of the *c-mos*^{Mo} open reading frame being designated + 1. Deletions in the mouse cellular DNA sequence (pMST7 and pMST30) are indicated on the diagram, and the 5′ site within the nucleotide sequence for each deletion mutant is indicated.

To test this hypothesis, c-mos[Hu] recombinants were constructed in which the Mo-MSV proviral LTR was inserted at varying positions 5′ to the start of the c-mos[Hu] sequence (Fig. 7). While analogous constructs of c-mos[Mo] efficiently transform NIH-3T3 cells, none of the c-mos[Hu] constructs induced detectable transformation (Woodworth et al. 1983). Two proviral constructs, in which v-mos was replaced by c-mos[Hu] sequences, were tested. In the first, designated pm1h, the 5′ portion of the Mo-MSV provirus was joined to c-mos[Hu] at a common *Bgl*I site located 144 bp 3′ to the start of the common open reading frame. In the second, pHT1h, HT1MSV v-mos sequences (Fig. 1) from the *Bgl*I to *Hind*III restriction sites were replaced with a homologous fragment from c-mos[Hu] (Watson et al. 1982). We detected p30 antigen expression in cells transfected by pm1h. These antigens are encoded by Mo-MSV-derived *gag* sequences of m1 (Robey et al. 1977). Furthermore, a 4.7-kb *mos*-specific polyadenylated RNA was detected in cells cotransfected with pm1h and pSV2-*gpt* (Mulligan and Berg 1981) and selected for mycophenolic acid resistance (Fig. 8, lane 2). The size of this RNA is consistent with it being transcribed from the transfected pm1h sequences. However, even though the pm1h was apparently expressed after transfection, neither the pm1h nor the analogous construct pHT1h produced foci. The failure of all c-mos[Hu] constructs (Fig. 7) to transform

NIH-3T3 cells suggested that a region within the c-mos[Hu] open reading frame prevented activation.

To determine if a specific region of c-mos[Hu] prevented transformation, we constructed a series of *mos* gene hybrids in which v-mos/c-mos[Hu] recombinations had taken place at various points within the homologous *mos* open reading frame. Evolutionary divergence had resulted in the loss of all but a few conserved six-base recognition restriction sites (Watson et al. 1982); therefore, it was necessary to generate the *mos* gene hybrids in *E. coli* using the πVX miniplasmid recombination system (Seed 1983). A series of reciprocal recombinant pairs were generated. One of each pair contained the 5′ portion of Mo-MSV with a hybrid *mos* gene consisting of 5′ or aminoterminal v-mos and 3′ or carboxyterminal c-mos[Hu] open reading frame (referred to as Vh recombinants). The reciprocal hybrid *mos* gene obtained from the recombination event consisted of aminoterminal c-mos[Hu] and carboxyterminal v-mos (hV recombinants) open reading frame followed by 3′ Mo-MSV sequences. All Vh recombinants contained the Mo-MSV-derived 5′ LTR and Mo-MSV sequences through v-mos, whereas all hV recombinants contained the 3′ Mo-MSV LTR.

Table 1 summarizes the results obtained when four of these pairs were analyzed for biological activity. Several of the hybrid *mos* clones induced foci on DNA transfection, but where activity was detected, both pairs of re-

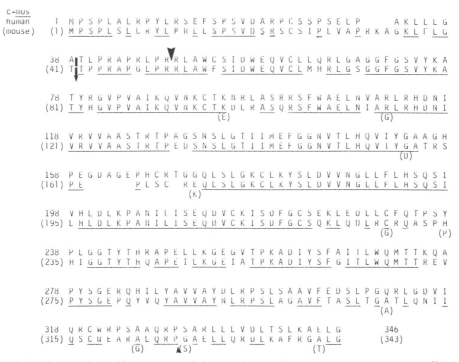

Figure 6 Comparison of the amino acid sequences of the proteins predicted to be encoded by c-mos[Mu] and c-mos[Hu]. Amino acid residues are both numbered from the common ATG initiation codon in the two cellular open reading frames (see text). Amino acids common to both sequences are underlined, and those different in the v-mos sequence of MoMSV124 are in parentheses. The c-mos[Mu] and v-mos sequences are from Van Beveren et al. (1981). The c-mos[Hu] sequence is from Watson et al. (1982). The letter code for the amino acids is: (A) alanine; (C) cysteine; (D) aspartic acid; (E) glutamic acid; (F) phenylalanine; (G) glycine; (H) histidine; (I) isoleucine; (K) lysine; (L) leucine; (M) methionine; (N) asparagine; (P) proline; (Q) glutamine; (R) arginine; (S) serine; (T) threonine; (V) valine; (W) tryptophan; (Y) tyrosine. (▮) Site of the in vivo insertion into c-mos[Mu] observed by Rechavi et al. (1982). (▼) Site of *Bgl*I restriction site. (▲) Position where the carboxyterminal open reading frame sequence of Reddy et al. (1980) differs from that of Van Beveren et al. (1981).

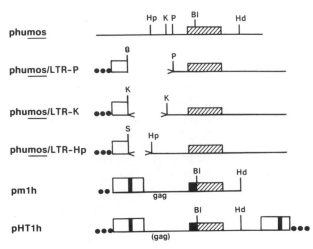

Figure 7 Mo-MSV-*c-mos*[Hu] recombinants. The top drawing represents the parental cloned fragment of *c-mos*[Hu] (Watson et al. 1982). The hybrids below were constructed using portions of the cloned Mo-MSV (Vande Woude et al. 1980). (▨) *c-mos*[Hu]; (■) *v-mos*; (▭) LTR sequences; (Hp) *Hpa*I; (K) *Kpn*I; (P) *Pvu*II; (B1) *Bgl*I; (Hd) *Hind*III; (●●) mink flanking sequences. *gag* sequences encoding the p60 polyprotein expressed in m1MSV-transformed cells but not expressed (*gag*) in HT1MSV-transformed cells. Biological activity of these constructs is discussed in the text.

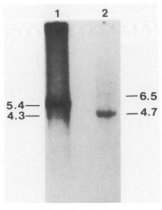

Figure 8 Analysis of polyadenylated RNA expressed in pm1h transfectants. RNA was prepared from NIH-3T3 cells cotransfected with *Ecogpt* and pm1h DNA and hybridized with *mos* probe, as described (Wood et al. 1983) (lane *1*). An identical analysis of NIH-3T3 cells cotransfected with pSV2-*gpt* (Mulligan and Berg 1981) and m1MSV proviral DNA is shown in lane *2*.

ciprocal Vh and hV recombinants were active. The most active pair, pVh02 and phV02, which have recombined between codons 82 and 95 (Table 1, Fig. 6), is approximately one-fifth as active as analogous Mo-MSV-derived plasmids containing *v-mos* and a single LTR (i.e., pHT22 or phT25, Table 1). As an independent confirmation of these results, two additional pairs of *mos* recombinants (05 and 42, data not shown) that have recombined within the same region as the 02 pairs are also active. The recombinants pVh 39 and phV 39, which have recombined between codons 108 and 136 (Table 1, Fig. 6) and carboxyterminal or 3' to the site of the 02 recombination, were also active. The level of biological activity of the 39 pair is lower than that observed for the 02 hybrids. Hybrids that have undergone recombination distal to the site of the 39 pair appear to be inactive. Only a single focus (of three detected) in the hV04 DNA transfection assays could be established as a cell line. This cell line does not contain new *mos* DNA fragments (Fig. 9B, lane 4), and it is possible that this recombinant does not stably transform cells or the original focus represented a spontaneous transformation event.

Southern blot analysis of other pVh- and phV-transformed cell DNA revealed that all transformants contained additional *mos* DNA fragments. *Bgl*II digestion of pVh02 generates a characteristic 1.5-kb fragment derived from a *Bgl*II site in front of *v-mos* and the *Bgl*II in *c-mos*[Hu]. DNA from cells transformed by pVh02 (Fig. 9A, lanes 2–5) and pVh05, an independent hybrid that has recombined within the same region as 02 (lanes 6 and 7), contain a band of approximately 1.5 kb in size, demonstrating that Vh02 and 05 were the source of the transfected DNA. A second *mos*-containing DNA fragment of 3.5 kb was detected in two of the pVh02 tumors (Fig.

Table 1 Biological Activity of *Hu-mos/v-mos* Recombinants

Recombinant[a]	Crossover position[b]	Foci/μg[c]
pVh02	82–95	235 (13)
phV02	82–95	124 (9)
pVh39	108–136	15 (5)
phV	108–136	16 (4)
pVh04	168–185	<4 (5)
phV04	168–185	6 (5)[3]
pVh17	229–248	<4 (5)
pm1-control	—	1400 (13)
pHT22-control	—	900 (1)
pHT25-control	—	880 (1)

[a]Clones containing recombinant hybrid *mos* sequences are designated Vh if sequences 5' to the crossover point are derived from the HT1 MSV provirus, whereas sequences 3' to the crossover are derived from p*Hu-mos*. Clones designated hV contain sequences 3' to the crossover are derived from HT1 MSV, whereas sequences 5' to the crossover are derived from p*Hu-mos*. 5' *Hu-mos* sequences in these constructs extend to an *Eco*RI restriction site 200 bp upstream from the first ATG of the open reading frame (Fig. 2), whereas 3' *Hu-mos* sequences extend to the *Hind*III site several hundred bases downstream (Fig. 8). Pm1 is the intact provirus of the m1 strain of Mo-MSV, whereas pHT22 and pHT25 are *mos*-containing subgenomic fragments containing LTR sequences 3' and 5', respectively, to *v-mos* (Blair et al. 1980).
[b]The position of the recombination in each hybrid was mapped by restriction analysis and is given in terms of the *Hu-mos* peptide sequence shown in Fig. 7. In each case, the crossover has occurred between the indicated codons.
[c]Biological activity is given as foci induced per microgram of transfected plasmid DNA and is the average of (*n*) determinations. Transfections were performed as previously described (Blair et al. 1980).

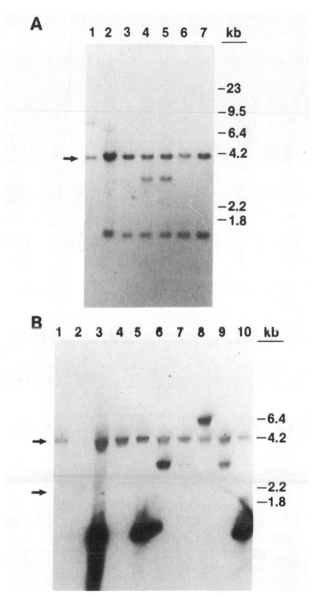

Figure 9 Detection of transfected *mos* DNA fragments in cells transformed with *v-mos*/*c-mos*^{Hu} recombinant DNA. Foci of cells transfected with various *mos* hybrid recombinants were picked, expanded, and injected into athymic nude mice. Tumors that arose were excised and high-molecular-weight DNA was prepared (Blair et al. 1983), digested with restriction nucleases, and separated on 0.7% agarose gels. Fragments were analyzed by the Southern technique (Southern 1975), using a *mos*-specific DNA probe (Oskarsson et al. 1980). (*A*) DNA was digested with *Bgl*II. (Lane *1*) pHT25-transformed (Fig. 4) cell DNA; (lanes *2, 3* and *4, 5*) replicate tumors induced by two independently derived pVh02-transformed cell lines; (lanes *6* and *7*) DNA from two tumors induced by a single pVh05-transformed cell line. The arrow indicates the position of the endogenous *c-mos* fragment. The 1.5-kb *Bgl*II fragment is evidence that the cell possesses the hybrid *mos* gene (see text). (*B*) DNA was digested with *Eco*RI and *Hind*III. (Lane *1*) NIH-3T3; (lane *2*) human placenta; (lanes *3, 8,* and *10*) DNA from tumors induced by independent phV02-transformed cell lines; (lane *4*) phV04-transformed cell line; (lane *5*) phV39-transformed cell line; (lane *6*) pVh42-transformed cell line; (lanes *7* and *9*) pVh02-transformed cell lines. The arrows indicate the position of the endogenous *c-mos*^{Mu} (upper) and *c-mos*^{Hu} (lower) DNA fragments. The significance of the new *mos*-hybridizing bands is discussed in the text.

9A, lanes 4 and 5) derived from a single focus. This fragment appears to be rearranged. As shown in Fig. 9B (lanes 7 and 9), *Eco*RI–*Hind*III digestion of pVh02-transformed cell DNA generates a 3.2-kb *mos*-containing fragment that is again characteristic of the transfecting pVh02 plasmid. A similar fragment is detected in cells transformed by pVh42, an analogous recombinant (Fig. 9B, lane 6). It should be noted that the intensity of hybridization of all new *mos*-containing fragments is approximately equivalent to that of the endogenous 4.2-kb (Fig. 9A) or 4.4-kb (Fig. 9B) *c-mos* bands, suggesting that they are present as single copies.

The hybridization pattern of cells transformed by phV recombinants (Fig. 9B, lanes 3, 5, 8, 10) is more complex and reveals several interesting features. A characteristic 1.2-kb *Eco*RI–*Hind*III fragment is generated from the hV recombinants and is derived from the *Eco*RI site 200 bp upstream from the *c-mos*^{Hu} ATG at position 1 (Fig. 2) and the *Hind*III site 3′ to the *v-mos* open reading frame. A 1.2-kb unrearranged *mos*-containing *Eco*RI–*Hind*III fragment is detected in DNA from cells transformed by phV39 (Fig. 9B, lane 5) and phV02 (Fig. 9B, lanes 3 and 10). The intensity of these bands suggests that multiple copies, estimated to be from 20 to 50 per genome equivalent, are present in these cells. In contrast, a larger *mos* DNA fragment is detected in another tumor induced by phV02 (Fig. 9B, lane 8). The altered size of this band indicates that the insert has undergone rearrangements affecting either one or both of the *Eco*RI and *Hind*III sites in the transfected DNA. It seems likely that the *Eco*RI site approximately 200 bp 5′ to the start of the *c-mos*^{Hu} open reading frame is affected since removal of the 3′ *Hind*III site would dissociate *mos* from the LTR. It is tempting to speculate that these two classes of recombinants, one with amplified *mos* hybrid sequences and the other with a low copy number, rearranged *mos* hybrid locus, represent two alternative pathways of cell transformation by phV recombinants. Sequences 5′ to *c-mos*^{Hu} could act like the UMS region in the *c-mos*^{Mo} locus to suppress the activity of a 3′ LTR enhancer (Figs. 3 and 4; Table 1). This could be overridden by either a large number of copies of the *mos* hybrid or by deleting these 5′ sequences and substituting a new promoter (Wood et al. 1983). Alternatively, the phV *mos* hybrid product may be less efficient as a transforming protein, and the presence of a large number of copies of the unrearranged phV sequences, or the substitution of an efficient promoter 5′ to the hybrid *mos* gene DNA derived from cell, vector, or carrier may be required for sufficient expression of the hybrid *mos* product to induce cell transformation.

The analysis of the *v-mos*/*c-mos*^{Hu} hybrid clones shows a complex pattern of activities that suggest multiple factors are involved in the transformation by these hybrid oncogenes. Our data is consistent with the hypothesis that the *mos* oncogene contains multiple domains which interact to produce an active gene product. Evolutionary alterations in the *c-mos*^{Hu} sequence relative to *c-mos*^{Mu} may have altered these domains in ways that no longer allow mouse domains and human domains to interact in

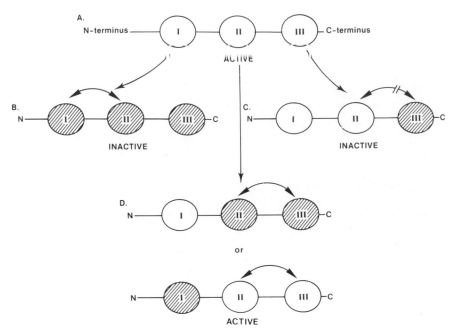

Figure 10 Schematic model of the domains of the *mos* polypeptide and their interactions as suggested by the biological activity of *v-mos/c-mos*^Hu recombinants (Table 1). The domains are designated I, II, and III and are not drawn to scale. Shading indicates that these regions were derived from *v-mos*-(-○-) or *c-mos*^Hu- (⊘) coding sequences. Arrows ( ) indicate that structural interactions are implied in activation of transforming potential. This symbol ( ) indicates the interaction is unfavorable to elicit transforming potential.

a functional way. Our analysis of the *mos* hybrid recombinants suggests that there are three domains that are essential for biological activity (Fig. 10). We postulate that in the *c-mos*^Hu product (Fig. 10B) residues in domain I interact with those in domain II to prevent transformation by *c-mos*^Hu. Thus, both pairs of the 02 and 39 hybrid *mos* recombinants (Fig. 10D) are active, and in these proteins, domains I and II of the *c-mos*^Hu are segregated. The inactivity of the pVh04, and especially the pVh17 hybrid (Table 1), which is 72% *v-mos*, suggests a third domain, i.e., interactions are required between domains II and III of *v-mos* for the protein to be biologically active, and this only occurs when both domains are from the same parent (Fig. 10D). Differences between *c-mos*^Hu and *v-mos* protein structures must prevent hybrids with the structure shown in Figure 10C (pVh17) from attaining an active configuration.

Our results map the first of these domains between the *Bgl*I site in *c-mos*^Hu (shown by the arrow in Fig. 6) and the site of the crossovers in the 02 hybrids (residues 82–95). The second domain would include the region between the 39 hybrid crossover (residues 108–136) and the 04 hybrid crossover (residues 168–185) and include a highly nonhomologous region of the open reading frame (residues 155–171) in which only 3 of 17 residues are conserved. The third domain is defined by the region between the site of pVh/hV17 recombination (residues 229–248) and the carboxyl terminus of *mos* at residue 346. By analyzing *mos* hybrid recombinants that occur carboxyterminal or 3' to codon 248, it should be possible to define the carboxyterminal position of the third domain.

The polypeptide sequence comparison of *c-mos*^Hu and *c-mos*^Mu (Fig. 6) reveals several features that suggest how domains I and II may interact in *c-mos*^Hu, but fail to interact in heterologous recombinants. One of the five amino acid differences between *c-mos*^Hu and *v-mos*^Mu in domain I is a cysteine in *c-mos*^Hu at residue 53. Since the area defined as domain II also contains a cysteine at residue 167, it is possible that interactions between these two residues may be responsible for the failure of *c-mos*^Hu constructs (Fig. 7) and pm1h and pHT1h to transform. In addition, the area between residues 136 and 168 represents a region of maximum divergence between the two *mos* genes. Thus, the new codons in the *c-mos*^Hu open reading frame are consistent with functional differences between the two proteins within domain II and may be related to evolutionary pressures to prevent oncogenic activation. Specific mutagenesis of these codons should allow us to determine whether the changes in these domains are responsible for the inactivity of *c-mos*^Hu.

The biological studies of these hybrid *mos* plasmids indicate that despite the high degree of conservation of the *mos* regions in mouse and man, significant differences have arisen in the requirements for oncogenic activation of these sequences. Although provirus insertion with the resulting quantitative changes in the level of *mos* expression have been shown both in vitro (Blair et al. 1981) and in vivo (Rechavi et al. 1982) to be sufficient to activate *c-mos*^Mo, our data here would suggest that additional qualitative changes in the *c-mos*^Hu gene are necessary to activate the oncogenic potential of this sequence. We have suggested the term "quantic"(i.e., quantic math, the function of two or more variables) to describe the situation in which two or more changes are required to effect oncogene activation. Since the frequency of a quantical oncogene activation is the product of the frequency of a quantitative or qualitative event, oncogenes requiring quantical activation would have a low probability of participating in cancer during the life span of an animal. Thus, the number of oncogenes in an animal requiring activation by a quantical event might influence the life span of the animal.

The study of the *mos* oncogene and its normal role has been hampered by the inability to detect expression from this locus in normal cells. However, the identification of a second region of homology upstream to *c-mos* in mouse and human, designated MUH, indicates that, structurally, *c-mos*^{Hu} and *c-mos*^{Mo} resemble a functional locus. It may be that *c-mos* is normally expressed at low levels in specific tissues or at specific developmental stages, and has therefore escaped detection. The UMS region of *mos*^{Mo} may relate to this problem since it is possible that this locus is involved in the normal regulation of *mos* expression.

We have observed that even in certain *v-mos* 3′ LTR transformants the level of *mos* gene RNA expression is from 1 to 10 copies per cell (Wood et al. 1983). This low level of RNA expression is consistent with the level of protein detected in murine sarcoma virus (MSV)-transformed cells by Papkoff et al. (1982) and would suggest that the protein is especially active as a transforming protein. However, this makes the study of the *mos* protein and its targets a formidable task. For this reason, it has been especially useful to study the *mos* gene *v-mos*/*c-mos*^{Hu} hybrid recombinants. These analyses have allowed us to identify what appear to be functional domains of the *mos* gene protein, and we may be able to determine structural features of the protein that are important to the transforming process when this information is used in conjunction with site-specific mutagenesis and transfection assays.

References

Bishop, J.M. 1978. Retroviruses. *Annu. Rev. Biochem.* **47**: 35.
———. 1981. Enemies within: The genesis of retrovirus oncogenes. *Cell* **23**: 5.
———. 1983. Cellular oncogenes and retroviruses. *Annu. Rev. Biochem.* **52**: 301.
Blair, D.G., C.S. Cooper, M.K. Oskarsson, L.A. Eader, and G.F. Vande Woude. 1983. A new method for detecting cellular transforming genes. *Science* **218**: 1122.
Blair, D.G., W.L. McClements, M.K. Oskarsson, P.J. Fischinger, and G.F. Vande Woude. 1980. Biological activity of cloned Moloney sarcoma virus DNA: Terminally redundant sequences may enhance transformation efficiency. *Proc. Natl. Acad. Sci.* **77**: 3504.
Blair, D.G., M. Oskarsson, T.G. Wood, W.L. McClements, P.J. Fischinger, and G.F. Vande Woude. 1981. Activation of the transforming potential of a normal cell sequence: A molecular model for oncogenesis. *Science* **212**: 941.
Frankel, A.E. and P.J. Fischinger. 1976. Nucleotide sequences in mouse DNA and RNA specific for Moloney sarcoma virus. *Proc. Natl. Acad. Sci.* **73**: 3705.
Gattoni, S., P. Kirschmeier, I.B. Weinstein, J. Escobedo, and D. Dina. 1982. Cellular Moloney murine sarcoma (c-*mos*)

sequences are hypermethylated and transcriptionally silent in normal and transformed rodent cells. *Mol. Cell. Biol.* **2**: 42.
Jelinek, W.R., T.P. Toomey, L. Leinwood, C.H. Duncan, P.A. Biro, P.V. Choudary, S.M. Weissman, C.M. Rubin, C.M. Houck, P.L. Deininger, and C.W. Schmid. 1980. Ubiquitous, interspersed repeated sequences in mammalian genomes. *Proc. Natl. Acad. Sci.* **77**: 1398.
Krayev, A.S., D.A. Kramerov, A.P. Ryskov, A.A. Bayev, and G.P. Georgiev. 1980. The nucleotide sequence of the ubiquitous repetitive DNA sequence B1 complementary to the most abundant class of mouse fold-back RNA. *Nucleic Acids Res.* **8**: 1201.
Maxam, A.M. and W. Gilbert. 1980. Sequencing end-labelled DNA with base-specific chemical cleavages. *Methods Enzymol.* **65**: 499.
McClements, W.L., R. Dhar, D.G. Blair, L. Enquist, M. Oskarsson, and G.F. Vande Woude. 1981. The long terminal repeat of Moloney sarcoma provirus. *Cold Spring Harbor Symp. Quant. Biol.* **45**: 699.
Moloney, J.B. 1966. Biological studies on a lymphoid leukemia virus extracted from sarcoma S37. I. Origin and introductory investigations. *Natl. Cancer Inst. Monogr.* **22**: 139.
Mulligan, R.C. and P. Berg. 1981. Selection from animal cells that express the *Escherichia coli* gene coding for xanthine-guanine phosphoribosyl-transferase. *Proc. Natl. Acad. Sci.* **78**: 2072.
Oskarsson, M., W.L. McClements, D.G. Blair, J.V. Maizel, and G.F. Vande Woude. 1980. Properties of a normal mouse cell DNA sequence (sarc) homologous to the *src* sequence of Moloney sarcoma virus. *Science* **207**: 1222.
Papkoff, J., I.M. Verma, and P. Hurter. 1982. Detection of a transforming gene product in Moloney murine sarcoma virus transformed cells. *Cell* **29**: 417.
Rechavi, G., D. Givol, and E. Canaani. 1982. Activation of a cellular oncogene by DNA rearrangement: Possible involvement of an IS-like element. *Nature* **300**: 607.
Reddy, E.P., M.J. Smith, E. Canaani, K.C. Robbins, S.R. Tronick, S. Zain, and S.A. Aaronson. 1980. Nucleotide sequence analysis of the transforming region and large terminal redundancies of Moloney murine sarcoma virus. *Proc. Natl. Acad. Sci.* **77**: 5234.
Robey, W.G., M.K. Oskarsson, G.F. Vande Woude, R.B. Naso, R.B. Arlinghaus, D.K. Haapala, and P.J. Fischinger. 1977. Cells transformed by certain strains of Moloney sarcoma virus contain murine p60. *Cell* **10**: 79.
Seed, B. 1983. Purification of genomic sequences from bacteriophage libraries by recombination and selection *in vivo*. *Nucleic Acids Res.* **11**: 2427.
Southern, E.M. 1975. Detection of specific sequences among DNA fragments separated by gel electrophoresis. *J. Mol. Biol.* **98**: 503.
Van Beveren, C., F. van Straaten, J.A. Galleshaw, and I.M. Verma. 1981. Nucleotide sequence of the genome of a murine sarcoma virus. *Cell* **27**: 97.
Vande Woude, G.F., M. Oskarsson, W. McClements, L. Enquist, D. Blair, P. Fischinger, J. Maizel, and M. Sullivan. 1980. Characterization of integrated Moloney sarcoma provirus and flanking sequences cloned in bacteriophage lambda. *Cold Spring Harbor Symp. Quant. Biol.* **44**: 735.
Watson, R., M. Oskarsson, and G.F. Vande Woude. 1982. Human DNA sequence homologous to the transforming gene (mos) of Moloney murine sarcoma virus. *Proc. Natl. Acad. Sci.* **79**: 4078.
Wood, T.G., M.L. McGeady, D.G. Blair, and G.F. Vande Woude. 1983. Long terminal repeat enhancement of v-*mos* transforming activity: Identification of essential regions. *J. Virol.* **46**: 726.
Woodworth, A., M. Oskarsson, D.G. Blair, M.L. McGeady, M. Tainsky, and G.F. Vande Woude. 1983. Biological properties of the human DNA sequence homologous to the *mos* transforming gene of Moloney sarcoma virus. In *Genes and proteins in oncogenes* (ed. I.B. Weinstein and H.J. Vogel), p. 233. Academic Press, New York.

An Homologous Domain between the *c-mos* Gene Product and a Papilloma Virus Polypeptide with a Putative Role in Cellular Transformation

O. Danos and M. Yaniv

Département de Biologie Moléculaire, Institut Pasteur, Paris, France

Papilloma viruses belong to the Papovaviridae family of DNA tumor viruses together with the polyoma viruses (SV40, BK virus, polyoma), which form a second genus. Papilloma virus infection of epithelial cells leads, under certain conditions, to malignant transformation. These virally induced neoplasias occur in natural conditions both in animals and in men.

The cottontail rabbit papilloma virus (CRPV), isolated from skin papillomas of wild cottontail rabbits, induces carcinomas at a high frequency when injected into domestic rabbits (Rous and Beard 1935). Such carcinomas have been transplanted for many generations in laboratory animals and still contain a high copy number of the viral genome (Favre et al. 1982). These tumors do not produce viruses, but the viral genome is transcribed (Wettstein and Stevens 1981). Frequent malignant conversions of bovine papilloma virus type-4-induced gastroesophageal lesions have also been reported in areas where cattle are fed on bracken fern (Campo et al. 1980).

Several types of human papilloma virus are associated with a rare disease, epidermodysplasia verruciformis, in which benign skin lesions frequently evolve into carcinomas (Orth et al. 1980). More recently, Dürst et al. (1983) have shown that a specific human papilloma virus DNA (HPV-16) is present in many biopsies of cervical carcinomas.

These facts clearly suggest that papilloma viruses play an important role in the establishment of naturally occurring epithelial carcinomas. The malignant transformation may well be the result of a synergy between cell-virus interaction and environmental factors (Orth et al. 1977, 1980).

The molecular basis of papilloma virus-mediated morphological transformation and interaction with epithelial cells is not currently understood. Such studies have been hampered in the past, due to the lack of a permissive tissue culture system. Recently, the ability of bovine papilloma virus 1 (BPV-1) DNA to transform established mouse fibroblasts lines (NIH-3T3 or C127) (Dvoretzky et al. 1980) has been used as a functional assay to define the viral sequences required for transformation. In fact, a 69% BPV-1 subgenomic fragment (5.6 kb) has been shown to be sufficient (Lowy et al. 1980). Furthermore, recent experiments indicate that a smaller EcoRI–BamHI (2.3 kb) fragment can efficiently transform

mouse fibroblasts when *cis*-activated by the enhancer element present on mouse sarcoma virus long terminal repeat (LTR) or SV40 early promoter (N. Sarver and P. Howley, pers. comm.). The major transcripts detected in BPV-1-transformed cells and in induced hamster tumors map within this 2.3-kb fragment. Correlatively, two CRPV-specific transcripts are found in the VX2 transplantable carcinomas (Nasseri et al. 1982; George et al. 1984) and correspond to two discontinuous regions of the viral genome, as revealed by electron microscopy heteroduplex mapping (George et al. 1984). The 3'-proximal exons of these mRNAs correspond to sequences homologous to the *Eco*RI–*Bam*HI BPV-1 fragment mentioned above, namely the E2 region (Chen et al. 1982; Danos et al. 1982; Schwartz et al. 1983; see Fig. 1).

We have determined the complete nucleotide sequence of the CRPV DNA (I. Giri et al., unpubl.), and the organization of the open reading frames is depicted in Figure 1. The L region bears the information for the virion structural proteins. The E region, which is transcribed in CRPV-induced carcinomas and is the ho-

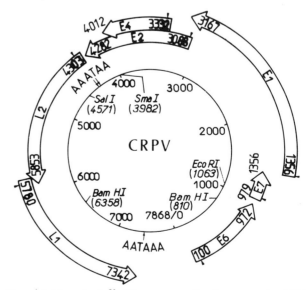

Figure 1 Organization of the open reading frames on the CRPV genome. Numbers in the arrows refer to the start and to the end of the open reading frames. The first methionine is depicted as a bar over each arrow.

molog of the BPV-1 69% transforming fragment, is composed of several exons likely to encode virus repli cation and transformation functions. CRPV transcripts detected in VX2 carcinomas correspond to E6 and/or E7 joined to the carboxyterminal half of E2. The large E1-coding region is spliced out of these mature transcripts.

To obtain further indications on E-coding segments that might play a role in cellular transformation, we used the straightforward approach of comparing each of the deduced amino acid sequences to the Protein Data Bank of the National Biomedical Research Foundation (NBRF). We discuss here the possible relevance of the homology we found between the *c-mos* gene product and the carboxyterminal portion of the E2-encoded polypeptide.

Computing Methods

Papilloma virus-encoded peptides were screened against the NBRF protein data bank using a simple and rapid scanning program originally developed by J.M. Claverie (Centre de Calcul, Institut Pasteur, unpubl.). This method searches for homologies between 80-amino-acid-long, successive overlapping strings from the papilloma virus putative protein sequences and the protein sequences present in the bank. The lower limit of detection was set at 20% (16/80) identical amino acids, and the searching program did not allow any gaps.

Homologies of interest were further analyzed using a Needleman-Wunsh-derived algorithm (Needleman and Wunsh 1970) to obtain optimal alignments allowing gaps (penalty for a gap was set to 2.5). Indications on their statistical significance were drawn from 50 reiterated comparisons to randomized sequences (see Table 1). A score value of 3.0 or more standard deviations above the mean score of randomized sequences was considered as statistically significant (Doolittle 1981).

Local hydrophilicity estimation was performed using a program similar to the one described by Hopp and Woods (1981). Prediction of secondary structure was obtained with the program designed by Garnier et al (1978).

Results

In the course of this systematic screening, several interesting homologies were observed. One of them, which will not be discussed here and was also observed by others (P. Clertant and I. Seif, in prep.), concerned a region of the papilloma virus E1 gene product found to be homologous to the proposed nucleotide binding site of ATP synthetases, polyoma and SV40 large T antigen, and p21 *ras* gene product. This homology shows how such a procedure can be helpful in predicting a testable biochemical activity for yet uncharacterized proteins of known sequence.

Another appealing homology to come out of the first "sliding segment procedure" was between the carboxyterminal part of the E2 putative protein of papilloma viruses and a segment of the human *c-mos* proto-oncogene-encoded protein (positions 164–245). Homologous amino acid sequences were optimally aligned and statistical significance was estimated (Table 1). The alignment between the segments of papilloma virus E2 protein and *c-mos* gene product is shown in Figure 2.

The alignment depicted here has been finally achieved by hand, in order to fit the four papilloma virus sequences together with the *c-mos* sequence. Three gaps have been introduced in the *c-mos* sequence and this alignment shows that 24 positions over 86 (29%) are identical between *c-mos* and E2 of at least two papilloma viruses. Only the human *c-mos* sequence is shown here, but the closely related sequences of mouse *c-mos* or Moloney sarcoma virus *v-mos* gene products (Van Beveren et al. 1981; Watson et al. 1982) would also match the E2 sequences. Analysis of the local hydrophilicity along the sequences also revealed a conserved pattern, with two hydrophilic peaks and one hydrophobic peak (Fig. 2). In addition, the predicted secondary structure shown here for the first 20 amino acids is strikingly conserved, with

Table 1 Alignment Scores (in S.D.) for Comparison of Protein Fragments Shown in Figure 2

	Sequence 1				
	CRPV	HPV-1a	HPV-6b	BPV-1	RSV-*src*
Sequence 2					
CRPV	—				
HPV-1a	28.0	—			
HPV-6b	10.0	10.0	—		
BPV-1	10.5	6.5	6.5	—	
c-mos	5.5	7.6	6.0	0.2	6.7

Values are given in standard deviations above the mean of shuffled sequences. The standard deviation was estimated each time by 50 reiterated comparisons of sequence 1 to shuffled sequence 2. Penalty for a gap was 2.5 (1.5 + *n*; *n* = gap size). Using these parameters, the *c-mos* segment was aligned with the corresponding segment of RSV-*src* product (residues 350–431) and the 6.7 S.D. value agrees with the previously reported one (Van Beveren et al. 1981). The nonsignificant value found in these conditions for BPV-1 E2 probably arises from the additional gap present in this alignment (see Fig. 2).

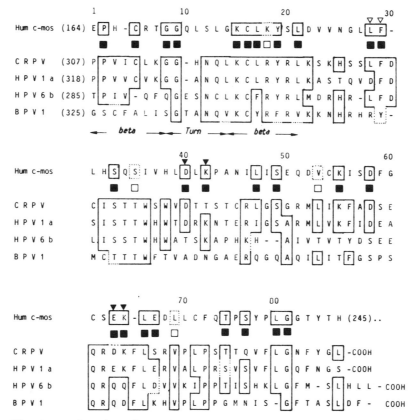

Figure 2 Papilloma viruses E2 and *c-mos* homology. Comparison of the deduced amino acid sequences of papilloma virus E2 protein carboxyl terminal and the segment of the human *c-mos* gene product between residues 164 and 245. Identical amino acids are boxed and a dotted line indicates a conservative change. *c-mos* residues identical (■) or analogous (□) to residues of at least two papilloma virus sequences are shown. Regions of highest local hydrophobicity (▽) or hydrophilicity (▼) are also shown, and the predicted secondary structure for positions 1–20 is outlined. (A) alanine; (G) glycine; (T) threonine; (C) cysteine; (P) proline; (M) methionine; (V) valine; (I) isoleucine; (L) leucine; (Y) tyrosine; (F) phenylalanine; (W) tryptophan; (D) aspartic acid; (E) glutamic acid; (R) arginine; (K) lysine; (H) histidine; (S) serine; (N) asparagine; (Q) glutamine.

two regions in the β sheet separated by a turn centered on the conserved glycine at position 9.

No other significant homology was detected outside this conserved domain between human *c-mos* (346 amino acids long) and papilloma viruses E2 proteins (368–410 amino acids long).

Discussion

A good statistical significance of the similarity described here (Table 1) does not imply per se biological relevance, and uncautious interpretation of such data may be hazardous (Doolittle 1981). First, one should note that only part of the proteins are taken into account for the alignment, and, as the surrounding regions are not homologous, considering them would dramatically lower the significance. Yet, we believe that consideration of the 85 carboxyterminal amino acids of papilloma virus E2 proteins as a functional domain is supported by the following facts: (1) it corresponds to the transcribed part of the E2 open reading frame in CRPV-induced carcinomas; (2) the E2-encoded polypeptides of all four papillomaviruses have an homologous aminoterminal domain of 200 amino acids followed by a variable segment of 80–100 residues and are terminated by a conserved

carboxyterminal domain. This conserved carboxyterminal domain corresponds precisely to the segment homologous to the *c-mos* gene product.

There is no experimental evidence for a biological role of this defined domain in the protein encoded by *mos* genes. Homologies between *v-mos* and RSV *src* gene products have been reported (Van Beveren et al. 1981), suggesting that they evolved from a common ancestor. This alignment with pp60[src] allows the observation that part of the *mos* domain homologous to E2 (positions 38–86, Fig. 2) corresponds to the segment surrounding the phosphotyrosine acceptor site common to a number of retroviral oncogenes (Groffen et al. 1983). However, the *v-mos* gene product has no detectable protein kinase activity (Papkoff et al. 1983). Altogether, our data suggest that this region of the *mos* and E2 proteins may play a role in the yet uncharacterized catalytic activity or binding of a substrate.

Obviously, the similarity discussed here does not directly shed light on papilloma virus-mediated cellular transformation. It only supports the idea that the carboxyterminal part of E2 open reading frame carries important information for the transformation process and should be chosen as a target for experiments regarding site-directed mutagenesis. It also pinpoints the presence of a somewhat peculiar papilloma virus transforming protein, perhaps similar to the *v-mos* product, which is a soluble cytoplasmic protein (Papkoff et al. 1983) expressed at very low level in Mo-MSV-transformed cells and against which no antisera can be obtained from tumor-bearing animals (Papkoff et al. 1982).

Finally, this analogy could suggest that remote events that led to the formation of these DNA tumor viruses have possibly included incorporation of host cellular sequences into the viral genome.

Acknowledgments

We thank E. George and E. Schwartz for communication of their data prior to publication, J.M. Claverie for making the search program available to us, and F. Francfort for preparation of the manuscript. This work was supported by grants from INSERM (PRC 118011 and 134018), CNRS (LA 270), and the Fondation pour la Recherche Médicale Française.

References

Campo, M.S., M.H. Moar, W.F.H. Jarrett, and H.M. Laird. 1980. A new papillomavirus associated with alimentary cancer in cattle. *Nature* **286:** 180.

Chen, E.Y., P.M. Howley, A.D. Levinson, and P.H. Seeburg. 1982. The primary structure and genetic organization of the bovine papillomavirus type 1 genome. *Nature* **299:** 529.

Danos, O., M. Katinka, and M. Yaniv. 1982. Human papillomavirus 1a DNA sequence: A novel type of genome organization among Papovaviridae. *EMBO J.* **1:** 231.

Doolittle, R.F. 1981. Similar amino acid sequences: Chance or common ancestry? *Science* **214:** 231.

Dürst, M., L. Gissmann, H. Ickenberg, and H. zur Hausen. 1983. A papillomavirus DNA from a cervical carcinoma and its prevalence in cancer biopsy samples from different geographic regions. *Proc. Natl. Acad. Sci.* **80:** 3812.

Dvoretzky, I., R. Shober, S.K. Chattopadhyay, and D.R. Lowy. 1980. A quantitative *in vitro* focus assay for bovine papillomavirus. *Virology* **103:** 369.

Favre, M., N. Jibard, and G. Orth. 1982. Restriction mapping and physical characterization of the cottontail rabbit papillomavirus genome in transplantable VX2 and VX7 domestic rabbit carcinomas. *Virology* **119:** 298.

Garnier, J., D.J. Osguthorpe, and B. Robson. 1978. Analysis of the accuracy and implications of simple methods for predicting the secondary structure of globular proteins. *J. Mol. Biol.* **120:** 97.

Georges, E., O. Croissant, N. Bonneau, and G. Orth. 1984. Physical state and transcription of the genome of the cottontail rabbit papilloma virus in the domestic rabbit papillomas and in the transplantable VX2 and VX7 carcinomas. *J. Virol.* (in press).

Groffen, J., N. Heisterkamp, F.H. Reynolds, and J.R. Stephenson. 1983. Homology between phosphotyrosine acceptor site of human c-abl and viral oncogene products. *Nature* **304:** 167.

Hopp, T.P. and K.R. Woods. 1981. Prediction of protein antigenic determinants from amino acid sequences. *Proc. Natl. Acad. Sci.* **78:** 3824.

Lowy, D.R., I. Dvoretzky, R. Shober, M.F. Law, L. Engel, and P.M. Howley. 1980. *In vitro* tumorigenic transformation by a defined subgenomic fragment of bovine papillomavirus DNA. *Nature* **287:** 72.

Nasseri, M., F.O. Wettstein, and S.G. Stevens. 1982. Two colinear and spliced viral transcripts are present in non-virus-producing benign and malignant neoplasms induced by the Shope (rabbit) papillomavirus. *J. Virol.* **44:** 263.

Needleman, S.B. and C.D. Wunsh. 1970. A general method applicable to the search of similarities in the amino acid sequence of two proteins. *J. Mol. Biol.* **48:** 443.

Orth, G., F. Breitburd, M. Favre, and O. Croissant. 1977. Papillomaviruses: A possible role in human cancer. *Cold Spring Harbor Conf. Cell Proliferation* **4:** 1043.

Orth, G., M. Favre, F. Breitburd, O. Croissant, S. Jablonska, S. Obalek, M. Jenzabek-Chozelska, and G. Rzesa. 1980. Epidemodysplasia verruciformis: A model for the role of papillomavirus in human cancer. *Cold Spring Harbor Conf. Cell Proliferation* **7:** 259.

Papkoff, J., E.A. Nigg, and T. Hunter. 1983. The transforming protein of Moloney murine sarcoma virus is a soluble cytoplasmic protein. *Cell* **33:** 161.

Papkoff, J., I.M. Verma, and T. Hunter. 1982. Detetion of a transforming gene product in cells transformed by Moloney murine sarcoma virus. *Cell* **29:** 417.

Rous, P. and J.W. Beard. 1935. The progression to carcinoma of virus-induced rabbit papillomas (Shope). *J. Exp. Med.* **62:** 523.

Schwartz, E., M. Durst, C. Demankowski, O. Lattermann, R. Zech, E. Wolfsperger, S. Suhai, and H. zur Hausen. 1983. DNA sequence and genome organization of genital human papillomavirus type 6b. *EMBO J.* **2:** 2361.

Van Beveren, C., J.A. Galleshow, V. Lonos, A.J.M. Berns, R.F. Doolittle, D.J. Donaghue, and I.M. Verma. 1981. Nucleotide sequence and formation of the transforming gene of mouse sarcoma virus. *Nature* **289:** 258.

Watson, R., M. Oskarsson, and G.F. Vande Woude. 1982. Human DNA sequence homologous to the transforming gene (mos) of Moloney murine sarcoma virus. *Proc. Natl. Acad. Sci.* **79:** 4078.

Wettstein, F.O. and J.G. Stevens. 1981. Transcription of the viral genome in papillomas and carcinomas induced by the Shope virus. *Virology* **109:** 448.

Transposition of Endogenous Intracisternal A-particle Genomes into the *c-mos* Oncogene

E. Canaani, J.B. Cohen, O. Dreazen, M. Horowitz, T. Unger, A. Klar,
G. Rechavi, and D. Givol
Department of Chemical Immunology, The Weizmann Institute of Science, Rehovot 76100, Israel

During the last several years, a group of cellular genes, termed oncogenes, was implicated in the spontaneous development of tumors (for reviews, see Cooper 1982; Weinberg 1982; Duesberg 1983). These genes, of which nearly 20 were so far identified, are evolutionarily conserved (Stehelin et al. 1976; Shilo and Weinberg 1981) and are the progenitors for the transforming genes within the genomes of RNA tumor viruses. Structural and functional (some of the genes code for proteins with tyrosine kinase activity) similarities between certain of the oncogenes suggest that they originated from common ancestral genes (e.g., Reddy et al. 1983). The oncogenes can be activated and trigger or enhance a malignant process by one of several ways: (1) integration of an exogenous retroviral genome near a cellular oncogene resulting in increased transcription of the latter (Hayward et al. 1981; Payne et al. 1982); (2) generation of a point mutation and subsequent production of an altered gene product (Reddy et al. 1982; Tabin et al. 1982); (3) amplification of an oncogene and consequent increased expression (Collins and Groudine 1982; Dalla-Favera et al. 1982a,b); (4) translocation of the oncogene to another chromosome (Shen-Ong et al. 1982; Dalla-Favera et al. 1982b; Taub et al. 1982), or insertion of another piece of cellular DNA near it (Rechavi et al. 1982; Canaani et al. 1983), resulting in both cases in enhanced expression of the oncogene.

The cellular DNA of all higher organisms contains repeated elements with the structure of retroviral genomes (Chattopadhyay et al. 1975; Todaro et al. 1975). Those were termed endogenous viruses and may or may not be expressed (e.g., Aaronson and Stephenson 1975). The mouse genome contains several such families, including endogenous intracisternal A-particle (IAP) genes. These genes, which number about 1000 per haploid mouse genome (Lueders and Kuff 1977), are present abundantly in every mouse plasmacytoma (Dalton et al. 1961) and in other mouse tumors (Kuff et al. 1972). Transcripts of some of these genes are about 9 kb and are encapsidated to form noninfectious retrovirallike entities (Paterson et al. 1978). In this article, we review our recent studies concerning the transposition of endogenous IAP genes into the *c-mos* oncogene in two murine plasmacytomas. One of these events resulted in activation of the oncogene.

Methods

Restriction enzyme analysis

High-molecular-weight cellular DNA and phage DNA were digested with restriction enzymes (New England BioLabs) according to the protocols of the manufacturer. Aliquots (20 μg) of cellular DNA were electrophoresed on 0.7% agarose gels and analyzed by hybridization to a *v-mos*-specific DNA fragment radiolabeled by nick-translation (Rigby et al. 1977) to a specific activity of 10^8 cpm/μg DNA. Conditions of electrophoresis, blotting, and hybridization are detailed in published work (Rechavi et al. 1982).

Northern blotting

RNA was extracted from tumor and normal tissues by the urea-lithium chloride method (Auffray and Rougeon 1980). Poly(A)-tagged RNA was selected on oligo(dT)-cellulose columns, and species containing *mos* sequences were identified by electrophoresis on formaldehyde gels, blotting onto nitrocellulose sheets, and hybridization to *mos*-specific radiolabeled probes (Rechavi et al. 1982).

Molecular cloning and DNA sequencing

Cellular DNA fragments desired to be cloned were enriched by preparative agarose gel electrophoresis (Rechavi et al. 1982) and cloned into λ Charon 4A (Blattner et al. 1977) or λ Wes B (Leder et al. 1977) vectors. Fragments to be sequenced were end-labeled using reverse transcriptase, and after strand separation or internal cleavage were sequenced by standard procedures (Maxam and Gilbert 1977).

Results

Rearrangement of the *c-mos* gene in two plasmacytomas

We screened the DNA of several BALB/c mouse myelomas by Southern blot analysis using a *v-mos*-specific fragment as a probe. Two of the tumors—XRPC24 and NSI—appeared by initial analysis to contain a rearranged *c-mos* gene and were studied in detail. The rearranged genes, as well as their normal counterparts, were compared by hybridization of various DNA digests with two probes. The first one contained sequences bounded by the *Bgl*I and *Hind*III sites in *v-mos* (Fig. 1, bottom) and detects the 3' 293 codons of *c-mos* (Van Beveren et al. 1981). The second probe was the *Xba*I–*Hind*III *v-mos* fragment (Fig. 1, bottom) which detects the 3' 368 codons of *c-mos* (out of 390 codons spanning the entire coding region). Therefore, cellular *mos* DNA fragments detected only by the second probe must originate from the 5' region of the oncogene. A typical analysis is shown in Figure 1. It demonstrates, for example, that by probing with the *Bgl*–*Hind*III fragment, a 14-kbp band was de-

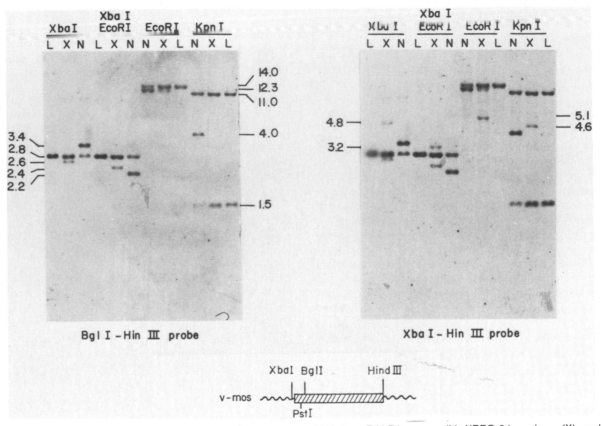

Figure 1 Restriction enzyme analysis of the *c-mos* gene in cellular DNA from BALB/c mouse (L), XRPC-24 myeloma (X), and NSI myeloma (N). The two probes used are described in the text and schematically shown at the bottom on the partial map of *v-mos* of Moloney murine sarcoma viral DNA. Numbers correspond to kbp. (▨) *v-mos*. (Data from J.B. Cohen et al., in prep.)

tected in *Eco*RI-digested BALB/c DNA as well as in the two tumors. This band represents the normal gene. An additional 12-kbp fragment was apparent in XRPC24 and NSI DNA and corresponded to rearranged *c-mos*. Using the *Xba*I–*Hind*III fragment as a probe, an additional 5.1-kbp fragment showed only in XRPC24 DNA. This experiment indicates that the two plasmacytomas carry a rearranged *c-mos*, that the rearrangement is not identical in both cases, and that at least in XRPC-24 it involves the 5' terminus of the gene. The rearranged genes in XRPC-24 and NSI tumors were termed *rc-mos*^{X24} and *rc-mos*^{NSI}, respectively. Hybridoma NSI-103, which was generated by fusion of NSI with BALB/c spleen cells (Parhami-Seren et al. 1983), and hybridoma X63-160, generated by fusion with a related MOPC-21-derived myeloma line P3-X63-Ag8 (Kearney et al. 1979), contained *rc-mos*^{NSI}.

c-mos transcription has never been observed in all normal and tumor tissues examined so far (Gattoni et al. 1982), therefore, it was of interest to determine whether the oncogene's rearrangement is correlated with its transcriptional activation. RNA was extracted from myeloma MPC-11 (representing myelomas which do not contain rearranged *c-mos*), myeloma XRPC-24, myeloma NSI, and the two hybridomas, and was analyzed for *mos* transcripts by the Northern technique. Figure 2 shows that

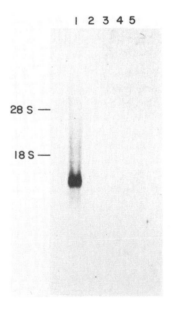

Figure 2 Northern blot analysis of *c-mos* transcripts in myeloma XRPC-24 (1), hybridoma 160 (2), hybridoma 103 (3), myeloma NSI (4), and myeloma MPC-11 (5). The positions of ribosomal RNA markers are indicated. (Data from J.B. Cohen et al., in prep.)

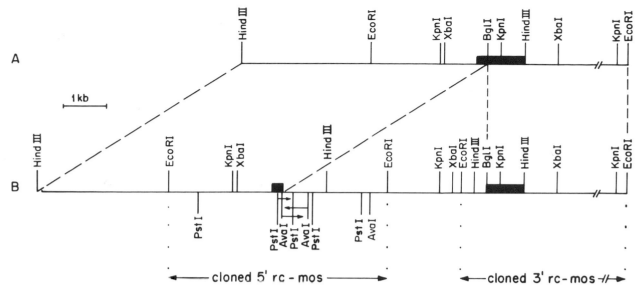

Figure 3 Physical maps of normal *c-mos* (*top*) and *rc-mos*^{X24} (*bottom*). (■) Coding regions; (→) strategy of DNA sequencing. (Data from Canaani et al. 1983.)

mos-specific RNA of 1.2 kb is synthesized in the XRPC-24 tumor. No homologous RNA could be detected in any of the other samples. These results indicate that in XRPC-24 *c-mos* rearrangement resulted in turning on of the oncogene's transcription.

Organization of *rc-mos*^{X24} and *rc-mos*^{NSI}

Using the two probes described in the previous section and by performing several double digestions, it became apparent that in both tumors the rearrangements involved the 5′ region of *mos*. To compare in detail the normal and rearranged gene, we molecularly cloned the normal *c-mos* 14-kbp *Eco*RI DNA fragment from BALB/c tissue, the rearranged 12-kbp and 5.0-kbp corresponding *Eco*RI fragments from XRPC-24 tumor, and the rearranged 12-kbp *rc-mos Eco*RI DNA of NSI myeloma. The cloned genes were analyzed by restriction enzymes and their physical maps are shown in Figures

3 and 4. *rc-mos*^{X24} originated by the insertion of a novel cellular DNA element of 4.7 kbp into the coding region near the *Bgl*I site. This resulted in splitting of the gene into two regions and the shifting upstream of 5′-flanking mouse sequences away from the main coding body of the gene.

c-mos in the NSI tumor has undergone a similar but not identical DNA rearrangement. Here, a 4.5-kbp DNA split the oncogene-coding region very close to its 5′ terminus (Fig. 4). The two novel DNA elements inserted within *c-mos* in XRPC-24 and NSI tumors show remarkable similarity in size. Moreover a constellation of three restriction enzyme sites (*Kpn*I, *Xba*I, and *Eco*RI) at the 3′ end of the element in *rc-mos*^{X24} appears to resemble closely a similar constellation at the 5′ end of the element in *rc-mos*^{NSI}. This suggests that similar cellular elements were inserted in opposite orientation into *c-mos* in the two myelomas.

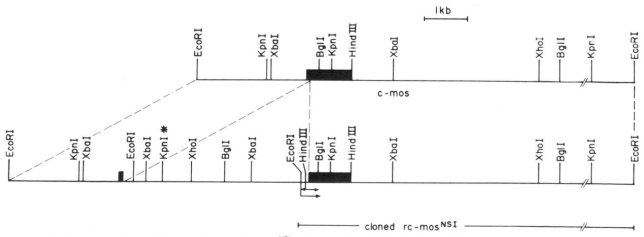

Figure 4 Physical map of normal *c-mos* (*top*) and *rc-mos*^{NSI} (*bottom*). (■) Coding regions; (→) strategy of DNA sequencing. (Data from J.B. Cohen et al., in prep.)

Cellular elements inserted within *c-mos* are endogenous IAP genes

To define precisely the points of insertion and further characterize the cellular elements interjected within *c-mos*, we determined the nucleotide sequence at the junctions between the main bodies of *c-mos*-coding regions and the inserted cellular elements (sequences near the *Bgl*I site at the *c-mos*-coding region in the two rearranged genes). The sequence of the *rc-mos*[X24] junction (Rechavi et al. 1982) indicated that the element was inserted at nucleotide 513 and codon 88 of the *c-mos* presumed coding sequence (Van Beveren et al. 1981). The cellular DNA fragment contained an open reading frame of 28 codons which joined in phase the rest of the *c-mos* open reading frame (302 codons). The sequence of *rc-mos*[NSI] junction (J.B. Cohen et al., in prep.) shows that *c-mos* was split at nucleotide 151 or codon 30. The two cellular DNA elements terminate at the junction points with the tetranucleotide AACA, which is identical to the terminus of the *Drosophila* transposable element *copia* (Dunsmuir et al. 1980), yeast Ty*1* mobile element (Farabough and Fink 1980; Gafner and Philippsen 1980), and spleen necrosis virus DNA (Shimotohno et

al. 1980). This last finding immediately suggested that the inserted cellular DNAs are related to transposable elements, and, indeed, it was found that a 349-bp segment of the cellular DNA immediately adjacent to the retained main body of *c-mos* sequences in *rc-mos*[X24] has close homology with the long terminal repeat (LTR) of a known IAP gene (Kuff et al. 1983). Comparison of the two sequences (Fig. 5) indicates 88% homology between the sequence of the inserted element and the "antisense" strand of the 5′ LTR of the IAP gene MIA 14. This means that a 5′ IAP LTR was inserted into *c-mos* in a head-to-head (5′-to-5′) configuration. Similar comparison with *rc-mos*[NSI] (J.B. Cohen et al., in prep.) showed that in this case a 3′ IAP LTR was inserted in a head-to-tail (3′-to-5′) orientation.

The sequence data have indicated that in XRPC-24 and NSI tumors a IAP LTR integrated within *c-mos*. To study whether a complete IAP gene was inserted, we used the 5.1-kbp *Eco*RI fragment that we have cloned molecularly from XRPC-24 DNA (termed "cloned 5′ *rc-mos*[NSI]" in Fig. 3). This fragment was partially sequenced according to the scheme depicted in Figure 3. The analysis showed that the 5′ end of the element integrated

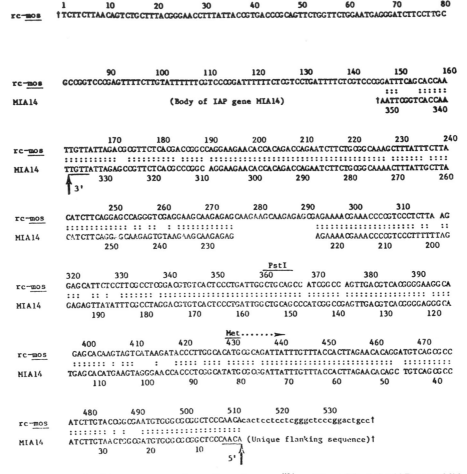

Figure 5 Comparison of the nucleotide sequences of a portion of *rc-mos*[X24] and the LTR of the IAP gene MIA 14. Arrows indicate the boundaries of IAP LTR. Short inverted repeats at the LTR termini are underlined. The *rc-mos* sequence is presented in the direction of transcription of *c-mos* and it is aligned with the antisense strand of IAP LTR. "Met" indicates the beginning of an open reading frame extending into the retained *c-mos* sequence. (Data from Kuff et al. 1983.)

within *c-mos* in XRPC-24 myeloma is an IAP LTR (Canaani et al. 1983). Therefore, both the 3' and 5' termini of the cellular element in *rc-mos*[x24] are IAP LTRs. To examine if the non-LTR sequences within the 4.7-kbp elements are also of IAP origin, we tested a non-LTR segment of the 5.1-kbp *Eco*RI fragment for hybridization to endogenous IAP sequences distributed within the mouse genome (Lueders and Kuff 1980; Shen-Ong and Cole 1982). Southern blots of *Eco*RI- and *Hind*III-digested BALB/c DNA were probed for IAP-specific fragments by hybridization to non-LTR probes derived from a typical IAP genome, pMIA1, and from the 5.1-kbp fragment. The pMIA1 probe detected an extensive array of IAP fragments ranging in size from 0.5 kbp to 6 kbp (Fig. 6, lane a). The *rc-mos*[x24] probe cross-hybridized with most of these fragments (Fig. 6, lane b). These results indicate that *rc-mos*[x24] contains a genuine IAP genome. Although a similar experiment was not done with the element inserted into *c-mos* in NSI myeloma, the similarity in size and restriction enzyme pattern of the two elements makes it highly probable that *rc-mos*[NSI] also contains an entire IAP genome.

Biological activity of the rearranged *c-mos* genes

Extensive experiments have shown that the molecularly cloned 14-kbp *Eco*RI frgment corresponding to the normal *c-mos* gene was inactive in transfection experiments, unless an LTR from Moloney sarcoma virus was attached to it in vitro (Oskarsson et al. 1980). We asked whether the rearranged genes cloned from the two myelomas are active by themselves when assayed by transfection. Two tested clones of the *Eco*RI 12-kbp fragments of *rc-mos*[x24] induced a large number of foci on NIH-3T3 monolayers with specific activities of 3100 and 4900 focus-forming units (ffu) per gram of DNA, respectively (Table 1). Molecularly cloned 12-kbp *Eco*RI *rc-mos*[NSI] DNA induced a small number of foci (E. Shtivelman, unpubl.). No foci were observed when the cloned 14-kbp *Eco*RI fragment of normal *c-mos* was assayed. Two recombinant phages containing integrated Moloney sarcoma viral DNA pro-

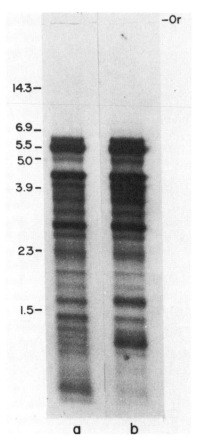

Figure 6 Southern blot analysis of *Hind*III + *Eco*RI-digested BALB/c mouse DNA examining hybridization to non-LTR probes derived from the pMIA1 IAP genome (Lueders and Kuff 1980) (lane *a*) and the IAP genome in *rc-mos*[x24] (lane *b*). Size of DNA markers are denoted in kbp. (Data from Canaani et al. 1983.)

duced 10,200 and 13,200 ffu per gram of DNA and served as a positive control. These results demonstrate that the rearrangement of *c-mos* in the XRPC-24 tumor resulted in a striking biological activation of the gene. The situation is not clear with regard to *rc-mos*[NSI] where

Table 1 Biological Activity of Molecularly Cloned *c-mos* and *rc-mos* DNAs

Clone	Insert DNA (ng)	Number of foci	Specific infectivity (ffu per pmole DNA)
λ-MSV 26	50	150	10,200
λ-MSV 3-3	100	220	13,200
λ-c-mos IA	125	0	<67
λ-rc-mos[x24]2B	100	43	3,100
λ-rc-mos[x24]2F	100	68	4,900
λ-rc-mos[NSI]26	700	8	90

Intact recombinant phage DNA was transfected into NIH-3T3 fibroblasts by the calcium phosphate method. The cultures were kept in medium containing 5% fetal calf serum and were scored for focus formation 2 weeks after transfection. λ-MSV 26 and λ-MSV 3-3 represent Mo-MSV molecules integrated within normal rat kidney cell DNA and molecularly cloned in λ Wes B vector. λ-c-mos and λ-rc-mos are molecular clones of the *c-mos* and *rc-mos* genes, respectively.

a significant but very low activity was observed. This low activity might reflect the true situation wherein *rc-mos*[NSI] in NSI is only marginally activated (which correlates with our inability to detect transcription of the gene), but could also be due to the fact that the 12-kbp *Eco*RI *rc-mos*[NSI] fragment cloned and examined for biological activity contained only 150 bases of IAP LTR, precluding the region with Z-DNA structure postulated to play a major role in LTR-induced transcriptional activation (see Discussion). A bigger fragment containing the entire *rc-mos*[NSI] gene is now being cloned and will be tested for biological activity.

Discussion

This work presents the first example of spontaneous activation of the *mos* oncogene. In addition, it provides a striking demonstration of an oncogene's activation through transposition of endogenous virus. In both cases, the IAP gene was inserted at the 5' terminus of *c-mos*, albeit not in identical sequences. This raises the possibility that *c-mos* provides a preferred target for IAP integration. The phenomenon of preferred target regions has been described in studies on transposable elements in bacteria (Calos and Miller 1980) and yeast (Farabough and Fink 1980) and was termed "regional specificity." The mode of IAP insertion was typical of retroviruses and transposable elements in that it occurred at the termini of the IAP genome and involved a duplication of the target site (6 nucleotides). The two IAP elements show great similarity in size and recognition sites for various restriction enzymes, and in these two aspects they differ from a variety of IAP genomes analyzed, including the minor population of endogenous elements reported to be transcribed and amplified in myeloma tumors (Shen-Ong and Cole 1982).

The mechanism of IAP relocation could involve a direct DNA transposition or the successive steps of transcription, reverse transcription into cDNA, and integration. The retroviruslike properties of these elements argue for the second mechanism. Furthermore, the recent demonstration that RNA transcripts of *copia* transposable elements are associated with virionlike structures in *Drosophila* cells (Shiba and Saigo 1983), and the striking similarity in the mode of transcription between yeast Ty1 transposable elements and retroviral DNA (Elder et al. 1983) suggests that synthesis of the RNA intermediate might be the general mechanism for relocation of eukaryotic moveable elements.

The activation of *c-mos* in XRPC-24 myeloma probably involved more than one factor. The integration of IAP resulted in relocation of 5' coding and flanking DNA to a position of 4.7 kbp upstream. Since *c-mos* appears to be under the regulation of a *cis*-acting control element located around 1 kbp upstream of the coding region (G. Vande Woude et al., pers. comm.), the insertion of the IAP genome has removed this element away and could have eliminated its effect on transcription of the oncogene. The activation most likely is associated with the introduction of a IAP LTR near the main body of the coding region. Like other LTRs of retroviral genomes, it probably contains a transcriptional enhancer element.

In fact, the stretches of alternating purines and pyrimidines in positions 425–435 and 491–501 of the *rc-mos*[X24] sequence (Fig. 5) show a structure of Z-DNA (Wang et al. 1979) suggested to be the critical component in enhancer elements (A. Rich, pers. comm.). It is still necessary to characterize both the *c-mos* transcript in XRPC-24 cells and the transforming protein presumably translated from it, in order to understand the activation in fine detail.

IAP integration in a head-to-tail orientation did not induce detectable *mos* transcription in NSI tumor. The cloned gene appears to have acquired a low transforming activity in transfection assays but the significance of this activity could be assessed only after further experiments are done (see Results). The absence of detectable *c-mos* transcription in NSI myeloma is unexpected, because it has been shown that exogenous retroviral LTRs may activate a neighboring oncogene when positioned upstream to it and in the same transcriptional orientation (Hayward et al. 1981; Payne et al. 1982). The failure of IAP integration to turn on transcription in this case might reflect mutations in critical sequences essential for transcriptional activation within the particular LTR inserted in *rc-mos*[NSI]. In this regard, it is noteworthy that unlike the LTRs of retroviral proviruses (Temin 1981; Varmus 1982) and the direct repeats at the ends of several *Drosophila* (Dunsmuir et al. 1980) and yeast (Farabough and Fink 1980; Gafner and Philippsen 1980) transposable elements, the two LTRs of a single IAP gene are not identical. Multiple differences were found between the two LTRs of the IAP gene in *rc-mos*[X24] (Canaani et al. 1983), and the LTRs of MIA 14 (Kuff et al. 1983). However, it is possible that the success or failure in turning on *c-mos* transcription is correlated with the orientation of the IAP gene with respect to *c-mos*. Such a correlation would emphasize the similarities between IAP genetic entities and the yeast Ty1 transposable elements, since activation of neighboring genes upon Ty1 insertion occurs only when the transposon is inserted head to head (Scherer et al. 1982; Elder et al. 1983).

Acknowledgments

This work was supported by grants from the Leukemia Research Foundation of Chicago, Israel Cancer Research Fund, Edith C. Blum Foundation, Israel-DKFZ cancer grant, and U.S.-Israel Binational Fund.

References

Aaronson, S.A. and J.R. Stephenson. 1975. Differential cellular regulation of three distinct classes of type C RNA viruses endogenous to mouse cells. *Cold Spring Harbor Symp. Quant. Biol.* **39**: 1129.

Auffray, C. and F. Rougeon. 1980. Purification of mouse immunoglobulins heavy chain messenger RNAs from total myeloma tumor RNA. *Eur. J. Biochem.* **107**: 303.

Blattner, F.R., B.G. Williams, A.E. Bleche, K. Denniston-Thompson, H.E. Faber, L.-A. Furlong, D.J. Grunvald, D.O. Kiefer, D.D. Moore, J.W. Schumm, E.L. Sheldon, and O. Smithies. 1977. Charon phages: Safer derivatives of bacteriophage lambda for DNA cloning. *Science* **196**: 161.

Calos, M.D. and J.H. Miller. 1980. Transposable elements. *Cell* **20**: 579.

Canaani, E., O. Dreazen, A. Klar, G. Rechavi, D. Ram, J.B. Cohen, and D. Givol. 1983. Activation of the *c-mos* oncogene in a mouse plasmacytoma by insertion of an endogenous intracisternal A-particle genome. *Proc. Natl. Acad. Sci.* **80:** 7118.

Chattopadhyay, S.K., D.R. Lowy, N.M. Teich, A.S. Levine, and W.P. Rowe. 1975. Qualitative and quantitative studies of AKR-type murine leukemia virus sequences in mouse DNA. *Cold Spring Harbor Symp. Quant. Biol.* **39:** 1085.

Collins, S. and M. Groudine. 1982. Amplification of endogenous myc-related DNA sequences in a human myeloid leukemia cell line. *Nature* **298:** 679.

Cooper, G.M. 1982. Cellular transforming genes. *Science* **218:** 801.

Dalla-Favera, R., F. Wong-Staal, and R.C. Gallo. 1982a. Onc gene amplification in promyelocytic leukaemia cell line HL-60 and primary leukaemic cells of the same patient. *Nature* **299:** 61.

Dalla-Favera, R., M. Bregni, J. Erikson, D. Paterson, R. Gallo, and C.M. Croce. 1982b. Human c-myc onc gene is located on the region of chromosome 8 that is translocated in Burkitt lymphoma cells. *Proc. Natl. Acad. Sci.* **79:** 7824.

Dalton, A.J., M. Potter, and R.M. Merwin. 1961. Some ultrastructural characteristics of a series of primary and transplanted plasma-cell tumors of the mouse. *J. Natl. Cancer Inst.* **26:** 1221.

Duesberg, P.H. 1983. Retroviral transforming genes in normal cells? *Nature* **304:** 219.

Dunsmuir, P., W.J. Brorein, Jr., M.A. Simon, and G.M. Rubin. 1980. Insertion of the Drosophila transposable element copia generates a 5 base pair duplication. *Cell* **21:** 575.

Elder, R.T., E.Y. Loh, and R.W. Davis. 1983. RNA from the yeast transposable element Ty1 has both ends in the direct repeats, a structure similar to retrovirus RNA. *Proc. Natl. Acad. Sci.* **80:** 2432.

Farabough, D.J. and G.R. Fink. 1980. Insertion of the eukaryotic transposable element Ty1 creates a 5-base pair duplication. *Nature* **286:** 352.

Gafner, J. and P. Philippsen. 1980. The yeast transposon Ty1 generates duplications of target DNA on insertion. *Nature* **286:** 414.

Gattoni, S., P. Kirschmeir, I.B. Weinstein, J. Escobedo, and D. Dina. 1982. Cellular Moloney murine sarcoma (*c-mos*) sequences are hypermethylated and transcriptionally silent in normal and transformed rodent cells. *Mol. Cell. Biol.* **2:** 42.

Hayward, W.S., B.G. Neel, and S.M. Astrin. 1981. Activation of a cellular *onc* gene by promoter insertion in ALV-induced lymphoid leukosis. *Nature* **290:** 475.

Kearney, J.F., A. Radbruch, B. Liesegang, and K. Rajewsky. 1979. A new mouse myeloma cell line that has lost immunoglobulin expression but permits the construction of antibody-secreting hybrid cell lines. *J. Immunol.* **123:** 1548.

Kuff, E.L., K.K. Lueders, K.L. Ozer, and N.A. Wivel. 1972. Some structural and antigenic properties of intracisternal A particles occurring in mouse tumors. *Proc. Natl. Acad. Sci.* **69:** 218.

Kuff, E.L., A. Feenstra, K. Lueders, G. Rechavi, D. Givol, and E. Canaani. 1983. Homology between an endogenous viral LTR and sequences inserted in an activated cellular oncogene. *Nature* **302:** 547.

Leder, P., D. Tiemeier, and L. Enquist. 1977. EK2 derivatives of bacteriophage lambda useful in the cloning of DNA from higher organisms: The λ gt WES system. *Science* **196:** 175.

Lueders, K.K. and E.L. Kuff. 1977. Sequences associated with intracisternal A particles are reiterated in the mouse genome. *Cell* **12:** 963.

———. 1980. Intracisternal A-particle genes: Identification in the genome of *Mus musculus* and comparison of multiple isolates from a mouse gene library. *Proc. Natl. Acad. Sci.* **77:** 357.

Maxam, A.M. and W. Gilbert. 1977. A new method for sequencing DNA. *Proc. Natl. Acad. Sci.* **74:** 560.

Oskarsson, M., W.L. McClements, D.G. Blair, F.V. Maizel, and G.F. Vande Woude. 1980. Properties of a normal mouse cell DNA sequence (sare) homologous to the src sequence of Moloney sarcoma virus. *Science* **207:** 1222.

Parhami-Seren, B., Z. Eshhar, and E. Mozes. 1983. Fine specificity and idiotypic expression of monoclonal antibodies directed against poly(Tyr,Glu)-poly(de Ala)-poly(Lys) and its ordered analogue (Tyr-Tyr-Glu-Glu)-poly(de Ala)-poly(Lys). *Immunology* **49:** 9.

Paterson, B.M., S. Segal, K.K. Lueders, and E.L. Kuff. 1978. RNA associated with murine intracisternal type A particles codes for the main particle protein. *J. Virol.* **27:** 118.

Payne, G.S., J.M. Bishop, and H.E. Varmus. 1982. Multiple arrangements of viral DNA and an activated host oncogene in bursal lymphomes. *Nature* **295:** 209.

Rechavi, G., D. Givol, and E. Canaani. 1982. Activation of a cellular oncogene by DNA rearrangement: Possible involvement of an Is-like element. *Nature* **300:** 607.

Reddy, E.P., R.K. Reynolds, E. Santos, and M. Barbacid. 1982. A point mutation is responsible for the acquisition of transforming properties by the T24 human bladder carcinoma oncogene. *Nature* **300:** 149.

Reddy, E.P., R.K. Reynolds, E. Santos, and M. Barbacid. 1982. A point mutation is responsible for the acquisition of transforming properties by the T24 human bladder carcinoma oncogene. *Nature* **300:** 149.

Reddy, E.P., M. Smith, and A. Srinivasan. 1983. Nucleotide sequence of Abelson murine leukemia virus genome. *Proc. Natl. Acad. Sci.* **80:** 3623.

Rigby, P.W.J., M. Dieckman, C. Rhodes, and P. Berg. 1977. Labeling deoxyribonucleic acid to high specific activity in vitro by nicktranslation with DNA polymerase I. *J. Mol. Biol.* **113:** 237.

Scherer, S., C. Mann, and R.W. Davis. 1982. Revision of a promoter deletion in yeast. *Nature* **298:** 815.

Shen-Ong, G.L.C. and M.D. Cole. 1982. Differing populations of intracisternal A-particles genes in myeloma tumors and mouse subspecies. *J. Virol.* **42:** 411.

Shiba, T. and K. Saigo. 1983. Retrovirus-like particles containing RNA homologous to the transposable elements copia in *Drosophila melanogaster*. *Nature* **302:** 119.

Shilo, B.Z. and R.A. Weinberg. 1981. DNA sequences homologous to vertebrate oncogenes are conserved in *Drosophila melanogaster*. *Proc. Natl. Acad. Sci.* **78:** 6789.

Shimotohno, K., S. Mizutani, and H.M. Temin. 1980. Sequence of retrovirus provirus resembles that of bacterial transposable element. *Nature* **285:** 550.

Stehelin, D., H.E. Varmus, J.M. Bishop, and P.K. Vogt. 1976. DNA related to the transforming gene(s) of avian sarcoma viruses is present in normal avian DNA. *Nature* **260:** 170.

Tabin, C.J., S.M. Bradley, C.I. Bargmann, R.A. Weinberg, A.G. Papageorge, E.M. Scolnick, R. Dhar, D.R. Lowy, and E.H. Chang. 1982. Mechanism of activation of a human oncogene. *Nature* **300:** 143.

Taub, R., I. Kirsch, C. Morton, G. Lenoir, D. Swan, S. Tronick, S. Aaronson, and P. Leder. 1982. Translocation of the c-myc gene onto the immunoglobulin heavy chain locus in human Burkitt lymphoma and murine plasmacytoma cells. *Proc. Natl. Acad. Sci.* **79:** 7837.

Temin, H.M. 1981. Structure, variation and synthesis of retrovirus long terminal repeat. *Cell* **27:** 1.

Todaro, G.J., R.E. Benveniste, R. Callahan, M.M. Lieber, and C.J. Sherr. 1975. Endogenous primate and feline type C viruses. *Cold Spring Harbor Symp. Quant. Biol.* **39:** 1159.

Van Beveren, C., F. van Staaten, J.A. Galleshaw, and I.M. Verma. 1981. Nucleotide sequence of the genome of a murine sarcoma virus. *Cell* **27:** 97.

Varmus, H.E. 1982. Form and function of retroviral proviruses. *Science* **216:** 812.

Wang, A.H.J., G.T. Quigley, F.T. Koplak, J.L. Crawford, J.H. Van Boom, G. Van der Marel, and A. Rich. 1979. Molecular structure of a left-handed double helical DNA fragment at atomic resolution. *Nature* **282:** 680.

Weinberg, R.A. 1982. Oncogenes of spontaneous and chemically induced tumors. *Adv. Cancer Res.* **36:** 149.

Identification of Some of the Parameters Governing Transformation by Oncogenes in Retroviruses

K.C. Wilhelmsen, W.G. Tarpley, and H.M. Temin
McArdle Laboratory for Cancer Research, University of Wisconsin, Madison, Wisconsin 53706

Retroviruses require cis- and trans-acting sequences for replication. The required cis-acting sequences include the long terminal repeats, the primer binding site, the polypurine tract, and the encapsidation sequences (Watanabe and Temin 1982). gag, pol, and env code for the trans-acting functions necessary for virus replication. The sequences that code for trans-acting functions can be removed or replaced if the defective virus or vector is grown in the presence of a helper virus or in a helper cell

Inserted sequences can affect the viability of retrovirus vectors. If the inserted sequences contain a transcriptional termination signal, so that the virion RNA transcript is prematurely terminated, infectious virus will not be made (Shimotohno and Temin 1981). The presence of a promoter in the inserted sequence can also interfere with the transcription from the viral promoter, especially if it is in the opposite orientation (Bandyopadhyay and Temin 1984a).

There is also variation in the sequences inserted in retroviral vectors during virus propagation, especially if an inserted promoter is directing transcription of a gene that is under positive selective pressure (Emerman and Temin 1984). If DNA containing intervening sequences is inserted into a retrovirus vector, the intervening sequences are lost during virus propagation (Shimotohno and Temin 1982; Sorge and Hughes 1982).

The level of expression of a coding sequence inserted in a retrovirus vector is determined by the structure and amount of the RNA transcripts. When an inserted sequence is transcribed using the virus promoter, the level of expression is determined by the distance between the transcriptional start in the LTR and the translational initiation signal of the inserted sequences, as well as by the number and the sequence of translational initiation signals 5' to the translational initiation signal of the inserted sequence (Bandyopadhyay and Temin 1984b). In In replication-competent retroviruses, the env gene coding sequences are at the 3' end of the virus. To express the env sequences efficiently, the many translational initiation sequences between the viral promoter in the LTR and the beginning of the env coding sequences must be removed from the env mRNA. However, the splicing to form the env transcript is not efficient (Hayward 1977). An inserted gene can be expressed like env, using a spliced transcript, but expression of this inserted sequence will be less than if it is placed closer to the viral promoter.

Highly oncogeneic retroviruses are natural retrovirus vectors that contain inserted sequences called oncogenes. Oncogenes are sequences inserted into highly oncogenic retroviruses that are not necessary for virus replication and are necessary for the transformation of infected target cells. Oncogenes are derived from normal cellular sequences called proto-oncogenes. Since viral oncogene and cellular proto-oncogene sequences when expressed in the same cells give rise to different phenotypes, there must be some qualitative or quantitative difference(s) between them. To determine parameters that govern transformation by oncogenes and not by in situ proto-oncogenes, we are using two approaches. The first approach is to identify the structural differences between the oncogene in reticuloendotheliosis virus strain T (Rev-T), v-rel, and its proto-oncogene, c-rel (turkey). In the second approach, we constructed by molecular techniques recombinants between spleen necrosis virus and v-src, c-src, v-Ha-ras, and c-Ha-ras and recovered virus after transfection of chicken cells. The differences in transformation of chicken embryo fibroblasts by these viruses were determined, and inferences have been made as to which parameters affect transformation by oncogenes.

Methods

Cells

The sources and procedures for propagating chicken embryo fibroblasts from SPAFAS embryos have been described previously (Fritsch and Temin 1977). BRL tk⁻ and chicken tk⁻ cells were propagated and used for the tk transformation assay as previously described (Shimotohno and Temin 1981). DNA transfection was done as previously described (Shimotohno and Temin 1981).

Sources of DNA

Rev-A, Rev-T, and c-rel (turkey) have been previously described (Chen et al. 1981, 1983; Chen and Temin 1982; Wilhelmsen et al. 1983; Wilhelmsen and Temin 1984). SNV-tk was described previously (Watanabe and Temin 1982).

pGT8, pGT10, pGT12, pGT22, pGT24, pGT26, and pSW212 were constructed using standard molecular genetic techniques and will be described elsewhere (W.G. Tarpley and H.M. Temin, in prep.).

Results

Analysis of molecular clones of proviruses of Rev-T and Rev-A (Rev-A is the nondefective helper virus of Rev-T) shows that in Rev-T, *v-rel* is substituted for most of *env* in Rev-A (see Fig. 1). Rev-T also has a large deletion relative to Rev-A of sequences that encode much of *gag* and *pol*. This deletion is necessary to express *rel* transformation (Chen and Temin 1982). There are two viral RNA transcripts that contain *v-rel* sequences in Rev-T-infected cells; a full-length genomic size transcript and a subgenomic RNA transcript which is similar in size to the *env* mRNA of Rev-A (Watanabe and Temin 1983; K.C. Wilhelmsen, unpubl.). The subgenomic transcript is thought to be translated to make the *v-rel* gene product.

v-rel

Nucleic acid sequence analysis of Rev-A and Rev-T indicates that *v-rel* contains one large open reading frame which is 1518 bp from the initiation codon to the stop codon. This open reading frame extends from the methionine that begins the *env*-coding sequences, which are in common with Rev-A, continues through the *v-rel* sequences, and ends out of frame with *env* within the 3′ *env*-coding sequences (see Fig. 1). There are 11 *env* amino acids (3 mutant), 474 *v-rel* amino acids, and 18 amino acids from out-of-frame *env*-coding sequences in the *env-v-rel*–out-of-frame *env* fusion product. The *env-v-rel*–out-of-frame *env* fusion product is predicted to be 59.5 kD, based on DNA sequence data. The predicted *env-v-rel*–out-of-frame *env* protein product does not have any large domains that are hydrophobic. The net charge for the predicted product is plus 4. *v-rel* is predicted to have an above average mole percentage of serine (9.1%) and of proline (8.7%). *v-rel* has no strong homology to *v-src*, *v-Ki-ras*, *v-mos*, *v-myc*, *v-fps*, *v-myb*, *v-fos*, *v-G-fes*, and *v-ST-fes* as detected by inspection of the best alignment of predicted peptide sequences (Needleman and Wunsch 1970; Smith and Waterman 1981; R. Doolittle, pers. comm.).

c-rel to *v-rel*

Rev-T was first isolated from a turkey in 1956 (Thelien et al. 1966). It is thought that Rev-T arose when a virus similar to Rev-A infected a turkey and recombined with *c-rel* from that turkey. There is one large *c-rel* locus that contains all of the sequences homologous to *v-rel* in turkeys (Wilhelmsen and Temin 1984). There are nine regions in the *c-rel* (turkey) locus that are homologous to

v-rel. The 5′-most region of *c-rel* that is homologous to *v-rel* is 23 kbp from the 3′-most region of *c-rel* that is homologous to *v-rel*. *v-rel*, in contrast, is only 1.5 kbp.

Each of the boundary regions of *c-rel* that is homologous to *v-rel* is bounded by plausible splice donor or acceptor sequences except for the 3′ boundary of region 7. The 3′ boundary of region 7 is the junction site between Rev-A and *c-rel*.

c-rel is transcribed in normal chicken cells as a 4-kb polyadenalated transcript (Chen et al. 1983). The *c-rel* RNA transcript found in chickens is known to extend 3′ to the 3′-most region of homology of *c-rel* to *v-rel*. It appears that *c-rel* transcription begins somewhere 5′ to region 0 in the *c-rel* locus. The 5′ junction of *v-rel* appears to correspond to the 5′ boundary of an exon within the *c-rel*-coding sequences. The 3′ junction of *v-rel* appears to correspond to coding sequences within an exon. It is not possible to determine where the coding sequences begin and end in *c-rel* at this time, since the transcriptional structure and the sequences flanking *c-rel* are not known.

Comparison of the restriction enzyme cleavage site map of the regions of *c-rel* with homology to *v-rel* and the restriction enzyme cleavage site map of *v-rel* indicates that there are sequence differences between *c-rel* and *v-rel* (see Fig. 2). Additional sequence differences have been detected in *c-rel*. The differences between *v-rel* and *c-rel* include seven silent transitions, nine missense transitions, four missense transversions, and three places where Rev-T has a small in-frame deletion of sequences relative to *c-rel*. Most of the coding sequence differences between *c-rel* and *v-rel* are nonconservative amino acid changes. It is not known if any of these sequence differences have functional consequences in the *v-rel* gene product.

Figure 3 shows nucleotide sequences at the 5′ and 3′ junctions of Rev-A and *c-rel*. Both 5′ and 3′ sequences show small regions of homology between Rev-A, Rev-T, and *c-rel*, indicating that homologous recombination may have been involved in the formation of Rev-T. In addition, at one site in the 5′ junction sequences between *c-rel* and the parental retrovirus, there is the remnant of a possible splice donor and acceptor in Rev-T (AGGG). *c-rel* at this site has the sequence TTTTGTTTTGTTAAG/G which is similar to the consen-

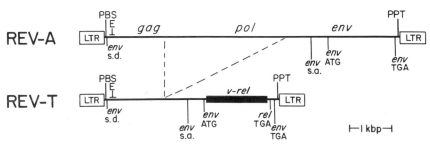

Figure 1 Rev-A and Rev-T structure. The organization of Rev-A and Rev-T DNAs. Abbreviations: (LTR) long terminal repeat; (PBS) primer binding site; (env s.d.) *env* transcript splice donor; (E) *cis*-acting encapsidation sequences; (env s.a.) *env* transcript splice acceptor; (PPT) polypurine tract. Also indicated are the relative positions of the *gag*-, *pol*-, and *env*-coding sequences, and the *v-rel* substitution. The position of the translational initiation and termination codons for *env* and the *env-v-rel* fusion product are shown. The dotted lines indicate the position of the large deletion of Rev-T relative to Rev-A.

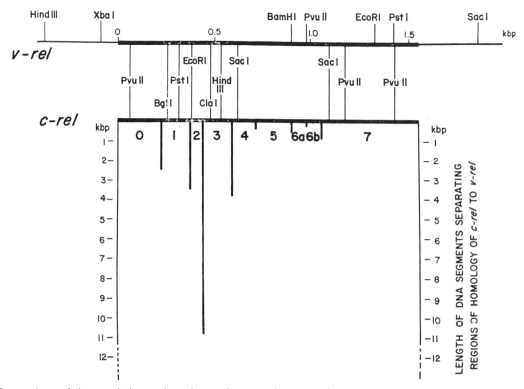

Figure 2 Comparison of the restriction endonuclease cleavage site maps of *v-rel* and *c-rel* (turkey). A restriction endonuclease cleavage site map of *v-rel* and flanking sequences and a restriction endonuclease cleavage site map of the regions of *c-rel* that are homologous to *v-rel* are shown. Each of the restriction endonuclease cleavage sites of Rev-T indicated has been verified by nucleic acid sequencing. The *Pst*I restriction enzyme cleavage site at 1.4 kbp in Rev-T is present in allele 2 of *c-rel* (turkey 7) but not in allele 1. The location of boundaries of the regions of *c-rel* that are homologous to *v-rel* are indicated by vertical lines below the restriction endonuclease cleavage site map of *c-rel*. The lengths of the lines at the boundaries between regions of *c-rel* are proportional to the lengths of the presumed intervening sequences.

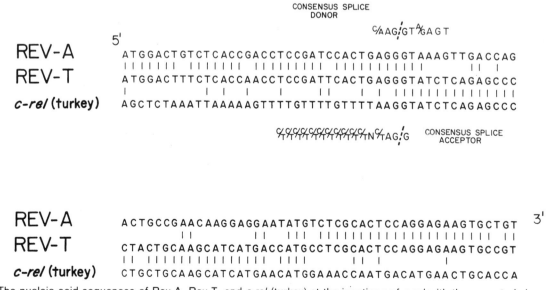

Figure 3 The nucleic acid sequences of Rev-A, Rev-T, and *c-rel* (turkey) at the junctions of *c-rel* with the ancestral virus of Rev-T. The upper three sequences in this figure show the 5′ junction site used to form Rev-T from *c-rel* and an ancestral virus. Rev-A is believed to be similar to the ancestral virus of Rev-T. Above and below the sequences of Rev-A, Rev-T, and *c-rel* (turkey) are consensus sequences for RNA splice donors and acceptor, respectively. The cleavage site used in RNA splicing is indicated by a dotted slash in the consensus sequences. Sequence identities between Rev-A and Rev-T or Rev-T and *c-rel* (turkey) are indicated with a "I" between the respective lines. The lower sequences in this figure show the 3′ junction site used to form Rev-T from *c-rel* (turkey) and an ancestral virus.

sus sequence for a splice acceptor (Y$_{11}$NYAG/G) (Mount 1982). A plausible, presumably cryptic, splice donor can also be identified at the recombination site in Rev-A. The sequence in Rev-A at the junction is AGG/ GTAA, which is similar to the consensus sequence for a splice donor (MG/GTRT). It is possible that Rev-T was formed using the cellular RNA splicing machinery to generate the recombinant between the parental virus and *c-rel*. This process would be analogous to the loss of sequences between regions of *c-rel* that are homologous to *v-rel*.

The models for acquisition of proto-oncogenes by retroviruses (Weiss et al. 1982) include: integration followed by deletion between viral and cell DNA sequences; virus integration 5' to the target sequences with a large readthrough transcript being spliced; and RNA-RNA recombination. The structural relationships of Rev-A, Rev-T, and *c-rel* do not allow any discrimination between the various models for acquisition of sequences by retroviruses.

Insertion of oncogenes or proto-oncogenes into retrovirus vectors

To investigate the relationship between oncogene and proto-oncogene expression and the morphological transformation of normal cells in culture, we inserted these genes into spleen necrosis virus (SNV) expression vectors. Bacterial plasmids containing all the viral sequences required in *cis* for virus propagation, an oncogene or proto-oncogene, and the herpes simplex virus type-I thymidine kinase (*tk*) gene were constructed by recombinant DNA methodology. Chicken embryo fibroblasts were cotransfected with the appropriate plasmid DNA and Rev-A proviral DNA, and virus was recovered. The recovered virus was used to infect tk⁻ cells (to assay for the titer of recombinant virus and morphological transformation of the tk⁺ clones) and chicken embryo fibroblasts (to assay for morphological transformation).

We constructed SNV-tk recombinants containing the *v-Ha-ras* or the *c-Ha-ras* II (rat) genes at the 5' end of the viral genome in a position that should allow high levels of expression. Insertion of *v-Ha-ras* into a 5' position in an SNV-vector (GT10) yielded a virus that transforms chicken embryo fibroblasts at high efficiencies (see Fig. 4 and Table 1). The analogous construction with *c-Ha-ras* II (rat), GT26, is not transforming (Fig. 4 and Table 1). These data indicate that there is an important qualitative difference between *v-Ha-ras* and *c-Ha-ras* II (rat) with respect to their transformation potential.

When *v-src* or *c-src* was inserted into an SNV-vector at the 5' end in a position that should allow high levels of *src* expression (GT8 and GT12), only relatively low titers of *tk* transforming virus were obtained (Fig. 4). Furthermore, no significant morphological transformation was obtained after infection of rat tk⁻ cells or chicken embryo fibroblasts with these viruses. We reasoned that inserting these genes into viruses in a position that enhances their expression may be toxic to cells as a result of an increased concentration of their gene prod-

ucts. To investigate this hypothesis, we cotransfected another SNV-tk vector that we knew yielded a high titer of *tk* transforming virus (SNV-tk) with an excess of either the *v-src* or *c-src* constructs. As seen in Table 1, the presence of GT8 or, to a lesser extent, GT12 during cotransfection inhibited the recovery of SNV-tk. These data indicate that expression of *v-src* or *c-src* is toxic to fibroblasts and that this toxicity may in part be responsible for the lack of transforming activity by these viruses. (This toxicity is also reflected by the relative amounts of *src*-containing virus recovered from chicken cells after transfection of these DNAs. Thus, GT12 is formed at 10-fold higher levels than GT8 after transfection, and GT12 is also about 10-fold less toxic to fibroblasts.)

In avian sarcoma viruses, *v-src* is always located at the 3' end of the viral genome and is expressed as a subgenomic RNA whose concentration is much less than full-length viral RNA (Weiss et al. 1982). Substitution of *v-src* into the *env* gene of SNV resulted in a virus (SW212) that transformed at very low efficiencies (Fig. 4), perhaps indicating a suppression of viral oncogene expression similar to that described by Chen and Temin (1982) for transformation by Rev-T. Insertion of *v-src* into an SNV-vector at the 3' end, such that it is expressed from a subgenomic message (GT22 and GT24), yielded a virus that is less toxic than GT8 (Fig. 4 and Table 1) and that also transformed both avian and rat cells. These data indicate that the formation of an active transforming virus requires the careful control of the quantity of the *src* gene product. Moreover, since GT22 and GT12 are formed at similar levels after transfection and are equally toxic to fibroblasts, the data indicate that the expression of *c-src* is not transforming in normal cells.

Discussion

Viral oncogene and in situ cellular proto-oncogene sequences when expressed in cells give rise to different phenotypes. Therefore, there must be some qualitiative or quantitative difference(s) between oncogenes and proto-oncogenes. There are many possible explanations of the apparent difference in phenotype of normal cells where *c-rel* is expressed and transformed cells where *v-rel* is expressed. The *c-rel* and *v-rel* gene products could have a qualitative difference in their function: *v-rel* contains a subset of the coding sequences of *c-rel*; the *v-rel* gene product, predicted on the basis of nucleic acid sequence, is expressed as a fusion product with 5' *env* sequences and 3' out-of-frame *env*-coding sequences; and there are nucleic acid coding sequence differences between the homologous portions of *v-rel* and *c-rel* which are predicted to cause amino acid sequence differences between the corresponding *c-rel* and *v-rel* gene products.

An alternative explanation for the difference in phenotype of normal cells that express *c-rel* and cells transformed by Rev-T that express *v-rel* is that there is a quantitative difference in the level of a functionally similar gene product. Possible reasons why *v-rel* is expressed at a different level than *c-rel* are: in contrast to *c-rel*, *v-*

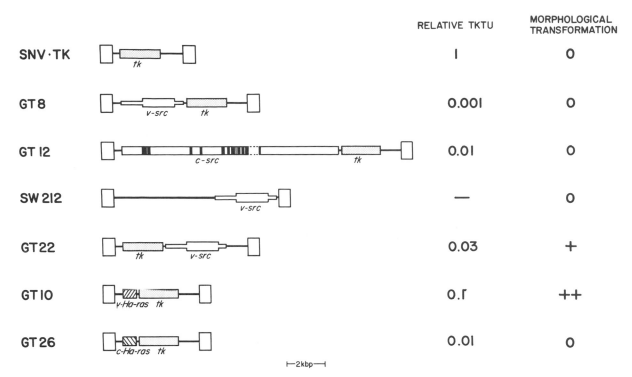

	RELATIVE TKTU	MORPHOLOGICAL TRANSFORMATION
SNV·TK	I	0
GT 8	0.001	0
GT 12	0.01	0
SW 212	—	0
GT 22	0.03	+
GT 10	0.Γ	++
GT 26	0.01	0

Figure 4 Structure and biological activity of several SNV-recombinant viruses. Chick embryo fibroblasts in 60-mm dishes were transfected with 1–5 μg of the indicated plasmid DNA and 0.1 μg of Rev-A DNA as described in Methods. BRL tk⁻ cells (to assay for morphological transformation) were infected with virus recovered 5 days after transfection. tk⁺ colonies were selected in HAT medium and morphological transformants were scored 5–7 days after infection.

rel is under viral transcriptional control, which is presumed to be insensitive to factors regulating *c-rel* transcription, and *v-rel*, when integrated as part of Rev-T, is in a different chromatin environment than *c-rel*.

The analysis of the structural differences between *c-rel* and *v-rel* has not enabled us to determine the basis for transformation by *v-rel*, because there are too many structural differences between *c-rel* and *v-rel*. An alternative approach to explain why oncogenes transform

cells and proto-oncogenes do not is to place different oncogenes and proto-oncogenes in the same transcriptional and translational environment in retrovirus vectors. SNV vectors with *v-Ha-ras* inserted near the viral promoter can transform chicken embryo fibroblasts with high efficiency. Virus with the proto-oncogene *c-Ha-ras* from rat inserted at the same position does not cause transformation. When *v-src* and *c-src* are placed in SNV vectors at their 5′ end, a position that should enable a high level of expression, the *v-src* gene product is toxic and the *c-src* gene product is nontransforming in chicken cells. Placement of *v-src* at the 3′ end of the virus, such that the gene product should be expressed from a subgenomic RNA transcript at lower levels, causes transformation of chicken cells. These data indicate that there is a functional difference between the *v-src* and *c-src* gene products and that the level of expression of *v-src* is important in transformation.

Thus, both qualitative and quantitative considerations are important in transformation by oncogenes and proto-oncogenes.

Table 1 Recovery of SNV-tk Virus after Cotransfection with DNA of SNV-oncogene or SNV-proto-oncogene Recombinants

	Relative tkTU of recovered SNV-tk
SNV-tk	1.0
SNV-tk + GT8	0.01
SNV-tk + GT12	0.1
SNV-tk + SW212	1.0
SNV-tk + GT22	0.1
SNV-tk + GT10	0.1
SNV-tk + GT26	0.4

Chicken embryo fibroblasts in 60-mm dishes were transfected with 1 μg of SNV-tk, 5 μg of the indicated construction, and 0.1 μg of Rev-A DNA as described in Methods. BRL tk⁻ cells were infected with virus harvested 3 days after transfection. tk⁺ cells were selected in HAT media and the number of colonies was determined 5–7 days after infection.

Acknowledgments

We would like to thank Susan Hellenbrand and Ann Troup for excellent technical assistance. We would also like to thank Katie Eggleton for the sequence of Rev-A.

This investigation was supported by U.S. Public Health Service Research Grants CA-07175 and CA-22443 from the National Cancer Institute. K.C.W. is a predoctoral trainee supported by U.S. Public Health

Service Training Grant CA-09135. W.G.T. is a post-doctoral trainee supported by U.S. Public Health Service Research Grant CA-09075. H.M.T. is an American Cancer Society Research Professor.

References

Bandyopadhyay, P.K. and H.M. Temin. 1984a. Expression of complete chicken thymidine kinase gene inserted in a retrovirus vector. *Mol. Cell. Biol.* **4:** (in press).

———. 1984b. Expression from an internal AUG codon of herpes simplex thymidine kinase gene inserted in a retrovirus vector. *Mol. Cell. Biol.* **4:** (in press).

Chen, I.S.Y. and H.M. Temin. 1982. Substitution of 5' helper sequences into non-*rel* portion of reticuloendotheliosis virus strain T suppresses transformation of chicken spleen cells. *Cell* **31:** 111.

Chen, I.S.Y., K.C. Wilhelmsen, and H.M. Temin. 1983. Structure and expression of c-rel, the cellular homologue to the oncogene of reticuloendotheliosis virus strain T. *J. Virol.* **45:** 104.

Chen, I.S.Y., T.W. Mak., J.J. O'Rear, and H.M. Temin. 1981. Characterization of reticuloendoetheliosis strain T DNA and isolation of a novel variant of reticuloendotheliosis virus strain T by molecular cloning. *J. Virol.* **40:** 800.

Emerman, M. and H.M. Temin. 1984. High frequency deletion in recovered retrovirus vectors containing exogenous DNA with promoters. *J. Virol.* **50:** (in press).

Fritsch, E. and H.M. Temin. 1977. Formation and structure of infectious DNA of spleen necrosis virus. *J. Virol.* **21:** 119.

Hayward, W.S. 1977. Size and genetic content of viral RNAs in avian oncovirus-infected cells. *J. Virol.* **24:** 47.

Mount, S.M. 1982. A catalogue of splice junction sequences. *Nucleic Acids Res.* **10:** 459.

Needleman, S.B. and C.D. Wunsch. 1970. A general method applicable to the search for similarities in the amino acid sequence of two proteins. *J. Mol. Biol.* **48:** 443.

Ohmotolino, K. and H.M. Temin. 1981. Formation of infectious progeny virus after insertion of herpes simplex thymidine kinase gene into DNA of an avian retrovirus. *Cell* **26:** 67.

———. 1982. Loss of intervening sequences in genomic mouse α-globin DNA inserted in an infectious retrovirus vector. *Nature* **299:** 265.

Smith, T.F. and M.S. Waterman. 1981. Comparison of biosequences. *Adv. Appl. Math.* **2:** 482.

Sorge, J. and S.H. Hughes. 1982. Splicing of intervening sequences introduced into an infectious retroviral vector. *J. Mol. Appl. Genet.* **1:** 547.

Thelien, G.H., R.F. Zeigel, and M.J. Twiehaus. 1966. Biological studies with RE virus (strain T) that induces reticuloendotheliosis in turkeys, chickens and Japanese quail. *J. Natl. Cancer Inst.* **37:** 731.

Watanabe, S. and H.M. Temin. 1982. Encapsidation sequences for spleen necrosis virus, an avian retrovirus, are between the 5' long terminal repeat and the start of the *gag* gene. *Proc. Natl. Acad. Sci.* **79:** 5986.

———. 1983. Construction of a helper cell for avian reticuloendotheliosis virus cloning. *Mol. Cell. Biol.* **3:** 2241.

Weiss, R., N. Teich, H. Varmus, and J. Coffin, eds. 1982. *Molecular biology of tumor viruses*, 2nd edition: *RNA tumor viruses*. Cold Spring Harbor Laboratory, Cold Spring Harbor, New York.

Wilhelmsen, K.C. and H.M. Temin. 1984. Structure and dimorphism of c-rel (turkey), the cellular homolog to the oncogene of reticuloendotheliosis virus strain T. *J. Virol.* **49:** 521.

Wilhelmsen, K.C., I.S.Y. Chen, and H.M. Temin. 1983. The organization of c-rel in chicken and turkey DNAs. In *Oncogenes and retroviruses: Evaluation of basic findings and clinical potential* (ed. T.E. O'Connor and F.J. Rauscher, Jr.), p. 43. A.R. Liss, New York.

The *fos* Gene: Organization and Expression

I.M. Verma, T. Curran, R. Müller,* F. van Straaten,† W.P. MacConnell,
A.D. Miller, and C. Van Beveren

Molecular Biology and Virology Laboratory, The Salk Institute for Biological Studies, San Diego, California
92138

Acutely oncogenic retroviruses induce a broad spectrum of malignant tumors (for review, see Graf and Beug 1978; Teich et al. 1982). They all contain sequences in their genomes that are responsible for neoplasms in vivo and cellular transformation in vitro. These sequences, termed viral oncogenes (*v-onc*), have their progenitors in the normal cellular genome (Bishop and Varmus 1982). Cellular homologs (*c-onc*) of 18 different retroviral oncogenes have now been identified in the genomes of a variety of vertebrate species (Stehelin et al. 1976; Bishop and Varmus 1982). Sequences homologous to some *c-onc* genes have even been identified in invertebrates (Shilo and Weinberg 1982). Another category of *c-onc* genes has been identified from the DNA of malignant cells by virtue of their ability to induce neoplastic transformation when "transfected" into a mouse fibroblastic cell line in vitro (for review, see Cooper 1982). In several cases, however, it has been shown that such sequences are, in fact, the cellular homologs of *v-onc* genes (Der et al. 1982; Parada et al. 1982; Santos et al. 1982; McCoy et al. 1983). Identification and isolation of novel *v-onc* genes, thus, offer a unique opportunity for the experimental manipulation of specific cellular genes, the perturbation of which can result in neoplastic growth.

Our laboratory is primarily interested in two questions: (1) What is the mechanism by which *v-onc* genes induce transformation, since their cellular progenitor, *c-onc*, generally does not transform cells? and (2) What role do the *c-onc* genes play in the normal metabolism of the cell? We have used Finkel-Biskis-Jinkins murine sarcoma virus (FBJ-MSV) as a model system to approach these questions. The FBJ murine osteosarcoma virus complex (FBJ-MSV) was isolated in 1966 from a spontaneous osteosarcoma in a CF1 mouse by Finkel et al. (1966). Serial passage of cell-free tumor extracts in newborn mice resulted in virus that induces osteosarcomas with a latency as short as 3 weeks (Finkel et al. 1966). The tumors can arise anywhere along the bones, although they appear occasionally in the abdominal peritoneum and the diaphragm, and they appear first as a cortical thickening or as small areas of increased density in the soft tissue adjacent to the bone (Finkel et al. 1966; Ward and Young 1976). Proliferation appears to begin at the periosteum, and growth proceeds peripherally,

with late involvement of the deep cortex. The FBJ virus complex consists of a replication-competent helper murine leukemia virus (FBJ-MLV) and a replication-defective transforming murine sarcoma virus (FBJ-MSV) (Levy et al. 1973, 1978). The two components of the FBJ virus complex have been isolated separately in tissue culture—FBJ-MLV by end-point dilution and FBJ-MSV by the establishment of nonproducer transformed rat cells (Curran and Teich 1982a). A 55,000-dalton phosphoprotein (p55), which is a potential product of the FBJ-MSV oncogene (*v-fos*), was identified by employing sera from rats bearing tumors induced by inoculation of nonproducer cells (Curran and Teich 1982b). In addition to p55, tumor-bearing rat sera also precipitated a 39-kD protein, presumably of host origin. It has recently been found that FBR murine osteosarcoma virus (FBR-MSV), which originated from a radiation-induced mouse osteosarcoma (Finkel et al. 1975; Lee et al. 1979), also contains the *fos* oncogene. The transforming protein of FBR-MSV, however, appears to be expressed as a *gag-fos* fusion protein of 75 kD (P75) (T. Curran et al., unpubl.). Cellular homologs (*c-fos*) of *v-fos* have been identified in the genomes of various vertebrates (Curran et al. 1982) as well as in *Drosphila* (I.M. Verma, unpubl.).

In this article, we describe the structure of the *v-fos* gene and its cellular homologs isolated from mouse or human DNA. We also describe the stage- and tissue-specific expression of the *c-fos* gene during mouse pre- and postnatal development.

Results

Organization of the *fos* gene

The FBJ-MSV proviral DNA obtained from FBJ-MSV-transformed nonproducer rat cells was molecularly cloned in bacteriophage Charon 30 and subsequently subcloned in pBR322 (Curran et al. 1982). The plasmid pFBJ-2 was biologically active and *fos*-specific sequences were further subcloned to generate p-*fos*-1 (Curran et al. 1982). The *fos* gene cellular progenitor from mouse and human cells was also molecularly cloned in bacteriophage Charon 30. Figure 1 (A–D) shows the heteroduplexes formed between pFBJ-2 DNA and molecular clones containing mouse *c-fos* and human *c-fos* gene sequences. The organization of *v-fos* and *c-fos* genes based upon the heteroduplex data and restriction enzyme analysis is shown in Figure 1E.

v-fos and *c-fos* genes have altered carboxyl termini

One of the major questions in which we were interested was to determine if the *v-fos* and *c-fos* gene products

---

*Present address: European Molecular Biology Laboratory, Postfach 10.2209, D-6900 Heidelberg, Federal Republic of Germany.

†Present address: MRC Laboratory of Molecular Biology, Cambridge, England.

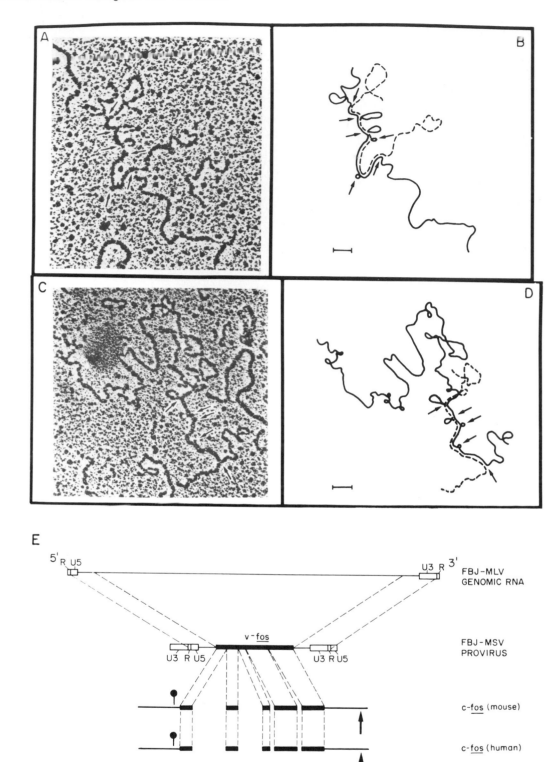

Figure 1 Organization of *fos* gene sequences. (*A–D*) Heteroduplex mapping of recombinant DNA clones. (*A*) DNA:DNA duplex between *Hind*III insert of pFBJ-2 DNA (Curran et al. 1983) and *Eco*RI insert of pc-*fos* (human)-1 (Curran et al. 1983). (*B*) Schematic drawing of *A*. (— — —) single-stranded pFBJ-2 DNA; (———), single-stranded *Eco*RI insert of p.λ-*c-fos* (human)-1, (═══) double-stranded) hybrid DNA. Arrow indicates the position of the DNA loops. (*C*) DNA:DNA duplex between the *Hind*III insert of pFBJ-2 DNA and λ-*c-fos* (mouse)-2 DNA (Curran et al. 1983). (*D*) Schematic of *C*, with symbols as described in *B*. (*E*) *v-fos/c-fos* gene organization. (□) LTR regions containing the U_3, R, and U_5 sequences; (■) regions of homology between FBJ-MSV and the *c-fos* (mouse) and *c-fos* (human) clones; (♀) the approximate 5′-cap nucleotide; (♦) putative poly(A)-addition signal.

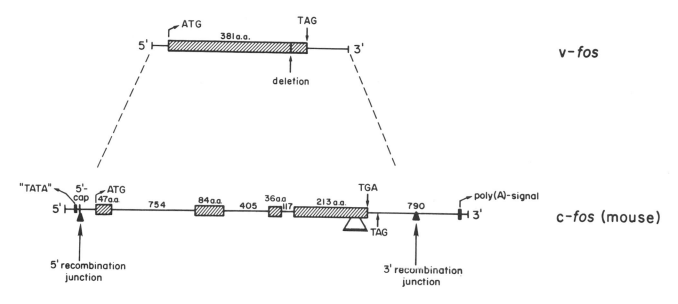

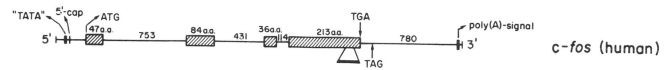

Figure 2 Sequence comparison of *v-fos* and *c-fos* genes. Broken lines indicate the acquired *c-fos* sequences, with the 104 bp deleted in *v-fos* shown. The amino acid sequences to the right of the deletion are in a different frame from that of *c-fos*. The 104 bp in *c-fos* are indicated by a triangle. The putative promoter and termination signals are shown. For details of the nucleotide sequences, see Van Beveren et al. (1983) and van Straaten et al. (1983).

are homologous or have undergone a change. To pursue this aim, we determined the complete nucleotide sequence of the *v-fos* gene and its cellular homolog, the mouse *c-fos* and human *c-fos* genes. Figure 2 depicts the salient features of the *v-fos* and mouse and human *c-fos* genes. The following general points can be noted:

1. The FBJ-MSV proviral DNA is 4026 nucleotides long and contains long terminal repeats of 617 nucleotides each.

2. The *v-fos* substitution encompasses 1639 nucleotides and replaces the entire *gag*, *pol*, and a large portion of the *env* gene of parental FBJ-MLV.

3. The *v-fos* sequences have a single open reading frame of 1143 nucleotides that is capable of encoding a protein of 381 amino acids.

4. From the TATA box to the putative poly(A)-addition signal, the *c-fos* mouse gene is 3397 nucleotides long. When compared with the *v-fos* sequences, the *c-fos* gene has four discontinuous regions. The first three discontinuities have features characteristic of introns found in most eukaryotic genes, since they all contain sequences that agree with the consensus donor splice sites at the 5′ ends and the acceptor sites at their 3′ ends (Van Beveren et al. 1983).

5. The 104-bp-long fourth discontinuity (Fig. 2) does not have an appropriate splice donor or acceptor site. Nucleotide sequence analysis of the human *c-fos* gene indicates that the sequence of the human

c-fos gene is colinear with that of the mouse *c-fos* genes, not the *v-fos* gene, across the fourth discontinuity. Thus, it is unlikely that the discontinuity is due to an insertion in the mouse or human *c-fos* clones. The nucleotide sequence of *c-fos* mRNA is the same as that of the mouse *c-fos* gene (Van Beveren et al. 1983). Furthermore, the 104-bp discontinuity has an open reading frame.

6. The mouse and human *c-fos* gene transcript encode a protein of 380 amino acids.

7. The amino acid sequences of the predicted gene products encoded by the *v-fos* and *c-fos* genes are shown in Figure 3. Despite the additional 104 bp in the *c-fos* gene transcripts, the predicted sizes of viral and cellular *fos* proteins are remarkably similar. A comparison of *v-fos* and mouse *c-fos* protein reveals that the first 332 amino acids have only five amino acid changes; however, the sequence of the remaining 49 amino acids is totally different. Since the additional 104 bp in the *c-fos* gene are immediately after the nucleotides encoding amino acid 332, and since 104 is not a multiple of 3, the remaining 49 amino acids of the *v-fos* gene product are encoded in a different reading frame of the *fos* sequence. The stop codon used for the *v-fos* gene product is present in the 3′ untranslated region of the mouse or human *c-fos* gene sequence (Van Beveren et al. 1983; van Straaten et al. 1983).

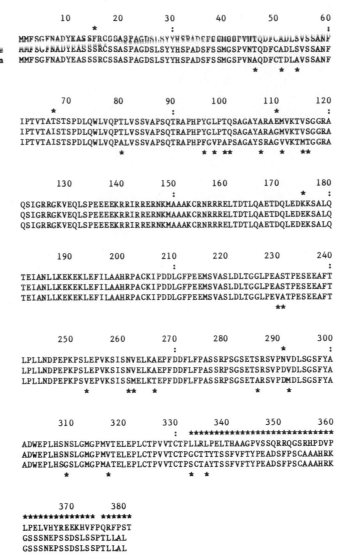

Figure 3 Amino acid sequence comparisons between *v-fos* and *c-fos* proteins. Amino acids are indicated with a single-letter code. Those that differ between *c-fos* (mouse) and *v-fos* gene are shown above the sequences, whereas those that differ between *c-fos* (mouse) and *c-fos* (human) are indicated below the sequence. The carboxyterminal 48 amino acids of *c-fos* gene products are totally different from those of *v-fos* protein.

8. A comparison of the deduced amino acid sequences of the *v-fos* and mouse *c-fos* gene products with the predicted amino acid sequence of the human *c-fos* gene product reveals that in the first 332 amino acids there are 27 amino acid differences between the human *c-fos* and *v-fos* gene products and 22 differences between human *c-fos* and mouse *c-fos* gene products. The remaining 48 amino acids of both the human and mouse *c-fos* protein differ at only two positions.

9. The *v-fos* and *c-fos* proteins are very hydrophilic with a net negative charge.

10. The coding regions of the human and mouse *c-fos* genes appear to be over 90% conserved.

Human *c-fos* gene has two *Alu* family sequences adjacent to its 3′ end

Approximately 570 nucleotides downstream from the 3′ poly(A)-addition signal, there are two *Alu* family se-

quences (van Straaten et al. 1983) separated by 827 nucleotides (Fig. 4). The first *Alu* repeat sequence of 98 nucleotides (positions 4087–4385) is bounded by a 6-nucleotide direct repeat. The second *Alu* repeat of 170 nucleotides (positions 5240–5410) has a 16-bp direct repeat. At least one and possibly both *Alu* repeat sequences can be transcribed in vitro by RNA polymerase III to yield appropriately sized transcripts (S. Fuhrman and C. Van Beveren, unpubl.). The significance of *Alu* repeat sequences for biological activity is not known.

Recombinant junction of *v-fos* substitution

To study the mechanism of biogenesis of FBJ-MSV, we have also molecularly cloned the parent FBJ-MLV DNA (Curran et al. 1983). Figure 5 shows the sequences of FBJ-MLV, FBJ-MSV, and mouse *c-fos* at the 5′ and 3′ extremities of the *v-fos* substitution. The putative parents of FBJ-MSV share a 5-nucleotide sequence at the 5′ end and 10 out of 11 nucleotides at the 3′ end of the *v-fos*

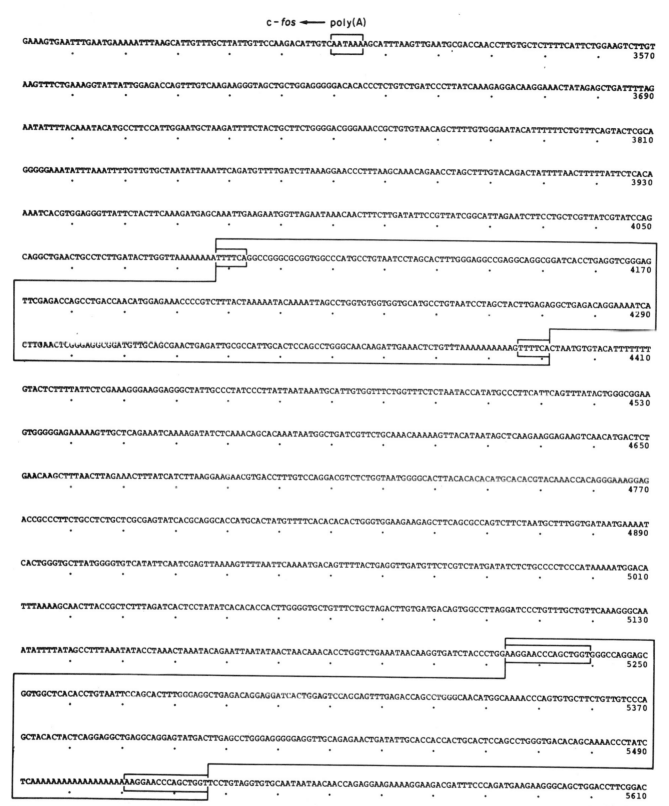

Figure 4 *Alu* sequences adjacent to human *c-fos* gene. Nucleotide sequences adjacent to the putative poly(A)-addition signal of human *c-fos* gene are shown. The two *Alu* family sequences are shown in large boxed areas. The direct repeats at the beginning and end of each *Alu* repeat sequence are also shown with small boxes. The sequence of the human *c-fos* gene upstream of the poly(A)-addition signal is given in van Straaten et al. (1983).

region. Sequences involved in the recombination at the 5′ end lie in the untranslated region of both FBJ-MLV

and mouse *c-fos*. Inspection of the mouse *c-fos* sequences reveals that recombination occurred immedi-

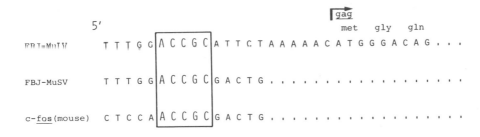

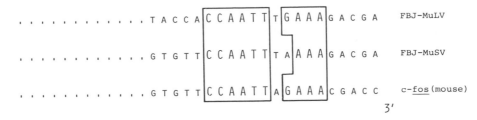

Figure 5 Recombination junctions of acquired *fos* sequences. The 5' and 3' extremities of the *fos* substitution in FBJ-MSV are compared with the sequences at equivalent positions in FBJ-MLV and the *c-fos* (mouse) gene. Nucleotides shared by the parental sequences are shown in open boxes. The beginning of FBJ-MLV is indicated by an arrow. (Reprinted, with permission, from Van Beveren et al. 1983.)

ately downstream from the region encoding the 5' end of mouse *c-fos* mRNA. The sequences that recombined at the 3' end of the *v-fos* were the 3' portion of the FBJ-MLV *env* gene and 3' untranslated region of the mouse *c-fos* gene.

The *fos* protein has an anomalous behavior on SDS-PAGE

The predicted molecular weight of the 381-amino acid-long *v-fos* protein is 41,601, yet it migrates on SDS-PAGE with a molecular weight of 55 kD (Curran and Teich 1982b). This anomalous mobility may be a reflection of its amino acid composition, which has high content of proline (10%) and a net negative charge (15% aspartic and glutamic acids versus 12% arginine, histidine, and lysine). It is, however, possible that the primary *v-fos* gene product is posttranslationally modified. To reconcile the differences between the predicted and apparent molecular weights of *v-fos* protein, we expressed it in *E. coli* under the control of the tryprophan operon regulatory region (Fig. 6). The 381-amino-acid protein was identified by synthesis in minicells isolated from bacteria containing the expression vector plasmid. A 52,000-dalton protein was made in these minicells along with the proteins encoded by the β-lactamase gene present in the expression vector plasmid. The tryptic peptide map of the 52-kD bacterial protein labeled with [35S]methionine was compared with that of the 35S-labeled protein immunoprecipitated from FBJ-MSV-transformed rat cells using tumor-bearing rat sera. The peptide map of the p55 *fos* protein matches exactly that of the bacterial 52-kD protein. The small difference in the electrophoretic mobility in SDS-PAGE gels (52 kD vs. 55 kD) is most likely due to posttranslational modification which does not occur in bacteria.

Biological activity of molecularly cloned FBJ-MSV, *c-fos* gene, and FBJ-MLV

Table 1 shows that molecularly cloned pFBJ-2 DNA induced transformation in rat 208F cells when introduced by calcium phosphate precipitation. The efficiency of transformation was approximately 150 ffu/pmole (Table 1). The morphology of the transformed 208F cells resembled closely that observed with FBJ-MSV. To determine if the viral genome in the pFBJ-2-transformed cells could be rescued, we isolated an individual focus of FBJ-2-transformed 208F cells (TX.F1) by micromanipulation and superinfected it with FBJ-MLV. Transforming virus could be readily detected in virus harvests of this culture (Table 1). The rescue efficiency was comparable to that obtained by superinfection of FBJ-MSV-transformed nonproducer cells (Table 1). The *c-fos* gene obtained from either mouse or human cells did not transform rat 208F cells or NIH-3T3 cells.

The molecularly cloned pFBJ-MLV-1 DNA containing the entire copy of the FBJ-MLV sequences was biologically active. Since this clone contained the FBJ-MLV genome permuted by cleavage at the *Hind*III site, the insert was removed by digestion with *Hind*III, purified by agarose gel electrophoresis, and self-ligated. The major products of the ligation were dimeric molecules, approximately one-half of which should have represented an entire copy of the FBJ-MLV provirus flanked by long terminal repeat (LTR) sequences. This DNA was introduced into NIH-3T3 cells by calcium phosphate precipitation. The next day, cells were seeded at 1:20 dilutions, allowed to grow to confluence, and overlaid with XC cells. Table 2 shows that the ligated DNA was infectious and had a titer of approximately 10^4 pfu/µg of ligated DNA. In a parallel experiment, cloned Moloney MLV proviral DNA had a titer of 3×10^3 pfu/µg. The large, dark-staining XC cell syncytia induced were typical of FBJ-

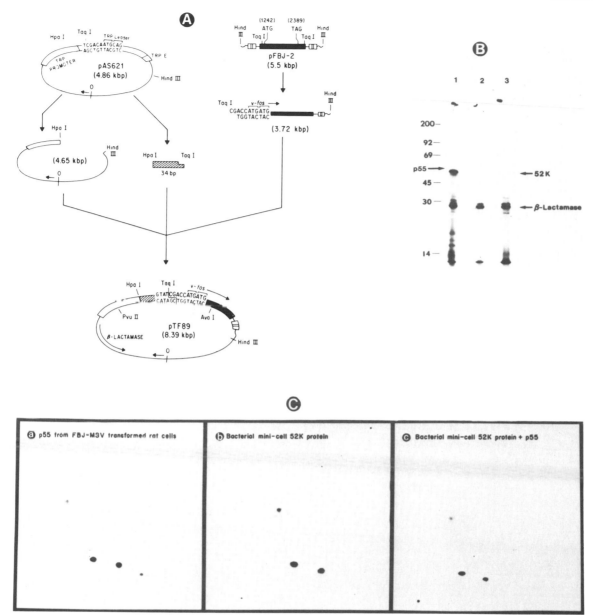

Figure 6 (*A*) Construction of the *v-fos* expression plasmid pTF89. The 5.5-kb fragment resulting from digestion of the plasmid pFBJ-2 with *Hind*III was purified by agarose gel electrophoresis and extracted by the glass powder procedure. From this DNA, the fragment spanning from *Taq*I and *Hind*III containing the *v-fos* was obtained by partial digestion with *Taq*I. The plasmid pAS621 was separately digested to completion in one case with the enzymes *Hpa*I and *Hind*III and in another case with *Hpa*I and *Taq*I. The 34-bp fragment spanning from *Hpa*I and *Taq*I was purified by polyacrylamide gel electrophoresis. The 4026-bp *Hpa*I–*Hind*III fragment was also purified by agarose gel electrophoresis. The three fragments of DNA were ligated together and transformed onto competent DH1 bacteria which were subsequently selected for ampicillin resistance. Colonies hybridizing to *v-fos* DNA were grown and DNA was prepared from them and analyzed by restriction enzyme digestion. The restriction endonuclease sites shown in the figure were used for constructing pTF89. (*B*) Expression in bacterial minicells. Minicells prepared from bacteria containing plasmids pTF89 and pAS621 were pulse-labeled with [^{35}S]methionine in media containing 100 μg/ml of tryptophan and analyzed by SDS gel electrophoresis and autoradiography. (Lane *1*) Labeled minicells from *trp*R⁻ bacteria containing the plasmid pTF89; (lane *2*) labeled minicells from *trp*R⁺ bacteria containing the plasmid pTF89; (lane *3*) labeled minicells from *trp*R⁻ bacteria containing the plasmid pAS621. (*C*) Autoradiograms of [^{35}S]methionine-containing peptides of p55 from FBJ-MSV-transformed rat cells and 52-kD protein from bacterial minicells. (*a*) Tryptic peptides of p55 from FBJ-MSV-transformed rat cells; (*b*) tryptic peptides from the 52-kD protein from *trp*R⁻ bacterial minicells; (*c*) the two sets of peptides described above which were run together.

MSV. Thus, pFBJ-MLV-1 contains an entire, functional copy of the FBJ-MLV genome.

Expression of cellular oncogenes

In recent years, major research efforts have focused on elucidating the physiological role of *c-onc* sequences in the normal cell. The ability of acutely oncogenic retroviruses to interfere with normal cell proliferation and differentiation has led to the postulation that the normal cellular homologs of *v-onc* gene products may fulfill certain physiological functions in these processes. In a sys-

Table 1 Biological Activity of Cloned FBJ-MSV Provirus

DNA	ffu/pmole[a]	
	Transfection	
Carrier	<1	
pFBJ-2[b]	150	
pH1[c]	20	
Mouse c-fos[d]	<1	
Human c-fos[e]	<1	
Supernatant	ffu/ml	pfu/ml[f]
	Infection	
TX.F1[g]	<10	—
TX.F1 (L1)[h]	1.4 × 10⁵	3.7 × 10⁶

[a]Focus-forming units on 208F cells.
[b]The entire recombinant plasmid DNA containing FBJ-MSV provirus was used for transfection.
[c]This clone contains Ha-MSV circular DNA permuted by cleavage at the EcoRI site.
[d]Mouse c-fos gene (Curran et al. 1983).
[e]Human c-fos gene (Van Straaten et al. 1983).
[f]XC plaque-forming units on NIH-3T3 cells.
[g]Harvest taken from a subconfluent culture of pFBJ-2 transformed cells (TX.F1).
[h]Harvest taken from a subconfluent culture of TX.F1 cells 1 week after superinfection with FBJ-MLV (clone L1) (multiplicity of infection 0.1–0.5).

Table 2 Biological Activity of pFBI-MLV 1

DNA	Number of XC plaques[a]	Number of plaques per μg[b]
Carrier (NIH-3T3)	0, 0	—
pMLVint-48[c]	77, 62	3 × 10³
Ligated FBJ-MLV insert (0.2 μg)	102, 110	1 × 10⁴

[a]Cells were seeded at 1:20 dilution in duplicate 1 day after transfection.
[b]Calculated as number of plaques per microgram of applied DNA.
[c]This clone contains the integrated Moloney-MLV clone, subcloned into the EcoRI site of pBR322 (A.D. Miller and I.M. Verma, unpubl.).

tematic study to understand the role of *c-onc* genes during pre- and postnatal development of the mouse, we have addressed two issues: (1) Are c-*onc* genes expressed during embryogenesis, and (2) Is there a differential expression of c-*onc* genes? Figure 7 displays that many *c-onc* genes are expressed during prenatal development, and, furthermore, a differential pattern of

expression can be witnessed (Müller et al. 1982). These observations lend support to the widely held notion that *c-onc* gene products participate in developmental processes (Chen 1980; Gonda et al. 1982; Müller et al. 1982, 1983a,b,c; Shiubuya et al. 1982; Vennström and Bishop 1982).

Both the *c-fos* and *c-fms* genes appear to be specifically expressed in extraembryonic tissue (Müller et al. 1982; 1983a,b,c). We have extensively analyzed the expression of these *c-onc* genes during development of the mouse fetus, placenta, and extraembryonal membranes (also referred to as fetal membranes, i.e., visceral yolk sac [VYS] and amnion) as well as in a variety of postnatal mouse tissues. A diagramatic sketch of a midgestation conceptus (i.e., fetus plus all extraembryonal tissues [placenta and membranes]) is shown in Figure 8. The results of these studies are summarized as follows:

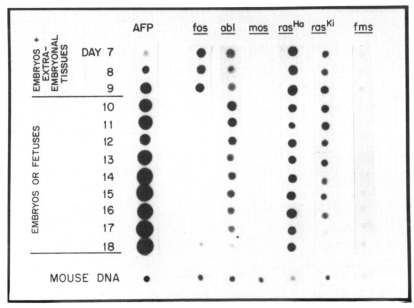

Figure 7 Expression of cellular oncogenes during mouse prenatal development. Probes used are AFP (α-fetoprotein obtained from S. Tilghman); *abl* (Abelson leukemia virus, obtained from S. Goff and D. Baltimore); Ha-*ras*, Ki-*ras* (Harvey and Kirsten MSV, obtained from E. Scolnick and colleagues); and *fms* (SM-FeSV, obtained from C. Sherr). For experimental details see Müller et al. (1982).

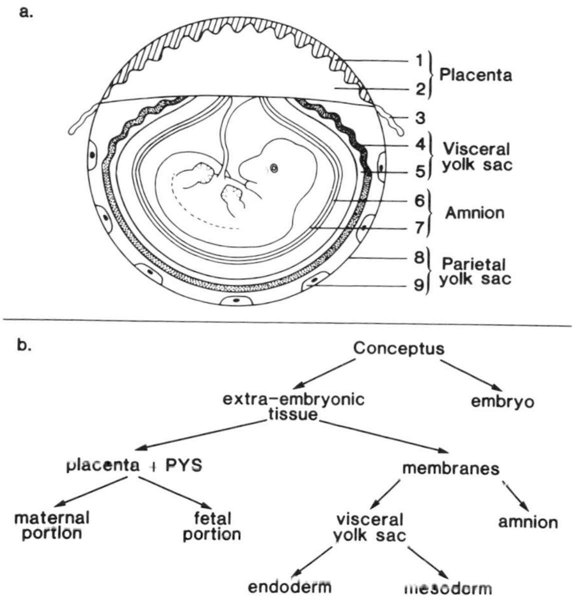

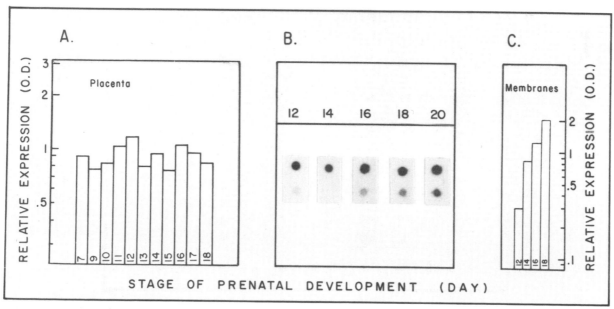

Figure 8 Dissection of midgestation concepts. Diagrammatic sketch of sectioned conceptus at days 12–18 of gestation. (Reprinted, with permission, from Müller et al. 1983a.)

Expression of c-fos *during development of the mouse placenta*

c-fos gene transcripts were observed at relatively high, but nearly constant levels in the undissected placenta throughout the gestational period and in day-6 to day-9 conceptuses (which consist largely of tissues participating in the formation of the placenta) (Müller et al. 1982, 1983a). Analysis of surgically dissected placentas, however, revealed that transcripts from the *c-fos* gene were approximately 15-fold more abundant in the outer portion of the midgestation placenta (primarily fetus-derived undifferentiated cytotrophoblast and maternal decidua) relative to the inner moiety (predominantly differentiated syncytiotrophoblast) (Fig. 9B). This finding suggests that the majority of *c-fos* transcripts in the midgestation placenta originate either from the maternally derived decidua basalis or from the fetal cytotrophoblast. In the inner placenta, the level of *c-fos* transcripts was found to increase gradually as gestation proceeds, and to reach a level that is approximately 50% of that found in the outer moiety. This increase in *c-fos* expression may be correlated with the differentiation of chorionic tissue, which in the mouse is fused with the inner placenta (Müller et al. 1983a).

Expression of c-fos *in mouse extraembryonal membranes*

The level of *c-fos* transcripts was found to be low in day-10 to day-12 extraembryonal membranes (Müller et al. 1982, 1983a), but increased approximately six-fold between days 12–18 of gestation to a level that is slightly higher than that observed in the placenta (Fig. 9). A detailed analysis of the microsurgically isolated components of the late-gestation extraembryonal membranes showed that the levels of *c-fos* transcripts were high in VYS endoderm and mesoderm, as compared with the placenta. Furthermore, the highest levels of expression of *c-fos* were observed in amnion (Fig. 10). The level of *c-fos* transcripts in the day-18 amnion was found to be close to the level of *v-fos* transcripts in cells transformed by FBJ-MSV.

The size of the *c-fos* (mouse) gene transcripts has been determined to be 2.2 kb in all tissues and cells analyzed (Fig. 11A) (Müller et al. 1982, 1983b). The

Figure 9 Quantification of the levels of the *c-fos* transcripts during prenatal development. (*A*) Placenta, days 7–18. (*B*) Outer and inner placenta. The upper lane is outer placenta while the lower lane is inner placenta. (*C*) Extraembryonal membranes (including amnion and visceral yolk sac).

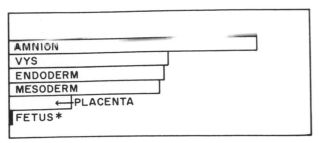

Figure 10 Relative levels of *c-fos* transcripts in surgically isolated extraembryonal tissues. The level of cross-contamination was about 10% (Müller et al. 1983a). (∗) Barely detectable levels.

sequence analysis of the *c-fos* gene would predict the *c-fos* RNA transcript to be about 2.2 kb following the removal of introns (Van Beveren et al. 1983). In some instances, a second *c-fos*-related RNA species of approximately 3.5 kb could be identified (Fig. 11, lane 2; Müller et al. 1983a), which presumably represents an unspliced mRNA precursor.

Expression of c-fos *in mouse fetuses and postnatal tissues*

Expression of *c-fos* was found to be low in fetuses throughout the gestational period from the tenth to the seventeenth day, but increased more than fivefold at later stages of prenatal development (Fig. 7). Analyses of a variety of tissues from newborn or 10-day-old mice showed elevated levels of *c-fos* expression only in "bone" (rib cage and vertebra; including bone marrow, muscles, and part of the pleura) and "skin" tissue (including the subcutaneous connective tissues, muscles, and part of the peritoneum) (Müller et al. 1982, 1983a). This finding is interesting since the *fos* sequences in FBJ-MSV have been implicated in the induction of osteosarcomas in newborn mice (Finkel et al. 1966; Finkel and Biskis 1968; Curran et al. 1982). The fact that significant levels of *c-fos* transcripts could also be detected in "skin," but not in any hematopoietic tissue (Müller et al. 1982), suggests that enhanced *c-fos* expression could occur in cells of mesenchymal origin that participate in the formation of connective tissues. Thus, the increase in the level of *c-fos* transcripts at late stages of fetal development (Fig. 7) may originate from cells present in "bone" and "skin" tissues.

Expression of c-fos *in human tissues*

The results obtained from an analysis of *c-fos* expression in human tissues and cells closely resembled that described above for mouse tissues (Müller et al. 1983b). The highest levels of *c-fos* transcripts were detected in

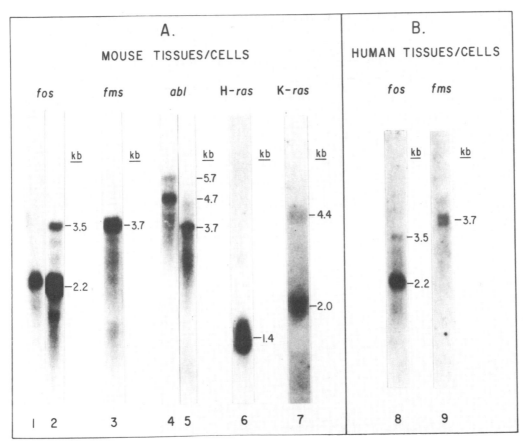

Figure 11 Molecular size of *c-onc* transcripts. Northern blot analysis of total poly(A)⁺ RNA from various prenatal and postnatal tissues from mouse (*A*) and human (*B*) cells. (Lane *1*) Neonatal "bone"; (lane *2*) day-17 membranes; (lane *3*) day-16 placenta; (lane *4*) day-11 embryo; (lane *5*) adult testes; (lane *6*) 12-day embryo; (lane *7*) day-12 membranes; (lane *8*) term placenta; and (lane *9*) BeWo cells.

human term chorion and amnion. Elevated concentrations of *c-fos* transcripts were also observed in term placenta and in a trophoblastic cell line (BeWo) derived from a human gestational choriocarcinoma relative to a number of other tissues and cells, including embryonal carcinoma cells, fetal fibroblasts, and a variety of postnatal tissues. The size of the transcripts from the *c-fos* (human) gene were found to be very similar to those from its murine counterpart (Fig. 11B). Thus, it appears that not only the structure of the *c-fos* gene but also the control mechanisms regulating its expression have been conserved during evolution.

Expression of c-fms

The expression pattern of the *c-fms* gene observed during mouse prenatal development bears some conspicuous similarities with that of the *c-fos* gene (Fig. 7, Müller et al. 1983c). For instance, the level of *c-fms* transcripts was found to be very low in fetuses of any developmental stage, but high in late-gestation placenta and extraembryonal membranes (Müller et al. 1983c). As in the case of *c-fos*, the concentration of transcripts from the *c-fms* gene gradually increased during development of the extraembryonal membranes. However, *c-fos* and *c-fms* are not expressed concordantly. In contrast to *c-fos*, the concentration of *c-fms* transcripts increased in the undissected placenta during mouse prenatal development (approximately 15-fold relative to day-7 to day-9 conceptuses) before reaching a plateau at days 14–16 of gestation (Müller et al. 1983c). The levels of *c-fms* transcripts were relatively unchanged in late-gestational amnion, VYS, and both moieties of the placenta (Müller et al. 1983c). No significant expression of *c-fms* could be detected in any postnatal tissue (Müller et al. 1983c). When human tissues and cells were analyzed, high levels of *c-fms* transcripts were found only in term placenta and fetal membranes as well as in the trophoblastic BeWo cell line (Müller et al. 1983b). Transcripts from both *c-fms* (mouse) and *c-fms* (human) were determined to be 3.7 kb in size (Fig. 11B).

Discussion

Viral oncogenes have been directly implicated in the onset of neoplastic transformation. In some instances, their cellular progenitors also have the potential to induce transformation. Thus, a study of the kinship of viral and cellular oncogenes is essential to understand their role in oncogenesis.

The *fos* gene

FBJ-MSV originated by recombination between FBJ-MLV and *c-fos* gene. Acquisition of *fos* sequences occurred at the expense of most of the viral structural genes. The FBJ-MSV genome contains 1639 nucleotides of cellular sequences, 2372 nucleotides that originate from FBJ-MLV, and 16 nucleotides that represent the regions shared at the junction of cellular sequences with those of helper MLV. The open reading frame that encodes the predicted *v-fos* gene product is totally contained within the *fos* substitution. A single transcript of about 3.5 kb that reacts with *fos*-specific sequences has been identified in FBJ-MSV-transformed cells. Since there is no evidence of subgenomic mRNAs, we assume that the 3.5-kb genomic RNA is the sole RNA transcribed from FBJ-MSV proviral DNA.

The *v-fos* sequences have a coding capacity of 381 amino acids which would have a predicted molecular weight of 41,600. However, the *v-fos* gene product identified in FBJ-MSV-transformed cells migrates as a 55-kD protein on SDS-PAGE. The anomalous behavior of the protein on SDS-PAGE may be due to its high proline content and distribution of charged amino acids, as has been proposed for the transforming proteins of SV40 (Fiers et al. 1978; Reddy et al. 1978), human adenovirus 5 (van Ormondt et al. 1978), and polyoma virus (Hunter et al. 1979). It is also possible that posttranslational modification of the primary *v-fos* gene translation product is responsible for some of the size discrepancy. Although p55 is a phosphoprotein (Curran and Teich 1982a), it does not appear that the phosphorylation of the *v-fos* gene product is solely responsible for its anomalous size. The product of in vitro cell-free translation of FBJ-MSV RNA also migrates as a protein with an approximate molecular weight of 55,000 (Curran and Teich 1982a). In addition, a *v-fos* gene fragment containing the entire coding region can be expressed in bacteria, and the resulting gene product has a mobility commensurate with a 52-kD protein (Fig. 6) which has similar tryptic peptides as observed with p55. The ability to make p52 in bacterial cells authenticates the identification of the *v-fos*-coding region.

The nucleotide sequence of the *c-fos* (mouse) gene indicates that it contains the signals for initiation of transcription (TATA-box) by DNA-dependent RNA polymerase II (Corden et al. 1980) and for polyadenylation (Proudfoot and Brownlee 1976). In vitro transcription of DNA fragments containing portions of the 5′ end of the *c-fos* (mouse) gene indicates that the 5′ end of the mouse *c-fos* mRNA is approximately at the position specified in Figure 2 (S.A. Fuhrman, pers. comm.). The size of *c-fos* transcripts, from the proposed 5′ cap to the canonical polyadenylation signal, after removal of introns, would be 2.2 kb. This is in close agreement with the size of *fos*-specific transcripts detected by Northern blot analysis in mouse cells (Müller et al. 1982; Fig. 11). In some cases, a *fos*-specific RNA approximately 3.5 kb in length, presumably representing the unspliced primary *c-fos* transcript, has been observed.

When compared with the 3′ end of the *c-fos* (mouse) gene, the *v-fos* gene has suffered a deletion of 104 bp. Consequently, the products of the *v-fos* and *c-fos* genes are predicted to have different carboxyl termini (Fig. 3). Inspection of the *c-fos* gene sequences reveals that there is a 5-nucleotide inverted repeat (GGGCT/AGCCC) that overlaps the borders of the deletion. A plausible explanation for the deletion would be that the 104-nucleotide segment was looped out, either during or after the recombination of the progenitors of FBJ-MSV.

c-fos gene expression

The role of c-onc genes in the normal cellular metabolic processes has been a subject of intense interest, but remains poorly understood. Availability of molecular clones of a variety of oncogenes has allowed the investigation of c-onc expression patterns in various tissues and cells from chicken (Chen 1980; Gonda et al. 1982; Shibuya et al. 1982; Vennström and Bishop 1982) and humans (Westin et al. 1982; Müller et al. 1983c). Expression of c-fos mouse genes during prenatal development is observed only in the extraembryonal tissues (i.e., placenta, visceral yolk sac, and membranes). Higher, but relatively constant, levels of expression of c-fos can be observed in the outer portion of placenta (primarily fetus-derived undifferentiated cytotrophoblast and maternal decidua) during entire gestational periods. In contrast, the levels of c-fos expression in the inner moiety of placenta (nonproliferating syncytiotrophoblast) are 10- to 14-fold lower than the outer moiety of the placenta in the early midgestation period (day 12, 17; Fig. 9B) and increase during the late-gestation period. By far the highest accumulation of c-fos transcripts occurs in the day-18 amnion. In the postnatal tissues, only the "bone" and "skin" tissues exhibit elevated levels of c-fos transcripts. In the human tissues, high levels of c-fos transcripts can be observed only in the extraembryonal tissues (placenta, amnion, and chorion). In all tissues expressing the c-fos gene, transcripts of 2.2 kb can be identified.

Differential expression of c-onc genes combined with their extensive phylogenetic conversation lends credence to the widely held notion of their role in normal cell metabolism. The present data, however, cannot unequivocally assign to c-onc genes a role in the natural developmental processes. Two types of experimental approaches are needed: (1) Identification of a function of the c-onc gene product. Recent findings that c-sis gene may be platelet-derived growth factor (PDGF) (Doolittle et al. 1983; Waterfield et al. 1983) offer an excellent opportunity to study the function of c-sis gene. Similarly, protein kinase activity associated with c-src product should be helpful in delineating its role in normal cellular processes. (2) Introduction of a mutated c-onc gene in the animal to study its role in development and normal cell metabolism. Unfortunately, this approach requires availability of a functional c-onc gene and sophisticated technology of introduction of the altered c-onc gene into the animal. A very promising development has been the identification of several c-onc homologs in Drosophila and yeast. It has recently been demonstrated that c-src (Drosophila)-specific sequences are expressed only at specific stages of larval development (M. Simon and J.M. Bishop, pers. comm.). A 21,000-dalton protein can be identified in yeast by immunoprecipitation with antisera raised against v-Ha-ras p21 protein (E. Scolnick, pers. comm.). The genomes of Drosophila and yeast can be genetically manipulated to study the role of mutated c-onc genes.

Mechanism of oncogenesis: Implications for c-fos gene

The precise mechanism of activation of c-onc genes in the induction of neoplastic transformation is not understood, but three viewpoints are currently prevalent. The proposed mechanisms include enhanced levels of the gene product (Bishop 1981), expression in an inappropriate cell type (Graf and Beug 1978), and expression of an aberrant form of the c-onc protein (Reddy et al. 1982; Tabin et al. 1982). Any one or a combination of these mechanisms could cause cellular transformation. The nucleotide sequence data reported here indicate that the v-fos- and c-fos-encoded proteins are nearly identical over the first 332 amino acids (with only 5 amino acid changes), but that the remaining 48 amino acids (49 amino acids in v-fos) at the carboxyl termini are entirely different. Thus, it appears that the viral fos gene product is an aberrant form of the c-fos gene product. Recent experiments in our laboratory indicate that the c-fos protein can transform fibroblasts. However, c-fos requires two manipulations before manifestation of its transforming potential. These include (1) linkage of transcription enhancer elements, and (2) disruption of interacting sequences at the 3' end of the c-fos gene. We have also recently observed that both the v-fos and c-fos gene products are located in the nucleus. Furthermore, in the day-18 amnion, which accumulates the highest concentration of c-fos transcripts, the c-fos protein is also located in the nucleus. The levels of expression of c-fos gene product in amnion are nearly similar to the levels of the v-fos protein in FBJ-MSV-transformed cells. The c-fos protein can induce transformation in fibroblasts, yet similar levels of c-fos protein do not transform normal amnion cells. These observations support the hypothesis that the normal cellular genetic complement harbors genes that are capable of inducing oncogenesis when expresed outside the natural constraints of cell growth and differentiation.

Acknowledgments

We thank Liza Zokas and Joanne Tremblay for excellent assistance during this work, which was supported by funds from the National Institutes of Health and the American Cancer Society. We are grateful to Jan Littrell for preparation of this manuscript.

References

Bishop, J.M. 1981. Retrovirus oncogenes. In *Developmental biology using purified genes* (ed. D.D. Brown), p. 515. Academic Press, New York.

Bishop, J.M. and H.E. Varmus. 1982. Functions and origins of retroviral transforming genes. In *Molecular biology of tumor viruses*, 2nd edition: *RNA tumor viruses* (ed. R. Weiss et al.), p. 999. Cold Spring Harbor Laboratory, Cold Spring Harbor, New York.

Chen, J.H. 1980. Expression of endogenous avian myeloblastosis virus information in different chicken cells. *J. Virol.* **36**: 162.

Cooper, G.M. 1982. Cellular transforming genes. *Science* **218**: 801.

Corden, J., B. Wasylyk, A. Buchwalder, P. Sassone-Corsi, C. Kedinger, and P. Chambon. 1980. Promoter sequences of eukaryotic protein-coding genes. *Science* **209**: 1406.

Curran, T. and N.M. Teich. 1982a. Identification of a 39,000-dalton protein in cells transformed by the FBJ murine osteosarcoma virus. *Virology* **116**: 221.

————. 1982b. Candidate product of the FBJ murine osteosarcoma virus oncogene: Characterization of a 55,000 dalton phosphoprotein. *J. Virol.* **42**: 114.

Curran, T., W.P. MacConnell, F. van Straaten, and I.M. Verma. 1983. Structure of FBJ murine osteosarcoma virus genome: Molecular cloning of its associated helper virus and the cellular homolog of the v-*fos* gene from mouse and human cells. *Mol. Cell. Biol.* **3**: 914.

Curran, T., G. Peters, C. Van Beveren, N.M. Teich, and I.M. Verma. 1982. The FBJ murine osteosarcoma virus: Identification and molecular cloning of biologically active proviral DNA. *J. Virol.* **44**: 674.

Der, C.J., T.G. Krontiris, and G.M. Cooper. 1982. Transforming genes of human bladder and lung carcinoma cell lines are homologous to the *ras* genes of Harvey and Kirsten sarcoma viruses. *Proc. Natl. Acad. Sci.* **79**: 3637.

Doolittle, R.F., M.W. Hunkapiller, L.E. Hood, S.G. Devare, K.C. Robbins, S.A. Aaronson, and H.N. Antoniades. 1983. Simian sarcoma virus *onc* gene, v-*sis*, is derived from the gene (or genes) encoding a platelet-derived growth factor. *Science* **221**: 275.

Fiers, W., R. Contreras, G. Haegman, R. Rogiers, A. Van de Voorde, H. Van Heuverswyn, J. Van Herreweghe, G. Volckaert, and M. Ysabaert. 1978. Complete nucleotide sequence of SV40 DNA. *Nature* **273**: 113.

Finkel, M.P. and B.O. Biskis. 1968. Experimental induction of osteosarcomas. *Prog. Exp. Tumor Res.* **10**: 72.

Finkel, M.P., B.O. Biskis, and P.B. Jinkins. 1966. Virus induction of osteosarcomas in mice. *Science* **151**: 698.

Finkel, M.P., C.A. Reilly, Jr., and B.O. Biskis. 1975. Viral etiology of bone cancer. *Front. Radiat. Ther. Oncol.* **10**: 28.

Gonda, T.J., D.K. Sheiness, and J.M. Bishop. 1982. Transcripts from the cellular homolog of retroviral oncogenes: Distribution among chicken tissues. *Mol. Cell. Biol.* **2**: 617.

Graf, T. and H. Beug. 1978. Avian leukemia viruses: Interaction with their target cells in vivo and in vitro. *Biochim. Biophys. Acta* **516**: 269.

Hunter, T., M.A. Hutchinson, W. Eckhart, T. Friedmann, A. Esty, P. LaPorte, and P. Deininger. 1979. Regions of the polyoma genome coding for T antigens. *Nucleic Acids Res.* **7**: 2275.

Lee, C.K., E.W. Chan, C.A. Reilly, Jr., V.A. Pahnke, G. Rockus, and M.P. Finkel. 1979. *In vitro* properties of FBR murine osteosarcoma virus (40650). *Proc. Soc. Exp. Biol. Med.* **162**: 214.

Levy, J.A., J.W. Hartley, W.P. Rose, and R.J. Huebner. 1973. Studies of FBJ osteosarcoma virus in tissue culture. I. Biologic characteristics of the "C"-type viruses. *J. Natl. Cancer Inst.* **51**: 525.

Levy, J.A., P.L. Kazan, C.A. Reilly, Jr., and M.P. Finkel. 1978. FBJ-osteosarcoma virus in tissue culture. III. Isolation and characterization of non-virus producing FBJ-transformed cells. *J. Virol.* **26**: 11.

McCoy, M.S., J.J. Toole, J.M. Cunningham, E.H. Chang, D.R. Lowy, and R.A. Weinberg. 1983. Characterization of a human colon/lung carcinoma oncogene. *Nature* **302**: 79.

Müller, R., I.M. Verma, and E.D. Adamson. 1983a. Expression of c-*onc* genes: c-*fos* transcripts accumulate to high levels during development of mouse placenta, yolk sac and amnion. *EMBO J.* **2**: 679.

Müller, R., J.M. Tremblay, E.D. Adamson, and I.M. Verma. 1983b. Tissue and cell type-specific expression of two human c-*onc* genes. *Nature* **304**: 454.

Müller, R., D.J. Slamon, J.M. Tremblay, J.M. Cline, and I.M. Verma. 1982. Differential expression of cellular oncogenes during pre- and postnatal development of the mouse. *Nature* **299**: 640.

Müller, R., D.J. Slamon, E.D. Adamson, J.M. Tremblay, D.M. Müller, M.J. Cline, and I.M. Verma. 1983c. Expression of c-*onc* genes c-*ras*[Ki] and c-*fms* during mouse development. *Mol. Cell. Biol.* **3**: 1062.

Parada, L.F., C.J. Tabin, C. Shih, and R.A. Weinberg. 1982. Human EJ bladder carcinoma oncogene is homologue of Harvey sarcoma virus *ras* gene. *Nature* **297**: 474.

Proudfoot, N.J. and G.G. Brownlee. 1976. 3' non-coding region sequences in eukaryotic messenger RNA. *Nature* **263**: 211.

Reddy, E.P., R.K. Reynolds, E. Santos, and M. Barbacid. 1982. A point mutation is responsible for the acquisition of transforming properties by the T24 human bladder carcinoma oncogene. *Nature* **300**: 149.

Reddy, V.B., B. Thimmappaya, R. Dhar, K.N. Subramanian, B.S. Zain, J. Pan, P.K. Ghosh, M.L. Celma, and S.M. Weissman. 1978. The genome of simian virus 40. *Science* **200**: 494.

Santos, E., S.R. Tronick, S.A. Aaronson, S. Pulciani, and M. Barbacid. 1982. T24 human bladder carcinoma oncogene is an activated form of the normal human homologue of BALB- and Harvey-MSV transforming genes. *Nature* **298**: 343.

Shibuya, M., H. Hanafusa, and P.C. Balduzzi. 1982. Cellular sequences related to three new *onc* genes of avian sarcoma virus (*fps, yes* and *ros*) and their expression in normal and transformed cells. *J. Virol.* **42**: 143.

Shilo, B.Z. and R.A. Weinberg. 1982. DNA sequences homologous to vertebrate oncogenes are conserved in *Drosophila melanogaster. Proc. Natl. Acad. Sci.* **78**: 6789.

Stehelin, D., H.E. Varmus, J.M. Bishop, and P.K. Vogt. 1976. DNA related to the transforming gene(s) of avian sarcoma viruses is present in normal avian DNA. *Nature* **260**: 170.

Tabin, C.J., S.M. Bradley, I. Bargmann, R.A. Weinberg, A.G. Papageorge, E.M. Scolnick, R. Dhar, D.R. Lowy, and E.H. Chang. 1982. Mechanism of activation of a human oncogene. *Nature* **300**: 143.

Teich, N.M., J. Wyke, T. Mak, A. Bernstein, and W. Hardy. 1982. Pathogenesis of retrovirus-induced disease. In *Molecular biology of tumor viruses*, 2nd edition: *RNA tumor viruses* (ed. R. Weiss et al.), p. 785. Cold Spring Harbor Laboratory, Cold Spring Harbor, New York.

Van Beveren, C., F. van Straaten, T. Curran, R. Müller, and I.M. Verma. 1983. Nucleotide sequence analysis of FBJ-MuSV provirus and c-*fos* (mouse) gene reveals that viral and cellular *fos* gene products have different carboxy termini. *Cell* **32**: 1241.

Van Ormondt, H., J. Maat, A. de Waard, and A.J. van der Eb. 1978. The nucleotide sequence of the transforming *HpaI-E* fragment of adenovirus type 5 DNA. *Gene* **4**: 309.

van Straaten, F., R. Müller, T. Curran, C. Van Beveren, and I.M. Verma. 1983. Nucleotide sequence of a human c-*onc* gene: Deduced amino acid sequence of human c-*fos* protein. *Proc. Natl. Acad. Sci.* **80**: 3183.

Vennström, B. and J.M. Bishop. 1982. Isolation and characterization of chicken DNA homologous to the two putative oncogenes of avian erythroblastosis virus. *Cell* **28**: 135.

Ward, J.M. and D.M. Young. 1976. Histogenesis and morphology of periosteal sarcomas induced by FBJ virus in NIH Swiss mice. *Cancer Res.* **36**: 3985.

Waterfield, M.D., G.T. Scrace, N. Whittle, P. Stroobant, A. Johnsson, A. Wasteson, B. Westermark, C.-H. Heldin, J.S. Huang, and T.F. Deuel. 1983. Platelet-derived growth factor is structurally related to the putative transforming protein p28[sis] of simian sarcoma virus. *Nature* **304**: 35.

Westin, E.H., R.C. Gallo, S.K. Arya, A. Eva, L.M. Souza, M.A. Baluda, S.A. Aaronson, and F. Wong-Staal. 1982. Differential expression of the *amv* gene in human hematopoietic cells. *Proc. Natl. Acad. Sci.* **79**: 2194.

Growth Regulation of Murine B Lymphoid Cells with and without the *v-abl* Oncogene

O. Witte,* C. Whitlock,† D. Robertson,* J. Kurland,* S. Swanson,* L. Treiman,* K. Denis,* and J. Stafford*

*Department of Microbiology and Molecular Biology Institute, University of California, Los Angeles, Los Angeles, California 90024;†Department of Pathology and School of Medicine, Stanford University, Stanford, California 94305

Abelson murine leukemia virus (Ab-MLV) has provided a useful tool for examining the effects of a particular oncogene on a developmental system (for review, see Baltimore et al. 1979; Rosenberg and Baltimore 1980; Witte 1983). Although the *v-abl* oncogene, a member of the tyrosine kinase group (Witte et al. 1980), can stimulate growth in or transform a variety of cell types including fibroblasts (Scher and Siegler 1975) and erythroid precursors (Waneck and Rosenberg 1981), it prefers target cells of the B-cell lineage both in vitro and in vivo. Abelson virus-transformed cell lines representing a wide range of B-lymphoid developmental stages have been key reagents used to dissect the molecular events of immunoglobulin gene rearrangements, RNA expression, and message structure.

To understand the fundamental mechanism Ab-MLV uses in lymphoid transformation, we have concentrated our efforts on the growth regulation of murine B lymphoid cells in the absence or presence of *v-abl* expression (Whitlock and Witte 1982; Whitlock et al. 1983a, b). We hope that a detailed analysis of the cellular and intercellular factors necessary to maintain B-cell growth in vitro will provide a better framework to observe the qualitative and quantitative effects of *v-abl* expression. By using defined populations of cells, we can observe both changes in growth phenotype and differentiation status that can accompany Ab-MLV transformation.

Methods

Detailed methodology for the in vitro bone marrow cultures is found in Whitlock and Witte (1982), Whitlock et al. (1983b), C.A. Whitlock et al. (in prep.), or the unpublished "B-cell cookbook" available from our laboratory. Other methods are noted in the relevant figure legends and tables.

Results and Discussion

Requirements for B-cell growth in long-term culture

Our initial approach to establishing long-term cultures of B cells utilized the observations of Dexter et al. (1977) in their work on marrow cultures producing cells of the granulocytic and erthyroid lineages. The crucial role of an adherent stromal cell feeder layer was documented. By confirming their observations with media conditions more appropriate to B lymphoid cells, we could selectively maintain B-lymphoid viability and eventually con-

tinous growth (Whitlock and Witte 1982; Whitlock et al. 1983b).

After an initial period of cell death and adaptation, cultures develop a feeder layer of cells and in most cases proliferation of nonadherent B lymphoid cells (Fig. 1). These cultures produce sufficient cells (1×10^6/ml to 2×10^6/ml) for biochemical and functional analysis. Several lines of evidence suggested that progenitors of pre-B and B cells were developing and rearranging immunoglobulin genes in culture. First, two-dimensional isoelectric focusing, SDS-polyacrylamide gel electrophoresis of metabolically labeled immunoglobulin species demonstrated heterogeneity of expressed variable regions for both μ and κ chains (Whitlock and Witte 1982). Second, we were able to clone successfully both pre-B, B-cell, and putative pre-pre-B-cell types from such cultures (Whitlock et al. 1983b; Table 1).

Our mass cultures of B cells and their progenitors can function in the in vivo reconstitution of immunodeficient mice. The CBA/N strain carries an X-linked mutation that renders it incapable of responding to certain antigens like TNP-Ficoll or forming in vitro B-cell colonies (Kincade and Paige 1979). F_1 (CBA/N $\times$ BALB/c) males

Table 1 Distribution of Phenotypes among Clonal Cell Lines Derived from B-Cell Cultures

Experiment	Number of clones		
	pre-pre B	pre-B	B
I	1	3	2
II	1	3	4

Clonal lines were derived from mass populations of B cells and their precursors by limiting dilution onto adherent feeder layers in 96-well culture dishes, as described by Whitlock et al. (1983b). Each clone was expanded and then analyzed for immunoglobulin protein synthesis and immunoglobulin gene rearrangements. Pre-pre-B cells are defined as lymphoid cells with partial immunoglobulin μ heavy-chain rearrangements but no μ synthesis. These clones can be induced to rearrange further and sometimes express μ protein (Whitlock et al., 1983b). Pre-B cells express μ protein but not light chain. B-cell clones express both μ and light chain and hence are surface immunoglobulin-positive. No other class of heavy-chain expression has been observed.

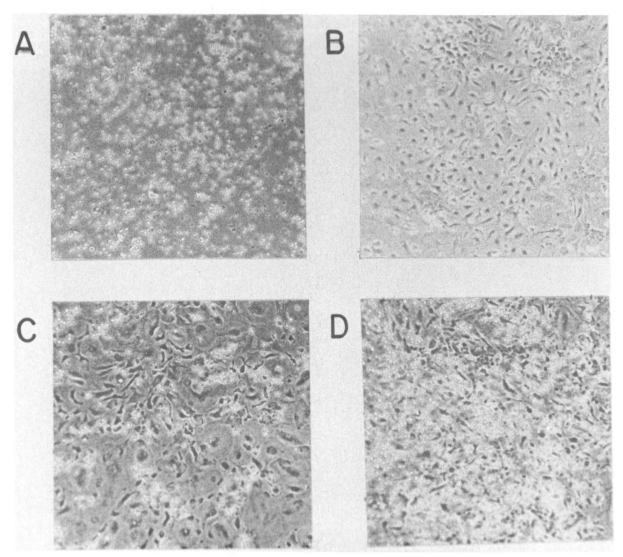

Figure 1 Time course of development of normal bone marrow B-cell cultures. Total bone marrow elements flushed from the femurs of 3- to 4-week-old mice are plated and maintained at 37°C in an RPMI-1640-based medium with 5% fetal calf serum at 2×10^6 cells/ml as described (Whitlock and Witte 1982; Whitlock et al. 1983b). (*A*) Low-power (100×) field at 1 day showing few adherent cells and mixed population of nonadherent elements. (*B*) Cultures at 1–2 weeks showed loss of most nonadherent elements and development of an adherent feeder layer. (*C*) Cultures at 3–5 weeks show regrowth of B cells and progenitors as foci of nonadherent cells. (*D*) Cultures from 4 weeks to 1 year or longer show higher density growth of B cells to 10^6/ml with doubling times of 24–48 hr.

also show this defect but can be reconstituted with bone marrow from the BALB/c parental strain. Recently, we have completed a series of reconstitution experiments using our long-term cultured populations of BALB/c B cells (J. Kurland and O. Witte, in prep.). These cultured cells required moderately long periods in vivo (6–8 weeks) to repopulate effectively a measurable TNP-specific plaque-forming cell and hemagglutination response after primary immunization. The precise nature and frequency of the cells functioning in this reconstitution remain to be determined. Clearly, such cells could provide a useful environment for the insertion and monitoring of genes that may regulate lymphoid development, since they can differentiate in vivo and do not induce tumors even after long latent periods.

Feeder layer cells secrete a soluble B-cell growth factor

The crucial role of an adherent feeder layer-soluble factor in the successful growth of B cells has been established by several criteria. Attempts to culture our B-cell populations in the absence of the adherent layer results in rapid cell death over a 24-hour interval. The B-cell populations can be separated by an agar layer from the adherent layer without a major decrease in B-cell viability or growth rate. Finally, conditioned media harvested from monolayers of adherent cells can support B-cell growth as monitored in short (24–30 hr) thymidine uptake studies, or longer if conditioned media is replenished daily (C. Whitlock et al., unpubl. observ.).

To understand better the nature of the cell producing

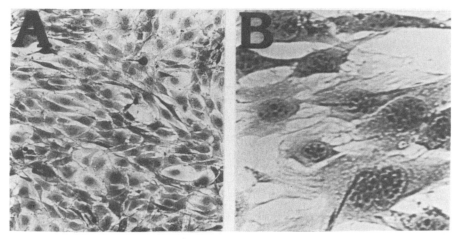

Figure 2 Morphology of clonal feeder layer cells. (A) Low-power (100×) view of Wright's-stained adherent feeder layer clonal cell line. (B) Higher power (400×) of same preparation. Some cells in the population are multinucleate.

the factor or factors and to provide a reproducible source for characterization, we have isolated clonal lines from the adherent cell populations (D. Robertson and O. Witte, in prep.).

A modified collagenase-DNA protocol (Dorshkind and Phillips 1982) was used to transfer the adherent population in a series of pauci-clonings to select first for rapid cell growth and maintenance of growth factor production. Finally, a true cloning protocol by microwell technique (1 cell plated per 5 wells) was used to isolate cellular clones. Characterization of these adherent cell clones revealed a dendritic cell-like morphology (Fig. 2). Conditioned media from these lines support growth of mass B-cell populations as well as pre-B- and B-cell clonal lines. Our preliminary observations using serum-free conditioned media suggest that the factor activity is a protein.

The availability of such cloned feeder cells enables us to overcome a major technical block. We can now produce large members of feeder layers of uniform quality at short notice on which to transfer B-cell populations or clones we wish to grow in large quantity.

Development of long-term cultures of fetal liver B cells and precursors

The early phases of B-cell development are the least well understood. Good tumor cell models now exist for the stages of pre-pre-B, pre-B, mature B, and plasma cells but the very early stem cell or B-cell progenitor is not available for molecular analysis.

Progenitor cells might show no evidence of immunoglobulin gene rearrangement and their morphology and surface antigen phenotype is unknown. They can now only be conclusively identified by their ability to repop-

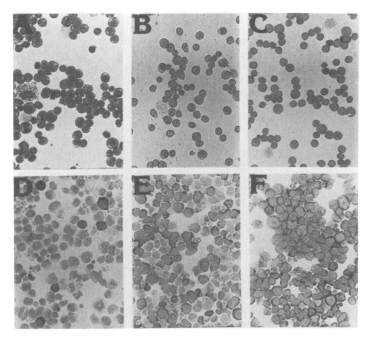

Figure 3 Morphology and immunoglobulin expression by cultured fetal liver lymphoid cells. (A) Wright's-stained cytocentrifuge preparation of cells harvested from 10-week-old fetal liver culture (400×) showing lymphoid morphology. (B) Same cell population as A with control staining protocol for immunoperoxidase reagents. (C) Same population as A and B with immunoperoxidase staining for cytoplasmic μ-positive cells using a primary anti-mouse μ antibody (Hofman et al. 1982) showing a low percentage of positive cells (≤10%). (D, E, and F) Individual Abelson virus-transformed subclones (see Fig. 5 and text) stained for cytoplasmic μ protein. Individual clones range from ≤10% to nearly 100% positive. Many subclones (not shown) have no detectable μ-positive cells.

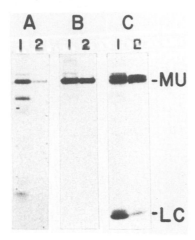

Figure 4 Biosynthesis of μ heavy chain by cultured fetal liver cells. Approximately 5 × 10⁶ cells of 12-week-old cultured fetal liver cells (*A*), a pre-B cell Abelson virus transformant (*B*), and a *B*-cell Abelson virus transformant (*C*) were labeled with [³H]leucine (100 μCi for 1 hr in leucine-free media) and extracted and immunoprecipitated with a polyvalent rabbit anti-mouse immunoglobulin (lanes *1*) with affinity-purified rabbit anti-μ heavy-chain-specific antibody (lanes *2*) (from R. Coffman). Samples were analyzed on SDS 10% polyacrylamide gels developed by fluorography. Details are given in Whitlock et al. (1983b).

ulate the B-cell compartment of genetic or radiation immunodeficient mice. An additional criteria for identification of such progenitor cells would be to induce in vitro the earliest known μ heavy-chain gene rearrangements (D-J joining) in a clonal cell population.

Fetal liver is the first site of B-cell development in the mouse and might be rich in these early cell types. We have modified our culture system to grow lymphoid elements from midgestation fetal liver. When a 14- to 17-day fetal liver cell suspension is plated onto an established feeder layer derived from bone marrow stromal elements, lymphoid elements grow out over a 3- to 4-week period (Fig. 3A). Only a small proportion of the cells (~10%) express μ heavy chain as monitored by immunoperoxidase staining (Fig. 3C) and small amount of μ heavy chain is detected by immunoprecipitation (Fig. 4).

To evaluate the molecular structure of the immunoglobulin loci in these cells, we have used the *v-abl* oncogene to transform them and allow us to isolate clonal sublines we can grow to high cell density in simple tissue culture media. Our preliminary results by immunoperoxidase staining (Fig. 3D–F) and by immunoprecipitation (Fig. 5) screening of a number of clonal isolates derived from single-cell-initiated agar colonies showed a low number of μ protein-expressing clones (6 of 40 total tested). Among the positive clones, the frequency of μ-expressing cells measured by immunoperoxidase staining varied widely (Fig. 3D–F). We are currently screening these clones for rearrangements at the μ and κ loci. If cells with germline organization can be found, they might potentially serve as useful models for early events in B-cell differentiation.

Future directions

Several technical goals occupy a major portion of our current efforts. We hope to derive clonal cell lines that represent very early portions of the B-cell pathway and clonal lines that represent later stages capable of binding and responding to a specific antigen. Such reagents would provide the opportunity to examine the early stages of immunoglobulin gene rearrangements and the interaction of specific antigen, T-cell help and other factors in B-cell triggering, and, perhaps, isotype switching. We are concentrating our efforts on cloning from the fetal liver-derived cultures as described above and systematically varying our culture conditions to enrich for early-stage cells. Our attempts to isolate antigen-specific cells take advantage of the in vivo TNP response reconstituted with BALB/c cultured B-cells in (CBA/N × BALB/c) F₁ male mice. We have recently been able to culture spleen cells from such animals on established feeder layer cells and will attempt to enrich and culture hapten-specific cells (J. Kurland and O. Witte, unpubl. observ.).

The role of the adherent feeder layer and the soluble factor it secretes must be further analyzed. Both protein purification and eventually gene isolation will be required to relate it to the increasing number of growth factors and hormones described for lymphoid cells. The inter-

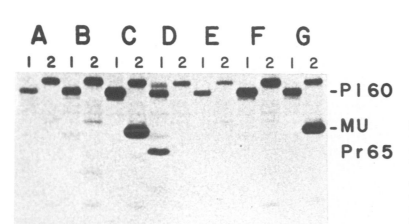

Figure 5 Screen of Abelson virus-transformed fetal liver cells for viral proteins and immunoglobulin in synthesis. Individual single-cell-derived agar colony transformants (*A–G*) derived by Ab-MLV (P160 strain) infection of cultured fetal liver cells were expanded in liquid culture and then labeled, extracted, immunoprecipitated, and analyzed as in Fig. 4 with anti-*gag* gene-specific monoclonal antibody (lanes *1*) or a polyvalent rabbit anti-mouse Ig (lanes *2*).

action of this factor with cells of other lineages has not yet been examined in any detail.

Finally, the role of both *v-abl* and *c-abl* must be tested for both growth alteration and differentiation induction on these defined cell populations. Our results to date (Whitlock et al. 1983b and unpubl.) suggest that a wide range of B-lineage cells can be transformed by *v-abl*, and coincident with this growth stimulation we often observe changes in the differentiation phenotype. What we do not know is whether this relates simply to a faster growth rate or a more specific effect of the *v-abl* gene product. A number of experiments using *v-abl* mutants and other *v-onc* genes inserted into mouse ectotropic retrovirus vectors are in progress to examine this point.

Acknowledgments

This work was supported by research grants from the National Institutes of Health and March of Dimes, and a Faculty Scholar Award from the American Cancer Society to O.N.W. Postdoctoral support for C.W. (ACS-California Division), J.K. (Leukemia Society of America), L.T. (Comprehensive Epilepsy Program), and K.D. (Immunology Training grant) and predoctoral support for D.R. (Carcinogenesis Training grant) is greatly appreciated.

References

Baltimore, D., N. Rosenberg, and O.N. Witte. 1979. Transformation of immature lymphoid cells by Abelson murine leukemia virus. *Immunol. Rev.* **48**: 35.

Dexter, T.M., T.D. Allen, and L.G. Lajtha. 1977. Conditions controlling the *in vitro* proliferation of hemopoietic stem cells in vitro. *J. Cell. Physiol.* **91**: 335.

Dorshkind, K. and R.A. Phillips. 1982. Maturational state of lymphoid cells in long term bone marrow cultures. *J. Immunol.* **129**: 2444.

Hofman, F.M., R.J. Billing, J.W. Parker, and C.R. Taylor. 1982. Cytoplasmic as opposed to surface Id antigens expressed on human peripheral blood lymphocytes and monocytes. *Clin. Exp. Immunol.* **49**: 355.

Kincade, P.W. and C.J. Paige. 1979. B-cell development in immunodeficient CBA/N mice. In *B lymphocytes in the immune response* (ed. M. Cooper et al.), p. 349. Elsevier North-Holland, New York.

Rosenberg, N. and D. Baltimore. 1980. Abelson virus. In *Viral oncology* (ed. G. Klein), p. 187. Raven Press, New York.

Scher, C.D. and R. Siegler. 1975. Direct transformation of 3T3 cells by Abelson murine leukemia virus. *Nature* **253**: 729.

Waneck, G. and N. Rosenberg. 1981. Abelson leukemia virus induces lymphoid and erythroid colonies in infected fetal cell cultures. *Cell* **26**: 79.

Whitlock, C.A. and O.N. Witte. 1982. Long-term culture of B lymphocytes and their precursors from murine bone marrow. *Proc. Natl. Acad. Sci.* **79**: 3608.

Whitlock, C.A., S.F. Ziegler, and O.N. Witte. 1983a. Progression of the transformed phenotype in clonal lines of Abelson virus infected lymphocytes. *Cell. Mol. Biol.* **3**: 596.

Whitlock, C.A., S.F. Ziegler, L.J. Treiman, J.I. Stafford, and O.N. Witte. 1983b. Differentiation of cloned populations of immature B cells after transformation with Abelson murine leukemia virus. *Cell* **32**: 903.

Witte, O.N. 1983. Molecular and cellular biology of Abelson virus transformation. *Curr. Top. Microbiol. Immunol.* **103**: 127.

Witte, O.N., A. Dasgupta, and D. Baltimore. 1980. Abelson Murine leukemia virus protein is phosphorylated in vitro to form phosphotyrosine. *Nature* **283**: 826.

The Oncogenes *fes* and *fms*

C.J. Sherr, S.J. Anderson, C.W. Rettenmier, and M.F. Roussel

Division of Human Tumor Cell Biology, St. Jude Children's Research Hospital, Memphis, Tennessee 38101

Oncogenes (*v-onc* sequences) of acutely transforming retroviruses have been acquired by genetic recombination between a retroviral vector and cellular proto-oncogene (*c-onc*) sequences (Bishop 1982, 1983). Because *c-onc* genes are highly conserved in evolution, molecularly cloned *v-onc* sequences have proven useful in identifying and isolating the homologous proto-oncogene sequences from normal cells of many species. This approach has afforded the first opportunity for detailed studies of cellular genes implicated in transformation and tumor formation. Comparisons of the *v-onc* and *c-onc* genes suggest mechanisms by which proto-oncogene sequences are recombined with vector sequences and placed under new regulatory control. Experimental manipulations of cloned *c-onc* genes that recapitulate these natural events have unleashed their latent transforming potential in vitro (Blair et al. 1981; DeFeo et al. 1981; Hanafusa et al., this volume) and have supported the view that proto-oncogenes can serve as natural determinants of malignancy (Huebner and Todaro 1969). Similarly, the ability to detect and characterize *c-onc* gene products based on their structural homology to *v-onc*-encoded proteins has revealed that *c-onc* polypeptides are synthesized in certain normal cells. An understanding of the functions of retroviral transforming proteins should provide parallel insights into the role of their cellular homologs and the manner by which they may regulate normal cellular growth and differentiation.

Results and Discussion

Feline sarcoma viruses are genetic recombinants

The feline leukemia virus (FeLV) is horizontally transmitted in domestic cats and is a natural etiological agent of leukemia (Hardy 1980). Many outbred cat populations have been exposed to FeLV, even though only a minority of infected animals ever develop viremia or frank disease. The high incidence of FeLV exposure in cats and the fact that the viral DNA intermediate can integrate at many sites in host cellular DNA suggest that FeLV may recombine at relatively high efficiency with cat cellular genes. Indeed, FeLV has recombined with at least five different cellular "proto-oncogenes," resulting in the formation of different feline sarcoma virus (FeSV) strains (Snyder and Theilen 1969; Gardner et al. 1970; McDonough et al. 1971; Irgens et al. 1973; Rasheed et al. 1982). These viruses, unlike FeLV, morphologically transform cells in culture and induce the rapid development of sarcomas in cats, dogs, and other susceptible species (Hardy 1980). Table 1 lists the currently characterized FeSV strains, their different *v-onc* genes, and the apparent molecular weights of their encoded products.

The most extensively studied of the FeSV isolates include the Snyder-Theilen (ST) and Gardner-Arnstein (GA) strains, both of which contain the viral oncogene *v-fes*, and the Susan McDonough (SM) strain, which contains the viral oncogene *v-fms* (Frankel et al. 1979). More recently characterized FeSV strains carry three other genes that include *v-sis* and *v-abl* (Besmer et al. 1983a, b), also found in acutely transforming retroviruses of monkeys and mice, respectively, and *v-fgr* (Naharro et al. 1983), a homolog of the avian *v-yes* and actin genes (Naharro et al. 1984) (see Table 1). Each of these sarcoma viruses is replication-defective, having acquired *v-onc* sequences at the expense of portions of the three FeLV-derived genes (*gag*, *pol*, and *env*) required for autonomous retroviral replication. In every case, the *v-onc*

Table 1 Oncogenes of Feline Sarcoma Viruses

v-onc gene	FeSV strain	Primary translation product
v-fes	Snyder-Theilen (ST)	$P85^{gag\text{-}fes}$
	Gardner-Arnstein (GA)	$P110^{gag\text{-}fes}$
	Hardy-Zuckerman-1 (HZ-1)	$P95^{gag\text{-}fes}$
v-fms	Susan McDonough (SM)	$P160^{gag\text{-}fms}$[a]
v-fgr	Gardner-Rasheed (GR)	$P70^{gag\text{-}fgr}$
v-sis	Parodi-Irgens (PI)	$P75^{gag\text{-}sis}$
v-abl	Hardy-Zuckerman-2 (HZ-2)	$P95^{gag\text{-}abl}$

[a]Whereas, $P160^{gag\text{-}fms}$ is predicted by nucleotide sequencing analysis (Hampe et al. 1984) and can be experimentally detected after tunicamycintreatment (Anderson et al. 1982), the polypeptides released from polyribosomes appear to be cotranslationally glycosylated to form $gP180^{gag\text{-}fms}$ (see text).

gene has been inserted in frame into the viral *gag* gene so that the order of sequences in each viral genome is 5'-*gag-onc-env*-3' (Sherr et al. 1979, 1980a; Fedele et al. 1981; Donner et al. 1982). Transcription of integrated FeSV proviruses generates full genome-length mRNAs that encode polyproteins specified by the truncated *gag* and acquired *v-onc* sequences (Stephenson et al. 1977; Sherr et al. 1978a,b; Barbacid et al. 1980b; Ruscetti et al. 1980; Van de Ven et al. 1980b). Hence, the amino-terminal portions of the polyprotein molecules are specified by FeLV-derived *gag* sequences, whereas the carboxyterminal portions are encoded by *v-onc* genes. Production of these polyproteins in FeSV-infected cells leads to morphological transformation in vitro, and is responsible for tumor formation in vivo.

Transduction of *c-fes* sequences by different viral vectors

Three different FeSV strains contain *v-onc* genes derived from the cat proto-oncogene *c-fes* (Table 1). The DNA proviruses of two of these strains have been molecularly cloned (Sherr et al. 1980a; Fedele et al. 1981) and the nucleotide sequences of major portions of the proviruses have been determined (Hampe et al. 1982, 1984). Approximately 1.2-kbp at the 3' end of the *v-fes* sequences are identical in the two FeSV strains, whereas sequences near the *gag-fes* junction are different; this accounts for the distinct sizes of the polyproteins encoded by ST- and GA-FeSV (Table 1).

When radiolabeled *v-fes* clones were used to characterize homologous sequences in normal cat cellular DNA, the *c-fes* proto-oncogene was found to be more complex than the transduced *v-fes* gene, due to interruption of the coding regions by intervening sequences (Franchini et al. 1981). Thus, transduction of the *c-fes* gene must have involved excision of these introns prior to recombination of processed *c-fes* sequences with an FeLV vector. The formation of recombinant FeSV strains probably occurred as a consequence of FeLV integration into or in the vicinity of *c-fes* proto-oncogene sequences (see Varmus 1982). Deletion or rearrangement of proviral DNA might have favored the formation of hybrid RNA transcripts containing 5' *gag* gene sequences fused to *c-fes* information. After processing of the hybrid transcripts, this *gag-fes* RNA would be packaged into virions and could serve as a template for reverse transcription in a second round of viral replication. Recombination with FeLV transcripts during reverse transcription could restore 3' viral regulatory sequences necessary for the perpetuation of *v-fes* sequences in a moveable FeSV element.

Nucleic acid hybridization experiments have generally failed to detect any sequence homology between different viral oncogenes. A notable exception was the sequence homology detected between the avian *v-onc* gene *v-fps* found in the Fujinami and PRCII strains of avian sarcoma virus, and the RNA of the ST- and GA-FeSV strains (Shibuya et al. 1980). As expected, the products encoded by *v-fes* and *v-fps* were found to be biochemically, antigenically, and functionally related

(Barbacid et al. 1981b; Beemon 1981). Nucleotide sequencing of Fujinami sarcoma virus (FSV) showed that *v-fps* and *v-fes* had more than 70% overall nucleotide sequence homology (Hampe et al. 1982; Shibuya and Hanafusa 1982), suggesting that they were derived from cognate *c-onc* loci of mammals and birds.

The *v-fps* gene of FSV is more complex than the *v-fes* sequences of either ST- and GA-FeSV, and is able to encode a 95-kD portion of the 130-kD *gag-fps* fusion polyprotein P130*gag-fps*. Because the product of the *c-fes/c-fps* proto-oncogene sequences is also 95–98 kD (see below), FSV appears to have transduced most, if not all, of the *c-fes/c-fps* coding region. Figure 1 shows a schematic comparison of the *v-onc* sequences of FSV and the two FeSV strains. At the junction between their *gag* and *v-onc* sequences, ST- and GA-FeSV contain different portions of the *c-fes/c-fps* genes, both of which are represented in FSV. In addition, FSV contains *c-fes/c-fps*-derived sequences not present in either FeSV strain. The sequences shared in common between all these viruses should be the ones required for transformation.

Independent transduction events between different retroviral vectors and the same *c-onc* gene would not be expected to duplicate the exact sites of recombination between viral and cellular genes (see Varmus 1982). This is because (1) integration of the transducing provirus can occur at many sites in the vicinity of *c-onc* sequences; (2) deletions within the integrated provirus can involve different viral genes; (3) the transduced RNA can recombine with helper viral sequences at many sites during reverse transcription. Although the 5' sites of recombination between *gag* and *v-fes* sequences are in fact different in ST- and GA-FeSV, the 3' sites of recombination are identical in both strains. The latter finding suggests that ST- and GA-FeSV arose from a single recombinational event and that deletions near the *gag-fes* junction led to the subsequent formation of two proviral DNA variants, each retaining different portions of

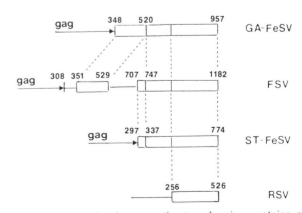

Figure 1 Homologies between the transforming proteins of FeSV, FSV, and RSV. The numbers refer to the position of residues from the amino termini of the predicted proteins. The domains showing homology are marked by the vertical dashed lines. The FeSV and FSV products are polyproteins encoded by both *gag* and *v-onc* sequences; RSV pp60*src* contains only *v-onc*-coded residues. (Data from Hampe et al. 1982.)

the *gag* and *v-fes* genes. An FeSV strain with a structure similar to that of FSV could have been the progenitor of both ST- and GA-FeSV.

The tyrosine kinase gene family

The *v-fes/v-fps* gene products each exhibit an associated tyrosine-specific protein kinase activity (Barbacid et al. 1980a; Feldman et al. 1980; Reynolds et al. 1980; Van de Ven et al. 1980a). In studies using temperature-sensitive mutants of FSV (Pawson et al. 1980; Hanafusa et al. 1981), and nonconditional transformation-defective mutants of ST-FeSV (Donner et al. 1980; Barbacid et al. 1981a; Reynolds et al. 1981a), enzyme activity was necessary for initiation and maintenance of the transformed phenotype. In this respect, the *v-fes/v-fps* genes encode enzymes functionally similar to those of several other viral oncogenes including *v-src* (Collett and Erikson 1978; Levinson et al. 1978; Sefton et al. 1980), *v-abl* (Witte et al. 1980), *v-yes* (Kawai et al. 1980), *v-ros* (Feldman et al. 1982), and *v-fgr* (Rasheed et al. 1982). The proteins specified by each of these genes induce phosphorylation of heterologous substrates in transformed cells, leading to a marked increase in the total levels of phosphotyrosine. In addition, each of the viral transforming proteins is itself phosphorylated in tyrosine, generally at a preferred site (Blomberg et al. 1981; Patchinsky et al. 1982).

Nucleotide sequence analyses of many of these genes predict that, despite their inability to cross-hybridize, they encode structurally related proteins. For example, third base-pair differences in virtually all respective codons prevent hybridization between *v-src* and *v-yes*, even though the two genes encode products with 80% overall amino acid sequence homology (Kitamura et al. 1982). Although these different *v-onc* genes originate from different proto-oncogene loci present in all mammalian and avian cells, the functionally conserved portions of the cellular genes must be descended from a single primordial sequence. The related coding regions of the *v-onc* genes (see schematic, Fig. 1) include the putative catalytic sites of the enzymes as well as the sites for nucleotide triphosphate binding (Barker and Dayhoff 1982). The divergence of other regions of these genes could possibly affect their differential expression in cells, the catalytic efficiencies of their encoded enzymes, or the subcellular localization of the proteins. Moreover, the *c-onc* genes may be members of a more extended gene family that also includes genes encoding tyrosine kinases associated with cell-surface receptors for the extracellular growth factors epidermal growth factor (EGF), platelet-derived growth factor (PDGF), and insulin (Ushiro and Cohen 1980; Ek et al. 1982; Kasuga et al. 1982). The association of tyrosine-specific protein kinase activities with these receptors suggests that the mechanism by which some *v-onc* gene products transform cells could involve subversion of hormonally regulated pathways controlling normal cell proliferation.

The *c-fes/c-fps* gene product

Antisera to *gag*-coded antigens can be used to precipitate the ST- and GA-FeSV polyproteins from lysates of transformed cells. The immune complexes containing either ST-FeSV P85$^{gag-fes}$ or GA-FeSV P110$^{gag-fes}$ can catalyze the transfer of phosphate from ^{32}P-labeled ATP to the polyproteins themselves, to immunoglobulin heavy chains coprecipitated in the immune complex, or to admixed heterologous substrates, such as casein (Barbacid et al. 1980a; Reynolds et al. 1980; Van de Ven et al. 1980a). Antisera to *v-fes*-coded antigenic determinants have previously been raised by immunizing with partially purified polyproteins (Sherr et al. 1978b; Barbacid et al. 1980a) or with FeSV-induced tumor cells inoculated into syngeneic recipients (Ruscetti et al. 1980). Unlike the antisera to *gag*-coded antigens, antisera to *v-fes*-coded determinants are sometimes inactive in immune complex kinase assays, presumably because they bind to critical regions of the enzymes and inhibit kinase activity (Sen et al. 1982; Veronese et al. 1982).

Since only low levels of *c-fes/c-fps* mRNA are detected in most normal cells (Shibuya et al. 1982), metabolic labeling and immunoprecipitation have not proven to be sufficiently sensitive in detecting the products encoded by the *c-fes* sequences. Utilizing a subset of antisera to *v-fes*-coded epitopes that do not inhibit the kinase reaction in immune complex assays affords a more sensitive means of detecting the normal cellular gene products. With such sera, Barbacid et al. (1980a) detected a 95-kD kinase in normal cells. More detailed studies in the avian system showed that *c-fps* mRNA is expressed at relatively high levels in bone marrow cells of the granulocytic lineage (Shibuya et al. 1982). A protein of 98-kD that was immunologically and biochemically similar to the *v-fps*-coded product was similarly detected in granulocytic cells (Mathey-Prevot et al. 1982). Expression of the *c-fps*-coded protein appears to be associated with normal granulocytic differentiation and has not been implicated in hematopoietic malignancy.

The human *c-fes/c-fps* proto-oncogene

Using plasmids derived from molecularly cloned ST-FeSV (Sherr et al. 1980a; Franchini et al. 1981), several laboratories have cloned homologous cellular proto-oncogene sequences from human DNA libraries (Franchini et al. 1982; Groffen et al. 1982; Trus et al. 1982). A map of the human *c-fes* gene in comparison with viral *v-fes* sequences is shown in Figure 2. As expected, molecular clones of *v-fps* also detect the same proto-oncogene sequences in the human genome (Groffen et al. 1983a). All exons homologous to GA-FeSV *v-fes* appear to be distributed on a single 12-kb *Eco*RI fragment of human DNA. The blocks of homologous sequences detected by nucleic acid hybridization (Fig. 2) are additively more complex than either GA-FeSV *v-fes* or FSV *v-fps*; hence, the actual number of exons must be greater than that shown in the figure. Attempts to produce a transforming recombinant by preparing chimeric constructions between proviral and cellular *c-fes* DNA have so far been unsuccessful (Groffen et al. 1982). Determination of the nucleotide sequence of the cellular gene would define the exact distribution of homologous se-

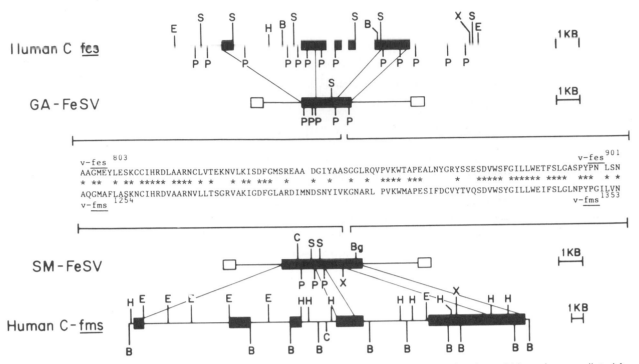

Figure 2 Restriction maps of human *c-fes* and *c-fms*, their viral counterparts, and regions of amino acid homology predicted from the sequenced *v-onc* genes. Restriction sites for several endonucleases include: (B) *Bam*HI; (Bg) *Bgl*II; (C) *Cla*I; (E) *Eco*RI; (H) *Hind*III; (P) *Pst*I; (S) *Sac*I/*Sst*I; and (X) *Xho*I. Shaded regions designate restriction fragments containing blocks of homologous sequences; they do not indicate the sizes or locations of the actual exons included therein. (Sequencing data is from Hampe et al. 1982, 1984; maps of GA-FeSV and SM-FeSV are from Fedele et al. 1981, and Donner et al. 1982; and maps of *c-onc* genes are from Franchini et al. 1982, Trus et al. 1982, Groffen et al. 1982, Heisterkamp et al. 1983, and Roussel et al. 1983.)

quences and may be critical in the design of experiments to "activate" the gene.

The *c-fes* locus has been mapped to the long arm of human chromosome 15 (Dalla-Favera et al. 1982; Heisterkamp et al. 1982). Rearrangements of chromosome 15 have been observed in acute promyelocytic leukemia, and involve a reciprocal translocation between chromosomes 15 and 17 (t[15:17] [q22.2:q21]) (Sheer et al. 1983). The *c-fes* locus is localized distal to the breakpoint on 15q22.2 and is presumed to be moved to the 17q− chromosome. The data suggest, however, that 15q+ is the most consistent cytogenetic marker in acute promyelocyte leukemia; in agreement, alterations of *c-fes* gene expression have not been detected in acute promyelocytic leukemia in man. To date, then, the *c-fes* gene has not been directly implicated in processes of tumor formation in any animal species.

The *v-fms* gene encodes a glycoprotein

The SM-FeSV genome was the first feline sarcoma virus isolate found to contain *v-onc* sequences different from *v-fes* (Frankel et al. 1979). The transforming gene of this strain, now designated *v-fms*, has not been found in any acutely transforming retrovirus other than SM-FeSV, leaving open the possibility that it is functionally distinct from other known oncogenes. Molecular cloning of the SM-FeSV provirus (Donner et al. 1982) and nucleotide sequence analysis (Hampe et al. 1984) predict that the primary translation product of SM-FeSV RNA is a 160-

kD *gag-fms* polyprotein. When cells transformed by SM-FeSV were metabolically labeled with amino acid precursors and the polyprotein precipitated with appropriate antisera, the earliest detectable protein labeled in vivo was 180 kD (Barbacid et al. 1980b; Ruscetti et al. 1980; Van de Ven et al. 1980b). The discrepancy in the molecular weights between the predicted and experimentally detected polyproteins is due to glycosylation (Sherr et al. 1980b; Anderson et al. 1982). The polyprotein molecules can be metabolically labeled with radioactive sugars, and glycosylation is sensitive to the antibiotic tunicamycin, which inhibits the linkage of sugar to asparaginyl residues in the polypeptide backbone. The first steps of glycosylation occur so rapidly that in metabolic labeling experiments performed with amino acid precursors, the nonglycosylated polyprotein is generally not observed. The SM-FeSV polyprotein is synthesized exclusively on membrane-bound polyribosomes, and the nascent chains are vectorially transported across the membrane into the cisternae of the endoplasmic reticulum (ER) where glycosylation takes place. Cotranslational addition of sugars within the ER is consistent with the observed kinetics of glycosylation and is in agreement with the observation that metabolically labeled polyproteins are quantitatively sedimented with membranous organelles in the absence of detergent treatment (Barbacid and Lauver 1981; Anderson et al. 1982).

The glycosylated SM-FeSV polyprotein (gP180*gag-fms*)

is posttranslationally cleaved near the *gag-fms* junction to yield two distinct polypeptide products. These include a protein of about 55 kD which contains only *gag*-coded antigenic determinants, and a glycoprotein of 120 kD (gp120^{fms}) which is precipitated only with antibodies directed to *v-fms*-coded epitopes (Barbacid et al. 1980b; Ruscetti et al. 1980; Sherr et al. 1980b). The fact that gp120^{fms} contains carbohydrate residues while p55^{gag} does not shows that all glycosylation occurs within the *v-fms*-coded portion of gP180$^{gag-fms}$. The mechanism and site(s) of proteolytic cleavage are not known. In fact, in metabolic labeling experiments, gP180$^{gag-fms}$ and gp120^{fms} appear to be labeled simultaneously, and it has not been possible to demonstrate formally a precursor-product relationship between the proteins by pulse-chase analyses (Barbacid et al. 1980b; Ruscetti et al. 1980).

Antisera to both gP180$^{gag-fms}$ and gp120^{fms} can be raised by inoculating normal rat kidney (NRK) cells nonproductively transformed by SM-FeSV into syngeneic Osborn-Mendel recipients. Four- to six-week-old animals receiving subcutaneous injections of approximately 1×10^6 transformed cells develop progressively growing tumors that kill most of the animals within 3 to 4 weeks. Many of these animals produce antibodies that precipitate the SM-FeSV gene products. By fusing spleen cells from a responding animal with a rat myeloma cell line, hybridomas were generated that produced monoclonal IgGs and IgM against *v-fms*-coded epitopes (Anderson et al. 1982). As expected, each of these antibodies precipitated gP180$^{gag-fms}$ and gp120^{fms} from metabolically labeled lysates of SM-FeSV-transformed mink, rat, or mouse cells, but did not react with p55^{gag} or other cellular polypeptides. Following production of monoclonal IgGs in serum-free medium and their subsequent biochemical purification, the antibodies were labeled with ^{125}I and used for immunoblotting experiments. The advantage of the latter technique is that it does not rely on incorporation of precursors and permits an assay of the steady-state levels of transforming glycoproteins in SM-FeSV-transformed cells. Surprisingly, a higher-molecular-weight form of the *v-fms*-coded glycoprotein (gp140^{fms}) that had not been previously recognized in pulse-labeling experiments was detected. Indeed, the latter protein was subsequently labeled only after prolonged pulse times, and was best detected using ^{3}H-labeled sugar precursors (Anderson et al. 1982). Recent experiments indicate that gp120^{fms} contains mannose-rich *N*-oligosaccharide side-chains characteristic of molecules within the cisternae of the rough endoplasmic reticulum; in contrast, gp140^{fms} contains complex carbohydrate chains which include terminal fucose and sialic acid residues added within the Golgi complex (S.J. Anderson et al., unpubl.). The simplest model relating the appearance of the various *v-fms*-coded glycoproteins in SM-FeSV-transformed cells proposes that the primary translation product, P160$^{gag-fms}$, is glycosylated (gP180$^{gag-fms}$) and rapidly cleaved to yield an aminoterminal peptide, p55^{gag}, and a carboxyterminal glycoprotein, gp120^{fms}. At least some of the latter product is subsequently modified by further glycosylation to generate gp140^{fms}. Immunoblotting analyses show that the incompletely processed molecule, gp120^{fms}, represents the major form of transforming glycoprotein in SM-FeSV-infected cells.

Subcellular localization of *v-fms*-coded glycoproteins

Fixed-cell immunofluorescence of SM-FeSV-transformed cells using either polyvalent or monoclonal antibodies to *v-fms*-encoded antigens localized the majority of the transforming glycoproteins to the juxtanuclear region of the cell cytoplasm (Anderson et al. 1982). No antigen was detected at the cell surface using conditions of fixation and staining that readily demonstrate the surface localization of the *v-ras*-coded protein p21 (Furth et al. 1982). It appeared, then, that although the majority of the *v-fms* gene products entered the cisternae of the ER, most of the proteins were not transported beyond the Golgi complex. The possibility that the glycoproteins were physically associated with sedimentable components of the cytoskeletal network was therefore investigated.

Double immunofluorescence experiments were performed using antisera to filament proteins together with anti-*fms* sera to look for a topological association of both classes of antigens. Although no relationship was seen between the distribution of *v-fms*-coded antigens and the microfilament protein actin, a good correlation was observed between the localization of the transforming glycoproteins and the intermediate filament proteins, keratin and vimentin, in both SM-FeSV-transformed rat kidney or mink lung cells (S.J. Anderson et al., in prep). Figure 3 shows a representative experiment performed with transformed mink cells. The intermediate filaments of these transformants were rearranged and condensed into juxtanuclear aggregates (Fig. 3A). Dual fluorescence staining using antibodies to *v-fms*-coded antigens showed that the latter antigens were localized in the same structures (Fig. 3B).

Subcellular fractionation procedures for the purification of the intermediate filament protein desmin (Granger and Lazarides 1980) were adapted to purify intermediate filaments from SM-FeSV-transformed cells. In brief, the cells were homogenized in a hypotonic buffer, and the nuclei and juxtanuclear cytoskeletal mass were recovered by low-speed centrifugation. By immunoblotting analysis, the majority of *v-fms*-coded glycoproteins were sedimented with the "nuclei" even though more than half of the cytoplasmic protein was released into the cytosol. The pelleted material was subjected to a series of extractions that eliminated DNA, contaminating membranes, and most nonfilament proteins; in particular, actin-containing microfilaments were extracted using 600 mM potassium iodide under conditions in which intermediate filaments remain insoluble. When the final filament preparation was denatured and subjected to immunoblotting analysis, it was found to be greatly enriched for *v-fms*-coded glycoproteins.

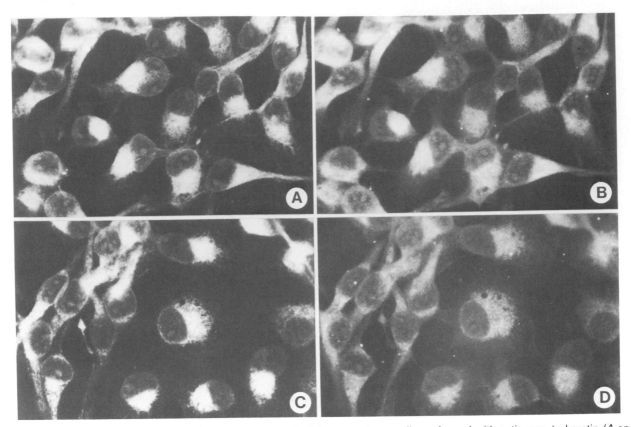

Figure 3 Dual immunofluorescence of SM-FeSV-transformed mink nonproducer cells performed with antiserum to keratin (*A* and *C*) and to *v-fms*-coded antigens (*B* and *D*). Note the distribution of the two antigens in the same fields of cells (*A* versus *B*; *C* versus *D*) simultaneously visualized with fluorescein- (*left panels*) and rhodamine- (*right panels*) conjugated antiglobulins. (Photos courtesy of M.A. Gonda, and taken from S.J. Anderson et al., in prep.)

The ability of gp120^{fms} to associate with intermediate filaments was further studied by in vitro assembly experiments. Intermediate filament preparations containing *v-fms*-coded antigens were denatured in SDS-urea, and the solubilized material was subjected to ion-exchange chromatography to remove SDS (Weber and Kuter 1971). The intermediate filaments were then self-assembled in vitro following removal of urea by dialysis. The reassembled material was seen by electron microscopy to be composed of purified 10–12-nm filaments. Assays for *v-fms*-coded antigens by immunoblotting again showed that the *v-fms* glycoproteins copurified with intermediate filaments assembled in vitro. These data suggest, then, that a portion of the *v-fms*-coded glycoprotein has an intermediate filament-associating domain (S.J. Anderson et al., in prep.).

A prerequisite for carbohydrate addition is the transport of proteins into the cisternae of the rough endoplasmic reticulum (ER) (for review, see Blobel 1980). If glycosylation occurs within the cisternal space, how can glycoproteins associate with filament proteins located on the cytoplasmic side of the ER membrane? One possibility is that the glycoproteins are transmembrane proteins oriented with their filament-associating domain on the cytoplasmic surface of the membrane.

Proteins that gain access to the ER contain aminoterminal hydrophobic "signal peptides" that direct nascent chains to binding sites on the ER membrane (see Blobel 1980). For secretory proteins like immunoglobulin, the signal sequences are proteolytically removed prior to completion of translation. In the case of glycoproteins that remain physically associated with membranes, additional hydrophobic "anchor" sequences interrupt translocation across the ER leaving the distal carboxyterminal residues on the cytoplasmic side of the membrane.

Nucleotide sequence analysis of the SM-FeSV polyprotein coding region (Hampe et al. 1984) predicts that gP180$^{gag-fms}$ has two strongly apolar peptides that fulfill the criteria for signal and anchor sequences (Segrest and Feldman 1974). The first, in the *gag* leader region, appears to represent the aminoterminal signal peptide for directing nascent chains to the ER membrane. A second hydrophobic anchor sequence was identified near the middle of the *v-fms*-coded moiety. Assuming that this latter sequence of amino acids would stop translocation across the ER membrane, approximately 400 amino acids at the *v-fms*-coded carboxyl terminus would protrude from the cytoplasmic surface of the membrane and would have the potential to interact with cytoplasmic target molecules.

A simple model for the processing and orientation of

the *v-fms*-coded gene products is shown in Figure 4. The model assumes that the precursor-product relationships between the various *v-fms*-specified molecules is as follows:

$$P160^{gag\text{-}fms} \rightarrow gP180^{gag\text{-}fms} \rightarrow p55^{gag} + gp120^{fms} \rightarrow gp140^{fms}$$

The aminoterminal signal peptide is postulated to direct nascent polypeptide chains to binding sites in the ER after which synthesis continues on membrane-bound polyribosomes. The nascent chains are vectorially transported across the ER membrane into the cisternae where glycosylation takes place and the *gag*-coded aminoterminal fragment p55*gag* is removed. Translation of the *v-fms* polypeptide continues until the hydrophobic anchor sequence is encountered, after which the nascent chains become immobilized in the membrane and translocation across the ER is terminated. Polyribosomes complete the synthesis of the *v-fms*-coded moiety by detaching from the ER and "running off" in the cytoplasm. The resulting protein is predicted to have a transmembrane orientation with the carboxyterminal *v-fms*-coded residues extending into the cytoplasm. The latter portion of the protein is proposed to include the filament-asso-ciating domain. Although the majority of *v-fms*-coded polypeptides remain internally sequestered within transformed cells, the molecules that are transported through the Golgi complex (gp140*fms*) could be targeted to other membranous organelles or to the plasma membrane.

Homology of *v-fms* to the tyrosine kinase gene family

Immune complex kinase assays performed using antisera to *v-fms*-coded antigens showed that gP180*gag-fms* and gp120*fms* were phosphorylated in tyrosine residues (Barbacid and Lauver 1981). In vivo, however, the same *v-fms* gene products were very poorly phosphorylated (Sherr et al. 1980b), and SM-FeSV transformants did not exhibit an elevation in phosphotyrosine (Barbacid and Lauver 1981; Reynolds et al. 1981b). Monoclonal antibodies that precipitated gP180*gag-fms* were found to yield immune complexes lacking in vitro tyrosine-specific protein kinase activity (Veronese et al. 1982). In our hands, immune complexes prepared with either polyvalent or monoclonal antibodies to *v-fms*-coded molecules are active in in vitro assays (C.W. Rettenmier et al., unpubl.). One possibility is that only a minority of *v-fms*-coded polypeptides are active as kinases in vivo.

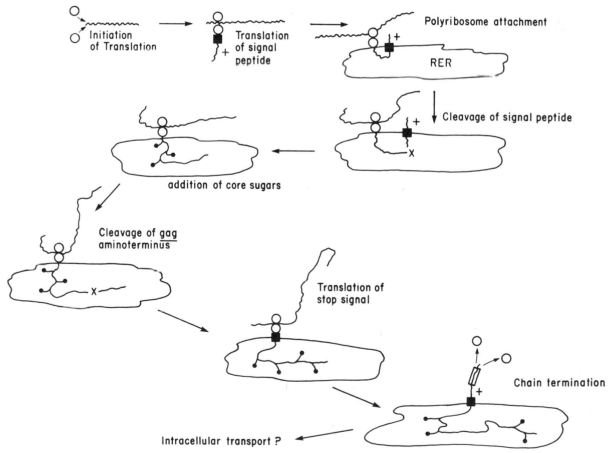

Figure 4 Model for translation, cotranslational glycosylation, and transmembrane insertion of *v-fms*-coded glycoproteins. (X) Sites of proteolytic cleavage; (■, +) hydrophoblic signal sequences (■) preceded or followed by positively charged amino acids(+); (●) core sugars attached to the polypeptide backbone; (▭) defines the carboxyl terminus of the *v-fms* glycoprotein (this region shows homology to *v-fes* [Fig. 2] and is proposed to be oriented on the cytoplasmic side of the membrane).

Alternatively, the situation could be similar to cells infected with polyoma virus in which the middle T antigen is coprecipitated with pp60 (Courtneidge and Smith 1983).

Nucleotide sequencing predicted that the *v-fms* gene encodes a product with marked homology to the *v-onc* genes specifying tyrosine-specific protein kinases (Hampe et al. 1984). Figure 2 shows a region of amino acid sequence homology predicted near the carboxy-terminal ends of the *v-fms* and *v-fes* gene products. Interestingly, the homologous regions of these proteins include the apparent sites of tyrosine phosphorylation within the proteins themselves, but do not include an upstream lysine residue that has been implicated in ATP binding (Barker and Dayhoff 1982). A feature of the model shown in Figure 4 is that, like pp60^{src}, the "kinase" domain of the *v-fms* glycoprotein would be oriented at the cytoplasmic surface of the membrane (Willingham et al. 1979).

Other viral oncogenes, including *v-mos* (Van Beveren et al. 1981) and *v-erb* (Yamamoto et al. 1983; J.M. Bishop, pers. comm.) which were not thought to encode kinases, are now also known to exhibit homology to members of the tyrosine kinase gene family. These data suggest that portions of all of these genes have descended from a single primordial sequence and have now evolved to be functionally distinct. The possibility that *v-fms*, *v-mos*, and *v-erb*-B specify tyrosine-specific protein kinases that show minimal activity in vivo cannot be formally excluded. Alternatively, other cryptic "transforming functions" could reside in the same regions of these molecules that do not critically depend on tyrosine phosphorylation per se. Previous studies with transformation-defective viral mutants do not rule out the latter possibility, since lesions affecting enzyme activity might conjointly affect other functions necessary for transformation.

The human c-fms locus

The complexity of *v-fms* sequences in the SM-FeSV genome is 3.0 kb. Subgenomic fragments derived from this region hybridize to a far more extensive region of cat DNA, showing that the *c-fms* proto-oncogene contains many intervening sequences (Donner et al. 1982). In human DNA, probes derived from the *v-fms* gene hybridize to a single genetic locus more than 30 kb in length (see Fig. 2) (Heisterkamp et al. 1983; Roussel et al. 1983). This is a minimal estimate of the size of the human *c-fms* proto-oncogene since the complete *c-fms*-coding region may not have been transduced in SM-FeSV. Muller et al. (1983a,b) have detected a 3.7-kb *c-fms* mRNA species in human placental tissues and in at least one choriocarcinoma cell line. The size of this spliced *c-fms* RNA (3.7 kb minus poly[A]) is close to that of the transduced *v-fms* gene (3.0 kb). The human *c-fms* locus maps to the long arm of human chromosome 5 (Groffen et al. 1983b; Roussel et al. 1983) and could potentially be deleted in the "5q − syndrome" which is associated with refractory anemia and predisposes to the development of acute myelogenous leukemia (Wisniewski and Hirschhorn 1983).

Future perspectives

The ability of viral oncogene products to transform cells and render them tumorigenic shows that these proteins can dramatically subvert processes that regulate normal growth. It seems likely that viral oncogene products mirror the functions of their normal cellular analogs but provide more abundant signals for proliferation. If the *c-onc* products define key points in a metabolism for growth, studies concerning mechanisms of malignant transformation by *v-onc* proteins should ultimately render corresponding insights about the biochemical mechanisms that regulate normal cell proliferation. For example, oncogene products that encode tyrosine-specific protein kinases may utilize the same pathways in regulating cell growth as some normal receptors for growth factors that exhibit this enzymatic activity. In the latter case, phosphorylation of the receptor is a consequence of binding an extracellular ligand that initiates a series of events leading to cell division. Phosphorylation mediated by high levels of a similar enzyme, or by an enzyme that is catalytically more efficient, might provide a constitutive stimulus for division utilizing the same cellular machinery. Oncogene products whose functions remain obscure seem likely to provide profound clues to the metabolism of cell growth. The presently incomplete mosaic provides more room for thought and investigation.

Acknowledgments

We thank the many investigators who have worked with us on the *fes* and *fms* genes over the last 5 years. In particular, we are most grateful to our French collaborators, Drs. Francis Galibert and Annie Hampe, Hôpital St. Louis, Paris, who performed the nucleotide sequence analysis of the cloned oncogenes, and continue to provide invaluable information; and to Dr. Matthew A. Gonda for collaborative studies on subcellular localization of *v-fms* antigens and for photomicrographs.

References

Anderson, S.J. M. Furth, L. Wolff, S.K. Ruscetti, and C.J. Sherr. 1982. Monoclonal antibodies to the transformation-specific glycoprotein encoded by the feline retroviral oncogene v-*fms*. *J. Virol.* **44:** 696.

Barbacid, M. and A.V. Lauver. 1981. The gene products of McDonough feline sarcoma virus have an *in vitro* associated protein kinase that phosphorylates tyrosine residues: Lack of detection of this enzymatic activity *in vivo*. *J. Virol.* **40:** 812.

Barbacid, M., K. Beemon, and S.G. Devare. 1980a. Origin and functional properties of the *src* gene product of the Snyder-Theilen strain of feline sarcoma virus. *Proc. Natl. Acad. Sci.* **77:** 5158.

Barbacid, M., A.V. Lauver, and S.G. Devare. 1980b. Biochemical and immunological characterization of polyproteins coded for by the McDonough, Gardner-Arnstein, and Snyder-Theilen strains of feline sarcoma virus. *J. Virol.* **33:** 196.

Barbacid, M., L. Donner, S.K. Ruscetti, and C.J. Sherr. 1981a. Transformation defective mutants of Snyder-Theilen feline sarcoma virus lack tyrosine specific protein kinase activity. *J. Virol.* **39:** 246.

Barbacid, M., M.L. Brietman, A.V. Lauver, L.K. Long, and P.K. Vogt. 1981b. The transformation-specific proteins of avian (Fujinami and PRCII) and feline (Snyder-Theilen and Gardner-Arnstein) sarcoma viruses are immunologically related. *Virology* **110:** 411.

Barker, W.C. and M.O. Dayhoff. 1982. Viral *src* gene products are related to the catalytic chain of mammalian cAMP-dependent protein kinase. *Proc. Natl. Acad. Sci.* **79**: 2836.

Beemon, K. 1981. Transforming proteins of some feline and avian sarcoma viruses are related structurally and functionally. *Cell* **24**: 145.

Besmer, P., H.W. Snyder, J.R. Murphy, W.D. Hardy, and A. Parodi. 1983a. The Parodi-Irgens feline sarcoma virus and simian sarcoma virus have homologous oncogenes. *J. Virol.* **46**: 606.

Besmer, P., W.D. Hardy, E. Zuckerman, L. Lederman, and H.W. Snyder. 1983b. The Hardy-Zuckerman-2 FeSV and Abelson MuLV have homologous oncogenes. *Nature* **303**: 825.

Bishop, J.M. 1982. Oncogenes. *Sci. Am.* **246**: 81.

———. 1983. Cancer genes come of age. *Cell* **32**: 1018.

Blair, D.G., M. Oskarsson, T.G. Wood, W.L. McClements, and G.F. Vande Woude. 1981. Activation of the transforming potential of a normal cell sequence: A molecular model for oncogenesis. *Science* **212**: 941.

Blobel, G. 1980. Intracellular protein topogenesis. *Proc. Natl. Acad. Sci.* **77**: 1496.

Blomberg, J., W.J.M. Van de Ven, F.H. Reynolds, R.P. Nalewaik, and J.R. Stephenson. 1981. Snyder-Theilen feline sarcoma virus P85 contains a single phosphotyrosine acceptor site recognized by its associated protein kinase. *J. Virol.* **38**: 886.

Collett, M.S. and R.L. Erikson. 1978. Protein kinase activity associated with the avian sarcoma virus *src* gene product. *Proc. Natl. Acad. Sci.* **75**: 2020.

Courtneidge, S.A. and A.E. Smith. 1983. Polyomavirus transforming protein associates with the product of the c-*src* cellular gene. *Nature* **303**: 434.

Dalla-Favera, R., G. Franchini, S. Martinotti, F. Wong-Staal, R.C. Gallo, and C.M. Croce. 1982. Chromosomal assignment of the human homologues of feline sarcoma virus and avian myeloblastosis virus *onc* genes. *Proc. Natl. Acad. Sci.* **79**: 4714.

DeFeo, D., M. Gonda, H.A. Young, E.H. Chang, D. Lowy, E.M. Scolnick, and R.W. Ellis. 1981. Analysis of two divergent rat genomic clones homologous to the transforming gene of Harvey murine sarcoma virus. *Proc. Natl. Acad. Sci.* **78**: 3328.

Donner, L., L.A. Fedele, C.F. Garon, S.J. Anderson, and C.J. Sherr. 1982. McDonough feline sarcoma virus: Characterization of the molecularly cloned provirus and its feline oncogene v-*fms*. *J. Virol.* **41**: 489.

Donner, L., L.P. Turek, S.K. Ruscetti, L.A. Fedele, and C.J. Sherr. 1980. Transformation defective mutants of feline sarcoma virus which express a product of the viral src gene. *J. Virol.* **35**: 129.

Ek, B., B. Westermark, A. Wasteson, and C.H. Heldin. 1982. Stimulation of tyrosine-specific phosphorylation by platelet-derived growth factor. *Nature* **295**: 419.

Fedele, L.A., J. Even, C.F. Garon, L. Donner, and C.J. Sherr. 1981. Recombinant bacteriophages containing the integrated transforming provirus of Gardner-Arnstein feline sarcoma virus. *Proc. Natl. Acad. Sci.* **78**: 4036.

Feldman, R.A., T. Hanafusa, and H. Hanafusa. 1980. Characterization of protein kinase activity associated with the transforming gene product of Fujinami sarcoma virus. *Cell* **22**: 757.

Feldman, R.A., L.H. Wang, H. Hanafusa, and P.C. Balduzzi. 1982. Avian sarcoma virus UR2 encodes a transforming protein which is associated with a unique protein kinase activity. *J. Virol.* **42**: 228.

Franchini, G., J. Even, C.J. Sherr, and F. Wong-Staal. 1981. *Onc* sequences (v-*fes*) of Snyder-Theilen feline sarcoma virus are derived from noncontiguous regions of a cat cellular gene (c-*fes*). *Nature* **290**: 154.

Franchini, G., E.P. Gelmann, R. Dalla-Favera, R.C. Gallo, and F. Wong-Staal. 1982. Human gene (c-*fes*) related to the *onc* sequences of Snyder-Theilen feline sarcoma virus. *Mol. Cell. Biol.* **2**: 1014.

Frankel, A.E., J.H. Gilbert, K.T. Porzig, E.M. Scolnick, and S.A. Aaronson. 1979. Nature and distribution of feline sarcoma virus nucleotide sequences. *J. Virol.* **30**: 821.

Furth, M.E., L.J. Davis, B. Fleurdelys, and E.M. Scolnick. 1982. Monoclonal antibodies to the p21 products of the transforming gene of Harvey murine sarcoma virus and of the cellular *ras* gene family. *J. Virol.* **43**: 294.

Gardner, M.B., R.W. Rongey, P. Arnstein, J.D. Estes, P. Sarma, R.J. Huebner, and C.J. Rickard. 1970. Experimental transmission of a feline fibrosarcoma to cats and dogs. *Nature* **226**: 807.

Granger, B.L. and E. Lazarides. 1980. Synemin: A new high molecular weight protein associated with desmin and vimentin filaments in muscle. *Cell* **22**: 727.

Groffen, J., N. Heisterkamp, F. Grosveld, W. Van de Ven, and J.R. Stephenson. 1982. Isolation of human oncogene sequences (v-*fes* homology) from a cosmid library. *Science* **216**: 1136.

Groffen, J., N. Heisterkamp, M. Shibuya, H. Hanafusa, and J.R. Stephenson. 1983a. Transforming genes of avian (v-*fps*) and mammalian (v-*fes*) retroviruses correspond to a common cellular locus. *Virology* **125**: 480.

Groffen, J., N. Heisterkamp, N. Spurr, S. Dana, J.J. Wasmuth, and J.R. Stephenson. 1983b. Chromosomal localization of the human c-*fms* oncogene. *Nucleic Acids Res.* **11**: 6331.

Hampe, A., M. Gobet, C.J. Sherr, and F. Galibert. 1984. Nucleotide sequence of the v-*fms* oncogene shows unexpected homology to oncogenes encoding tyrosine-specific protein kinases. *Proc. Natl. Acad. Sci.* **81**: 85.

Hampe, A., I. Laprevotte, F. Galibert, and C.J. Sherr. 1982. Nucleotide sequence of feline retroviral oncogenes (v-*fes*) provide evidence for a family of tyrosine-specific protein kinase genes. *Cell* **30**: 775.

Hampe, A., M. Gobet, J. Even, C.J. Sherr, and F. Galibert. 1983. Nucleotide sequences of feline sarcoma virus long terminal repeats and 5′ leaders show extensive homology to those of other mammalian retroviruses. *J. Virol.* **45**: 466.

Hanafusa, T., B. Mathey Prevot, R.A. Feldman, and H. Hanafusa. 1981. Mutants of Fujinami sarcoma virus which are temperature-sensitive for cellular transformation and protein kinase activity. *J. Virol.* **38**: 347.

Hardy, W.D., Jr. 1980. The virology, immunology, and epidemiology of the feline leukemia virus. In *Feline leukemia virus* (ed. W.J. Hardy, Jr. et al.), p. 79. Elsevier North Holland, Amsterdam.

Heisterkamp, N., J. Groffen, and J.R. Stephenson. 1983. Isolation of v-*fms* and its human cellular homolog. *Virology* **126**: 248.

Heisterkamp, N., J. Groffen, J.R. Stephenson, N.K. Spurr, P.N. Goodfellow, E. Solomon, B. Carritt, and W.F. Bodmer. 1982. Chromosomal locations of human cellular homologies of two viral oncogenes. *Nature* **299**: 747.

Huebner, R.J. and G.J. Todaro. 1969. Oncogenes of RNA tumor viruses as determinants of cancer. *Proc. Natl. Acad. Sci.* **64**: 1087.

Irgens, K., M. Wyers, A. Moraillon, A. Parodi, and V. Fortuny. 1973. Isolement d'un virus sarcomatogene felin a partir d'un fibrosarcome spontane du chat: Etude du pouvoir sarcomatogene *in vivo*. *C.R. Acad. Sci.* **26**: 1783.

Kasuga, M., Y. Zick, D.L. Blithe, M. Crettaz, and R. Kahn. 1982. Insulin stimulates tyrosine phosphorylation of the insulin receptor. *Nature* **298**: 667.

Kawai, S., M. Yoshida, K. Segawa, H. Sugiyama, R. Ishizaki, and K. Toyoshima. 1980. Characterization of Y73, a newly isolated avian sarcoma virus: A unique transforming gene and its product, a phosphoprotein with protein kinase activity. *Proc. Natl. Acad. Sci.* **77**: 6199.

Kitamura, N., A. Kitamura, K. Toyoshima, Y. Hirayama, and M. Yoshida. 1982. Avian sarcoma virus Y73 genome sequence and structural similarity of its transforming gene product to that of Rous sarcoma virus. *Nature* **297**: 205.

Levinson, A.D., H. Oppermann, L. Levintow, H.E. Varmus, and J.M. Bishop. 1978. Evidence that the transforming gene of avian sarcoma virus encodes a protein kinase associated with a phosphoprotein. *Cell* **15**: 561.

Mathey-Prevot, B., H. Hanafusa, and S. Kawai. 1982. A cellular protein is immunologically cross-reactive with and functionally homologous to the Fujinami sarcoma virus transforming protein. *Cell* **28**: 897.

McDonough, S.K., S. Larsen, R.S. Brodey, W.D. Stock, and W.D. Hardy, Jr. 1971. A transmissible feline fibrosarcoma of viral origin. *Cancer Res.* **31**: 953.

Muller, R., J. Tremblay, E.D. Adamson, and I.M. Verma. 1983a. Tissue and cell type-specific expression of two human c-*onc* genes. *Nature* **304**: 454.

Muller, R., D.L. Slamon, E.D. Adamson, J.M. Tremblay, D. Muller, M.J. Cline, and I.M. Verma. 1983b. Transcription of c-*onc* genes c-*ras*^{ki} and c-*fms* during mouse development. *Mol. Cell. Biol.* **3**: 1062.

Naharro, G., K.C. Robbins, and E.P. Reddy. 1984. Gene product of v-*fgr onc*: Hybrid protein containing a portion of actin and a tyrosine-specific protein kinase. *Science* **223**: 63.

Naharro, G., S.R. Tronick, S. Rasheed, M.B. Gardner, S.A. Aaronson, and K.C. Robbins. 1983. Molecular cloning of integrated Gardner-Rasheed feline sarcoma virus: Genetic structure of its cell-derived sequence differs from that of other tyrosine kinase-coding *onc* genes. *J. Virol.* **47**: 611.

Patchinsky, T., T. Hunter, F.S. Esch, J.A. Cooper, and B.M. Sefton. 1982. Analysis of the sequence of amino acids surrounding sites of tyrosine phosphorylation. *Proc. Natl. Acad. Sci.* **79**: 973.

Pawson, T., J. Guyden, T.H. Kung, K. Radke, T. Gilmore, and G.S. Martin. 1980. A strain of Fujinami sarcoma virus which is temperature-sensitive in protein phosphorylation and cellular transformation. *Cell* **22**: 767.

Rasheed, S., M. Barbacid, S.A. Aaronson, and M.B. Gardner. 1982. Origin and biological properties of a new feline sarcoma virus. *Virology* **117**: 238.

Reynolds, F.H., Jr., W.J. Van de Ven, and J.R. Stephenson. 1980. Feline sarcoma virus P115-associated protein kinase phosphorylates tyrosine. Identification of a cellular substrate conserved during evolution. *J. Biol. Chem.* **255**: 11040.

Reynolds, F.H., W.J.M. Van de Ven, J. Blomberg, and J.R. Stephenson. 1981a. Involvement of a high molecular weight protein translational product of Snyder-Theilen feline sarcoma virus in malignant transformation. *J. Virol.* **37**: 643.

———. 1981b. Differences in mechanisms of transformation by independent feline sarcoma virus isolates. *J. Virol.* **38**: 1084.

Roussel, M.F., C.J. Sherr, P.E. Barker, and F.H. Ruddle. 1983. Molecular cloning of the c-*fms* locus and its assignment to human chromosome 5. *J. Virol.* **48**: 770.

Ruscetti, S.K., L.P. Turek, and C.J. Sherr. 1980. Three independent isolates of feline sarcoma virus code for three distinct *gag*-x polyproteins. *J. Virol.* **35**: 259.

Sefton, B.M., T. Hunter, K. Beemon, and W. Eckhart. 1980. Evidence that the phosphorylation of tyrosine is essential for cellular transformation by Rous sarcoma virus. *Cell* **20**: 806.

Segrest, J.P. and R. Feldman. 1974. Membrane proteins: Amino acid sequence and membrane penetration. *J. Mol. Biol.* **67**: 835.

Sen, S., R.A. Houghton, C.J. Sherr, and A. Sen. 1982. Antibodies of predetermined specificity detect two retroviral oncogene products and inhibit their kinase activities. *Proc. Natl. Acad. Sci.* **80**: 1246.

Sheer, D., L. Hiorns, K.F. Stanley, P.N. Goodfellow, D.M. Swallow, S. Povey, N. Heisterkamp, J. Groffen, J.R. Stephenson, and E. Solomon. 1983. Genetic analysis of the 15;17 chromosome translocation associated with acute promyelocytic leukemia. *Proc. Natl. Acad. Sci.* **80**: 5007.

Sherr, C.J., L.A. Fedele, L. Donner, and L.P. Turek. 1979. Restriction endonuclease mapping of unintegrated proviral DNA of Snyder-Theilen feline sarcoma virus: Localization of sarcoma-specific sequences. *J. Virol.* **32**: 860.

Sherr, C.J., G.J. Todaro, A. Sliski, and M. Essex. 1978a. Characterization of a feline sarcoma virus-coded antigen (FOCMA-S) by radioimmunoassay. *Proc. Natl. Acad. Sci.* **75**: 4489.

Sherr, C.J., A. Sen, G.J. Todaro. A. Sliski, and M. Essex. 1978b. Pseudotypes of feline sarcoma virus contain an 85,000 dalton protein with feline oncornavirus-associated cell membrane antigen (FOCMA) activity. *Proc. Natl. Acad. Sci.* **75**: 1505.

Sherr, C.J., L.A. Fedele, M. Oskarsson, J. Maizel, and G. Vande Woude. 1980b. Molecular cloning of Snyder-Theilen feline leukemia and sarcoma viruses: Comparative studies of feline sarcoma virus with its natural helper virus and with Moloney murine sarcoma virus. *J. Virol.* **34**: 200.

Sherr, C.J., L. Donner, L.A. Fedele, L. Turek, J. Even, and S.K. Ruscetti. 1980b. Molecular structure and products of feline sarcoma and leukemia viruses: Relationship to FOCMA expression. In *Feline leukemia virus* (ed. W.D. Hardy, Jr. et al.), p. 293. Elsevier/North Holland, Amsterdam.

Shibuya, M. and H. Hanafusa. 1982. Nucleotide sequence of Fujinami sarcoma virus: Evolutionary relationship of its transforming gene with transforming genes of other sarcoma viruses. *Cell* **30**: 787.

Shibuya, M., H. Hanafusa, and P.C. Balduzzi. 1982. Cellular sequences related to three new onc genes of avian sarcoma virus (*fps, yes,* and *ros*) and their expression in normal and transformed cells. *J. Virol.* **42**: 143.

Shibuya, M., T. Hanafusa, H. Hanafusa, and J.R. Stephenson. 1980. Homology exists among the transforming sequences of the avian and feline sarcoma viruses. *Proc. Natl. Acad. Sci.* **77**: 6536.

Snyder, S.P. and G.H. Theilen. 1969. Transmissible feline fibrosarcoma. *Nature* **221**: 1074.

Stephenson, J.R., A.S. Khan, A.H. Sliski, and M. Essex. 1977. Feline oncornavirus-associated cell membrane antigen: Evidence for an immunologically cross-reactive feline sarcoma virus coded protein. *Proc. Natl. Acad. Sci.* **74**: 5608.

Trus, M.D., J.G. Sodroski, and W.A. Haseltine. 1982. Isolation and characterization of a human locus homologous to the transforming gene (v-*fes*) of feline sarcoma virus. *J. Biol. Chem.* **257**: 2730.

Ushiro, H. and S.J. Cohen. 1980. Identification of phosphotyrosine as a product of epidermal growth factor-activated protein kinase in A-431 cell membranes. *J. Biol. Chem.* **255**: 8363.

Van Beveren, C., J.A. Galleshaw, V. Jones, A.J.M. Berns, R.F. Doolittle, D.J. Donoghue, and I.M. Verma. 1981. Nucleotide sequence and formation of the transforming gene of a mouse sarcoma virus. *Nature* **289**: 258.

Van de Ven, W.J.M., F.H. Reynolds, and J.R. Stephenson. 1980a. The nonstructural components of polyproteins encoded by replication-defective mammalian transforming retroviruses are phosphorylated and have associated kinase activity. *Virology* **101**: 185.

Van de Ven, W.J.M., F.H. Reynolds, R.P. Nalewaik, and J.R. Stephenson. 1980b. Characterization of a 170,000 dalton polyprotein encoded by the McDonough strain of feline sarcoma virus. *J. Virol.* **35**: 165.

Varmus, H.E. 1982. Form and function of retroviral proviruses. *Science* **216**: 812.

Veronese, F., G.J. Kelloff, F.H. Reynolds, R.W. Hill, and J.R. Stephenson. 1982. Monoclonal antibodies specific to transforming polyproteins encoded by independent isolates of feline sarcoma virus. *J. Virol.* **43**: 896.

Weber, K. and D.J. Kuter. 1971. Reversible denaturation of enzymes by sodium dodecyl sulfate. *J. Biol. Chem.* **246**: 4505.

Willingham, M.C., G. Jay, and I. Pastan. 1979. Localization of the ASV *src* gene product to the plasma membrane of transformed cells by electronmicroscopic immunocytochemistry. *Cell* **18**: 125.

Wisniewski, L.P. and K. Hirschhorn. 1983. Acquired partial deletions of the long arm of chromosome 5 in hematologic disorders. *Am. J. Hematol.* **15**: 295.

Witte, O.N., A. Dasgupta, and D. Baltimore. 1980. Abelson murine leukemia virus protein is phosphorylated *in vitro* to form phosphotyrosine. *Nature* **283**: 826.

Yamamoto, T., T. Nishida, N. Miyajima, S. Kawai, T. Ooi, and K. Toyoshima. 1983. The *erbB* gene of avian erythroblastosis virus is a member of the *src* gene family. *Cell* **35**: 71.

Analysis of the Avian Erythroblastosis Virus *erb* Oncogene Products

M.J. Hayman*
Viral Leukaemogenesis Laboratory, Imperial Cancer Research Fund, London WC2A 3PX, England

H. Beug
EMB Laboratories, 6900 Heidelberg, West Germany

Avian erythroblastosis virus (AEV) is a replication-defective avian acute leukemia virus that can cause acute erythroid leukemia and sarcomas after injection into young chicks. Analysis of the genome of AEV revealed that it was 5.0 kb in length and that the gene order was 5'-*gag erb env*-poly(A)-3', where *gag* and *env* represent partially deleted structural genes and *erb* is a 3.25-kb sequence of nonviral origin (Bister and Duesberg 1979; Lai et al. 1979). Attempts to characterize these nonviral sequences showed that sequences homologous to *erb* could be found in cellular DNA from all vertebrate species tested (Roussel et al. 1979; Stehelin et al. 1980). These data suggested that the *erb* sequences represented the viral oncogene of AEV, and led to studies attempting to define the products of this gene.

These studies rapidly revealed that AEV was unique among avian retroviruses in that it contained an oncogene capable of coding for two gene products. Consequently, the *erb* gene was divided into two regions known as *erb*-A and *erb*-B. The first gene product identified was the *erb*-A protein, which is a 75,000-molecular-weight protein p75^{erb-A} that was found in cells transformed by AEV (Hayman et al. 1979). This protein was shown to be composed of aminoterminal *gag* sequences plus approximately 50,000 daltons of *erb*-A sequences. Recently, the *erb*-B protein has also been identified in AEV-transformed cells as a membrane glycoprotein (Hayman et al. 1983; Privalsky et al. 1983). This protein, initially synthesized as a 66,000-dalton glycoprotein, gp66^{erb-B}, is subsequently modified by further glycosylation to a 68,000-molecular-weight form, gp68^{erb-B} (Hayman et al. 1983).

Interest in the *erb*-B protein was heightened by several recent observations. First, site-directed mutagenesis experiments on the AEV genome demonstrated that it was primarily the *erb*-B gene that was responsible for the transformation of both erythroid cells and fibroblasts (Frykberg et al. 1983). However, the presence of the *erb*-A gene did play some role in the development of the fully transformed phenotype. Second, characterization of a new isolate of AEV, termed AEV-H, which was capable of causing both erythroblastosis and fibrosarcoma (Hihara et al. 1983), revealed that it only contained the

erb-B sequences in its genome. Finally, it was demonstrated that avian leukosis virus-induced erythroblastosis was caused by an insertional mutagenesis of the long terminal repeat (LTR) into the cellular *erb*-B locus resulting in the elevation of *c-erb*-B transcription (Fung et al. 1983). Thus, the central role of *erb*-B in erythroblastosis and fibrosarcoma induction has encouraged us to characterize the product of this gene in greater detail.

Methods

Cells and viruses
Erythroblast cell lines transformed by either wild-type AEV-ES4 or *ts*34 AEV were used in these studies. The isolation and characterization of these cell lines have been described previously (Beug et al. 1982). The A23 clone of Rous sarcoma virus transformed rat cells was described previously (Dyson et al. 1982).

Preparation of antisera
Antisera were prepared in (Fisher × Wistar) F$_1$ rats by injection of 10^6 rat fibroblasts transformed by AEV (Hayman et al. 1983). The clone used in these experiments was the AT1a clone described by Quade et al. (1983). Tumors developed after 6–8 weeks, at which time samples were taken and tested for antibodies against either *erb*-A or *erb*-B by immunoprecipitation.

Immune precipitation
Erythroblasts were labeled with [^{35}S]methionine; detergent lysates were prepared and immune precipitates were isolated and analyzed by SDS-polyacrylamide gel electrophoresis, as described previously (Hayman et al. 1979).

Endo H analysis
The state of maturation of the carbohydrate side chains was analyzed using the enzyme endo-β-*N*-acetylglucosaminidase H (endo H) (Tarentino and Maley 1974); this enzyme was a kind gift of Dr. M.J. Owen. Immune precipitates were treated with the enzyme as described in Owen et al. (1980).

Protein kinase assays
The immune complex assay described by Sefton et al. (1980) for determining protein kinase activity was used. The anti-*src* serum used as control was raised against the B77 strain and recognizes both *v-src* and *c-src* (Dyson et al. 1982).

---

*Present address: Imperial Cancer Research Fund Laboratories at St. Bartholomew's Hospital, London EC1A 7BE, England.

Results

Identification of the *erb*-B glycoproteins as membrane proteins

Using antisera obtained from rats carrying tumors induced by AEV-transformed fibroblasts, we have identified the *erb*-B gene product as a glycoprotein that is initially synthesized as a 66,000-molecular-weight protein that is modified into a 68,000-molecular-weight form (Hayman et al. 1983). These antisera contained antibodies against both the *erb*-A and *erb*-B products. Recently, we obtained an antiserum that reacts only with *erb*-B (M.J. Hayman and H. Beug, in prep.). This antiserum allowed us to reexamine both the cellular localization and the processing of the *erb*-B glycoprotein.

Our initial analysis had shown that the *erb*-B glycoproteins were located exclusively in the membrane fraction of transformed cells (Hayman et al. 1983). In contrast, the *erb*-A p75 protein was essentially a soluble cytoplasmic protein. However, a small percentage of p75 was also located in the microsomal fraction (Hayman et al. 1983). Since it is known that the *erb*-A gene augments the transformation induced by the *erb*-B gene (Frykberg et al. 1983), it was possible that this membrane-associated p75 was complexed to the *erb*-B proteins. Therefore, we repeated the membrane fractionation experiments using the *erb*-B-specific antiserum (Fig. 1). In confirmation of our previous results, essentially all of the *erb*-B proteins were found in the microsomal fraction (Fig. 1). However, there was now no p75 in any of the fractions, implying that the *erb*-B proteins were not physically associated with p75 (Fig. 1).

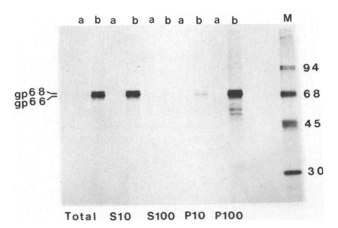

Figure 1 Localization of the *erb*-B proteins to the membrane. AEV-transformed erythroblasts were labeled for 1 hr with 500 µCi of [^{35}S]methionine, washed, resuspended into 10 mM Tris (pH 7.4) and 1 mM MgCl$_2$, and then disrupted by means of Dounce homogenization. An aliquot was then removed to provide a sample before fractionation (Total), and then the amount of cell breakage was assessed by preparing a solubilized fraction (S10), plus a nuclear fraction (P10). The S10 fraction was then subdivided into a cytoplasmic (S100) and microsomal fraction (P100) as described (Hayman et al. 1983). Detergent lysates were prepared and immune-precipitated with normal rat serum (lanes *a*) and rat anti-*erb*-B serum (lanes *b*). Track *M* is radioactively labeled molecular-weight markers (Amersham).

Endoglycosidase-H analysis of the *erb*-B glycoproteins

In our previous studies (Hayman et al. 1983) the *erb*-B proteins had been shown to be glycosylated using endo H, which specifically cleaves core sugars from glycoproteins (Tarantino and Maley 1974). However, in these initial experiments, only a short labeling time had been used and therefore the major protein examined was the gp66 form. To extend these studies, a pulse-chase analysis was performed and samples taken at different times and treated with endo H. The results of this analysis are shown in Figure 2. As reported previously, the gp66 form of the *erb*-B protein can be chased into a gp68 form as seen from the samples not treated with endo H. However, both of these proteins are digested with endo H to generate the p62 form of the *erb*-B protein. These data show that over a 4-hour time period neither gp66 or gp68 become resistant to endo H, although during this time period they turn over (Fig. 2). These data imply that either a form of the *erb*-B protein exists that is not being detected in these experiments or that the carbohydrate side chains on these proteins are not being modified to the usual complex forms.

To distinguish between these possibilities, we reexamined the *erb*-B proteins using the *erb*-B-specific serum. Figure 3B shows a similar pulse-chase analysis performed using this new antiserum. After a 4-hour chase period, a protein migrating as a diffuse band of molecular weight 74,000 was detected that could be shown to be resistant to digestion by endo H (Fig. 3B). (For these experiments, we used the *ts*34 isolate of AEV [Graf et al. 1978]; however, similar results were obtained with wild-type virus, [data not shown].) This protein would therefore be a candidate for the final product of the *erb*-B gene.

Conditional mutants of AEV have been isolated that are temperature-sensitive for transformation (Graf et al. 1978; Palmieri et al. 1982). To test whether this endo H-resistant form of the *erb*-B protein had any physiolog-

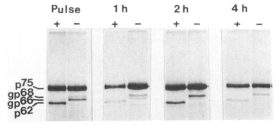

Figure 2 Endo H analysis of the *erb*-proteins. AEV-transformed erythroblasts were pulse-labeled for 30 min with 100 µCi of [^{35}S]methionine. The cells were then pelleted and resuspended in growth medium. An aliquot of cells was removed for time point zero (pulse) and subsequent aliquots were removed after 1, 2, and 4 hr. Immune precipitates were formed with anti-*erb* serum from tumor-bearing rats. The immune precipitates were then divided into two, and one-half was treated with endo H (+) as described previously (Owen et al. 1980) and the other half (−) was kept on ice. Both samples were then treated in exactly the same way and analyzed on a 10% SDS-polyacrylamide gel.

A. Pulse chase at 41°C   **B. Pulse chase at 35°C**

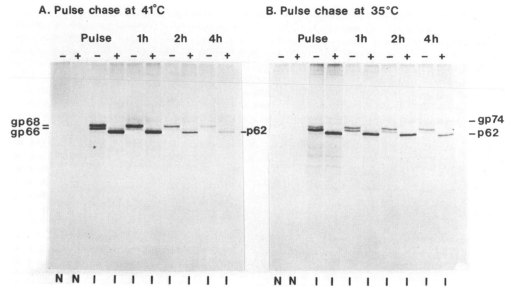

Figure 3 Endo-H analysis of temperature sensitive AEV *erb*-B proteins. *ts*34 AEV-transformed erythroblasts were pulse-chased and treated with endo H as described in Fig. 2. (*A*) Cells were grown for 3 days and labeled at 41°C; (*B*) cells were grown and labeled at 35°C. Immune precipitates were formed either with normal rat serum (N) or anti-*erb*-B-specific serum (I).

ical significance, we analyzed its synthesis in *ts*34 AEV-infected cells now grown at the nonpermissive temperature of 41°C. Figure 3A shows that at this temperature there is no endo H-resistant *erb*-B protein present in the cells, although the other forms are synthesized (cf. panels A and B), as is the *erb*-A p75 protein (data not shown). These data imply that it is the final processing of the *erb*-B glycoprotein that is temperature-sensitive in mutant virus and that it is the correct synthesis of gp74 that is important in the transformation process.

The *erb* proteins have no detectable kinase activity

Avian sarcoma viruses are divided into three main groups on the basis of the oncogenes found in their genomes (Neil 1983). However, the common feature that these three groups share is the ability of their gene products to function as tyrosine kinases. Sequence analysis of the oncogenes from these three groups has shown that they contain a region that is highly conserved, especially at the amino acid level, and it is this region that is responsible for the kinase activity of these proteins (Neil 1983). Recently, sequence analysis of the *erb*-B gene has revealed that it contains a region that is highly homologous to the kinase-specific region of the sarcoma viruses (M.L. Privalsky, pers. comm.). These data prompted us to test the *erb*-B protein for kinase activity in the standard immune complex assay (Sefton et al. 1980).

The results are shown in Figure 4. As a control, we included an anti-*src* serum that recognizes both v-*src* kinase activity in Rous sarcoma virus-transformed rat cells (Fig. 4A) and c-*src* activity in AEV-transformed erythroblasts (Fig. 4B). However, no kinase activity could be found associated with the *erb* gene products, either *erb*-A p75 alone or together with *erb*-B proteins (Fig. 4B).

Discussion

AEV is unique among avian retroviruses in that it contains an oncogene that is capable of coding for two gene products, both of which effect cell transformation. Although only one of these gene products, the *erb*-B protein, is necessary for transformation, the *erb*-A gene enhances the effect of this gene. Viruses containing both *erb*-A and *erb*-B genes are more leukemogenic in vivo, and the cells transformed in vitro display more phenotypic markers of transformation than those transformed by *erb*-B-only viruses (Frykberg et al. 1983). Recent experiments involving transfections of viral or cellular oncogenes onto primary or carcinogen-immortalized cells in tissue culture have implied that in certain cases more

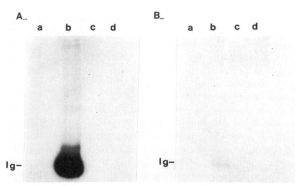

Figure 4 Analysis of *erb* proteins for protein kinase activity. Rous sarcoma virus-transformed rat cells, clone A 23 (*A*) and wild-type AEV-transformed erythroblasts were lysed in detergent and the immune precipitates were formed using normal rat serum (lanes *a*), anti-*gag* serum (lanes *b*), anti-*src* serum (lanes *c*), or anti-*erb* serum (lanes *d*). The complexes were then assayed for protein kinase activity as described (Sefton et al. 1980).

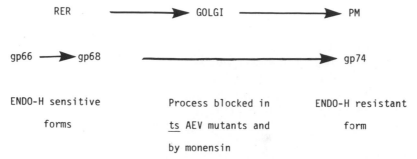

Figure 5 Schematic representation of the processing of the *erb*-B protein.

than one gene function may be required for tumorigenicity (Land et al. 1983; Newbold and Overell 1983; Ruley 1983). These effects seem to be important at the level of protein function rather than an enhancement effect on transcription (Land et al. 1983). Therefore, to see if there was any direct interaction between the *erb*-A and *erb*-B gene products, we determined the cellular location of the proteins and found that the *erb*-B proteins were located in the membranes and were not complexed with any *erb*-A p75. These data imply that if the functions of these two gene products are involved in a synergistic reaction, they do so via separate pathways rather than by acting directly upon each other.

Recent data on the isolation of a virus containing just the *erb*-B gene (Hihara et al. 1983), plus the demonstration that avian leukosis virus-induced erythroblastosis is caused by promoter insertion into the *c-erb*-B locus (Fung et al. 1983), confirms previous studies showing that the *erb*-B products alone are sufficient to induce both erythroid and fibroblast transformation (Frykberg et al. 1983). In an attempt to understand the function of these proteins, we have extended our previous characterization of these glycoproteins. These studies have demonstrated that the processing of these glycoproteins results in an endo H-resistant form of 74 kD, which presumably represents the final form of the *erb*-B gene product. Moreover, in an AEV conditional mutant *ts*34, which is temperature-sensitive for transformation (Graf et al. 1978), this gp74 protein is made at the permissive temperature but not at the nonpermissive temperature. In addition, recent evidence suggests that gp74 is a plasma membrane form of the protein and there is no cell-surface expression of *erb*-B as judged by immunofluorescence in *ts* mutant-infected cells grown at the nonpermissive temperature (M.J. Hayman and H. Beug, unpubl. observ.). These data are shown schematically in Figure 5 and suggest that expression in the plasma membrane is crucial for the function of the *erb*-B proteins.

Sequence analysis of the *erb*-B gene has revealed the presence of a carboxyterminal domain of the protein with homology to the tyrosine kinase domains of the avian sarcoma viruses, that is, the *src, yes*, and *fps* oncogenes (M.L. Privalsky, pers. comm.). These data are intriguing since various growth factor receptors have also been shown to be associated with tyrosine kinase activity, for example, the epidermal growth factor receptor (Cohen et al. 1980), insulin receptor (Kasuga et al. 1983), and platelet-derived growth factor regulator (Ek et al. 1982). However, no kinase activity associated with the *erb*-B proteins could be detected in the standard immune com-

A) Erb B CODES FOR A GROWTH FACTOR RECEPTOR

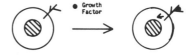

B) Erb B CODES FOR A MUTATED RECEPTOR THAT FUNCTIONS IN THE ABSENCE OF A GROWTH FACTOR

C) Erb B CODES FOR A RECEPTOR THAT FUNCTIONS ON INTERACTION WITH OTHER PLASMA MEMBRANE PROTEINS

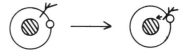

D) Erb B CODES FOR A SUBUNIT OF A GROWTH FACTOR RECEPTOR

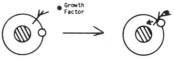

Figure 6 Hypothetical models for the mechanism of action of the *erb*-B protein.

plex assay. This does not mean that the *erb*-B protein could not function as a kinase under certain conditions, for example, in the presence of the correct growth factor. Even in the absence of any detectable kinase activity, these data strongly suggest that the *erb*-B gene product is related to some growth factor receptor, and they provide the possible models for function depicted in Figure 6. In model A, the gp74$^{erb\text{-}B}$ protein represents a growth factor receptor. In this case, the growth factor would come either from the serum in the tissue culture medium or would be released from the transformed cell. The target cell specificity of AEV could be addressed by this model: Perhaps only cells responsive to a second signal would be transformed by AEV, or, alternatively, only cells capable of synthesizing the correct growth factor would be transformed. In model B, the *erb*-B protein is a mutated form of a growth factor receptor that signals continued growth even in the absence of the correct growth factor. Mutation could either be caused by truncation of the protein or by single-base changes. Only cells that respond to this signal are transformed. In the third model, *erb*-B codes a receptor that functions only following interaction with another plasma membrane protein. This cellular protein would provide for the target cell specificity observed and could be either an intrinsic membrane protein or an extrinsic protein, perhaps on the cytoplasmic face of the membrane. Finally, in model D, which is a combination of models A and C, the *erb*-B protein interacts with another membrane protein to form a growth factor receptor, which subsequently interacts with the growth factor itself. Target cell specificity could be explained as in models A and C. We are currently devising experiments that hopefully will distinguish between these four models. In addition, we are trying to determine the role of *erb*-A in this process since presently none of these models addresses the role of this protein.

Acknowledgments

We are indebted to Gay Kitchener for her technical assistance and to Joyce Newton for typing the manuscript.

References

Beug, H., G. Doederlein, C. Freudenstein, and T. Graf. 1982. Erythroblast cell lines transformed by a temperature-sensitive mutant of avian erythroblastosis virus: A model system to study erythroid differentiation *in vitro*. *J. Cell. Physiol.* (suppl.) **1**: 195.

Bister, K. and P.H. Duesberg. 1979. Structure and specific sequences of avian erythroblastosis virus RNA; evidence for multiple classes of transforming genes among avian tumor viruses. *Proc. Natl. Acad. Sci.* **76**: 5023.

Cohen, S., G. Carpenter, and L.E. King. 1980. Epidermal growth factor-receptor protein kinase interactions. *J. Biol. Chem.* **255**: 4834.

Dyson, P.J., K. Quade, and J.A. Wyke. 1982. Expression of the ASV *src* gene in hybrids between normal and virally transformed cells: Specific suppression occurs in some hybrids but not others. *Cell* **30**: 491.

Ek, B., B. Westermark, A. Wasteson, and C-H. Heldin. 1982. Stimulation of tyrosine-specific phosphorylation by platelet-derived growth factor. *Nature* **295**: 419.

Frykberg, L., S. Palmieri, H. Beug, T. Graf, M.J. Hayman, and B. Vennstrom. 1983. Transforming capacities of avian erythroblastosis virus mutants deleted in the *erb* A or *erb* B oncogenes. *Cell* **32**: 227.

Fung, Y.K.T., W.G. Lewis, H-J. Kung, and L.B. Crittenden. 1983. Activation of the cellular oncogene c-*erb* B by LTR insertion: Molecular basis for induction of erythroblastosis by avian leukosis virus. *Cell* **33**: 357.

Graf, T., N. Ade, and H. Beug. 1978. Temperature sensitive mutant of avian erythroblastosis virus suggests a block of differentiation as mechanism of leukaemogenesis. *Nature* **257**: 496.

Hayman, M.J., B. Royer-Pokora, and T. Graf. 1979. Defectiveness of avian erythroblastosis virus: Synthesis of a 75K *gag*-related protein. *Virology* **92**: 31.

Hayman, M.J., G. Ramsay, K. Savin, G. Kitchener, T. Graf, and H. Beug. 1983. Identification and characterization of the avian erythroblastosis virus *erb* B gene product as a membrane glycoprotein. *Cell* **32**: 579.

Hihara, H., H. Yamamoto, H. Shimohira, K. Arai, and T. Shimizu. 1983. Avian erythroblastosis virus isolated from chicken erythroblastosis induced by lymphatic leukemia virus subgroup A. *J. Natl. Cancer Inst.* **70**: 891.

Kasuga, M., Y. Fijita-Yamaguchi, D.L. Blithe, and C.R. Kahn. 1983. Tyrosine-specific protein kinase activity is associated with the purified insulin receptor. *Proc. Natl. Acad. Sci.* **80**: 2137.

Lai, M.M.C., S.S.F. Hu, and P.K. Vogt. 1979. Avian erythroblastosis virus: Transformation-specific sequences form a contiguous segment of 3.25 kb located in the middle of the 6 kb genome. *Virology* **97**: 366.

Land, H., L.F. Parada, and R.A. Weinberg. 1983. Tumorigenic conversion of primary embryo fibroblasts requires at least two co-operating oncogenes. *Nature* **304**: 596.

Neil, J.C. 1983. Defective avian sarcoma viruses. *Curr. Top. Microbiol. Immunol.* **103**: 51.

Newbold, R.F. and R.W. Overell. 1983. Fibroblast immortality is a prerequisite for transformation by EJ.c-Ha-ras oncogene. *Nature* **304**: 648.

Owen, M.J., A.M. Kissonerghis, and H.F. Lodish. 1980. Biosynthesis of HLA-A and HLA-B antigens *in vivo*. *J. Biol. Chem.* **255**: 9678.

Palmieri, S., H. Beug, and T. Graf. 1982. Isolation and characterization of four new temperature-sensitive mutants of avian erythroblastosis virus (AEV). *Virology* **123**: 296.

Privalsky, M.L., L. Sealy, J.M. Bishop, J.P. McGrath, and A.D. Levinson. 1983. The product of the avian erythroblastosis virus *erb* B locus is a glycoprotein. *Cell* **32**: 1257.

Quade, K., S. Saule, D. Stehelin, G. Kitchener, and M.J. Hayman. 1983. Viral gene expression in rat cells transformed by avian myelocytomatosis MC29 and avian erythroblastosis virus. *J. Gen. Virol.* **64**: 83.

Roussel, M., S. Saule, C. Lagrou, C. Rommens, H. Beug, T. Graf, and D. Stehelin. 1979. Three new types of viral oncogene of cellular origin specific for haematopoietic cell transformation. *Nature* **281**: 452.

Ruley, H.E. 1983. Adenovirus early region 1A enables viral and cellular transforming genes to transform primary cells in culture. *Nature* **304**: 602.

Sefton, B.M., T. Hunter, and K.L. Beemon. 1980. Temperature-sensitive transformation by Rous sarcoma virus and temperature-sensitive protein kinase activity. *J. Virol.* **33**: 220.

Stehelin, D., S. Saule, M. Roussel, A. Sergeant, C. Lagrou, C. Rommens, and M.B. Raes. 1980. Three new types of viral oncogenes in defective avian leukemia viruses. 1. Specific nucleotide sequences of cellular origin correlate with specific transformation. *Cold Spring Harbor Symp. Quant. Biol.* **44**: 1215.

Tarentino, A.L. and F.L. Maley. 1974. Purification and properties of an endo-β-*N*-acetylglucosaminidase from *Streptomyces griseus*. *J. Biol. Chem.* **249**: 811.

Viral Integration and Early Gene Expression Both Affect the Efficiency of SV40-induced Transformation of Murine Cells: Biochemical and Biological Characterization of an SV40 Retrovirus

M. Kriegler, C. Perez, C. Hardy, and M. Botchan

Department of Molecular Biology, University of California, Berkeley, California 94720

The murine sarcoma viruses oncogenically transform rodent cells with very high efficiency. Indeed, transformation follows single-hit kinetics: One can readily transform an entire population of infected cells at low multiplicities of infection. In striking contrast, it is impossible to transform an entire population of infected cells with SV40 virus, even at multiplicities exceeding 10,000 plaque-forming units per cell, although, in stably transformed lines, a single integrated copy of the SV40 early region is sufficient for maintenance of the transformed phenotype.

It has been known for some time that infection of rodent cells with SV40 virus causes a large fraction of those cells to divide, transiently manifesting a morphological and characteristically oncogenic phenotype. Such cells are known to contain virally encoded T antigen as well. Therefore, we know that virtually all of the nuclei of the infected cells contain viral DNA. However, upon suspension in soft agar, the vast majority of these infected cells cease to retain the transformed phenotype and are termed abortive transformants. Abortive transformation is thought to occur as the result of the loss of the infecting viral genome. It is believed that the infecting viral genome of abortively transformed cells exists as an episome for a limited number of cell divisions and expresses the early-region genes, after which the episomal viral DNA is lost through dilution and degradation (Stoker 1968; Tooze 1973). However, a subpopulation of infected cells, usually less than 0.1%, continues to divide and form visible macrocolonies after a few weeks incubation in soft agar. These stable transformants have been shown to express the SV40 early gene products and are known to contain at least one complete copy of the SV40 early region (Botchan et al. 1976). In this paper, we have designed experiments to determine which parameters serve to limit the ability of SV40 to transform rodent cells in culture. We sought to determine if the following factors were responsible for the abortive phenotype: (1) stabilization of the viral genome in the nucleus of the infected cell via integration, (2) inefficient expression of the SV40 early genes, (3) cell competence, or (4) the fact that the SV40 early antigens were poor transforming proteins. Our initial studies employed an infectious SV40 recombinant virus containing a retroviral enhancer element inserted into the viral late region (SVLTR) and indicate that ineffective expression of the integrated intact SV40 early region(s) may be the cause of the abortive phenotype in approximately 10% of abortive transformants (Kriegler and Botchan 1982, 1983). We obtained further information about the biology of abortive transformation from cotransformation experiments with selectable and nonselectable marker DNAs. The experiments of ourselves and others (Wigler et al. 1979; Kriegler et al. 1983) indicate that cointegration, or genotypic cotransformation, occurs at a very high frequency (~80%). However, we and others observed that coexpression of the tk⁺ phenotype and the morphologically transformed phenotype (phenotypic cotransformation) occurred with low frequency (~5%) in cells cotransfected with both HSV-*tk* and SV40 DNAs (Hanahan et al. 1980; Perucho and Wigler 1980; Kriegler et al. 1983). In fact, 90–95% of the tk⁺ cotransfectants fail to express the SV40 early proteins when examined for T antigen immunofluoresence. Many of these T antigen-negative cotransfectants contain at least one, but in several cases multiple, intact copies of the SV40 early region (Hanahan et al. 1980; Kriegler et al. 1983).

These nontransformed tk⁺ cells, termed "cryptic transformants," serve to demonstrate that stable integration of an intact SV40 early transcription unit into the genome of the host cell is insufficient to insure stable expression of the SV40 early gene products. From these results, we concluded that abortive transformation is, in part, the consequence of a similar effect. We suggest that efficient expression of the integrated copy of the SV40 early region is an important factor that determines whether a cell becomes an abortive or a stable transformant. Our data strongly support the notion that the host chromosomal site of integration of the SV40 genome plays a vital role in determining whether or not the early genes are expressed in that cell. In addition, our results indicate that such "position effects" can be overcome through either the substitution of the endogenous SV40 promoter with a murine retroviral promoter or the supplementation of the endogenous SV40 enhancer-promoter assembly with a murine retroviral enhancer element (Kriegler et al. 1983). Although it is clear from our cotransfection studies that enhancer augmentation can serve to eliminate "cryptic transformation" during co-transfection of rodent cells. It is also clear from our studies of an infectious SV40 recombinant virus containing a retroviral enhancer element (SVLTR) that promoter enhancement alone was insufficient to entirely abolish abortive transformation. From these data, we concluded that during SV40 transformation of murine cells a second factor, probably viral integration, might be rate-limiting as well. To test this hypothesis, we employed a unique retrovirus vector and converted SV40 into an infectious, transforming retrovirus and thus exploited the highly efficient integration mechanism of the murine retroviruses. We now report the engineering of an SV40 retrovirus (MV40) with which we are able to abolish abortive transformation of rodent cells. The parental retroviral vector contains virtually no *gag-*, *pol-*, or *env*-encoding sequences and thus the transforming functions of the new retrovirus are solely SV40 derived. Transformation of both rat and mouse cells by MV40 is highly efficient, and foci are readily visible 6 days postinfection. Thus, it appears that: (1) the highly efficient integration mechanism of the murine retroviruses serves to stabilize the MV40 early-region genes into the host genome and (2) the promotion of the SV40 early region, lacking its own promoter, from a highly efficient retroviral promoter enables MV40 to transform tissue culture cells as efficiently as the murine sarcoma viruses. These data taken in toto indicate that both inefficient early gene expression and inefficient proviral integration are responsible for the abortively transformed phenotype and therefore for the poor transforming ability of SV40 virus.

Materials and Methods

Cells and viruses
Rat-2 (tk⁻) cells and Rat-1 Moloney leukemia virus producer cells were grown in Dulbecco's modified Eagle's essential medium (DMEM) containing 10% fetal calf serum (FCS) in a 5% CO^2-containing atmosphere. NIH-3T3 cells were grown in DMEM containing 10% calf serum (CS) in a 5% CO_2-containing atmosphere.

Generation of recombinant plasmid DNAs
Recombinant plasmid DNAs were transformed into *Escherichia coli* strains HB101 or DH1. Bacteria were grown in X-broth 50 μ/ml in ampicillin. Plasmid DNA was prepared according to the procedure of Birnboim and Doly (1979), banded twice in cesium chloride, and dialyzed into TE buffer (10 mM Tris [pH 7.4], 1 mM EDTA; see Kriegler and Botchan 1983).

Generation of recombinant SV40 virus stocks
Recombinant SV40 virus stocks were generated as described in Kriegler and Botchan (1983).

DNA transformation and cotransformation of Rat-2 (tk⁻) cells and Rat-1 Moloney leukemia virus producer cells
Calcium phosphate-mediated gene transfer was carried out by using the modification of the method of Graham and van der Eb developed by Wigler et al. (1978) for

preparing the DNA calcium phosphate coprecipitate as described in Kriegler et al. (1983). Drug selection of cells transfected with selectable marker genes was carried out as described in Kriegler et al. (1983).

T antigen immunofluorescence analysis of cotransfected cells
Cell colonies surviving exposure to selective media were stained in situ as described previously (Kriegler and Botchan 1983).

Quantitative immunoprecipitation analysis of in vivo-labeled SV40 T antigens
Quantitative immunoprecipitation analysis of in vivo labeled SV40 T antigens was carried out as described in Kriegler and Botchan (1983).

Results

An SV40 recombinant virus containing a retroviral enhancer element inserted into the late region transforms NIH-3T3 cells 10–20× as efficiently as SV40 wild type
In our first attempt to determine if viral integration is a rate-limiting step in SV40-induced morphological transformation of murine cells, we constructed a recombinant SV40 DNA containing a single permuted copy of the Harvey murine sarcoma virus (Ha-MSV) long terminal repeat (LTR) (Kriegler and Botchan 1983). This recombinant viral DNA was converted into an infectious SV40 viral particle through cotransfection of CV-1 (permissive) cells with cloned helper viral d1001 DNA (pd13). Our intent was to determine if the DNA sequence information within the LTR (permuted around the 3'–5' joint of a cloned, closed circular provirus containing two LTRs) was sufficient to drive proviral integration at the joint of the LTR. We postulated that more efficient proviral integration would result in more efficient transformation of murine cells by the new recombinant virus. We found that this hybrid virus, SVLTR1, transforms cells with 10–20 times the efficiency of SV40 wild type (Table 1). Unexpectedly, Southern blot analysis of SVLTR1 virus-transformed cell genomic DNAs revealed that simple integration of the viral DNA within the retroviral LTR could not account for the enhanced transformation capability of the recombinant virus (Kriegler and Botchan 1983). In fact, a restriction fragment derived from the SVLTR1 virus that contains an intact LTR was readily identified in a majority of the transformed cell DNAs. These results suggest that the LTR fragment that contains the attachment sites and flanking sequences for the proviral DNA duplex derived from a circular provirus may be insufficient to facilitate correct retrovirus integration and that some other functional element of the LTR, perhaps the promoter, was responsible for the increased transformation potential of this virus. To test this hypothesis, we found that a complete copy of the Ha-MSV LTR linked to well-defined structural genes lacking their own promoters (SV40 early region, thymidine kinase, G418 resistance, and dihydrofolate reductase) can be used effectively to promote marker gene expression. To de-

Table 1 Quantitation of Transforming Potential of SVLTR1 Virus on NIH-3T3 Cells

Virus	Colonies (no.) in soft agar		Increase relative to SV40 control (fold)
Experiment 1			
SV40 wild type	19		1
SVLTR1	121		6.37
Mock	1		0.05
Experiment 2			
SV40 wild type	9		1
SVLTR1	94		10.44
Mock	0		
Experiment 3[a]			
SV40 wild type	9	(10, 7, 4, 13, 11)	1
SVLTR1	163	(145, 184, 160)	18.1
SVLTRΔPRO	154.25	(154, 140, 175, 148)	17.13
Mock	3.6	(9, 1, 3, 2, 3)	0.43
Experiment 4[a]			
SV40 wild type	21.55	(24, 30, 11)	1
SVLTR1	207.6	(201, 207, 193, 224, 213)	9.58
SVLTRΔPRO	242.75	(242, 238, 251, 240)	11.20
Mock	4.5	(3, 5, 3, 7)	0.20

NIH-3T3 cells were plated at a density of 10^5 cells per 60-mm petri plate and infected with SV40 wild-type virus, SVLTR1 virus, or SVLTRΔPRO virus at equivalent multiplicities. At 24 hr postinfection, the cells were trypsinized, counted, and suspended in soft agar at 10^5 cells per dish. Four weeks later, the plates were photographed and the colonies were counted. The numbers of colonies counted on separate plates are shown for each experiment as is the average colony count of all the plates. (Reprinted, with permission, from Kriegler and Botchan 1983.)

[a] For experiments 3 and 4, the value given is the average colony count of plates shown in parentheses.

termine if the promoter element of the LTR served to enhance the biological activity of the recombinant virus described above, we deleted DNA sequences essential for promoter activity (between Xbal and Sac I; see Kriegler and Botchan 1983) within the LTR. SV40 virus stocks reconstructed with this mutated copy of the Harvey murine sarcoma virus LTR, lacking an effective promoter (SVLTRΔPRO), still transform murine cells at an enhanced frequency (Table 1). From these data, we speculate that when the LTR is placed more than 1.5 kb from the SV40 early promoter, a cis-acting enhancer element within the LTR can increase the ability of the SV40 promoter to operate effectively when integrated into a murine chromosome.

To analyze further the effects of a heterologous enhancer and/or promoter on SV40 gene expression, we employed a carefully characterized cotransformation assay.

Absolute and relative concentrations of selectable marker DNAs have a dramatic effect on the cotransformation index of the phenotypes conferred by those DNAs

Previous reports served to establish the analomous behavior of HSV-tk + SV40 DNA in cotransformation stud-

ies. When one seeks to determine the frequency of phenotypic cotransformation of the two marker genes at equimolar concentrations of HSV-tk and SV40 DNA, approximately 5% of the tk[+] colonies manifest the morphologically transformed phenotype (Hanahan et al. 1980; Perucho and Wigler 1980; Kriegler et al. 1983).

Early in our studies of this phenomenon, we determined that variation of two experimental parameters has a dramatic effect on the phenotypic cotransformation of HSV-tk and SV40 DNA in calcium phosphate-mediated gene transfer. The first parameter is the molar ratio of the two transfected marker DNAs. For example, transfection with a 20-fold molar excess of SV40 DNA relative to HSV-tk DNA will result in a high percentage of tk[+] colonies that manifest the morphologically transformed phenotype. Within a limited range, the significance of these ratios is independent of absolute concentrations. The second parameter is the absolute amount of the selectable marker DNAs transfected into the cells, even if both marker DNAs are present in equimolar amounts. For example, cotransfection of Rat-2 cells with a large amount (i.e., 10 μg) of each selectable marker DNA (essentially an equimolar ratio) also results in a high percentage of the cotransfected cells manifesting both the the tk[+] and the morphologically transformed phenotypes. These results imply that, in cell lines containing many independent insertions of SV40 DNA, cryptic phenotypic expression is low. We have found that the anomalous expression pattern of the SV40 genome in cotransfection experiments is highly reproducible under the following conditions. First, the studies must be conducted under conditions in which the transformation of Rat-2 (tk⁻) cells to the tk⁺ phenotype is linear with respect to plasmid input. This occurs within the range of 50–200 ng of input marker gene in the precipitates added to each plate. Second, in all experiments, input plasmid DNAs containing selectable marker genes were transfected in equimolar amounts. Therefore, none of our studies were done under conditions in which those cells competent for efficient DNA uptake were saturated for input DNA. Under these conditions, one can measure the effect of *cis*-acting elements that affect the level of stable transformation of selected marker DNAs.

Rat-2 cells cotransfected with three marker DNAs reveal an equivalent index of cotransformation

Rat-2 (tk⁻) cells were cotransfected under the nonsaturating conditions described above with various combinations of either cloned HSV-*tk* DNA, cloned G418 resistance DNA promoted from either the HSV-*tk* promoter or the Ha-MSV LTR (Kriegler and Botchan 1983; Kriegler et al. 1983), and/or a cloned, reconstructed Ha-MSV provirus (Kriegler et al. 1983). In our first experiment, those plates containing cells transfected with both HSV-*tk* DNA and the G418 resistance marker were first placed under HAT selection to measure the frequency of transformation to the tk⁺ phenotype. Once all the HAT-sensitive cells had been cleared from the transfected plate, the number of tk⁺ colonies was counted and recorded and the surviving colonies were tested for their ability to grow in media containing 400 μ/ml of G418. Ten to fourteen days later, those colonies that were both HAT resistant and G418 resistant were counted and recorded. The number of G418 + HAT-resistant colonies divided by the number of HAT-resistant colonies × 100 yielded the cotransformation index—in this experiment, 75% (Table 2). In our second experiment, cells transfected with HSV-*tk* DNA, the G418 resistance marker, and the complete cloned unpermuted Ha-MSV proviral DNA, pBVX (*ras*) (Kriegler et al. 1983), were first placed under HAT selection to measure the frequency of transformation to the tk⁺ phenotype. Once HAT selection was complete, the number of resistant

colonies was counted and recorded, after which the cells were placed under selection for G418 resistance. Ten to fourteen days later, the number of surviving colonies was counted and recorded, and 10% of the surviving colonies were picked randomly. Those colonies remaining on the dish were stained to ease visualization of those cells that were both HAT resistant, G418 resistant, and morphologically transformed. Visualization of the stained colonies indicated that approximately 80% of the HAT-resistant, G418-resistant cells were morphologically transformed (Table 2). However, this was not the case with HSV-*tk* + SV40 DNA cotransfection of Rat-2 cells where, under the same conditions, the index of phenotypic cotransformation is approximately 5–10%.

Promoter substitution and enhancer augmentation increase the phenotypic cotransformation index of HSV-*tk* + SV40 DNA to levels equivalent to those of HSV-*tk* + Ha-MSV proviral DNA

Rat-2 (tk⁻) cells were cotransfected with HSV-*tk* DNA and various SV40 recombinant plasmid DNAs, including (1) SV40 wild-type DNA cloned into pBR322 or pML (pJYI, pJYM), (2) a *Bgl*I – *Bam*HI linear of SV40 DNA promoted from either one or three retroviral LTRs (pRETRO T III, pRETRO T I), and (3) a *Hpa*II – *Bam*HI fragment of SV40 DNA containing an intact SV40 early transcription unit inserted into a Ha-MSV subgenomic clone in which a region known to be essential for efficient transcription from the retroviral LTR contained within this clone had been deleted, leaving behind a fragment of the LTR known to contain "enhancer" activity. In these plasmid subclones, the intact SV40 transcription unit was inserted either 5' or 3' to the retroviral enhancer element (pSVTE 5' LTR, pSVTE 3' LTR) (Kriegler et al. 1983).

The phenotypic cotransformation index of each of these SV40 recombinant plasmids was determined under the conditions described above. The results of five experiments are shown in Table 3. We summarize these results as follows: promotion of the SV40 early region from the promoter within the Ha-MSV LTR is sufficient to increase the index of cotransformation from approximately 5% to approximately 80%. Insertion of a fragment containing an intact SV40 early transcription unit (containing an intact SV40 enhancer-promoter assembly) either 5' or 3' to a retroviral enhancer element results in a similar increase in the cotransformation index (~ 80%). Thus, in this nonselective assay, we were able

Table 2 Cotransformation Analysis of Rat-2 Cells Cotransfected with HSV-*tk*, G418 Resistance, and Ha-MSV Proviral DNAs

	tk⁺ Colonies	Cotransformed colonies	Cotransformation percentage
tk⁺ DNA	135	N.A.	N.A.
tk⁺ DNA + pG418ʳ	124	93[a]	75.0
tk⁺ DNA + pG418ʳ + pBVX (*ras*)	115	83[a]/64[b]	72.17[a]/55.65[b]

[a]HAT- and G418-resistant colonies.
[b]HAT- and G418-resistant and morphologically transformed colonies.

Table 3 Cotransformation Analysis of Rat-2 Cells Cotransfected with Retro T and HSV-*tk* DNAs

	tk + Colonies	Morphologically transformed tk +	Cotransformation percentage
Experiment I			
SV40 + *tk* DNA	>100	5	<5
pBVX (Ha-MSV provirus) + *tk* DNA	93	76	81.7
pRETRO T + *tk* DNA	86	73	84.8
Experiment II			
SV40 + *tk* DNA	>100	7	<7
pBVX (Ha-MXV provirus) + *tk* DNA	85	75	88.2
pRETRO T + *tk* DNA	78	63	80.7
Experiment III			
SV40 + *tk* DNA	>100	9	<9
pBVX (Ha-MXV provirus) + *tk* DNA	113	88	77.8
pRETRO T + *tk* DNA	107	80	74.7
Experiment IV			
SV40 + *tk* DNA	>100	10	<10
pBVX (Ha-MXV provirus) + *tk* DNA	76	66	86.8
pRETRO T + *tk* DNA	74	57	77.0
pSVTE LTR 5′ + *tk* DNA	67	51	76.1
pSVTE LTR 3′ + *tk* DNA	64	47	73.4
Experiment V			
SV40 + *tk* DNA	>100	7	<7
pBVX (Ha-MSV provirus) + *tk* DNA	82	70	85.3
pRETRO T + *tk* DNA	78	67	85.8
pSVTE LTR 5′ + *tk* DNA	80	63	78.0
pSVTE LTR 3′ + *tk* DNA	85	72	84.7

to increase the efficiency of early-region transformation to levels equivalent to the Ha-MSV proviral DNA.

An infectious SV40 retrovirus transforms rodent cells with high efficiency and appears to abolish abortive transformation

An infectious SV40 retrovirus was generated as described below. *Bam*HI linkers were ligated to the *Bgl*I to *Hpa*I fragment lacking the SV40 promoter, spanning the SV40 early region through the stop codon but lacking the early-region polyadenylation signal. This *Bam*HI fragment was cloned into the unique *Bgl*II site of an 1197-bp retrovirus vector pEVX lacking virtually all *gag*-, *pol*-, and *env*-encoding sequences but containing many useful restriction sites for inserting genes of interest (Fig. 1; Kriegler et al., in prep.). The resultant construction, pEVX-T (Fig. 1) which fails to morphologically transform Rat-1 cells, was cotransfected into Rat-1 Moloney murine leukemia virus (Mo-MLV) producer cells with the retrovirus vector pEVX-G418 (Fig. 1) which confers resistance to the drug G418 and can be readily rescued as an infectious retrovirus itself (Kriegler et al., in prep.). G418-resistant colonies were isolated, expanded, and analyzed for T antigen production via immunofluorescence analysis. The supernatant from these G418-resistant, T

antigen-positive Mo-MLV producer Rat-1 cell lines was filtered and transferred to uninfected Rat-2 (tk⁻) cells and these cells were allowed to incubate for 10–14 days. Numerous foci were readily visible after 14 days. These foci were isolated, expanded, and analyzed for T antigen immunofluoresence. All were found to be brillantly positive and to exhibit classical nuclear fluoresence with nucleolar sparing and, unlike the parental cell line of the virus, HAT sensitive.

We next analyzed the ability of the transforming retrovirus, termed MV40, produced by this cell line to transform murine cells. We infected 1×10^4 NIH-3T3 cells with 1 ml of MV40 supernatant fluid derived from a 12-hour harvest. We concurrently infected 1×10^4 NIH-3T3 cells with SV40 wild-type virus at a multiplicity of infection (moi) of 1000 and suspended both populations of cells in soft agar. These soft agar suspensions were monitored for the appearance of microcolonies (abortive transformants) and macrocolonies (stable transformants). In the SV40-infected cultures, only 0.01–0.1% of the infected cells manifested the stably transformed phenotype. However, the majority of the cells in the MV40-infected culture were stably transformed. Therefore, the MV40 retrovirus transforms murine cells over two orders of magnitude more efficiently than the SV40

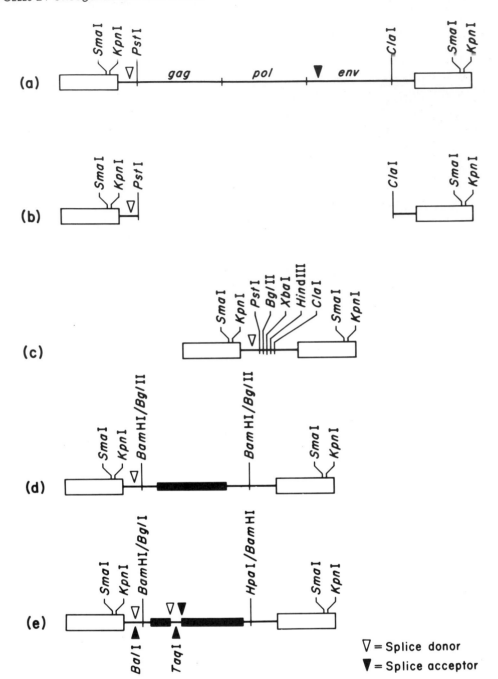

Figure 1 Schematic diagram detailing the assembly of retrovirus vector pEVX and the prototype proviral derivatives encoding the retroviruses EVX/G418 and EVX/T (MV40). (*A*) Schematic diagram of the Mo-MLV indicating the positions of *gag*-, *pol*-, and *env*-encoding sequences. (*B*) Restriction endonuclease digestion of the Mo-MLV provirus at *Pst*I and *Cla*I to assemble the retroviral vector pEVX. (*C*) Generation of pEVX through the insertion of a polylinker fragment (derived from plasmid πvx) into the *Pst*I and *Cla*I sites of the deleted Mo-MLV above to generate unique restriction sites permitting the insertion of genes and gene clusters of interest to obtain efficient expression and rescue of the retroviral chimeras as infectious viral particles. (*D*) Provirus EVX/G418: Insertion of a prototypical single exon-containing gene (the *Bgl*II fragment of the kanamycin-resistance marker derived from Tn5) inserted into the unique *Bgl*II site of pEVX. The inserted gene lacks its own promoter or polyadenylation signal (these signals are provided by the the retroviral vector itself). (*E*) Provirus EVX/T (MV40): Insertion of a prototypical multiple exon gene (the *Bgl*I to *Hpa*I fragment of the SV40 early region spanning the entire SV40 early region but lacking the SV40 promoter, T antigen-binding sites I and II, and the SV40 polyadenylation signal. Again, the promoter and polyadenylation signals are provided by the retrovirus vector itself inserted into the unique *Bgl*II site of pEVX.

DNA virus even when the DNA virus is applied at an moi of 1000. When one isolated Rat-2 (tk⁻) cell line (EVXπ2) transformed by MV40 was subjected to Southern blot analysis, it was found to contain a single copy of the integrated MV40 retrovirus provirus (Kriegler et al., in prep.). Quantitative immunoprecipitation analysis of the large T antigen in this cell line indicated that this cell line contains large T antigen that is virtually indistinguishable from that of SV40-transformed cells and that MV40-transformed cell lines contain 5–10× the amount of large T antigen present in cells transformed by SV40 virus (Fig. 2).

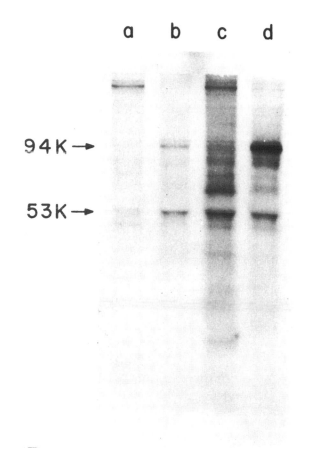

Figure 2 Quantitative immunoprecipitation analysis of T antigens encoded by SV40- and MV40-transformed rodent cells. Various cell lines were plated at 1×10^5 cells per 60-mm petri plate, incubated for 1 hr in methionine minus free medium, and labeled for 2 hr with 100 μCi of [^{35}S]methionine (400 Ci/mM). The labeled cells were harvested and lysed in immunoprecipitation buffer (Kriegler and Botchan 1983). Incorporated counts were measured and equivalent amounts of trichloracetic acid-precipitable counts were treated with anti-hamster tumor antiserum and protein A-Sepharose beads (Pharmacia). Immunoprecipitated proteins were eluted and subjected to electrophoresis in a 12% polyacrylamide gel. An autoradiogram of that gel is shown above. (Lane a) Rat-2 (tk⁻); (lane b) SV40-1 (an SV40 virus-transformed NIH-3T3 cell line containing a single copy of the SV40 genome); (lane c) MLV3B (the parental cell line of the original MV40 virus isolates); and (lane d) EVXπ2 (a RAT-2 [tk⁻] cell line transformed by the MV40 retrovirus (containing a single proviral insertion of the MV40 genome). The arrows indicate the position of stained protein markers. Authentic large T antigen migrates at 94K. The intensity of the 94K bands directly reflects the relative percentage of the total amount of radioactive methionine actually incorporated into large T antigen in one cell line relative to the others indicated the position of authentic 94K SV40 large T antigen.

Discussion

Our initial experiments were designed to determine if, during nonproductive infection of rodent cells, stabilization via integration of the SV40 viral genome into the genome of the host cell was a rate-limiting step in SV40-induced morphologic transformation. We attempted to incorporate the specialized integration apparatus of the murine retroviruses into the genome of a recombinant SV40 virus. To accomplish this, we inserted a single copy of a retroviral LTR permuted around the 5′–3′ joint derived from a cloned circular provirus containing two LTRs into the late region of an SV40 recombinant molecule. We rescued this defective virus with the appropriate nontransforming helper viral DNA. If viral integration were rate limiting and if the DNA duplex retroviral LTR joint fragment were sufficient to drive proviral integration, then we might expect to observe more efficient morphologic transformation of murine cells by the SV40/LTR (SVLTR) recombinant virus when compared with wild type. In fact, the SV40/LTR (SVLTR) recombinant virus does transform cells with higher efficiency. However, the enhanced transformation phenotype was not due to retroviruslike integration within the LTR (Kriegler and Botchan 1982, 1983). It appears to be due to an enhancer element within the LTR (Kriegler and Botchan 1982, 1983; Laimins et al. 1982; Luciw et al. 1983), a contention that was strongly supported by calcium phosphate-mediated gene transfer experiments. These experiments were designed to characterize more completely calcium phosphate-mediated cotransfection in an attempt to use the assay to determine why SV40 + HSV-*tk* cotransfection of murine cells gives a high index of genotypic cotransformation but a surprisingly low index of phenotypic cotransformation.

Initially, we observed that the variation of two experimental parameters can have a dramatic effect on the efficiency of phenotypic cotransformation of a variety of selectable marker DNAs (HSV-*tk*, G418 resistance, various retrovirus proviruses, etc.). First, the molar ratios of the cotransfected DNAs are very important. A high molar excess of one DNA relative to the other can dramatically skew the cotransformation index in favor of the overrepresented DNA. Second, saturation of the transfection potential of a given plate of Rat-2 (tk⁻) cells with microgram quantities of two selectable marker DNAs, even if they are present in equimolar amounts, will insure a cotransformation index of 80%, minimizing the effect of any *cis*-acting control element linked to the structural gene of interest. Because we set out to study such *cis*-acting control elements, all experiments were designed to eliminate the effect of these variables.

Under such conditions, with all but one selectable marker plasmid DNA we have studied, the absolute number of cells phenotypically transformed is linear with respect to plasmid input. Under these conditions, we found that phenotypic cotransformation of cells with two selectable marker DNAs present in equimolar amounts is roughly 80% and that phenotypic cotransformation with three selectable marker DNAs is roughly 80% of 80%, or 60% (Kriegler et al. 1983). Thus, it was surprising that we and others (Hanahan et al. 1980; Kriegler et al. 1983) found that, under identical conditions, whereas genotypic cotransformation of murine cells with HSV-*tk* and SV40 DNA is quite high, phenotypic cotransformation of the cells is very low with 5–10% of the tk⁺ transformants manifesting the morphologically transformed phenotype. From unpublished data based upon virus rescue (J. Miller et al.) and blot data previously reported (Hanahan et al. 1980), essentially all SV40 + *tk* cotransfected lines contain integrated SV40 DNA. Why is SV40 DNA different from other marker DNAs? Evidence from our laboratory suggests that specific marker genes require more efficient transcription than other marker genes to manifest their phenotype. For example, conversion of a given cell from the tk⁻ or G418-sensitive phenotype to the tk⁺ (HAT-resistant) or G418-resistant phenotype requires the presence of but a few RNA molecules per cell. In contrast, relatively high amounts of SV40 T antigen protein and its appropriate RNA are necessary to manifest the morphologically transformed phenotype (Kriegler et al., in prep.). We believe that herein lies the essential difference between SV40 DNA and other marker DNAs. Because we have demonstrated that during calcium phosphate-mediated gene transfer integration of cotransfected marker DNAs occurs at high efficiency, in these studies we were able to eliminate the effect of those factors that serve to stabilize integration of the viral DNA on phenotypic transformation and focus on the roles that gene expression and cell competence play. The observation that genotypic cotransformation occurs at much higher frequency than phenotypic cotransformation (as measured by Southern blot analysis and T antigen immunofluorescence) supports the notion that inefficient SV40 transformation of murine cells is the result of inefficient gene expression. The observation that substitution of the retroviral promoter for the SV40 promoter or augmentation of the SV40 enhancer with the retroviral enhancer serves to increase the level of phenotypic cotransformation by the SV40 *A* gene to levels equivalent to those of other selectable marker genes further strengthens this argument. These enhancer elements may (1) alter the expression of linked genes by either providing a site for entry of factors that are required for efficient promotion of transcription or (2) provide a *cis*-acting signal that actively prevents a promoter from being shut off. In either case, markers that require relatively high levels of transcription to manifest their phenotype would be more likely to work in a given chromosomal domain when linked to a potent enhancer than would such a marker lacking the enhancer element.

These results may serve to explain, in part, the biology of SV40 abortive transformation of murine cells. It has long been assumed that infected cells appear to be abortively transformed because the unintegrated infective viral DNA is lost through dilution and degradation and therefore fails to establish itself through stable integration into the genome of the host cell (Tooze 1973). Such a mechanism would explain why SV40 is such a poor transforming virus. In contrast, the transforming retro-

viruses are more efficient transforming agents because they contain a highly efficient integration mechanism. If this notion is correct, then stable integration of an intact SV40 early region into the host genome of an infected or transfected cell should be sufficient to transform a cell. The effect of retroviral enhancer sequences upon SV40 cotransformation argues that, in at least a fraction of the abortively transformed cells, effective expression of the early antigens plays a role as well.

We and others (Hanahan et al. 1980; Kriegler et. al. 1983) have shown that genotypic cotransformation of cells occurs with high efficiency. In most cases, high genotypic cotransformation is associated with a high phenotypic transformation index. However, the high index of genotypic cotransformation of HSV-*tk* and SV40 DNA is not associated with a high index of phenotypic cotransformation and therefore appears to mimic the phenomenon of abortive transformation in that a high percentage of infected or transfected cells pick up the infected or transfected viral DNA but only a minority of those cells stably express the transformed phenotype. As the phenotypic cotransformation index goes up relatively by a factor of 10 upon insertion of a retroviral enhancer element into the SV40 constructions, we argue that only one in ten random insertions of SV40 lead to effective gene expression. Therefore, stable integration of wild-type SV40 DNA into the host genome is by itself insufficient to insure that the cell carrying the integrated DNA will become transformed. Efficient gene expression is necessary since *cis*-acting elements that promote efficient gene expression enhance the penetration of the *A* gene in these transfection studies.

Efficient expression and rescue of multiple exon-containing genes such as the SV40 *A* gene is dramatically affected by the choice of retroviral vector as well. For example, we have found that our Ha-MSV-derived expression-rescue vectors function far more efficiently than our seemingly identical Mo-MLV- or Mo-MSV-derived retroviral vectors. We have found that this difference appears to be due to the fact that, unlike the Mo-MLV or the Mo-MSV, the Ha-MSV no longer carries a functional splice donor. The sequence AGGT has been altered to AGGC in the Ha-MSV (Kriegler et al., in prep.). We hypothesize that in our Mo-MLV- and Mo-MSV-derived vectors aberrant splicing between the Moloney-derived splice donor and the splice acceptor(s) of the multiple exon genes to be expressed and rescued occurs and effectively lowers the yield of biologically active RNA. However, in our Ha-MSV-derived vectors, aberrant splicing between the mutated, nonfunctional Ha-MSV splice donor and the splice acceptors of the multiple exon gene to be expressed and rescued cannot occur. The result is a higher yield of biologically active translational templates and more efficient expression (Kriegler et al., in prep.).

In Ha-MSV, it appears as if the splice donor has been destroyed as the result of a completed splicing event between Mo-MLV sequences carrying a functional splice donor (AGGT) and cell-derived (VL30) sequences. Furthermore, the sequence AGGC characteristic of a completed splice donor-splice acceptor interaction, is found in the Ha-MSV (Kriegler et al., in prep.). In support of this contention, we have found that DNA sequences upstream of the mutated splice donor are derived from the Mo-MLV, whereas DNA sequences downstream of the mutated splice donor appear to be cell derived. In other studies, we have found that sequences essential for efficient rescue of the Ha-MSV lie within these cell-derived sequences. Deletion of these sequences destroys the ability of Mo-MLV to rescue the mutated Ha-MSV but has no effect on the ability of this deleted Ha-MSV proviral DNA to transform rodent cells by DNA transfection (Kriegler et al., in prep.).

However, as described above, it is possible to rescue a high-titer recombinant retrovirus containing a multiple exon gene with our Mo-MLV derived vector. We postulate that the appearance of this transforming virus in the supernatant of a nontransformed cell line is the result of a point mutation or rearrangement that occurred during transcription or reverse transcription of the viral RNA. Such a rearrangement would destroy the Mo-MLV-derived splice donor, thus eliminating aberrant splicing events, and allow for efficient expression of the early region. Our studies with such an engineered SV40 retrovirus, MV40, show that the SV40 *A* gene is capable of complete acute transformation of 100% of the cells receiving the gene by an appropriate vector. Indeed, MV40 transforms murine cells at least two orders of magnitude more efficiently than SV40. From our earlier studies of the SV40/LTR recombinant DNA viruses (SVLTR1 and SVLTRΔPRO), it is clear that only 1% of the enhanced transformation property of MV40 can be attributed to so-called enhancer effects. The major effect of conversion of SV40 into an infectious retrovirus may be due to more efficient stabilization via integration as a retrovirus of the proviral genome in the nucleus of the infected cell or to more efficient transcription, or both. The observation that MV40-transformed cells form foci 2–3× more rapidly than SV40-transformed cells may be due to the fact that MV40-infected cells produce 5–10× the amount of SV40 large T antigen when compared with their SV40-transformed counterparts. In any case, it is clear from the data presented above that both inefficient proviral integration and inefficient early gene expression are responsible for the abortively transformed phenotype and therefore for the poor transforming ability of SV40 virus.

References

Birnboim, H.C. and J. Doly. 1979. A rapid alkaline extraction procedure for screening recombinant plasmid DNA. *Nucleic Acids Res.* **7:** 1513.

Botchan, M., W.C. Topp, and J. Sambrook. 1976. The arrangement of simian virus 40 sequences in the DNA of transformed cells. *Cell* **9:** 269.

Hanahan, D., D. Lane, L. Lipsich, M. Wigler, and M. Botchan. 1980. Characteristics of an SV40-plasmid recombinant and its movement into and out of the genome of a murine cell. *Cell* **21:** 127.

Kriegler, M. and M. Botchan. 1982. A retroviral LTR contains a new type of eukaryotic regulatory element. In *Eukaryotic viral vectors* (ed. Y. Gluzman), p. 171. Cold Spring Harbor Laboratory, Cold Spring Harbor, New York.

———. 1983. Enhanced transformation by a simian virus 40 recombinant virus containing a Harvey murine sarcoma virus long terminal repeat. *Mol. Cell. Biol.* **3:** 325.

Kriegler, M., C. Perez, and M. Botchan. 1983. Promoter substitution and enhancer augmentation increases the penetrance of the SV40 A gene to levels comparable to that of the Harvey murine sarcoma virus *ras* gene in morphologic transformation. *UCLA Symp. Mol. Cell. Biol.* **8:** 107.

Laimins, L.A., G. Khoury, C. Gorman, B. Howard, and P. Gruss. 1982. Host specific activation of transcription by tandem repeats from simian virus 40 and Moloney murine sarcoma virus. *Proc. Natl. Acad. Sci.* **79:** 6453.

Luciw, P.A., J.M. Bishop, H.E. Varmus, and M.R. Capecchi. 1983. Location and function of retroviral and SV40 sequences that enhance biochemical transformation after microinjection of DNA. *Cell* **33:** 705.

Perucho, M. and M. Wigler. 1980. Linkage and expression of foreign DNA in cultured animal cells. *Cold Spring Harbor Symp. Quant. Biol.* **44:** 829.

Stoker, M. 1968. Abortive transformation by polyoma virus. *Nature* **218:** 234.

Tooze, J. 1973. *The molecular biology of tumor viruses.* Cold Spring Harbor Laboratory, Cold Spring Harbor, New York.

Wigler, M.A., A. Pellicer, S. Silverstein, and R. Axel. 1978. Biochemical transfer of single copy eukaryotic genes using total cellular DNA as a donor. *Cell* **14:** 729.

Wigler, M., R. Sweet, G.K. Sim, B. Wold, A. Pellicer, E. Lacy, T. Maniatis, S. Silverstein, and R. Axel. 1979. Transformation of mammalian cells with genes from procaryotes. *Cell* **16:** 777.

Influence of Genetic, Cellular, and Hormonal Factors on Simian Virus 40-induced Transformation

J.M. Pipas, L.C. Chiang, and D.W. Barnes
Department of Biological Sciences, University of Pittsburgh, Pittsburgh, Pennsylvania 15260

The large T antigen of SV40 is capable of inducing neoplastic transformation in different cell types of a variety of species (Tooze 1981). A number of assays have been developed to probe the effects of this protein on cell biology and to ascertain which parameters are critical to the process of neoplastic transformation. These assays have led to the definition of a series of biological activities that have been ascribed to T antigen. Among these are the ability to stimulate cellular DNA synthesis, to activate the transcription of silent rRNA genes, and to help human adenoviruses grow in monkey cells. In addition, T antigen is responsible for initiating, and in many cases for maintaining, the multiple alterations in cellular physiology that accompany transformation. These include: a lowered serum dependence in culture; acquisition of the ability to form foci on a monolayer of normal cells; acquisition of the ability to form colonies in soft agar; and increased tumorigenic potential in test animals. In addition, T antigen is capable of "immortalizing" cells from primary cultures.

The mechanism by which this single protein induces such varied and profound effects on cellular functions has been the subject of intense study by several laboratories. Our initial approach to this problem was to isolate a series of viral deletion mutants that synthesize altered T antigens and to assess their biological and biochemical activities (Clark et al. 1983; Pipas et al. 1983; Soprano et al. 1983). These studies demonstrated that some of T antigen's activities were lost coordinately with mutation whereas others retained a degree of independence. For example, the ability to stimulate cellular DNA synthesis requires only the aminoterminal 272 residues (there are 708 in the wild-type protein), and a fragment 509 amino acids long is capable of activating rRNA gene transcription. On the other hand, three T antigen functions, namely, the ATPase activity, the viral DNA replication function, and the ability to transform the rat cell line REF52, require all but the carboxyterminal region of T antigen and were inactivated coordinately by mutation. In other studies, several groups have reported the isolation of mutants that have lost the ability to replicate viral DNA but are still competent for transformation, indicating that these activities too can be uncoupled (Gluzman and Ahrens 1982; Stringer 1982; S. Pearson-White and D. Nathans, pers. comm.; K. Peden, pers. comm.). This type of analysis has led to the hypothesis that T antigen possesses multiple biochemical activities, some of which act independently to initiate specific changes in cellular physiology.

The availability of a series of T antigen mutations, each expressing a different set of activities, allows new approaches to the problem of virus-cell interactions. Two such approaches are described in this paper. First, we have begun to examine the ability of T antigen mutants to transform a number of different cell lines. The goal here is to identify cell types that by virtue of their genetic background, state of differentiation, or passage history, require only a subset of T antigen's activities to be transformed. In the second approach, we have initiated studies on the response to SV40 infection of cells maintained in serum-free media. These studies are designed to define the manner in which viral infection and transformation alter the responses of cells to environmental factors and the manner in which the hormonal environment of the cells affects its ability to express a transformed phenotype.

Materials and Methods

SV40 viral stocks
The growth and titrating of the small-plaque strain of SV40 on BSC40 cells has been described (Brockman et al. 1973). Serum-free stocks were prepared by passaging the virus on BSC40 cells, maintained in a basal nutrient medium consisting of a one to one mixture of Ham's F12 and Dulbecco's modified Eagle's medium, supplemented with 15 mM HEPES (pH 7.4), 1.2 g/liter sodium bicarbonate, and antibiotics (F12:DME). The serum-free stock was titered as usual.

SV40 mutants
The isolation and characterization of T antigen deletion mutants has been described (Pipas et al. 1983). Mutant DNA was molecularly cloned into pBR322 via the BamHI site and propagated in Escherichia coli as the chimeric plasmid. pSVB3 is the wild-type parental SV40 strain cloned in pBR322 (Peden et al. 1980).

Cell culture
The established rat embryo fibroblast cell line REF52 was the gift of W. Topp (Cold Spring Harbor Laboratory). The C3H 10T1/2 line was originally established in the laboratory of Dr. C. Heidelberger (Reznikoff et al. 1973) and was kindly supplied by Dr. L. Sompayrac (University of Colorado).

Procedures for the development of the serum-free media for the 10T1/2 line, routine growth of cells in these media, and maintenance and storage of medium supplements are essentially as described for other media and lines and have been reviewed previously (Barnes and Sato 1980a,b). For the initiation of experiments, cells grown in serum-containing medium (F12:DME supplemented with 10% fetal calf serum) were trypsinized, treated with trypsin inhibitor, and replated in the indicated media at 2×10^4 cells per 35-mm plate. Final concentrations of bovine insulin (Sigma), human transferrin (Sigma), human plasma fibronectin (Meloy Laboratories), and mouse epidermal growth factor (Collaborative Research) were 10 μg/ml, 30 μg/ml, 10 μg/ml, and 10 ng/ml, respectively. For determination of cell number, cells were trypsinized and suspensions were counted in a Coulter particle counter.

Transformation

REF52 cells or 10T1/2 cells were seeded into 5-cm dishes at approximately 2×10^4 cells per dish. The calcium phosphate procedure of Graham and van der Eb (1973) was used for transfection of cells with mutant DNAs. Triplicate dishes were treated with 1 μg or 20 μg of recombinant plasmid and fed every 4 days with minimum essential medium plus 10% fetal bovine serum. Foci were generally visible by 2 weeks posttransfection. In cases where the results were negative, dishes were observed for an additional 4 weeks to score any slowly developing foci.

Indirect immunofluorescence

Cells growing in chamber slides were fixed in ice-cold ethanol and stained with hamster anti-T serum (Pope and Rowe 1964).

Results

Transformation by SV40 T antigen mutants is cell-line dependent

Our previous studies with SV40 deletion mutants indicated that the transformation function was sensitive to mutation in nearly all portions of the molecule (Pipas et al. 1983). Mutations near the carboxyl terminus left this activity intact, but in-frame deletions near the amino terminus as well as the central portion of the molecule were inactive as were frameshift mutations that synthesized altered T antigens of 590 residues or less. Many of these transformation-negative mutants retained other activities of T antigen. These results were not consistent with a report by Sompayrac et al. (1983) which indicated F8dl, a deletion mutant that expresses a fragment less than 40% the size of wild-type T antigen, transforms the C3H mouse 10T1/2 line with a low but measurable frequency. To determine if these disparate results were due to differences in the cell lines used, we performed parallel transformation assays on REF52 and 10T1/2 cells using the deletion mutants listed in Table 1.

Wild-type SV40 (pSV-B3) transforms the two cell types with comparable frequencies (Table 1). However, several mutants that synthesize T antigens shortened from the carboxyl terminus or internally transform 10T1/2 but not REF52 cells (dl1138, dl1001, dl1055, dl1061, dl1135, dl1047, dl1151). Finally mutants that produce a short (39-residue) aminoterminal fragment of T antigen (dl1042), or alter the early-region mRNA splice signals (dl1136) fail to transform either REF52 or 10T1/2 cells, indicating that expression of a T antigen fragment may be necessary for the transformation of 10T1/2 cells.

Several of the wild-type and mutant-induced foci were picked using a cloning cylinder and then twice recloned. Immmunofluorescent staining of these lines with anti-T hamster serum revealed two types of staining patterns. Cells transformed with wild-type, dl1066, or dl1140 showed the typical strong nuclear fluorescence with little or no staining of the cytoplasm (Fig. 1a). Note that these same mutants are also capable of transforming REF52 where a similar fluorescent pattern is seen (data not shown). On the other hand, cells transformed by dl1138,

Table 1 Transformation of REF52 and 10T1/2 Cells by SV40 T Antigen Mutants

Plasmid	Nucleotides deleted[a]	Amino acid residues deleted	Efficiency of transformation (foci/μg)	
			REF52	10T1/2
Mock	—	—	< 0.05	<0.05
pBR322	—	—	< 0.05	<0.05
pSV-B3	—	—	49.6	63.4
pdl1136	5067–4262	33–708[c]	< 0.05	<0.05
pdl1042	5046–4980	40–708[c]	< 0.05	<0.05
pdl1138	4339–4311	161–708	< 0.05	6.9
pdl1001	4002–3476	273–708	< 0.05	1.6
pdl1055	3620–3566	400–708	< 0.05	0.7
pdl1061	3048–2907	591–708	< 0.05	5.2
pdl1066	2809–2730	671–708	51.7	4.8
pdl1135	5114–5082	17– 27	< 0.05	14.0
pdl1047	4007–3570	271–416	< 0.05	8.7
pdl1151	3798–3472	341–449	< 0.05	4.1
pdl1140	2792–2763	676–685	54.0	6.8

[a]Data from Pipas et al. (1983).
[b]Predicted from DNA sequence.
[c]The predicted peptide has not been detected.

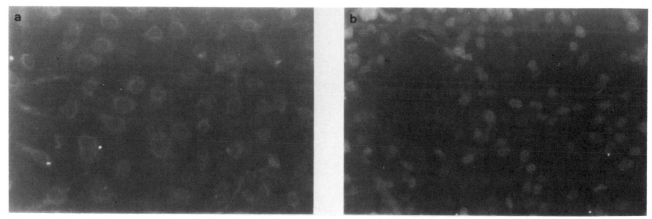

Figure 1 Immunofluorescent staining for T antigen of SV40 wild-type (*a*) or *dl*1135 transformed (*b*) 10T1/2 cells.

*dl*1001, *dl*1055, *dl*1061, *dl*1135, *dl*1047, and *dl*1151 show a pattern similar to that seen in Figure 1b. The nucleus is dark, but there is intense staining of the cytoplasm. We are currently undertaking experiments to determine whether this cytoplasmic fluorescence is due to the mutant large T antigen fragment, or to an overproduction of small T antigen. In any event, the ability of SV40 T antigen mutants to transform, as measured by the dense-focus assay, is clearly dependent on the cell line assayed.

C3H 10T1/2 cells grown in serum-free medium

To study the manner in which SV40 infection and transformation alter cellular growth factor requirements, we developed a serum-free medium capable of supporting the growth of 10T1/2 cells. This medium consists of basal salts and nutrients supplemented with four factors: insulin, transferrin, fibronectin, and epidermal growth factor (EGF) (Fig. 2). 10T1/2 cells plated in this medium reach the same saturation density as those growing in medium supplemented with 10% FCS, but do so with a

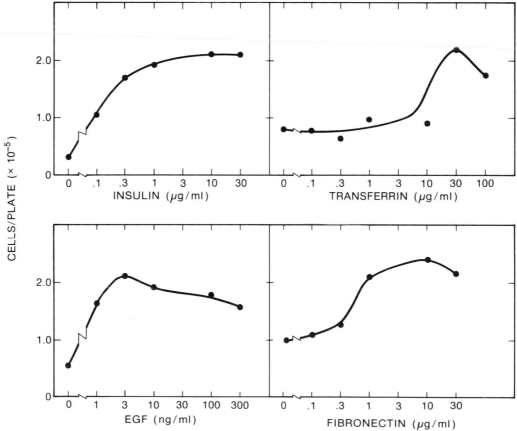

Figure 2 Dose-response of 10T1/2 cells to basal nutrient medium supplements. Cells were plated (2 × 10⁴ cells/35-mm dish) in media containing constant amounts of three factors while the concentration of the fourth was varied. Optimum concentrations of insulin, transferrin, EGF, and fibronectin were determined by a 6-day growth-response assay.

slower doubling time. The medium will not support the growth of 10T1/2 cells at clonal density.

Optimal mitogenic dose for each of the four factors was determined by measuring the response of 10T1/2 cells to different concentrations of each of the four supplements. Thus, insulin and fibronectin were used at 10 μg/ml, transferrin at 30 μg/ml, and EGF at 10 ng/ml. The relative importance of each factor to the growth of 10T1/2 cells can be determined by experiments in which each supplement is omitted individually from the complete serum-free medium. The results of such an experiment are shown in Figure 3. Cells growing in the presence of all four factors reach saturation after 11 days (initial plating density of 2×10^4 cells/35-mm dish) versus 7 days for cells growing in medium supplemented with 10% FCS. At this initial density, cells plated in the absence of any supplements do not survive. Furthermore, cell growth is severely restricted by the absence of either insulin or EGF. Less dramatic, but measurable, restrictions also occur in the absence of transferrin or fibronectin.

Response of 10T1/2 cells maintained in serum-free medium to SV40 infection

We next measured the response to SV40 infection of 10T1/2 cells maintained in serum-free medium with all four supplements or its growth-restrictive, "minus-one supplement" derivatives. Cells were seeded to 35-mm dishes (2×10^4 cells/dish), infected with serum-free virus stock (moi = 100), and maintained in the appropriate test medium. The results of such an experiment are shown in Figure 4. Viral infection does not improve the growth or survival of cells plated in basal nutrient medium in the absence of all of the four supplements, these being severely growth restricted as in the case of mock-infected cells. When the effects are examined of the in-

dividual deletion of various supplements on SV40-infected and mock-infected cells, it is seen that the relative order of importance of individual factors does not change, but that in each case more cells are present in the infected dishes. Furthermore, the degree to which viral infection overcomes the growth restriction of cells in the absence of a given factor varies depending on the factor deleted. These points are illustrated in Figure 5, which compares cell number for mock- and virus-infected dishes at day 11 after infection for each of the media used. In most cases, viral infection results in a two- to three-fold increase in cell number over mock-infected cultures. The largest difference in growth response between SV40-infected and mock-infected cultures was obtained with cells maintained in the absence of EGF where an eightfold difference in cell number was observed following SV40 infection.

The mechanism by which SV40 infection increases cell number in these various media is not clear. Nor is it clear why the relative effect of infection is greater with media lacking EGF. One possibility is that some SV40 gene product, perhaps T antigen, either possesses an activity that replaces EGF, or converts the cell to a state in which it requires little or no EGF for growth. In any event, these observations raised the possibility that individual deletions of each of these four supplements from complete serum-free medium could be used as growth-restrictive conditions to allow the selection of SV40 transformants following viral infection.

Cell populations selected following SV40 infection

To determine if the growth-restrictive conditions described above would allow the selection of SV40 transformants, we performed the following experiment. 10T1/2 cells were infected with serum-free virus stock (moi = 100) or mock-infected and maintained in complete or

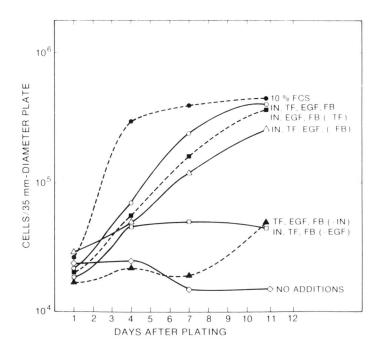

Figure 3 Growth curves of 10T1/2 cells in basal nutrient media containing various supplements. Cell number was determined periodically following plating in media supplemented with 10% fetal calf serum (●); the four required factors (○) insulin (IN), fibronectin (FB), transferrin (TF), and epidermal growth factor (EGF); three of the four factors: −FB (△), −TF (■), −IN (▲), and −EGF (□); or no supplements (◇).

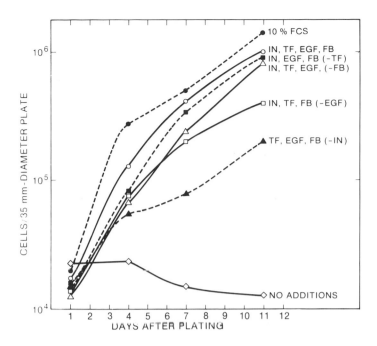

Figure 4 Growth curves of SV40-infected 10T1/2 cells in media containing various supplements. Same as Fig. 3 except cells were infected with SV40 serum-free virus stock (moi = 100) at initiation of the experiment.

growth-restrictive, serum-free media devised by the individual deletion of each of the four supplements for 3 months with periodic passaging.

This resulted in the establishment of six independent cell populations, each derived under different selection conditions. These included: SV (4F), SV40-infected cells selected in serum-free medium containing all four supplements; SV(−FB), SV40-infected cells maintained in the absence of fibronectin; SV(−TF), SV40-infected cells maintained in the absence of transferrin; SV(−EGF), infected cells maintained in the absence of EGF; M(−FB), mock-infected cells maintained in the absence of fibronectin; M(−TF), mock-infected cells maintained without transferrin; and mock-infected cells carried in the presence

of all four factors, M(4F). Viral or mock-infected cells carried in the absence of insulin, as well as mock-infected cells carried without EGF, failed to yield surviving cell populations upon extended culture.

The properties of these cell populations, as determined after 3 months of serum-free culture, are compared with the parental line (10T1/2) or a prototype wild-type SV40 transformant originally isolated as a dense focus in 10% FCS (SV10T1/2-1) in Table 2. No T antigen-positive cells were detected among the SV40-infected cell population maintained in the absence of transferrin, or in any of the mock-infected cell populations. All of the cells in the SV(−EGF) population gave a uniformly weak but positive nuclear fluorescence (Fig.

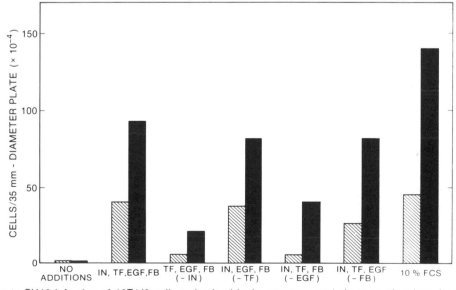

Figure 5 Response to SV40 infection of 10T1/2 cells maintained in the presence and absence of various factors. Data are taken from day 11 of Figs. 3 and 4.

6). The SV(4F) and SV(−FB) populations contained 81% and 39% T antigen-positive cells. In these cases, the fluorescent staining was indistinguishable from the prototype line SV10T1/2-1.

The saturation densities in 1% and 10% FCS as well as the plating efficiency in agarose are also listed for each cell population in Table 2. All of the populations maintained for 3 months in serum-free media grew to higher saturation densities in both 1% and 10% FCS than the parental 10T1/2 line. In comparing these results to the parental line or to the prototype SV40 transformant, one must keep in mind that these cell lines are uncloned from the time of infection and the saturation densities listed in at least some cases are the result of a mixed population of cells with regard to T antigen expression and, probably, with regard to growth characteristics also. Nevertheless, passage through serum-free media seems to select for cells with higher saturation densities, and this phenomenon is not related to

viral infection. When these cell populations were tested for the ability to grow independently of anchorage, it was found that only the SV(1F) and SV(−FB) were capable of doing so. In these two cases, the plating efficiency in 0.25% agarose roughly correlated with the percentage of T antigen-positive cells in the population. However, the SV(−EGF) line, which is 100% T antigen-positive, failed to grow in agarose.

Discussion

Transformed cells acquire a new array of properties that are reflected in their ability to grow under conditions that are restrictive for the multiplication of normal cells. Such restrictive conditions have been used both as a means of selecting for transformants and as a way of gauging the transformed phenotype. Thus, transformed cells are capable of growth in 1% FCS, form foci on a monolayer of normal cells, and grow when suspended in a semisolid

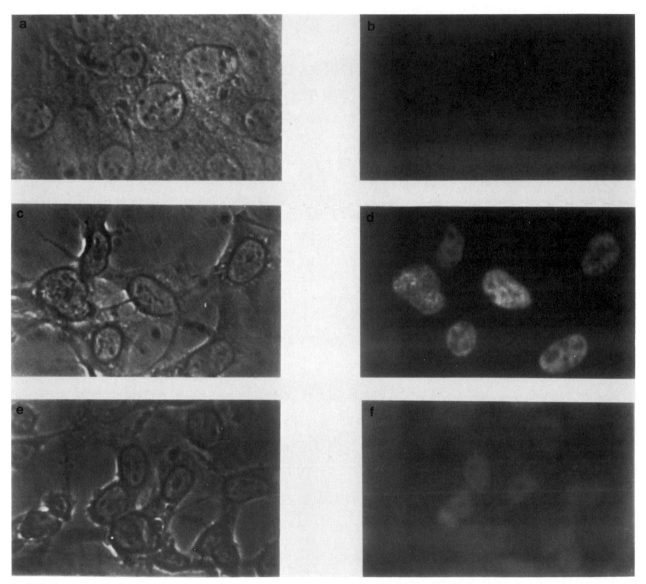

Figure 6 Phase-contrast and immunofluorescence microscopy of a cell population selected by growth in serum-free medium and examined for immunolocalization of T antigen. Shown are the parental 10T1/2 line (*a, b*), SV10T1/2-1 (*c, d*), and SV(−EGF) (*e, f*).

Table 2 Properties of Cell Populations Selected by Growth in Serum-free Media

Cells[a]	T antigen (%)	Saturation density (cells/35-mm dish)		Growth in agarose (colonies/ dish)
		10% FCS	1% FCS	
10T1/2	<0.5	5.4×10^5	2.9×10^5	0,0,0
SV10T1/2-1	100	3.4×10^6	1.6×10^6	114,127,161
SV(4F)	81	2.2×10^6	9.8×10^5	146,166,170
SV(−FB)	39	2.1×10^6	1.1×10^6	62,41
SV(−TF)	<0.5	1.7×10^6	5.0×10^5	0,0,0
SV(−EGF)	100(weak)	2.8×10^6	1.2×10^6	1,2,0
M(4F)	<0.5	1.7×10^6	7.9×10^5	0,0,0,
M(−FB)	<0.5	1.5×10^6	6.8×10^5	1,0,0,0
M(−TF)	<0.5	1.1×10^6	5.0×10^5	1,0,0

[a]SV and M refers to SV40 and mock-infected cell populations, respectively. The selection conditions are indicated in parenthesis. 4F indicates all four factors were present.

[b]2000 cells/dish were plated.

medium such as agarose. The large T antigen of SV40 is capable of coordinately inducing all these properties in cells to which it has been introduced (Tooze 1981). However, the abilities to grow in each of these different environments can be expressed independently (Risser and Pollack 1974). Thus, each of these assays may reflect the switch-on of a series of cellular functions whose net result is a specific expansion of the cell's growth potential. We have studied the influence of three broad parameters that affect transformation by SV40; namely, the genetic background of the infecting virus, the cell type infected, and the hormonal environment in which the infection and subsequent selection occur. Our studies with regard to the first point have led us to conclude that T antigen is a multifunctional protein and that some of its activities may be dissociated by mutation (Clark et al. 1983; Pipas et al. 1983; Soprano et al. 1983). This paper addresses the latter two parameters.

Our conclusions may be summarized as follows: First, the transforming activity of SV40 mutants is cell-line-dependent. T antigen deletion mutants fall into three classes with respect to their ability to transform REF52 and 10T1/2 cells. Mutants that do not synthesize T antigen, or synthesize only a short aminoterminal fragment of 39 amino acids, fail to transform either cell type. Mutants in the carboxyterminal region of T antigen (*dl*1066, *dl*1140) transform both cell types. Finally, several mutants are capable of transforming 10T1/2 cells but not the REF52 line. Transformed cells of this latter class do not stain positive for nuclear T antigen. Rather a protein reactive with anti-T tumor sera is seen in the cytoplasm. At this time, we do not know if this is small T antigen or a truncated large T. These results imply that either 10T1/2 cells produce a product capable of complementing the mutant T antigen for transformation or that transformation of these cells occurs by a different mechanism than in most cell types. Such cell-type differences may explain the observations that aminoterminal fragments of T antigen are capable of transforming primary

rat cells or the Rat-1 cell line (Clayton et al. 1982; Colby and Shenk 1982).

Second, 10T1/2 cells grow in a serum-free basal nutrient medium supplemented with fibronectin, transferrin, insulin, and EGF. Removal of any one of these supplements adversely affects the growth of these cells, with the absence of insulin or EGF being the most critical. Thus, media lacking any one supplement can be used as selective, growth-restrictive environments.

Third, SV40 infection enhances cell growth under such restrictive conditions. The fact that SV40 infection could induce cell division in medium lacking some serum factors has been known for some time (Smith et al. 1971). In addition, several workers have reported that viral transformation leads to a change in the response of transformed cells to factors required for optimal growth of untransformed cells, such as insulin or EGF (Cherington et al. 1979; Kaplan et al. 1982; McClure et al. 1982; McClure 1983) implying that some viral gene product is capable of alleviating the cell's need for certain factors for survival or growth in culture (Pledger et al. 1982). Consistent with these reports is our observation that the effect on cell growth of the deletion of EGF from the complete serum-free medium is reduced in SV40-infected cell populations when compared with mock-infected populations. This led us to attempt to use such growth-restrictive conditions as a selection for SV40-transformed cells.

A total of seven cell populations was generated by viral or mock-infecting cells and then maintaining them in complete serum-free medium or in media from which each of the four supplements had been individually deleted. The cell population selected in the absence of EGF was 100% positive for T antigen, as assayed by indirect immunofluorescence. These cells grow to the highest saturation density of the lines selected in serum-free media, but fail to grow in 0.25% agarose. The SV(−EGF) cell population retained the ability to respond fully to EGF, while SV10T1/2-1, a focus-derived transformant, exhibited a reduced response to EGF compared with the response of untransformed 10T1/2 (data not shown). Populations selected from infected cells placed in the absence of fibronectin or in the presence of all factors contained a high percentage of T antigen-positive cells and were capable of growth in 0.25% agarose. All of the cell populations passed long-term in serum-free medium, including the mock-infected, grew to higher saturation densities than the parental line.

Finally, we point out that studies such as these should lead to the development of methods for selecting previously undetected classes of transformed cells. SV(−EGF) is one such example. Analysis of the growth factor requirements and growth properties of this and similarly selected lines should aid in the identification of the cellular targets of viral oncogenes and allow the correlation of their functions with the tumorigenic potential of the cell.

Acknowledgments

This work was supported by grants GC-368 from the American Cancer Society and CA 35214-01 from the National Institutes of Health to D.B.; PCM 80-21649 from the National Science Foundation and MV-182 from the American Cancer Society to J.P. The authors wish to express their appreciation to J. Silnutzer for her help and advice. Dr. L.C. Chiang is a Visiting Research Scientist from PPG Industries, Inc.

References

Barnes, D. and G. Sato. 1980a. Methods for growth of cultured cells in serum-free medium. *Anal. Biochem.* **102:** 255.

———. 1980b. Serum-free cell culture: A unifying approach. *Cell* **22:** 649.

Brockman, W.W., T.N.H. Lee, and D. Nathans. 1973. The evolution of new species of viral DNA during serial passage of simian virus 40 at high multiplicity. *Virology* **54:** 384.

Cherington, P.V., B.L. Smith, and A.B. Pardee. 1979. Loss of epidermal growth factor requirement and malignant transformation. *Proc. Natl. Acad. Sci.* **76:** 3937.

Clark, R., K. Peden, J.M. Pipas, D. Nathans, and R. Tjian. 1983. Biochemical activities of T-antigen proteins encoded by simian virus 40 A gene deletion mutants. *Mol. Cell. Biol.* **3:** 220.

Clayton, C.E., D. Murphy, M. Lovett, and P.W.J. Rigby. 1982. A fragment of the SV40 large T antigen gene transforms. *Nature* **299:** 59.

Colby, W.W. and T. Shenk. 1982. Fragments of the simian virus 40 transforming gene facilitate transformation of rat embryo cells. *Proc. Natl. Acad. Sci.* **79:** 5189.

Gluzman, Y. and B. Ahrens. 1982. SV40 early mutants that are defective for viral DNA synthesis but competent for transformation of cultured rat and simian cells. *Virology* **123:** 78.

Graham, F.L. and A.J. van der Eb. 1973. A new technique for the assay of infectivity of human adenovirus 5 DNA. *Virology* **52:** 456.

Kaplan, P.L., M. Anderson, and B. Ozanne. 1982. Transforming growth factor(s) production enables cells to grow in the absence of serum: An autocrine system. *Proc. Natl. Acad. Sci.* **79:** 485.

McClure, D.B. 1983. Anchorage-independent colony formation of SV40 transformed BALB/c-3T3 cells in serum-free medium: Role of cell- and serum-derived factors. *Cell* **32:** 999.

McClure, D.B., M.J. Hightower, and W.C. Topp. 1982. Effect of SV40 transformation on the growth-factor requirements of the rat embryo cell line REF52 in serum-free medium. *Cold Spring Harbor Conf. Cell Proliferation* **9:** 345.

Peden, K.W.C., J.M. Pipas, S. Pearson-White, and D. Nathans. 1980. Isolation of mutants of an animal virus in bacteria. *Science* **290:** 1392.

Pipas, J.M., K.W.C. Peden, and D. Nathans. 1983. Mutational analysis of simian virus 40 T antigen: Isolation and characterization of mutants with deletions in the T-antigen gene. *Mol. Cell. Biol.* **3:** 203.

Pledger, W.J., E.B. Leof, B.B. Chou, N. Olashaw, E.J. O'Keefe, J.J. Van Wyk, and W.R. Wharton. 1982. Initiation of cell-cycle traverse by serum-derived growth factors. *Cold Spring Harbor Conf. Cell Proliferation* **9:** 259.

Pope, J.H. and W.P. Rowe. 1964. Detection of specific antigen in SV40-transformed cells by immunofluorescence. *J. Exp. Med.* **120:** 121.

Reznikoff, C.A., D.W. Brankow, and C. Heidelberger. 1973. Establishment and characterization of a cloned line of C3H mouse embryo cells sensitive to postconfluence inhibition of division. *Cancer Res.* **33:** 323.

Risser, R. and R. Pollack. 1974. A nonselective analysis of SV40 transformation of mouse 3T3 cells. *Virology* **59:** 477.

Smith, H.S., C.D. Scher, and G.J. Todaro. 1971. Induction of cell division in medium lacking serum growth factor by SV40. *Virology* **44:** 359.

Sompayrac, L.M., E.G. Gurney, and K.J. Danna. 1983. Stabilization of the 53,000-dalton nonviral tumor antigen is not required for transformation by simian virus 40. *Mol. Cell. Biol.* **3:** 290.

Soprano, K.J., N. Galanti, G.J. Jonak, S. McKercher, J.M. Pipas, K.W.C. Peden, and R. Baserga. 1983. Mutational analysis of simian virus 40 T antigen: Stimulation of cellular DNA synthesis and activation of rRNA genes by mutants with deletions in the T-antigen gene. *Mol. Cell. Biol.* **3:** 214.

Stringer, J.R. 1982. Mutant of simian virus 40 large T-antigen that is defective for viral DNA synthesis, but competent for transformation of cultured rat cells. *J. Virol.* **42:** 854.

Tooze, J., ed. 1981. *Molecular biology of tumor viruses*, 2nd edition, revised: *DNA tumor viruses*. Cold Spring Harbor Laboratory, Cold Spring Harbor, New York.

The ATPase Activity of SV40 Large T Antigen

R. Clark,* ‡ M.J. Tevethia,† and R. Tjian†

*Department of Biochemistry, University of California, Berkeley, California 94720
†Department of Microbiology, The Pennsylvania State University College of Medicine, Hershey,
Pennsylvania 17033

Although a growing number of proteins have been implicated in the induction of neoplastic transformation, there are indications that many of these may induce transformation through common pathways. Thus, it is hoped that the elucidation of these pathways will lead to a general understanding of growth control in eukaryotic cells. We believe that further progress in this area will require the characterization of oncogenic proteins on a molecular level. Accordingly, we have focused our attention on the biochemistry of large T antigen, the transforming protein of SV40 (Tooze 1981). This multifunctional protein is thought to encode more than one oncogenic activity because it is sufficient to initiate and maintain the transformation of primary cells in culture. In addition, T antigen is the key regulatory protein of the lytic cycle of SV40 in permissive monkey cells. The functions of this 92-kD phosphoprotein include: the induction of SV40 DNA replication (Tegtmeyer 1972); the autoregulation of SV40 early-region transcription (Tegtmeyer et al. 1975; Rio et al. 1980); the activation of late-region transcription (Alwine and Khoury 1980); the induction of host-cell DNA synthesis (Chou and Martin 1975; Galanti et al. 1981); the stimulation of rRNA transcription (Pöckel and Wintersberger 1980; May et al. 1976); the ability to allow adenovirus 2 to grow in monkey cells (helper function) (Rabson et al. 1964; Kimura 1974; Cole et al. 1979); and possibly a role in the assembly of infectious virions (Cosman and Tevethia 1981). There is considerable evidence that these functions are genetically distinct and can be mapped to different portions of the *A* gene (Tooze 1981). This suggests that T antigen may possess a variety of biochemical activities that carry out these functions and that T antigen may be composed of several protein domains that have some degree of independent function.

T antigen has been shown to possess at least three biochemical activities. It binds specifically to SV40 DNA at multiple sites near the origin of viral DNA replication (Tjian 1978), possesses an ATPase activity (Giacherio and Hager 1979; Tjian and Robbins 1979; Clark et al. 1981), and binds tightly to a 53K host protein (Lane and Crawford 1979). Genetic and biochemical evidence indicate that the DNA-binding activity is required for the induction of viral DNA synthesis (Shortle et al. 1979; Myers and Tjian 1980) and for the regulation of viral transcription (Rio et al. 1980; Hansen et al. 1981; Myers

‡Present address: Cetus Corporation, 1400 53rd Street, Emeryville, California 94608.

et al. 1981b). The other two activities, however, have not yet been linked to a T antigen function. This paper describes our efforts to show that the ATPase activity is intrinsic to T antigen, to determine the relationship of this activity to the biological functions of T antigen, and to identify a protein domain that is required for this activity.

Purification and properties of T antigen

The ATPase activity of T antigen was originally detected in highly purified preparations of a T antigen-related protein (D2 T antigen) produced by the naturally occurring adeno-SV40 hybrid virus Ad2 + D2 (Tjian and Robbins 1979). Ad2 + D2 is a convenient source of T antigen because it is produced at very high levels in easily cultured HeLa cells. However, D2 T antigen is a fusion protein in which about 10% of the amino terminus of T antigen is replaced by an adenovirus-coded peptide (Hassel et al. 1978). Therefore, the possibility remained that the activity resulted from the adeno-coded portion of D2 T antigen or from trace amounts of other viral or cellular proteins contaminating the D2 T preparations. Accordingly, we set out to determine whether the ATPase was intrinsic to T antigen or an activity indirectly associated with it. When T antigen was purified from alternative sources (lytically infected monkey cells and SV40-transformed human cells), the ATPase activity was found to copurify strictly with T antigen through several chromatographic steps, and comparable specific activities were observed for T antigen from all three sources (Tjian et al. 1980). Furthermore, both hamster anti-T and rabbit anti-D2T sera were found to inhibit specifically the ATPase activities of these T antigen preparations. These results provide strong evidence that the ATPase activity is intrinsic to T antigen. Additional evidence that confirms this observation is presented below. In contrast, a protein kinase activity that was detected in some T antigen preparations met none of the criteria used to establish the intrinsic nature of the ATPase (Clark et al. 1980). The kinase activity, therefore, appears to arise from a T antigen-associated cellular protein.

After isolating the ATPase activity and demonstrating that it was directly attributable to T antigen, we sought to characterize this activity biochemically with respect to its substrates and potential activators. Kinetic analysis showed T antigen to be a fairly typical ATPase (V_{max} = 18 nmole/min · mg, K_m = 4 μM). The enzyme, however, prefers dATP as a substrate (K_m = 0.5 μM) and is activated about fivefold by poly(dT) but not by other polynucleotides (Giacherio et al. 1979; Tjian et al. 1980). By analogy to prokaryotic replicases, the occurrence of both ATPase and sequence-specific DNA binding in T antigen suggested that it might function as an ATP-dependent DNA unwinding enzyme during the initiation of viral DNA replication. The topological state of SV40 origin-containing plasmids is not, however, affected by the binding of T antigen to the origin in either the presence or absence of ATP (Myers et al. 1981a). Furthermore, the ATPase activity is not altered when bound to the origin (R. Clark, unpubl.). These results indicate that T antigen does not act as an ATP-dependent DNA-unwinding protein in isolated form, but do not exclude the possibility that T antigen may contribute to such an activity when in association with host cellular proteins or other components of SV40 chromatin. Association of T antigen with a cellular protein is discussed in the final section of this paper.

We have recently constructed several adeno-SV40 hybrid viruses (Thummel et al. 1983) that serve as a rich source of wild-type T antigen. These viruses (e.g., AdSVR284) provide the advantages of producing high levels of T antigen in HeLa cells, without the liability of an altered amino terminus. We have purified the SVR284 protein both by conventional chromatography and by monoclonal antibody-affinity chromatography (Fig. 1). The latter procedure, which takes advantage of the stability of T antigen at high pH, produces higher yields, greater purity, and is much easier than the conventional purification scheme. On the other hand, the ATPase and origin DNA-binding-specific activities of conventionally purified T antigen are approximately twofold higher than those of the affinity-purified preparations.

Antibodies as ATPase probes

As noted above, both hamster anti-T and rabbit anti-D2T were found to inhibit the ATPase activities of the various T antigen preparations. However, the use of polyclonal sera in these experiments allows the possibility that the inhibition results from antibodies that are directed against trace amounts of cellular ATPases in the preparations or, alternatively, that essentially covering the surface of the T antigen molecule with a large number of antibodies might indirectly alter the activity of a cellular protein that is tightly associated with T antigen. Therefore, we tested the ability of monoclonal anti-T antibodies to inhibit the T antigen ATPase. Several monoclonal antibodies (e.g., PAb204) were found to inhibit strongly the ATPase activity. The binding sites of these antibodies were localized on the primary sequence of T antigen by testing their ability to immunoprecipitate different mutant T antigens. These sites were found to be within or overlapping the region indicated as the binding site for monoclonal antibody PAb204 in Figure 2. Antibodies that bind outside of this region, however, have no effect on the activity (Fig. 2). One antibody, PAb205, has a unique effect on the ATPase activity; it inhibits weakly (~ 20%) at high ATP concentrations and more strongly at low concentrations, apparently by increasing the K_m of T antigen for ATP (and dATP). This antibody does not bind to SDS-denatured T antigen and requires a large intact

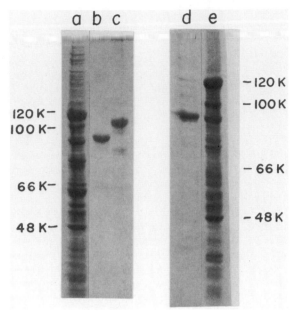

Figure 1 SDS-polyacrylamide gel electrophoresis of purified T antigen preparations. Crude lysate of AdSVR284-infected HeLa cells (lane *a*), monoclonal antibody affinity-purified Ad-SVR284 T antigen (lane *b*), conventionally purified D2 T antigen (lane *c*), conventionally purified AdSVR284 T antigen (lane *d*), and crude lysate of Ad2 + D2-infected cells (lane *e*) were analyzed on SDS-polyacrylamide gels (7–15% acrylamide gradient; Studier et al. 1973). The bands were visualized by staining with Coomassie brilliant blue. A description of the monoclonal antibody affinity purification procedure follows. AdSVR284-infected HeLa cells were harvested 34 hr postinfection, washed once in PBS, and lysed by suspending in 10 packed cell volumes of lysis buffer (20 mM Tris [pH 8.0], 200 mM LiCl, 0.5% NP-40, 1 mM EDTA, 0.02% PMSF, and 0.5 mM DTT) for 15 min on ice; the lysate was centrifuged for 15 min at 90,000*g* to remove cellular debris and incubated for 30 min at 4°C with a slurry of Reacti-gel 6X beads (Pierce) which had been coupled to monoclonal antibody PAb419 (Harlow et al. 1981b). The Reacti-gel beads were packed into a column and washed with 3 column volumes of a buffer containing 20 mM Tris (pH 8), 1 M LiCl, and 0.5% NP-40 followed by 2 volumes of a buffer containing 20 mM Tris (pH 8), 100 mM NaCl, and 0.5% NP-40. The column was successively eluted with elution buffer (50 mM NaHCO₃, 100 mM NaCl, 0.05% NP-40, 1 mM EDTA, 10% glycerol) at pHs 9.5, 10.0, and 10.6: the fractions eluting at pH 10.6, which contained the majority of the T antigen, were immediately neutralized (to ~pH 8) with 1 M acetic acid and pooled according to protein concentration. A brief description of the conventional purification of AdSVR284 T antigen follows: A cytoplasmic lysate of AdSVR284-infected HeLa cells was prepared by Dounce homogenization as described previously (Tjian and Robbins 1979), clarified by centrifugation (20 min at 90,000*g*), and concentrated by precipitation with 60% ammonium sulfate; further purification was achieved by chromatography on (in order) phosphocellulose, Ultrogel AcA 34, and DEAE-cellulose, essentially as described previously (Tjian and Robbins 1979).

portion of T antigen for binding. This region, indicated on Figure 2, includes the area where strongly inhibitory monoclonal antibodies bind. These results, in addition to providing additional evidence that the ATPase is intrinsic to T antigen, suggest that a protein domain required for the activity may reside near the binding site of PAb204.

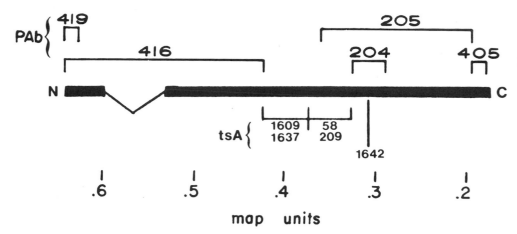

Figure 2 Map positions of monoclonal antibody-binding sites and *tsA* mutations on the coding sequence of T antigen. Monoclonal antibody-binding sites were determined by testing the ability of the antibodies to immunoprecipitate the mutant T antigens listed in Table 2 and by consideration of results obtained previously (Clark et al. 1981; Harlow et al. 1981b). The map positions of the *tsA* mutants were determined previously (Lai and Nathans 1975; Cosman and Tevethia 1981).

The identification of monoclonal antibodies with differential effects on the ATPase activity has allowed us to develop a highly specific assay for T antigen ATPase in crude cellular extracts. This assay, the monoclonal antibody-bound ATPase (MBA) assay (Clark et al. 1981), eliminates the need for conventional purification when determining the ability of novel T antigen-related proteins to hydrolyze ATP. In the MBA assay, a noninhibitory monoclonal antibody is added to a crude extract of infected or transformed cells and the resulting immune complexes are immobilized on Sepharose beads that have been chemically cross-linked to *Staphylococcus aureus* protein A or anti-mouse IgG. Contaminating cellular ATPases are efficiently removed from the immobilized T antigen by washing the beads in a suitable buffer so that T antigen activity that is retained on the beads can be assayed for ATPase activity directly. The specificity of the assay is monitored by determining the proportion of immobilized ATPase activity that is inhibitable by an anti-T antigen monoclonal IgG such as PAb204. Thus, the protein responsible for the measured activity must be recognized by two monoclonal antibodies. To determine specific activities, T antigen can be eluted from the beads with SDS sample buffer, analyzed by electrophoresis on SDS-polyacrylamide gels, and quantified by Coomassie blue staining. This assay is sensitive enough to detect as little as 2 ng of T antigen or about 0.4% of the T antigen on a 9-cm plate of SV40-infected monkey cells ($\sim 2 \times 10^6$ cells).

Our studies using monoclonal antibodies lead us to suggest that these highly specific immunological reagents may be generally useful for characterizing enzymes, particularly those whose functions are not clearly established. Their most important uses include: (1) the identification of an enzymatic activity as being intrinsic to a particular protein; (2) their use as highly specific enzyme inhibitors for both in vitro and in vivo studies; (3) the construction of structure-function maps of proteins; and (4) the rapid isolation of active enzymes or complexes from crude extracts.

ATPase of *tsA* T antigens

The development of the MBA assay has allowed us to determine the effect of various SV40 mutations on the ATPase activity. SV40 *tsA* mutants contain lesions that alter T antigen such that viral growth can occur only at reduced temperature (32–33°C). In addition, initiation and maintenance of cellular transformation by these viruses is defective at high temperatures. Analogous mutations in the *sarc* gene of Rous sarcoma virus have been used effectively to link an enzymatic activity to the transforming function of the *sarc* protein. We therefore wanted to see how the *tsA* mutations affected T antigen ATPase activity. Five mutants that have been mapped to three different regions of the *A* gene were chosen for analysis (Fig. 2). Lysates of CV1 cells infected at the permissive temperature with these viruses were analyzed for T antigen-specific ATPase using either PAb205 or PAb419 to immobilize T antigen (Table 1). When the PAb419 antibody was used for immobilization, T antigen from the *tsA*1609 and *tsA*1637 mutants showed no activity, whereas the T antigen ATPase activity from mutants *tsA*1642, *tsA*209, and *tsA*58 was comparable to that of wild type (*tsA*209 was somewhat lower than wild type). However, when antibody PAb205 was used, the T antigen isolated from *tsA*1609 and *tsA*1637 exhibited nearly wild-type specific activities. Moreover, the ATPase activity from these mutants was not inhibited by the subsequent binding of PAb419, indicating that the extremely labile activity of these proteins is stabilized by the binding of PAb205. This unexpected result suggests that the tertiary structure recognized by PAb205 (encoded between 0.37 and 0.20 map units) may be related to the conformation that is required for ATPase activity.

The T antigens of the *tsA* T antigens were also tested for temperature sensitivity in vitro by incubating them at the nonpermissive temperature (39°C) prior to assay. The ATPase of T antigen from mutants *tsA*1642, *tsA*209, and *tsA*58 were as stable at 39°C as that of wild-type T antigen. In contrast, the ATPase of T antigen from *tsA*1609 and *tsA*1637 was thermolabile relative to wild-

Table 1 Specific Activities of *tsA* T Antigens

Virus	Immobilizing antibody	
	PAb419	PAb205
Wild-type SV40	1.0	1.0
*tsA*1642	1.3	1.0
*tsA*1637	<0.05	0.9
*tsA*1609	<0.05	0.7
*tsA*209	0.3	0.3
*tsA*58	1.0	1.8

Initial rate of dATP hydrolysis per mg of T antigen relative to wild-type T antigen. The activities were determined as described previously (Clark et al. 1983).

type T antigen, despite the presence of PAb205 (Fig. 3). These results provide a final piece of evidence that the ATPase activity is intrinsic to T antigen and suggest that amino acid residues coded within 0.43–0.38 map units contribute to the ATPase activity. A similar finding was reported for conventionally purified T antigen from *tsA*30 (Griffin et al. 1980), which contains a lesion in the same region as *tsA*1609 and *tsA*1637 (the *Hind*II + III H fragment).

The *tsA*1642 mutant differs from the other mutants in that it is not defective in inducing viral DNA replication or late viral protein synthesis and is only partially defective for transformation, but nevertheless produces a low

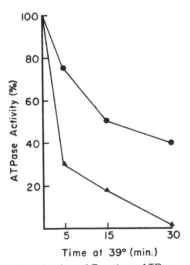

Figure 3 Heat inactivation of T antigen ATPase activity. Wild-type (●) and *tsA*1637 (▲) T antigen was bound to polyacrylamide beads with monoclonal antibody PAb205 as described previously (Clark et al. 1983). The beads were incubated for the indicated times at 39°C in ATPase assay buffer and immediately assayed for ATPase activity at 22°C (Clark et al. 1983). The activity is given as the percentage of ATPase activity remaining relative to initial activity (no incubation at 39°C) corrected for background activity detected on control beads prepared using mock-infected cell lysates. The initial activities as a percentage of total dATP hydrolyzed in 30 min were: 6.6% for wild-type, 4.0% for *tsA*1637, and 0.5% for the mock-infection. The ATPase activities of the wild-type and *tsA*1637 T antigens were inhibitable by PAb204 (> 70%). Similar results were obtained for *tsA*1609.

yield of infectious virus at the nonpermissive temperature. Because the T antigen from this mutant is wild-type for ATPase activity, it is unlikely that ATPase activity is involved in this unusual phenotype. Similarly, the presence of heat-stable ATPase activity in T antigens from *tsA*58 and *tsA*209 suggests that the biological defects in these proteins, which include viral DNA replication and transformation, are not directly related to the ATPase activity. In the case of 1609 and 1637, however, the temperature sensitivity of the ATPase activity does correlate with the defect in the ability of these viruses to induce viral DNA replication at the nonpermissive temperature, suggesting that the defect may be due, at least in part, to the lack of ATPase activity. It should be pointed out, however, that these proteins have also been found to lack origin-binding activity (Wilson et al. 1982; R. Clark, unpubl.).

Deletion mutants

To define further the region of T antigen required for ATPase activity and to determine how the activity is related to the biological functions of T antigen, we examined a set of *A* gene deletion mutants (Clark et al. 1983; Pipas et al. 1983). Because many of the mutations were found to be nonconditionally lethal, we faced the problem of obtaining virus stocks that were free of helper virus. This was done by transfecting the cloned DNA into COS7 cells, a permissive, SV40-transformed line that produces wild-type T antigen and thus complements SV40 *A* gene mutants (Gluzman 1981).

The expression of T antigen in CV1 cells infected with deletion mutants was detected by immunoprecipitation of T antigens from ^{35}S-methionine-labeled extracts. The molecular weights of the immunoprecipitated proteins, as determined by polyacrylamide gel electrophoresis, corresponded to the molecular weights predicted from the mutant DNA sequence. The map positions of the mutant proteins on the SV40 early coding sequence were determined by immunoprecipitation with monoclonal antibodies specific for the aminoterminal, carboxyterminal, and central portions of the T antigen molecule.

The ATPase activities of the mutant T antigens were determined with the MBA assay, using lysates of mutant-infected CV1 cells as a source of protein. The molar specific activities of selected mutant T antigens are listed in Table 2. These results, taken together with the antibody inhibition results, show that three or more sites in the region of T antigen encoded between 0.2 and 0.4 map units are required for the ATPase activity. Most of this region is not, however, required for origin DNA-binding activity. It is not clear from these results whether the protein sequence encoded between 0.4 and 0.5 map units is also required. An in-frame deletion in this region (*dl*2411, Tornow and Cole 1983) does not, however, reduce the ATPase activity of the corresponding mutant protein (R. Clark et al., in prep.). The amino terminus of T antigen (0.60–0.65 map units) is absent from D2 T antigen and therefore is not required for ATPase activity. Thus, it is surprising that *dl*1135 T antigen, which lacks amino acids 17–27, is greatly reduced in ATPase activ-

Table 2 Activities of Mutant T Antigens

Virus	Coding sequence	ATPase[a]	Origin binding[b]	Viral DNA replication[c]	Transformation[c]
SV40		1.0	+	+	+
dl1140		1.0	+	+	+
dl1066		1.1	+	+	+
dl1061		<0.02	+	−	−
dl1058		<0.01	+	−	−
dl1055		<0.02	+	−	−
dl1151		<0.05	−	−	−
dl1047		<0.04	−	−	−
dl1135		0.1	−	−	−
Ad2+D2		1.1	+		
Ad-SVR280		1.1	+		

Map Units: .6 .5 .4 .3 .2

[a]Initial rate of dATP hydrolysis per mole of T antigen relative to wild-type T antigen.
[b]Results of Clark et al. (1983).
[c]Results of Pipas et al. (1983).

ity. In this case, it appears likely that the conformation of the region required for ATPase activity is somehow disrupted in dl1135 by its interactions with the altered aminoterminal region.

To help establish the role of the ATPase activity in T antigen function, we have correlated the biological properties of the mutants with the ATPase activity of the mutant T antigens they produce. As shown in Table 2, there is a strong correlation between ATPase activity and two biological functions: transformation of an established cell line (REF52) and viral DNA replication. The correlation between the ATPase activity and viral DNA replication has been further strengthened by the observation that deletion of a single amino acid near 0.29 map units (dl2462, Tornow and Cole 1983) greatly reduces both the ATPase and viral replication functions without significantly affecting the origin binding ability or stability of the protein (R. Clark et al., in prep.). In contrast, the ATPase activity does not correlate with the ability of mutant T antigen to activate silent rRNA genes, stimulate host-cell DNA synthesis, or localize in the nucleus (Clark et al. 1983; Soprano et al. 1983), thus indicating that the ATPase activity is not involved in these three functions.

ATPase activity of the T-p53 complex

An understanding of the mechanism of action of T antigen and the role of the ATPase in different biochemical processes will likely include the interactions of T antigen with various cellular proteins. An obvious subject for the study of this kind of interaction is the p53 protein of mammalian cells (for review, see Crawford 1982). This protein is found at elevated levels in cells that have been transformed by a variety of viruses and carcinogens and appears to be induced by T antigen (Linzer et al. 1979). In SV40-transformed cells, up to half the T antigen exists in a stable complex with p53 that is resistant to disruption by 2 M urea and 4 M NaCl (McCormick and Harlow 1980). A similar complex is formed in productively in-

fected cells that is somewhat less stable and includes a smaller portion of the total T antigen present (Harlow et al. 1981a).

If the 53K protein is involved in coupling the ATPase activity to a biological process, one would expect the T-p53 complex to exhibit an ATPase activity that differs in some way from that of uncomplexed T antigen. Accordingly, we purified the complex from SV40-transformed mouse cells by both conventional and affinity chromatography and tested it for ATPase activity. The specific activity of the T-p53 complex was found to be approximately the same as the free form of T antigen. In addition, both forms respond similarly to the presence of polydeoxythymidine or the SV40 origin of replication DNA sequences. These results suggest that p53 does not directly mediate ATPase-related T antigen function. If the p53 protein is involved in the DNA replication or transformation functions of T antigen, it may affect other T antigen activities such as interaction with chromatin. Alternatively, the activities of p53 itself may be modified by binding to T antigen.

Acknowledgments

We thank Frank McCormick, Alan Robbins, and Kathy Jones for helping with T antigen purification, Satvir Tevethia for helpful discussions, and Karen Erdley for preparation of this manuscript. This work was funded by the National Institutes of Health (CA 25417 and CA24694) and partially by a National Institutes of Environmental Health Sciences Center grant.

References

Alwine, J.C. and G. Khoury. 1980. Effect of a tsA mutation on simian virus 40 late gene expression: Variation between host cell lines. J. Virol. 33: 920.

Chou, J.Y. and R.G. Martin. 1975. DNA infectivity and the induction of host DNA synthesis with temperature-sensitive mutants of simian virus 40. J. Virol. 15: 145.

Clark, R., D.P. Lane, and R. Tjian. 1981. Use of monoclonal antibodies as probes of simian virus 40 T antigen ATPase activity. *J. Biol. Chem.* **256:** 11854.

Clark, R., A. Robbins, and R. Tjian. 1980. Intrinsic and associated enzymatic activities of SV40 large T antigen. In *Protein phosphorylation and bio-regulation* (ed. G. Thomas et al.), p. 209. Karger, Basel.

Clark, R., K. Peden, J.M. Pipas, D. Nathans, and R. Tjian. 1983. Biochemical activities of T antigen proteins encoded by simian virus 40 A gene deletion mutants. *Mol. Cell. Biol.* **3:** 220.

Cole, C.N., L.V. Crawford, and P. Berg. 1979. Simian virus 40 mutants with deletions at the 3' end of the early region are defective in adenovirus helper function. *J. Virol.* **30:** 683.

Cosman, D.J. and M.J. Tevethia. 1981. Characterization of a temperature-sensitive, DNA-positive, nontransforming mutant of simian virus 40. *Virology* **112:** 605.

Crawford, L. 1982. The origins of p53 in relation to transformation. *Adv. Viral Oncol.* **2:** 3.

Galanti, N., G.J. Jonak, K.J. Soprano, J. Floros, L. Kaczmarek, S. Weissman, V.B. Reddy, S.M. Tilghman, and R. Baserga. 1981. Characterization and biological activity of cloned simian virus 40 DNA fragments. *J. Biol. Chem.* **256:** 6469.

Giacherio, D. and L.P. Hager. 1979. A poly dT stimulated ATPase activity associated with SV40 large T antigen. *J. Biol. Chem.* **254:** 8113.

Gluzman, Y. 1981. SV40-transformed simian cells support the replication of early SV40 mutants. *Cell* **23:** 175.

Griffin, J.D., G. Spangler, and D.M. Livingston. 1980. Enzymatic activities associated with the SV40 large T antigen. *Cold Spring Harbor Symp. Quant. Biol.* **44:** 113.

Hansen, U., D.G. Tenen, D.M. Livingston, and P.A. Sharp. 1981. T antigen repression of SV40 early transcription from two promoters. *Cell* **27:** 603.

Harlow, E., D. Pim, and L. Crawford. 1981a. Complex of SV40 large T antigen and host 53,000 molecular weight protein in monkey cells. *J. Virol.* **37:** 564.

Harlow, E., L.V. Crawford, D.C. Pim, and N.M. Williamson. 1981b. Monoclonal antibodies specific for the SV40 tumor antigens. *J. Virol.* **39:** 861.

Hassell, J.A., E. Lukanidin, G. Fey, and J. Sambrook. 1978. The structure and expression of two defective adenovirus 2/simian virus 40 hybrids. *J. Mol. Biol.* **120:** 209.

Kimura, G. 1974. Genetic evidence for SV40 gene function in enhancement of replication of human adenovirus in simian cells. *Nature* **248:** 590.

Lai, C.J. and D. Nathans. 1975. A map of temperature-sensitive mutants of simian virus 40. *Virology* **66:** 70.

Lane, D.P. and L.V. Crawford. 1979. T antigen is bound to a host protein in SV40-transformed cells. *Nature* **278:** 261.

Linzer, D., W. Maltzman, and A. Levine. 1979. The SV40 A gene product is required for the production of a 54,000 molecular weight cellular tumor antigen. *Virology* **98:** 308.

May, P., E. May, and J. Borde. 1976. Stimulation of cellular RNA synthesis in mouse kidney cell cultures infected with SV40 virus. *Exp. Cell Res.* **100:** 433.

McCormick, F. and E. Harlow. 1980. Association of a murine 53,000-dalton phosphoprotein with simian virus 40 large T antigen in transformed cells. *J. Virol.* **4:** 213.

Myers, R.M. and R. Tjian. 1980. Construction and analysis of SV40 origins defective in T antigen binding and DNA replication. *Proc. Natl. Acad. Sci.* **77:** 6491.

Myers, R.M., M. Kligman, and R. Tjian. 1981a. Does simian virus 40 T antigen unwind DNA? *J. Biol. Chem.* **256:** 10156.

Myers, R.M., D.C. Rio, A.K. Robbins, and R. Tjian. 1981b. SV40 gene expression is modulated by the cooperative binding of T antigen to DNA. *Cell* **25:** 373.

Pipas, J.M., K.W.C. Peden, and D. Nathans. 1983. Mutational analysis of SV40 T antigen: Isolation and characterization of mutants with deletions in the T antigen gene. *Mol. Cell. Biol.* **3:** 203.

Pöckl, E. and E. Wintersberger. 1980. Increased rate of RNA synthesis: Early reaction of primary mouse kidney cells to infection with polyoma virus or simian virus 40. *J. Virol.* **35:** 8.

Rabson, A.S., G.T. O'Conor, I.K. Berezesky, and F.J. Paul. 1964. Enhancement of adenovirus growth in African green monkey cell cultures by SV40. *Proc. Soc. Exp. Biol. Med.* **116:** 187.

Rio, D., A. Robbins, R. Myers, and R. Tjian. 1980. Regulation of simian virus 40 early transcription in vitro by a purified tumor antigen. *Proc. Natl. Acad. Sci.* **77:** 5706.

Shortle, D.R., R.F. Margolskee, and D. Nathans. 1979. Mutational analysis of the simian virus 40 replicon; pseudorevertants of mutants with a defective replication origin. *Proc. Natl. Acad. Sci.* **76:** 6128.

Soprano, K.J., N. Galanti, G.J. Jonak, J.M. Pipas, K.W.C. Peden, and R. Baserga. 1983. Mutational analysis of SV40 T antigen: Stimulation of cellular DNA synthesis and activation of ribosomal RNA genes by mutants with deletions in the T antigen gene. *Mol. Cell. Biol.* **3:** 214.

Studier, F.W. 1973. Analysis of bacteriophage T7 early RNAs and proteins on slab gels. *J. Mol. Biol.* **79:** 237.

Tegtmeyer, P. 1972. Simian virus 40 deoxyribonucleic acid synthesis: The viral replicon. *J. Virol.* **10:** 591.

Tegtmeyer, P., M. Schwartz, J.K. Collins, and K. Rundell. 1975. Regulation of tumor antigen synthesis by simian virus 40 gene A. *J. Virol.* **16:** 168.

Thummel, C., R. Tjian, S. Hu, and T. Grodzicker. 1983. Translational control of T antigen expressed from the adenovirus late promoter. *Cell* **33:** 455.

Tjian, R. 1978. The binding site on SV40 DNA for a T antigen-related protein. *Cell* **13:** 165.

Tijan, R. and A. Robbins. 1979. Enzymatic activities associated with a purified SV40 T antigen-related protein. *Proc. Natl. Acad. Sci.* **76:** 610.

Tjian, R., A. Robbins, and R. Clark. 1980. Catalytic properties of the SV40 tumor antigen. *Cold Spring Harbor Symp. Quant. Biol.* **44:** 103.

Tooze, J., ed. 1981. *Molecular biology of tumor viruses*, 2nd edition, revised: *DNA tumor viruses*, p. 125. Cold Spring Harbor Laboratory, Cold Spring Harbor, New York.

Tornow, J. and C.N. Cole. 1983. Intracistronic complementation in the simian virus 40 A gene. *Proc. Natl. Acad. Sci.* **80:** 6312.

Wilson, V.G., M.J. Tevethia, B.D. Lewton, and P. Tegtmeyer. 1982. DNA binding properties of simian virus 40 temperature-sensitive A proteins. *J. Virol.* **44:** 458.

Nuclear and Cytoplasmic Localization of the SV40 Small T Antigen

M. Ellman, I. Bikel, J. Figge, T. Roberts, R. Schlossman, and D.M. Livingston

The Dana-Farber Cancer Institute and the Departments of Medicine and Pathology,
Harvard Medical School, Boston, Massachusetts 02115

The early region of SV40 encodes two known proteins, large T antigen and small T antigen. Both of these elements are active in the process of virus-induced neoplastic transformation, although the mechanisms by which they operate in this regard are wholly unknown. Unlike large T, it appears that small T is dispensable during productive infection (Shenk et al. 1976), although under some conditions both proteins play essential, albeit complementary, roles in the transforming process (Sleigh et al. 1978; Fluck and Benjamin 1979; Martin et al. 1979; Tooze 1980; Rubin et al. 1982). Large T can be readily identified in infected cells by a variety of techniques, including indirect immunofluorescence which shows it to be largely a nuclear constituent. By contrast, it has not been possible to detect small T immunofluorescence in the past. The cellular location of this protein could, therefore, be assessed only by biochemical extraction studies which suggested that it was largely a constituent of the postnuclear soluble fraction and might, therefore, be largely, if not wholly, a cytoplasmic constituent (Prives et al. 1978; Spangler et al. 1980). Comparable results were obtained for polyoma small T antigen (Silver et al. 1978). However, in view of the indirect nature of the analytic approach employed in all of these studies, a detailed understanding of the intracellular geography of small T was not possible. In an effort to address this problem, we have raised an antibody against homogeneous SV40 small T, synthesized in *Escherichia coli* (Roberts et al. 1979; Bikel et al. 1983), and used it to decorate cells that synthesize substantial levels of small T but no readily detectable intact or truncated large T by indirect immunofluorescence. Results of these experiments reveal that small T fluorescence can be readily identified in both the nucleus and the cytoplasm of two different cell types. As expected, in the same types of experiments, large T fluorescence was noted to be largely, if not exclusively, nuclear.

We have recently described a plasmid (pHR402) and a derivative, infectious SV40 viral mutant (SV402) that, upon introduction into rodent or monkey cells, lead to the synthesis of small T but not clearly or reproducibly detectable quantities of large T or a truncated derivative thereof (Rubin et al. 1982). The 402 genome contains two tandemly oriented viral replication origins upstream of an intact small T coding unit. The 402 early region has also sustained a $\simeq 1.5$ kb deletion of large T unique coding sequences. Furthermore, when this plasmid was cotransfected onto NIH-3T3 cells in the presence of pSV2 *Ecogpt* (Mulligan and Berg 1981), some of the

clones that grew in medium containing mycophenolic acid also synthesized intact SV40 20-kD small T antigen and failed to accumulate readily detectable quantities of intact or truncated large T, as assayed by specific immunoprecipitation of ^{35}S-methionine-labeled cell extracts. One such example is shown in Figure 1. The rabbit antiserum used in these experiments was raised against SDS gel band-purified small T synthesized in *E. coli* (Bikel et al. 1983). This serum recognized both small T and large T, but failed to bind small T after its absorption to an extract of monkey cells infected by a T$^+$/t$^-$ virus (*dl*884) (Shenk et al. 1976; Bikel et al. 1983). Hence, the vast majority, if not all, of the relevant antibody molecules in this serum recognize an antigen(s) contained within the common T/t sequence. In an experiment analogous to that reported above, CV-1P cells were acutely infected with SV402, and extracts of these cells were exposed to anti-T/t immunoprecipitation (Fig. 1). No cytopathic effect or production of large T were observed in such SV402-infected cultures, and, in keeping with this observation, only small T was clearly identified by specific immunoprecipitation. In this regard, others have shown that mouse Ltk cells transformed by a recombinant genome (pVBtTK-1), which contains an analogously deleted SV40 early region, also failed to accumulate readily detectable truncated large T protein with the sera employed in the relevant immunoprecipitation assays (Reddy et al. 1982). As an indication that expression of the 402 genome did not lead to a truncated large T antigen which comigrated with small T in SDS-polyacrylamide gels, extracts of NIH-3T3 clone 5-4 (one of the above-noted t$^+$/T$^-$, gpt$^+$ cotransformants) and of COS1 cells (a T$^+$/t$^+$ monkey cell line) were immunoprecipitated with the above-noted serum. An aliquot of the eluted products was then reduced with dithiothreitol and alkylated with *N*-ethylmaleimide (Crawford and O'Farrell 1979). As noted in Figure 1, comigrating small T bands were noted in these two extracts before and after reduction/alkylation, and, in each case, the migration rate of small T slowed to the same degree after chemical modification, in keeping with the original observation of Crawford and O'Farrell (1979). By contrast, no major alteration in COS1 large T migration was detected and no new immunoreactive bands were seen after the above-noted treatment. Since the putative truncated large T molecule, encoded by the 402 early region (Rubin et al. 1982), would lack small T unique sequences and be expected to have a different cysteine content than small T (5 vs. 11), the failure to detect a previously "hidden" 20K band after reduction and alkylation is consistent

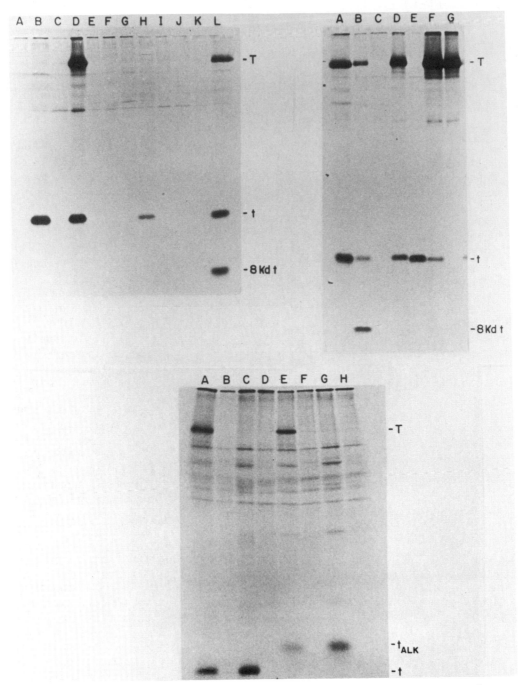

Figure 1 Immunoprecipitation of ³⁵S-methionine-labeled SV40 large T and small T antigens from various cell extracts. All cells were grown in Dulbecco's modification of Eagle's minimal essential medium in a 10% CO_2-containing atmosphere. The conditions for virus production, titering, cell labeling with [³⁵S]L-methionine, cell lysis, the raising of anti-SV40 small T antibody against SDS gel-purified protein, specific immunoprecipitation, SDS-polyacrylamide gel electrophoresis, and autoradiography have been described previously (Spangler et al. 1980; Rubin et al. 1982; Bikel et al. 1983). SDS gel electrophoresis was routinely performed in 15% polyacrylamide running gels cast beneath 4% stacking segments. (*Upper left*) (lanes *B, D, F, H, J, L*) Rabbit anti-small T immunoprecipitates; (other lanes) preimmune rabbit serum precipitates. Extracts employed were: SV402-infected CV-1P cells (*A,B*); SV40 (strain 776, clone 1)-infected CV-1P cells (*C,D*); CV-1P cells (*E,F*); NIH-3T3/Ecogpt⁺ cells (Mulligan and Berg 1981) that were cotransformed with pHR402 (Rubin et al. 1982) (clone 5-4) (*G,H*); NIH-3T3/Ecogpt⁺ clone 2-1 cells which lack SV40 sequences (cf. below) (*I,J*); and SV80 cells (*K,L*). SV80 synthesizes large T, small T, and an 8-kD truncated large T which is largely composed of SV40 T/t common sequences (Spangler et al. 1980; Tooze 1980). (*Upper right*) (all lanes) Rabbit anti-small T serum precipitates of [³⁵S]methionine-labeled cell extracts. The extracts used were those of: COS1 cells (Gluzman 1981) (*A*), SV80 cells (*B*), uninfected CV-1P (*C*), SV40 (strain 776)-infected CV-1P (*D*); SV402-infected CV-1P (*E*); *dl*883-infected CV-1P (Shenk et al. 1976; Khoury et al. 1979) (*G*); and *dl*883 + SV402-infected CV-1P (*F*). The slight migration difference between SV40 (776) small T in lane *D* and the other small T species here was specific to this clone of virus. (*Bottom panel*) (lanes *A, B, E,* and *F*) COS1 cell extract; (lanes *C, D, G,* and *H*) SV402-infected CV-1P extract. (Lanes *A, C, E,* and *G*) Rabbit anti-small T serum precipitates; (lanes *B, D, F,* and *H*) preimmune rabbit serum precipitates. The SDS-eluted antigen(s) in lanes *E–H* had been exposed to 20 mM dithiothreitol and 40 mM *N*-ethylmaleimide prior to electrophoresis, as described previously (Crawford and O'Farrell 1979).

with the notion that expression of the 402 genome does not lead to the intracellular accumulation of a truncated form of large T which normally comigrates with small T. Furthermore, a one-dimensional isoelectric focusing gel analysis of ^{35}S-methionine-labeled pHR402 small T from the NIH-3T3 gpt$^+$ cotransformant clone 5-4 revealed that all of the specifically immunoprecipitated radioactivity that was detected appeared to comigrate with authentic SV40 small T synthesized from an intact small T-coding unit in *E. coli* (Roberts et al. 1979; Bikel et al. 1983) (data not shown). Hence, by these criteria, all of the radioactivity in the anti-small T-reactive 20-kD band in cells bearing the 402 genome is SV40 small T.

With the availability of a monospecific antibody that recognized one or more segments of the common T/t sequence and cells that, as characterized with this reagent, appear to accumulate small T and not large T, it was possible to search for this protein in fixed cells by indirect immunofluorescence. Thus, as shown in figures 2 and 3, t$^+$/T$^-$ Ecogpt$^+$-cotransformed NIH-3T3 cells and CV-1P cells acutely infected with SV402 were sequentially fixed in 3.7% formaldehyde followed by absolute methanol and then incubated with this antibody. Following a reaction with fluoresceinated goat anti-rabbit IgG, distinct, bright fluorescence was noted in the nuclei and cytoplasm of both cell types. The intranuclear fluorescence was found to be diffuse and to spare evident nucleoli. Cytoplasmic fluorescence in many cells was noted to be "lacy" and, in part, to decorate a tight, albeit irregular, network of particulate material. Additional examples of these effects are noted in Figure 3. No fluorescence was noted in NIH-3T3 cells transformed only with pSV2 *Ecogpt* (Fig. 2B), in uninfected CV-1P cells reacted with anti-small T serum (Fig. 2E), or in SV40-infected CV-1P cells reacted with preimmune rabbit serum (data not shown). By contrast, CV-1P cells infected by *dl*883 (a t$^-$/T$^+$ viral mutant [Shenk et al. 1976; Khoury et al. 1979]) contained only large T (cf. Fig. 1, upper right panel, lane G) and revealed bright nuclear fluorescence without detectable cytoplasmic staining under the conditions employed (Fig. 2C). This result is in keeping with the widely appreciated observation that $\geq$ 90% of large T in such cells is a nuclear constituent. Results qualitatively similar to those noted in the small T-containing cells described here were obtained with the above-noted t$^+$/Ecogpt$^+$ NIH-3T3 clone 5-4 after fixation with methanol alone or with 3.7% formaldehyde followed by 1% Triton X-100 or acetone. In addition, identical results to those noted in Figures 2 and 3 were obtained with the two other t$^+$/Ecogpt$^+$ NIH-3T3 clones (5-1 and 5-10) available in our laboratory. Hence, the nuclear and cytoplasmic staining effect is a reproducible finding in more than one cell type that synthesizes SV40 small T antigen in the absence of large T. Moreover, similar, although less intense staining of fixed, 402 genome-containing t$^+$/T$^-$ cells was obtained after incubation with one lot of pooled, hamster anti-SV40 tumor serum. In keeping with the contention that the observed fluorescence is due to an immune reaction with small T antigen and not the predicted, $\approx$20-kD truncated species of large T, which can, in theory, be encoded by the 402 genome, only small T was detected by specific immunoprecipitation, under the conditions employed, with the same serum used in the indicated immunofluorescence experiments; and others have found that, with hamster anti-SV40 tumor serum, large T antigens extending less than 272 amino acids from the normal amino terminus failed to score in immunofluorescence assays (Pipas et al. 1983).

In an independent test of the suggestion that small T is present in both the nuclear and the cytoplasmic cell compartments, clone 5-4 cells were fractionated into nuclei and a postnuclear soluble fraction following hypotonic swelling at 80 mM NaCl and Dounce homogenization performed by a modification of a previously described procedure (Abrams et al. 1982). Nuclei were purified by differential centrifugation and washing. By phase-contrast microscopy, the final pellet fraction was found to be composed of $\geq$ 95% intact nuclei; $\leq$ 2% intact cells were identified after examining 100 intact nuclei. Purified nuclei were extracted in RIPA buffer (0.05 M Tris-HCl [pH 7.4], 1% Triton X-100, 1% sodium deoxycholate, and 0.1% SDS), and the resulting fractions were subjected to excess anti-SDS gel band small T immunoprecipitation. The results depicted in Figure 4 show that small T was present in both the nuclear and postnuclear soluble fractions. Densitometric tracing of the small T gel bands revealed that $\approx$78% of the total immunoreactive small T extracted in these two fractions was in the latter fraction, whereas $\approx$22% was in the nuclear fraction. No small T was detected in the nuclear wash, and the finding of nucleus and soluble fraction-specific gel bands strongly suggests that little or no significant cross-contamination of these three fractions had occurred (Fig. 4, right panel). It should also be noted that when the same cells or SV402-infected CV-1P were swollen at 10 mM Na$^+$ prior to homogenization, $\leq$ 5% of the extracted small T was present in the nuclear fraction (data not shown), suggesting that retention of small T in the nucleus during and/or after cell disruption is, at least in part, a salt-sensitive phenomenon.

Thus, by two criteria—indirect immunofluorescence and biochemical extraction analysis—small T appears to be distributed in two major cell compartments. The quantitative distribution between these locations in vivo is difficult to establish accurately, as the relative in vivo immunoreactivities of nuclear and cytoplasmic small T may not prove to be the same as they are in vitro. Moreover, it seems likely that some small T leaks from the nucleus during hypotonic swelling and/or Dounce homogenization, and this may also have occurred during the experiment described in Figure 4. In a similar experiment performed on SV40 or *dl*883-infected CV-1P cells, little or no large T antigen was detected in the postnuclear soluble fraction, and nearly all of the antigen was present in the nuclear fraction (data not shown). Hence, the cell fractionation technique per se does not lead to indiscriminant loss of another known nuclear constituent.

In many cells, cytoplasmic small T appeared to be distributed in a tightly packed, inhomogeneous pattern.

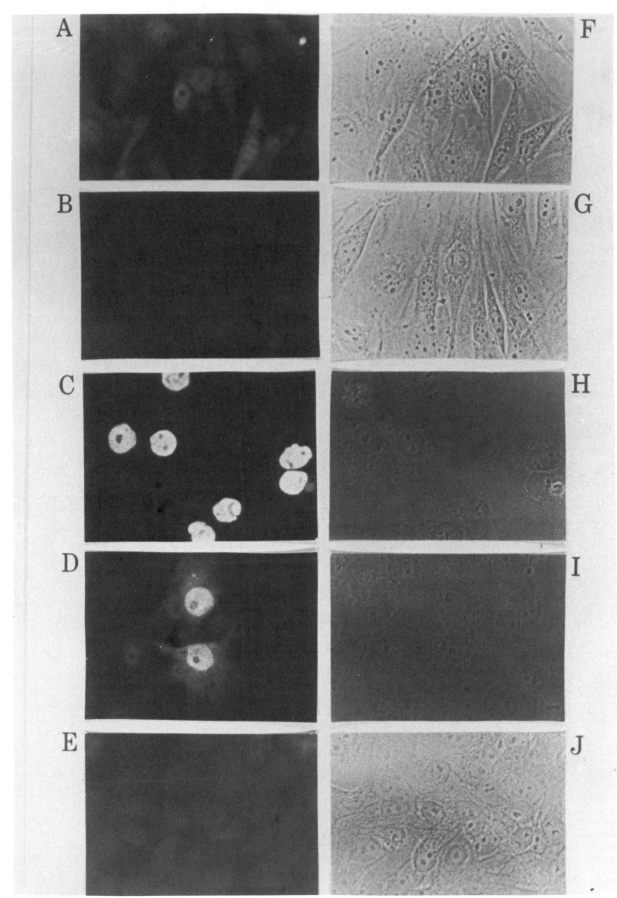

Figure 2 (*See facing page for legend.*)

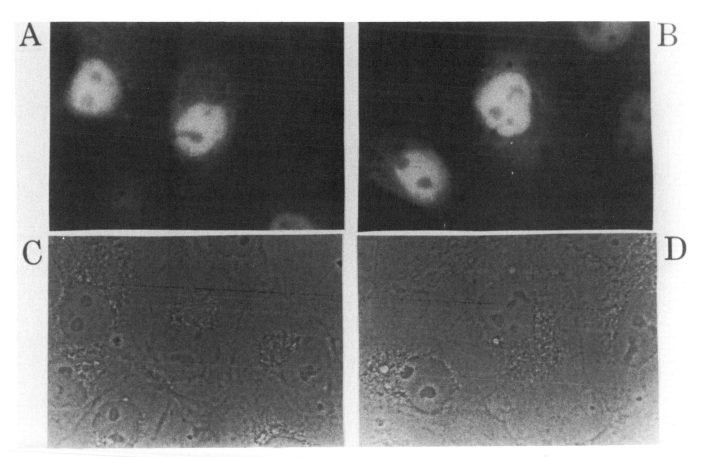

Figure 3 Anti-small T immunofluorescent analysis of SV402-infected CV-1P cells. The same absorbed rabbit anti small T serum described in the legend to Fig. 2 was employed here. Cells were fixed and reacted with antibody, as noted previously (see legend to Fig. 2). SV402/CV-1P cells were viewed at a 63× magnification. UV fluorescent images (*top panels*); phase-contrast bright-field images (*bottom panels*).

This raises the possibility that it might, at least in part, be bound to one or more organized cell structures—for example, a cytoskeletal component and/or to a structure like the Golgi or endoplasmic reticulum. The protein has been shown to be able to bind to at least two cell proteins in vitro (Yang et al. 1979; C. Murphy et al., in prep.). Whether either or both of these are associated with such structures is unknown, although recent evidence suggests that small T can also form tight and specific complexes with tubulin in vitro (C. Murphy et al., unpubl.).

The data presented here represent the first in situ demonstration of SV40 small T antigen and lead to the surprising conclusion that, in addition to existing in the cytoplasm, small T is also a nuclear component. Recently, a similar conclusion has been drawn from immunofluorescent experiments in other laboratories for polyoma (R. Kamen, pers. comm.) and BK (D. McCance and A.E. Smith, pers. comm.) small T antigens, two papova viral proteins that are closely related to SV40 small T. Large T is also present and functions in the nucleus, but since small T was detected there in cells lacking large T, its entry into that compartment is not a large T-dependent process.

The significance of the dual distribution of small T is unclear, but certain relevant possibilities can be cited: (1) Perhaps small T is biologically active only in the nu-

Figure 2 Immunofluorescence of SV40 large T and small T antigen in various cell lines. Cells were grown on glass coverslips, as noted in the legend to Fig. 1. They were then rinsed in phosphate-buffered saline (PBS) (0.01 M sodium phosphate [pH 7.4]; 0.14 M NaCl) and immersed in 3.7% formaldehyde in PBS for 20 min at room temperature. Coverslips were again rinsed three times in PBS and then immersed in ice-cold absolute methanol for 2 min at −23°C. After three more rinses in room-temperature PBS, coverslips were drained of obvious surface fluid and then incubated with rabbit anti-SDS gel band purified small T serum (1:40 dilution) for 30 min at 37°C in a humidified atmosphere. Subsequently, they were rinsed three times in PBS and then incubated with fluoresceinated goat anti-rabbit F(ab')$_2$ IgG (1:100) (Cappel Labs, Downingtown, Pa.), rinsed again three times in PBS, and then dried and mounted in 50% glycerol in PBS. Cells were viewed and photographed at 40× magnification with a Zeiss inverted UV microscope under oil immersion. (*Left panels*) Fluorescent images. (*Right panels*) Bright-field/phase-contrast images. All panels indicate cells after incubation with rabbit anti-SDS gel band-purified small T serum described in the legend to Fig. 1. Cells: (*A*) NIH-3T3/Ecogpt$^+$/t$^+$ clone 5-4; (*B*) NIH-3T3/Ecogpt$^+$ clone 2-1, a cell line that was transfected only with pSV$_2$ Ecogpt; (*C*) dl883-infected CV-1P cells; (*D*) SV402-infected CV-1P cells; (*E*) uninfected CV-1P cells. The rabbit serum employed was the same one used in the experiments described in Fig. 1 and was serially adsorbed at a 1:1 dilution (in PBS) against CH$_3$OH-fixed monolayers of NIH-3T3 cells (5 successive incubations of 1 hr at 23°C with confluent monolayers seeded on 60-mm plates).

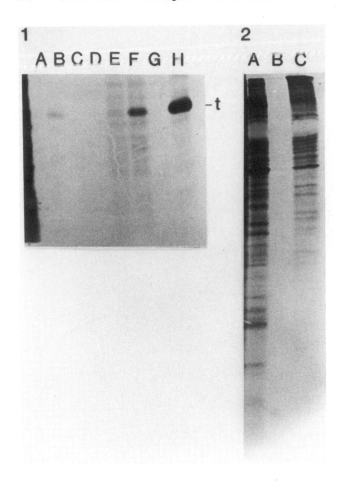

Figure 4 Anti-small T immunoprecipitation of various ^{35}S-labeled subcellular fractions of clone 5-4 cells. Two 100-mm dishes of NIH-3T3/Ecogpt$^+$/t$^+$ (clone 5-4) cells ($\approx 2 \times 10^6$ cells/dish) were labeled for 3.5 hr with [35S]methionine (60 μCi/ml) and then washed three times in PBS. One dish was then lysed with 1.2 ml of modified RIPA buffer (50 mM Tris [pH 7.4], 1% sodium deoxycholate, 0.1% SDS, 1% Triton X-100, 1 mg/ml bovine serum albumin [BSA]), and this lysate was centrifuged in an Eppendorf microfuge for 10 min at 4°C. The supernatant was labeled extract A. Cells on the other dish were scraped into 1.2 ml of 10 mM Mes (pH 6.2), 80 mM NaCl, 1.5 mM MgCl$_2$, and 1 mg/ml BSA with a rubber policeman and were then swollen on ice for 40 min. After 25 strokes of Dounce homogenization, ≥95% of cells were broken as defined by phase-contrast microscopic inspection. The suspension was centrifuged at 1600 rpm for 10 min at 4°C in a Beckman J6B centrifuge. The supernatant was labeled extract B (postnuclear soluble fraction). The pellet was suspended in 1.2 ml of 10 mM Mes (pH 6.2), 80 mM NaCl, 3 mM MgCl$_2$, and 1 mg/ml BSA and after extensive, gentle mixing, this fraction was again centrifuged at 1600 rpm for 10 min at 4°C. The supernatant was labeled extract C (nuclear wash). An aliquot ($\approx 5\%$) of the pellet was suspended in PBS and was found to be composed of ≥95% intact nuclei. The remainder of the nuclear pellet was dissolved in 1.2 ml of RIPA buffer containing 1 mg/ml BSA (extract D – nuclear extract). Again, all fractions were centrifuged at 1600 rpm for 10 min. A 25-μl aliquot of each fraction was removed for direct electrophoretic analysis (*right panel*), and the rest was immunoprecipitated with either rabbit anti-SV40 small T serum or preimmune rabbit serum, as noted previously. All samples were electrophoresed through a 15% SDS-polyacrylamide gel bearing a 4% stacking gel as described previously (Rubin et al. 1982). Siliconized plastic centrifuge tubes that had been subsequently immersed in a 1 mg/ml solution of BSA in water were used throughout to inhibit nonspecific binding of radioactive small T antigen. (*Left panel*) Immunoprecipitates: (lanes *B, D, F,* and *H*) anti-small T serum precipitates; (lanes *A, C, E,* and *G*) preimmune rabbit serum precipitates. Extracts employed were A (whole-cell lysate, lanes *G, H*); B (postnuclear soluble fraction, lanes *E, F*); C (nuclear wash, lanes *C, D*); D (nuclear extract, lanes *A, B*). (*Right panel*) Direct electrophoretic analysis of: (lane *A*) postnuclear extract (extract B); (lane *B*) nuclear wash (extract C); (lane *C*) nuclear extract (extract D).

cleus and is transported there slowly or inefficiently, thereby creating a sizeable pool of nonfunctioning cytoplasmic small T; (2) small T may exist largely in the nucleus and leak out into the cytoplasm during cell fixation and/or immunofluorescent manipulations; (3) perhaps small T functions in both the nucleus and the cytoplasm and, if so, in at least partially different ways in the two cell compartments; (4) it is theoretically possible that small T moves from the cytoplasm to the nucleus in the course of performing a discrete function(s) and/or at a special point in the cell cycle. Clearly, without more information, it is impossible to conclude which, if any, of the above are correct. However, resolution of these possibilities might shed new light on how small T functions in the SV40 transforming process (see Ellman et al. 1984).

References

Abrams, H.D., L.R. Rohrschneider, and R.N. Eisenman. 1982. Nuclear location of the putative transforming protein of avian myelocytomatosis virus. *Cell* **29**: 427.

Bikel, I., T. Roberts, M.L. Bladon, R. Green, E. Amann, and D.M. Livingston. 1983. Purification of biologically active SV40 small t antigen. *Proc. Natl. Acad. Sci.* **80**: 906.

Crawford, L.V. and P.Z. O'Farrell. 1979. Effect of alkylation on the physical properties of simian virus 40 T-antigen species. *J. Virol.* **29**: 587.

Ellman, M., I. Bikel, J. Figge, T. Roberts, R. Schlossman, and D.M. Livingston. 1984. SV40 small tumor antigen is localized in the nucleus and cytoplasm. *J. Virol.* (in press).

Fluck, M. and T.L. Benjamin. 1979. Comparisons of two early gene functions essential for transformation in polyoma virus and SV40. *Virology* **96**: 205.

Gluzman, Y. 1981. SV40-transformed simian cells support the replication of early SV40 mutants. *Cell* **23**: 175.

Khoury, G., P. Gruss, R. Dhar, and C.-J. Lai. 1979. Processing and expression of early SV40 mRNA: A role for RNA conformation in splicing. *Cell* **18**: 85.

Martin, R., V. Setlow, C. Edwards, and D. Vembu. 1979. The roles of the simian virus 40 tumor antigens in transformation of Chinese hamster lung cells. *Cell* **17**: 635.

Mulligan, R. and P. Berg. 1981. Selection for animal cells that express the *E. coli* gene coding for xanthine-guanine phosphoribosyltransferase. *Proc. Natl. Acad. Sci.* **78**: 2072.

Pipas, J., K. Peden, and D. Nathans. 1983. Mutational analysis of simian virus 40 T antigen: Isolation and characterization of mutants with deletions in the T-antigen gene. *Mol. Cell. Biol.* **3**: 203.

Prives, C., E. Gilboa, M. Revel, and E. Winocour. 1977. Cell-free translation of simian virus early messenger RNA coding for viral T-antigen. *Proc. Natl. Acad. Sci.* **74**: 457.

Reddy, V.B., S.S. Tevethia, M.J. Tevethia, and S.M. Weissman. 1982. Nonselective expression of simian virus 40 large tumor antigen fragments in mouse cells. *Proc. Natl. Acad. Sci.* **79**: 2064.

Roberts, T., I. Bikel, R. Yocum, D.M. Livingston, and M.

Ptashne. 1979. Synthesis of small t antigen in *E. coli. Proc. Natl. Acad. Sci.* **76:** 5596.

Rubin, H., J. Figge, M.T. Bladon, L.-B. Chen, M. Ellman, I. Bikel, M.P. Farrell, and D.M. Livingston. 1982. Role of small t antigen in the acute transforming activity of SV40. *Cell* **30:** 469.

Shenk, T., J. Carbon, and P. Berg. 1976. Construction and analysis of viable deletion mutants of simian virus 40. *J. Virol.* **18:** 664.

Silver, J., B. Schaffhausen, and T.L. Benjamin. 1978. Tumor antigens induced by nontransforming mutants of polyoma virus. *Cell* **15:** 485.

Sleigh, M., W.C. Topp, R. Hanich, and J. Sambrook. 1978. Mutants of SV40 with an altered small t protein are reduced in their ability to transform cells. *Cell* **14:** 79.

Spangler, G., J. Griffin, H. Rubin, and D.M. Livingston. 1980. Identification and initial characterization of a new low molecular weight, virus-encoded T antigen in a line of SV40-transformed cells. *J. Virol.* **36:** 488.

Tooze, J., ed. 1980. *Molecular biology of tumor viruses*, 2nd edition: *DNA tumor viruses*. Cold Spring Harbor Laboratory, Cold Spring Harbor, New York.

Yang, Y.-C., P. Hearing, and K. Rundell. 1979. Cellular proteins associated with simian virus 40 early gene products in newly infected cells. *J. Virol.* **32:** 147.

The p53 Protein and Cell Proliferation

W.E. Mercer, C. Avignolo, H. Liu,* and R. Baserga

Department of Pathology and Fels Research Institute, Temple University School of Medicine, Philadelphia, Pennsylvania 19140

The term p53 protein designates a family of cellular proteins that vary in size from 48 kD to 55 kD in different species and are frequently present in higher amounts in transformed cells (Crawford et al. 1981; Rotter et al. 1981), especially SV40-transformed cells (Lane and Crawford 1979; Linzer et al. 1979), or in actively dividing cells (DeLeo et al. 1979; Linzer and Levine 1979; Milner and McCormick 1980; Milner and Milner 1981). Although the evidence suggests a close relationship between levels of p53 protein and actively dividing cells (Linzer and Levine 1979; Carroll et al. 1980; Dippold ot al. 1981; Milner and Milner 1981), very little information is available on the function that this protein has in mammalian cells. We have investigated the function of the p53 protein in mammalian cells by microinjecting directly into the nuclei of cells in culture monoclonal antibodies against the p53 protein and determining the effect that these antibodies have on cell proliferation. This paper will discuss four aspects of our approach, namely: (1) the basis for the use of microinjected monoclonal antibodies to study cell functions; (2) the effect of microinjected monoclonal antibodies against the p53 protein on cell proliferation; (3) the effect of microinjected monoclonal antibodies against p53 protein on RNA accumulation in cells; and (4) the domain of the SV40 T antigen-coding gene responsible for the induction of the p53 protein, because it relates to the role that the p53 protein may have on the transition of cells from G_0 to S phase.

Basis for the use of microinjected monoclonal antibodies to study cell functions

The studies to be related, dealing with the role of the p53 protein in cell proliferation, depend on the demonstration that antibodies microinjected into the nuclei of mammalian cells are nontoxic and preserve their specificity of action. The evidence is now substantial that antibodies microinjected into mammalian cells can, indeed, be used to study the function of the antigens against which they are directed. The evidence includes:

1. Antibodies can be microinjected into cells without any detectable toxicity (Zavortink et al. 1979; Antman and Livingston 1980; Floros et al. 1981; Mercer et al. 1983).
2. Microinjected antibodies against SV40 T antigen inhibit the replication of SV40 DNA (Antman and Livingston 1980).
3. Microinjected antibodies against the SV40 T antigen

inhibit SV40-induced cellular DNA synthesis but not serum-stimulated DNA synthesis (Floros et al. 1981; Mercer et al. 1983).
4. An antibody against RNA polymerase I inhibits, when microinjected into Swiss-3T3 cells, nucleolar RNA synthesis but not nucleoplasmic RNA synthesis or serum-stimulated DNA synthesis (Mercer et al. 1984).
5. Control IgGs microinjected into the nuclei of mammalian cells do not inhibit RNA synthesis (Mercer et al. 1984), nor serum-stimulated DNA synthesis (Floros et al. 1981; Mercer et al. 1982, 1984).

The specificity and lack of toxicity of microinjected antibodies is illustrated in the experiments summarized in Table 1. In the first experiments, an antibody against RNA polymerase I (Rose et al. 1981) or a control IgG were microinjected into cells. Their effect on nucleolar RNA synthesis was determined by labeling cells with [³H]uridine and autoradiographically counting the number of grains over the nucleolus. The results of Table 1 (2nd column) show that the antibody against RNA polymerase I produces a 65% inhibition of nucleolar RNA synthesis, whereas the control IgG does not cause any inhibition. In a second experiment, the same antibody was comicroinjected with the recombinant plasmid pC2, which contains both the entire SV40 genome and a frag-

Table 1 Specificity of Action of Antibodies Microinjected into Mammalian Cells

Antibody	Nucleolar RNA synthesis (no. of grains)	T⁺ cells (%)	tk⁺ cells (%)
Anti-RNA pol I	9	48	150
Control IgG	25	45	152
None	26	46	133

Anti-RNA pol I is the antibody against RNA polymerase I described by Rose et al. (1981). Control IgG was prepared from serum of a nonimmunized rabbit. Both IgGs were microinjected into the nuclei of exponentially growing cells. Nucleolar RNA synthesis was determined by labeling the cells with [³H]uridine and counting the number of grains after autoradiography. For unique-copy gene transcription, anti-rat RNA pol I was comicroinjected with pC2, a recombinant plasmid that contains both the entire SV40 genome and the fragment of HSV that contains the gene for thymidine kinase (Linnenbach et al. 1980). T⁺ = cells positive for SV40 T antigen. tk⁺ = cells capable of incorporating [³H]thymidine (the tk⁻ ts13 cells used in this experiment have a background of virtually 0).

*On leave from: Biology Dept., Beijing Normal University, Beijing, People's Republic of China.

ment of the herpes simplex virus (HSV) that includes the gene for thymidine kinase (*tk*) (Linnenbach et al. 1980). It is known that transcription of these two genes depends not on RNA polymerase I but on RNA polymerase II. The tk⁻ ts 13 cells that were used in the comicroinjection experiments (Shen et al. 1982) have a low background, virtually 0. Whether one investigates the expression of the SV40 T antigen (3rd column), or the ability of the microinjected cells to incorporate [^{3}H]thymidine (last column), Table 1 clearly shows that neither the antibody against RNA polymerase I, nor the control IgG affect the expression of these two genes. Incidentally the number of cells capable of incorporating [^{3}H]thymidine is above 100% because the cells microinjected were growing exponentially and gene expression in microinjected cells was determined 24 hours after microinjection. These experiments confirm that microinjected antibodies are nontoxic and preserve an exquisite specificity of action.

Having established that microinjected antibodies can be used to study cellular functions, we have investigated the function of the p53 protein by microinjecting cells with two different monoclonal antibodies to the p53 protein, namely Pab 122, a monoclonal antibody described by Gurney et al. (1980), and 200-47, a monoclonal antibody described by Dippold et al. (1981).

Effect of microinjected antibodies against the p53 protein on cell proliferation

In a previous paper from our laboratory (Mercer et al. 1982), we had microinjected a monoclonal antibody against the p53 protein into the nuclei of quiescent Swiss-3T3 mouse cells. The cells were subsequently stimulated with 10% fetal calf serum. Microinjection of the p53 antibody at the time of serum stimulation (± 2 hr) clearly inhibited the subsequent entry of Swiss-3T3 cells into the S phase of the cell cycle. The p53 antibody had no effect on serum-stimulated DNA synthesis when it was microinjected 4 hours or later after serum stimulation. Control antibodies had no effect on serum-stimulated DNA synthesis regardless of the time at which they were microinjected. We stated at that time that "these experiments, while not defining the role of p53 in the initiation of cell proliferation, do suggest that p53 is a key factor in the transition of cells from a resting to a growing stage." Table 2 confirms these results. When a monoclonal antibody against a p53 protein (Pab 122) is microinjected into serum-stimulated Swiss-3T3 cells at the time of stimulation, it inhibits their entry into S phase. If the antibody is microinjected 6 hours or 17 hours after stimulation, no inhibition is observed. The microinjection of a control antibody Lyt 2.2 or of an antibody against rat RNA polymerase I at the same times after serum stimulation has no effect on the entry of Swiss-3T3 cells into DNA synthesis. It is especially important to note that the antibody against RNA polymerase I is totally ineffective on serum-stimulated DNA synthesis. This antibody strongly inhibits nucleolar RNA synthesis and cellular RNA accumulation (Mercer et al. 1984 and Table 1), and, since its action is definitely located in the nucleus, it serves as an ideal control for the in-

hibitory effect of the monoclonal antibody against the p53 protein.

In subsequent experiments from our laboratory, we have shown that the monoclonal antibody 200-47, which recognizes the p53 protein of mouse and hamster cells but not of human cells, inhibits serum-stimulated DNA synthesis only when microinjected into mouse or hamster cells, but not when microinjected into human cells. Conversely, monoclonal antibody Pab 122, which recognizes the p53 of mouse and human cells, but not of hamster cells, exerts an inhibitory effect only when microinjected into mouse or human cells (W.E. Mercer et al., unpubl.).

Because the microinjected antibody against the p53 protein inhibited serum-stimulated DNA synthesis only when microinjected at the time of stimulation, we thought that if this protein were truly related to the exit of cells from G_0 then its monoclonal antibody would have no effect when microinjected into G_1 cells. We did, in fact, carry out a series of experiments by microinjecting Pab 122 into Swiss-3T3 cells that were progressing through G_1. One of these experiments is shown in Figure 1 in which cells were collected by mitotic detachment, replated, and microinjected with Pab 122 or with a control IgG within 1.5 hours after replating. The cells were then followed for 11.5 hours, fixed, and stained with acridine orange, and their DNA amount was determined by a computer-operated microspectrofluorimeter. The technique used for acridine orange staining and its validity for measuring DNA amounts have already been discussed in previous papers (Darzynkiewicz et al. 1976, 1979; Ashihara et al. 1978). The results of Figure 1 clearly indicate that microinjection of Pab 122 has no effect on the progression of Swiss-3T3 cells from mitosis to S phase, but is capable of inhibiting the progression of the same cells from G_0 to S phase. Similar experiments were carried out on exponentially growing cells (W.E. Mercer et al., unpubl.) and again clearly indicated that microinjection of Pab 122 had no effect on the progression of G_1 cells into S phase. In all these experiments, the time interval between the microinjection of the antibody and the termination of the experiments was

Table 2 Effect of Microinjected Antibodies on Serum-stimulated DNA Synthesis in Swiss-3T3 Cells

Time of microinjection	Antibody (% of labeled cells)			
	Lyt 2.2	αp53	αRNA pol I	none
0	48	10	54	51
6	50	45	48	50
17	50	52	53	49

Quiescent Swiss-3T3 cells were serum-stimulated and microinjected at the times indicated in the first column. The antibodies microinjected were: Lyt 2.2, a control monoclonal antibody; αp53, monoclonal Pab 122, described by Gurney et al. (1980); and αRNA pol I, an antibody against rat RNA polymerase I, described by Rose et al. (1981). Cells were continuously labeled with [^{3}H]thymidine and fixed 18 hr after serum stimulation.

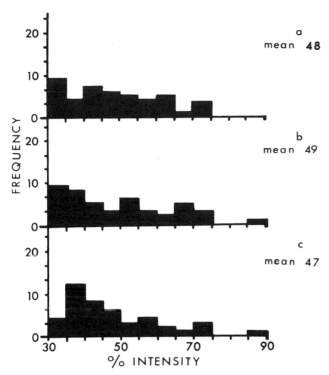

Figure 1 Histogram of DNA amounts in Swiss-3T3 cells growing in 10% fetal calf serum. Cells collected by mitotic detachment were replated and fixed 11.5 hr later. The amount of DNA in individual cells was determined by measuring the green fluorescence of acridine orange-stained cells using a computer-operated microspectrofluorimeter. Fluorescence intensity is expressed in arbitrary units (*abscissa*). (*a*) Untreated cells; (*b*) cells microinjected with Pab 122; (*c*) cells microinjected with a control IgG.

well within the limits of the half-life (~24 hr) of microinjected antibodies (Yamaizumi et al. 1979; Zavortink et al. 1979; Mercer et al. 1982).

It seems, therefore, that the p53 protein plays a role in the transition of cells from G_0 to S, but not from mitosis to S. Two alternative explanations that promptly come to mind are: (1) p53 is not needed for G_1 progression, or (2) G_1 cells have more p53 than G_0 cells (Milner and Milner 1981), and the amount of microinjected antibody

is not sufficient to neutralize the increased amount of p53 protein. Incidentally, we are already microinjecting the maximum amount of antibody that can be delivered to a cell and it is not possible for us to increase further the amount of antibody delivered. Regardless of the explanation, one has to conclude that the p53 protein does play a role, qualitative or quantitative, in the transition of Swiss-3T3 cells from a resting to a growing stage.

Effect of microinjected monoclonal antibodies against the p53 protein on the amount of cellular RNA

It is well known that the amount of cellular RNA rapidly increases when cells are stimulated to proliferate (for review, see Baserga 1981). Although there are exceptions, the amount of cellular RNA (85% of which is rRNA) seems to correlate strongly with the ability of cells to enter into the S phase (Darzynkiewicz et al. 1979; Singer and Johnston 1982). Therefore, we investigated the effect that microinjected Pab 122 may have on the amount of cellular RNA in Swiss-3T3 cells. The results are summarized in Table 3. The amount of cellular RNA was measured in fixed cells stained with acridine orange using a computer-operated microspectrofluorimeter. The mean amount of cellular RNA in arbitrary units in quiescent Swiss-3T3 cells was 21. Seventeen hours after serum stimulation, the mean amount of cellular RNA was 42, that is, doubled, which is in agreement with all the reports in the literature. If the serum-stimulated cells were microinjected with the control IgG, the mean amount of cellular RNA was 39 arbitrary units, which is essentially undistinguishable from the control, nonmicroinjected serum-stimulated cells. However, when the cells were microinjected with Pab 122, the mean amount of cellular RNA increased only to 27, that is, there was a 66% inhibition in the accumulation of cellular RNA in serum-stimulated cells. These experiments have been repeated with the same results. It seems therefore that a monoclonal antibody against the p53 protein, when microinjected into serum-stimulated cells, inhibits the accumulation of cellular RNA that usually occurs after cells make their transition from a resting to a growing stage.

Table 3 Microinjected Pab 122 Inhibits the Accumulation of Cellular RNA

Treatment	Antibody microinjected	Mean cellular RNA (arbitrary units per cell)
None	none	21
10% fetal calf serum	none	42
	control IgG	39
	Pab 122	27

Swiss-3T3 cells were made quiescent and left as such or stimulated with fetal calf serum. For the stimulated cells, the controls are the cells on the same coverslips outside the circle of microinjection. The amount of RNA was determined on fixed, acridine orange-stained cells using a computer-operated microspectrofluorimeter. The stimulated cells were fixed 17 hr after stimulation, when ~50% of the cells have reached S phase.

SV40 domains for the p53 protein and their relationship to cellular RNA accumulation

In previous experiments, we have shown that the ability to induce cell DNA replication maps on different domains of the SV40 genome than its ability to stimulate RNA synthesis, that is, growth in size (Soprano et al. 1983). We have therefore investigated the induction of the p53 protein by a deletion mutant of SV40 that is known to induce DNA synthesis but not growth in size. For this purpose we used deletion mutant *dl*1001, described by Pipas et al. (1983), whose deletion limits extend from nucleotide residue 4001 to nucleotide residue 3476 (out of phase). This deletion mutant was then introduced into the pTK plasmid, i.e., a pBR322 plasmid containing the *tk* gene of HSV. The transfection technique used was the one described by Shen et al. (1982). To avoid selection based on the expression of T antigen, the transfected tk⁻ ts13 cells were selected for their ability to grow in gHAT medium. A number of clones were obtained and a few clones were selected for further stud-

ies. One cell line HR8 was transformed with a wild-type SV40 cloned in pTK and produced a regular size T antigen (Fig. 2, lane a). EM83 cells transformed by *dl*1001 cloned pTK produced a 33K T antigen (Fig. 2, lane a) in agreement with the prediction based on Pipas et al.'s (1983) determination of the deletion boundaries. The sizes of the T antigens are visible in Figure 2, where the autoradiographs of the immunoprecipitates also show the ability of the various antibodies to precipitate the p53 protein. It will be noticed that antibodies against T antigen, or against the p53 protein, will immunoprecipitate the p53 protein in HR8 cells (lanes a and c). However, in EM83 cells the antibody against T antigen is not capable of precipitating a p53 protein (lane a). The results, therefore, seem to indicate that the deletion mutant of SV40, *dl*1001 (Pipas et al. 1983), coding for a 33K T antigen is incapable of inducing or binding p53 protein. This is further confirmed in Figure 3 where we have measured by computer-operated microspectrofluorimetry the amount of p53 protein in tk⁻ ts13 cells (untransformed) and in EM83 and HR8 cells. The p53 protein was stained by indirect immunofluorescence using the monoclonal antibody 200-47 and anti-mouse IgG. Figure 3 shows that in HR8 cells the amount of p53 protein is sixfold the amount detectable in tk⁻ ts13 cells. In EM83 cells, it is only doubled.

The SV40 genome is interrupted in *dl*1001 at nucleotide 4001 and the deletion brings the nucleotide se-

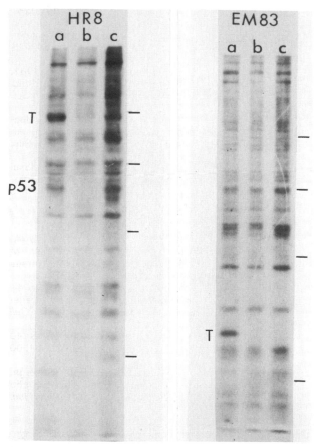

Figure 2 Autoradiography of immunoprecipitated proteins labeled with [³⁵S]methionine from HR8 and EM83 cells. (Lanes a) Hamster anti-T antiserum; (lanes b) normal hamster serum; (lanes c) monoclonal antibody 200-47. The methods for the labeling and extraction of proteins, immunoprecipitation, and electrophoresis have been described in the papers by Shen et al. (1982). Molecular-weight markers are indicated by horizontal lines and, from top to bottom, are: phosphorylase B, 92,500 daltons; bovine serum albumin, 68,000 daltons; ovalbumin, 43,000 daltons; and β-lactoglobulin, 18,400 daltons.

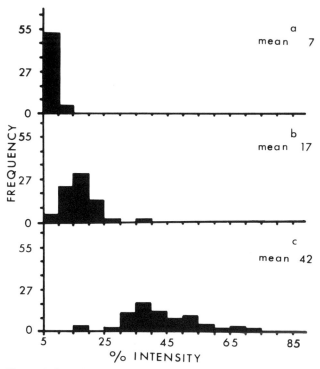

Figure 3 Quantitation of p53 protein amounts in cells stained by indirect immunofluorescence. The antibody used was monoclonal 200-47 (Dippold et al. 1981). The cells were tk⁻ ts13 (Shen et al. 1982) untransformed and their derivative, EM83 (transformed with *dl*1001) and HR8 (transformed with wild-type SV40). Fluorescence intensity (on the abscissa) is expressed in arbitrary units.

quence out of phase. It seems, therefore, that for the induction of the p53 protein some DNA sequences 3' to nucleotide 4001 are necessary. These results are of interest because the sequences for the reactivation of rRNA genes, that is for growth in size, on the SV40 T antigen-coding gene also map 3' to nucleotide 4001 (Soprano et al. 1983). Therefore, this reinforces our interpretation that the p53 protein may be somehow involved in the regulation of growth in size of the cell.

Conclusions

The technique of microinjecting monoclonal antibodies to study the function of the antigens against which they are directed seems to be reliable and to have a high degree of specificity. Using this technique, we have been able to show that the p53 plays a role in cell proliferation. More specifically, our results indicate that the p53 protein plays an important role, either qualitative or quantitative, in the transition of cells from a resting to a growing stage. It does not seem to be as important in cell-cycle progression when cells go from mitosis to S phase. If this is correct, then the p53 protein will actually be the first protein in the literature that can really be implicated in the exit of cells from G_0. Whether the p53 protein is actually the triggering protein for cell proliferation remains to be seen. However, the data do seem to indicate that p53 plays a major role in bringing noncyclic cells back into the cell cycle.

If the p53 protein is important in the exit of cells from G_0, it would be interesting to know the mechanism by which it exerts its function. At the present moment, very little information is available on this topic. However, the fact that a microinjected antibody against a p53 protein inhibits the accumulation of RNA suggests that the mechanism by which the p53 protein regulates cell proliferation is to control the size of the cell. This is further supported by the fact that an SV40 deletion mutant that can induce cellular DNA synthesis but not growth in size is not capable of inducing the appearance of p53 protein. The p53 protein, by regulating growth in size, could prime the cells, so to speak, to respond to growth factors that regulate cell DNA replication. This finding is compatible with results already published in the literature. Oren et al. (1981) have shown that the cellular amounts of the p53 protein in 3T3 cells are regulated at the post-transcriptional level. We also know that growth in size of the cells is independent of unique copy gene transcription (Ashihara et al. 1978; Baserga et al. 1982), whereas cell DNA replication requires transcription of unique copy genes (Baserga et al. 1982). Therefore, we would like to offer as conclusions the following: (1) the p53 protein is one of the major proteins regulating the exit of cells from G_0 into the cell cycle, and (2) the p53 protein may regulate cell proliferation by regulating the growth in size of the cells.

Acknowledgments

This work was supported by grants from the National Cancer Institute (CA25898) and the National Institute of Aging (AG00378).

References

Antman, K.H. and D.M. Livingston. 1980. Intracellular neutralization of SV40 tumor antigens following microinjection of specific antibodies. *Cell* **19**: 627.

Ashihara, T., F. Traganos, R. Baserga, and Z. Darzynkiewicz. 1978. A comparison of cell cycle related changes in post mitotic and quiescent AF8 cells, as measured by cytofluorimetry after acridine orange staining. *Cancer Res.* **38**: 2514.

Baserga, R. 1981. Introduction to cell growth. In *Tissue growth factors* (ed. R. Baserga), p.1. Springer-Verlag, Berlin.

Baserga, R., D.E. Waechter, K.J. Soprano, and N. Galanti. 1982. Molecular biology of cell division. *Ann. N.Y. Acad. Sci.* **397**: 110.

Carroll, R.B., O.K. Muello, and J.A. Melero. 1980. Coordinate expression of the 48K host nuclear phosphoprotein and SV40 T Ag upon primary infection of mouse cells. *Virology* **102**: 447.

Crawford, L.V., D.C. Pim, E.G. Gurney, P. Goodfellow, and J. Taylor-Papadimitriou. 1981. Detection of a common feature in several human tumor cell lines. A 53000 dalton protein. *Proc. Natl. Acad. Sci.* **78**: 41.

Darzynkiewicz, Z., F. Traganos, T. Sharpless, and M.R. Melamed. 1976. Lymphocyte stimulation. A rapid multiparameter analysis. *Proc. Natl. Acad. Sci.* **73**: 2881.

Darzynkiewicz, Z., D.P. Evanson, L. Staiano-Coico, T.K. Sharpless, and M.L. Melamed. 1979. Correlation between cell cycle duration and RNA content. *J. Cell. Physiol.* **100**: 425.

DeLeo, A.B., G. Jay, E. Appella, G.C. Dubois, L.W. Law, and L.J. Old. 1979. Detection of a transformation related antigen in chemical induced sarcomas and other transformed cells of the mouse. *Proc. Natl. Acad. Sci.* **76**: 2420.

Dippold, W.J.G., A.B. DeLeo, G. Khoury, and L.J. Old. 1981. p53 transformation related protein. Detection by monoclonal antibodies in mouse and human cells. *Proc. Natl. Acad. Sci.* **78**: 1695.

Floros, J., G. Jonak, N. Galanti, and R. Baserga. 1981. Induction of cell DNA replication in G_1 specific ts mutants by microinjection of recombinant SV40 DNA. *Exp. Cell Res.* **132**: 215.

Gurney, E.G., R.O. Harrison, and J. Fenno. 1980. Monoclonal antibodies against simian virus 40 T antigens. Evidence for distinct subclasses of large T antigen and for similarities among nonviral T antigens. *J. Virol.* **34**: 752.

Lane, D.P. and L.V. Crawford. 1979. T antigen is bound to a host protein in SV40 transformed cells. *Nature* **278**: 261.

Linnenbach, A., K. Huebner, and C.M. Croce. 1980. DNA-transformed murine teratocarcinoma cells regulation of expression of simian virus 40 tumor antigen in stem versus differentiated cells. *Proc. Natl. Acad. Sci.* **77**: 4875.

Linzer, D.I.H. and A.J. Levine. 1979. Characterization of a 54K dalton cellular SV40 tumor antigen present in SV40 transformed cells and uninfected embryonal carcinoma cells. *Cell* **17**: 43.

Linzer, D.I.H., W. Maltzman, and A.J. Levine. 1979. The SV40 A gene product is required for the production of a 54000 MW cellular tumor antigen. *Virology* **98**: 308.

Mercer, W.E., D. Nelson, A.B. DeLeo, L.J. Old, and R. Baserga. 1982. Microinjection of monoclonal antibody to protein p53 inhibits serum-induced DNA synthesis in 3T3 cells. *Proc. Natl. Acad. Sci.* **79**: 6309.

Mercer, W.E., D. Nelson, J.K. Hyland, C.M. Croce, and R. Baserga. 1983. Inhibition of SV40 induced cellular DNA synthesis by microinjection of monoclonal antibodies. *Virology* **127**: 149.

Mercer, W.E., C. Avignolo, N. Galanti, K.M. Rose, J.K. Hyland, S. Jacob, and R. Baserga. 1984. Cellular DNA replication is independent from the synthesis or accumulation of ribosomal RNA. *Exp. Cell Res.* **118**: 118.

Milner, J. and F. McCormick. 1980. Lymphocyte stimulation: Concanavalin A induces the expression of a 53K protein. *Cell Biol. Int. Rep.* **4**: 663.

Milner, J. and S. Milner. 1981. SV40 53K antigen: A possible role of 53K in normal cells. *Virology* **112**: 785.

Oren, M., W. Maltzman, and A. Levine. 1981. Post-translational regulation of the 54K cellular tumor antigen in normal and transformed cells. *Mol. Cell. Biol.* **1:** 101.

Pipas, J.M., K.W.C. Peden, and D. Nathans. 1983. Mutational analysis of simian virus 40 T antigen: Isolation and characterization of mutants with deletions in the T antigen gene. *Mol. Cell. Biol.* **3:** 203.

Rose, K.M., D.A. Stetler, and S.T. Jacob. 1981. Protein kinase activity of RNA polymerase I purified from a rat hepatoma: Probable function of M$_r$ 42000 and 24600 polypeptides. *Proc. Natl. Acad. Sci.* **78:** 2833.

Rotter, V., M.A. Boss, and D. Baltimore. 1981. Increased concentration of an apparently identical cellular protein in cells transformed by either Abelson murine leukemia virus or other transforming agents. *J. Virol.* **38:** 336.

Shen, Y.M., R.R. Hirschhorn, W.E. Mercer, E. Surmacz, Y. Tsutsui, K.J. Soprano, and R. Baserga. 1982. Gene transfer: DNA microinjection compared with DNA transfection with a very high efficiency. *Mol. Cell. Biol.* **2:** 1145.

Singer, R.A. and G.C. Johnston. 1982. Transcription of rRNA genes and cell cycle regulation in the yeast *Saccharomyces cerevisiae*. In *Genetic expression in the cell cycle* (ed. G.M. Padilla and K.S. McCarty, Sr.), p. 181. Academic Press, New York.

Soprano, K.J., N. Galanti, G.J. Jonak, S. McKercher, J.M. Pipas, K.W.C. Peden, and R. Baserga. 1983. Mutational analysis of simian virus 40 T antigen: Stimulation of cellular DNA synthesis and activation of rRNA genes by mutants with deletions in the T antigen gene. *Mol. Cell. Biol.* **3:** 214.

Yamaizumi, M., T. Uchida, E. Mekada, and Y. Okada. 1979. Antibodies introduced into living cells by red cell ghosts are functionally stable in the cytoplasm of cells. *Cell* **18:** 1009.

Zavortink, M., T. Thacher, and M. Rechsteiner. 1979. Degradation of proteins microinjected into cultured mammalian cells. *J. Cell. Physiol.* **100:** 175.

Molecular Analysis of the Gene for the p53 Cellular Tumor Antigen

S. Benchimol
The Ontario Cancer Institute, Toronto, Ontario, Canada

J.R. Jenkins
Marie Curie Foundation Research Institute, Surrey, England

L.V. Crawford, K. Leppard, P. Lamb, N.M. Williamson, and D.C. Pim
Imperial Cancer Research Fund Laboratories, London, England

E. Harlow
Cold Spring Harbor Laboratory, Cold Spring Harbor, New York 11724

p53 is a cellular protein that is present in a wide variety of transformed cell lines, whether they be spontaneously, virally, or chemically derived, but is present in very low amounts in normal cells (DeLeo et al. 1979; Crawford et al. 1981; Dippold et al. 1981; Rotter et al. 1981; Benchimol et al. 1982). This has led many workers to speculate on a possible role for p53 in at least some types of neoplastic transformation. Supporting evidence comes from the following observations; (1) p53 synthesis is increased in many induced and spontaneous mouse tumor cell lines (Rotter 1983); (2) sera from animals bearing tumors, including human patients, often contain antibodies specific for p53, whereas normal sera do not (DeLeo et al. 1979; Lane and Crawford 1979; Linzer and Levine 1979; Rotter et al. 1980; Crawford et al. 1982; P. May and K. Chandrasekaran, pers. comm.); (3) in cells transformed by SV40 or adenovirus, p53 is specifically associated with the virus-coded tumor antigen that is required for transformation (Lane and Crawford 1979; Linzer and Levine 1979; McCormick and Harlow 1980; Sarnow et al. 1982). In addition, several studies have suggested that p53 may play an obligatory role in the steps between mitogen stimulation and the initiation of cellular DNA synthesis, thus suggesting some regulatory role during normal cell growth (Milner and Milner 1981; Mercer et al. 1982).

An understanding of how synthesis of this protein is regulated may provide insight into the control of cell proliferation. Toward this goal we have isolated a cDNA clone for p53. In this communication, we describe the construction and isolation of this p53-specific cDNA clone. We have used this cDNA clone to identify two genomic loci that are homologous to the p53 coding region. One of these loci is a processed pseudogene and the other is apparently the authentic p53 gene.

Materials and Methods

Purification of p53 mRNA by polysome immunoselection

The SV40-transformed mouse fibroblast cell line SVA31E7 was grown in Dulbecco's modified Eagle's medium with 10% fetal calf serum. Confluent cell monolayers were rinsed with Tris-buffered saline containing cycloheximide (1 μg/ml) and the cells were collected by scraping. Polysomes were isolated as described by MacGillivray et al. (1979). All solutions contained cycloheximide (1 μg/ml). The polysomes were stored frozen at −80°C.

The immunoselection of polysomes followed the procedure of Kraus and Rosenberg (1982) and is outlined below. The monoclonal antibody RA3 2C2 (Rotter et al. 1980; Coffman and Weissman 1981) was made RNase-free by passage of the hybridoma supernatant over protein A-Sepharose CL-4B (Pharmacia) in 0.1 M potassium phosphate (pH 8.0), and elution with 0.1 M potassium phosphate (pH 3.0) followed by neutralization of the eluate with 0.1 volume of 1 M potassium phosphate (pH 8.0).

Polysomes were diluted to 15 A_{260}/ml with a solution containing 10 mM HEPES (pH 7.5), 0.15 M NaCl, and 5 mM $MgCl_2$. The purified monoclonal antibody RA3 2C2 was added at a ratio of 250 A_{260} units of polysomes per mg of antibody. Heparin and cycloheximide were added at a final concentration of 0.1 mg/ml and 1 μg/ml, respectively. The final $MgCl_2$ concentration was maintained at 5 mM. The polysome-antibody mixture was incubated for 16 hours at 10°C prior to passage over a column of protein A-Sepharose CL-4B that was previously equilibrated with polysome buffer (25 mM Tris [pH7.5], 150 mM NaCl, 5 mM $MgCl_2$, 0.1% NP-40, 1 μg/ml cycloheximide, 0.2 mg/ml heparin). The flow-through was passed over once again, and the column was then washed extensively (100 column volumes) with the same buffer. The polysomes were dissociated and the ribosomal subunits and the specific mRNA were eluted from the column with a solution containing 25 mM Tris (pH 7.4), 20 mM EDTA, and 0.2 mg/ml heparin. The EDTA eluate was immediately adjusted to 0.5 M NaCl and 0.1% SDS and applied to a column of oligo(dT)-cellulose (type 3, Collaborative Research Inc.). The flow-through was passed over once again. The column was washed and the bound poly(A)+ mRNA eluted as described (Maniatis et al. 1982). The eluted RNA was precipitated at −20°C with 2 volumes of ethanol and 0.1 volume of 2 M potassium acetate in the presence of calf liver tRNA (Boehringer Mannheim).

The extent of enrichment for p53-specific mRNA was estimated by translation of the RNA preparation in a mRNA-dependent cell-free protein-synthesizing system derived from rabbit reticulocytes (Pelham and Jackson 1976). The translated polypeptides were fractionated on an SDS/10% polyacrylamide gel either directly or after immunoprecipitation. Immunoprecipitations with formalin-fixed *Staphylococcus aureus* (Kessler 1975) were performed as described previously (Benchimol et al. 1982) using a cocktail of monoclonal antibodies directed against p53: PAb421 (Harlow et al. 1981), RA3 2C2 (Rotter et al. 1980; Coffman and Weissman 1981), and 200-47 (Dippold et al. 1981). The gels were fixed, dried, and fluorographed (Bonner and Laskey 1974).

Synthesis of double-stranded cDNA

Reverse transcriptase was used to synthesize single-stranded DNA under the conditions described by Retzel et al. (Retzel et al. 1980). Immunoselected RNA was used as template. The second strand was prepared by self-priming with the Klenow fragment of *Escherichia coli* polymerase followed by reverse transcriptase. S1 endonuclease and T4 DNA polymerase were used to cleave the hairpin loop and generate blunt ends, respectively. BglII and PstI synthetic oligonucleotide linkers were added simultaneously to the cDNA to generate dissimilar cohesive ends in a reaction catalyzed by T4 DNA ligase as described by Kurtz and Nicodemus (1981). After digestion with BglII and PstI, the cDNA was size-selected and separated from the linkers by gel electrophoresis through low-melting-point agarose. cDNA was extracted from the agarose and ligated to a plasmid vector derived from pAT153 containing BglII and PstI acceptor sites (J. Jenkins and E. Harlow, unpubl.). The ligated DNA was used to transform *E. coli* strain LE 392. The transformed colonies were plated directly onto nitrocellulose (HATF, Millipore) and prepared for hybridization by treatment with alkali and neutralization (Maniatis et al. 1982).

Preparation of probes

Random calf thymus oligonucleotides were used as primers to synthesize ^{32}P-labeled cDNA probes from p53-enriched and p53-depleted RNA templates in a reaction catalyzed by reverse transcriptase (Maniatis et al. 1982). After 90 minutes at 37°C, the reaction was stopped by addition of an equal volume of phenol-chloroform. The mixture was blended in a Vortex mixer, centrifuged, and the upper aqueous phase containing the cDNA was recovered. The cDNA was precipitated with ethanol, alkali treated, reprecipitated, and hybridized to the filters carrying the transformed colonies treated as described above.

Identification of p53 cDNA clones by hybridization-selection and cell-free translation

Clones to be tested were grown in LB containing tetracycline (10 μg/ml) and amplified in the presence of chlor-amphenicol (150 μg/ml). Plasmid DNAs were isolated as described (Maniatis et al. 1982), digested with BglII to linearize the molecules, heat-denatured in the presence of 0.3 M NaOH, neutralized with ammonium acetate, and bound to squares (5 mm × 5 mm) of nitrocellulose membrane (HATF, Millipore). The bound DNA was hybridized to total poly(A)$^+$ mRNA from E7 cells (450 μg/ml) in a volume of 0.1 ml hybridization solution (Ricciardi et al. 1979) at 45°C for 4 hours. The filters were then washed at 60°C and the RNA eluted thermally as described (Maniatis et al. 1982). The eluted RNAs were subsequently analyzed by cell-free translation and immunoprecipitation. Total poly(A)$^+$ mRNA was isolated by the guanidinium isothiocyanate procedure described by Chirgwin et al. (1979) followed by oligo(dT)-cellulose chromatography.

Determination of nucleotide sequence

Plasmid p53-clone 9 was treated with PstI, and subjected to electrophoresis on a preparative low-melting-point agarose gel. The PstI fragment (see text) was extracted from the gel (Maniatis et al. 1982) and ligated into PstI-cut, phosphatase-treated bacteriophage M13 mp9 vector (Messing and Vieira 1982). Both orientations of the PstI fragment were obtained. In addition, the DNA was reduced to smaller size and subcloned into M13 mp9 vector as follows: (1) digestion of cDNA insert with TaqI followed by ligation into AccI/PstI-cut vector, and (2) digestion of cDNA insert with RsaI followed by ligation into a SmaI-cut vector and a SmaI/PstI-cut vector. The ligated mixtures were used to transfect *E. coli* JM 101 (Messing 1979). Single-stranded template was prepared from colorless M13 plaques and used for sequence determination by the dideoxy chain-termination procedure (Sanger et al. 1977, 1980).

Similar methodology was used for the subcloning and sequencing of the genomic DNA.

DNA blot hybridization

DNA was extracted from mouse and human cells, digested with restriction endonucleases, and fractionated by electrophoresis on a 0.8% agarose gel in 40 mM Tris/ 5 mM sodium acetate/1 mM EDTA (pH 7.8). The gels were denatured, neutralized, and transferred to nitrocellulose paper (Maniatis et al. 1982). The digested DNA on the nitrocellulose paper was then hybridized with ^{32}P-labeled p53 cDNA clone 9, as described by Maniatis et al. (1982). Mouse DNA was hybridized to the probe at 68°C. The hybridized blots were washed in a solution of 0.1 × SSC at 68°C (1 × is 0.15 M NaCl/0.015 M sodium citrate). Optimal conditions for detection of human p53 nucleotide sequences were found to be hybridization in 6 × SSC at 62°C and washing in three changes of 6 × SSC, 1% SDS at 62°C. This protocol is referred to as reduced stringency in the text.

Results

Enrichment of p53 mRNA

As a first step in developing a strategy to construct and isolate a cDNA clone for p53, it was necessary to estimate the abundance of p53-specific mRNA in the cell. Total poly(A)$^+$ mRNA was isolated by the guanidinium isothiocyanate procedure from the SV40-transformed mouse cell line SVA31E7 that was previously shown by radioimmunoassay to contain more p53 protein than other mouse cell lines that were examined (Benchimol et al. 1982). The RNA was translated in a cell-free system containing [^{35}S]methionine, and translated polypeptides were immunoprecipitated with monoclonal antibody directed against p53 and fractionated by polyacrylamide gel electrophoresis. The autoradiograph presented in Figure 1 shows that p53 mRNA can be detected by in vitro translation. Furthermore, from the amount of radioactivity specifically immunoprecipitated with anti-p53 monoclonal antibody relative to the total acid-precipitable radioactivity incorporated into protein by cell-free translation, we estimate that p53 mRNA constitutes approximately 0.01% of total poly(A)$^+$ mRNA.

To facilitate cloning of cDNA copies corresponding to p53-specific mRNA sequences, enrichment of p53 mRNA was performed by immunoselection of polysomes using monoclonal antibodies directed against p53. The immunoselection of polysomes, described under Mate-

rials and Methods, followed the procedure of Kraus and Rosenberg (1982). The extent of enrichment was estimated by cell-free translation followed by SDS gel electrophoresis and fluorography (Fig. 2). Comparison of lane A (translation of immunoselected p53 mRNA) with lane B (translation with no added RNA) indicated that a polypeptide of 53 kD is the major product of the in vitro translation. Figure 2 also demonstrates that this 53-kD polypeptide can be immunoprecipitated by monoclonal antibodies specific for p53. We estimate that the p53 mRNA is enriched about 1000-fold by this procedure.

Synthesis and identification of cDNA clones for p53

The p53-enriched poly(A)$^+$ mRNA preparation was used to construct a cDNA library in *E. coli* as described under Materials and Methods. Approximately 300 colonies were generated when immunoselected RNA obtained from 100 A_{260} units of polysomes was used as template for first-strand cDNA synthesis. This library was screened in duplicate for the presence of p53 sequences by differential hybridization to cDNA probes made from either p53-enriched or p53-depleted poly(A)$^+$ mRNA.

Twenty-two colonies showing preferential hybridization to the p53-enriched cDNA probe were selected for further characterization by hybridization selection and in vitro translation of the eluted RNA. DNA from each of these clones was linearized by restriction enzyme diges-

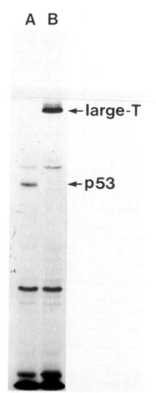

Figure 1 Cell-free translation of total poly(A)$^+$ mRNA from an SV40-transformed mouse cell line analyzed by immunoprecipitation and SDS-polyacrylamide gel electrophoresis. Poly(A)$^+$ mRNA was isolated from the SV40-transformed mouse cell line SVA31E7 and translated in a cell-free system derived from rabbit reticulocytes. (Lane A) Translated polypeptides were immunoprecipitated with a cocktail of monoclonal antibodies directed against p53: PAb421, RA3 2C2, and 200-47. (Lane B) Translated polypeptides were immunoprecipitated with a cocktail of monoclonal antibodies directed against the SV40 large T antigen: PAb416 and PAb419 (Harlow et al. 1981).

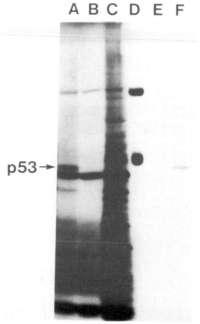

Figure 2 SDS-polyacrylamide gel analysis of polypeptides translated from total SVA31E7 poly(A)$^+$ and from immunoselected mRNA. (Lane A) Translation with immunoselected mRNA; (lane B) translation with no added mRNA; (lane C) translation of total mRNA; (lane D) protein markers phosphorylase a, 94 kD, and glutamate dehydrogenase, 54 kD; (lane E) translation products shown in lane A after immunoprecipitation with monoclonal antibodies against the SV40 large-T antigen (PAb416 and PAb419); (lane F) translation products shown in lane A after immunoprecipitation with a cocktail of monoclonal antibodies against p53 (PAb421, RA3 2C2, and 200-47).

tion, bound to small squares of nitrocellulose, and used in a hybridization selection assay with total poly(A)+ mRNA. The bound RNA was eluted, translated in vitro, and the polypeptide products immunoprecipitated with monoclonal antibody directed against p53 prior to fractionation by SDS gel electrophoresis. The results presented in Figure 3 demonstrate that seven plasmid DNAs (lanes b,h,i,k–n) were capable of hybridizing p53 mRNA. For purposes of comparison, vector DNA alone was included in the hybridization selection assay (lane w). A faint band migrating with the same mobility as p53 can be seen in some of the tracks in Figure 5. Because this band is also present in lane w (plasmid vector DNA alone), it is thought to arise nonspecifically. These results, therefore, serve to identify seven plasmids that contain sequences that are homologous to p53 mRNA.

Subsequent characterization of the inserts present in the seven plasmids by size (560 bp) and HaeIII restriction enzyme digestion (data not shown) indicated that all were identical. The most likely explanation is that the seven colonies are sibling clones derived from a single transformed bacterial colony prior to plating.

Nucleotide sequence of p53 cDNA
One of the plasmids (designated p53-clone 9) was chosen for further characterization by nucleotide sequenc-

ing. It should be noted that *Pst*I and *Bgl*II synthetic oligonucleotide linkers were used to generate dissimilar cohesive ends in the cDNA prior to ligation into the plasmid vector. The insert present in p53-clone 9, however, can be excised from the plasmid by digestion with *Pst*I alone whereas digestion with *Bgl*II serves only to linearize the plasmid (data not shown). The following type of insert is consistent with these observations: *Pst*I end–cDNA–*Pst*I linker–*Bgl*II end. This orientation was confirmed by nucleotide sequencing described below.

The complete nucleotide sequence of the p53 cDNA was determined by the dideoxy chain-termination procedure (Sanger et al. 1977, 1980) using the bacteriophage M13 vector mp9 (Messing 1979). The strategy employed to obtain the complete sequence of both strands is described under Materials and Methods. Examination of the nucleotide sequence identifies a single reading frame that is open throughout its entire length. The nucleotide sequence together with the inferred amino acid sequence of the encoded polypeptide is presented in Figure 4. Recently, Leppard et al. (1983) determined the amino acid sequence of a tryptic peptide from p53. Comparison of the peptide sequence, shown boxed in Figure 4, with the predicted polypeptide translation product shows a precise match and serves to confirm the correct reading frame. Most importantly, the

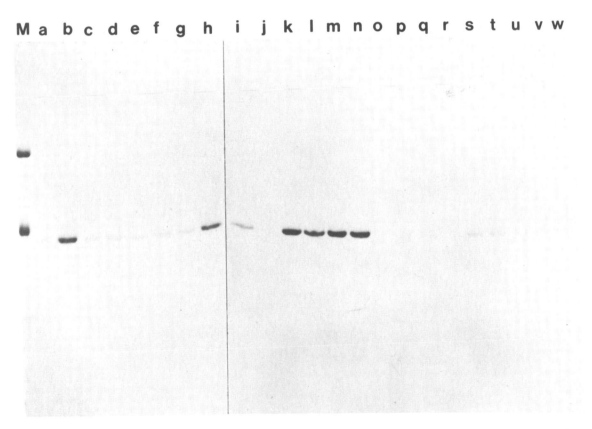

Figure 3 Identification of p53 cDNA clones by hybridization-selection and cell-free translation. Plasmid DNAs from putative recombinant clones were bound to nitrocellulose membrane filters and hybridized to total poly(A)+ mRNA from SVA31E7 cells. Bound RNA was eluted thermally and analyzed subsequently by cell-free translation. Lane *M* contains protein size markers phosphorylase a, 94 kD, and glutamate dehydrogenase, 54 kD. Lanes *a–w* contain the translated products immunoprecipitated with a cocktail of monoclonal antibodies against p53 (PAb421, RA3 2C2, and 200-47). DNAs used for hybridization-selection are: 22 cDNA clones in lanes *a–v*; plasmid vector DNA alone in lane *w*.

```
            20                        40
G TAT CCC GAG TAT CTG GAA GAC AGG CAG ACT TTT CGC CAC AGC GTG GTG GTA CCT
  Tyr Pro Glu Tyr Leu Glu Asp Arg Gln Thr Phe Arg His Ser Val Val Val Pro

        60                        80                        100
TAT GAG CCA CCC GAG GCC GGC TCT GAG TAT ACC ACC ATC CAC TAC AAG TAC ATG
Tyr Glu Pro Pro Glu Ala Gly Ser Glu Tyr Thr Thr Ile His Tyr Lys Tyr Met

            120                        140                        160
TGT AAT AGC TCC TGC ATG GGG GGC ATG AAC CGC CGA CCT ATC CTT ACC ATC ATC
Cys Asn Ser Ser Cys Met Gly Gly Met Asn Arg Arg Pro Ile Leu Thr Ile Ile

                    180                        200
ACA CTG GAA GAC TCC AGT GGG AAC CTT CTG GGA CGG GAC AGC TTT GAG GTT CGT
Thr Leu Glu Asp Ser Ser Gly Asn Leu Leu Gly Arg Asp Ser Phe Glu Val Arg

220                        240                        260
GTT TGT GCC TGC CCT GGG AGA GAC CGC CGT ACA GAA GAA GAA AAT TTC CGC AAA
Val Cys Ala Cys Pro Gly Arg Asp Arg Arg Thr Glu Glu Glu Asn Phe Arg Lys

            280                        300                        320
AAG GAA GTC CTT TGC CCT GAA CTG CCC CCA GGG AGC GCA AAG AGA GCG CTG CCC
Lys Glu Val Leu Cys Pro Glu Leu Pro Pro Gly Ser Ala Lys Arg Ala Leu Pro

                340                        360
ACC TGC ACA AGC GCC TCT CCC CCG CAA AAG AAA AAA CCA CTT GAT GGA GAG TAT
Thr Cys Thr Ser Ala Ser Pro Pro Gln Lys Lys Lys Pro Leu Asp Gly Glu Tyr

380                        400                        420
TTC ACC CTC AAG ATC CGC GGG CGT AAA CGC TTC GAG ATG TTC CGG GAG CTG AAT
Phe Thr Leu Lys Ile Arg Gly Arg Lys Arg Phe Glu Met Phe Arg Glu Leu Asn

        440                        460                        480
GAG GCC TTA GAG TTA AAG GAT GCC CAT GCT ACA GAG GAG TCT GGA GAC AGC AGG
Glu Ala Leu Glu Leu Lys Asp Ala His Ala Thr Glu Glu Ser Gly Asp Ser Arg

            500                        520            538
GCT CAC TCC AGC TAC CTG AAG ACC AAG AAG GGC CAG TCT ACT TCC CGC CAT
Ala His Ser Ser Tyr Leu Lys Thr Lys Lys Gly Gln Ser Thr Ser Arg His
```

Figure 4 Nucleotide sequence of p53 cDNA clone 9 together with its predicted translation product. The p53 tryptic peptide K9 isolated and sequenced by Leppard et al. (1983) is shown boxed. In addition to the sequence shown, clone 9 contains a sequence A_{18} at its 3' end, derived from the oligo(dT) used to prime cDNA synthesis (see text), and has PstI linker sequences at each end.

agreement between peptide sequence (Leppard et al. 1983) and inferred amino acid sequence establishes the authenticity of p53-clone 9. In addition, it appears that p53-clone 9 consists entirely of coding sequences.

Analysis of p53-specific cellular DNA

p53-specific sequences in cellular DNA were examined by the Southern blot hybridization technique (Southern 1975) using p53 cDNA clone 9 as the hybridization probe (Fig. 5). Cellular DNA was isolated from SVA31E7 mouse cells and digested with: EcoRI (lane a); HindIII (lane b); EcoRI and HindIII (lane c). Southern blot analysis reveals two EcoRI fragments approximately 18 kb and 3.3 kb in length (Fig. 5A, lane a) and two HindIII fragments approximately 7.6 kb and 2.0 kb long (Fig. 5A, lane b) that hybridize to the cDNA probe.

Detection of p53-specific nucleotide sequences in human DNA was more difficult. When human DNA was hybridized to p53 cDNA clone 9 under the same hybridization conditions used to detect p53-specific sequences in mouse DNA, no hybridization was observed. Adjustment of the conditions, however, allowed us to detect human p53 sequences. The blot shown in Figure 5B was hybridized to p53 cDNA clone 9 under reduced stringency as described in Materials and Methods. Southern blot analysis reveals two HindIII fragments ap-

proximately 7.0 kb and 2.5 kb in size, the larger fragment being cut by EcoRI to give a 5.0-kb fragment. With BamHI, a single fragment of approximately 8.0 kb was seen.

To study more thoroughly the organization of the mouse genomic DNA that was homologous to the p53 cDNA, cellular DNA from the mouse SVA31E7 cell line was digested with HindIII and run on a low-gelling-temperature agarose gel. Using autoradiographs from Southern transfers as templates, DNA from the region corresponding to the size of the two HindIII fragments was excised and purified. These DNAs were cloned into λ NM1147. Plaques containing sequences homologous to p53 were identified by hybridization with p53 clone-9 cDNA probe. The inserts from these phage were purified and analyzed by dideoxynucleotide sequencing. Figure 6 shows the sequence of the corresponding regions of the clone 9 cDNA, the 7.6-kb HindIII fragment (p53MG1), and the 2.0-kb HindIII fragment (p53MG2).

Discussion

This communication describes the purification of the mRNA for the cellular tumor antigen p53, the cloning of its cDNA, and the determination of the cDNA nucleotide sequence. p53 mRNA is a low-abundance message that represents approximately 0.01% of the total mRNA in a

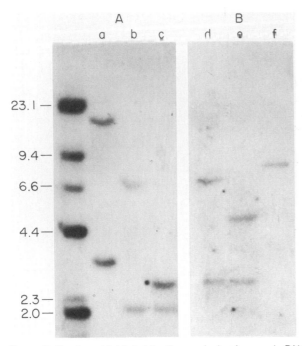

Figure 5 Southern blot hybridization analysis of genomic DNA. Aliquots (20 μg) of DNA were digested with *Eco*RI (lane *a*), *Hind*III (lane *b*), *Eco*RI plus *Hind*III (lane *c*), *Hind*III (lane *d*), *Hind*III plus *Eco*RI (lane *e*), and *Bam*HI (lane *f*) endonucleases, fractionated by electrophoresis through a 0.8% agarose gel, blotted onto nitrocellulose paper, and probed with ^{32}P-labeled p53 cDNA clone 9. DNA-length markers (*Hind*III digest of phage λ DNA) were run as markers, and their sizes are given in kb. (*A*) Digests of high-molecular-weight DNA isolated from the SV40-transformed mouse cell SVA31E7. (*B*) Digests of high-molecular-weight human fetal liver DNA.

mouse cell. The availability of monoclonal antibodies for p53 has enabled us to employ the technique of polysome immunoselection to isolate p53-specific mRNA. We estimate that p53 mRNA is enriched about 1000-fold by this procedure. Our success, together with that of others (Kraus and Rosenberg 1982; Korman et al. 1982; Robson et al. 1982; Lee et al. 1983; Oren and Levine 1983), suggests that the technique of polysome immunoselection will become increasingly important as a means of purifying low-abundance mRNA species.

We have used the enriched mRNA to isolate a cDNA for p53. Agreement between the nucleotide sequence of the cDNA and the amino acid sequence of a p53 tryptic peptide (Leppard et al. 1983) provides definitive identification of the cDNA clone. Moreover, the amino acid sequence data confirm the correct reading frame predicted from the nucleotide sequence and indicate that the entire cDNA sequence is translated. Thus, we have isolated a cDNA copy of an internal region of the p53 mRNA. This is surprising because oligo(dT) priming of cDNA synthesis is normally heavily biased towards sequences at the 3′ end of an mRNA template. It is possible that an internal stretch of adenine residues on the mRNA has competed with the poly(A) tail of the mRNA for binding to oligo(dT) in the priming step of first-strand cDNA synthesis. A stretch of adenine residues that could serve as this type of priming sequence is present in the region of genomic DNA adjacent to the 3′ end of the cDNA clone-9 sequences.

We have used the cDNA clone 9 to examine p53-specific nucleotide sequences in human and mouse cellular DNA. These analyses have shown that in mice there

```
  1                                                  gaattcctaaacagaactccaatgactcaggctttaagatctagaattgataaataggac  P53MB1

 61  cacatgaaactgaaagacttctgtaaggaaaaggacatagtcaataggacaaataggcaatctatagattggggaaagcatcctcactaatcccacatcc  P53MB1

                5'DR >>>>>>>>>>>>
161  aatagagggctaatatccaaactctatAAAGAACTCAAGAGGTAGAGTTAGGGGGCACCTAGCATTCAGGCCCTCATCCTCCTCCTTCCCAGCAGGGTGT  p53MB1

261  CACGCTTCCCGAAGACTGGATGACTGCCATGGAGGAGTCACAGTCGGATATCAGCCTCGAGCTCCCTCTGAGTCAGGAGACATTTTCAGGCTTATGGAAA  p53MB1

361  CTACTTCCTCCAGAAGATATCCTGCCATCACCTCACTCCATGGACGATCTGTTGCTGCCCCAGGATGTTGAGGAGTTTTTTGAAGGCCCAAGTGAAGCCC  p53MB1

461  TCCAAGTGTCAGGAGCTCCTGCAGCACAGGACCCTGTCACTGAGACCCCTGGGCCAGTGGCCCCTGCCCCAGCTACTCCATGGCCCCCGTCATCTTTTGT  p53MB1

                                                             ‡   ‡‡‡‡‡‡
561  CCCTTCTCAAAAAAACTTACCAGGGCAACTATGGCTTCCACCTGGGCTTGCTGCAGTCTGGGACAGCCAAGTCTGTTACTGT------ACTCTCCTCCCCT  p53MB1

                                                     ‡                                             ‡
655  CAATAAGCTATTCTGCCAGCTGGCGAAGACGTGCCCTGTGCAGTTGTGAGTCAGCGCCACACCTCCAGCTGGGAGCCGTGTCCGCGCCATGGCCATCTTC  p53MB1

           ‡  ‡‡‡                                   ‡                                      ‡
755  AAGAAGTCACAGCATATTCTGGAGGTCGTGAGACGCTGCCCCCACCATGAGTGCTGCTCCGATGGTGATGGCCTGGCTCCTCCCCAGCATCTTATCAGGG  p53MB1
```

Figure 6 (*See facing page for legend.*)

```
                 ‡   ‡                              ‡           ‡              ‡
 855 TGGAAGGAAATTTGTATGCCGAATATCTGGAAGACAGGCAGACTTTTCGCCACAGTGTGGTGGTACCTTACGAGCCACCCGAGGTCGGCTCTGAGTATAC  p53M81
   1       GTATCCCGAGTATCTGGAAGACAGGCAGACTTTTCGCCACAGCGTGGTGGTACCTTATGAGCCACCCGAGGCCGGCTCTGAGTATAC  p53c19

                       ‡     ‡            ‡
 955 CACCATCCACTACAAGTACATGTGTAGTAGCTCTTGCATGGGGGGCATAAACCGCCGACCTATCCTTACCATCATCACACTGGAAGACTCCAGTGGGAAC  p53M81
  88 CACCATCCACTACAAGTACATGTGTAATAGCTCCTGCATGGGGGGCATGAACCGCCGACCTATCCTTACCATCATCACACTGGAAGACTCCAGTGGGAAC  p53c19

            ‡                              ‡ ‡‡     ‡         ‡    ‡    ‡
1055 CTTCTGGGACCGGACAGCTTTGAGGTTCGTGTTTGTGCCTGCCCTGGGAGAGACTGGAGTACAGAGGAAGAAAATTTCCCCAAAAAAGGAAGTCCCTTGC  p53M81
 188 CTTCTGGGACGGGACAGCTTTGAGGTTCGTGTTTGTGCCTGCCCTGGGAGAGACCGCCGTACAGAAGAAGAAAATTTCCGCAAAAA-GGAAGTCCTTTGC  p53c19

        ‡  ‡     ‡ ‡     ‡‡              ‡ ‡    ‡    ‡ ‡‡‡‡‡‡          ‡
1155 CCTGATCTGACCCCAGGTAGTGCAAAGA--GCGCTGCCCACCTGCACA-GTGCCTCCCCCCCCCAAAAAAAAAAGAAAAAAACACTTGATGGAGAGTATT  p53M81
 287 CCTGAACTGCCCCCAGGGAGCGCAAAGAGAGCGCTGCCCACCTGCACAAGCGCCTCTCCCCGC------AAAAGAAAAAACCACTTGATGGAGAGTATT  p53c19
   1                aagcttgttgtacacgttctactg-< 176 nucleotides >-catctcacttcat  p53M82

                     ‡            ‡
1252 TCACCCTCAAGATCCGCGGGCGTGAACGCTTTGAGATGTTCCGGGAGCTGAATGAGGCCTTAGAGTTAAAGGATGCCCATGCTACAGAGGAGTCTGGAGA  p53M81
 381 TCACCCTCAAGATCCGCGGGCGTAAACGCTTCGAGATGTTCCGGGAGCTGAATGAGGCCTTAGAGTTAAAGGATGCCCATGCTACAGAGGAGTCTGGAGA  p53c19
 214 ctctgctgcagATCCGCGGGCGTAAACGCTTCGAGATGTTCCGGGAGCTGAATGAGGCCTTAGAGTTAAAGGATGCCCATGCTACAGAGGAGTCTGGAGA  p53M82

                <----------------------intervening sequence---------------------->
1352 CAGCAGGGCTCACTCCAG-----------------------------------------------------------CTACCTGAAGACCAA  p53M81
 481 CAGCAGGGCTCACTCCAG-----------------------------------------------------------CTACCTGAAGACCAA  p53c19
 314 CAGCAGGGCTCACTCCAGgtaagtggcctggggcagcgcc-< 543 nucleotides >-cccctttctgtcttcctatagCTACCTGAAGACCAA  p53M82

        ‡           ‡            ‡                                     ---       ‡    ‡
1385 GAAGGACCAGTCTACTTCCCCCCCATAAAAAAAAACAATGGTCAAGAAAGTGGGGCCTGACTCAGACTGACTGCCTCTGTATCCTGTCCCCATCACCAGCCT  p53M81
 514 GAAGGGCCAGTCTACTTCCCGCCCAT  p53c19
 934 GAAGGGCCAGTCTACTTCCCGCCCATAAAAAAA-CAATGGTCAAGAAAGTGGGGCCTGACTCAGACTGACTGCCTCTGCATCCCGTCCCCATCACCAGCCT  p53M82

                                                                       ---
                                                                       STOP

        ‡           ‡            ‡         ‡‡‡‡‡‡‡‡‡‡‡‡‡‡‡‡‡‡‡‡‡‡‡‡‡‡‡‡‡‡‡‡‡‡‡‡‡‡‡‡‡‡‡          ‡
1485 CTCCCTCTCCTTGCTGTCTCATGACTTCAAGGCTGAGAG-------------------------------------------AGGGCTCAGCCCTCTCT  p53M81
1033 CCCCCTCTCCTTGCTGTCTTATGACTTCAGGGCTGAGACACAATCCTCCCGGTCCCTTCTGCTGCCTTTTTTACCTTGTAGCTAGGGCTCAGCCCCCTCT  p53M82

                                 ‡         ‡          ‡    ‡    ‡                          ‡
1541 CTGAGTAGTGGTTCCTGGCCCAAGTTGGGGAATAGGTTGGTAGTTGCCAGGTCTCTGCTGACCCAGTGAAATCCTATCCAGCCAGTTGTTGGACCCTAGC  p53M81
1133 CTGAGTAGTGGTTCCTGGCCCAAGTTGGGGAATAGGTTGATAGTTGTCAGGTCTCTGCTGGCCCAGCGAAATTCTATCCAGCCAGTTGTTGGACCCTGGC  p53M82

                  ‡                                              ‡
1641 ACCTACAATGAAATATCACCCTACCCCACACCCTGTAAGATTCTATCTTGGGCCCTCATAGGGTCCATATCCTCCAGGACCTACTTTCCTTCCATTCTGC  p53M81
1233 ACCTACAATGAAATCTCACCCTACCCCACACCCTGTAAGATTCTATCTTGGGCCCTCATAGGGTCCATATCCTCCAGGGCCTACTTTCCTTCCATTCTGC  p53M82

              ‡           ‡          ‡‡‡‡‡‡ ‡                                     ------
1741 AAAGCCTGTCTGCATTTATCCACCCTCCACCCTGCCTCCCTCTTTTTTTT----AAACTCCTTTTTATATATCAATTTCCTATTTTACAATAAAATTTTG  p53M81
1333 AAAGCCTGTCTGCATTTATCCACCCCCCACCCTGTCTCCCTCTTTTTTTTTTTTTACCCCTTTTTATATATCAATTTCCTATTTTACAATAAAATTTTG  p53M82

         (----- poly A -----)>>>>>>>>>>>>>> 3'DR
1837 TTATCACTAAAAAAAAAAAAAAAAAAAAAAAAAAAAAGAACTCAAGAaactaacctccaaaaaagcaa-< 653 nucleotides >-gaactcaagaagctt  p53M81
1433 TTATCACTtatatggttttgagaggttgatatcagcataagctgtctgggcccccaggggca-< 492 nucleotides >-aatgaatcgaagctt  p53M82
```

Figure 6 Nucleotide sequence comparisons of genomic and cDNA p53 sequences. Explanation of symbols: (> > > >) 5′ direct repeat or 3′ direct repeat. Nonhomologous nucleotides are marked by an asterisk or are shown in lowercase if they are from flanking regions or introns.

are at least two loci that are complementary to the p53 coding region. One of these loci has all the characteristics of a processed pseudogene. This genetic element appears to be a cDNA copy of the p53 mRNA that has been integrated into the genome. It is flanked by direct repeats and has a polyadenylic acid stretch directly 3′ to a consensus poly(A) addition site. In addition, this genomic DNA has a number of stop codons within the region that would correspond to the coding region. Taken together, these data suggest that this DNA does not code for a polypeptide, and we favor the hypothesis that this region was formed by the synthesis of a cDNA copy of the p53 mRNA followed by integration into the genomic DNA.

In contrast, the second locus appears to have all the expected properties of the functional gene. Comparisons between the sequence of the genomic DNA and cDNA show that these sequences are identical for several long stretches and that the regions of identity within the genomic DNA are bounded by consensus sequences for splice acceptors and donors. There is a polyadenylation signal downstream from the predicted stop codon within the genomic DNA. Although the actual demonstration that this DNA codes for the p53 protein must await further work, it seems likely that this locus will prove to be the functional allele.

Similar results to the data presented here have also been reported recently by Chumakov et al. (1982) and Oren and his colleagues (Oren and Levine 1983; Oren et al., this volume). Those studies in conjunction with the studies presented here are the initial steps in determining the complete structure of the p53 gene. Hopefully, this experimental approach will establish not only the organization of the p53 gene but will also allow us to determine the primary amino acid sequence of p53, to begin studies to identify the regions important in the control of p53 expression, and eventually will lead to experiments that will help to ascertain the function of this protein.

Acknowledgments

We would like to thank Kit Osborn for her invaluable help with cell culture.

References

Benchimol, S., D. Pim, and L. Crawford. 1982. Radioimmunoassay of the cellular protein p53 in mouse and human cell lines. *EMBO J.* **1**: 1055.

Bonner, W.M. and R.A. Laskey. 1974. A film detection method for tritium-labeled proteins and nucleic acids in polyacrylamide gels. *Eur. J. Biochem.* **46**: 83.

Chirgwin, J.M., A.E. Przybyla, R.J. Macdonald, and W.J. Rutter. 1979. Isolation of biologically active ribonucleic acid from sources enriched in ribonuclease. *Biochemistry* **18**: 5294.

Chumakov, P.M., V.S. Iotsova, and G.P. Georgiev. 1982. Isolation of plasmid clone containing sequence of messenger-RNA for murine non-viral T antigen. *DAN USSR* **267**: 1272.

Coffman, R.L. and I.L. Weissman. 1981. A monoclonal antibody that recognizes B cells and B cell precursors in mice. *J. Exp. Med.* **153**: 269.

Crawford, L.V., D.C. Pim, and R.D. Bulbrook. 1982. Detection of antibodies against the cellular protein p53 in sera from patients with breast cancer. *Int. J. Cancer* **30**: 403.

Crawford, L.V., D.C. Pim, E.G. Gurney, P. Goodfellow, and J. Taylor-Papadimitriou. 1981. Detection of a common feature in several human tumor cell lines—A 53,000-dalton protein. *Proc. Natl. Acad. Sci.* **78**: 41.

DeLeo, A.B., G. Jay, E. Appella, G.C. Dubois, L.W. Law, and L.J. Old. 1979. Detection of a transformation-related antigen in chemically induced sarcomas and other transformed cells of the mouse. *Proc. Natl. Acad. Sci.* **76**: 2420.

Dippold, W.G., G. Jay, A.B. DeLeo, G. Khoury, and L.J. Old. 1981. p53 transformation-related protein: Detection by monoclonal antibody in mouse and human cells. *Proc. Natl. Acad. Sci.* **78**: 1695.

Harlow, E., L.V. Crawford, D.C. Pim, and N.M. Williamson. 1981. Monoclonal antibodies specific for the SV40 tumor antigens. *J. Virol.* **39**: 861.

Kessler, S.W. 1975. Rapid isolation of antigens from cells with a staphylococcal protein A-antibody adsorbent: Parameters of the interaction of antibody-antigen complexes with protein A. *J. Immunol.* **115**: 1617.

Korman, A.J., P.J. Knudsen, J.F. Kaufman, and J.L. Strominger. 1982. cDNA clones for the heavy chain of HLA-DR antigens obtained after immunopurification of polysomes by monoclonal antibody. *Proc. Natl. Acad. Sci.* **79**: 1844.

Kraus, J.P. and L.E. Rosenberg. 1982. Purification of low-abundance messenger RNAs from rat liver by polysome immunoadsorption. *Proc. Natl. Acad. Sci.* **79**: 4015.

Kurtz, D.T. and C.F. Nicodemus. 1981. Cloning of alpha$_{2u}$ globulin cDNA using a high efficiency technique for the cloning of trace messenger RNAs. *Gene* **13**: 145.

Lane, D.P. and L.V. Crawford. 1979. T antigen is bound to a host protein in SV40-transformed cells. *Nature* **278**: 261.

Lee, D.C., D.F. Carmichael, E.G. Krebs, and G.S. McKnight. 1983. Isolation of a cDNA clone for the type I regulatory subunit of bovine cAMP-dependent protein kinase. *Proc. Natl. Acad. Sci.* **80**: 3608.

Leppard, K., N. Totty, M. Waterfield, E. Harlow, J. Jenkins, and L. Crawford. 1983. Purification and partial amino acid sequence analysis of the cellular tumour antigen, p53, from mouse SV40-transformed cells. *EMBO J.* **2**: 1993.

Linzer, D.I.H. and A.J. Levine. 1979. Characterization of a 54K dalton cellular SV40 tumor antigen present in SV40-transformed cells and uninfected embryonal carcinoma cells. *Cell* **17**: 43.

MacGillivray, R.T.A., D.W. Chung, and E.W. Davie. 1979. Biosynthesis of bovine plasma proteins in a cell-free system; amino-terminal sequence of preproalbumin. *Eur. J. Biochem.* **98**: 477.

Maniatis, T., E.F. Fritsch, and J. Sambrook, eds. 1982. *Molecular cloning: A laboratory manual.* Cold Spring Harbor Laboratory, Cold Spring Harbor, New York.

McCormick, F. and E. Harlow. 1980. Association of a murine 53,000 dalton phosphoprotein with simian virus 40 large-T antigen in transformed cells. *J. Virol.* **34**: 213.

Mercer, W.E., D. Nelson, A.B. DeLeo, L.J. Old, and R. Baserga. 1982. Microinjection of monoclonal antibody to protein p53 inhibits serum-induced DNA synthesis in 3T3 cells. *Proc. Natl. Acad. Sci.* **79**: 6309.

Messing, J. 1979. *Recombinant DNA Tech. Bull.* **2**: 43.

Messing, J. and J. Vieira. 1982. A new pair of M13 vectors for selecting either DNA strand of double-digest restriction fragments. *Gene* **19**: 269.

Milner, J. and S. Milner. 1981. SV40-53K antigen: A possible role for 53K in normal cells. *Virology* **112**: 785.

Oren, M. and A. Levine. 1983. Molecular cloning of a cDNA specific for the murine p53 cellular tumor antigen. *Proc. Natl. Acad. Sci.* **80**: 56.

Pelham, H.R.B. and R.J. Jackson. 1976. An efficient mRNA-dependent translation system from reticulocyte lysates. *Eur. J. Biochem.* **67**: 247.

Retzel, E.F., M.S. Collett, and A.J. Faras. 1980. Enzymatic synthesis of deoxyribonucleic acid by the avian retrovirus reverse transcriptase in vitro: Optimum conditions required for transcription of large ribonucleic acid templates. *Biochemistry* **19**: 513.

Ricciardi, R.P., J.S. Miller, and B.E. Roberts. 1979. Purification and mapping of specific mRNAs by hybridization-selection and cell-free translation. *Proc. Natl. Acad. Sci.* **76:** 4927.

Robson, K.J.H., T. Chandra, R.T.A. MacGillivray, and S.L.C. Woo. 1982. Polysome immunoprecipitation of phenylalanine hydroxylase mRNA from rat liver and cloning of its cDNA. *Proc. Natl. Acad. Sci.* **79:** 4701.

Rotter, V. 1983. p53, a transformation-related cellular-encoded protein, can be used as a biochemical marker for the detection of primary mouse tumor cells. *Proc. Natl. Acad. Sci.* **80:** 2613.

Rotter, V., M.A. Boss, and D. Baltimore. 1981. Increased concentration of an apparently identical cellular protein in cells transformed by either Abelson murine leukemia virus or other transforming agents. *J. Virol.* **38:** 336.

Rotter, V., O.N. Witte, R. Coffman, and D. Baltimore. 1980. Abelson murine leukemia virus-induced tumors elicit antibodies against a host cell protein, P50. *J. Virol.* **36:** 547.

Sanger, F., S. Nicklen, and A.R. Coulson. 1977. DNA sequencing with chain-terminating inhibitors. *Proc. Natl. Acad. Sci.* **74:** 5463.

Sanger, F., A.R. Coulson, B.G. Barrell, A.J.H. Smith, and B.A. Roe. 1980. Cloning in single-stranded bacteriophage as an aid to rapid DNA sequencing. *J. Mol. Biol.* **143:** 161.

Sarnow, P., Y.S. Ho, J. Williams, and A.J. Levine. 1982. Adenovirus E1b-58kd tumor antigen and SV40 large tumor antigen are physically associated with the same 54kd cellular protein in transformed cells. *Cell* **28:** 387.

Southern, E.M. 1975. Detection of specific sequences among DNA fragments separated by gel electrophoresis. *J. Mol. Biol.* **98:** 503.

Structure and Expression of the Genes Encoding the Murine p53 Cellular Tumor Antigen

R. Zakut-Houri, D. Givol, B. Bienz, A. Rogel, and M. Oren

Department of Chemical Immunology, The Weizmann Institute of Science, Rehovot 76100, Israel

The cellular tumor antigen p53 is a phosphoprotein detectable in elevated levels in many types of transformed cells (for review, see Klein 1982). The protein can be found in very low amounts in nontransformed cells (Linzer et al. 1979; Simmons 1980; Dippold et al. 1981), where it possesses an unusually short half-life, on the order of 20–30 minutes (Oren et al. 1981; Mora et al. 1982). In such nontransformed cells, p53 levels appear to increase upon substantial cell proliferation (Dippold et al. 1981; Milner and Milner 1981) and to decrease markedly upon cessation of cell division (Dippold et al. 1981). Furthermore, p53 synthesis in normal cells appears to be cell cycle related (Milner and Milner 1981; Mercer et al. 1982; N. Reich and A. Levine, cited in Winchester 1983), and there is an indication that p53 activity may be required for the reentry of quiescent cells into the G_1 or S phase following serum stimulation (Mercer et al. 1982). Increased levels of p53 have been reported in cells transformed by a wide variety of agents, such as DNA tumor viruses (Chang et al. 1979; Lane and Crawford 1979; Linzer and Levine 1979; Melero et al. 1979; Sarnow et al. 1982), RNA tumor viruses (Rotter et al. 1980), chemical carcinogens (DeLeo et al. 1979; Maltzman et al. 1981), ionizing radiation (DeLeo et al. 1979), as well as in embryonal carcinoma cells (Linzer and Levine 1979; Linzer et al. 1979) and in spontaneous transformants (DeLeo et al. 1979; Maltzman et al. 1981). In addition, p53 has been reported to be produced in significant amounts in primary cells from midgestation embryos (Mora et al. 1980; Chandrasekaran et al. 1981). Although initially described in the mouse system, similar p53-like proteins were also reported in several other mammalian species; particularly, increased levels of such a protein were observed in cells derived from a series of human tumors (Crawford et al. 1981). In at least two systems studied so far, a close correlation could be established between experimental modulation of the transformed phenotype and cellular p53 levels (Oren et al. 1981, 1982). All these findings are compatible with a model suggesting that p53 plays a role in regulating the proliferation of normal cells, probably by controlling their ability to go through a certain step of the cell cycle. This model, however, is still very far from proven, and much pertinent information should be obtainable by elucidating the mechanisms involved in the control of p53 expression in normal as well as transformed systems. Although some important information along this line could be obtained by methods employing the analysis and quantitation of the protein, it is obvious that a more profound understanding of the molecular biology and bioregulation of p53 depends greatly on our ability to explore the structure and function of the pertinent genes.

To facilitate the study of the p53-related genes and the corresponding mRNA species, a cDNA clone specific for murine p53 was isolated (Oren and Levine 1983). To that end, polyadenylated RNA from SVT2 cells was fractionated over a sucrose gradient, and fractions enriched for p53-specific mRNA were identified by in vitro translation combined with immunoprecipitation. The enriched mRNA was used to construct a cDNA library in pBR322, consisting of approximately 10^4 clones. To screen this library for p53-specific clones, SVT2 polysomes were immunoprecipitated employing anti-p53 monoclonal antibodies, and the polyadenylated RNA derived from this material served as a template for making radiolabeled cDNA. Using such highly enriched probes, we were able to isolate a single recombinant clone specific for p53. The identity of this clone, pp53-208, was confirmed by its ability specifically to select p53 mRNA in a hybrid-selection in vitro translation assay. Using this first clone as a source for hybridization probes, several additional p53-specific cDNA clones were isolated and further characterized (Oren et al. 1983; Zakut-Houri et al. 1983). In addition, these clones were utilized to study the murine p53-related mRNA species and to isolate and characterize the corresponding genes. The major findings emerging from this analysis are described in the following sections.

Methods of Experimental Procedures

Construction and screening of cDNA libraries

Poly(A)$^+$ RNA from transformed cells was fractionated over a sucrose gradient, translated in vitro, and tested for the presence of p53 mRNA as described (Oren and Levine 1983). The fractions displaying the best enrichment for p53 messenger were used for making cDNA, which was then cloned into pBR322 employing *Escherichia coli* RR1 as the host strain (Oren and Levine 1983). Colonies were grown to a diameter of 1–2 mm, blotted onto nitrocellulose (Thayer 1979), and hybridized to either the cDNA insert of pp53-208 (released with *Pst*I) or the 3.3-kb fragment of Ch53-11. Positive clones were finally verified by the hybrid-selection/translation method, as described before (Oren and Levine 1983).

Extraction and analysis of mRNA

RNA was extracted from tumors by a modification of the guanidine-thiocyanate method (Chirgwin et al. 1979). Prior to extraction, deep-frozen tissue pieces were pulverized in liquid nitrogen employing a Waring Blendor. The RNA was chromatographed over two consecutive oligo(dT)-cellulose columns and ethanol precipitated. Aliquots of the desired samples (7 μg per lane) were loaded on a 1% formaldehyde gel (Rave et al. 1979) and electrophoresed for 4 hours at 80 mA. The RNA was transferred onto nitrocellulose (Thomas 1980) in 10× SSC, and hybridized at 42°C for 48 hr in 50% formamide, 5× SSC, 1× Denhardt's solution, 50 mM sodium phosphate (pH 6.8), and 100 μg/ml denatured salmon DNA. The probe employed was pp53-271 DNA (Oren et al. 1983), nick-translated to a specific activity of 1×10^8 to 2×10^8 cpm/μg. The reacted blots were washed at room temperature with 2× SSC, 0.5% SDS, and 20 mM sodium pyrophosphate, followed by 30 minutes at 50°C with 0.1× SSC, 0.5% SDS, and 20 mM sodium pyrophosphate.

Analysis of genomic DNA

High-molecular-weight genomic DNA was extracted from deep-frozen tissues by the method of Blin and Stafford (1976), and digested with the indicated enzymes. The digestion products were separated on a 0.7% agarose gel, blotted onto nitrocellulose (Southern 1975), and hybridized to nick-translated plasmid DNA. Hybridization with homologous probes (mouse cDNA and mouse genomic DNA) was conducted at 42°C in 50% formamide, 5× SSC, 5× Denhardt's solution, 50 mM sodium phosphate (pH 6.5), 5% dextran sulfate, and 100 μg/ml salmon DNA, and the blots were consequently washed in 3× SSC at 65°C, followed by washing in 0.5× SSC at the same temperature. Hybridization of mouse cDNA with human genomic DNA was at 42°C in 35% formamide, 5× SSC, 5× Denhardt's solution, 50 mM sodium phosphate, 5% dextran sulfate, and 100 μg/ml salmon DNA. The blots were then washed in 3× SSC at 60°C for 1 hour and used to expose X-ray film.

Isolation of genomic clones

Recombinant phage clones containing the 3.3-kb *Eco*RI fragment were isolated from a BALB/c embryo partial *Eco*RI library (Zakut et al. 1980). To isolate clones carrying the 16-kb *Eco*RI fragment, BALB/c liver DNA was digested to completion with *Eco*RI and fractionated over a 10–40% sucrose gradient (Maniatis et al. 1978). Fraction aliquots were electrophoresed on a 0.7% agarose gel, blotted, and hybridized to nick-translated pp53-176 DNA (Zakut-Houri et al. 1983). The reactive fractions were combined and the DNA cloned in Charon 4A. Resultant phage plaques were screened by standard procedures (Benton and Davis 1977).

Heteroduplex analysis

For the analysis, the 16-kb *Eco*RI insert of Ch53-16 was purified from a 0.6% agarose gel; pCh 53-11 was linearized with *Bam*HI and pp53-176 was linearized with *Eco*RI. The 16-kb insert was then reannealed with either pCh53-11 or pp53-176 DNA, and the products spread on a 10% formamide hypophase. Samples were analyzed in a Philips EM 410 microscope, employing the procedure of Davis et al. (1971). Single-stranded φX174 and double-stranded SV40 DNA served as internal length markers.

Primer extension and nucleic acid sequencing

For primer extension, polyadenylated IB-9 RNA (260 μg) was reannealed with 1.5×10^6 cpm (approximately 1.5 pmole) of 5′ end-labeled *Xho*I–*Hae*III fragment. The reaction was in 75% formamide, 10 mM HEPES (pH 6.4), 0.4 M NaCl, and 1 mM EDTA at 50°C for 6 hours. Reaction products were chromatographed over oligo(dT)-cellulose, and the bound material was used as a primer-template for the synthesis of cDNA, essentially as described by Snyder et al. (1982). Products were separated on a 6% polyacrylamide gel containing 8 M urea. Nucleic acid sequencing was according to Maxam and Gilbert (1980).

Results

Analysis of murine p53 mRNA

Polyadenylated RNA from a variety of cells and tissues was fractionated on formaldehyde-agarose gels, blotted onto nitrocellulose, and hybridized with a probe prepared from clone pp53-271. This cDNA clone contains a p53-specific cDNA insert of approximately 0.6 kb (Oren et al. 1983). The results of one such experiment are shown in Figure 1. It is obvious that the p53-specific probe detects a rather broad RNA band, possessing an average size of approximately 2 kb. In addition, substantial differences exist in the relative abundance of p53 mRNA in different systems, since equal amounts of poly(A) RNA were applied to each lane. Generally, there was a good correlation between the intensity of the signal in the RNA experiments and the levels of p53 protein in the corresponding system. Thus, IB-9 cells, which displayed the strongest reaction with the p53-specific cDNA probe (Fig. 1), are also substantial overproducers of the protein (data not shown). Similar observations were made in several other systems (Reich et al. 1983). Furthermore, relatively high levels of p53 mRNA were detected both in tissue culture IB-9 cells (Oren et al. 1983) and in the corresponding tumors (Fig. 1), indicating that p53 overproduction is not an in vitro artifact. An additional feature implied by Figure 1 is that p53 mRNA may be heterogeneous and consist of more than a single species. This is most obvious in the sample derived from NSI mouse plasmacytoma cells, where the shape of the band is suggestive of a doublet. The question whether this possible heterogeneity has any functional significance still remains to be answered.

The mouse genome contains two distinct p53-specific genes

High-molecular-weight DNA from various mouse strains and tissues was digested with several restriction enzymes and tested for hybridization with p53-specific cDNA probes (Fig. 2). As seen in Figure 2a, the probe

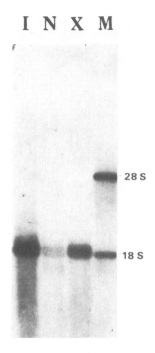

I N X M

28 S

18 S

Figure 1 Analysis of p53 mRNA. Equal amounts (7 μg) of polyadenylated RNA from several different mouse tumors were separated electrophoretically, blotted, and hybridized with nick-translated pp53-271 DNA. The tumors analyzed were: IB-9 methylcolanthrene-induced fibrosarcoma (*I*), NSI plasmacytoma (*N*), and XRPC-24 plasmacytoma (*X*). *M* denotes the positions of ^{32}P-labeled 28S and 18S rRNA markers.

reacts with a very small number of fragments in each case. Particularly, one should note that *Eco*RI-digested DNA displays two p53-specific bands, possessing approximate sizes of 16 kb and 3.3 kb. This suggests that at most there are two p53-specific genes in the mouse genome. However, both these genomic fragments could also be derived from a single gene containing an internal *Eco*RI site. To explore this possibility, a basically similar experiment was performed, employing clones pp53-208 and pp53-271 as probes. As seen in Figure 2b, both probes detect exactly the same *Eco*RI bands: the aforementioned 16 kb and 3.3 kb, and an additional band of 5.6 kb, which is probably a product of incomplete digestion (see below). Since clones pp53-208 and pp53-271 are absolutely nonoverlapping (Oren et al. 1983), one must conclude that the 16-kb and 3.3-kb bands represent two distinct p53-specific genes. This conclusion is further confirmed by the finding that the 16-kb and the 3.3-kb fragments are derived from different mouse chromosomes (H. Czosnek et al., in prep.). The restriction patterns of p53-specific DNA were next studied in different mouse strains and tissues. As seen in Figure 2a, two different mouse strains displayed identical patterns. The same picture was obtained with DNA from several other strains (D. Wolf et al., in prep.) and no p53-related strain-dependent, restriction-site polymorphism has been observed so far. Comparison of DNA from BALB/c liver and from three BALB/c plasmacytomas did not reveal any tissue-specific rearrangements (Fig. 2c). Inter-

estingly enough, though, the liver DNA exhibited a much stronger 5.6-kb *Eco*RI band. This band most likely represents a partial digestion product, which consists of the 3.3-kb fragment and a neighboring 2.3-kb one, and which can also be generated by incomplete cleavage of the corresponding recombinant phage clone with *Eco*RI (Oren et al. 1983). Failure to cleave the genomic DNA completely at this site was repeatedly observed with several preparations of liver DNA, whereas DNA prepared from a variety of tissue culture cells and tumors could usually be digested to completion with *Eco*RI under identical conditions. It is therefore tempting to speculate that the presence of the 5.6-kb band may be due to a tissue-specific or growth state-specific chemical modification of the DNA.

Detection of p53-specific sequences in other mammals

The previous section presented evidence that the mouse genome contains two p53-specific genes. Similar experiments were performed employing DNA from several other species. Human DNA (Fig. 3) displays a very simple pattern, compatible with the existence of a single p53-specific gene (or at most two genes). Simple patterns were also obtained with DNA from rat and hamster, although in these species the results suggest the existence of at least two genes (data not shown). It should be noted that the hybrids between the human DNA and the murine p53-specific probes do not survive high-stringency washes (B. Bienz and O. Pinhasi, unpubl.), suggesting that the p53 genes are not very highly conserved between those species.

Isolation of murine p53-specific genomic clones

As noted above, the mouse genome contains two p53-specific genes. To characterize those genes further, it was necessary to clone each of them molecularly. To begin with, a preexisting mouse genomic library was screened with the cDNA clone pp53-208. Three different genomic clones were obtained, all containing the 3.3-kb *Eco*RI fragment (Zakut-Houri et al. 1983). Since this library did not yield any recombinant phage containing the 16-kb fragment, this piece was cloned directly from BALB/c liver DNA, employing sucrose-gradient centrifugation as a preliminary enrichment step. In addition, use was made of a clone similarly obtained from Abelson virus-transformed C57L/J mouse cells, generously provided to us by D. Wolf and V. Rotter (The Weizmann Institute of Science, Rehovot) and designated here Ch53-16. The structural relationship between each of the two mouse p53 genes and the corresponding mRNA was explored by heteroduplex analysis. To that end, DNA of the largest cDNA clone pp53-176, was linearized with *Eco*RI and reannealed with the purified 16-kb *Eco*RI fragment of Ch53-16. In parallel, the 3.3-kb p53-specific *Eco*RI fragment was isolated from the corresponding genomic clone and subcloned in pBR322. The DNA of this subclone (designated pCh53-11) was linearized with *Bam*HI and also reannealed with the 16-kb insert of Ch53-16. Typical electronmicrographs are shown in

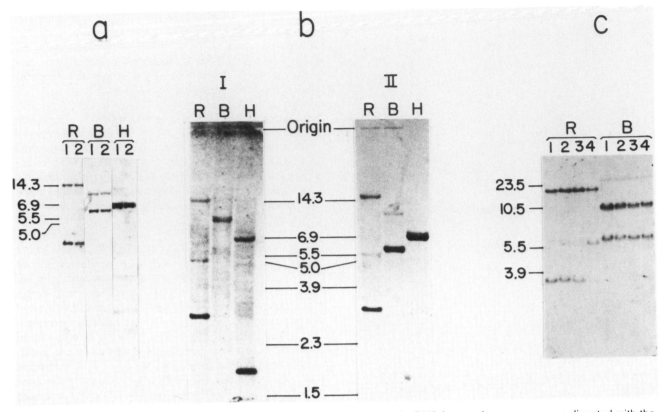

Figure 2 Detection of p53-specific mouse genomic DNA. High-molecular-weight DNA from various sources was digested with the restriction enzymes indicated below, electrophoresed, blotted, and reacted with p53-specific cDNA probes. (*a*) Liver DNA from BALB/c (lane *1*) or C57/BL (lane *2*) mice, digested with either *Eco*RI (R), *Bam*HI (B), or *Hind*III (H) and probed with pp53-176. (*b*) BALB/c liver DNA digested with either *Eco*RI (lane *1*), *Bam*HI (lane *2*), or *Hind*III (lane *3*) and probed with pp53-208 (I) or pp53-271 (II). (*c*) DNA from plasmacytomas MPC11 (lane *1*), 104E (lane *2*), XRPC24 (lane *3*), and from BALB/c liver digested with *Eco*RI (R) or *Bam*HI (B) and probed with pp53-176. Numerical values refer to the sizes (in kb) of molecular-weight markers (panels *a* and *b*, Charon 4A DNA digested with *Eco*RI and *Bam*HI; panel *c*, Charon 4A DNA digested with *Bam*HI). (Panel *b* is reprinted, with permission, from Oren et al. 1983.)

Figure 4, together with interpretive drawings. Several conclusions can be drawn from these data. The heteroduplex formed between the 16-kb insert and the cDNA (panels A and B) suggests the existence of at least 7 introns and 8 exons in the gene. The approximate lengths of these exons and introns were determined relative to internal standards, and are shown schematically at the bottom of Figure 4. The pattern displayed by the hybrids between the 16-kb insert and the 3.3-kb fragment (panels C and D) is essentially identical to that obtained with the cDNA clones, except for differences in the lengths of the first and last exons. This implies that the 3.3-kb fragment contains no detectable introns and is thus probably a processed pseudogene. Hence, the 16-kb fragment must represent the only true gene, the total size of which is at least 12 kb. Further evidence supporting the conclusions made here is presented in the following section.

Sequence analysis of p53-specific cDNA and genomic clones

To characterize further the p53-specific clones, nucleic acid sequencing was performed employing the Maxam and Gilbert (1980) procedure. Figure 5 displays the re-

sults of this analysis. The sequence derived from the cDNA clones (cDNA) is shown in parallel to the corresponding regions in the 3.3-kb *Eco*RI genomic fragment (ψ gene) and in the 5′ end of the 16-kb genomic fragment (gene). The predicted amino acid sequence dictated by the largest open reading frame is also shown. Overall, the presented cDNA sequence spans 1715 nucleotides, whereas the length of the entire p53 mRNA, including the poly(A), is about 2 kb (see Fig. 1). The orientation of the presented sequence is the same as that of the mRNA, as determined by S1 analysis (Oren et al. 1983). Inspection of the data discloses that the only large open reading frame is located between nucleotides 1 and 1170, specifying a polypeptide of 390 amino acids. This value is markedly less than the apparent molecular weight of p53 on SDS-polyacrylamide gels (Klein 1982). This discrepancy could theoretically reflect a cloning or sequencing error. However, the multiple terminators found upstream to position 1, defining the 5′ end of the open reading frame, are found in both pp53-176 and pp53-271, derived from different cDNA libraries, as well as in the corresponding region of the genomic clone Ch53-16. The 3′ end of the reading frame is determined by the terminator codon TGA at positions 1171–1173.

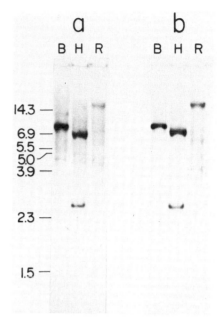

Figure 3 Detection of p53-related human genomic DNA. High-molecular-weight human placenta DNA was digested with either *Bam*HI (lanes *B*), *Hind*III (lanes *H*), or *Eco*RI (lanes *R*) and analyzed essentially as described for Fig. 2. The radiolabeled probes employed were either whole pp53-176 DNA (*a*) or a purified *Pst*I fragment comprising the 3' 840 bp of the insert from that plasmid (*b*).

Again, this triplet is found in both pp53-422 and pp53-176, derived from different libraries. Thus, it is possible, although not proven, that the p53 protein is indeed shorter than suggested by its SDS-polyacrylamide gel mobility. It should be noted, though, that elimination of the terminator at positions 1171–1173 would extend the open reading frame by another 80 amino acids, creating a polypeptide of 470 amino acids, a size compatible with the apparent molecular weight of the protein. Inspection of the relevant sequence from the 3.3-kb genomic fragment (ψ gene) reveals some interesting structural features. First, in agreement with the heteroduplex study, it is colinear with the cDNA and possesses no introns. Second, it contains a long (28 bp) poly(A) tract starting at nucleotide 1614, preceded by a consensus poly-adenylation signal (positions 1594–1599, underlined in Fig. 5). This poly(A) tract is located 55 bp downstream to the end of pp53-208, the most 3' of the cDNA clones analyzed by us. Finally, the part of the 3.3-kb fragment that is homologous to p53 mRNA is bounded by a pair of 13-bp direct repeats (D.R., boxed in Fig. 5). All these features are indicative of a processed pseudogene (Bernstein et al. 1982; Hollis et al. 1982; Lemischka and Sharp 1982; Lee et al. 1983). Hence, we conclude that the 3.3-kb *Eco*RI fragment carries a processed p53 gene, probably generated by reverse transcription of p53 mRNA followed by insertion into a new chromosomal location.

It is noteworthy that the pseudogene lacks part of the p53-specific sequences found in the cDNA clones (upstream to position −75). Hence, it cannot encode the complete p53 mRNA. Since there is only one additional p53-specific murine gene—the one harbored in the 16-kb fragment—the latter must, by elimination, constitute the functional p53 gene. This conclusion is also supported by the limited sequence data available (Fig. 5), as well as by the heteroduplex studies (Fig. 4).

Primer-extension analysis of p53 mRNA

The sequence information pertaining to the processed gene enables the determination of the 3' end of the p53 mRNA. However, this does not define the 5' end of the gene, since the processed gene apparently lacks this part (see previous section). In an attempt to overcome this problem, primer extension analysis was performed, employing the 5' end-labeled *Xho*I–*Hae*III fragment of pp53-176 (nucleotides 41 to −50) and mRNA from IB-9 cells. The result is shown in Figure 6. A short exposure (Fig. 6a) revealed a major extension product (denoted X), possessing a size of 155 ± 5 nucleotides (lane 1). This major band was prepared in relatively large amounts, employing 260 μg of polyadenylated RNA, and subjected to sequence analysis. The resultant sequence (Fig. 6c) was identical to that of nucleotides −51 to −114 shown in Figure 5. Since the cDNA clone pp53-176 extends further upstream to that region, it is obvious that the reverse transcription did not proceed all the way to the 5' end of the mRNA. Repeated experiments consistently yielded this same extended band (data not shown); hence, this most likely reflects the existence of a major reverse transcriptase stop signal. It should be noted that the extension reaction was specific; a primer derived from the other strand of the cDNA clone did not yield anything, except for a small amount of a product of the same size as X, probably due to a contamination of P1 with minute amounts of P2 or an analogous partial *Hae*III digestion product. Prolonged exposure of the same gel (Fig. 6b, picture size somewhat reduced relative to a) revealed a series of additional bands, the biggest of which possessed a length of 200 ± 5 bp (Fig. 6b, lane 1). Unless this represents another reverse transcriptase stop site, the data may be taken to imply that the mRNA extends approximately 200 nucleotides 5' to the *Xho*I site (position 41), reaching a point that is only a few nucleotides upstream to the beginning of clone pp53-176.

Discussion

The murine genome contains two p53-specific genes. One of these possesses distinctive features of a processed pseudogene and probably results from the integration of a reverse transcript of p53 mRNA. This pseudogene lacks the 5' portion of the p53-specific sequence, possibly due to the integration of an incomplete reverse transcript or to a postintegrational deletion event. One might have considered the possibility that this pseudogene is still involved in the production of p53, since it contains the whole putative coding region and a consensus TATA box (nucleotide −96). This, however, is ruled out by the presence of several deletions that

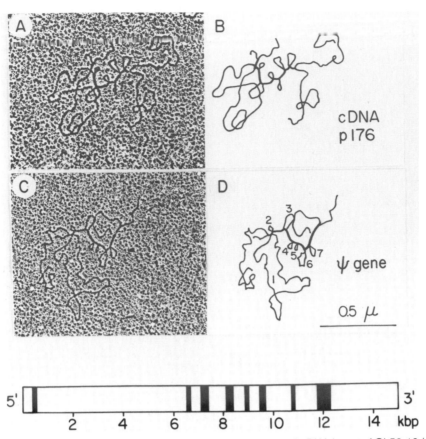

Figure 4 Heteroduplex analysis of p53-specific clones. The purified *Eco*RI genomic DNA insert of Ch53-16 (see text) was denatured and reannealed either with the cDNA clone pp53-176 (*A,B*) or with a plasmid subclone containing the 3.3-kb *Eco*RI fragment of genomic clone Ch53-11 (*C,D*). The numbers in *D* indicate the introns in a 5' → 3' order. The inferred organization of the functional p53 gene is presented at the bottom; dark areas represent exons, white areas represent introns and flanking regions. Note that the total size of the *Eco*RI fragment, as suggested by these data, is somewhat smaller than that determined by gel electrophoresis (15 kb v. 16 kb).

modify the reading frame so that it contains in-phase terminators. The finding of a p53-processed gene suggests that the functional gene is expressed, at least at a certain stage, in germ-line cells. This is not surprising, since the protein seems to be found, albeit at low amounts, almost in all cell types examined so far (Klein 1982). The conclusion that there is only a single functional p53 gene implies that all different forms of the protein observed experimentally (see, for instance, Crawford 1982) must be products of the same gene, probably reflecting posttranslational or posttranscriptional events.

The p53 mRNA possesses an approximate length of 2 kb, which is several hundreds of nucleotides more than needed to encode the entire protein. The sequence data suggests the existence of a single large open reading frame, encoding 390 amino acids. The assignment of

this reading frame rests upon the presence of multiple termination codons both 5' and 3' to it. However, there may still be a possibility that, due to some experimental problem, one of the boundaries of the coding region may have been misplaced, resulting in an underestimate of the protein size. An intriguing possibility is that there is more than a single splicing pattern of p53-specific transcripts, and that another mRNA, somewhat different from the one represented by our cDNA clones, is indeed the one encoding the actual protein. Despite these reservations, it still seems more likely that the reading frame assignment is correct and that the p53 polypeptide indeed contains only 390 residues. In that case, the apparent discrepancy with the value predicted from SDS-polyacrylamide gels may be, in part, related to the high proline content of this protein.

The predicted p53 protein has a distinct domained

Figure 5 Nucleotide sequences of p53-specific clones. The composite sequence of the several cDNA clones analyzed (cDNA) is shown in parallel with that of the pertinent region of the genomic clone Ch53-11, which harbors the pseudogene (ψ gene), and with a partial sequence of the 5'-proximal region of Ch53-16, which corresponds to the functional gene (gene). The amino acids predicted from the large open reading frame are also shown. Termination codons 5' to the putative first ATG are underlined; those in phase with the open reading frame are double-underlined (see text for further details).

```
                                                    -530      -520       -510      -500
                                           GGCTTACAAA GACTCTGTCT TAAAAATCCA AAAAGA        GENE

    -490      -480       -470      -460       -450      -440       -430      -420       -410      -400       -390
TGGC TATGACTATC TAGCTGGATA GGAAAGAGCA CAGAGCTCAG AACAGTGGCG GTCCACTTAC GATAAAAACT TAATTCTTTC CACTCTTTAT ACTTGACACA GAGG        GENE

    -380      -370       -360      -350       -340      -330       -320      -310       -300      -290       -280
CAGGAG TCCTCCGAAT CGGTTTCCAC CCATTTTGCC CTCACAGCTC TATATCTTAG ACGACTTTTC ACAAAGCGTT CCTGCTGAGG GCAACATCTC AGGGAGAATC CT        GENE

        -270      -260       -250      -240       -230      -220       -210      -200       -190      -180
          C CAATGACTCA GGCCCCAAGA TCTAGAATTG ATAAATAGGA CCACATGAAA CTGAAAGACT TCTGTAAGAA AAGGACATAG TCAATAGGAC       ♦-GENE
GACTCTGC AAGTCCCCGC CTCCATTTCT TACCCTCAAC CCACGGAAGG ACTTGCCCTT ACTTGTTATG GCGACTATCC AGCTTTGTGC CAGGAGTCTC GCGGGGGTTG         GENE

   -160      -150       -140      -130       -120      -110       -100       -90 D.R.    -80            -70
AAATAGGCAA TCTATAGATT GGGGAAAGCA TCCTCACTAA TCCCAGATCC AATAGAGGGC TAATATCCAA ACTCTAT[AAA GAACTCAAGA] GGTAG----- ---------        ♦-GENE
CTGGGATTGG GAC------- --------- --------- --------- --------- --------- --------- --------- ---------        GENE
           TTTCCCC TCCCACGTGC TCACCCTCTG TAAAGTTCTG TAGCTTCAGT TCATTGGGAC CATCCTGGCT GTAGGTACGC ACTACAGTTA GGGGGCACC        CDNA

  -60       -50        -40       -30        -20       -10        1         10         20         30
- --------- --------- --------- --------- --------- --------- GTA AGT AAT TGA TGA GCG TGA CGA --- --- ---   ...........INTRON        ♦-GENE
                                                                                                                                  GENE
T AGCATTCAGG CCCTCATCCT CCTCCTTCCC AGCAGGGTGT CACGCTTCTC CGAAGACTGG ATG ACT GCC ATG GAG GAG TCA CAG TCG GAT ATC AGC CTC        CDNA
                                                             MET THR ALA MET GLU GLU SER GLN SER ASP ILE SER LEU  13

40         50         60         70         80         90         100        110        120
--- --- --- --- --T --- --- --- --- --- --- --- --- --- --- --- --- --- --- --- --- -C- --- --- --- ---        ♦-GENE
GAG CTC CCT CTG AGC CAG GAG ACA TTT TCA GGC TTA TGG AAA CTA CTT CCT CCA GAA GAT ATC CTG CCA TCA CCT CAC TGC ATG GAC GAT        CDNA
GLU LEU PRO LEU SER GLN GLU THR PHE SER GLY LEU TRP LYS LEU LEU PRO PRO GLU ASP ILE LEU PRO SER PRO HIS CYS MET ASP ASP  43

130        140        150        160        170        180        190        200        210
--- --- --- --- --- --- --- --- --- --- --- --- --- --- --- --- --A --- --- --- --- --- --- --- --- ---        ♦-GENE
CTG TTG CTG CCC CAA GAT GTT GAG GAG TTT TTT GAA GGC CCA AGT GAA GCC CTC CGA GTG TCA GGA GCT CCT GCA GCA CAA GAC CCT GTC        CDNA
LEU LEU LEU PRO GLN ASP VAL GLU GLU PHE PHE GLU GLY PRO SER GLU ALA LEU ARG VAL SER GLY ALA PRO ALA ALA GLN ASP PRO VAL  73

220        230        240        250        260        270        280        290        300
--T --- --- --- --- --- --- --- --- --- --C --- --- --- --- --- --- --- --- --- --- --- --- --- --- ---        ♦-GENE
ACC GAG ACC CCT GGG CCA GTG GCC CCC GCC CCA GCC ACT CCA TGG CCC CTG TCA TCT TTT GTC CCT TCT CAA AAA ACT TAC CAG GGC AAC        CDNA
THR GLU THR PRO GLY PRO VAL ALA PRO ALA PRO ALA THR PRO TRP PRO LEU SER SER PHE VAL PRO SER GLN LYS THR TYR GLN GLY ASN  103

310        320        330        340        350        360        370        380        390
--- --- --- --- --- --- --- --- --G --- --- --- --- --CT --- --- --- --- --- --- --- --- --- --- ---        ♦-GENE
TAT GGC TTC CAC CTG GGC TTC CTG CAG TCT GGG ACA GCC AAG TCT GTT ATG TGC ACG TAC TCT CCT CCC CTC AAT AAG CTA TTC TGC CAG        CDNA
TYR GLY PHE HIS LEU GLY PHE LEU GLN SER GLY THR ALA LYS SER VAL MET CYS THR TYR SER PRO PRO LEU ASN LYS LEU PHE CYS GLN  133

400        410        420        430        440        450        460        470        480
--- --- --- --- --- --- --- --- --- --- --- --- --- --- --- --- --- --- --- --- --- --- TT- --- --- ---        ♦-GENE
CTG GCG AAG ACG TGC CCT GTG CAG TTG TGG GTC AGC GCC ACA CCT CCA GCT GGG AGC CGT GTC CGC GCC ATG GCC ATC CAC AAG AAG TCA        CDNA
LEU ALA LYS THR CYS PRO VAL GLN LEU TRP VAL SER ALA THR PRO PRO ALA GLY SER ARG VAL ARG ALA MET ALA ILE HIS LYS LYS SER  163

490        500        510        520        530        540        550        560        570
--- --T --T CT --A --- --- --- --- --- --- --- T-- --- --- --- --- --- --- --- --- --- --- --- --- A--        ♦-GENE
CAG CAC ATG ACG GGG GTC GTC AGG AGG TGC CCC CAC CAT GAG AGG TGC TCC GAT GGT GAT GGC CTG GCA CCC CAG CAT CTT ATC AGG        CDNA
GLN HIS MET THR GLY VAL VAL ARG ARG CYS PRO HIS HIS GLU ARG CYS SER ASP GLY ASP GLY LEU ALA PRO GLN HIS LEU ILE ARG  193

580        590        600        610        620        630        640        650        660
--- --- --- --- --- G-- --A --- --- --- --- --- --- --- --- --- --T --- --- --- --- --C --- --- -T- --- ---        ♦-GENE
GTG GAA GGA AAT TTG TAT CCC GAG TAT CTG GAA GAC AGG CAG ACT TTT CGC CAC AGC GTG GTG GTA CCT TAT GAG CCA CCC GAG GCC GGC        CDNA
VAL GLU GLY ASN LEU TYR PRO GLU TYR LEU GLU ASP ARG GLN THR PHE ARG HIS SER VAL VAL VAL PRO TYR GLU PRO PRO GLU ALA GLY  223

670        680        690        700        710        720        730        740        750
--- --- --- --- --- --- --- --- --- --G --- -G- --- --- --- --- --- --- --- --- --- --- --- --- ---        ♦-GENE
TCT GAG TAT ACC ACC ATC CAC TAC AAG TAC ATT TGT AAT AGC TCC TGC ATG GGG GGC ATG AAC CGC CGA CCT ATC CTT ACC ATC ATC ACA        CDNA
SER GLU TYR THR THR ILE HIS TYR LYS TYR ILE CYS ASN SER SER CYS MET GLY GLY MET ASN ARG ARG PRO ILE LEU THR ILE ILE THR  253

760        770        780        790        800        810        820        830        840
--- --- --- --- --- --- --- --- --- --C --- --- --- --- --- --- --- --- --- --- --- T-G A-- --- --G ---        ♦-GENE
CTG GAA GAC TCC AGT GGG AAC CTT CTG CTG GGA CGG GAC AGC TTC GAG GTT CGT GTT TGT GCC TGC CCT GGG AGA GAC CGC CGT ACA GAA GAA        CDNA
LEU GLU ASP SER SER GLY ASN LEU LEU LEU GLY ARG ASP SER PHE GLU VAL ARG VAL CYS ALA CYS PRO GLY ARG ASP ARG ARG THR GLU GLU  283

850        860        870        880        890        900        910        920        930
--- --- --C- --- --- --- --- --- --T --- --- --- --C --- --- --- --- --- --- --- --T --- --C --- ---        ♦-GENE
GAA AAT TTC CGC AAA AAG GAA GTC CTT TGC CCT GAA CTG CCC CCA GGG AGC GCC CTG AGG AGA GCC CTG CCC ACA CGC TCT ACA TCT CCC        CDNA
GLU ASN PHE ARG LYS LYS GLU VAL LEU CYS PRO GLU LEU PRO PRO GLY SER ALA LYS ARG ALA LEU PRO THR CYS THR SER ALA SER PRO  313

940        950        960        970        980        990        1000       1010       1020
--C --- --- --- --- A-- --- --- --- --- --- --- --- --- --- --- --- --- --- --- --- --- --- --- ---        ♦-GENE
    CAAAAA
CCG CAA AAG AAA AAA CCA CTT GAT GGA GAG TAT TTC ACC CTC AAG ATC CGC GGG CGT AAA CGC TTC GAG ATG TTC CGG GAG CTG AAT GAG        CDNA
PRO GLN LYS LYS LYS PRO LEU ASP GLY GLU TYR PHE THR LEU LYS ILE ARG GLY CGT LYS ARG PHE GLU MET PHE ARG GLU LEU ASN GLU  343

1030       1040       1050       1060       1070       1080       1090       1100       1110
--- --- --- --- --- --- --- --- --- --- --- --- --- --- --- --- --- --- --- --- --- --- --A --- --- ---        ♦-GENE
GCC TTA GAG TTA AAG GAT GCC CAT GCT ACA GAG GAG TCT GGA GAC AGC AGG GCT CAC TCC AGC TAC CTG AAG ACC AAG AAG GGC CAG TCT        CDNA
ALA LEU GLU LEU LYS ASP ALA HIS ALA THR GLU GLU SER GLY ASP SER ARG ALA HIS SER SER TYR LEU LYS THR LYS LYS GLY GLN SER  373

1120       1130       1140       1150       1160       1170       1180       1190       1200       1210
--- ---C-- --- --A --- --- --- --- --- --- --- --- --- --- --- --T---T-- --- --- --T --- --- ---        ♦-GENE
ACT TCC CGC CAT AAA AAA ACA ATG GTC AAG AAA GTG GGG CCT GAC TCA GAC TGA CTGCCTC TGCATCCCGT CCCCATCACC AGCCTCCCCC TCTCCT        CDNA
THR SER ARG HIS LYS LYS THR MET VAL LYS LYS VAL GLY PRO ASP SER ASP END  390

          1220      1230       1240      1250       1260      1270       1280      1290       1300      1310      1320
          ---- --C--- -------A------ --G---        ♦-GENE
TGCT GTCTTATGAC TTCAGGGCTG AGACACAATC CTCCCGGTCC CTTCTGCTGC CTTTTTTACC TTGTAGCCTG GGCTCAGCCC CCTCTCTGAG TAGTGGTTCT CGGC        CDNA

     1330      1340       1350      1360       1370      1380       1390      1400       1410      1420
     --GT--- ---A--- ---CTA--- ---A        ♦-GENE
CCAAGT TGGGGAATAG GTTGAAAGTT GTCAGGTCTC TGCTGGCCCA GCGAAATTCT ATCCAGCCAG TTGTTGGACC TCGGCACCTA CAATGAAATC TCACCCTACC CC        CDNA

        1440      1450       1460      1470       1480      1490       1500      1510       1520      1530
                                                                                              T---------        ♦-GENE
ACACCCTG TAAGATTCTA TCTTGGGCCC TCATAGGGTC CATATCCTCC AGGGCCTACT TTCCTTCCAT TCTGCAAAGC CTGTCTGCAT TTATCCACCC CCCACCCTGT        CDNA

1540       1550       1560       1570       1580       1590       1600       1610       1620       1630       1640 D.R.
---------- --------- ------A AACTCCTTTT TTATATACTA ATTCCTTATT TTAC[AATAAA] ATTTCGTTAT CACTAAAAAA AAAAAAAAAA AAAAAAAA[A AAGAACTCA        ♦-GENE
CTCCCTCTTT TTTTTTTT        CDNA

     1650      1660       1670      1680       1690      1700       1710      1720       1730      1740      1750
A GA]AACTAACC TCCAAAAAAG CAAACAACCT AATTACAAAT CGAGTATAGA ACTGAACAGA GAAAATCGAA AACAAAGGAA TCTCAAATGG CCAAGAAGCA CTTAAAG        ♦-GENE

1760       1770       1780       1790       1800       1810       1820       1830       1840       1850       1860
AAA TGTTCAAAGT CCTTAATCAT CAGGGAAATA TAAATCAAAC AACCCTAAGA TTCCACTTTA TACCATTCAG AATGTCTAAG ATCCAAACCT CATGTGACAA CACAC        ♦-GENE

1870       1880       1890       1900       1910
ATTGG TGAGGATGTA GAGAAAGGGG AATACTCCAC AACTGCTAGT GATATTGC        ♦-GENE
```

Figure 5 (*See facing page for legend.*)

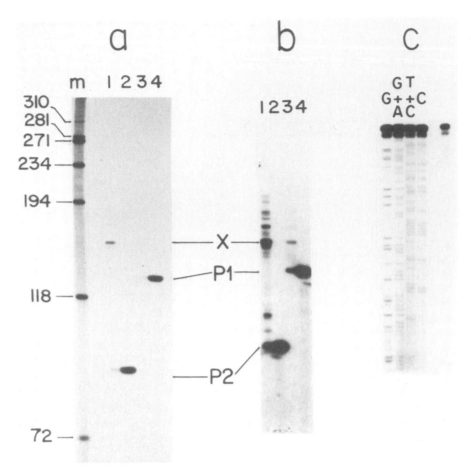

Figure 6 Primer-extension analysis of p53 mRNA. Denatured 5′ end-labeled *Xho*I–*Hae*III fragments of pp53-176, derived either from the transcribed strand (P2) or the nontranscribed strand (P1) were reannealed with poly(A)⁺ IB-9 RNA and the primer was extended as described under Methods. (*a* and *b*) Short and long exposures of the gel, respectively. The lanes represent the extension products of P2 (lanes *1*), unreacted P2 (lanes *2*), extension products of P1 (lanes *3*), and unextended P1 (lanes *4*). X refers to the position of the major extended product. Numbers denote the size in base pairs of fragments generated by *Hae*III cleavage of single-stranded φX174 DNA (*m*). Product X was prepared in relatively large amounts and subjected to Maxam-Gilbert sequence analysis (*c*).

structure. Thus, its carboxyterminal part has a high proportion of Arg and Lys. Since p53 is a DNA-binding protein (D. Lane, pers. comm.), this may be the region involved in DNA-protein interaction. The center of the molecule contains a substantial amount of hydrophobic residues, whereas the aminoterminal part is markedly acidic. The significance of these features is still unknown, but it may contain some hints as to the mode of action of p53. Further studies are still required to produce answers to some of the major questions in the field, namely: What are the normal functions of p53, how is the expression of p53 regulated, and how is it all related to cellular transformation?

Acknowledgments

The expert technical assistance of S. Hazum and O. Pinhasi is gratefully acknowledged. The authors wish to thank D. Wolf and V. Rotter for gifts of clone Ch53-16 and of MethA mRNA, V. Lavie for performing the heteroduplex analysis, and J.B. Cohen for help with sequencing and for illuminating discussions. This work was supported in part by a grant from the Leukemia Research Foundation of Chicago and a M. Ulinky memorial grant from the Israel Cancer Association (to M.O.) and by a grant from the Henry Gutwirth Fund (to D.G.). M.O. is a fellow of the Bat-Sheva de Rothschild Fund for the Advancement of Science.

References

Benton, D.W. and R.W. Davis. 1977. Screening λgt recombinant clones by hybridization to single plaques in situ. *Science* **196:** 180.

Bernstein, L.B., S. Mount, and A.M. Weiner. 1982. Pseudogenes for human small nuclear RNA U3 appear to arise by integration of self-primed reverse transcripts of the RNA into new chromosomal sites. *Cell* **32:** 461.

Blin, N. and D.W. Stafford. 1976. A general method for isolation of high molecular weight DNA from eukaryotes. *Nucleic Acids Res.* **3:** 2303.

Chandrasekaran, K., W.V. MacFarland, D.T. Simmons, M. Dziadek, E.G. Gurney, and P.T. Mora. 1981. Quantitation and characterization of a species-specific and embryo-stage dependent 55-kilodalton phosphoprotein also present in cells transformed by simian virus 40. *Proc. Natl. Acad. Sci.* **78:** 6953.

Chang, C., D.T. Simmons, M.A. Martin, and P.T. Mora. 1979. Identification and partial characterization of new antigens from simian virus 40-transformed mouse cells. *J. Virol.* **31:** 463.

Chirgwin, J.M., A.E. Przybyla, R.J. MacDonald, and W.J. Rutter. 1979. Isolation of biologically active ribonucleic acid from sources enriched in ribonuclease. *Biochemistry* **18:** 5294.

Crawford, L.V. 1982. The origins of p53 in relation to transformation. *Adv. Viral Oncol.* **2:** 3.

Crawford, L.V., D.C. Pim, E.G. Gurney, P. Goodfellow, and J. Taylor-Papadimitriou. 1981. Detection of a common feature in several human tumor cell lines — A 53,000-dalton protein. *Proc. Natl. Acad. Sci.* **78:** 41.

Davis, R.W., M. Simon, and N. Davidson. 1971. Electron microscope heteroduplex methods for mapping regions of base sequence homology in nucleic acids. *Methods Enzymol.* **21:** 413.

DeLeo, A.B., G. Jay, E. Appella, G.C. Dubois, L.W. Law, and L.J. Old. 1979. Detection of a transformation-related antigen in chemically induced sarcomas and other transformed cells of the mouse. *Proc. Natl. Acad. Sci.* **76:** 2420.

Dippold, W.G., G. Jay, A.B. DeLeo, G. Khoury, and L.J. Old. 1981. p53 transformation-related protein: Detection by monoclonal antibody in mouse and human cells. *Proc. Natl. Acad. Sci.* **78:** 1695.

Hollis, G.F., P.A. Hieter, O.W. McBride, D. Swan, and P. Leder. 1982. Processed genes: A dispersed human immunoglobulin gene bearing evidence of RNA-type processing. *Nature* **296:** 321.

Klein, G., ed. 1982. The transformation-associated cellular p53 protein. *Adv. Viral Oncol.* **2.**

Lane, D.P. and L.V. Crawford. 1979. T antigen is bound to a host protein in SV40-transformed cells. *Nature* **278:** 261.

Lee, M.G.S., S.A. Lewis, C.D. Wilde, and N.J. Cowan. 1983. Evolutionary history of a multigene family: An expressed human β-tubulin gene and three processed pseudogenes. *Cell* **33:** 477.

Lemischka, I. and P.A. Sharp. 1982. The sequences of an expressed rat α-tubulin gene and a pseudogene with an inserted repetitive element. *Nature* **300:** 330.

Linzer, D.I.H. and A.J. Levine. 1979. Characterization of a 54K dalton cellular SV40 tumor antigen present in SV40-transformed cells and uninfected embryonal carcinoma cells. *Cell* **17:** 43.

Linzer, D.I.H., W. Maltzman, and A.J. Levine. 1979. The SV40 A gene product is required for the production of a 54,000 MW cellular tumor antigen. *Virology* **98:** 308.

Maltzman, W., M. Oren, and A.J. Levine. 1981. The structural relationships between 54,000 molecular weight cellular tumor antigens detected in viral and nonviral transformed cells. *Virology* **112:** 145.

Maniatis, T., R.C. Hardison, E. Lacy, J. Lauer, C. O'Connell, D. Quon, D.K. Sim, and E. Efstratiadis. 1978. The isolation of structural genes from libraries of eucaryotic DNA. *Cell* **15:** 687.

Maxam, A.M. and W. Gilbert. 1980. Sequencing end-labeled DNA with base-specific chemical cleavages. *Methods Enzymol.* **65:** 499.

Melero, J.A., D.T. Stitt, W.F. Mangel, and R.B. Carroll. 1979. Identification of new polypeptide species (48–55K) immunoprecipitable by antiserum to purified large-T antigen and present in SV40-infected and transformed cells. *Virology* **93:** 466.

Mercer, W.E., D. Nelson, A.B. DeLeo, L.J. Old, and R. Baserga. 1982. Microinjection of monoclonal antibody to protein p53 inhibits serum-induced DNA synthesis in 3T3 cells. *Proc. Natl. Acad. Sci.* **79:** 6309.

Milner, J. and S. Milner. 1981. SV40-53K antigen: A possible role for 53K in normal cells. *Virology* **112:** 785.

Mora, P.T., K. Chandrasekaran, and V.W. McFarland. 1980. An embryo protein induced by SV40 virus transformation of mouse cells. *Nature* **288:** 722.

Mora, P.T., K. Chandrasekaran, J.C. Hoffman, and V.W. McFarland. 1982. Quantitation of a 55K cellular protein: Similar amount and instability in normal and malignant mouse cells. *Mol. Cell. Biol.* **2:** 763.

Oren, M. and A.J. Levine. 1983. Molecular cloning of a cDNA specific for the murine p53 cellular tumor antigen. *Proc. Natl. Acad. Sci.* **80:** 56.

Oren, M., W. Maltzman, and A.J. Levine. 1981. Post-translational regulation of the 54K cellular tumor antigen in normal and transformed cells. *Mol. Cell. Biol.* **1:** 101.

Oren, M., N. Reich, and A.J. Levine. 1982. Regulation of the cellular p53 tumor antigen in teratocarcinoma cells and their differentiated progeny. *Mol. Cell. Biol.* **2:** 443.

Oren, M., B. Bienz, D. Givol, G. Rechavi, and R. Zakut. 1983. Analysis of recombinant DNA clones specific for the murine p53 cellular tumor antigen. *EMBO J.* **2:** 1633.

Rave, N., R. Crkvenjakov, and J. Boedtker. 1979. Identification of procollagen mRNAs transferred to diazobenzyloxymethyl paper from formaldehyde agarose gels. *Nucleic Acids Res.* **6:** 3559.

Reich, N.C., M. Oren, and A.J. Levine. 1983. Two distinct mechanisms regulate the levels of a cellular tumor antigen, p53. *Mol. Cell. Biol.* **3:** 2143.

Rotter, V., O.N. Witte, R. Coffman, and D. Baltimore. 1980. Abelson murine leukemia virus-induced tumors elicit antibodies against a host protein, P50. *J. Virol.* **36:** 547.

Sarnow, P., Y.S. Ho, J. Williams, and A.J. Levine. 1982. Adenovirus E1b-58kd tumor antigen and SV40 large tumor antigen are physically associated with the same 54kd cellular protein in transformed cells. *Cell* **28:** 387.

Simmons, D.T. 1980. Characterization of tau antigens isolated from uninfected and simian virus 40-infected monkey cells and papovavirus-transformed cells. *J. Virol.* **36:** 519.

Snyder, M., M. Hunkapiller, D. Yuen, D. Silvert, J. Fristrom, and N. Davidson. 1982. Cuticle protein genes of *Drosophila*: Structure, organization and evolution of four clustered genes. *Cell* **29:** 1027.

Southern, E.M. 1975. Detection of specific sequences among DNA fragments separated by gel electrophoresis. *J. Mol. Biol.* **98:** 503.

Thayer, R.E. 1979. An improved method for detecting foreign DNA in plasmids of *Escherichia coli. Anal. Biochem.* **98:** 60.

Thomas, P.S. 1980. Hybridization of denatured RNA and small DNA fragments transferred to nitrocellulose. *Proc. Natl. Acad. Sci.* **77:** 5201.

Winchester, G. 1983. p53 protein and control of growth. *Nature* **303:** 660.

Zakut, R., D. Givol, and Y.Y. Mory. 1980. Structure of immunoglobulin γ2b heavy chain gene cloned from mouse embryo gene library. *Nucleic Acids Res.* **8:** 453.

Zakut-Houri, R., M. Oren, B. Bienz, V. Lavie, S. Hazum, and D. Givol. 1983. A single gene and a pseudogene for the cellular tumour antigen p53. *Nature* **306:** 594.

Modification of p53 Gene Expression by Integration of a Foreign DNA Element

D. Wolf and V. Rotter

Department of Cell Biology, The Weizmann Institute of Science, Rehovot, Israel

p53 is a cellular-encoded protein that is abundantly synthesized in a wide range of neoplastic transformed cell lines (Deleo et al. 1979; Lane and Crawford 1979; Linzer and Levine 1979; Rotter et al. 1980) and primary tumors in mice (Rotter 1983). Indistinguishable p53 molecules were detected in a variety of tissue types of tumors in several species (Simmons et al. 1980; Crawford et al. 1981; Dippold et al. 1981; Rotter et al. 1983b). It is a phosphoprotein (Melero et al. 1980, Jay et al. 1981; Rotter et al. 1981) capable of complexing with several viral tumor antigens (Lane and Crawford 1979; Linzer and Levine 1979; McCormick et al. 1981; Sarnow et al. 1982).

In addition to its wide distribution in malignant transformed cells, a limited occurrence of p53 was also observed in nontransformed cells including normal thymocytes (Rotter et al. 1980), primary embryonic cells (Mora et al. 1980), and 3T3 fibroblasts (Oren et al. 1981). The amount of p53 synthesized in these cells is reduced compared with that observed in transformed cells. The presence of p53 in nontransformed cells supports the idea that this protein is encoded by the cellular genome and may be involved in the normal cell cycle (Milner and Milner 1981; Mercer et al. 1982).

The fact that it is overproduced in a wide range of tumor cells suggests that accumulation of p53 may play a role in the neoplastic transformation. To elucidate the molecular mechanism controlling p53 expression, we made a comparative study of an Abelson murine leukemia virus (Ab-MLV)-transformed lymphoid cell line lacking the p53 protein (Rotter et al. 1980, 1983a) and cell lines expressing it abundantly. L12 is an Ab-MLV-transformed cell line that expresses the viral-encoded p120 Abelson oncogene product (abl) (Witte et al. 1979) but lacks the cellular-encoded p53 protein (Rotter et al. 1980, 1983a). Injection of L12 cells into syngeneic mice induces the development of local tumors that are subsequently rejected, whereas other Ab-MLV-transformed cells, overproducing both p120 and p53, develop into lethal tumors (Witte et al. 1979; Rotter et al. 1983a).

The experiments described here were aimed at elucidating the molecular mechanism controlling p53 expression in the above-mentioned transformed cell lines. It was found that the inability of L12 cells to produce p53 is due to the total absence of mature p53-specific mRNA (2.0 kb). Instead, these cells contain two major p53-specific mRNA species of a substantially larger size (3.5 kb and 6.5 kb) than the p53-specific mRNA in the p53-producing cells. Analysis of DNA sequences hybridizing with a p53-specific probe, revealed the existence of a DNA insert in the active p53 gene, unique to the L12 cell line.

Methods of Experimental Procedures

Cell lines

The Ab-MLV-transformed lymphoid cell lines used were: 2M3/M also containing the Moloney helper/virus (Mo-MLV); 2M3, a Moloney nonproducer cell line derived from 2M3/M (both of BALB/c origin), and L12 and 230-23-8 (a gift from N. Rosenberg, Tufts University), of $C_{57}L/J$ origin. Lymphoid cells were grown in RPMI-1640 medium enriched with 10% heat-inactivated fetal calf serum (Biolab, Israel) and 2×10^5 M β-mercaptoethanol. 3T3-NIH fibroblasts and Meth A chemically transformed cells of BALB/c origin were grown in RPMI supplemented with 10% heat-inactivated calf serum. Hybridoma cell lines RA3-2C2 (Rotter et al. 1980; Coffman and Weissman 1981), PAb122 (Gurney et al. 1980), and PAb421 (Harlow et al. 1981) were grown in RPMI-1640 medium enriched with 20% heat-inactivated fetal calf serum supplemented with 20 mM L-glutamine and 20 mM sodium-pyruvate.

Antibodies

Monoclonal anti-p53 antibodies were obtained from established hybridoma cell lines (described above). Antibodies were purified and concentrated by binding to Sepharose-protein A columns (Sigma). Goat anti-Moloney virus protein antibodies were obtained from the Division of Cancer Cause and Prevention, National Cancer Institute (NIH, Bethesda, Md.). The latter antibodies immunoprecipitate the p120 Abelson-encoded protein as well as the Moloney virus-related product.

In vivo labeling of proteins and their immunoprecipitations

Cells (10^7) were washed several times in phosphate-buffered saline and resuspended in 1.5 ml RPMI-1640 medium without methionine supplemented with 10% dialyzed heat-inactivated fetal calf serum and 250 μCi of [^{35}S]methionine (purchased from Amersham, England). Cells were incubated for 1 hour at 37°C, washed in phosphate-buffered saline, and extracted into 5 ml of lysis buffer (10 mM NaH_2PO_4-Na_2HPO_4 [pH 7.5], 500 mM NaCl, 1% Triton X-100, 0.5 sodium deoxycholate, 0.1% SDS) at 0°C. Cell lysates were precleared by repeated absorption onto *Staphylococcus aureus* and non-immune serum. Equal amounts of radioactive protein were immunoprecipitated with various antibodies. Antigen-antibody complexes were collected by *S. aureus*

(Kessler 1975). SDS-polyacrylamide gel electrophoresis was performed according to Laemmli (1970).

RNA and DNA blot analysis

RNA was prepared according to Auffray and Rougeon (1980) and selected for polyadenylated molecules by oligo(dT)-cellulose chromatography (Aviv and Leder 1972). Aliquots of 5 µg polyadenylated RNA prepared from various cell lines were heated for 10 minutes at 60°C in 50% formamide, 6% formaldehyde, and running buffer (20 mM MOPS [pH 7.0], 5 mM NaAc, and 1 mM EDTA). The samples were electrophoresed through a 1% agarose gel containing 6% formaldehyde. The RNA was transferred onto a nitrocellulose sheet (Thomas 1980) and hybridized to nick-translated (Rigby et al. 1977) whole plasmid pp53-271 (see text for description of the probe; specific activity = 1×10^8 cpm/µg). Hybridization was for 16 hours at 43°C in 50% formamide, $5\times$ SSC, $5\times$ Denhardt's solution (Denhardt 1966), 20 mM sodium phosphate (pH 7.0), and 100 µg/ml salmon sperm DNA, and 10% dextran sulfate. Hybridized filters were washed extensively at 50°C with $0.1\times$ SSC and 1% SDS, and autoradiographed. Aliquots of restriction enzyme digested high-molecular-weight DNA (5 µg) were electrophoresed on 0.8% agarose gels, blotted onto nitrocellulose filters (Southern 1975), and hybridized to nick-translated pp53-271 DNA (Rigby et al. 1977). Autoradiography was performed at −70°C with an intensifier screen.

Results

Absence of p53 in L12 cells and its presence in 230-23-8 cells

p53 was immunoprecipitated from [^{35}S]methionine-labeled Ab-MLV-transformed cell extracts by either polyvalent or monoclonal anti-p53 antibodies (Rotter et al. 1980). Figure 1 illustrates the specific products detected when L12 and 230-23-8 Ab-MLV-transformed cell lysates were immunoprecipitated with normal serum, RA3-2C2, PAb122, PAb421, and goat anti-Moloney. Lanes b–d in the figure represent the specific products immunoprecipitated with anti-p53 monoclonal antibodies. Lane e represents the Abelson virus-encoded p120 and the Moloney-related products. It is clear that L12 cells lack a p53 product that is seen clearly in Ab-MLV-transformed 230-23-8 cells. L12 is a unique Ab-MLV-transformed cell line that lacks an immunoprecipitable [^{35}S]methionine-labeled p53 product. The absence of this protein in L12 cells was also confirmed in cells labeled by [^{3}H]leucine or orthophosphate. The last two radioactive isotopes were shown to be efficiently incorporated into newly synthesized p53 molecules (Rotter et al. 1980, 1981). L12 cells, however, contain a virus-encoded p120 that immunoprecipitates with specific antibodies, suggesting that they have already acquired some malignant characteristics. The p120 of these cells seems to be a functional oncogene product. Addition of radioactive γ-ATP to the in vitro immunoprecipitated molecule yielded a tyrosine phosphorylated p120 product

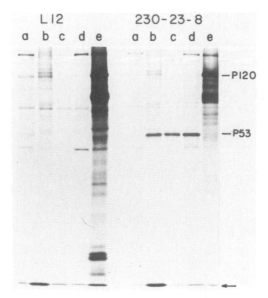

Figure 1 Absence of p53 in L12 and its presence in the 230-23-8 Ab-MLV-transformed cell lines. Equal amounts of [^{35}S]methionine-labeled proteins of L12 or 230-23-8 cell lysates were immunoprecipitated with the following antibodies: (lane *a*) normal serum; (lane *b*) RA3-2C2; (lane *c*) PAb122; (lane *d*) PAb421; and (lane *e*) goat anti-Moloney-containing antiviral-encoded p120 and anti-Moloney-related products (Rotter et al. 1983a).

(Rotter et al. 1983a) as detected in other Ab-MLV-transformed cell lines (Witte et al. 1980).

Ab-MLV-transformed cell lines were established by infecting bone marrow cells with a mixture of Ab-MLV and Mo-MLV stocks (Rosenberg and Baltimore 1976). As expected, therefore, both cell lines exhibited Moloney-related products immunoprecipitating with goat anti-Moloney serum (Fig. 1, lane e), most prominently detected were the envelope and the *gag* Moloney precursor molecules.

Immunoprecipitation of in vitro translated products with anti-p53 antibodies has indicated that L12 cells do not contain a polyadenylated mRNA molecule capable of directing the translation of a p53 molecule under in vitro conditions (Wolf et al. 1984).

All these findings support the conjecture that lack of p53 in L12 cells results from the absence of specific polyadenylated mRNA coding for this protein. Previously analyzed systems displayed a quantitative regulation of cellular p53 levels, due to their modulation of the amount of translatable p53 mRNA (Oren et al. 1982) or to post-translational mechanisms (Oren et al. 1981). The L12 cells represent a unique system in which p53 synthesis is completely absent, apparently due to an absolute lack of mature p53 mRNA.

Survey of p53-specific polyadenylated mRNA

Recently, p53-specific cDNA was cloned in pBR322 (Oren and Levine 1983), permitting the direct study of p53 mRNA by nucleic acid hybridization. This clone, pp53-208 (Oren and Levine 1983), was used to derive additional larger p53-specific cDNA clones from a similar cDNA library. One such clone, pp53-271, was analyzed by the hybrid selection assay and was clearly shown to be p53-specific (Oren et al. 1983). Radioactive clone pp53-271 DNA was next used as a probe to analyze polyadenylated RNA from the above-described cell lines. We tested mRNA of the following cell lines: L12 and 230-23-8, the two of which are of C57L/J mouse origin; 2M3, an Ab-MLV-transformed lymphoid cell line of BALB/c mouse origin; and 2M3/M, which is superinfected with Moloney helper virus (both of these lines are high p53 producers); Meth A, a chemically transformed fibrosarcoma of BALB/c origin, synthesizing high levels of p53 (DeLeo et al. 1979; Rotter et al. 1981); and NIH-3T3 (Oren et al. 1981), a low in vivo producer of this protein. Polyadenylated mRNA of each cell line was separated through a formaldehyde agarose gel, transferred to nitrocellulose paper, and hybridized with a radioactive p53 cDNA probe.

The results of this experiment are illustrated in Figure 2a. All cell lines except L12 contained a p53-specific mRNA of apparently identical size (2.0 kb). This species was virtually absent in the L12 cells. Instead, L12 cells displayed substantial levels of two larger polyadenylated RNA species, of approximately 6.5 kb and 3.5 kb, that hybridized the p53 cDNA. Very low amounts of a 6.5-kb mRNA were also detected in all p53 producers. This product may represent a precursor mRNA molecule, which is not unexpected, since total (nuclear and cytoplasmic) RNA was used in these experiments. It is unclear whether this putative precursor is identical to the major 6.5-kb RNA found in L12 cells. The 3.5-kb mRNA hybridizing with the p53 cDNA probe is unique to the L12 cell line and is not detected in other transformed cells studied here.

To define further the specific regions of homology between the pp53-271 probe and the various polyadenylated mRNA species observed above, pp53-271 DNA

was digested with *Pst*I into three fragments: *Pst* A, B, and C (see Fig. 2b; the order of the *Pst*I fragments corresponds to their 5′ and 3′ orientation within the pp53-271 plasmid). These fragments were labeled and utilized for RNA hybridization. A representative result is illustrated in Figure 2b. Clearly, the 5′ *Pst* A fragment (320 bp) contains most of the sequences homologous to the aberrant polyadenylated mRNA unique to the L12 cell line. Furthermore, an internal *Xho*I–*Pvu*II fragment of pp53-271 (approximately 350 bp) spanning between the middle of *Pst* A through *Pst* C (see Fig. 2b) *only* hybridizes to the p53 2.0-kb polyadenylated mRNA. This suggests that the extreme 5′ end of pp53-271 (approximately 130 bp) corresponds to the novel polyadenylated mRNA found in the L12 cell line. The fragments of *Pst* B (120 bp) and C (160 bp) appear to be specific for mature polyadenylated p53 mRNA. Under prolonged exposure, those fragments occasionally showed weak hybridization to the larger mRNA species recognized by *Pst* A. This is probably due to a contamination of fragments B and C with small amounts of fragment A.

Primer extension assay of mature p53 mRNA

The observation that clone pp53-271 contains at least two discrete regions of homology to the various p53 polyadenylated mRNA species necessitated the localization of this cDNA clone relative to the mature mRNA. This was performed by a primer extension assay. Fragments *Pst* B and C but not *Pst* A were selected for primer extension due to the G–C tails created by the particular cloning technique employed (Oren et al. 1983).

The selected fragments were labeled at their 3′ ends with the Klenow fragment of *Escherichia coli* polymerase I, strand-separated, and both strands were initially used independently for RNA hybridization followed by cDNA extension with unlabeled deoxynucleoside triphosphates

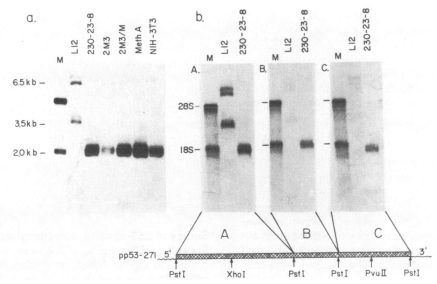

Figure 2 Analysis of polyadenylated mRNA from various cellular sources for p53-specific sequences. RNA was hybridized to either (a) whole plasmid pp53-271 or (b) restriction enzyme-digested fragments. ³²P-labeled 18S and 28S rRNA were used as molecular-weight markers (M).

by reverse transcriptase (Treisman et al. 1983). Total polyadenylated mRNA used for the assay was obtained from the following cell sources; Meth A, L12, and 2M3/M. Only one strand of each fragment was an effective primer in this assay, establishing the identity of the sense and anti-sense strands. The representative results of primer extension employing the anti-sense strands of fragments *Pst* B and C are shown in Figure 3. Primer extension products generated by both 3′ and labeled anti-sense strands from fragments *Pst* B and C indicated the same major 5′ stop in either Meth A or 2M3/M cell lines. Fragment *Pst* B yielded a final extension product of approximately 440 bp (Fig. 3B). Fragment *Pst* C in turn yielded a terminal extension product of approximately 600 bp (Fig. 3C). In accordance with our previous hybridization results (Figs. 2a,b), neither fragment produced primer extension products from L12 total polyadenylated mRNA. The products generated by L12 RNA were found to be similar to those obtained in the control where no external total polyadenylated mRNA was added (Fig. 3; compare lanes L12 with control lanes).

Taking into account a G–C tail length of roughly 30 bp at the 5′ and 3′ ends of clone pp53-271 (Oren et al. 1983), it can be calculated that the final extension product extends to approximately 40 bp 5′ to the end of the *Pst* A fragment. This suggests that clone pp53-271 is derived from the 5′ proximal region of the p53 mRNA. This is also in agreement with the results obtained from the study of a series of cDNA clones covering a total of 1700 bp of p53 mRNA (Oren et al. 1983).

Altered p53 genomic DNA pattern in L12 nonproducer cells

In an attempt to elucidate further the complex molecular mechanisms responsible for the altered p53 mRNA patterns observed, an analysis of the genomic DNA fragments hybridizing to the p53-specific probes was performed. DNA from a variety of cell lines was digested with several restriction enzymes and hybridized to nick-translated clone pp53-271 DNA. Examination of *Eco*RI digests reveals that all p53-producing cell lines (of both BALB/c and C57L/J genetic origin) display the same 3.3-kb and 16-kb *Eco*RI fragments. However, nonproducer L12 cells contain an apparently identical 3.3-kb band and a larger fragment—approximately 23.0 kb—hybridizing with the p53-specific probes (Fig. 4I). The fact that *Eco*RI, *Hin*dIII, and *Bam*HI do not cut within clone pp53-271 implies that the genomic region related to the cDNA is duplicated or represents two independent p53-related genes. The different size of the *Eco*RI fragment is not due to strain-specific restriction site polymorphism, since 230-23-8 cells of the same C57L/J genetic background display the usual 16-kb band (Wolf et al. 1984). To characterize in more detail the alteration of L12 DNA, extensive restriction enzyme digestion and double digestion of genomic DNA from p53 producer and nonproducer cell lines was performed, using fragments *Pst* A, *Xho*I–*Pvu*II, and *Pst* C of pp53-271 as probes. The results obtained indicated the existence of two noncontiguous p53 genes, one contained within the 3.3-kb *Eco*RI fragment and the second within the 16-kb *Eco*RI fragment. We have mapped approximately 20 kb around the 3.3 *Eco*RI fragment which does not overlap the 16-kb fragment and found no variations between the p53 producer and nonproducer cells. Employing fragment *Pst* A derived from the 5′ end of the mRNA (see above), we found an altered restriction enzyme pattern in the 5′ region of the p53 *Eco*RI 23.0-kb genomic DNA segment in L12 cells (Fig. 4II, A.5′). However, no difference was observed between the p53 gene contained in the 23-kb *Eco*RI fragment of the L12 cell line and that in the 16-kb *Eco*RI fragment of the p53 producer cell line hybridizing with the *Xho*I–*Pvu*II or *Pst* C probes (Fig. 4II, C.3′). Hybridization of digested and double-digested DNA of L12 and 230-23-8 cells with either 3′ or 5′ end cDNA probes revealed an absolute homology in the p53 genomic sequences (16-kb fragment) spanning from beyond the 3′ distal end of the gene to a *Hin*dIII restriction site contained within 5′ proximal region of the first intron. The alteration in the p53 gene of the L12 cells maps therefore to the 5′ proximal part of the gene, starting upstream to the *Hin*dIII restriction site contained in the first intron. (For details see Fig. 5, gene No. 2.) To localize and characterize the rearranged region, DNA probes corresponding to the first intron rather than cDNA probes were required. For that purpose we cloned the 16-kb DNA fragment of the 230-23-8 p53 producer cell line. Clone 8-1 lambda, containing the 16-kb DNA fragment was isolated from an *Eco*RI library prepared in a Charon 4A lambda. Next we restricted clone 8-1 with *Hin*dIII, generating five fragments that were subcloned

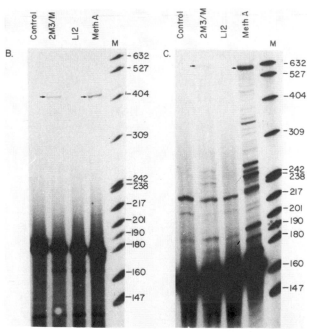

Figure 3 Primer extension analysis of total polyadenylated RNA from p53 producer cell lines. The primer extension cDNA products generated by the antisense strand of *Pst* B are shown in Fig. 3B, and those of *Pst* C are given in Fig. 3C. The 5′ end-labeled *Hpa*II fragments of pBR322 were used as size markers as indicated.

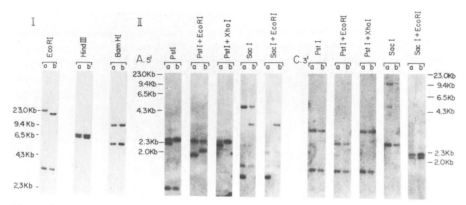

Figure 4 Southern blot analysis of p53 specific sequences in Ab-MLV-transformed mouse lymphoid cells. Aliquots (5 μg) of high-molecular-weight DNA from Ab-MLV-transformed mouse lymphoid cell lines L12 (lanes *a*) and 230-23-8 (lanes *b*) were electrophoresed and hybridized with (*I*) the whole clone pp53-271 DNA and (*II*) *Pst* A and *Pst* B fragments. The *Hind*III digests of λ DNA were used as molecular-weight markers.

into pBR322 plasmid. The clones obtained corresponded to exon and intron regions of the p53 gene (D. Wolf and V. Rotter, in prep.). The clones generated in their order from the 5′ end to the 3′ end of the p53 gene were: H-1, 600 bp; H-2, 2500 bp; H-3, 7000 bp; H-4, 2000 bp; and H-5, 2000 bp.

When genomic DNA blots obtained from L12 or 230-23-8 origin were probed with each of the following clones, H-1, H-3, H-4, and H-5, similar restriction enzyme maps were derived. However, major differences were observed when the same genomic DNA blots were probed with clone H-2, which corresponds to the 5′ of the first intron. In accordance with these results, we reached the conclusion that L12 cells contain a DNA insert of about 13.5 kb in the first intron of the p53 gene. The summary of the results and the predicted map of the rearranged p53 gene are illustrated in Figure 5.

Detailed analysis of the inserted DNA fragment revealed close homology to the Mo-MLV situated in a 5′ to 3′ transcription orientation similar to that of the p53 gene (D. Wolf and V. Rotter, in prep.).

Discussion

The present results define a unique system in which p53 production is controlled by the presence or absolute

absence of the corresponding mature 2.0-kb mRNA. All p53 producer cell lines including the nontransformed NIH-3T3 fibroblasts contain a 2.0-kb mRNA consisting of the mature p53-coding species. L12 cells that are devoid of p53 protein fail to produce this 2.0-kb mRNA but exhibit two major p53-specific mRNA species, 3.5 kb and 6.5 kb. The aberrant polyadenylated p53 mRNA species produced in the L12 cell line is homologous only in part to the normal mature polyadenylated p53 mRNA. Employing the cDNA clone pp53-271, the homologous region was located at the 5′ end of the normal p53 mRNA. Our results indicated the presence of two potential noncontiguous p53 genes, one contained in a 3.3-kb *Eco*RI fragment and the second in a 16-kb *Eco*RI fragment. Analysis of p53 genomic sequences in L12 cells indicated an apparent reorganization in only the p53-related gene contained in the 23-kb *Eco*RI fragment. The lack of the 16.0-kb p53-specific *Eco*RI fragment in L12 cells implies that the normal homolog is not present in those cells. Therefore, in addition to the rearrangement in one of the p53 genes, those cells must have undergone a chromosomal event resulting in the deletion of normal p53-specific sequences. These results imply that the 16-kb *Eco*RI fragment represents the principal active p53 gene. Since this gene is structurally altered in the L12 cells, it is conceivable that this alteration is

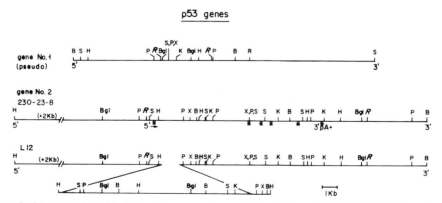

Figure 5 Comparison of p53 genes found in L12 p53 nonproducer cell line to those in 230-23-8 p53 producer cell line.

the principle cause for the existence of the aberrant nonproductive p53 mRNA in those cells (Wolf et al. 1984; D. Wolf and V. Rotter, in prep.). Detailed genomic analysis using defined fragments of pp53-271 cDNA indicated that the rearrangement of a p53 gene in the nonproducer L12 cell line maps to its 5' region. The localization and the characterization of the rearrangement observed was further pursued by using DNA probes obtained from cloned genomic p53 DNA sequences. We found that the principal 23-kb p53 gene of L12 nonproducer cells and that of 16-kb 230-23-8 producer cells share homology upstream and downstream from the rearranged region, located at the 5' proximal part of the first intron. Analysis of genomic DNA blots using clone H-2, which corresponds to the 5' proximal part of the first p53 intron, indicated the presence of a DNA insert of about 13.5 kb in the 5' proximal region of the first intron of the L12 p53 gene. We concluded that the L12 p53 gene contains all the exons and principal introns of the normal p53 16-kb gene and its function was interrupted by the insertion of a novel DNA insert into the noncoding intervening sequences. Analysis of the inserted DNA fragment has shown close homology to the Mo-MLV (D. Wolf and V. Rotter, in prep.). It is therefore possible that the initial step of establishing the L12 cell line, which involved the infection of bone marrow cells with a stock containing the Ab-MLV and Mo-MLV (Rosenberg and Baltimore 1976), included a genetic event where a Mo-MLV was integrated into the first intron of the p53 gene.

Inactivation of cellular genes by retrovirus insertion has been reported recently in several instances. Kuff et al. (1983) have demonstrated the presence of A-type particle proviral genomes in mutated immunoglobulin genes. Jenkins et al. (1981) had shown that insertion of a retroviral genome into a germ line of mice was associated with spontaneous mutations. In tissue culture, Varmus et al. (1981) induced phenotypic reversion of transformed cells by infection with Mo-MLV. More recently, Schnieke et al. (1983) have shown that integration of proviral genomes into the alpha1(I) collagen gene leads to its complete block.

Acknowledgments

This work was supported by a grant from the Leukemia Research Foundation, Inc. V.R. is the incumbent of the Norman and Helen Asher Career Development Chair. The authors wish to thank Dr. M. Oren of the Department of Chemical Immunology, The Weizmann Institute of Science, for fruitful collaboration and discussion during the performance of these experiments, and Mrs. S. Admon for excellent technical assistance.

References

Auffray, C. and F. Rougeon. 1980. Purification of mouse immunoglobulin heavy-chain messenger RNAs from total myeloma tumor RNA. *Eur. J. Biochem.* **107:** 303.

Aviv, H. and P. Leder. 1972. Purification of biologically active globin messenger RNA by chromatography on oligothymidylic acid cellulose. *Proc. Natl. Acad. Sci.* **69:** 1408.

Coffman, R.L. and I.L. Weissman. 1981. A monoclonal antibody which recognizes B cells and B cell precursors in mice. *J. Exp. Med.* **153:** 269.

Crawford, L.V., D.C. Pim, E.G. Gurney, P. Goodfellow, and J. Taylor-Papadimitriou. 1981. Detection of a common feature in several human tumor cell lines—a 53,000 dalton protein. *Proc. Natl. Acad. Sci.* **78:** 41.

Deleo, A.B., E. Jay, G.C. Appella, C.G. Dubois, L.W. Law, and L.J. Old. 1979. Detection of a transformation-related antigen in chemically-induced sarcoma and other transformed cells of the mouse. *Proc. Natl. Acad. Sci.* **76:** 2420.

Denhardt, D. 1966. A membrane-filter technique for the detection of complementary DNA. *Biochem. Biophys. Res. Commun.* **23:** 641.

Dippold, W.G. G. Jay, A.B. Deleo, G. Khoury, and L.J. Old. 1981. p53 transformation related protein. Detection by monoclonal antibody in mouse and human cells. *Proc. Natl. Acad. Sci.* **78:** 1695.

Gurney, E.G., R.O. Harrison, and J. Fenno. 1980. Monoclonal antibodies against simian virus 40 T antigens: Evidence for distinct subclasses of large T antigen for similarities among non-viral antigens. *J. Virol.* **34:** 752.

Harlow, B., L.V. Crawford, D.C. Pim, and N.H. Williamson. 1981. Monoclonal antibodies specific for simian virus 40 tumor antigens. *J. Virol.* **39:** 861.

Jay, G., G. Khoury, A.B. Deleo, G. Wolfgang, W.G. Dippold, and L.J. Old. 1981. p53 transformation-related protein: Detection of an associated phosphotransferase activity. *Proc. Natl. Acad. Sci.* **78:** 2932.

Jenkins, N.A., N.G. Copeland, B. A. Taylor, and B.K. Lee. 1981. Dilute (d) coat color mutation of DBA-2J mice is associated with the site of integration of an isotropic MuLv genome. *Nature* **293:** 370.

Kessler, S.W. 1975. Rapid isolation of antigens from cells with a staphylococcal protein A antibody adsorbent: Parameters of the interaction of antibody-antigen complex with protein A. *J. Immunol.* **115:** 1617.

Kuff, E.L., A. Feenstra, K. Lueders, L. Smith, R. Hawley, N. Hozumi, and M. Shulman. 1983. Intracisternal A-particle genes as movable elements in the mouse genome. *Proc. Natl. Acad. Sci.* **80:** 1992.

Laemmli, U.K. 1970. Cleavage of structural proteins during the assembly of the head of bacteriophage T4. *Nature* **227:** 680.

Lane, D.P. and L.V. Crawford. 1979. T antigen is bound to a host protein in SV40 transformed cells. *Nature* **278:** 261.

Linzer, D.I.H. and A.J. Levine. 1979. Characterization of a 54K dalton cellular SV40 tumor antigen present in SV40 transformed cells and uninfected embryonal carcinoma cells. *Cell* **17:** 43.

McCormick, F., R. Clark, E. Harlow, and R. Tjian. 1981. SV-40 T antigen binds specifically to a cellular 53K protein in vitro. *Nature* **23:** 63.

Melero, J.A., S. Tur, and R.B. Carroll. 1980. Host nuclear proteins expressed in simian virus 40 transformed and infected cells. *Proc. Natl. Acad. Sci.* **77:** 97.

Mercer, W.E., D. Nelson, A.B. Deleo, L.J. Old, and R. Baserga. 1982. Microinjection of monoclonal antibodies to protein p53 inhibits serum induced DNA synthesis in 3T3 cells. *Proc. Natl. Acad. Sci.* **79:** 6309.

Milner, J. and S. Milner. 1981. SV40-53K antigen: A possible role of 53k normal cells. *Virology* **112:** 785.

Mora, P.T., K. Chandrasekaran, and W. McFarland. 1980. An embryo protein induced by SV40 virus transformation of mouse cells. *Nature* **288:** 722.

Oren, M. and A.J. Levine. 1983. Molecular cloning of cDNA specific for the murine p53 cellular tumor antigen. *Proc. Natl. Acad. Sci.* **80:** 56.

Oren, M., W. Malzman, and A.J. Levine. 1981. Posttranslational regulation of the 54K cellular encoded tumor antigen in normal and transformed cells. *Mol. Cell. Biol.* **1:** 101.

Oren, M., N.C. Reich, and A.J. Levine. 1982. Regulation of the cellular p53 tumor antigen in teratocarcinoma cells and their differentiated progeny. *Mol. Cell. Biol.* **2:** 443.

Oren, M., B. Bienz, D. Givol, G. Rechavi, and R. Zakut. 1983. Analysis of recombinant DNA clones specific for the murine p53 cellular tumor antigen. *EMBO J.* **2**: 1633.

Rigby, P.W., M. Dieckmann, C. Rhodes, and P. Berg. 1977. Labeling deoxyribonucleic acid to high specific activity in vitro by nick translation with DNA polymerase I. *J. Mol. Biol.* **113**: 237.

Rosenberg, N. and D. Baltimore. 1976. A quantitative assay for transformation of bone marrow cells by Abelson murine leukemia virus. *J. Exp. Med.* **143**: 1453.

Rotter, V. 1983. p53, a transformation-related cellular encoded protein, can be used as a biochemical marker for the detection of primary mouse tumor cells. *Proc. Natl. Acad. Sci.* **80**: 2613.

Rotter, V., H. Abutbul, and D. Wolf. 1983a. The presence of p53 transformation related protein in Ab-Mulv transformed cells is required for their development into lethal tumors in mice. *Int. J. Cancer* **31**: 315.

Rotter, V., M.A. Boss, and D. Baltimore. 1981. Increased concentration of an apparently identical cellular protein in cells transformed by either Abelson-murine leukemia virus or other transforming agents. *J. Virol.* **38**: 336.

Rotter, V., O.N. White, R. Coffman, and D. Baltimore. 1980. Abelson-murine leukemia virus-induced tumors elicit antibodies against a host cell protein, p50. *J. Virol.* **36**: 547.

Rotter, V., H. Friedman, A. Katz, K. Zerivitz, and D. Wolf. 1983b. Variation in antigenic determinants of p53 transformation-related protein obtained from various species. *J. Immunol.* **181**: 329.

Sarnow, P., Y.S. Ho, J. Williams, and A.J. Levine. 1982. Adenovirus E1b-58 kd tumor antigen and SV40 large tumor antigen are physically associated with the same 54 K alpha cellular protein in transformed cells. *Cell* **28**: 387.

Schnieke, A., K. Harbers, and R. Jaenisch. 1983. Embryonic lethal mutation in mice induced by retrovirus insertion into the alpha1(I) collagen gene. *Nature* **304**: 315.

Simmons, D.T., M.A. Martin, P.T. Mora, and C. Chang. 1980. Relationship among tau antigens isolated from various lines of simian 40-transformed cells. *J. Virol.* **34**: 650.

Southern, E.J. 1975. Detection of specific sequences among DNA fragments separated by gel electrophoresis. *J. Mol. Biol.* **98**: 503.

Thomas, P.S. 1980. Hybridization of denatured RNA and small DNA fragments transferred to nitrocellulose. *Proc. Natl. Acad. Sci.* **77**: 5201.

Triesman, R.H., S.H. Orkin, and T. Maniatis. 1983. Specific transcription and RNA splicing defects in five cloned beta-thalassaemia genes. *Nature* **302**: 591.

Varmus, H.E., N. Quintrell, and S. Ortiz. 1981. Retrovirus as mutagens: Insertion and excision of a nontransforming provirus alter expression of resident transforming provirus. *Cell* **25**: 23.

Witte, O.N., A. Dasgupta, and D. Baltimore. 1980. Abelson murine leukemia virus protein is phosphosylated in vitro to form phosphotyrosine. *Nature* **283**: 826.

Witte, O.N., N. Rosenberg, and D. Baltimore. 1979. Preparation of syngeneic tumor regressor serum reactive with the unique determinants of the Abelson MuLV encoded p120 protein at the cell surface. *J. Virol.* **31**: 776.

Wolf, D., S. Admon, M. Oren, and V. Rotter. 1984. Abelson murine leukemia virus-transformed cells that lack p53 protein synthesis express aberrant p53 mRNA species. *Mol. Cell. Biol.* (in press).

Expression and Mapping of an Epstein-Barr Virus Nuclear Antigen, EBNA

J. Hearing and A.J. Levine

State University of New York at Stony Brook, Department of Microbiology, School of Medicine, Stony Brook, New York 11794

Epstein-Barr virus (EBV) is the etiological agent of infectious mononucleosis (Henle and Henle 1979) and is associated with Burkitt's lymphoma in Africa (de The et al. 1978) and nasopharyngeal carcinoma in China (Klein 1979). The viral genome is maintained in Burkitt's lymphoma cell lines as a circular episome (Lindahl et al. 1976) in copy numbers varying between 2–100 per cell (nonproducer cell lines) (Adams 1979). Similarly, nasopharyngeal carcinoma cells contain circular episomal EBV DNA (Kaschka-Dierich et al. 1976). EBV is able to convert nondividing B cells into continuous cell lines in vitro (immortalization) (Henle et al. 1967). In most EBV-positive lymphoblastoid cell lines, the virus remains latent with less than 10% of the viral genome expressed as stable, polyribosome-associated mRNA (Orellana and Kieff 1977). Transcription maps of the EBV genome in latently infected lymphocytes are at a preliminary stage. At the present time, six polyadenylated EBV-specific transcripts have been identified (van Santen et al. 1981). In addition, these cells express two polymerase III EBV transcripts called EBER-1 and EBER-2 (Rosa et al. 1981; van Santen et al. 1981). Thus, only a small percentage of the viral genome is expressed in growth-transformed cells (latent state).

Several EBV-associated antigens have been described using antisera from patients with Burkitt's lymphoma, nasopharyngeal carcinoma, or infectious mononucleosis. An EBV-associated nuclear antigen, EBNA, is invariably present in all EBV-positive cells (Pope et al. 1969; Reedman and Klein 1973). Recently polypeptides ranging from 65,000 to 73,000 m.w. were identified in latently infected lymphoblastoid cell lines using human sera containing anti-EBNA antibodies (Strnad et al. 1981). In addition, the BamHI K restriction fragment of EBV has been demonstrated to induce the expression of an EBNA in mouse cells (Summers et al. 1982). The BamHI K fragment varies in molecular weight between different EBV isolates and this variation has been localized to a repeat sequence within this fragment (Hennessy et al. 1983). Based upon a correlation between the size of the EBNA-associated polypeptide and the size of the BamHI K fragment in a given cell line, it was suggested that this protein is encoded in part or entirely by the BamHI K fragment (Hennessy et al. 1983).

In the experiments described here, the BamHI K fragment from the B95-8 strain of EBV has been introduced into a polyoma virus expression vector. The resulting plasmids are able to replicate after transfection into mouse cells and an 88,000-m.w. protein is detected with human sera containing antibodies to EBNA. A similar-sized protein is also detected in a B-cell line established in vitro with the same EBV strain (B95-8). Sera previously characterized as not containing antibodies directed against EBNA fail to detect these proteins. EBNA-positive sera identify a new nuclear antigen in mouse cells transfected with the vector containing the BamHI K fragment. Deletion and insertion mutations have been introduced into the BamHI K fragment to determine if the 88,000-m.w. protein is encoded by this fragment. These mutations result in the synthesis of proteins of lower molecular weight that also react with EBNA-positive sera. These data provide good evidence that an EBV nuclear antigen is encoded by the BamHI K fragment, and the mutants provide a genetic map of the coding regions of this genomic DNA.

Materials and Methods

Cells

The NIH-3T3 cells used in the transfection experiments were provided by M. Wigler (Cold Spring Harbor Laboratory). These cells were maintained at low passage number in Dulbecco's modified Eagle's medium supplemented with 10% fetal bovine serum (Flow Laboratories). The lymphoblastoid cell lines BJAB and Jijoye were obtained from G. Miller (Yale University). Loucks and IB4 were a gift of E. Kieff (University of Chicago), Namalwa was provided by J. Pagano (University of North Carolina), Ramos was from I. Ernberg (University of Chicago), and Raji was from C. Anderson (Brookhaven National Laboratory). All lymphoid lines were maintained in RPMI-1640 supplemented with 10% fetal bovine serum.

Plasmids and construction of mutations

All plasmids used in these experiments were carried in Escherichia coli HB101 (rec A⁻). The vector pMLPyA2 consists of a 4576-bp BamHI–HindIII fragment of polyoma virus A2 strain (nucleotides 4632–3918) (Griffin et al. 1981) inserted between the BamHI and HindIII sites of pML2 (Lusky and Botchan 1981). The EBV B95-8 strain BamHI K fragment was isolated from pDF225 (Dambaugh et al. 1980; kindly provided by E. Kieff) and inserted at the unique BamHI site of pMLPyA2 in both possible orientations.

Insertion mutations at the HindIII sites in the BamHI K fragment were constructed by partially digesting pMLPyA2K' with HindIII, repairing the ends with the Klenow fragment of E. coli DNA polymerase I (Corden et al. 1980), gel-purifying the full-length linear molecules, and recircularizing the molecules with T4 DNA ligase. *E. coli* HB101 transformed with these molecules were screened for plasmids that had lost a *Hind*III site within *Bam*HI K. Insertion mutations at *Sma*I sites in *Bam*HI K were constructed by partially digesting pMLPyA2K' with *Sma*I and ligating with *Bgl*II linkers (Collaborative Research, Inc.) using T4 DNA ligase. Excess linkers were removed by digestion with *Bgl*II and full-length linear molecules were purified by agarose gel electrophoresis. These linear molecules were recircularized with T4 DNA ligase and used to transform *E. coli* HB101. Transformed bacteria were screened for plasmids that had lost a *Sma*I restriction site and gained a *Bgl*II site at the position of the former *Sma*I site. Plasmids were also constructed that lacked sequences between the various *Sma*I sites.

Transfections

Cells were transfected using a modification of the procedure of Luthman and Magnusson (1983). NIH-3T3 cells were seeded at 0.7×10^6 cells per 10-cm dish and incubated at 37°C. The following day the monolayers were washed twice with Tris-buffered saline (TBS) (pH 7.4) and incubated with 0.5 ml of TBS containing 0.5 mg/ml DEAE-dextran (molecular weight 2×10^6; Pharmacia Fine Chemicals) and 2 μg of the appropriate plasmid for 8 minutes at room temperature. Longer incubations with these cells resulted in significant cell death. The cells were washed once with TBS and incubated for 2.5 hours at 37°C with medium containing 100 μM chloroquine diphosphate (Sigma). The cells were then washed twice with TBS, fed with medium, and incubated at 37°C.

Immunofluorescence

Cells were prepared for immunofluorescence as described (Luthman and Magnusson 1983). The fixed cells were incubated with a 1:40 dilution of different human sera with anti-EBNA antibody titers of greater than 1:80 (kindly provided by W. Henle) at 37°C for 45 minutes. After washing the coverslips with phosphate-buffered saline (PBS), the cells were incubated with goat anti-human IgG, IgA, and IgM (FITC-conjugated; Cappel Laboratories) diluted 1:20 for 45 minutes at 37°C. The coverslips were rinsed with PBS, mounted in Aquamount (Lerner Laboratories), and visualized by fluorescence microscopy. Cells were stained for polyoma tumor antigens, as described above, using polyoma tumor serum (hamster) (a generous gift of C. Prives) and FITC-conjugated rabbit anti-hamster immunoglobulin (Grand Island Biological Company).

RNA isolation and Northern hybridization analysis

Total cytoplasmic RNA and cytoplasmic polyadenylated RNA were isolated by the procedure of McGrogan and Raskas (1977) and digested with RNase-free DNase (Worthington). The RNA was separated on formaldehyde-agarose gels (Rave et al. 1979) and transferred to nitrocellulose filters (Schleicher and Schuell, BA85). The filters were prehybridized and hybridized as described by Alwine et al. (1977) and washed as recommended by Schleicher and Schuell (technical bulletin no. 352-354).

Radioimmunoelectrophoresis

Cell extracts were prepared by sonicating washed cell pellets in a small volume of 2% (w/v) SDS, 1% (v/v) 2-mercaptoethanol, and 8 mM Tris-HCl (pH 6.8). The samples were heated at 100°C for 5 minutes and centrifuged at 12,800g for 5 minutes. The supernatants were stored at −20°C. The protein concentrations of the samples were determined by a Bio-Rad protein assay. Samples were subjected to SDS-polyacrylamide gel electrophoresis by a modification of the procedure of Laemmli (1970). The separating gel was composed of 12.5% acrylamide and 0.1% bisacrylamide; the buffers were as described (Laemmli 1970). The conditions for the electrophoretic transfer of the proteins to nitrocellulose and probing with antiserum and radioiodinated protein A were as described by Burnette (1981). [^{125}I]-labeled protein A was purchased from New England Nuclear. The dilution factor for the human sera is indicated in the figure legends.

Results

A polyoma expression vector for EBV DNA

The goal of these studies was to identify those EBV sequences responsible for the expression of viral proteins detected in the latent state. For these experiments, an expression vector was constructed that consists of the entire early region, origin of replication, and leader sequences for late mRNA of polyoma virus (nucleotides 4632–3918) (Griffin et al. 1981) inserted into pML2. This vector, pMLPyA2 (Fig. 1a), expresses the polyoma T antigens (as determined by indirect immunofluorescence) and replicates when transfected into mouse cells. The EBV *Bam*HI K fragment was subcloned into this vector at the *Bam*HI site in both possible orientations termed pMLPyA2K and pMLPyA2K' (Fig. 1b,c). In latently infected lymphocytes, the *Bam*HI K fragment of EBV DNA is transcribed to produce a 3.7-kb mRNA (van Santen et al. 1981). In the pMLPyA2K' plasmid, the polyoma late promoter and late leader sequence are 5' and on the same DNA strand as the coding strand for this EBV transcript whereas the opposite orientation is termed pMLPyA2K (Fig. 1b,c).

The transcripts produced by pMLPyA2K and pMLPyA2K'

The expression of the EBV *Bam*HI K fragment in the polyoma vector was examined by Northern hybridization analysis. pMLPyA2, pMLPyA2K, and pMLPyA2K' were transfected into NIH-3T3 cells using DEAE-dextran (Luthman and Magnusson 1983). Forty-eight hours after transfection, total cytoplasmic RNA was extracted from these cells and analyzed by Northern hybridization analysis using either the EBV *Bam*HI K DNA fragment or polyoma late leader sequence as a probe (Fig. 2). Both pMLPyA2K and pMLPyA2K' gave rise to a variety of stable cytoplasmic transcripts. Cells transfected with the K' orientation plasmid synthesized a prominent 3.7–3.9-kb doublet of RNAs; the higher-molecular-weight species was also detected with the polyoma late leader

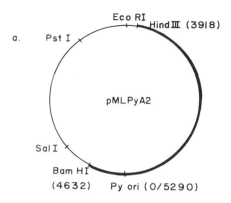

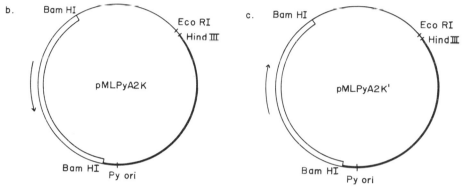

Figure 1 Organization of the vector pMLPyA2 and its derivatives pMLPyA2K and pMLPyA2K'. (a) Vector pMLPyA2 consists of a *Bam*HI–*Hind*III fragment of polyoma virus (A2 strain) inserted into the large *Bam*HI–*Hind*III fragment of pML2. The numbers in parentheses refer to polyoma virus nucleotide numbers (Griffin et al. 1981). (*b* and *c*) Plasmids pMLPyA2K and pMLPyA2K' were constructed by inserting the 5.0-kb *Bam*HI K fragment of EBV DNA (B95-8 strain) into pMLPyA2 in both possible orientations. The arrows refer to the direction of transcription of a 3.7-kb mRNA which is detected in an EBV growth-transformed lymphoblastoid cell line (van Santen et al. 1981).

probe (Fig. 2). A similar-size transcript was also found in cells transfected with pMLPyA2K but at much reduced levels. Polyadenylated cytoplasmic RNA (5 μg) from an EBV-positive lymphoblastoid cell line (IB4 cells) was compared with total cytoplasmic RNA (15 μg) derived from pMLPyA2K- or pMLPyA2K'-transfected mouse cells. Cells transfected with pMLPyA2K and pMLPyA2K' produced 50- to 100-fold more *Bam*HI K-specific RNA than observed in IB4 cells.

The expression of EBV proteins

The Western blot immunotransfer procedure (Burnette 1981) was used to determine if NIH-3T3 cells transfected with pMLPyA2K or pMLPyA2K' were also synthesizing EBV-associated proteins. As a comparison and control for these studies, several EBV-positive and -negative lymphoblastoid cell lines were tested for antigens using sera with or without antibodies directed against EBNA. Total cellular proteins were subjected to electrophoresis on SDS-polyacrylamide gels. The proteins were transferred to nitrocellulose filters, incubated with the appropriate serum, and then probed with ^{125}I-labeled protein A to detect bound antibody (Fig. 3). The EBV-positive lymphoblastoid cell lines (Raji, Namalwa, Jijoye,

IB4) each contained a prominent antigen whose molecular weight varied between 65,000 (Raji) and 92,000 (Namalwa). These data are in good agreement with observations made by Strnad et al. (1981) and Hennessy et al. (1983). These polypeptides were not detected in EBV-negative lymphoblastoid cell lines (BJAB, Loucks, Ramos) and were not detected in any of the cell lines when probed with sera lacking antibodies to EBNA (Fig. 3; data not shown). Mouse cells transfected with pMLPyA2K and pMLPyA2K' both produced an 88,000-m.w. antigen detected with EBNA antibody-positive sera. Cells transfected with pMLPyA2K' contained about 10-fold more antigen than cells transfected with the opposite orientation plasmid. Diluting the 3T3:pMLPyA2K' extract 10-fold provided a signal of antibody bound to antigen that was roughly equivalent to the 3T3:pMLPyA2K extract (Fig. 3) indicating that approximately 10 times more antigen is present in cells transfected with pMLPyA2K'. The molecular weight of the polypeptide detected in transfected mouse cells was the same as the antigen produced in IB4 cells. The *Bam*HI K fragment in these plasmids was derived from the B95-8 virus, the strain that was used to establish the IB4 cell line. These data suggest EBV strain differences

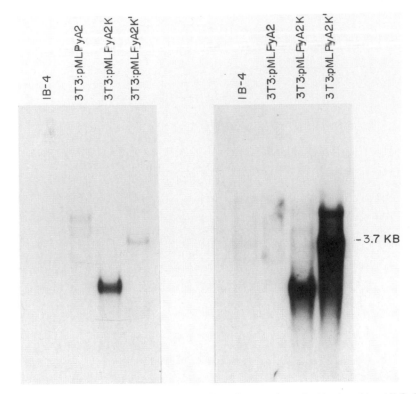

Figure 2 Northern hybridization analysis of RNA synthesized in NIH-3T3 cells transfected with plasmids pMLPyA2, pMLPyA2K, and pMLPyA2K'. Total cytoplasmic RNA (15 μg) from transfected 3T3 cells (DNase-treated) was separated in the lanes indicated. Polyadenylated RNA (5 μg) from IB4 cells was examined. The filter on the left was probed with a *Bam*HI–*Pvu*II fragment of polyoma virus (nucleotides 4632–5128) (Griffin et al. 1981) that contains the reiterated late leader sequence. The filter on the right was probed with the *Bam*HI K fragment. The position of a 3.7-kb RNA observed in IB4 cells is noted.

may result in antigen size variations, in good agreement with the observations of Hennessy et al. (1983).

When the murine cells transfected with pMLPyA2K' were fixed and stained with sera containing antibodies against EBNA, approximately 1% of the cells in the culture showed a bright nuclear fluorescent stain (Fig. 4b) demonstrating the nuclear location of this antigen. Human sera, known not to contain antibodies directed against EBNA, failed to detect this antigen in mouse cells transfected with pMLPyA2K' (Fig. 4a). Based upon the nuclear location of this antigen and the detection (by Western blots and fluorescent antibody staining) only with antisera known to contain antibodies directed against EBNA, the 88,000-m.w. antigen can be classified as an Epstein-Barr virus nuclear antigen.

EBNA is encoded by the EBV *Bam*HI K DNA fragment

EBNA detected in the previous experiments could be encoded by the *Bam*HI K DNA fragment or could be a virus-induced cellular protein that elicits an antibody response in humans. An example of the latter type of antigen is the nonviral p53 antigen whose levels are increased in transformed cells; animals bearing SV40-induced tumors often produce antibodies directed against p53 (Linzer and Levine 1979). To determine if the 88,000-m.w. EBNA was encoded by the EBV *Bam*HI

K fragment, a series of insertion and deletion mutants were introduced into this fragment at selected sites (Fig. 5). Partial digestion of pMLPyA2K' with *Sma*I followed by the insertion of a *Bgl*II restriction site linker (10 bp) should produce frameshift mutations at those locations (mutant S2). Partial digestion of pMLPyA2K' with *Hind*III, repairing the ends with the Klenow fragment of *E. coli* DNA polymerase I and subsequent blunt end ligations should produce four base-pair insertion mutations (mutants H1, H2). A set of deletions in *Bam*HI K DNA was obtained by restriction enzyme digestion and by the removal of an internal restriction DNA fragment within the EBV sequences (mutant S6). The mutations S3 and S7 resulted from the deletion of EBV sequences between the *Sma*I sites indicated and addition of a *Bgl*II linker at the site of the deletions. Mutant S8 lacks approximately 500 bp to the right of IR3 (Fig. 5). The precise ends of this deletion are presently unknown.

Figure 5 presents a map of these restriction enzyme sites in the 5.0-kb *Bam*HI K fragment and indicates the mutants generated by these procedures. Each of these mutants was transfected into NIH-3T3 cells. The polypeptides synthesized in these transfected cells were analyzed by Western immunoblots using sera containing anti-EBNA antibodies and are shown in Figure 5. Both the insertion and deletion mutations in the *Bam*HI K fragment resulted in altered molecular-weight forms of the

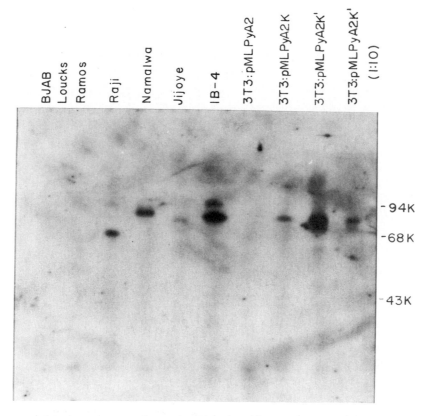

Figure 3 Proteins detected by EBNA-positive human sera in EBV-positive lymphoblastoid cell lines and transfected NIH-3T3 cells. Total cellular proteins from the sources indicated above each lane were examined by radioimmunoelectrophoresis. The filter was probed first with a 1:100 dilution of human serum (EBNA-positive) and then radioiodinated *Staphylococcus aureus* protein A. BJAB, Loucks, and Ramos are EBV-negative Burkitt's lymphoma cell lines. Raji, Namalwa, Jijoye, and IB4 are EBV-positive B cell lines. The rightmost lane contains a 1:10 dilution of the extract 3T3:pMLPyA2K .

EBNA indicating the coding and noncoding regions of EBV *Bam*HI K DNA. It is clear from this analysis that the *Bam*HI K DNA fragment encodes an EBNA.

Discussion

EBV is capable of infecting primary B lymphocytes in culture, resulting in the production of permanent cell lines. This immortalization, or transformation, of B cells (Henle et al. 1967) results in cell lines containing 2–100 copies of EBV DNA per cell in a circular episomal form (Lindahl et al. 1976) of which less than 10% is expressed (Orellana and Kieff 1977). At present, little or nothing is known about the viral functions that may be required for transformation, replication, and maintenance of the viral DNA, DNA copy number control, and regulation of EBV gene expression in these cells. All lymphoblastoid cell lines examined thus far that contain EBV DNA express a nuclear antigen (Pope et al. 1969; Reedmann and Klein 1973), termed EBNA, which can be detected with antibodies from the serum of patients recovering from infectious mononucleosis. The size of one EBNA component varies between different strains of EBV (Strnad et al. 1981; Hennessy et al. 1983) and Summers et al. (1982) demonstrated that the EBV *Bam*HI K fragment is able to encode or induce an EBNA in mouse

cells. There are several reasons why progress in characterizing EBV-encoded or -induced proteins in latent infections has been slow. First, specific antibody reagents to these proteins are not readily available and only unique and diverse human sera from different patients have been used to date. Second, these sera are known to contain autoantibodies, heterophile antibodies, and antibodies directed against a variety of infectious agents. Therefore, the molecular nature of EBV-associated antigens and their origin remains unclear. Third, the levels of EBV-encoded or -induced antigens in lymphoblastoid cells appear to be quite low (Strnad et al. 1981) and, finally, only a few spontaneous EBV mutants are available to correlate genetic alterations with structural changes in protein.

To address these problems, a polyoma expression vector, pMLPyA2, was constructed (Fig. 1) and the EBV *Bam*HI K fragment was introduced into the late region of polyoma. The design of this expression vector permits plasmid DNA replication in mouse cells (template amplification) and takes advantage of the polyoma virus late promoter and late leader sequences for efficient transcription and translation of exogenous sequences. When the *Bam*HI K fragment was inserted in this vector such that the polyoma promoter and late leader sequence are 5′ to and on the same DNA strand as the DNA encoding

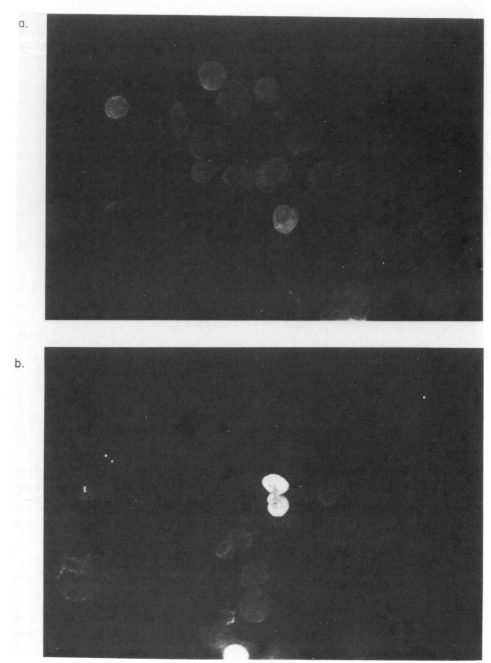

Figure 4 Indirect immunofluorescence of NIH-3T3 cells transfected with pMLPyA2K'. NIH-3T3 cells were transfected with pMLPyA2K' and analyzed 40 hr later for EBV-associated proteins by indirect immunofluorescence. The cells in *a* were incubated with EBNA-negative human serum whereas the cells in *b* were incubated with EBNA-positive serum. Bound antibodies were detected by fluorescein-labeled goat anti-human IgG, IgM, and IgA.

the EBV transcript, increased levels of a 3.9-kb EBV-specific mRNA (Fig. 2) and an EBV 88,000-m.w. protein (Fig. 3) are obtained when compared with the same *Bam*HI K fragment placed in the opposite orientation. NIH-3T3 cells transfected with pMLPyA2K' contain approximately 100 times more 88,000-m.w. EBNA when compared with EBV-positive lymphoblastoid cell lines. The fact that the 88,000-m.w. EBNA is synthesized in cells transfected with the vector containing *Bam*HI K in either of the two orientations demonstrates that this EBV

DNA fragment contains most or all of the signals required for transcription and translation of this protein. The 88,000-m.w. protein produced by transfection of mouse cells with pMLPyA2K' is a nuclear antigen (Fig. 4).

Proof that the EBV *Bam*HI K DNA fragment encodes the 88,000-m.w. EBNA comes from a series of insertion and deletion mutations the *Bam*HI K fragment. These mutations alter the size of this EBNA and allow the coding sequences for this protein to be predicted. It remains possible that additional proteins encoded by the *Bam*HI

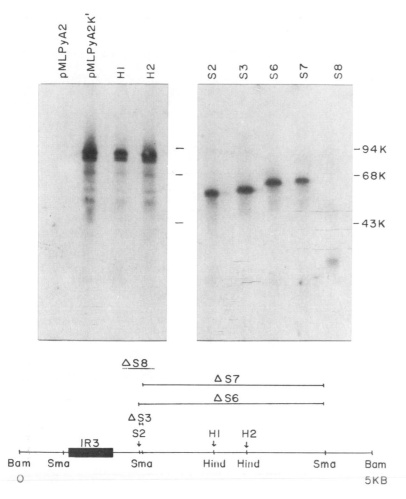

Figure 5 Deletion and insertion mutations in the *Bam*HI K fragment of pMLPyA2K' and the EBV-specific proteins synthesized in cells transfected with these mutants. The map at the bottom of the figure indicates relevant restriction endonuclease sites in the EBV *Bam*HI K fragment. The direction of transcription of a 3.7-kb RNA encoded by the *Bam*HI K fragment is from left to right. The positions of insertion mutations are indicated by arrows. The sequences deleted in mutants S3, S6, and S7 are indicated above the map. The ends of the deletion S8 have not yet been determined. The EBV-specific proteins synthesized in NIH-3T3 cells transfected with these plasmids were detected by radioimmunoelectrophoresis (*top*). IR3 is an internal repeated nucleotide sequence described by Hennessy et al. (1983).

K fragment exist and were not recognized by the anti-EBNA antibody-positive antisera used in these experiments. The availability of wild-type and mutant proteins in increased quantities should now allow studies of the function of this Epstein-Barr virus protein.

Acknowledgments

The assistance of R. Pashley, A.K. Teresky, and G. Urban is appreciated. This research was supported by a grant from the American Cancer Society. J.H. is a predoctoral fellow of the National Cancer Institute training grant 2 T 32 CA9176-08.

Note Added in Proof

Results similar to those reported here have been obtained with an SV40 expression vector and *Bam*HI K DNA by Fischer et al. (1984).

References

Adams, A. 1979. The state of the viral genome in transformed cells and its relationship to host cell DNA. In *The Epstein-Barr virus* (eds. M.A. Epstein and B.G. Anchong), p. 155. Springer-Verlag, Berlin.

Alwine, J.C., D.J. Kemp, and G.R. Stark. 1977. Method for detection of specific RNAs in agarose gels by transfer to diazobenzyloxymethyl-paper and hybridization with DNA probes. *Proc. Natl. Acad. Sci.* **74**: 5350.

Burnette, W.N. 1981. "Western blotting": Electrophoretic transfer of proteins from sodium dodecyl sulfate-polyacrylamide gels to unmodified nitrocellulose and radiographic detection with antibody and radioiodinated protein A. *Anal. Biochem.* **112**: 195.

Corden, J., B. Wasylyk, A. Buchwalder, P. Sassone-Corsi, C. Kedinger, and P. Chambon. 1980. Promoter sequences of eukaryotic protein-coding genes. *Science* **209**: 1406.

Dambaugh, T., C. Beisel, M. Hummel, W. King, S. Fennewald, A. Cheung, M. Heller, N. Raab-Traub, and E. Kieff. 1980. Epstein-Barr virus (B95-8) DNA VII: Molecular cloning and detailed mapping. *Proc. Natl. Acad. Sci.* **77**: 2999.

de The, G., A. Geser, N.E. Day, P.M. Tukei, E.H. Williams, D.P. Beri, P.G. Smith, A.G. Dean, G.W. Bornkamm, P. Feorino, and W. Henle. 1978. Epidemiological evidence for causal relationship between Epstein-Barr virus and Burkitt's lymphoma: Results of the Ugandan prospective study. *Nature* **272**: 756.

Fischer, D.K., M.F. Robert, D. Shedd, W.P. Summers, J.E. Robinson, J. Wolak, J.E. Stefano, and G. Miller. 1984. Identification of Epstein-Barr nuclear antigen polypeptide in mouse and monkey cells after gene transfer with a cloned 2.9-kilobase-pair subfragment of the genome. *Proc. Natl. Acad. Sci.* **81**: 43.

Griffin, B.E., E. Soeda, B.G. Barrell, and R. Staden. 1981. Sequence and analysis of polyoma virus DNA. In *Molecular biology of tumor viruses*, 2nd edition: *DNA tumor viruses*, p.

843. Cold Spring Harbor Laboratory, Cold Spring Harbor, New York.

Henle, W. and G. Henle. 1979. The virus as the etiologic agent of infectious mononucleosis. In *The Epstein-Barr virus* (eds. M.A. Epstein and B.G. Anchong), p. 297. Springer-Verlag, Berlin.

Henle, W., V. Diehl, G. Kohn, H. zur Hausen, and G. Henle. 1967. Herpes-type virus and chromosome marker in normal leukocytes after growth with irradiated Burkitt cells. *Science* **157:** 1064.

Hennessy, K., M. Heller, V. van Santen, and E. Kieff. 1983. Simple repeat array in Epstein-Barr virus DNA encodes part of the Epstein-Barr nuclear antigen. *Science* **220:** 1396.

Kaschka-Dierich, C., A. Adams, T. Lindahl, G.W. Bornkamm, G. Bjursell, G. Klein, B.C. Giovanella, and S. Singh. 1976. Intracellular forms of Epstein-Barr virus DNA in human tumour cells *in vivo*. *Nature* **260:** 302.

Klein, G. 1979. The relationship of the virus to nasopharyngeal carcinoma. In *The Epstein-Barr virus* (eds. M.A. Epstein and B.G. Anchong), p. 339. Springer-Verlag, Berlin.

Laemmli, U.K. 1970. Cleavage of structural proteins during the assembly of the head of bacteriophage T4. *Nature* **227:** 680.

Lindahl, T., A. Adams, G. Bjursell, G.W. Bornkamm, C. Kaschka-Dierich, and U. Jehn. 1976. Covalently closed circular duplex DNA of Epstein-Barr virus in a human lymphoid cell line. *J. Mol. Biol.* **102:** 511.

Linzer, D.I.H. and A.J. Levine. 1979. Characterization of 54K dalton cellular SV40 tumor antigen present in SV40-transformed cells and uninfected embryonal carcinoma cells. *Cell* **17:** 43.

Lusky, M. and M. Botchan. 1981. Inhibition of SV40 replication in simian cells by specific pBR322 DNA sequences. *Nature* **293:** 79.

Luthman, H. and G. Magnusson. 1983. High efficiency polyoma DNA transfection of chloroquine treated cells. *Nucleic Acids Res.* **11:** 1295.

McGrogan, M. and H.J. Raskas. 1977. Species identification and genome mapping of cytoplasmic adenovirus type 2 RNAs synthesized late in infection. *J. Virol.* **23:** 240.

Orellana, T. and E. Kieff. 1977. Epstein-Barr virus-specific RNA II. Analysis of polyadenylated viral RNA in restringent, abortive and productive infections. *J. Virol.* **22:** 321.

Pope, J.H., M.K. Horne, and E.J. Wetters. 1969. Significance of a complement-fixing antigen associated with the herpeslike virus and detected in the Raji cell line. *Nature* **222:** 186.

Rave, N., R. Crkvenjakov, and H. Boedtker. 1979. Identification of procollagen mRNAs transferred to diazobenzyloxymethyl paper from formaldehyde agarose gels. *Nucleic Acids Res.* **6:** 3559.

Reedman, B.M. and G. Klein. 1973. Cellular localization of an Epstein-Barr virus (EBV)-associated complement-fixing antigen in producer and non-producer lymphoblastoid cell lines. *Int. J. Cancer* **11:** 499.

Rosa, M.D., E. Gottlieb, M.R. Lerner, and J.A. Steitz. 1981. Striking similarities are exhibited by two small Epstein-Barr virus-encoded ribonucleic acids and the adenovirus-associated ribonucleic acids VAI and VAII. *Mol. Cell. Biol.* **1:** 785.

Strnad, B.C., T.C. Schuster, K.F. Hopkins III, R.H. Neubauer, and H. Rabin. 1981. Identification of an Epstein-Barr virus nuclear antigen by fluoroimmunoelectrophoresis and radioimmunoelectrophoresis. *J. Virol.* **38:** 996.

Summers, W.P., E.A. Grogan, D. Shedd, M. Robert, C.-R. Liu, and G. Miller. 1982. Stable expression in mouse cells of nuclear neoantigen after transfer of a 3.4-megadalton cloned fragment of Epstein-Barr virus DNA. *Proc. Natl. Acad. Sci.* **79:** 5688.

van Santen, V., A. Cheung, and E. Kieff. 1981. Epstein-Barr virus RNA VII: Size and direction of transcription of virus-specified cytoplasmic RNAs in a transformed cell line. *Proc. Natl. Acad. Sci.* **78:** 1930.

Structure and Activation of *ras* Genes

M. Wigler, O. Fasano, E. Taparowsky, S. Powers, T. Kataoka, D. Birnbaum, K. Shimizu,* and M. Goldfarb

Cold Spring Harbor Laboratory, Cold Spring Harbor, New York 11724

Transforming genes have been found in the acutely pathogenic RNA tumor viruses and in some tumor cells (Cooper 1982). In general, they derive from normal cellular genes by a variety of processes, documented in this volume, which are still being analyzed. Among these processes, those that activate the transforming potential of the *ras* genes are the simplest. Transforming *ras* genes can differ from normal cellular *ras* genes by a single point mutation resulting in a single amino acid substitution in the encoded protein (Reddy et al. 1982; Tabin et al. 1982; Taparowsky et al. 1982, 1983; McGrath et al. 1983; Santos et al. 1983; Shimizu et al. 1983a; Sukumar et al. 1983; Yuasa et al. 1983). This and two other factors make study of the *ras* genes an especially attractive pathway for understanding the molecular mechanisms of cancer: first, *ras* genes are frequently activated in tumor cells (Der et al. 1982; Parada et al. 1982; Hall et al. 1983; Shimizu et al. 1983b); and second, genes highly homologous to *ras* are found in yeast, a simple eukaryotic organism which can be subjected to powerful genetic analysis (DeFeo-Jones et al. 1983; Powers et al. 1984). A little is already known about the *ras* proteins. They bind guanine nucleotides (Ellis et al. 1981) and are associated with the internal plasma membrane (Willingham et al. 1980). In this paper, we discuss the structure of the *ras* genes and their products, the structure of related genes found in yeast, and the mutations that can activate *ras* oncogenic potential.

Structure of the Human *ras* Gene Family and Their Proteins

The Ha-*ras* and Ki-*ras* genes were first identified as the oncogenes of the Harvey and Kirsten sarcoma viruses (Ellis et al. 1981). These genes arose by transduction of normal rat cellular genes (Ellis et al. 1981). Homologs of these genes are found in vertebrates, detectable by Southern hybridization (Ellis et al. 1981). A third member of the family, the N-*ras* gene, was first found as the transforming gene of certain tumor cell DNAs (Hall et al. 1983; Shimizu et al. 1983b). From the sequence of these genes and the cDNA copies of their mRNA transcripts, we and others have derived the predicted amino acid sequences of their proteins (see Fig. 1) (Capon et al. 1983; Fasano et al. 1983; McGrath et al. 1983; Shimizu et al. 1983a; Taparowsky et al. 1983). The coding sequences for each *ras* gene are interrupted by three intervening sequences at precisely analogous positions, from which we con-

clude that Ha-, Ki-, and N-*ras* have evolved from a common spliced ancestral gene (McGrath et al. 1983; Shimizu et al. 1983a; Taparowski et al. 1983). The Ki-*ras* gene has two fourth coding exons and alternate splicing patterns can specify either of two proteins (McGrath et al. 1983; Shimizu et al. 1983a). Alternate splicing pathways have not been described for Ha-*ras* or N-*ras*.

Comparison of the *ras* protein amino acid sequences reveals some interesting points (see Fig. 1). First, the three human *ras* genes are identical for the first 86 amino acid positions. From position 87 to 170, there is greater than 80% homology, with many differences being conservative amino acid changes. After this, they diverge radically for 15 amino acids. We call this the variable region. All four *ras* proteins then terminate with the sequence, CysAAX, where A is an aliphatic amino acid and X is the terminal amino acid.

We have speculated that the variable region is the domain of the *ras* protein that determines a unique physiologic specificity. Four pieces of circumstantial evidence point to this conclusion: (1) The variable region is the major region where the *ras* genes vary from each other; (2) this region has been highly conserved in evolution, at least from rat to man (Fasano et al. 1983; Shimizu et al. 1983a); (3) the alternate coding exons of the Ki-*ras* gene essentially specify alternate variable regions; (4) we observe analogous variable regions in two yeast *ras* genes (Powers et al. 1984).

Structure of the Yeast *ras* Genes and Their Proteins

The *ras* genes have been highly conserved in mammals, and homologous sequences in *Drosophila* have been found (Shilo and Weinberg 1981). We therefore looked for similar sequences in the yeast *Saccharomyces cerevisiae*. We observed two highly homologous genes in yeast by Southern hybridization and have cloned and sequenced both. We have called these genes *RAS1* and *RAS2* and their predicted amino acid sequence, alongside that of the human Ha-*ras* gene, is shown in Figure 2. The predicted proteins have a strikingly homologous structure to the mammalian *ras* proteins. After a short peptide leader, they have nearly 90% homology to the first 80 amino acid positions of Ha-*ras* and nearly 50% homology to the next 80 amino acids. Although the predicted yeast *ras* proteins are much larger than their mammalian counterparts, they too terminate with the conserved sequence CysAAX. Moreover, the yeast *ras* proteins also contain variable domains. *RAS1* and *RAS2* are highly homologous for the first 176 amino acid positions, but they then diverge radically after that, and are

*Present Address: Department of Biology, Faculty of Science, Kyushu University, Kukuoka 812, Japan.

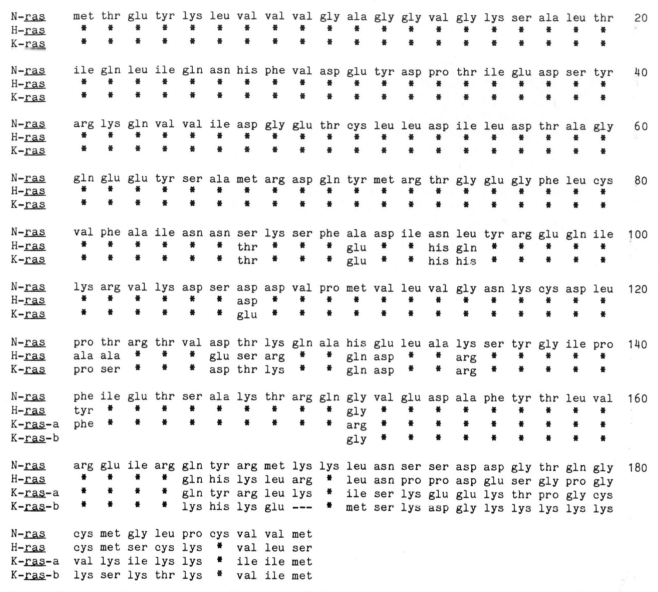

Figure 1 Comparison of human *ras* amino acid sequences. Predicted amino acid sequences for the normal human Ha-*ras*, Ki-*ras*, and N-*ras* genes are shown. Ki-*ras*-a and Ki-*ras*-b refer to proteins specified by mRNA utilizing exons IVa or IVb, respectively. Asterisks indicate where the same amino acid is specified by all *ras*. At positions where there is not complete agreement, all specified amino acids are indicated. Dashes indicate a frameshift in Ki-*ras*-b that results in improved sequence alignment. Numbers in the left-hand margin are the position of the last amino acid on the respective line.

homologous again only for the terminal eight amino acids. This variable region begins at the position precisely analogous to the beginning of the mammalian variable region.

We have speculated the conserved aminoterminal domain of the *ras* genes is an effector domain that carries out an enzymatic or regulatory function. Because of the sequence conservation, this biochemical function is probably similar in yeast and mammals. This hypothesis can be tested by the construction of chimeric mammal-

ian/yeast genes and a study of their function when introduced into cells. Moreover, it is likely that yeast and mammalian *ras* interact with proteins that have also been conserved in evolution. Identification of these proteins and their genes in yeast may facilitate their identification in mammals. It is also possible that the physiologic role for *ras* in cells has been conserved between yeast and mammals, but this is a harder hypothesis to test. In any event, it is clear that study of yeast *ras* genes may lead to valuable insights into mammalian *ras* function.

Figure 2 Comparison of yeast and human *ras* amino acid sequences. Predicted amino acid sequences for the *S. cerevisiae RAS1* and *RAS2* genes and the human Ha-*ras* genes are shown. Positions are underlined when two or more identical amino acids are specified. Positions differing by conservative amino acids changes are dotted. Gaps indicate frameshifts imposed to improve alignments. Asterisks mark positions where amino acid substitutions activate the transforming potential of Ha-*ras*.

```
RAS2                                                                        met pro leu asn lys ser asn     7
RAS1                                                                        met gln gly asn lys ser thr     7

RAS2    ile arg glu tyr lys leu val val val gly gly gly gly val gly lys ser ala leu thr    27
RAS1    ile arg glu tyr lys ile val val val gly gly gly gly val gly lys ser ala leu thr    27
H-ras   met thr glu tyr lys leu val val val gly ala gly*gly*val gly lys ser ala leu thr    20

RAS2    ile gln leu thr gln ser his phe val asp glu tyr asp pro thr ile glu asp ser tyr    47
RAS1    ile gln phe ile gln ser tyr phe val asp glu tyr asp pro thr ile glu asp ser tyr    47
H-ras   ile gln leu ile gln asn his phe val asp glu tyr asp pro thr ile glu asp ser tyr    40

RAS2    arg lys gln val val ile asp asp glu val ser ile leu asp ile leu asp thr ala gly    67
RAS1    arg lys gln val val ile asp asp lys val ser ile leu asp ile leu asp thr ala gly    67
H-ras   arg lys gln val val ile asp gly glu thr cys leu leu asp ile leu asp thr ala*gly    60

RAS2    gln glu glu tyr ser ala met arg glu gln tyr met arg asn gly glu gly phe leu leu    87
RAS1    gln glu glu tyr ser ala met arg glu gln tyr met arg thr gly glu gly phe leu leu    87
H-ras   gln*glu glu*tyr ser ala met arg asp gln tyr met arg thr gly glu gly phe leu cys    80

RAS2    val tyr ser ile thr ser lys ser ser leu asp glu leu met thr tyr tyr gln gln ile   107
RAS1    val tyr ser val thr ser arg asn ser phe asp glu leu leu ser tyr tyr gln gln ile   107
H-ras   val phe ala ile asn asn thr lys ser phe glu asp ile his gln tyr arg glu gln ile   100

RAS2    leu arg val lys asp thr asp tyr val pro ile val val val gly asn lys ser asp leu   127
RAS1    gln arg val lys asp ser asp tyr ile pro val val val val gly asn lys leu asp leu   127
H-ras   lys arg val lys asp ser asp asp val pro met val leu val gly asn lys cys asp leu   120

RAS2    glu asn glu lys gln val ser tyr gln asp gly leu asn met ala lys gln met asn ala   147
RAS1    glu asn glu arg gln val ser tyr glu asp gly leu arg leu ala lys gln leu asn ala   147
H-ras   ala ala arg thr val glu ser arg gln     ala gln asp leu ala arg ser tyr gly ile   139

RAS2    pro phe leu glu thr ser ala lys gln ala ile asn val glu glu ala phe tyr thr leu   167
RAS1    pro phe leu glu thr ser ala lys gln ala ile asn val asp glu ala phe tyr ser leu   167
H-ras   pro tyr ile glu thr ser ala lys thr arg gln gly val glu asp ala phe tyr thr leu   159

RAS2    ala arg leu val arg asp glu gly gly lys tyr asn lys thr leu thr glu asn asp asn   187
RAS1    ile arg leu val arg asp asp gly gly lys tyr asn ser met asn arg gln leu asp asn   187
H-ras   val arg glu ile arg gln his lys leu arg lys leu asn pro pro asp glu ser gly pro   179

RAS2    ser lys gln thr ser gln asp thr lys gly ser gly ala asn ser val pro arg asn ser   207
RAS1    thr asn glu ile arg asp ser glu leu thr ser ser ala thr ala asp ile glu lys lys   207
H-ras   gly cys met ser cys lys                                                            185

RAS2    gly gly his arg lys met ser asn ala ala asn gly lys asn val asn ser ser thr thr   227
RAS1    asn asn gly ser tyr val leu asp asn ser leu thr asn ala gly thr gly ser ser ser   227

RAS2    val val asn ala arg asn ala ser ile glu ser lys thr gly leu ala gly asn gln ala   247
RAS1    lys ser ala val asn his asn gly glu thr thr lys arg thr asp glu lys asn tyr val   247

RAS2    thr asn gly lys thr gln thr val arg thr asn ile asp asn ser thr gly gln ala gly   267
RAS1    asn gln asn asn asn asn glu gly asn thr lys tyr ser ser asn gly asn gly asn arg   267

RAS2    gln ala asn ala gln ser ala asn thr val asn asn arg val asn asn asn ser lys ala   287
RAS1    ser asp ile ser arg gly asn gln asn asn ala leu asn ser arg ser lys gln ser ala   287

RAS2    gly gln val ser asn ala lys gln ala arg lys gln gln ala ala pro gly gly asn thr   307
RAS1    glu pro gln lys asn ser ser ala asn ala arg lys glu ser                           301

RAS2    ser glu ala ser lys ser gly ser gly gly cys cys ile ile ser                       322
RAS1                            ser gly gly cys cys ile ile cys                           309
H-ras                                       cys val leu ser                               189
```

Figure 2 (*See facing page for legend.*)

Activating Mutations of the *ras* Genes

There have been multiple examples of activated *ras* genes found in tumor cells. In all cases that have been examined, these activated *ras* genes result from single point mutations in the *ras* coding regions, and in all cases either of two codons are involved, the 12th and 61st (Reddy et al. 1982; Tabin et al. 1982; Taparowsky et al. 1982, 1983; McGrath et al. 1983; Santos et al. 1983; Shimizu et al. 1983a; Sukumar et al. 1983; Yuasa et al. 1983). It appears that virtually any amino acid substitution at these positions results in the activation of the transforming potential of the *ras* proteins. To determine if these were the only sites for mutational activation of the *ras* genes, we randomly mutagenized the normal human Ha-*ras* gene by bisulfite treatment and tested pools of mutants for their ability to induce transformed foci of NIH-3T3 cells (Fasano et al. 1984). In this manner, we identified in vitro mutants with transforming ability, and by sequence analysis and chimeric gene construction we have found three other sites where amino acid substitution leads to activation of *ras* transforming potential: the 13th, 59th, and 63rd amino acid positions. At the 13th position, either serine or aspartic acid substitution for glycine results in a transforming allele; at the 59th, threonine for alanine; at the 63rd, lysine for glutamine. Not all these *ras* proteins have equal transforming ability (see Table 1).

Our results with random mutagenesis raise some new questions. First, it is no longer clear why only mutations in the 12th and 61st codons have been found in the *ras* genes of tumors. Second, it is curious that the viral *ras* genes found in Harvey and Kirsten sarcoma viruses each contain two activating mutations: one at position 12 and one at position 59 (Dahr et al. 1982; Tsuchida et al.

1982). We have no simple explanation for this at the moment.

The activating mutations are clearly clustered about two regions: region I, the codons 12 and 13; and region II, the codons 59–63. Others have argued from comparative sequence data that the region about the 12th amino acid is the guanine nucleotide binding site of the *ras* proteins (Wierenga and Hol 1983). We also argue that region II may also form part of the guanine nucleotide binding site since if threonine is encoded in position 59 it becomes phosphorylated when *ras* proteins are incubated in the presence of GTP (Shih et al. 1980, 1982; Papageorge et al. 1982). If these speculations are correct, amino acid substitutions that activate the transforming potential of *ras* may do so either by altering the kinetics of guanine nucleotide binding or by disrupting the conformational changes induced by guanine nucleotides.

The two regions where activating mutations cluster are regions that are conserved between mammalian and yeast *ras* genes (see Fig. 2). Preliminary results from our lab indicate that introduction of these mutations into the yeast *ras* genes has a discernible dominant phenotype (T. Kataoka et al., in prep.). Therefore, yeast may prove to be a workable model for understanding growth transformation induced by mutant *ras* genes.

References

Capon, D., Y. Ellson, A. Levinson, P. Seeburg, and D. Goeddel. 1983. Complete nucleotide sequences of the T24 human bladder carcinoma oncogene and its normal homologue. *Nature* **302:** 33.

Cooper, G. 1982. Cellular transforming genes. *Science* **217:** 801.

Dahr, R., R.W. Ellis, T.Y. Shih, S. Oroszlan, B. Shapiro, J.

Table 1 Amino Acid Changes that Activate the Transforming Potential of the Normal Ha-*ras* Gene

| Plasmids[a] | Amino acid at positions in the Ha-*ras*-encoded p21[a] | | | | Relative potency in focus induction[a] |
	12	13	59	63	
pTPT (negative control)	Gly	Gly	Ala	Glu	<0.0001
pT24 (positive control)	*Val*	Gly	Ala	Glu	1.0
BSS194	*Ser*	Gly	Ala	Glu	0.4
BSS176	*Asp*	*Glu*	Ala	Glu	0.5
BSC454	Gly	*Asp*	Ala	Glu	0.2
BSS197	Gly	*Ser*	Ala	Glu	0.001
TPO24	Gly	Gly	Ala	*Lys*	0.1
TPO87[b]	Gly	Gly	*Thr*	Glu	0.2
THR09[c]	Gly	Gly	*Thr*	Glu	0.6

[a]Plasmids pTPT and pT24 are genomic clones of normal and mutant *ras* genes, respectively. All other plasmids derive from pTPT by bisulfite mutagenesis and contain only point mutations. All transforming potencies are relative to that of pT24 in a standard NIH-3T3 focus induction assay. At least two assays were performed on each plasmid. The encoded amino acids that differ from the wild type are italicized. See Fasano et al. (1984) for more details.

[b]Additional mutations leading to amino acid change were present in positions 49 (Lys instead of Glu), 62 (Lys instead of Glu), and 73 (His instead of Arg).

[c]Additional amino acid changes were present in positions 42 (Arg instead of Lys), 47 (Asn instead of Asp), and 81 (Met instead of Val).

Maizel, D. Lowy, and E. Scolnick. 1982. Nucleotide sequence of the p21 transforming protein of Harvey murine sarcoma virus. *Science* **217**: 934.

DeFeo-Jones, D., E. Scolnick, R. Koller, and R. Dhar. 1983. *ras*-Related gene sequences identified and isolated from *Saccharomyces cerevisiae. Nature* **306**: 707.

Der, C., T. Krontiris, and G. Cooper. 1982. Transforming genes of human bladder and lung carcinoma cell lines are homologous to the *ras* genes of Harvey and Kirsten sarcoma viruses. *Proc. Natl. Acad. Sci.* **79**: 3637.

Ellis, R.W., D. Defeo, T.Y. Shih, M.A. Gonda, H.A. Young, N. Tsuchida, D.R. Lowy, and E.M. Scolnick. 1981. The p21 *src* genes of Harvey and Kirsten sarcoma viruses originate from divergent members of a family of normal vertebrate genes. *Nature* **292**: 506.

Fasano, O., E. Taparowsky, J. Fiddes, M. Wigler, and M. Goldfarb. 1983. Sequence and structure of the coding region of the human H-*ras*-1 gene from T24 bladder carcinoma cells. *J. Mol. Appl. Genet.* **2**: 173.

Fasano, O., T. Aldrich, F. Tamanoi, E. Taparowsky, M. Furth, and M. Wigler. 1984. Analysis of the transforming potential of the human H-*ras* gene by random mutagenesis. *Proc. Natl. Acad. Sci.* (in press).

Hall, A., C. Marshall, N. Spurr, and R. Weiss. 1983. Identification of the transforming gene in two human sarcoma cell lines as a new member of the *ras* gene family located on chromosome. *Nature* **303**: 396.

McGrath, J.P., D.J. Capon, D.H. Smith, E.Y. Chen, P.H. Seeburg, D.V. Goeddel, and A.D. Levinson. 1983. Structure and organization of the human Ki-*ras* proto-oncogene and a related processed pseudogene. *Nature* **304**: 501.

Papageorge, A., D. Lowy, and E. Scolnick. 1982. Comparative biochemical properties of p21 *ras* molecules coded for viral and cellular *ras* genes. *J. Virol.* **44**: 509.

Parada, L., C. Tabin, C. Shih, and R. Weinberg. 1982. Human EJ bladder carcinoma oncogene is homologue of Harvey sarcoma virus *ras* gene. *Nature* **297**: 474.

Powers, S., T. Kataoka, O. Fasano, M. Goldfarb, J. Strathern, J. Broach, and M. Wigler. 1984. Genes in *Saccharomyces cerevisiae* encoding proteins with domains homologous to the mammalian *ras* proteins. *Cell* **36**: 607.

Reddy, E., R. Reynolds, E. Santos, and M. Barbacid. 1982. A point mutation is responsible for the acquisition of transforming properties by the T24 human bladder carcinoma oncogene. *Nature* **300**: 149.

Santos, E., E.P. Reddy, S. Pulciani, R.J. Feldman, and M. Barbacid. 1983. Spontaneous activation of a human proto-oncogene. *Proc. Natl. Acad. Sci.* **80**: 5253.

Shih, T.Y., A.G. Papageorge, P.E. Stokes, M.O. Weeks, and E.M. Scolnick. 1980. Guanine nucleotide-binding and autophosphorylating activities associated with the p21*src* protein of Harvey murine sarcoma virus. *Nature* **287**: 686.

Shih, T., P. Stokes, G. Smythes, R. Dhar, and S. Oroszlan. 1982. Characterization of the phosphorylation sites and the surrounding amino acid sequences of the p21 transforming proteins coded for by the Harvey and Kirsten strains of murine sarcoma virus. *J. Biol. Chem.* **257**: 11767.

Shilo, B. and R. Weinberg. 1981. DNA sequences homologous to vertebrate oncogenes are conserved in *Drosophila melanogaster. Proc. Natl. Acad. Sci.* **78**: 6789.

Shimizu, K., D. Birnbaum, M. Ruley, O. Fasano, Y. Suard, L. Edlund, E. Taparowsky, M. Goldfarb, and M. Wigler. 1983a. The structure of the K-*ras* gene of the human lung carcinoma cell line Calu-1. *Nature* **304**: 497.

Shimizu, K., M. Goldfarb, Y. Suard, M. Perucho, Y. Li, T. Kamata, J. Feramisco, E. Stavnezer, J. Fogh, and M. Wigler. 1983b. Three human transforming genes are related to viral *ras* oncogenes. *Proc. Natl. Acad. Sci.* **80**: 2112.

Sukumar, S., V. Notario, D. Martin-Zanca, and M. Barbacid. 1983. Induction of mammary carcinomas in rats by nitrosomethylurea involves malignant activation of H-*ras*-1 locus by single point mutations. *Nature* **306**: 658.

Tabin, C., S. Bradley, C. Bargmann, R. Weinberg, A. Papageorge. E. Scolnick, R. Dhar, D. Lowy, and E. Chang. 1982. Mechanism of activation of a human oncogene. *Nature* **300**: 143.

Taparowsky, E., K. Shimizu, M. Goldfarb, and M. Wigler. 1983. Structure and activation of human N-*ras* gene. *Cell* **34**: 581.

Taparowsky, E., Y. Suard, O. Fasano, K. Shimizu, M. Goldfarb, and M. Wigler. 1982. Activation of the I24 bladder carcinoma transforming gene is linked to a single amino acid change. *Nature* **300**: 762.

Tsuchida, N., T. Ryder, and E. Ohtsubo. 1982. Nucleotide sequence of the oncogene encoding the p21 transforming protein of Kirsten murine sarcoma virus. *Science* **217**: 937.

Wierenga, R. and W. Hol. 1983. Predicted nucleotide-binding properties of p21 protein and its cancer-associated variant. *Nature* **302**: 842.

Willingham, M., I. Pastan, T. Shih, and E. Scolnick. 1980. Localization of the *src* gene product of the Harvey strain of MSV to plasma membrane of transformed cells by electron microscopy immunocytochemistry. *Cell* **19**: 1005.

Yuasa, Y., S. Srivastava, C. Dunn, J. Rhim, E. Ready, and S. Aaronson. 1983. Acquisition of transforming properties by alternative point mutations within c-bas/has human proto-oncogene. *Nature* **303**: 775.

A Common Mechanism for the Malignant Activation of *ras* Oncogenes in Human Neoplasia and in Chemically Induced Animal Tumors

V. Notario, S. Sukumar, E. Santos, and M. Barbacid

Laboratory of Cellular and Molecular Biology, National Cancer Institute, Bethesda, Maryland 20205

Identification and isolation of transforming genes in human tumors have made possible the investigation at the molecular level of some of the steps involved in the development of human neoplasia (Goldfarb et al. 1982; Pulciani et al. 1982b; Shih and Weinberg 1982). A large proportion of human transforming genes have been found to be members of the *ras* gene family (Der et al. 1902; Parada et al. 1982; Santos et al. 1982), a type of gene that can also acquire malignant properties upon recombination with certain retroviral sequences (Andersen et al. 1981; Ellis et al. 1981). So far, three different *ras* oncogenes, Ha-*ras*, Ki-*ras*, and N-*ras*, have been characterized (Goldfarb et al. 1982; Santos et al. 1982; Shih and Weinberg 1982; Hall et al. 1983; McGrath et al. 1983; Shimizu et al. 1983a, b). Although they exhibit different genetic structures and complexities, they code for highly related proteins of 189 amino acid residues generically known as p21 (Shih et al. 1979).

Comparative analysis of molecular clones containing human *ras* oncogenes and their corresponding normal alleles has led to the demonstration that these genes acquired malignant properties by single point mutations within two specific "hot spots," their twelfth and sixty-first codons (Reddy et al. 1982; Tabin et al. 1982; Taparowsky et al. 1982, 1983; Capon et al. 1983; Santos et al. 1983 and in prep.; Shimizu et al. 1983b; Yuasa et al. 1983; Santos et al. 1984). Some of these critical point mutations create restriction enzyme polymorphisms that can be utilized to distinguish between normal and transforming *ras* alleles (Reddy et al. 1982; Tabin et al. 1982). This experimental approach has been successfully utilized to demonstrate a specific association between activation of a Ki-*ras* oncogene by a single point mutation and tumor development in a patient with a squamous cell lung carcinoma (Santos et al. 1984).

Understanding the precise role that activated *ras* oncogenes play in the development of human tumors requires the utilization of appropriate model systems. Tumor induction by chemical and physical carcinogens in inbred animal strains has been envisioned for many years as a potentially adequate model for human cancer. We (Sukumar et al. 1983) and others (Balmain and Pragnell 1983; Eva and Aaronson 1983; Guerrero et al., this volume) have demonstrated that *ras* oncogenes can be activated reproducibly in tumors induced by a variety of chemical carcinogens. In this report, we describe that malignant activation of the rat Ha-*ras*-1 locus in mammary carcinomas induced by *N*-nitroso-*N*-methylurea (NMU) occurs by the same mutational mechanisms previously identified in human tumors.

Experimental Procedures

A detailed description of the experimental protocols utilized in these studies has been reported elsewhere. The protocols concern cell culture and maintenance (Pulciani et al. 1982b), isolation of high-molecular-weight DNA (Pulciani et al. 1982b), NIH-3T3 transfection assays (Graham and van der Eb 1973; Wigler et al. 1977), Southern blot analysis (Southern 1975), molecular cloning techniques (Maniatis et al. 1982), and nucleotide sequence analysis (Maxam and Gilbert 1977). Specific experimental details related to other techniques are given, when necessary, throughout the text.

Results

Transforming genes in human tumors

During the last 3 years, DNAs isolated from a variety of human tumor cell lines as well as human solid tumors have been tested in our laboratory for their ability to induce malignant transformation upon transfection into NIH-3T3 cells. Of a total of 60 tumor cell lines, 8 exhibited transforming activity, whereas 7 out of 44 solid tumors scored as positives in the NIH-3T3 assay (Table 1). Most of the transforming genes identified by this biological assay were found to be members of the *ras* gene family (Pulciani et al. 1982a). As shown in Table 1, the Ha-*ras* oncogene was found only in T24 human bladder carcinoma cells. In contrast, activated N-*ras* and Ki-*ras* genes were detected in a number of cell lines and solid tumors. Ki-*ras* was the oncogene most frequently detected, being present in 60% of the cases. Interestingly, Ki-*ras* was found in each of the four lung carcinomas known to contain transforming genes. Similar results have been reported also by other investigators (Perucho et al. 1981; Der et al. 1982; McCoy et al. 1983), thus suggesting a preferential, although not specific (Yuasa et al. 1983), activation of this particular oncogene in human lung carcinomas.

A transforming gene (*onc* D) present in a colon carcinoma (solid tumor #2033) did not hybridize with

Table 1 Summary of Human Oncogenes Detected in Our Laboratory

Type of tumor	Source of DNA	Oncogene
Carcinomas		
bladder	T24 cells	Ha-*ras*
bladder	A1698 cells	Ki-*ras*
colon	solid tumor #1665	N-*ras*
colon	solid tumor #2033	onc D[a]
colon	A2233 cells	Ki-*ras*
gall bladder	A1604 cells	Ki-*ras*
liver	solid tumor #2193	N-*ras*
liver	Hep G2 cells	N-*ras*
lung	A2182 cells	Ki-*ras*
lung	A427 cells	Ki-*ras*
lung	solid tumor #1615	Ki-*ras*
lung	solid tumor #LC-10	Ki-*ras*
pancreas	solid tumor #1189	Ki-*ras*
Sarcomas		
fibrosarcoma	HT-1080 cells	N-*ras*
rhabdomyosarcoma	solid tumor #1085	Ki-*ras*
Chemically transformed cells	MNNG-HOS cells	onc E[a]

The human origin and independent identity of above cell lines was determined by karyologic and isoenzyme analysis (Pulciani et al. 1982a).

[a]*onc* D and *onc* E did not hybridize to probes specific for each of the three known human *ras* genes even under relaxed hybridization conditions (20% formamide, 5×SSC, 42°C).

probes specific for each of the three human *ras* genes, even under relaxed hybridization conditions, suggesting that this gene may represent a different class of human oncogenes (Table 1). Another oncogene (*onc* E, Table 1), which did not share sequence homology with *ras* genes, was identified in MNNG-HOS cells, a chemically transformed human osteosarcoma cell line. This oncogene was not detected in the parental HOS osteosarcoma cells. Thus, activation of *onc* E must have been a direct consequence of treatment of HOS cells with *N*-methyl-*N*-nitro-*N*-nitrosoguanidine (MNNG), a potent chemical carcinogen. Blair et al. (1982) have also detected this oncogene utilizing a different experimental approach in which transforming genes are detected by their ability to induce tumors in nude mice. Both *onc* D and *onc* E are larger than 15 kbp, based on the size of human DNA fragments present in NIH-3T3 transformants. Thus, these oncogenes appear to be different from other non-*ras* oncogenes previously identified by Cooper and co-workers in human tumors of hematopoietic origin and MCF-7 mammary carcinoma cells (Lane et al. 1981, 1982).

Activation of a human Ki-*ras* oncogene by a single point mutation within its twelfth codon

Comparative analysis of molecular clones containing the T24 oncogene and its corresponding proto-oncogene present in normal human cells has led to the recent discovery that a single point mutation is responsible for its malignant properties (Reddy et al. 1982; Tabin et al. 1982; Taparowsky et al. 1982). A G → T transversion located at nucleotide 35 of the T24 oncogene coding sequences results in the incorporation of valine instead

of glycine as the twelfth amino acid residue of the p21 protein, the gene product of the T24 human oncogene. Since then, these observations have been extended to other *ras* transforming genes, including not only Ha-*ras* (Santos et al. 1983) but also Ki-*ras* oncogenes (Capon et al. 1983; Shimizu et al. 1983b; Nakano et al. 1984; Santos et al. 1984). Moreover, point mutations affecting the coding properties of the codon 61 of Ha-*ras* and N-*ras* oncogenes have also been shown to be sufficient to confer malignant properties to these genes (Taparowski et al. 1983; Yuasa et al. 1983).

In view of the frequent activation of the Ki-*ras* locus in human lung carcinomas, the most common of all human cancers, we examined whether this oncogene also became activated by mechanisms involving point mutations in this type of tumors. Given the large genetic complexity of the human Ki-*ras* locus (Capon et al. 1983; Shimizu et al. 1983b), we limited our cloning efforts to DNA segments containing exon sequences. For this purpose we subcloned domains of v-*kis*, the *onc* gene of the Kirsten strain of murine sarcoma virus (Ellis et al. 1981; Tsuchida et al. 1982), which contained sequences homologous to each of the Ki-*ras* exons. We utilized a 124-bp *Sst*II–*Sau*3A I DNA fragment of v-*kis*, expanding from nucleotides located at positions −24 to +120 from the initiator ATG, as a probe to identify the first exon of the human Ki-*ras* gene. This retroviral probe was used to screen a library of human fetal liver DNA partially digested with *Eco*RI and amplified in λ Charon 4A phages (Lawn et al. 1978). A recombinant phage containing 18 kbp of human DNA was isolated and an internal 6.6-kbp *Eco*RI DNA fragment was subcloned in pBR322. The corresponding 6.6-kbp *Eco*RI fragment was isolated from 118-41 cells, a third-cycle NIH-3T3 transformant derived from A2182 human lung carcinoma cells (Table 1). In this case, the 6.6-kbp EcoRI DNA fragment containing the first exon of the A2182 Ki-ras oncogene was subcloned from a cosmid that contained 32 kbp of transfected human DNA present in 118-41 cells (Santos et al. 1984). First-exon sequences, localized by hybridization to the 5′ end of v-kis, were mapped within a 1.0-kbp HincII DNA fragment. This DNA fragment obtained from both the normal Ki-ras proto-oncogene and its transforming allele was subsequently characterized by nucleotide sequence analysis.

Figure 1 shows the sequence of the first exon of the human Ki-ras proto-oncogene in comparison with the A2182 oncogene as well as with normal and transforming Ha-ras genes. A single base pair difference between the normal Ki-ras gene and the A2182 oncogene was observed. This mutation, a G→C transversion, occurred at nucleotide 34, that is, the first base pair of the twelfth codon, the same codon found to be mutated in the T24 human oncogene. As a consequence of this point mutation, the glycine residue that is incorporated into position 12 of normal Ki-ras p21 molecules will be substituted by an arginine residue in the A2182 oncogene-coded p21 transforming protein (Fig. 2).

Efforts aimed at determining whether this point mutation was indeed responsible for the malignant properties of the A2182 oncogene were hampered by the genetic complexity of the human Ki-ras locus. Thus, we decided to construct hybrid ras genes in which the first exon of the normal Ha-ras gene was substituted by either the first exon of the normal Ki-ras proto-oncogene or its transforming allele, the A2182 oncogene. EcoRI–XbaI DNA fragments of 4.1 kbp containing Ki-ras first-exon sequences were ligated to a 4.6-kbp XbaI–BamHI DNA fragment that contained the second, third, and fourth exons of the normal human Ha-ras gene (Santos et al. 1982). These hybrid ras genes were next tested in NIH-3T3 transfection assays. Whereas the hybrid gene containing the first exon of the normal Ki-ras gene had no detectable biological activity, that containing the first exon of the A2182 oncogene exhibited a transforming activity of about 100 ffu/μg of DNA. These results demonstrated that the G→C transversion observed in the twelfth codon of the A2182 lung carcinoma oncogene is responsible for its transforming properties.

Restriction enzyme polymorphisms can be utilized to identify ras transforming genes in human tumors

Single point mutations responsible for the malignant activation of the Ha-ras gene present in T24/EJ bladder carcinoma cells not only altered the coding properties of its twelfth codon, but also eliminated the tetranucleotide CCGG specifically recognized by the restriction endonucleases HpaII and MspI (Reddy et al. 1982; Tabin et al. 1982). These results provided the experimental basis to develop a simple biochemical assay capable of distinguishing between normal and transforming Ha-ras genes (Feinberg et al. 1983; Santos et al. 1983). In the case of the human Ki-ras proto-oncogene, neither of the two deoxyguanosines that determine the coding prop-

erties of its twelfth codon GGT were part of any nucleotide sequence specifically recognized by known restriction endonucleases. However, substitution of the first deoxyguanosine of this codon by a deoxycytidine creates the sequence GAGCTC (nucleotide positions 29 to 34) which is recognized by SacI. As shown above, this G→C mutation was found to be responsible for the malignant activation of the A2182 oncogene. These findings predict that this oncogene can be distinguished from its normal allele by SacI restriction endonuclease analysis.

Southern blot analysis of normal human DNA revealed that the first exon of the Ki-ras proto-oncogene is located in a 14-kbp SacI DNA fragment. In contrast, A2182 lung carcinoma cell DNA exhibited two SacI DNA fragments of 8.2 kbp and 5.8 kbp containing first-exon Ki-ras sequences. These results, shown schematically in Figure 3, indicate that specific restriction enzyme polymorphisms can be utilized as a simple assay to identify single point mutations that are responsible for the malignant activation of Ki-ras oncogenes.

Malignant activation of a Ki-ras gene occurs in tumor but not in normal tissue

We next investigated whether any of the additional eight transforming Ki-ras genes identified in our laboratory (Table 1) might have been activated by the same mutational event detected in the A2182 oncogene. Genomic DNAs from each of these tumors and tumor cell lines were digested with SacI and submitted to Southern blot analysis. Two of these eight human tumor DNAs, those isolated from the A1698 bladder carcinoma cell line and from the LC-10 squamous cell lung carcinoma, exhibited the same 8.2-kbp and 5.8-kbp SacI DNA fragments detected in A2182 lung carcinoma DNA, indicating that their respective Ki-ras oncogenes were activated by the same G→C mutational event in nucleotide 34 (Fig. 4).

A1698 cells were established from a bladder carcinoma and have been shown to be distinct from A2182 cells by karyological and isoenzyme analysis (Pulciani et al. 1982a). LC-10 was a tumor surgically removed from a 66-year-old male (P.G.) and obtained from Drs. M. Pierotti and G. della Porta (Istituto di Tumori, Milan) (Santos et al. 1984). P.G. is a heavy smoker and was not submitted to chemotherapy prior to surgery. The tumor was histologically classified as a moderately differentiated squamous cell carcinoma. It was located in the upper right lobe with a mass measuring 7 × 7 cm and it infiltrated the pleura as well as the thoracic wall. No evidence of metastasis was observed. The patient is currently under close clinical surveillance at the Istituto di Tumori and so far has not shown any symptoms of tumor recurrence.

Three types of normal tissue, including bronchia, parenchyma, and blood lymphocytes from the above patient were available for examination. As shown in Figure 4, none of these normal cells including the bronchia, which corresponds to the tissue from which the squamous cell carcinoma was derived, possessed the activating G→C mutation detected in tumor tissue. Moreover, DNA iso-

Figure 1 Comparative nucleotide sequence analysis of the first exon of normal and transforming *ras* genes isolated in our laboratory. Point mutations affecting the first or second nucleotides of the twelfth codon are shown in large characters. Shaded areas indicate differences between the first exon of the human Ha-*ras* genes (three top lines) and either the human Ki-*ras* genes or the Ha-*ras* and Ki-*ras* genes present in viral or rat genomes (NMU-*ras* gene). Asterisks correspond to differences between the viral Ki-*ras* gene and the human Ki-*ras* genes, normal and transforming (three bottom lines).

Gene		Sequence (reading from ATG; twelfth codon in **bold**)
H-ras	(normal human)	ATG ACG GAA TAT AAG CTG GTG GTG GTG GGC GCC **GGC** GGT GTG GGC AAG AGT GCG CTG ACC ATC CAG CTG ATC CAG AAC CAT TTT GTG GAC GAA TAC GAC CCC ACT ATA GAG
H-ras	(T24 bladder ca. oncogene)	ATG ACG GAA TAT AAG CTG GTG GTG GTG GGC GCC **GTC** GGT GTG GGC AAG AGT GCG CTG ACC ATC CAG CTG ATC CAG AAC CAT TTT GTG GAC GAA TAC GAC CCC ACT ATA GAG
H-ras	(spont. activated oncogene)	ATG ACG GAA TAT AAG CTG GTG GTG GTG GGC GCC **GAC** GGT GTG GGC AAG AGT GCG CTG ACC ATC CAG CTG ATC CAG AAC CAT TTT GTG GAC GAA TAC GAC CCC ACT ATA GAG
H-ras	(normal rat)	ATG ACA GAA TAC AAG CTT GTG GTG GTG GGC GCT **GGA** GGT GTG GGC AAG AGT GCC CTG ACC ATC CAG CTC ATC CAG AAC CAT TTT GTG GAC GAA TAT GAC CCC ACT ATA GAG
H-ras	(NMU-activated oncogene)	ATG ACA GAA TAC AAG CTT GTG GTG GTG GGC GCT **GAA** GGT GTG GGC AAG AGT GCC CTG ACC ATC CAG CTC ATC CAG AAC CAT TTT GTG GAC GAA TAT GAC CCC ACT ATA GAG
v-H-ras	(Harvey-MSV)	ATG ACA GAA TAC AAG CTT GTG GTG GTG GGC GCT **AGA** GGT GTG GGC AAG AGT GCC CTG ACC ATC CAG CTC ATC CAG AAC CAT TTT GTG GAC GAA TAT GAC CCC ACT ATA GAG
K-ras	(normal human)	ATG ACT GAA TAT AAA CTT GTA GTA GTT GGA GCT **GGT** GGC GTA GGC AAG AGT GCC TTG ACG ATA CAG CTA ATT CAG AAT CAT TTT GTA GAA TAT GAT CCA ACA ATA GAG
K-ras	(A2182 lung ca. oncogene)	ATG ACT GAA TAT AAA CTT GTA GTA GTT GGA GCT **CGT** GGC GTA GGC AAG AGT GCC TTG ACG ATA CAG CTA ATT CAG AAT CAT TTT GTA GAA TAT GAT CCA ACA ATA GAG
v-K-ras	(Kirsten-MSV)	ATG ACT GAA TAT AAA CTT GTA GTA GTT GGA GCT **AGT** GGC GTA GGC AAG AGT GCC TTG ACG ATA CAG CTA ATT CAG AAT CAT TTT GTA GAA TAT GAT CCT ACA ATA CTG*

Figure 2 Predicted amino acid sequences of p21 proteins coded for by the first exons of the normal and transforming *ras* genes described in Fig. 1. The critical twelfth amino acid residues are indicated in large characters. The letter codes for the amino acids are: A, alanine; D, aspartic acid; E, glutamic acid; F, phenylalanine; G, glycine; H, histidine; I, isoleucine; K, lysine; L, leucine; M, methionine; N, asparagine; P, proline; Q, glutamine; R, arginine; S, serine; T, threonine; V, valine, and Y, tyrosine.

Gene		Amino acid sequence (twelfth residue in **bold**)
H-ras	(normal human)	M T E Y K L V V V G A **G** G V G K S A L T I Q L I Q N H F V D E Y D P T I E
H-ras	(T24 bladder ca. oncogene)	M T E Y K L V V V G A **V** G V G K S A L T I Q L I Q N H F V D E Y D P T I E
H-ras	(spont. activated oncogene)	M T E Y K L V V V G A **D** G V G K S A L T I Q L I Q N H F V D E Y D P T I E
H-ras	(normal rat)	M T E Y K L V V V G A **G** G V G K S A L T I Q L I Q N H F V D E Y D P T I E
H-ras	(NMU-activated oncogene)	M T E Y K L V V V G A **E** G V G K S A L T I Q L I Q N H F V D E Y D P T I E
v-H-ras	(Harvey-MSV)	M T E Y K L V V V G A **R** G V G K S A L T I Q L I Q N H F V D E Y D P T I E
K-ras	(normal human)	M T E Y K L V V V G A **G** G V G K S A L T I Q L I Q N H F V D E Y D P T I E
K-ras	(A2182 lung ca. oncogene)	M T E Y K L V V V G A **R** G V G K S A L T I Q L I Q N H F V D E Y D P T I E
v-K-ras	(Kirsten-MSV)	M T E Y K L V V V G A **S** G V G K S A L T I Q L I Q N H F V D E Y D P T I Q

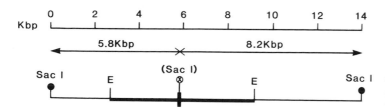

Figure 3 Schematic representation of the *Sac*I polymorphism created by a G→C mutation within the twelfth codon of the human Ki-*ras* proto-oncogene. As a consequence of this point mutation, first exon sequences of the Ki-*ras* oncogene are located in two *Sac*I DNA fragments of 5.8 kbp and 8.2 kbp, instead of the 14-kbp fragment present in their normal allele.

lated from these normal tissues failed to exhibit transforming activity in NIH-3T3 transfection assays. These results demonstrate, for the first time, a specific association between a mutational event responsible for the malignant activation of a *ras* transforming gene and the development of a human cancer.

Transforming genes in experimentally induced animal tumors

The above results confirm the role of point mutations in the activation of human *ras* proto-oncogenes and demonstrate a specific association between those mutational events and the development of human cancers. However, our progress in understanding the role played by activated *ras* genes in the development of human neoplasia is seriously limited by the impossibility of experimental manipulations with human subjects, the lack of well-defined preneoplastic stages, and the relatively low frequency with which active oncogenes are found in human tumors. Therefore, we felt that utilization of well-defined animal model systems will be required to understand fully the role of oncogene activation in carcinogenesis. Several chemically induced animal tumor systems have been explored to search for adequate models with which to study systematically the relationship between oncogene activation and neoplasia.

In the present report, we describe the detection and isolation of *ras* oncogenes from mammary carcinomas induced by NMU in Buf/N rats. Gullino and co-workers (1975) have reported that exposure of 50-day-old Buf/N female rats to NMU results in the induction of mammary carcinomas in 90% of the animals after variable latency periods. The specific carcinogenic action of this chem-

ical is limited to a short period of time during which Buf/N rats reach their sexual maturity. Hormonal influence during NMU-induced carcinogenesis has been well illustrated by Gullino and co-workers by showing that ovariectomized rats have a negligible incidence of tumor formation (Gullino et al. 1975). NMU, a compound of very short half-life, was always injected intravenously to allow its rapid distribution to all the organs of the body. Therefore, its exquisite carcinogenic specificity must be mandated by a very special stage of growth and/or differentiation of certain cell type(s) of the mammary gland during sexual development. We have modified Gullino's protocol by injecting a single dose of NMU (30 μg/g of body weight) to ensure that tumor induction would be the result of a single carcinogen insult. Under our experimental conditions, the exclusive induction of mammary carcinomas was observed (Sukumar et al. 1983).

DNAs isolated from nine mammary tumors were tested in transfection assays for their ability to transform NIH-3T3 mouse fibroblasts. Foci of morphologically transformed cells appeared in each case with frequencies ranging from 0.01 to 0.08 foci/μg of donor DNA. DNAs isolated from normal breast tissues of untreated control rats exhibited no transforming activity, demonstrating that activation of transforming genes was specifically associated with the development of the NMU-induced mammary carcinomas.

Reproducible activation of Ha-*ras* oncogenes by single point mutations in NMU-induced mammary carcinomas

High-molecular-weight DNAs isolated from representative NIH-3T3 transformants derived from each of the nine

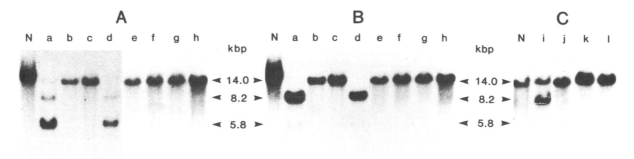

Figure 4 *Sac*I polymorphism in the Ki-*ras* locus of human tumor cell lines and solid tumors. DNA isolated from normal human foreskin (lanes *N*), A1698 bladder carcinoma cell line (*a*), A2233 colon carcinoma cell line (*b*), A1604 gall bladder carcinoma cell line (*c*), A2182 lung carcinoma cell line (*d*), A427 lung carcinoma cell line (*e*), lung carcinoma #1615 (*f*), pancreatic carcinoma #1189 (*g*), embryonal rhabdomyosarcoma #1085 (*h*), squamous cell lung carcinoma #LC-10 (*i*), and normal bronchia, parenchyma, and blood lymphocytes of the patient from whom LC-10 tumor was surgically removed (*j–l*), were digested with *Sac*I, electrophoresed in agarose gels, and blotted to nitrocellulose paper as described by Southern (1975). Blots were hybridized under stringent conditions to DNA fragments containing the following human Ki-*ras* gene sequences: (*A*) Ki-*ras* first exon and 370 bp 5′ upstream sequences, (*B,C*) Ki-*ras* first exon and 3.5 kbp 3′ downstream sequences. Migration of DNA fragments containing Ki-*ras* sequences is indicated by arrows. Their sizes (labeled in kilobase pairs) were deduced from their relative migration with respect to coelectrophoresed DNA fragments of *Hind*III-cleaved λ c1857 DNA.

mammary carcinomas were submitted to Southern blot analysis for detection of *ras*-related sequences. Each NIH-3T3 transformant analyzed exhibited a DNA fragment not present in control mouse DNA which hybridized strongly to a probe specific for the human Ha-*ras* oncogene. Cosegregation of these Ha-*ras*-related sequences with the malignant phenotype in subsequent cycles of transfection demonstrated that these *ras* sequences were responsible for the malignant phenotype of NIH-3T3 transformants (Sukumar et al. 1983).

We next proceeded to isolate a representative NMU-Ha-*ras* oncogene by molecular cloning techniques. DNA isolated from a NIH-3T3 transformant designated S2-72 was digested to completion with *Bam*HI and the Ha-*ras*-related 12-kbp DNA fragment was partially purified by sucrose gradient centrifugation. Bacteriophage λ 1059 was used as the cloning vector. Seventeen recombinant phages were isolated. Nine of the isolates contained the expected 12-kbp *Bam*HI DNA fragment of S2-72 DNA, whereas eight contained a 6.9-kbp *Bam*HI DNA insert. Both types of phages, however, were able to transform NIH-3T3 cells with similar efficiencies (3×10^3 to 8×10^3 ffu/pmole of phage DNA), suggesting that neighboring nontransforming sequences had been lost during cloning procedures. The 6.9-kbp *Bam*HI DNA fragment was then subcloned into pBR322. The resulting plasmid, designated pNMU-1, exhibited a specific transforming activity of 3×10^4 ffu/pmole of DNA. Detailed restriction enzyme and heteroduplex analysis of pNMU-1 established that the NMU-Ha-*ras* oncogene is a transforming allele of the normal rat Ha-*ras*-1 gene, instead of the Ha-*ras*-2 pseudogene also present in rat genomic DNA (De Feo et al. 1981).

The mechanism by which the rat Ha-*ras*-1 locus became activated in NMU-induced mammary carcinomas was next investigated. The nucleotide sequence of the first exon of the NMU-Ha-*ras* gene was determined and compared with that corresponding to the first exon of the normal Ha-*ras*-1 gene, which was molecularly cloned for this purpose from normal Buf/N rat DNA utilizing λ 1059 phage as the cloning vector (Sukumar et al. 1983). First-exon sequences of the NMU-Ha-*ras* gene and its normal allele were identified by the existence of a 52-bp *Hin*dIII–*Pvu*II DNA fragment that shared nucleotide sequence homology with the first exon of the T24 bladder carcinoma oncogene (Reddy et al. 1982; Tabin et al. 1982). The nucleotide sequence of the first exon of NMU-Ha-*ras* and its normal allele are depicted in Figure 1. A single nucleotide difference, consisting of the substitution of the second deoxyguanosine residue of the twelfth codon (nucleotide 35) by a deoxyadenosine, was observed. As a consequence of this point mutation, the glycine residue located at position 12 of the normal rat Ha-*ras*-1 p21 protein is substituted by glutamic acid in the gene product of the NMU-Ha-*ras* oncogene. (Fig. 2)

The predicted amino acid sequence of the first exon of the p21 protein coded for by the Buf/N Ha-*ras*-1 gene is identical to that of the gene products of human Ha-*ras* (Reddy et al. 1982; Tabin et al. 1982; Taparowsky et al. 1982) and Ki-*ras* (McGrath et al. 1983; Santos et al., in prep.) genes (Fig. 2), as well as to the corre-

sponding domains of the Harvey and BALB-MSV p21 retroviral proteins, with the exception of the critical twelfth amino acid residue (Dhar et al. 1982; E.P. Reddy, pers. comm.). At the nucleotide level, no differences were observed between Ha-*ras*-1 and the *onc* gene of Harvey-MSV, with the exception of a G→A transition at position 34 (Dhar et al. 1982), which is thought to be responsible for the malignant properties of this virus, although this point remains to be demonstrated. When comparisons between first exon sequences of rat and human Ha-*ras*-1 genes were made, only 11 (30%) third-base substitutions could be detected. In contrast, little homology was observed between the first-intron sequences of these two Ha-*ras* genes. These findings illustrate the strong evolutionary pressure exerted to conserve the amino acid sequence of the aminoterminal domain of p21 proteins.

Substitution of a glutamine residue located at position 61 of the Ha-*ras* gene-coded p21 protein has recently been shown to be sufficient for the malignant activation of this locus in a human lung carcinoma cell line (Yuasa et al. 1983). Because the sixty-first codon of the Ha-*ras* gene lies within its second exon, we also determined the nucleotide sequence of the second exon of the NMU-Ha-*ras* oncogene and its normal allele. In this case, no differences could be observed, both genes having glutamine residues at position 61 (Sukumar et al. 1983). Thus, a single point mutation is responsible for the malignant activation of the Ha-*ras*-1 locus in NMU-induced mammary carcinomas of Buf/N rats.

Discussion

Molecular characterization of human *ras* loci has led to the demonstration that these genes acquire malignant properties by single point mutations that affect the incorporation of the twelfth or sixty-first amino acid residue of their respective p21-coded proteins (Reddy et al. 1982; Tabin et al. 1982; Taparowsky et al. 1982; Capon et al. 1983; Santos et al. 1983, 1984; Shimizu et al. 1983b; Yuasa et al. 1983). Mutations within the twelfth codon of the Ha-*ras* gene alter the sequence CCGG, which is specifically recognized by certain restriction endonucleases, thus providing a simple biochemical assay for detection of transforming Ha-*ras* genes. Unfortunately, the potential use of these findings is hampered by the infrequent activation of this locus in human tumors (Pulciani et al. 1982a; Feinberg et al. 1983). In contrast, Ki-*ras* oncogenes have been frequently detected in a variety of human neoplasias.

In the present report, we have illustrated how restriction enzyme polymorphisms can be utilized as a diagnostic tool for the detection of activated Ki-*ras* oncogenes in human tumors. The possibility of distinguishing between Ki-*ras* transforming genes and their normal alleles simply by Southern blot analysis has enabled us to demonstrate unequivocally an association between the appearance of specific point mutations responsible for oncogene activation and development of human cancer. Moreover, this technique eliminates the need for the tedious and often insensitive NIH-3T3 transfection assays. Unfortunately, some of the critical mutations known to turn proto-oncogenes into transforming genes do not create or eliminate restriction endonuclease cleavage sites. New technical approaches such as those recently utilized by Conner et al. (1983) to identify mutated globin alleles in β-thalassemia might be useful to detect all possible point mutations that result in the generation of transforming genes.

The simplicity of the genetic changes leading to *ras* oncogene activation has also been instrumental in predicting their possible consequences at the gene product level. Exploitation of computer analysis of the amino acid sequence of normal and transforming p21 proteins has indicated that they exhibit basic conformational differences (Pincus et al. 1983; Santos et al. 1983). Substitution of the normal glycine residue of normal *ras* p21 proteins by any other amino acid will consistently cause the same structural alteration. A flexible hinge region that allows the aminoterminal domain of normal p21 proteins to fold into the central core of the molecule disappears in their mutated counterparts. As a consequence, transforming p21 proteins possess a more rigid configuration, independently of the point mutation that originates them, as long as it results in substitution of the critical glycine residue at position twelve (Pincus et al. 1983; Santos et al. 1983).

Recent theoretical studies on the primary structure of p21 proteins (Gay and Walker 1983; Wierenga and Hol 1983), along with their possible enzymatic activity (Scolnick et al. 1979), have suggested that the critical twelfth and sixty-first amino acid residues might be involved in guanine nucleotide binding. On such grounds, Taparowsky et al. (1983) have proposed a model of p21 activation similar to the adenyl cyclase regulatory complex found in rabbit liver plasma membranes. However, the actual occurrence of those conformational changes and the validity of the activation model remain to be demonstrated. Expression of large quantities of normal and transforming p21 proteins in microorganisms (J.C. Lacal et al., in prep.) should facilitate the biochemical characterization of these molecules and help to elucidate their role in normal cells as well as in tumor development.

Establishment of the detailed role played by oncogene activation in the multistep carcinogenic processes requires the existence of suitable animal model systems. We have described the specific and reproducible activation of the Ha-*ras*-1 locus in mammary carcinomas induced in Buf/N rats by a single injection of NMU (Sukumar et al. 1983). Moreover, we have shown that NMU-Ha-*ras* oncogenes acquired their malignant properties by single point mutations affecting the coding properties of their twelfth codon, the same genetic alterations previously identified in human *ras* oncogenes. These findings have two important consequences. First, they validate this animal system as an accurate model to study human carcinogenesis, and second, it provides the biochemical basis for the development of molecular assays that will allow the detailed investigation of the role of oncogenes in the multistep processes that lead to neoplasia.

Among the six possible point mutations that alter the coding properties of the normal twelfth codon of the Ha-*ras*-1 gene, GGA, five will originate a transforming gene. A G→T substitution in the first base pair will create a TGA terminator codon. Of the five viable mutations, four can be biochemically identified due to the creation of restriction enzyme polymorphisms similar to that described above for the human Ki-*ras* locus. Mutations affecting the second deoxyguanosine residue eliminate a *Mnl*I cleavage site ($G^{35}AGG$) present in the normal gene. Similarly, substitution of the first deoxyguanosine by a deoxycytosine will generate the sequence $CTC^{34}GAG$, which is specifically recognized by *Xho*I. Only the G^{34}→A transition will go undetected by Southern blot analysis. These observations illustrate how simple biochemical assays can be utilized to monitor the process of oncogene activation in model systems in which a specific locus can be reproducibly activated.

Transforming genes have also been identified in several other animal tumor systems induced by a variety of carcinogens. They include dimethylbenzanthracene (DMBA)-induced mouse skin carcinomas (Balmain and Pragnell 1983), methylcholanthrene (MCA)-induced fibrosarcomas (Eva and Aaronson 1983), and NMU- and X-ray-induced mouse thymomas (Guerrero et al., this volume). Moreover, we have recently reported (S. Sukumar et al., in prep.) the activation of a *ras* oncogene in guinea pig fetal cells treated either in vivo or in vitro with four different chemical carcinogens. The frequent detection of transforming genes in chemically induced tumors strongly suggests that these oncogenes must play an important role in tumor development. Moreover, the great similarity between results obtained in animal model systems and in a significant percentage (about 15%) of all human cancers suggests that both types of tumors might proceed through similar routes, some of which now can be dissected and studied at the molecular level.

Acknowledgments

We thank Anne V. Arthur and Linda K. Long for excellent technical assistance.

References

Andersen, P.R., S.G. Devare, S.R. Tronick, R.W. Ellis, S.A. Aaronson, and E.M. Scolnick. 1981. Generation of BALB-MuSV and Ha-MuSV by type C virus transduction of homologous transforming genes from different species. *Cell* **26**: 129.

Balmain, A. and I.B. Pragnell. 1983. Mouse skin carcinomas induced *in vivo* by chemical carcinogens have a transforming Harvey-*ras* oncogene. *Nature* **303**: 72.

Blair, D.G., C.S. Cooper, M.K. Oskarsson, L.A. Eader, and G.F. Vande Woude. 1982. New method for detecting cellular transforming genes. *Science* **218**: 1122.

Capon, D.J., P.H. Seeburg, J.P. McGrath, J.S. Hayflick, U. Edman, A.D. Levinson, and D.V. Goeddel. 1983. Activation of Ki-*ras* 2 gene in human colon and lung carcinomas by two different point mutations. *Nature* **304**: 507.

Conner, B.J., A.A. Reyes, C. Morin, K. Itacura, R.L. Teplitz, and R.B. Wallace. 1983. Detection of sickle cell β-globin allele by hybridization with synthetic oligonucleotides. *Proc. Natl. Acad. Sci.* **80**: 278.

De Feo, D., M.A. Gonda, H.A. Young, E.H. Chang, D.R. Lowy, E.M. Scolnick, and R.W. Ellis. 1981. Analysis of two divergent rat genomic clones homologous to the transforming gene of Harvey murine sarcoma virus. *Proc. Natl. Acad. Sci.* **78**: 3328.

Der, C., T. Krontiris, and G. Cooper. 1982. Transforming genes of human bladder and lung carcinoma cell lines are homologous to the *ras* genes of Harvey and Kirsten sarcoma viruses. *Proc. Natl. Acad. Sci.* **79**: 3637.

Dhar, R., R.W. Ellis, T.Y. Shih, S. Oroszlan, B. Shapiro, J. Maizel, D. Lowy, and E. Scolnick. 1982. Nucleotide sequence of the p21 transforming protein of Harvey murine sarcoma virus. *Science* **217**: 934.

Ellis, R.W., D. De Feo, T.Y. Shih, M.A. Gonda, H.A. Young, N. Tsuchida, D.R. Lowy, and E.M. Scolnick. 1981. The P21 *src* genes of Harvey and Kirsten sarcoma viruses originate from divergent members of a family of normal vertebrate genes. *Nature* **292**: 506.

Eva, A. and S.A. Aaronson. 1983. Frequent activation of c-*kis* as a transforming gene in fibrosarcomas induced by methylcholanthrene. *Science* **220**: 955.

Feinberg, A.P., B. Vogelstein, M.J. Droller, S.B. Baylin, and B.D. Nelkin. 1983. Mutation affecting the 12th amino acid of the c-Ha-*ras* oncogene product occurs infrequently in human cancer. *Science* **220**: 1175.

Gay, N.J. and J.E. Walker. 1983. Homology between human bladder carcinoma oncogene product and mitrochondrial ATP-synthase. *Nature* **301**: 262.

Goldfarb, M., K. Shimizu, M. Perucho, and M. Wigler. 1982. Isolation and preliminary characterization of a human transforming gene from T24 bladder carcinoma cells. *Nature* **296**: 404.

Graham, F.L. and A.J. Van der Eb. 1973. A new technique for the assay of infectivity of human adenovirus 5 DNA. *Virology* **52**: 456.

Gullino, P.M., H.H. Pettigrew, and F.H. Grantham. 1975. N-Nitrosomethylurea as mammary gland carcinogen in rats. *J. Natl. Cancer Inst.* **54**: 401.

Hall, A., C. Marshall, N. Spurr, and R. Weiss. 1983. Identification of the transforming gene in two human sarcoma cell lines as a new member of the *ras* gene family located on chromosome 1. *Nature* **303**: 396.

Lane, M.A., A. Sainten, and G. Cooper. 1981. Activation of related transforming genes in mouse and human mammary carcinomas. *Proc. Natl. Acad. Sci.* **78**: 5185.

———. 1982. Stage-specific transforming genes of human and mouse B- and T-lymphocyte neoplasms. *Cell* **28**: 873.

Lawn, R.M., E.F. Fritsch, R.C. Parker, G. Blake and T. Maniatis. 1978. The isolation and characterization of linked δ- and β-globin genes from a cloned library of human DNA. *Cell* **15**: 1157.

Maniatis, T., E.F. Fritsch, and J. Sambrook, eds. 1982. Molecular cloning. *A laboratory manual.* Cold Spring Harbor Laboratory, Cold Spring Harbor, New York.

Maxam, A.M. and W. Gilbert. 1977. A new method for sequencing DNA. *Proc. Natl. Acad. Sci.* **74**: 560.

McCoy, M.S., J.J. Toole, J.M. Cunningham, E.H. Chang, D.R. Lowy, and R.A. Weinberg. 1983. Characterization of a human colon/lung carcinoma oncogene. *Nature* **302**: 79.

McGrath, J.P., D.J. Capon, D.H. Smith, E.Y. Chen, P.H. Seeburg, D.V. Goeddel, and A.D. Levinson. 1983. Structure and organization of the human Ki-*ras* proto-oncogene and a related processed pseudogene. *Nature* **304**: 501.

Nakano, H., F. Yamamoto, C. Neville, D. Evans, T. Mizuno, and M. Perucho. 1984. Isolation of transforming sequences of two human lung carcinomas: Structural and functional analysis of the activated c-K-*ras* oncogenes. *Proc. Natl. Acad. Sci.* **81**: 71.

Parada, L.F., C.J. Tabin, C. Shih, and R.A. Weinberg. 1982. Human EJ bladder carcinoma oncogene is homologue of Harvey sarcoma virus *ras* gene. *Nature* **297**: 474.

Perucho, M., M. Goldfarb, K. Shimizu, C. Lama, J. Fogh, and M. Wigler. 1981. Human-tumor-derived cell lines contain common and different transforming genes. *Cell* **27**: 467.

Pincus, M.R., J. van Renswoude, J.B. Harford, E.H. Chang, R.P. Carty, and R.D. Klausner. 1983. Prediction of the three-dimensional structure of the transforming region of the EJ/T24 human bladder oncogene product and its normal cellular homologue. *Proc. Natl. Acad. Sci.* **80**: 5253.

Pulciani, S., E. Santos, A.V. Lauver, L.K. Long, S.A. Aaronson, and M. Barbacid. 1982a. Oncogenes in solid human tumors. *Nature* **300**: 539.

Pulciani, S., E. Santos, A.V. Lauver, L.K. Long, K.C. Robbins, and M. Barbacid. 1982b. Oncogenes in human tumor cell lines: Molecular cloning of a transforming gene from human bladder carcinoma cells. *Proc. Natl. Acad. Sci.* **79**: 2845.

Reddy, E.P., R.K. Reynolds, E. Santos, and M. Barbacid. 1982. A point mutation is responsible for the acquisition of transforming properties by the T24 human bladder carcinoma oncogene. *Nature* **300**: 149.

Santos, E., E.P. Reddy, S. Pulciani, R.J. Feldmann, and M. Barbacid. 1983. Spontaneous activation of a human proto-oncogene. *Proc. Natl. Acad. Sci.* **80**: 4679.

Santos, E., S.R. Tronick, S.A. Aaronson, S. Pulciani, and M. Barbacid. 1982. T24 human bladder carcinoma oncogene is an activated form of the normal human homologue of BALB- and Harvey-MSV transforming genes. *Nature* **298**: 343.

Santos, E., D. Martin-Zanca, E.P. Reddy, M.A. Pierotti, G. Della Porta, and M. Barbacid. 1984. Malignant activation of a K-*ras* oncogene in lung carcinoma but not in normal tissue of the same patient. *Science* **223**: 661.

Scolnick, E.M., A.G. Papageorge, and T.Y. Shih. 1979. Guanine nucleotide-binding activity as an assay for *src* protein of rat-derived murine sarcoma viruses. *Proc. Natl. Acad. Sci.* **76**: 5355.

Shih, C. and R.A. Weinberg. 1982. Isolation of a transforming sequence from a human bladder carcinoma cell line. *Cell* **29**: 161.

Shih, T.Y., M.O. Weeks, H.O. Young, and E.M. Scolnick. 1979. Identification of a sarcoma virus-coded phosphoprotein in nonproducer cells transformed by Kirsten or Harvey murine sarcoma virus. *Virology* **96**: 64.

Shimizu, K., M. Goldfarb, M. Perucho, and M. Wigler. 1983a. Isolation and preliminary characterization of the transforming gene of a human neuroblastoma cell line. *Proc. Natl. Acad. Sci.* **80**: 383.

Shimizu, K., D. Birnbaum, M. A. Ruley, O. Fasano, Y. Suard, L. Edlund, E. Taparowsky, M. Goldfarb, and M. Wigler. 1983b. Structure of the Ki-*ras* gene of the human lung carcinoma cell line Calu-1. *Nature* **304**: 497.

Southern, E. 1975. Detection of specific sequences among DNA fragments separated by gel electrophoresis. *J. Mol. Biol.* **98**: 503.

Sukumar, S., V. Notario, D. Martin-Zanca, and M. Barbacid. 1983. Induction of mammary carcinomas in rats by nitrosomethyl-urea involves the malignant activation of the H-*ras*-1 locus by single point mutations. *Nature* **306**: 658.

Tabin, C.J., S.M. Bradley, C.I. Bargmann, R.A. Weinberg, A.G. Papageorge, E.M. Scolnick, R. Dhar, D.R. Lowy, and E.H. Chang. 1982. Mechanism of activation of a human oncogene. *Nature* **300**: 143.

Taparowsky, E., K. Shimizu, M. Goldfarb, and M. Wigler. 1983. Structure and activation of the human N-*ras* gene. *Cell* **34**: 581.

Taparowsky, E., Y. Suard, O. Fasano, K. Shimizu, M. Goldfarb, and M. Wigler. 1982. Activation of the T24 bladder carcinoma transforming gene is linked to a single amino acid change. *Nature* **300**: 762.

Tsuchida, N., T. Ryder, and E. Ohtsubo. 1982. Nucleotide sequence of the oncogene encoding the p21 transforming protein of Kirsten murine sarcoma virus. *Science* **217**: 937.

Wierenga, R. and W. Hol. 1983. Predicted nucleotide binding properties of p21 protein and its cancer-associated variant. *Nature* **302**: 842.

Wigler, M., S. Silverstein, L.S. Lee, A. Pellicer, Y.C. Cheng, and R. Axel. 1977. Transfer of purified herpes virus thymidine kinase gene to cultured mouse cells. *Cell* **11**: 223.

Yuasa, Y., S.K. Srivastava, C.Y. Dunn, J.S. Rhim, E.P. Reddy, and S.A. Aaronson. 1983. Acquisition of transforming properties by alternative point mutations within c-*bas*/*has* human proto-oncogene. *Nature* **303**: 775.

ras-Related Oncogenes of Human Tumors

Y. Yuasa, A. Eva, M.H. Kraus, S.K. Srivastava, S.W. Needleman, J.H. Pierce,
J.S. Rhim, R. Gol, E.P. Reddy, S.R. Tronick, and S.A. Aaronson

Laboratory of Cellular and Molecular Biology, National Cancer Institute, Bethesda, Maryland 20205

Investigations of the genetic alterations that cause normal cells to become malignant have recently focused on a small set of cellular genes. Acute transforming retroviruses have substituted viral genes necessary for replication with these discrete segments of host genetic information. When incorporated within the retroviral genome, such transduced sequences derived from normal cellular genes (proto-oncogenes) acquire the ability to induce neoplastic transformation. Findings that independent virus isolates have often recombined with the same or closely related proto-oncogenes have implied that only a limited number of cellular genes are capable of acquiring transforming properties under these conditions (Weiss et al. 1982; Bishop 1983; Duesberg 1983).

Evidence has accumulated that proto-oncogenes can also be activated to become transforming genes by mechanisms independent of retroviral involvement. Genetic changes as small as point mutations, as well as DNA rearrangements such as transposition and chromosomal translocations, have all been implicated in this process. This review summarizes studies within our laboratory on members of the *ras* family of proto-oncogenes that appear to be frequent targets for genetic alterations leading normal human cells along the pathway toward malignancy.

Transforming genes of human tumors are frequently related to the *ras* family of retroviral *onc* genes

The development of DNA-mediated gene-transfer techniques has provided an approach for the detection of cellular transforming DNA sequences. DNAs from human tumors and tumor cell lines have been found to induce malignant transformation of NIH-3T3 cells (Cooper 1982; Weinberg 1982), a continuous murine cell line that is contact-inhibited and highly susceptible to DNA transfection. By using this assay, transforming genes have been detected in diverse human tumors, including sarcomas, carcinomas, and hematopoietic malignancies (Krontiris and Cooper 1981; Murray et al. 1981; Shih et al. 1981; Lane et al. 1981, 1982; Goldfarb et al. 1982; Marshall et al. 1982; Pulciani et al. 1982b; Shih and Weinberg 1982; Eva et al. 1983).

The first human oncogene to be cloned molecularly was derived from human bladder carcinoma cell line designated T24 (Goldfarb et al. 1982; Pulciani et al. 1982b; Shih and Weinberg 1982). The sequences of the T24 oncogene responsible for its transforming activity were shown to be related to those of the oncogenes of the BALB and Harvey strains of murine sarcoma virus (MSV)

(Der et al. 1982; Parada et al. 1982; Santos et al. 1982). The transforming genes of these viruses are members of a small family of retroviral oncogenes, designated Ha-*ras* (Coffin et al. 1981), whose cellular homologs (c-Ha-*ras*) are well conserved in the DNA of vertebrate species.

Frequency and distribution of *ras*-related oncogenes in human tumors

Findings that human oncogenes can be the activated forms of normal cellular homologs of retroviral oncogenes led us to analyze transforming genes isolated from a variety of human tumors and tumor cell lines. In one series of experiments, oncogenes from solid tumors have been examined for transforming DNA sequences (Pulciani et al. 1982a). Transforming DNAs were demonstrated in about 15% of the fresh tumors tested (5/28), including two colon carcinomas, carcinomas of the lung and pancreas, and an embryonal rhabdomyosarcoma. Transforming genes were also detected in cell lines established from carcinomas of the colon, lung, gall bladder, and urinary bladder, as well as from a fibrosarcoma.

Each of these DNAs was subjected to Southern blot analysis using a battery of retroviral *onc* gene probes. Eight tumors were found to possess oncogene-containing sequences related to the transforming gene of Kirsten (Ki-) MSV. This acute retrovirus possesses an oncogene that is another *ras* gene family member (Ellis et al. 1981). Although its nucleotide sequence is diverged from those of BALB and Harvey (Ha-) MSVs, the predicted amino acid sequence of its *ras* gene-coded 21,000-m.w. protein (p21) is closely related to the p21s of BALB and Ha-MSVs (Dhar et al. 1982; Tsuchida et al. 1982; E. Reddy et al., unpubl.).

Attempts to study oncogenes of hematopoietic tumors have resulted in the detection of transforming DNA sequences in a human promyelocytic cell line, HL60, and in lymphoid cell tumors of both human and murine origin (Murray et al. 1981; Lane et al. 1982). Lane et al. (1982) have reported that specific transforming genes are activated in lymphocyte neoplasms that exhibit distinct stages of differentiation.

In our studies of 22 DNAs isolated from established human hematopoietic tumor cell lines or primary tumors, 7 were positive in the DNA transfection assay (5/10 from cell lines, 2/12 from tumors) (Eva et al. 1983). The frequency at which transforming genes were detected in hematopoietic tumor cell lines and primary malignancies was similar to that observed with solid tumors. Moreover, activation of cellular oncogenes does not appear to be an artifact of tissue culture growth of tumor cells since primary human hematopoietic (Eva et al. 1983), as well as solid tumors (Pulciani et al. 1982a), can register as positive in the NIH-3T3 transfection assay. The relatively high frequency of detection of activated *ras* oncogenes in diverse carcinomas, sarcomas, and hematopoietic tumors suggests that these oncogenes may play important roles in processes leading normal cells to become malignant.

Using *v-onc* gene probes including *v-Ki-ras*, *v-Ha-ras*, *v-mos*, *v-abl*, *v-fes* ST, *v-sis*, *v-src*, *v-myc*, and *v-myb*, only DNA from an acute lymphocytic leukemic cell line (CCRF-CEM) was positive (Eva et al. 1983). However, in a search for additional members of the human *ras* oncogene family, we succeeded in isolating a *ras*-related clone from a library of normal human DNA that was equally diverged from either Ki-*ras* or Ha-*ras*. The structure of this clone was found to resemble closely that of an oncogene, designated N-*ras*, that had been isolated from a human neuroblastoma cell line (Shimizu et al. 1983a). Using a probe derived from this new *ras* gene family member, we detected related exogenous sequences in NIH-3T3 cells transformed by DNAs isolated from established ALL and CML cell lines and also from cells derived directly from a primary AML tumor. Thus, the N-*ras* gene appears to be the most frequently activated *ras* transforming gene in human hematopoietic neoplasms (Eva et al. 1983).

It is striking that a very high fraction of the transforming DNA sequences associated with solid and hematopoietic tumors analyzed to date are related to members of the *ras* gene family. Not only can a variety of tumor types contain the same activated *ras* oncogene, but the same tumor type can contain different activated *ras* oncogenes. Thus, in hematopoietic tumors, we observed different *ras* oncogenes (Ki-*ras*, N-*ras*) activated in lymphoid tumors at the same stage of hematopoietic cell differentiation, and as well as N-*ras* genes activated in tumors as diverse in origin as acute and chronic myelogenous leukemia. These findings strongly imply that *ras* oncogenes detected in the NIH-3T3 transfection assay are not specific to a given stage of cell differentiation or tissue type.

Retroviruses that contain *ras*-related *onc* genes are known to possess a wide spectrum of target cells for transformation in vivo and in vitro. In addition to inducing sarcomas and transforming fibroblasts (Gross 1970), these viruses are capable of inducing tumors of immature lymphoid cells (Pierce and Aaronson 1982). They also can stimulate the proliferation of erythroblasts (Hankins and Scolnick 1981) and monocyte/macrophages (Greenberger 1979) and can even induce alterations in the growth and differentiation of epithelial cells (Weissman and Aaronson 1983). Thus, the wide array of tissue types that can be induced to proliferate abnormally by these *onc* genes may help to explain the high frequency of detection of their activated human homologs in diverse human tumors.

Mechanism of activation of *ras* oncogenes
The availability of molecular clones of the normal and activated alleles of the Ha-*ras* genes made possible at-

tempts to determine the molecular mechanism responsible for the malignant conversion of Ha-*ras* (human). The genetic lesions responsible for the activation of a number of *ras* oncogenes have been localized to single-base changes in their p21 coding sequences (Reddy et al. 1982; Tabin et al. 1982; Capon et al. 1983a; Taparowsky et al. 1983b). In the T24/EJ bladder carcinoma oncogene, a transversion of G→T causes a valine residue to be incorporated instead of a glycine into position 12 of the predicted p21 primary structure. During our analyses of human cells for transforming DNA sequences, we were able to isolate and molecularly clone an oncogene from a human lung carcinoma, designated Hs242 (Yuasa et al. 1983). This gene was also identified as an activated Ha-*ras* (human) proto-oncogene, making it possible to compare the mechanisms by which the same human proto-oncogene has been independently activated in human tumor-derived cells.

The Hs242 transforming sequence was isolated and subjected to restriction enzyme analysis to compare its physical map with that of the previously reported T24/EJ bladder tumor oncogene (Yuasa et al. 1983), as well as c-Ha-*ras* cloned from a normal human fetal liver library (Santos et al. 1982). The restriction map of the Hs242 oncogene closely corresponded with both, diverging only outside the region previously shown to be required for the transforming activity of the T24 oncogene.

To map the position of the genetic lesion in Hs242 leading to its malignant activation, recombinants were constructed in which fragments of the Hs242 oncogene were substituted by the homologous sequences of Ha-*ras* (human) (Fig. 1). By this analysis, the genetic alteration that activated the Hs242 oncogene was localized to a 0.45-kbp region that encompassed its second coding exon. Nucleotide sequence analysis of this region revealed that the Hs242 oncogene and Ha-*ras* (human) differed at a single base within codon 61. The change of an A→T resulted in the replacement of glutamine by leucine in this codon. Thus, a single amino acid substitution seems sufficient to confer transforming properties on the product of the Hs242 oncogene. These results also established that the site of activation in the Hs242 oncogene was totally different from that of the T24/EJ oncogene (Yuasa et al. 1983).

In subsequent studies, we have assessed the generality of point mutations as the basis for acquisition of malignant properties by c-*ras* genes by molecularly cloning and analyzing other activated *ras* oncogenes (Table 1). Activation of an Ha-*ras* transforming gene of the Hs0578 human breast carcinosarcoma line has been localized to a point mutation at position 12 changing glycine to aspartic acid in the amino acid sequence (M.H. Kraus et al., in prep.). An N-*ras* transforming gene isolated from the human lung carcinoma cell line, SW1271, has also been subjected to similar genetic analyses (Y. Yuasa et al., in prep.). Restriction enzyme analysis of N-*ras* revealed that its *ras*-related coding sequences reside within adjacent 9-kbp and 7-kbp *Eco*RI fragments. The first two exons were localized to the larger fragment. By switching the corresponding *Eco*RI fragments between

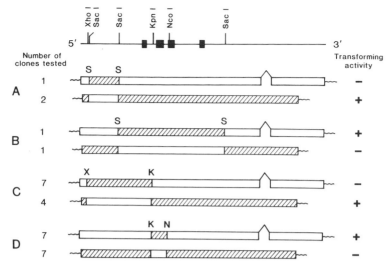

Figure 1 Location of the region of *c*-Ha-*ras* (human) that underwent the genetic alterations which led to activation of the Hs242 oncogene. The restriction map shows the cleavage sites for various enzymes within the insert in pBR322. Hybrid plasmids contained sequences from the Hs242 oncogene (▨) and *c*-Ha-*ras* (human) (☐). Constructs were made in *A* and *B* by mixing the three fragments simultaneously, and in *C* and *D* in bimolecular ligations. Replaced fragments were: *SacI*, 0.8 kbp (*A*); *SacI*, 2.9 kbp (*B*); *XhoI KpnI*, 1.8 kbp (*C*); and *KpnI–NcoI*, 0.45 kbp (*D*). Deletion (∧) and the locations of the four exons (■) are depicted. The left-hand column shows the number of independent clones transfected onto NIH-3T3 cells. Results of the transfections are shown at the right-hand side: (+) >10³ ffu/μg; (−) <10⁰ ffu/μg.

the SW1271 and N-*ras* genes, it was established that the transforming activity of the SW1271 oncogene must have resulted from lesions within either the first or second exons. The nucleotide sequences of the first two exons of the SW1271 and N-*ras* genes were determined and compared. The only change resulted from single point mutation of an A→G at position 61 in the coding sequence resulting in the substitution of arginine for glutamine.

Recently, Wigler and co-workers (Taparowsky et al. 1983a) reported that the lesion leading to activation of the N-*ras* oncogene in a neuroblastoma line was due to the alteration of codon 61 from CAA to AAA causing the substitution in this case of lysine for glutamine.

Investigators analyzing the activated forms of the Ki-*ras* oncogene (Capon et al. 1983b; Shimizu et al. 1983b)

have achieved strikingly similar results. In two Ki-*ras* transforming genes so far analyzed, single point mutations in codon 12 have been shown to be responsible for acquisition of malignant properties (Table 1). Thus, mutations at positions 12 or 61 appear to be the genetic lesions most commonly responsible for activation of *ras* oncogenes under natural conditions in human tumor cells.

Altered electrophoretic mobility of p21 proteins characteristic of position 12 or 61 substitutions

The translational products of human *ras* oncogenes have been identified using antisera directed against the Ha-MSV transforming gene product. Comparison of the migration of p21s coded for by T24 and Hs242 Ha-*ras* oncogenes revealed striking differences. Whereas the

Table 1 Mutations Leading to the Activation of *ras* Oncogenes in Human Tumors

Oncogenes	Origin	Codons affected	Base change	Amino acid change	References
Ha-*ras*					
T24	bladder carcinoma	12	G → T	Gly → Val	Tabin et al. (1982) Reddy et al. (1982) Taparowsky et al. (1983b) Capon et al. (1983a)
Hs0578	mammary carcinosarcoma	12	G → A	Gly → Asp	M.H. Kraus et al. (in prep.)
Hs242	lung carcinoma	61	A → T	Gln → Leu	Yuasa et al. (1983)
N-*ras*					
SK-N-SH	neuroblastoma	61	C → A	Gln → Lys	Taparowsky et al. (1983a)
SW-1271	lung carcinoma	61	A → G	Gln → Arg	Y. Yuasa et al. (in prep.)
Ki-*ras*					
Calu-1	lung carcinoma	12	G → T	Gly → Cys	Shimizu et al. (1983b) Capon et al. (1983b)
SW 480	colon carcinoma	12	G → T	Gly → Val	Capon et al. (1983b)

T24 gene product migrates with a slower mobility than that of the Ha-*ras* proto-oncogene, the Hs242 gene product migrates much faster (Fig. 2). Presumably this reflects different conformational changes in the molecule induced by point mutation at positions 12 and 61, respectively.

We have also analyzed the electrophoretic mobilities of the products of other *ras* oncogenes whose site of activation has been localized to one of these two positions. In each case, the migration of such p21s corresponds to the results shown in Figure 2. Thus, altered electrophoretic mobility not only appears to be a diagnostic marker of activated *ras* oncogenes but may be useful in tentatively assigning the site of the lesion.

Cancer risk syndromes

Although most forms of cancer occur sporadically, clinical observations have revealed the existence of certain familial aggregations of cancer involving specific target organs. Other familial syndromes are associated with a strikingly increased risk of cancer characterized by onset at an early age and tumors affecting tissues of more than one developmental type (Fraumeni 1982). Such clinical syndromes provide the opportunity to test whether the germline transmission of oncogenes capable of registering in the NIH-3T3 transfection assay might account for these patients' genetically determined high risk of cancer (Needleman et al. 1983).

High-molecular-weight DNA was prepared from fibroblast cultures derived from skin of patients with various clinical conditions associated with a high risk of cancer. The largest group comprised affected individuals from five families with Gardner's syndrome. This syndrome is associated with a dominant trait for susceptibility to colon cancer as well as a striking familial predisposition to benign neoplasms of bone, soft tissue, and skin (Gardner and Richards 1953). Essentially 100% of such affected individuals develop colon cancer in the absence of clinical intervention. In addition, we studied fibroblasts from tumor-bearing members of families with site-specific tumor aggregations with apparent autosomal transmission (Li and Fraumeni 1969; Miller 1971; Fraumeni 1982). Patients affected with other syndromes associated with strikingly increased cancer risk, including xeroderma pigmentosum and von Recklinghausen's syndrome, were studied as well (Fraumeni 1982).

Although transforming activity of DNAs isolated from tumor cells from patients with sporadically occurring cancers (colon, lung) could be readily detected (20% and 30% positive, respectively), transforming DNA sequences in any of the skin fibroblast lines from patients with the high cancer susceptibility syndromes could not be detected (Needleman et al. 1983). In addition to performing transfection assays, we examined the level of expression and electrophoretic mobility of the *ras* gene-encoded p21 molecule in each of the human fibroblast lines. No differences in p21 levels or electrophoretic mobility in these cells from the normal controls were observed.

These results argue strongly against the germline transmission of oncogenes capable of registering in the NIH-3T3 transfection assay and further support the concept that the germ-line transmission of oncogenes detectable in this assay does not account for these patients' high susceptibility to develop cancer.

Evidence that oncogenes activated in human tumors are involved in the neoplastic process

It is of critical importance to establish the relevance of an oncogene activated in a human tumor to the neoplastic process. Indirect evidence in support of this relationship derives from the close homology of human *ras* oncogenes to *ras* oncogenes present in retroviruses known to be capable of inducing a variety of malignancies in vivo. An even more telling argument derives from the analysis of normal cells from patients whose tumors contain *ras* oncogenes. In at least four independent cases where such normal cells have been available for analysis, the DNAs have lacked transforming activity (Pulciani et al. 1982a; M.H. Kraus et al., in prep.; Y. Yuasa et al., unpubl.).

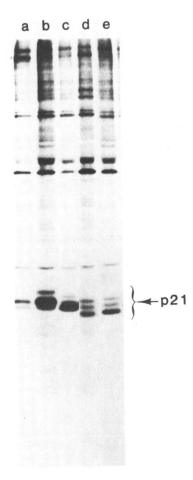

Figure 2 Detection of proteins antigenically related to the Ha-*ras* gene products in NIH-3T3 transfectants. Cells were labeled with [^{35}S]methionine at 37°C for 3 hr, and extracts were prepared and immunoprecipitated using anti-H-MSV p21 monoclonal antibody (Y13-259). (Lane *a*) NIH-3T3 cells. (Lanes *b–e*) Transformed NIH-3T3 cells with DNA from T24 (*b*), Hs0578 (*c*), Hs242 (*d*), and SW-1271 (*e*) cells. Migration of p21 is indicated by arrows.

In one case (M.H. Kraus et al., in prep.), that of the human breast carcinosarcoma line, Hs0578, a restriction polymorphism for *Msp*I is conferred by substitution within codon 12 of its activated Ha-*ras* oncogene. We have demonstrated the lack of this substitution in alleles present in normal cells from the same patient. These results establish that the mutations activating *ras* oncogenes are the result of a somatic event apparently selected for within the tumor.

To ascertain the importance of this selection process to the tumor itself, we have biologically cloned individual tumor cells from a mass population of Hs0578 breast carcinosarcoma cells. As shown in Figure 3, all tumor cell clones analyzed contained the activated allele, as demonstrated by the presence of a 411-bp fragment following *Msp*I digestion and Southern blotting analysis using a probe specific for this region of the Ha-*ras* oncogene (Yuasa et al. 1983). Some clones possessed, whereas others appeared to lack, the faster-migrating 355-bp DNA fragment characteristic of the normal allele

(Fig. 3). All of these findings establish a powerful selective advantage of the activated oncogene in each and every tumor cell. As such, these findings imply that activation of the oncogene very likely contributes to rather than is a result of the neoplastic process.

Implications

As summarized above, oncogenes of the *ras* family have been detected at high frequency in a wide variety of human tumors. Incredibly, these three oncogenes appear to be most commonly activated by point mutations at one of two major "hot spots" in the coding region of the genes. Accumulating evidence strongly supports the concept that their activation as oncogenes contributes to the processes leading to the malignant state. The number of independent steps necessary for the development of a frankly malignant cell remains to be determined. In fact, findings that simple point mutations can activate *ras* oncogenes have implied that this event alone cannot be responsible. The known frequency of spon-

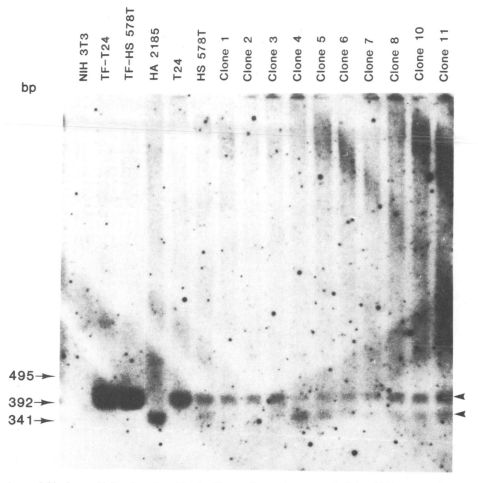

Figure 3 Comparison of *Msp*I sensitivity at codon 12 of c-Ha-*ras* (human) genes. Cellular DNAs were digested with *Msp*I, electrophoresed in a horizontal agarose (2% w/v) gel, blotted onto a nitrocellulose filter, and hybridized to the T24 *Msp*I 411-bp fragment. T24 cells and representative transformed cells by T24 (TF-T24) and Hs0578 DNA (TF-Hs578T), which lack the middle *Msp*I site, showed the large 411-bp fragment, as shown by the arrow. Representative human cells (A 2185) yielded the faster-migrating, 355-bp DNA fragment (also shown by the arrow), characteristic of the normal allele. Hs0578 cells and their cell clones were examined. Coelectrophoresed DNA fragments of *Hinc* II-digested φX174 RF DNA served as standards (labeled in base pairs). The *Msp*I 56-bp fragment was not observed in these experimental conditions.

taneous mutations is too high to be reconciled with such a conclusion (Perler et al. 1980; Miyata and Yasunaga 1981).

It remains to be determined what normal functions are served by *ras* proto-oncogenes as well as how point mutations at positions 12 or 61 can so markedly alter their biologic functions. In the meantime, it may be possible through development of monoclonal antibodies or appropriate anti-peptide antibodies to develop immunologic reagents capable of specifically recognizing the altered *ras*-coded p21 proteins. Alternatively, it may be possible to develop in situ hybridization techniques sensitive enough to detect specifically the altered alleles or transcripts. Such approaches may be useful in developing means of identifying cells with these genetic changes and, thus, determining whether such changes are predictive of a particular clinical course.

References

Bishop, J.M. 1983. Cellular oncogenes and retroviruses. *Annu. Rev. Biochem.* **52**: 301.

Capon, D.J., E.Y. Chen, A.D. Levinson, P.H. Seeburg, and D.V. Goeddel. 1983a. Complete nucleotide sequences of the T24 human bladder carcinoma oncogene and its normal homologue. *Nature* **302**: 33.

Capon, D.J., P.H. Seeburg, J.P. McGrath, J.S. Hayflick, U. Edman, A.D. Levinson, and D.V. Goeddel. 1983b. Activation of Ki-*ras* 2 gene in human colon and lung carcinomas by two different point mutations. *Nature* **304**: 507.

Coffin, J.M., H.E. Varmus, J.M. Bishop, M. Essex, W.D. Hardy, S.M. Martin, N.E. Rosenberg, E.M. Scolnick, R.A. Weinberg, and P.K. Vogt. 1981. Proposal for naming host cell-derived inserts in retrovirus genomes. *J. Virol.* **40**: 953.

Cooper, G.M. 1982. Cellular transforming genes. *Science* **218**: 801.

Der, C.J., T.G. Krontiris, and G.M. Cooper. 1982. Transforming genes of human bladder and lung carcinoma cell lines are homologous to the *ras* genes of Harvey and Kirsten sarcoma viruses. *Proc. Natl. Acad. Sci.* **79**: 3637.

Dhar, R., R.W. Ellis, T.Y. Shih, S. Oroszlan, B. Shapiro. J. Maize, D. Lowy, and E. Scolnick. 1982. Nucleotide sequence of the p21 transforming protein of Harvey murine sarcoma virus. *Science* **217**: 934.

Duesberg, P.H. 1983. Retroviral transforming genes in normal cells (?). *Nature* **304**: 219.

Ellis, R., D. DeFeo, T.Y. Shih, M.A. Gonda, H.A. Young, N. Tsuchida, D.R. Lowy, and E.M. Scolnick. 1981. The p21 *src* genes of Harvey and Kirsten sarcoma viruses originate from divergent members of a family of normal vertebrate genes. *Nature* **292**: 506.

Eva, A., S.R. Tronick, R.A. Gol, J.H. Pierce, and A.S. Aaronson. 1983. Transforming genes of human hematopoietic tumors: Frequent detection of *ras*-related oncogenes whose activation appears to be independent of tumor phenotype. *Proc. Natl. Acad. Sci.* **80**: 4926.

Fraumeni, J.F. 1982. Genetics of cancer. In *Cancer Medicine* (ed. J. Holland and E. Frei), chapt. 2, p. 5. Lea and Febiger, Philadelphia.

Gardner, E.J. and R.C. Richards. 1953. Multiple cutaneous and subcutaneous lesions occurring simultaneously with hereditary polyposis and osteomatosis. *Am. J. Hum. Genet.* **5**: 139.

Goldfarb, M., K. Shimizu, M. Perucho, and M. Wigler. 1982. Isolation and preliminary characterization of a human transforming gene from T24 bladder carcinoma cells. *Nature* **296**: 404.

Greenberger, J.S. 1979. Phenotypically distinct target cells for murine sarcoma virus and murine leukemia virus marrow transformation *in vitro*. *J. Natl. Cancer Inst.* **62**: 337.

Gross, L. 1970. *Oncogenic viruses*, 2nd edition. Pergamon Press, Oxford.

Hopkins, D.W. and E.M. Scolnick. 1981. Harvey and Kirsten sarcoma viruses promote the growth and differentiation of erythroid precursor cells *in vitro*. *Cell* **26**: 91.

Krontiris, T.G. and G.M. Cooper. 1981. Transforming activity of human tumor DNAs. *Proc. Natl. Acad. Sci.* **78**: 1181.

Lane, M.A., A. Sainten, and G.M. Cooper. 1981. Activation of related transforming genes in mouse and human mammary carcinomas. *Proc. Natl. Acad. Sci.* **78**: 5185.

———. 1982. Stage-specific transforming genes of human and mouse B- and T-lymphocyte neoplasms. *Cell* **28**: 873.

Li, F.P. and J.F. Fraumeni. 1969. Rhabdomyosarcoma in children: Epidemiologic study and identification of a familial cancer syndrome. *J. Natl. Cancer Inst.* **43**: 1365.

Marshall, C.J., A. Hall, and R.A. Weiss. 1982. A transforming gene present in human sarcoma cell lines. *Nature* **299**: 171.

Miller, R.W. 1971. Deaths from childhood leukemia and solid tumors among twins and other sibs in U.S., 1960-1967. *J. Natl. Cancer Inst.* **46**: 203.

Miyata, T. and T. Yasunaga. 1981. Rapidly evolving mouse α-globin-related pseudogene and its evolutionary history. *Proc. Natl. Acad. Sci.* **78**: 450.

Murray, M.J., B.Z. Shilo, C. Shih, D. Cowing, H. W. Hsu, and R.A. Weinberg. 1981. Three different human tumor cell lines contain different oncogenes. *Cell* **25**: 355.

Needleman, S.W., Y. Yuasa, S. Srivastava, and S.A. Aaronson. 1983. Normal cells of patients with high cancer risk syndromes lack transforming activity in the NIH/3T3 transfection assay. *Science* **222**: 173.

Parada, L.F., C.J. Tabin, C. Shih, and R.A. Weinberg. 1982. Human EJ bladder carcinoma oncogene is homologue of Harvey sarcoma virus *ras* gene. Nature **297**: 474.

Perler, F., A. Efstratiadis, P. Lomedico, W. Gilbert, R. Kolodner, and J. Dodgson. 1980. The evolution of genes: The chicken preproinsulin gene. *Cell* **20**: 555.

Pierce, J.H. and S.A. Aaronson. 1982. BALB- and Harvey-murine sarcoma virus transformation of a novel lymphoid progenitor cell. *J. Exp. Med.* **156**: 873.

Pulciani, S., E. Santos, A.V. Lauver, L.K. Long, S.A. Aaronson, and M. Barbacid. 1982a. Oncogenes in solid human tumors. *Nature* **300**: 539.

Pulciani, S., E. Santos, A.V. Lauver, L.K. Long, K.C. Robbins, and M. Barbacid. 1982b. Oncogenes in human tumor cell lines: Molecular cloning of a transforming gene from human bladder carcinoma cells. *Proc. Natl. Acad. Sci.* **79**: 2845.

Reddy, E.P., R.K. Reynolds, E. Santos, and M. Barbacid. 1982. A point mutation is responsible for the acquisition of transforming properties by the T24 human bladder carcinoma oncogene. *Nature* **300**: 149.

Santos, E., S.R. Tronick, S.A. Aaronson, S. Pulciani, and M. Barbacid. 1982. T24 human bladder carcinoma oncogene is an activated form of the normal human homologue of BALB- and Harvey-MSV transforming genes. *Nature* **298**: 343.

Shih, C. and R.A. Weinberg. 1982. Isolation of a transforming sequence from a human bladder carcinoma cell line. *Cell* **29**: 161.

Shih, C., L.C. Padhy, M. Murray, and R.A. Weinberg. 1981. Transforming genes of carcinomas and neuroblastomas introduced into mouse fibroblasts. *Nature* **290**: 261.

Shimizu, K., M. Goldfarb, M. Perucho, and M. Wigler. 1983a. Isolation and preliminary characterization of the transforming gene of a human neuroblastoma cell line. *Proc. Natl. Acad. Sci.* **80**: 383.

Shimizu, K., D. Birnbaum, M.A. Ruley, O. Fasano, Y. Suard, L. Edlund, E. Taparowsky, M. Goldfarb, and M. Wigler. 1983b. Structure of the Ki-*ras* gene of the human lung carcinoma cell line Calu-1. *Nature* **304**: 497.

Tabin, C.J., S.M. Bradley, C.I. Bargmann, R.A. Weinberg, A.G. Papageorge, E.M. Scolnick, R. Dhar, D.R. Lowy, and E.H. Chang. 1982. Mechanism of activation of a human oncogene. *Nature* **300**: 143.

Taparowsky, E., K. Shimizu, M. Goldfarb, and M. Wigler. 1983a. Structure and activation of the human N-*ras* gene. *Cell* **34**: 581.

Taparowsky, E., Y. Suard, O. Fasano, K. Shimizu, M. Goldfarb, and M. Wigler. 1983b. Activation of the T24 bladder carcinoma transforming gene is linked to a single amino acid change. *Nature* **300**: 762.

Tsuchida, N., R. Ryder, and E. Ohtsubo. 1982. Nucleotide sequence of the oncogene encoding the p21 transforming protein of Kirsten murine sarcoma virus. *Science* **217**: 937.

Weinberg, R.A. 1982. Fewer and fewer oncogenes. *Cell* **30**: 3.

Weiss, R.A., N. Teich, H. Varmus, and J. Coffin, eds. 1982. *Molecular biology of tumor viruses*; 2nd edition: *RNA tumor viruses*. Cold Spring Harbor Laboratory, Cold Spring Harbor, New York.

Weissman, B.E. and S.A. Aaronson. 1983. BALB and Kirsten murine sarcoma viruses alter growth and differentiation of EGF-dependent BALB/c mouse epidermal keratinocyte lines. *Cell* **32**: 599.

Yuasa, Y., S.K. Srivastava, C.Y. Dunn, J.S. Rhim, E.P. Reddy, and S.A. Aaronson. 1983. Acquisition of transforming properties by alternative point mutations within c-*bas/has* human proto-oncogene. *Nature* **303**: 775.

ras Genes and Cell Transformation

C.J. Marshall, K. Vousden, A. Hall, S. Malcolm,* R.F. Newbold, H. Paterson, and R.A. Weiss

Institute of Cancer Research, Chester Beatty Laboratories, Fulham Road, London SW3 6JB, England;
*Department of Biochemistry, Queen Elizabeth College, London, England

Many of the activated transforming genes detected in tumor cells by transfection of NIH-3T3 cells are the cellular homologs of the viral oncogenes of Harvey and Kirsten murine sarcoma viruses (Ha-MSV, Ki-MSV) (Der et al. 1982; Parada et al. 1982; Santos et al. 1982; McCoy et al. 1983). We have recently identified an activated transforming gene in two human sarcoma cell lines, HT1080 and RD (Marshall et al. 1982). Although no homology of this gene with any of the viral oncogenes could be detected by Southern blot analysis of transfectant DNA, subsequent hybridization of molecular clones showed it to be related to the viral ras genes (Hall et al. 1983). The same gene is activated in a neuroblastoma (Shimizu et al. 1983), a promyelocytic leukemia (Murray et al. 1983), an acute myeloid leukemia (C. Moroni and C. Gambke, pers. comm.), and a variety of T-cell acute lymphoblastic leukemia cell lines (Eva et al. 1983). This new member of the ras gene family has been called N-ras. We review here aspects of our studies of ras genes and their relevance to tumorigenesis.

Methods of Experimental Procedures

Transfection of cells was carried out with high-molecular-weight ($>30 \times 10^6$ bp) cellular DNA using the calcium phosphate coprecipitation technique as described by Wigler et al. (1979).

NIH-3T3 cells (2×10^5/10-cm dish) were transfected with 20 μg of cellular DNA for 18–22 hr, and the cells maintained by feeding with Dulbecco's modified Eagle's medium (DMEM) containing 5% calf serum every 3–4 days. Foci were scored at 15–17 days posttransfection.

Clone 11 cells (LMTK⁻, APRT⁻, HPRT⁻; R.F. Newbold, unpubl.) were seeded at 5×10^5 cells per 10-cm dish and then 1 day later treated with 1 ml of a calcium phosphate coprecipitate containing 20 μg of DNA. After overnight incubation, the cells were washed and fed with DMEM containing 10% calf serum. After a further 24 hr, this medium was changed to DMEM + 10% calf serum containing 4.5 μg/ml azaserine and 13.5 μg/ml adenine to select for APRT⁺ cells. This medium was changed every 3–4 days and colonies scored 14 days after transfection.

Revertant HT1080 1c cells were seeded at 2×10^5 cells/6-cm dish in DMEM + 10% fetal calf serum 1 day before transfection. Each dish received 20 μg of normal mouse DNA and either 1 μg of the methotrexate-resistance plasmid pHG (O'Hare et al. 1981) and 1 μg of the cloned EJ gene (pEJ 6.6, Shih and Weinberg 1982) or 1 μg of pSV2-neo/N-ras (a recombinant plasmid containing the N-ras gene cloned from HT1080 cells and the pSV2-neo vector of Southern and Berg (1982). Control plates received either pHG or pSV2-neo alone. Cells were incubated with the coprecipitate for 4 hours, washed, and fed with DMEM + 10% fetal calf serum. After 24 hours, the cells from each 6-cm plate were subcultured onto two 10-cm plates containing either 0.8 μM methotrexate or 1 mg/ml Geneticin (Gibco, U.K.) in DMEM + 10% fetal calf serum. The cells were fed after 1 week and transformed cells scored after 2 weeks.

Hamster dermal fibroblasts were seeded and transfected as described by Newbold and Overell (1983).

In situ hybridization was carried out as described in Davis et al. (1983).

Results and Discussion

The HT1080 N-ras gene

Figure 1a shows a restriction map of the cloned N-ras gene from HT1080 cells. The cloned gene transforms NIH-3T3 cells with an efficiency of approximately 2000 foci/μg DNA. This efficiency of transformation is very similar to that obtained with the cloned c-Ha-ras-1 gene from EJ/T24 bladder carcinoma cells (Goldfarb et al. 1982; Shih and Weinberg et al. 1982). Comparison of the restriction map of the N-ras transforming allele cloned from HT1080 cells with the normal nontransforming allele cloned from human fetal liver tissue shows no detectable differences, indicating that the gene is not grossly rearranged in HT1080 cells. Preliminary DNA sequence data indicate a coding change for amino acid 61 in the second exon from glutamine to lysine.

Chromosomal localization of N-ras

In a survey of 20 tumor cell lines, we have been unable to detect any amplification or rearrangement of the N-ras gene; furthermore, all tumor cell lines so far examined appear to express the same levels of the 2.2-kb RNA transcript from the N-ras gene. Murray et al. (1983) have shown that, in two tumor cell lines that have activated N-ras genes, the c-myc gene is altered either by amplification or rearrangement. However, the c-myc gene in HT1080 and in RD cells does not appear to be rearranged or amplified.

To investigate further whether the N-ras gene is involved in chromosomal rearrangements in some tumors, we have determined its chromosome localization. Using somatic cell hybrid techniques, the N-ras gene has been

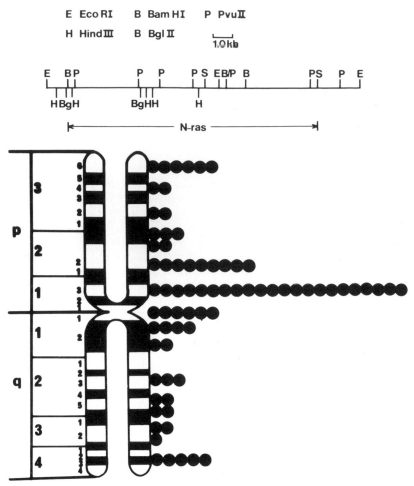

Figure 1 (*Top*) Restriction map of human N-*ras* gene locus. (*Bottom*) A diagram of chromosome 1 showing the distribution of silver grains from an analysis of 16 cells.

mapped to chromosome 1 (Hall et al. 1983). This chromosomal site is different from that of the other known members of the *ras* gene family: *c*-Ha-*ras*-1 (11); *c*-Ha-*ras*-2 (X); *c*-Ki-*ras*-1 (6); and *c*-Ki-*ras*-2 (12) (O'Brien et al. 1983). To localize the gene to a specific chromosomal region, we have used a 4.0-kb *Bgl*II fragment of the gene for in situ hybridization experiments. Figure 1b shows the distribution of silver grains on chromosome 1 from an analysis of 16 cells. The N-*ras* gene was found to be localized on the short arm of chromosome 1 between the centromere and band p21 (Davis et al. 1983). In a survey of 218 human tumors with aberrations of chromosome 1, Brito-Babapulle and Atkin (1981) have shown that about 6% of cases involve deletions occurring between the centromere of chromosome 1 and band p21. We currently are analyzing such material to determine whether the N-*ras* gene has been affected by such deletions in this subset of human tumors.

Activated *ras* genes transform only established cell lines and not primary cells
Considerable evidence suggests that neoplastic transformation is a multistage process (for review, see Cairns, 1978). However the transformation of NIH-3T3 cells by

cloned *ras* genes occurs in a single step. A plausible explanation for this apparent discrepancy is that NIH-3T3 cells have already undergone some of the genetic changes on the route to malignancy. NIH-3T3 cells differ from normal fibroblasts but resemble tumor cell lines in having an indefinite lifespan in culture. We therefore investigated whether a cloned *ras* oncogene (EJ *c*-Ha-*ras*-1) could transform nonestablished cell strains. Table 1 shows that this gene was unable to induce progressively growing foci of morphologically transformed cells even though the recipient cells, Syrian hamster dermal (SHD) fibroblasts, were competent to take up DNA (Newbold and Overell 1983). In contrast, established cell lines that had been derived from dermal fibroblasts using chemical carcinogens (Newbold et al. 1982) could be fully transformed by cloned *ras* genes by morphology, anchorage independence, and malignant growth in vivo (Newbold and Overell 1983). NIH-3T3 cells have undergone many cell divisions since escaping senescence, so that it could be argued that they can only be transformed by *ras* genes because they have undergone other changes in addition to establishment. However, the established hamster cells can be transformed after as few as three passages after escaping from senescence. These results, there-

Table 1 Transforming Effects of the EJ *c*-Ha-*ras*-1 Oncogene following Transfection into SHD Fibroblasts and Carcinogen-induced Immortal Variants.

Recipient cell (immortalizing agent)	Passage number following immortalization	Number of foci induced by cloned EJ *c*-HA-*ras*-1 DNA/number of dishes	Percent soft agar cloning efficiency of cells from isolated focus
4DH2 (DMS)	4	5440/10	41.2[a]
4XH1 (X-ray)	3	3372/10	52.0
4XH2 (X-ray)	5	4132/10	34.3
3M1 (MNU)[b]	10	3420/10	19.6
SHD	limited proliferative potential	0/25	—

For details, see Newbold and Overell 1983.
[a]Soft agar cloning efficiency of immortal cell lines transfected with carrier DNA only: $<10^{-6}$
[b]MNU, *N*-methyl-*N*-nitrosourea.

fore, argue that establishment per se is sufficient to render cells responsive to transforming *ras* genes and that additional changes are not required. Cotransfection of nonestablished, tertiary SHD cells with cloned EJ *c*-Ha-*ras* and *v-myc* showed that, while either oncogene alone caused little phenotypic change, the two oncogenes together induced progressively growing transformed foci. However, these foci still entered senescent crisis after an extended life span.

Tumor cells respond to their own transforming genes

Although the transformation of recipient cells with DNA isolated from a tumor demonstrates that the tumor cells contain an activated transforming gene, it does not prove that the transforming gene is responsible for the transformed phenotype of the tumor. It is possible that mutations that allow a transforming gene to be detected by the transfection assay have no relevance to the phenotype of the tumor. To determine whether tumor cells can respond to their own transforming gene, we have isolated flat revertants (Pollack et al. 1968) of human tumor cells and tested whether they can be retransformed with cloned *ras* genes. HT1080 revertants were isolated after treating cells with *N*-methyl-*N*-nitrosoguanidine (MNNG), plating the cells in low serum (1–2%), and then selecting against dividing cells with 5-fluorodeoxyuridine (FudR) and cytosine arabinoside (AraC). Table 2 shows that these revertants are anchorage dependent, unlike the parental HT1080 cells, and have greatly reduced tumorigenicity. When tumors do occur, they appear to arise from the selection of "rerevertants," since cells cultured from such tumors exhibit increased anchorage independence.

When one such revertant, 1c, was transfected with either the cloned *c*-Ha-*ras*-1 oncogene from EJ bladder carcinoma cells or the cloned N-*ras* oncogene from HT1080, foci of morphologically transformed cells were produced (see Fig. 2). The efficiency of transfection of the revertants is at least 100-fold less than that of NIH-3T3. Furthermore, the morphologically transformed cells were only apparent when the *ras* genes were transfected in the presence of selectable markers, either by cotransfection with a methotrexate resistance gene from the plasmid pHG (O'Hare et al. 1981) or by inserting the *ras* genes into the G418 resistance vector pSV2-*neo* (Southern and Berg 1982). Land et al. (1983) have shown that transformed cells arising from transfection with *ras* genes can sometimes only be discerned when the surrounding normal cells are eradicated by selection. The retransformed revertant cells contain the transfected *ras* genes (data not shown).

These experiments show that a revertant derived from HT1080 tumor cells can be transformed both by the same *ras* gene activated in HT1080 cells and by a *ras* gene that is not activated in HT1080 but is activated in other tumors. As we have been unable to transform normal human diploid fibroblasts with *ras* genes, these results provide the first demonstration that human cells can be transformed by *ras* cellular oncogenes. Furthermore, they show that a revertant cell line derived from a tumor that contains an activated transforming gene can be re-

Table 2 Properties of Revertants of HT1080 Cells

Cell line	Growth in agar	Tumorigenicity
HT1080	1.8%	14/14 (15 days)
Revertant 1c	0.005%	9/16 (53 days)
Revertant 10a	0.001%	0/4 (120 days)

Growth in agar was measured by plating serial dilutions of cells from 10^6 cells/plate into 0.3% agar over a base of 0.5% agar in Dulbecco's medium containing 10% fetal calf serum. Tumorigenicity was measured by inoculating 10^7 cells in culture medium subcutaneously into the flank of nude mice. The figure in parentheses gives the lag period in days before the emergence of a 0.8–1.0-cm tumor.

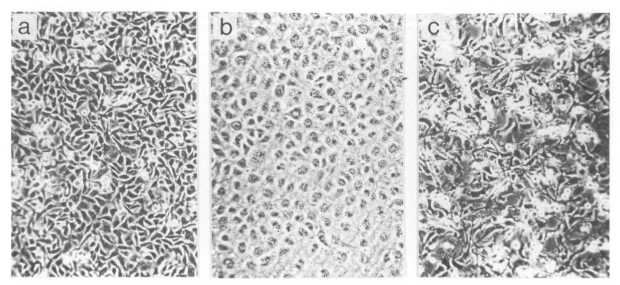

Figure 2 Phase-contrast photographs of HT1080 cells (*a*), revertant 1c (*b*), and revertant 1c retransformed by the N-*ras* (HT1080) oncogene (*c*).

transformed with the activated gene cloned from that tumor.

Activation of a transforming gene as an event in tumor progression

The phenotype of many naturally occurring and experimentally maintained tumors changes with time or passage. The biological basis of this phenomenon, known as tumor progression (Foulds 1969), is not understood but presumably reflects selection for changes in genes affecting the growth and behavior of tumor cells. To investigate whether such changes result from the activations of additional oncogenes in a cell that is already tumorigenic, we have used transfection experiments to study a model system of tumor progression.

The L5178Y-E tumor is a methylcholanthrene-induced T lymphoma which, like most mouse tumors (Kim 1970), does not metastasize in the syngeneic host. However, a number of years ago a spontaneous variant of this tumor arose, which very rapidly gave widely disseminated metastatic disease in subsequent in vivo passage (Parr

1972). This variant, L5178Y–ES, has been extensively characterized immunologically (Schirrmacher et al. 1982) and its derivation from L5178Y-E demonstrated by cytogenetic analysis (Dzarlieva et al. 1982). To determine whether the difference in behavior of L5178Y-E and L5178Y-ES could be due to the activation of a transforming gene, we used DNA from these two cell types in NIH-3T3 transfection experiments. Table 3 shows that DNA prepared from the 'metastatic' variant L5178Y-ES efficiently induced foci of morphologically transformed NIH-3T3 cells, whereas no foci were obtained from the parental L5178Y-E cells in a large number of experiments with three different DNA preparations from each tumor. As a control for the integrity of the DNA preparations, we found that the frequency of adenosine phosphoribosyl transferase (APRT) gene transfer to a tk⁻, APRT⁻, HPRT⁻ L- cell derivative, clone 11 was equivalent for each subline (Table 3).

These results show that a metastatic variant derived from a nonmetastatic tumor contains a transforming gene that can be detected by transfection, whereas the orig-

Table 3 Transforming Efficiencies of DNAs from L5178Y-E and L5178Y-ES Tumor Cell Lines

Donor DNA	Source of DNA	Efficiency of APRT transfer (azaserine-resistant colonies/μg DNA)	Efficiency of primary transfection[a] (number foci/μg DNA)	Efficiency of secondary transfection[b] (number foci/μg DNA)
L5178Y-E	tumor	N.D.[c]	<0.01 (0/21)	
	cultured cell	0.28	<0.01 (0/22)	—
	cultured cell	0.63	<0.01 (0/20)	—
L5178Y-ES	tumor	N.D.	0.07 (15/11)	0.11, 0.11, 0.15
	cultured cell	0.28	0.05 (18/17)	0.06
	cultured cell	0.23	0.02 (2/6)	—

[a]The number of foci scored/number of plates examined is shown in parentheses.
[b]Each value represents the transfection efficiency of a different primary focus.
[c]N.D., not done.

inal tumor does not. It is unclear whether the terminology nonmetastatic and metastatic is wholly appropriate for these cells, since they both produce metastases in immunodeficient nude mice (Eccles et al. 1980), although the variant produces a more aggressive disseminated disease in immunocompetent syngeneic hosts. It is unlikely that the presence of the activated transforming gene is a random event unlinked to the emergence of the metastatic variant, since we examined the L5178Y-ES at a passage level (83) that was close to the emergence of the variant (73). We therefore conclude that the difference in behavior of these two related tumors is due to the spontaneous activation of a transforming gene. In studies to be reported elsewhere, we have shown that the L5178Y-ES transforming gene is a cellular homolog of v-Ki-*ras*.

Our studies show that cellular *ras* genes may be activated at a number of different stages in tumorigenesis and progression, with perhaps different consequences for the cells. Cell transformation in vitro by *ras* genes depends on the establishment of cells for indefinite growth, which is an independent step in tumorigenesis. Flat revertants of human tumor cells that retain their capacity for indefinite growth can be retransformed by cloned *ras* genes, including one derived from the original tumor.

Acknowledgment

These studies were supported by the British Medical Research Council and Cancer Research Campaign.

References

Brito-Babapulle, V. and N.B. Atkin. 1981. Breakpoints in chromosome # 1 abnormalities of 218 human neoplasms. *Cancer Genet. Cytogenet.* **4:** 215.

Cairns, J. 1978. *Cancer science and society.* W.H. Freeman, San Francisco.

Davis, M., S. Malcolm, A. Hall, and C.J. Marshall. 1983. Localization of the human N-*ras* oncogene to chromosome 1cen-p21 by *in situ* hybridization. *EMBO J.* **2:** 228.

Der, C.J., T.G. Krontiris, and G.M. Cooper. 1982. Transforming genes of human bladder and lung carcinoma cell lines are homologous to the *ras* genes of Harvey and Kirsten sarcoma viruses. *Proc. Natl. Acad. Sci.* **79:** 3637.

Dzarlieva, S., V. Schirrmacher, and N.F. Fusenig. 1982. Cytogenetic changes during tumor progression towards invasion, metastasis and immune escape in the Eb/Esb model system. *Int. J. Cancer* **30:** 633.

Eccles, S.A., S.E. Heckford, and P. Alexander. 1980. Effect of Cyclosporin A on the growth and spontaneous metastasis of syngeneic animal tumors. *Br. J. Cancer* **42:** 252.

Eva, A., S.R. Tronick, R.A. Gol, J.H. Pierce, and S.A. Aaronson. 1983. Transforming genes of human hematopoietic tumors: Frequent detection of *ras*-related oncogenes whose activation appears to be independent of tumor phenotype. *Proc. Natl. Acad. Sci.* **80:** 4926.

Foulds, L. 1969. *Neoplastic development,* vol. 1. Academic Press, London.

Goldfarb, M., K. Shimizu, M. Perucho, and M. Wigler. 1982. Isolation and preliminary characterization of a human transforming gene from T24 bladder carcinoma cells. *Nature* **296:** 404.

Hall, A., C.J. Marshall, N. Spurr, and R.A. Weiss. 1983. The transforming gene in two human sarcoma cell lines is a new member of the *ras* gene family located on chromosome 1. *Nature* **303:** 396.

Kim, U. 1970. Metastasizing mammary carcinomas in rats: Induction and study of their immunogenicity. *Science* **167:** 72.

Land, H., L.F. Parada, and R.A. Weinberg. 1983. Tumorigenic conversion of primary embryo fibroblasts requires at least two co-operating oncogenes. *Nature* **304:** 596.

Marshall, C.J., A. Hall, and R.A. Weiss. 1982. A transforming gene present in human sarcoma cell lines. *Nature* **299:** 171.

McCoy, M.S., J.J. Toole, J.M. Cunningham, E.H. Chang, D.R. Lowy, and R.A. Weinberg. 1983. Characterization of a human colon/lung carcinoma oncogene. *Nature* **302:** 79.

Murray, M.J., J.M. Cunningham, L.F. Parada, F. Dautry, P. Leibowitz, and R.A. Weinberg. 1983. The HL60 transforming sequence: A *ras* oncogene co-existing with altered *myc* genes in hematopoietic tumors. *Cell* **33:** 749.

Newbold, R.F. and R.W. Overell. 1983. Fibroblast immortality is a prerequisite for transformation by EJ c-Ha-*ras* oncogene. *Nature* **304:** 648.

Newbold, R.F., R.W. Overell, and J.R. Connell. 1982. Induction of immortality is an early event in malignant transformation of mammalian cells by carcinogens. *Nature* **299:** 633.

O'Brien, S.J., W.G. Nash, J.L. Goodwin, D.R. Lowy, and E.H. Chang. 1983. Dispersion of the *ras* family of transforming genes to four different chromosomes in man. *Nature* **302:** 839.

O'Hare, K., C. Benoist, and R. Breathnach. 1981. Transformation of mouse fibroblasts to methotrexate resistance by a recombinant plasmid expressing a prokaryotic dihydrofolate reductase. *Proc. Natl. Acad. Sci.* **78:** 1527.

Parada, L.F., C.J. Tabin, C. Shih, and R.A. Weinberg. 1982. Human EJ bladder carcinoma oncogene is homologue of Harvey sarcoma virus *ras* gene. *Nature* **297:** 474.

Parr, I. 1972. Response of syngeneic murine lymphomata to immunotherapy in relation to the antigenicity of the tumor. *Br. J. Cancer* **26:** 174.

Pollack, R.E., H. Green, and G.J. Todaro. 1968. Growth control in cultured cells: Selection of sublines with increased sensitivity to contact inhibition and decreased tumor-producing ability. *Proc. Natl. Acad. Sci.* **60:** 126.

Santos, E., T. Tronick, S.A. Aaronson, S. Pulciani, and M. Barbacid. 1982. T24 human bladder carcinoma oncogene is an activated form of the normal human homologue of BALB and Harvey-MSV transforming genes. *Nature* **298:** 343.

Shih, C. and R.A. Weinberg. 1982. Isolation of a transforming sequence from a human bladder carcinoma cell line. *Cell* **29:** 161.

Shimizu, K., M. Goldfarb, M. Perucho, and M. Wigler. 1983. Isolation and preliminary characterization of the transforming gene of a human neuroblastoma cell line. *Proc. Natl. Acad. Sci.* **80:** 383.

Schirrmacher, V., M. Fogel, E. Russmann, K. Bosslet, and L. Beck. 1982. Antigenic variation in cancer metastasis; immune escape versus immune control; report from a tumor model system. *Cancer Metastasis Rev.* **1(3):** 241.

Southern, P.J. and P. Berg. 1982. Transformation of mammalian cells to antibiotic resistance with a bacterial gene under control of the SV40 early region promoter. *J. Mol. Appl. Genet.* **1:** 327.

Wigler, M., A. Pellicer, S. Silverstein, R. Axel, G. Urlaub, and L. Chasin. 1979. DNA-mediated transfer of the adenine phosphoribosyl transferase locus into mammalian cells. *Proc. Natl. Acad. Sci.* **76:** 1373.

Structure and Mechanisms of Activation of the c-Ki-*ras* Oncogene from Two Human Lung Tumors

H. Nakano, C. Neville, F. Yamamoto, J.L. Garcia,* J. Fogh,† and M. Perucho

Department of Biochemistry, State University of New York, Stony Brook, New York 11794
†Human Tumor Cell Laboratory, Sloan Kettering Institute for Cancer Research, Rye, New York 10580

Oncogenes activated in human tumors have been detected by DNA-mediated gene transfer using the growth-controlled mouse fibroblast cell line NIH-3T3 as recipient (Weinberg 1981; Cooper 1982). The majority of these oncogenes have been identified as members of the *ras* gene family (Der et al. 1982; Parada et al. 1982; Santos et al. 1982; Shimizu et al. 1983b). Activated human *ras* oncogenes have been isolated from some tumor cell lines, and the molecular nature of the mutations responsible for the acquisition of their transforming activities has been determined as single-base substitutions in the protein-coding regions of the oncogenes. Thus, the human c-Ha-*ras* oncogene has been detected in bladder carcinoma (the T24 line and the EJ line, which appears to be a contaminant of the T24 line) (Fogh et al. 1983) and in lung carcinoma (Hs242) cell lines. The c-Ha-*ras* proto-oncogene has been activated in the T24-EJ bladder carcinoma cells by a single point mutation in position 12 of the predicted amino acid sequence of the p21 protein, the gene product of the *ras* genes (Reddy et al. 1982; Tabin et al. 1982; Taparowsky et al. 1982; Capon et al. 1983a). A different mutation has occurred in the same proto-oncogene activated in the lung carcinoma cell line Hs242. In this case, a single-base change in the second exon of the oncogene is responsible for the structural alteration of the p21 protein which confers oncogenic capability in the NIH-3T3 assay (Yuasa et al. 1983).

In contrast with the human c-Ha-*ras* oncogene, which has been found so far activated in only these two examples, the human c-Ki-*ras* oncogene has been detected in an active form in a relatively large proportion of tumors (Murray et al. 1981; Perucho et al. 1981; Pulciani et al. 1982; Nakano et al. 1984). The difference in the frequency of activation of these two *ras* genes in human tumors is not clear at present. One obvious difference is their size. All the sequences required for the transforming activity of the c-Ha-*ras* oncogene are contained within a DNA fragment of about 3 kbp (Goldfarb et al. 1982; Parada et al. 1982; Santos et al. 1982). The minimum size of the c-Ki-*ras* oncogene was previously calculated as 30 kbp, and has been recently reported to be about 38–45 kbp (Shimizu et al. 1983a; McGrath et al. 1983). This larger size has made the isolation of this gene as well as the analysis of the structural alteration undergone in the tumors that resulted in its activation, more difficult.

We have molecularly cloned over 40 kbp of the c-Ki-*ras* oncogene activated in two human lung carcinomas, and the structure of the oncogene has been determined by restriction mapping and hybridization studies with the viral Kirsten sarcoma virus oncogene (v-Ki-*ras*) (Ellis et al. 1981). No clear differences were observed between the restriction maps of the cloned oncogene sequences of these two tumors, and Southern blot hybridization studies also revealed no gross alterations in the structure of the oncogenes relative to the normal proto-oncogene. DNA sequence analysis in concert with gene transfer experiments indicates that the genetic alteration of these two oncogenes is similar to those previously described for the c-Ha-*ras* oncogene: One lung tumor oncogene appears mutant in position 12 of the first exon, whereas the other cloned oncogene contains a base substitution at position 61 of the second coding exon. These results strongly suggest that the mechanism of activation of the same proto-oncogene (c-Ki-*ras*) can occur by different mutational events.

Experimental Procedures

The experimental procedures used in this work have been described in detail elsewhere (Perucho et al. 1981; Nakano et al. 1984). They include DNA transfection experiments, Southern blots, construction of partial phage libraries, and DNA sequencing experiments.

Results

Cloning the oncogenes of the human lung tumors PR310 and PR371

We previously found that DNA from two human lung (Calu-1 and SK-LU-1) and one colon carcinoma (SK-CO-1) cell lines was able to induce morphological transformation of NIH-3T3 mouse fibroblasts upon transfection with the calcium phosphate precipitate technique (Perucho et al. 1981). The *Alu* blot pattern of NIH-3T3 secondary transformants DNA indicated that the same or closely related oncogene was activated in these tumor cell lines. Another two human lung (PR310 and PR371) (Fogh et al. 1980) and one colon (PR135) (Fogh et al. 1979) tumors, maintained by successive passages in nude mice, also contained the same transforming gene,

*Present address: Antibioticos, S.A., Bravo Murillo, 38, Madrid-3, Spain.

which was detected by the ability of the tumor DNAs to induce foci of morphologically transformed cells in the NIH-3T3 assay and identified by Southern blot hybridization with the Blur 8 clone (Nakano et al. 1984, and data not shown). The oncogene activated in these lung and colon carcinoma cell lines has been identified (Shimizu et al. 1983b) as the human homolog of the Kirsten murine sarcoma virus oncogene (c-Ki-*ras*-2) (Chang et al. 1982).

A fragment of the Calu-1 oncogene had been previously isolated (Shimizu et al. 1983b). DNA from one NIH-3T3 secondary transformant was used to construct an EcoRI partial library in Charon 4A, and one phage clone, λL2-3.4, was isolated by screening the library with the Blur 8 clone containing a member of the human *Alu* family sequence. We have used this phage isolate to clone the sequences of the human oncogene activated in the human lung tumors PR371 and PR310 by walking along the genome of mouse NIH-3T3 secondary and tertiary transformants induced by DNA from these tumors.

DNA fragments from λL2-3.4 (Fig. 1) were subcloned in pBR322 and used as probes in Southern blot hybridization experiments of DNA from NIH-3T3 secondary and tertiary transformants to define the position of restriction sites located outside of the cloned fragment of the oncogene. We found that the next HindIII site of the c-Ki-*ras* oncogene was located approximately 14 kbp 5′ from the "left" HindIII site in λL2-3.4, using as probe the "left" EcoRI–HindIII 0.9-kb fragment of λL2-3.4 (PL-RHO.9). DNA from OS9 and OS10, tertiary transformants from PR371 and PR310, respectively, was digested to completion with HindIII, size-fractionated by agarose gel electrophoresis, and the 13–15-kbp fractions used to prepare recombinant phages by in vitro ligation to similarly gel-purified HindIII arms of λ47.1 phage DNA.

The resulting recombinant phages obtained after in vitro packaging of the ligated DNA were screened with PL-RHO.9 as probe. Eighty-eight phages were identified after screening about 150,000 total recombinant phages from the OS10 partial library. This result indicated that the enrichment obtained by size fractionation of HindIII-cleaved genomic DNA was approximately 100-fold (one positive clone every 2000 total packaged phages), thus simplifying considerably the screening procedure. In a similar way, 20,000 and 10,000 phages were screened, resulting in the isolation of six and two independent recombinant phages containing the 14-kbp HindIII fragment from the PR371 and Calu-1 oncogenes, respectively (λLD-H14 and λLC-H14)(Fig. 1a).

The same procedure was used to clone the 10.5-kbp HindIII fragments from OS9 and OS10 transformants using as probe the 3.1-kbp EcoRI fragment of the λL2-3.4 phage subcloned in pBR322 (Fig. 1). In this case, it was necessary to screen approximately 100,000 in vitro packaged phages to obtain two and three clones containing the 10.5-kbp HindIII fragment from OS9 and OS10 (λLD-H10 and λLN-H10), respectively. The lower yield obtained probably was due to the smaller size of the HindIII fragment as well as the presence of some sequences in this HindIII fragment that are relatively more difficult to clone in either plasmids or phages.

A restriction map was constructed from the inserted DNA of λLD-H14 and λLN-H14 (Fig. 1). The presence of a BamHI site, 250 bp 3′ from the left HindIII site allowed us to continue walking along the oncogene. The 250-bp HindIII–BamHI fragment was subcloned in pBR322 (PL-HBO.25) and used as hybridization probe in Southern blot experiments of DNA of several tertiary transformants derived from different lung and colon carcinomas DNA. The probe hybridized with a 10-kbp BamHI fragment present in all the transformant DNAs analyzed (Nakano et al. 1984).

DNA from OS10 was digested to completion with BamHI and electrophoresed through agarose gels, and the 8–12-kbp fragments were fractionated as described. These enriched restriction fragments were used to construct recombinant phages by in vitro ligation to BamHI-cleaved, purified λ47.1 arms, as before. The partial library was screened using PL-HBO.25 as probe and two recombinant phages isolated by two plating and screening cycles. These phages were called λLN-B10, and a restriction map was constructed (Fig. 1).

The 5′ end of the oncogenes was isolated in a similar way by cloning in λ47.1 the 15-kbp (λLD-H15) and 16-kbp (λLN-H16) HindIII fragments present in D2-2 and N2-4, which are NIH-3T3 secondary transformants derived from PR371 and PR310, respectively. By Southern blot experiments, we found, based on the conservation of these human DNA sequences in mouse transformants, that these HindIII fragments contained all the sequences at the 5′ end of the oncogene essential for its transforming activity (Nakano et al. 1984). The restriction maps of λLD-H15 and λLN-H16 were identical up to the SstI site located at 2.2 kbp of the BamHI site. From this site to the 5′ end, the restriction maps differed (Fig. 1). Southern blot experiments revealed that the λLD-H15 clone contained human sequences in this region of the insert, while the 5′ end of λLN-H16 contained mouse sequences (Nakano et al. 1984). These results suggest that the 5′ end sequences of the c-Ki-*ras* oncogene essential for its transforming activity in the NIH-3T3 cells are located between the two SstI sites of λLD-H15 (Fig. 1).

By similar analysis, we found that some NIH-3T3 transformants induced by DNA from different lung and colon carcinomas did not contain the last 3′ 1.1-kbp EcoRI fragment of λL2-R7 (Fig. 1) (Nakano et al. 1984). Therefore, we estimate the size of the DNA region essential for the transforming activity of the human c-Ki-*ras* oncogene as 43–46 kbp.

Structure of the c-Ki-*ras* oncogene of PR310 and PR371 human lung tumors

Restriction mapping analysis of the fragments of the c-Ki-*ras* oncogenes from PR310, PR371, and Calu-1 cloned in our recombinant phages revealed no differences, with the exception of the above-mentioned 5′ end sequences. Therefore, a composite restriction map of the 47-kbp region of human DNA comprising the entire c-Ki-*ras* oncogene was constructed (Fig. 1b).

The restriction map of the c-Ki-*ras* oncogene from the PR371 and PR310 human lung tumors is essentially

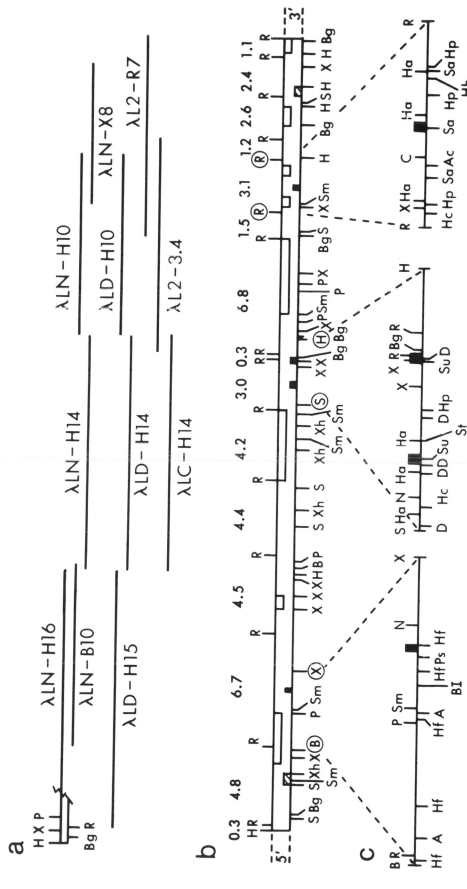

Figure 1 Physical map of the human c-Ki-*ras* oncogene. A composite restriction map of the human c-Ki-*ras* oncogene was derived from the restriction maps of the DNA fragments from the oncogenes of Calu-1, PR371, and PR310 human lung carcinomas cloned in overlapping and/or contiguous phage vectors. (*a*) The names of the recombinant λ47.1 phages containing fragments of the oncogenes of PR310 (λLN-), PR371 (λLD-), or Calu-1 (λLC-) are represented and their origin described in the text and in Nakano et al. (1984). λL2-3.4 and λL2-R7 are recombinant Charon 4A phages containing fragments of the Calu-1 transforming gene obtained by EcoRI partial digestion of NIH-3T3 secondary transformants (Shimizu et al. 1983b). (*b*) The restriction map of the c-Ki-*ras* oncogene is depicted in the diagram. The entire region has been mapped for the restriction endonucleases BamHI (B), BglII (Bg), EcoRI (R), HindIII (H), PvuII (P), SmaI (Sm), SstI (S), XbaI (X), and XhoI (Xh). There are no SalI sites in the entire region. The distances in kbp between the EcoRI fragments are indicated at the top of the map. The position of fragments containing human Alu repeat sequences is indicated by empty boxes. The black boxes indicate the position of the first four coding exons of the oncogene as determined by hybridization with the v-Ki-*ras* clone HiHi 3. Two hatched boxes represent the position of sequences hybridizing with the viral c-Ki-*ras* clone pKBE-2 but not with the HiHi 3. (*c*) The regions containing the coding exons of the c-Ki-*ras* oncogene were analyzed in greater detail for other restriction endonucleases. The BamHI–XbaI 4.6-kbp fragment and the SstI–HindIII 3.9-kbp fragment subcloned in pchtK-2 and the EcoRI 3.1-kbp fragment subcloned in pBR322 were mapped for the enzymes indicated. (A) AvaI, (Ac) AccI, (BI) BglI, (C) ClaI, (D) DdeI, (Ha) HaeIII, (Hc) HincII, (Hf) HinfI, (Hh) HhaI, (Hp) HpaII, (Nd) NdeI, (Ps) PstI, (Sa) Sau3A, (Su) Sau96.I, and (St) StuI. The restriction maps of the different fragments are complete for the enzymes indicated within the individual fragments.

coincident with the map reported for the Calu-1 oncogene (Shimizu et al. 1983a) and the human *c*-Ki-*ras*-2 proto-oncogene (McGrath et al. 1983). However, some differences are also noted. The Calu-1 oncogene contains a 3.7-kbp *Eco*RI fragment at the 5′ end of the cloned sequences, instead of the 4.7-kbp *Eco*RI fragment reported for the proto-oncogene and the 4.8-kbp *Eco*RI fragment that we have cloned from the PR371 oncogene. We predict that the 3.7-kbp *Eco*RI fragment of the Calu-1 cloned oncogene contains sequences unrelated to the oncogene upstream of the *Sma*I site. The *c*-Ki-*ras*-2 proto-oncogene contains a 3.4-kbp *Eco*RI fragment next to the 6.7-kbp *Eco*RI fragment containing the first exon, instead of the 4.4-kbp *Eco*RI fragment reported for the Calu-1 oncogene, and the 4.5-kbp *Eco*RI fragment that we found in both PR310 and PR371 oncogenes. We suggest that the isolated clone containing this region of the *c*-Ki-*ras*-2 proto-oncogene has suffered a deletion of about 1 kbp, thus losing an *Xba*I and a *Hind*III site.

The position of the regions of the oncogene containing human *Alu* sequences (Fig. 1) was determined by hybridization of cloned oncogene fragments with the Blur 8 clone. Eight *Eco*RI fragments of sizes 6.8, 6.7, 4.7., 4.5, 4.2, 3.1, 2.6, and 1.1 kbp, respectively, were found to contain *Alu* sequences confirming the previous results obtained by genomic blots of NIH-3T3 transformants (Perucho et al. 1981).

The coding exons of the oncogene were localized by cross-hybridization studies using the viral oncogene as probe. Four regions were identified that hybridized with the HiHi 3 clone (Ellis et al. 1981), which contains all the sequences of the viral oncogene necessary to encode for the p21 protein, and that represent the first four coding exons of the *c*-Ki-*ras* oncogene (Shimizu et al. 1983a; McGrath et al. 1983; Nakano et al. 1984, and our unpublished results). Another two regions in the oncogene were identified by hybridization with the clone pKBE-2, which contains extra sequences of the viral oncogene at both 5′ and 3′ ends of the coding sequences for the p21 protein (Ellis et al. 1981). These have been identified and characterized as a 5′ untranslated exon (McGrath et al. 1983) and a fifth alternative exon (Shimizu et al. 1983a; McGrath et al. 1983) of the human *c*-Ki-*ras* oncogene, respectively.

The oncogenes of PR371 and PR310 contain different point mutations in the protein-coding regions

We have sequenced the first three exons of the PR310 and PR371 oncogenes (Nakano et al. 1984; and F. Yamamoto et al., in prep.). These analyses have revealed that the PR371 oncogene presents a point mutation at position 12 of the predicted amino acid sequence of the first exon. A G→T transversion at position 34 of the PR371 oncogene-coding sequences has resulted in the incorporation of cysteine instead of glycine as the amino acid 12 of the p21 protein (Nakano et al. 1984). The nucleotide sequence of the second and third exons of the PR371 oncogene revealed no other changes relative

to the reported sequence of these exons of the normal *c*-Ki-*ras*-2 allele (McGrath et al., 1983) and the Calu-1 oncogene (Shimizu et al. 1983a).

On the other hand, the PR310 oncogene nucleotide sequence is normal in the first and third exons. This gene however contains a different point mutation at position 61 of the second coding exon. An A→T transversion at position 183, which corresponds to the third base of codon 61, results in the incorporation of histidine instead of glutamine in the predicted amino acid sequence of the p21 protein. The sequence data as well as the functional analysis of the mutation in the PR310 oncogene will be published in more detail elsewhere.

Functional analysis of the mutation of PR371 oncogene

We designed a functional assay to test if the presence of cysteine at codon 12 of the PR371 oncogene was sufficient for the acquisition of transforming activity of this gene. We constructed, by in vitro ligation, chimeric genes by substituting the first mutant exon of the bladder carcinoma oncogene (Goldfarb et al. 1982) with the exons of the two lung carcinomas. The purified 2.1-kbp *Xba*I–*Pvu*II fragment of PTB1 containing the last three exons of the T24 oncogene was ligated in vitro in equimolar ratio with the 5-kbp *Xba*I fragments of λLN-H16 and λLD-H15. The ligated DNA was added to NIH-3T3 cells as a calcium phosphate precipitate, and foci of morphologically transformed cells were scored after 15–17 days. Only the ligated DNA containing the 5-kbp *Xba*I fragment from the PR371 oncogene was capable of inducing foci in NIH-3T3 cells.

Several of these foci were isolated by the use of cloning cylinders, grown into mass culture, and analyzed by Southern blot experiments for the presence of chimeric genes. DNA of five transformants that we analyzed contained a 2.4-kbp *Stu*I–*Apa*I fragment that hybridized to both *c*-Ki-*ras* (*Stu*I–*Xba*I 1.35-kbp fragment of λLD-H15) and *c*-Ha-*ras* (*Xba*I–*Apa*I 0.95-kbp fragment of PBXP2.1) probes (Figs. 2A,B, lanes 3–7). NIH-3T3 transformants derived from either the bladder (lanes 1) or the lung (lanes 2) carcinoma oncogenes hybridized only with the probe corresponding to the specific oncogene. Other additional bands are also present in this blot. Some of them could be derived from extra copies of the lung or bladder purified fragments used in the ligation and others are probably the result of partial digestion. These results indicate that the malignant phenotype of these NIH-3T3 transformants appears to be dependent on the presence of PR371-T24 chimeric gene sequences in the host mouse cell genome.

Since it was difficult to compare transforming efficiencies using in vitro-ligated DNA fragments, we constructed recombinant plasmids containing *c*-Ki-*ras*–*c*-Ha-*ras* chimeric genes. The *Xba*I–*Pvu*II 2.1-kbp fragment of the T24 oncogene previously cloned in the recombinant plasmid PTBI (Goldfarb et al. 1982) was inserted into the *Xba*I–*Sma*I site of pchtk-2, a plasmid containing the chicken thymidine kinase gene (Perucho et al. 1980b). The resulting plasmid PBXP2.1 was used to

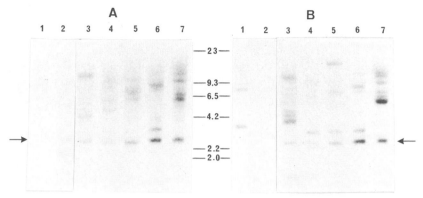

Figure 2 Presence of c-Ki-*ras*–c-Ha-*ras* chimeric sequences in NIH-3T3 transformants. The 2.1-kbp *Xba*I–*Pvu*II fragment of PTB1 was gel-purified and ligated in vitro to the 5-kbp *Xba*I fragments of λLD-H15 at a concentration of 100 µg/ml and at a molar ratio of 1:1. Ligated DNA (0.5 µg) was mixed with 20 µg of NIH-3T3 carrier DNA and applied as a calcium phosphate precipitate to a plate of NIH-3T3 cells as described (Perucho et al. 1981). Several foci of morphologically transformed cells were picked with cloning cylinders, grown into mass culture, and DNA was prepared as described (Perucho et al. 1981). DNA (6 µg each) of D3-9, PR371 tertiary transformant (lanes *1*), R2-1, a T24-derived secondary transformant (lanes *2*), and five independently cloned foci from the ligation experiment (lanes *3–7*) were digested with *Apa*I and *Stu*I, and electrophoresed in a 1% agarose gel. The probes were the gel-purified *Stu*I–*Xba*I 1.35-kbp fragment of λLD-H15 (*A*), or the *Xba*I–*Apa*I 0.95-kbp fragment of PTBG-1 (*B*), labeled by nick-translation to 10⁸cpm/µg, as described (Perucho et al. 1981). The position and molecular weights in kbp of λDNA *Hind*III fragments are indicated at the center of the figure. The arrows indicate the position of the 2.4-kbp *Stu*I–*Apa*I fragment.

construct chimeric genes by insertion of the *Xba*I 5-kbp fragment of PR310 and PR371 oncogenes (see Fig. 3). Two plasmids were obtained, PLDX2P and PLNX2P, each containing the *Xba*I 5-kbp fragment of the lung carcinoma oncogenes in the correct orientation.

These plasmids were tested for transforming activity in the NIH-3T3 assay (Table 1). Only PLDX2P showed transforming activity. Southern blot experiments also revealed that the foci induced by PLDX2P contained the 2.4-kbp *Stu*I–*Apa*I hybrid fragment which hybridized to both lung and bladder carcinoma oncogene probes (data not shown).

These results indicate that a chimeric gene containing the first exon of the human c-Ki-*ras* oncogene and the last three exons of the c-Ha-*ras* oncogene is functional, and at the same time, that the mutation in position 12 of the PR371 oncogene is most likely responsible for the activation of this oncogene in PR371 tumor cells.

Circular or *Bam*HI-cleaved PLDX2P transformed NIH-3T3 cells with efficiencies 20- to 40-fold lower than circular or *Bam*HI-linearized PTBG1, which contains the indigenous T24 oncogene (Fig. 3 and Table 1). This low efficiency could be explained by the absence of a promoter in the 5-kbp *Xba*I fragment of the lung carcinoma oncogene. The transforming activity of PLDX2P could be due to promoters present in the NIH-3T3 carrier DNA which became ligated to the gene during the transfection experiment (Perucho et al. 1980a). A similar observation has been made with the transforming region of polyoma virus deprived of its expression-enhancer sequences (Fried et al. 1983).

Alternatively, the transforming activity of the chimeric gene could be explained by the presence of sequences upstream of the first exon that could allow the transcription of the gene, but with lower efficiencies than the naturally occurring promoter in the c-Ki-*ras* oncogene, which most likely resides between the two *Sst*I sites of the λLDH-15 clone. This is supported by the presence

of a 5′ untranslated exon in this region of the oncogene (McGrath et al. 1983). The transforming activity of restriction endonuclease-cleaved chimeric plasmids (Table 1) argues in favor of this possibility. *Bam*HI- or *Eco*RI-cleaved PLDX2P showed similar transforming activities, whereas cleavage with *Pvu*II decreased the transforming efficiency of the plasmid. This suggests that the putative sequences that could be acting as secondary promoters reside between the *Eco*RI and *Pvu*II sites of the λLDH-15 clone. The foci induced by *Pvu*II-cleaved PLDX2P could be due to ligation to promoters from the carrier DNA. Construction of chimeric plasmids containing sequences upstream of the 5′ *Xba*I site of PLDX2P together with analysis of transforming efficiencies of DNA of NIH-3T3 cells transformed with these chimeric genes should provide additional information to decide between these possibilities.

Discussion

The advent of methodology to transform cultured cell lines with selected genes using total cellular DNA as donor has made possible the identification and isolation of oncogenes specific for some human tumors. The majority of these oncogenes have been identified as members of the human *ras* gene family, which is a family of evolutionarily well-conserved genes in eukaryotes encoding immunologically related proteins of 21 kD. Although the function of these proteins in physiological conditions is unknown, the genetic alteration that the *ras* proto-oncogenes undergo in these tumors confers oncogenic capabilities to the *ras* p21 proteins in the NIH-3T3 assay.

The comparison of the structure of the c-Ha-*ras* oncogene activated in some human tumors with its normal allele has revealed that the structural alteration suffered by the c-Ha-*ras* proto-oncogene resides in single-base substitutions in the protein-coding region.

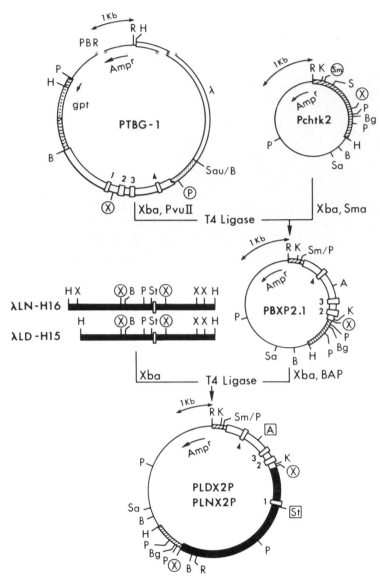

Figure 3 Construction of chimeric *c*-Ki-*ras*–*c*-Ha-*ras* genes. The *Xba*I–*Pvu*II 2.1-kbp fragment of the T24 bladder carcinoma oncogene contained in the recombinant plasmid PTBG-1 was inserted into the *Xba*I–*Sma*I site of pchtk-2 (Perucho et al. 1980b). The resulting plasmid PBXP2.1 therefore contains the last three exons of the human *c*-Ha-*ras* oncogene. PTBG-1 is a recombinant plasmid that was previously constructed by inserting the *Bam*HI-linearized pSV2-*gpt* plasmid (Mulligan and Berg 1980) into the *Bam*HI site of PTB1 (Goldfarb et al. 1982) which contains the T24 bladder carcinoma oncogene, followed by deletion of the *Eco*RI fragment containing the *Bam*HI–*Eco*RI 4-kbp fragment of pBR322 and the *Eco*RI–*Bam*HI 1-kbp fragment of pSV2-*gpt*. PBXP2.1 was cleaved with *Xba*I, treated with bacterial alkaline phosphatase (BAP), and the 5-kbp *Xba*I fragments of λLNH-16 or λLD-H15 containing the first exon of the *c*-Ki-*ras* oncogene of PR310 and PR371 human lung carcinomas, respectively, were inserted into the *Xba*I site of PBXP2.1. Two plasmids were isolated after transformation of *E. coli* DH1 with the ligated DNA, which contained a *c*-Ki-*ras*–*c*-Ha-*ras* chimeric gene composed of the first exon of the *c*-Ki-*ras* oncogene of PR310 (PLNX2P) or PR371 (PLDX2P) and the last three exons of the *c*-Ha-*ras* oncogene of T24, in the correct orientation. (▭▭) λ Sequences of PTB1; (▭▭) human sequences that became ligated to the 3′ end of the T24 oncogene during the transfection experiment which originated the NIH-3T3 transformant (a-2) that was used to clone the T24 oncogene (Goldfarb et al. 1982); (▭▭) SV40 sequences of pSV2-*gpt* plasmid; (▭▭) bacterial *gpt* gene of pSV2-*gpt*; (▱) pBR322 sequences; (▭▭) chicken thymidine kinase sequences of pchtk2; (▭▭) T24 bladder carcinoma oncogene sequences; and (▬) PR310 and PR371 oncogene sequences. The boxes indicate the exons of the *c*-Ki-*ras* and *c*-Ha-*ras* oncogenes. (R) *Eco*RI; (H) *Hin*dIII; (B) *Bam*HI; (P) *Pvu*II; (X) *Xba*I; (Bg) *Bgl*II; (Sau) *Sau*3A; (Sa) *Sal*I; (St) *Stu*I; (K) *Kpn*I; (Sm) *Sma*I; (A) *Apa*I; (S) *Sst*I.

Similar studies with the *c*-Ki-*ras* oncogene have been hampered by the large size of this gene. We have cloned in λ47.1 recombinant phages over 40 kbp of the *c*-Ki-*ras* oncogene activated in two human lung carcinomas from different individuals. This allowed us to perform a

comparative study of the structure of the oncogenes activated in different tumors, as well as to determine the nature of the mutation responsible for their activation.

We have found that the structure of the *c*-Ki-*ras* oncogene resembles that of the *c*-Ha-*ras* oncogene in its

Table 1 Transforming Efficiencies of c-Ki-*ras* Chimeric Genes

Plasmid[a]	Total number foci[b] (foci/ng)[c]					
	Circular	*Hind*III	*Bam*HI	*Eco*RI	*Pvu*II	*Stu*I
PBXP2.1	0 (<0.005)	0 (<0.005)	N.D.	N.D.	N.D.	N.D.
PLNX2P	0 (<0.005)	0 (<0.005)	0 (<0.005)	0 (<0.005)	0 (<0.005)	0 (<0.005)
PLDX2P	55, 46 (0.25)	35, N.D. (0.17)	126, 81 (0.51)	90, 105 (0.48)	6, 0 (0.03)	0, N.D. (<0.005)
PTBG-1	350 (7.02)	N.D.	560 (11.2)	N.D.	N.D.	N.D.

[a]200 ng each of PBXP2.1, PLNX2P, and PLDX2P, and 50 ng of PTBG-1, either in circular form or cleaved to completion with the restriction endonucleases indicated, were mixed with 60 µg of NIH-3T3 carrier DNA. Transfection assays were performed by the addition of 30 µg of DNA to each of two plates of semiconfluent NIH-3T3 cultures, as previously described (Perucho et al. 1981), and foci of morphologically transformed cells were scored after 14–20 days.

[b]Total number of foci obtained in the experiment. When two numbers are listed, they represent the values obtained in two independent experiments.

[c]The average values of foci per nanogram of recombinant plasmid in the experiments are indicated in parentheses.

[d]ND, not determined.

intron-exon organization, and also that the mechanism of activation of the oncogenes of these lung carcinomas is similar to that previously described for c-Ha-*ras* oncogenes—single amino acid substitutions at positions 12 and 61 of the p21 protein. Although the examples studied so far are limited in number, it has become clear from these studies that these two positions in c-Ha-*ras* (Reddy et al. 1982; Tabin et al. 1982; Taparowski et al. 1982; Capon et al. 1983a; Yuasa et al. 1983) and c-Ki-*ras* (Shimizu et al. 1983a; Capon et al. 1983b; Nakano et al. 1984; and this work) oncogenes are hot-spots for mutagenesis resulting in the acquisition of oncogenic capability by the encoded p21 proteins. These results also suggest that the p21 proteins encoded by the *ras* genes are functionally equivalent. Our observation of transforming activity of c-Ki-*ras*–c-Ha-*ras* chimeric genes supports this hypothesis.

However, although the activity of these two oncogenes mutated in analogous structural regions is identical with respect to their ability to transform NIH-3T3 cells, their physiological role in normal cells must be different, as indicated by the evolutive pressure which has maintained both genes as functional entities despite their marked divergence in size.

Acknowledgments

We thank the excellent technical help of C. Lama, Dr. R. Ellis, and E. Scolnick for providing the v-Ki-*ras* clones, J. Koenig for preparation of the manuscript, and M. Inouye for his support. This work was also supported by a grant from the National Cancer Institute (CA33021).

References

Capon, D.J., E.Y. Chen, A.D. Levinson, P.H. Seeburg, and D.V. Goeddel. 1983a. Complete nucleotide sequence of the T24 human bladder carcinoma oncogene and its normal homologue. *Nature* **302**: 33.

Capon, D.J., P.H. Seeburg, J.P. McGrath, J.S. Hayflick, U. Edman, A.D. Levinson, and D.V. Goeddel. 1983b. Activation of ki-*ras*-2 gene in human colon and lung carcinomas by two different point mutations. *Nature* **304**: 507.

Chang, E.H., M.A. Gonda, R.W. Ellis, E.M. Scolnick, and D.R. Lowy. 1982. Human genome contains four gene homologous to transforming genes of Harvey and Kirsten murine sarcoma viruses. *Proc. Natl. Acad. Sci.* **79**: 4848.

Cooper, G.M. 1982. Cellular transforming genes. *Science* **218**: 801.

Der, C.J., T.G. Krontiris, and G.M. Cooper. 1982. Transforming genes of human bladder and lung carcinoma cell lines are homologous to the *ras* genes of Harvey and Kirsten sarcoma virus. *Proc. Natl. Acad. Sci.* **79**: 3637.

Ellis, R.W., D. DeFeo, T.Y. Shih, M.A. Gonda, H.A. Young, N. Tsuchida, D.R. Lowy, and E.M. Scolnick. 1981. The p21 *src* genes of Harvey and Kirsten sarcoma viruses originate from divergent members of a family of normal vertebrate genes. *Nature* **292**: 506.

Fogh, J., N.C. Dracopoli, M.S. Pollack, and M.H. Wigler. 1983. Human bladder carcinoma lines *in vitro* and in athymic nude mice. In *Advances in bladder cancer research 2nd National Bladder Conference*, Sarasota, Florida, January ed. p. 94.

Fogh, J., T. Orfeo, J. Tiso, and F.E. Sharkey. 1979. Establishment of human colon carcinoma lines in nude mice. *Exp. Cell Biol.* **47**: 136.

Fogh, J., J. Tiso, T. Orfeo, F.E. Sharkey, W.P. Daniels, and J.M. Fogh. 1980. Thirty-four lines of six human tumor categories established in nude mice. *J. Natl. Cancer Inst.* **64**: 745.

Fried, M., M. Griffiths, B. Davies, G. Bjursell, G. LaMantia, and L. Lania. 1983. Isolation of cellular DNA sequences that allow expression of adjacent genes. *Proc. Natl. Acad. Sci.* **80**: 2117.

Goldfarb, M., K. Shimizu, M. Perucho, and M. Wigler. 1982. Isolation and preliminary characterization of a human transforming gene from T24 bladder carcinoma cell. *Nature* **296**: 404.

McGrath, J.P., D.J. Capon, D.H. Smith, E.Y. Chen, P.H. Seeburg, D.V. Goeddel, and A.D. Levinson. 1983. Structure and organization of the human Ki-*ras* protooncogene and a related processed pseudogene. *Nature* **304**: 501.

Mulligan, R.C. and P. Berg. 1980. Expression of a bacterial gene in mammalian cells. *Science* **209**: 1422.

Murray, M.J., B.Z. Shilo, C. Shih, D. Cowing, H.W. Hsu, and R.A. Weinberg. 1981. Three different human tumor cell lines contain different oncogenes. *Cell* **25**: 355.

Nakano, H., F. Yamamoto, C. Neville, D. Evans, T. Mizuno, and M. Perucho. 1984. Isolation of transforming sequences of two human lung carcinomas: Structural and functional analysis of the activated *c-K-ras* oncogenes. *Proc. Natl. Acad. Sci.* **81**: 71.

Parada, L., C. Tabin, C. Shih, and R. Weinberg. 1982. Human CJ bladder carcinoma oncogene is homologue of Harvey sarcoma virus *ras* gene. *Nature* **297**: 474.

Perucho, M., D. Hanahan, and M. Wigler. 1980a. Genetic and physical linkage of exogenous sequences in transformed cells. *Cell* **22**: 309.

Perucho, M., D. Hanahan, L. Lipsich, and M. Wigler. 1980b. Isolation of the chicken thymidine kinase gene by plasmid rescue. *Nature* **285**: 207.

Perucho, M., M. Goldfarb, K. Shimizu, C. Lama, J. Fogh, and M. Wigler. 1981. Human-tumor-derived cell lines contain common and different transforming genes. *Cell* **27**: 467.

Pulciani, S., E. Santos, A.V. Lauver, L.K. Long, S.A. Aaronson, and M. Barbacid. 1982. Oncogenes in solid human tumors. *Nature* **300**: 539.

Reddy, E.P., R. Reynolds, E. Santos, and M. Barbacid. 1982. A point mutation is responsible for the acquisition of transforming properties by the T24 human bladder carcinoma oncogene. *Nature* **300**: 149.

Santos, E., S.R. Tronick, S.A. Aaronson, S. Pulciani, and M. Barbacid. 1982. T24 human bladder carcinoma oncogene is an activated form of the normal human homologue of BALB- and Harvey-MSV transforming genes. *Nature* **298**: 343.

Shimizu, K., D. Birnbaum, M.A. Ruley, O. Fasano, Y. Suard, L. Edlund, E. Taparowsky, M. Goldfarb, and M. Wigler. 1983a. Structure of the Ki-*ras* gene of the human lung carcinoma cell line Calu-1. *Nature* **304**: 497.

Shimizu, K., M. Goldfarb, Y. Suard, M. Perucho, Y. Li, T. Kamata, J. Feramisco, E. Stavenzer, J. Fogh, and M.H. Wigler. 1983b. Three human transforming genes are related to the viral *ras* oncogenes. *Proc. Natl. Acad. Sci.* **80**: 2112.

Tabin, C.J., S.M. Bradley, C.I. Bargmann, R.A. Weinberg, A.G. Papageorge, E.M. Scolnick, R. Dhar, D.R. Lowy, and E.H. Chang. 1982. Mechanism of activation of a human oncogene. *Nature* **300**: 143.

Taparowsky, E., Y. Suard, O. Fasano, K. Shimizu, M. Goldfarb, and M. Wigler. 1982. Activation of the T-24 bladder carcinoma transforming gene is linked to a single amino acid change. *Nature* **300**: 762.

Weinberg, R.A. 1981. Use of transfection to analyze genetic information and malignant transformation. *Biochim. Biophys. Acta* **651**: 25.

Yuasa, Y., S.K. Srivastava, C.Y. Dunn, J.S. Rhim, E.P. Reddy, and S.A. Aaronson. 1983. Acquisition of transforming properties by alternative point mutations within c-bas/has human proto-oncogene. *Nature* **303**: 775.

Carcinogen- and Radiation-induced Mouse Lymphomas Contain an Activated *c-ras* Oncogene

I. Guerrero, A. Villasante, A. Mayer,* and A. Pellicer

Department of Pathology and Kaplan Cancer Center, New York University Medical Center, New York, New York 10016

The study of thymic lymphoma development in inbred strains of mice provides an excellent model system for tumor development in humans. Many human cancers are thought to result from exposure to radiation or chemical carcinogens occurring several years prior to onset of tumor growth. A defined set of protocols involving either radiation or various chemical carcinogens has been elaborated to induce reproducibly a very high incidence of thymic lymphoma in treated mice (Kaplan 1967; Joshi and Frei 1970; Ball and McCarter 1971; Duran-Reynals and Cook 1974; Meruelo et al. 1981; see Fig. 1). The use of inbred laboratory strains provides a reproducible genetic background for these studies. A long latent period intervenes between exposure to the carcinogen at a young age and outgrowth of the lymphoma many months later in middle age.

In the past few years, a powerful technique has been worked out to study the process of neoplasia. It was observed that high-molecular-weight DNA from several transformed cell lines and primary tumors has the ability to "transform" NIH-3T3 cells that are exposed to the DNA in the form of a calcium phosphate precipitate (Shih et al. 1979, 1981; Cooper and Neiman 1980; Cooper et al. 1980; Krontiris and Cooper 1981; Lane et al. 1981; Perucho et al. 1981). The transformation is observed as a low frequency of focus formation, that is, clonal outgrowth of morphologically altered cells with enhanced growth potential over the background of untransformed contact-inhibited NIH-3T3 cells. Transformation of recipient NIH-3T3 cells is due to uptake and incorporation of donor DNA that imparts, in dominant fashion, altered growth and morphologic properties. Attention has been focused on the molecular cloning of DNA sequences with "transforming" potential from a variety of tumors and transformed cell lines because of the widely held thesis that these genes may be responsible for the neoplastic phenotypes of the tumor cells from which they are derived (for review, see Cooper 1982).

Recently, several genes from human tumor cell lines have been isolated (Goldfarb et al. 1982; Pulciani et al.

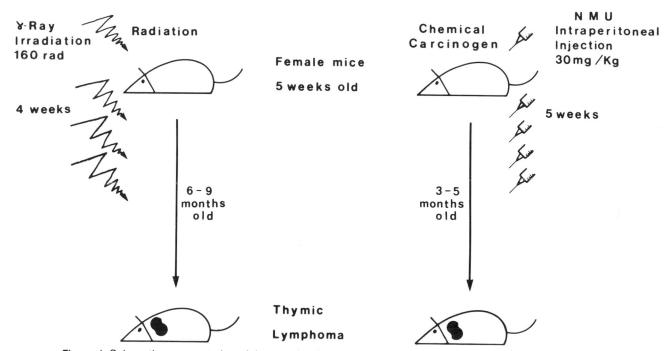

Figure 1 Schematic representation of the way thymic tumors are induced on mice by carcinogen and radiation.

*Present address: University of Miami Medical School, Miami, Florida 33101.

1982b; Shih and Weinberg 1982; Shimizu et al. 1983a) and the sequences responsible for transformation have been identified as cellular counterparts of the transforming genes of the *ras* family (Parada et al. 1982; Santos et al. 1982) that were previously found in certain rodent retroviruses.

During the last few months, a report appeared showing activation of the Ha-*ras* gene in carcinogen-induced (and subsequently transplanted) skin carcinomas (Balmain and Pragnell 1983). We have obtained activation of the N-*ras* and Ki-*ras* genes in murine tumors of the lympho-hemopoietic system induced by means of carcinogen or γ-radiation. These findings should be instrumental in studying the early stages of carcinogenesis in this model in vivo system.

Materials and Methods

Induction of the tumors

Thymic lymphomas were induced (see Fig. 1) by: (1) intraperitoneal injection of mice with 30 mg/kg body weight of the chemical carcinogen *N*-nitrosomethyl urea (NMU) once a week for 5 consecutive weeks, starting with 35–60 day-old animals and (2) exposure at similar ages to whole-body γ-radiation doses of 160 rads once a week for 4 consecutive weeks. The mice used, derived from crosses between the inbred AKR and RF strains, had very low incidences of spontaneous thymic lymphoma. The tumors appeared 3–5 months after injection of the carcinogen and between 5–8 months after radiation.

Transformation of cells

Stocks of NIH-3T3 and Rat-2 cells were obtained from M. Perucho (State University at Stony Brook, New York) and maintained at low density in Dulbecco's modified Eagle's medium (DMEM) with 10% calf serum. Every 2 months, new cells were thawed and extreme care was taken to prevent stock cells from becoming confluent.

DNA from tumors or primary foci was used to transform NIH-3T3 or Rat-2 cells by precipitation with calcium phosphate (Graham and Van der Eb 1973; Wigler et al. 1978; Pellicer et al. 1980). Two to three weeks later, transformed foci growing in 5% serum were picked up and expanded, and their DNAs were extracted.

Extraction of RNA and DNA, electrophoresis, and hybridization

RNA was extracted from normal and transformed cells by adding to the cell monolayer a solution of 4 M guanidine thiocyanate, 50 mM Tris-HCl (pH 7.6), 10 mM EDTA, 2% Sarkosyl, and 0.14 M β-mercaptoethanol. The viscous cell lysate was homogenized and heated at 65°C for 10 minutes. An equal volume of hot phenol was added, mixed, and maintained at 65°C for 10 minutes, with occasional shaking. After that, a volume equal to the original lysate was added of both 0.1 M NaAc (pH 5.0) and chloroform:isoamyl alcohol (24:1) and was kept for another 10 minutes at 65°C with intermittent shaking. The mixture was chilled on ice and spun to separate the

aqueous phase, which was extracted again in the same way with phenol:chloroform:isoamyl alcohol (50:48:2). After a final extraction with chloroform:isoamyl alcohol (24:1), the aqueous phase was precipitated with two volumes of ethanol. The poly (A)$^+$ RNAs were obtained by chromatography of the redissolved precipitates on oligo(dT)-cellulose columns and were electrophoresed in agarose-formaldehyde gels and transferred to nitro-cellulose filters (Corces et al. 1981).

Thymic tumors appeared in the induced mice after 3 to 9 months. After disruption of the tumors through a wire mesh, high-molecular-weight DNAs of these tissues were obtained as described (Corces et al. 1981).

DNAs were digested with restriction endonuclease under standard conditions, fractionated by electrophoresis through an agarose gel, and transferred to nitrocellulose using the technique of Southern (1975).

Filters containing DNA or RNA were blocked and hybridized in Denhardt's mixture (0.02% each of bovine serum albumin, Ficoll, and polyvinyl pyrrolidone), 5× SSC (0.15 M NaCl, 0.015 M sodium citrate), 50% formamide, 100 μg/ml of sonicated and denatured calf thymus DNA, 10 mM EDTA, and 0.1% SDS for 16 hours at 42°C. Filters were washed in 0.1% SDS and 2× SSC at room temperature and afterward in solutions of decreasing salt concentration (2×, 1×, and 0.4× SSC) at 65°C and autoradiographed.

Labeling of protein and immunoprecipitation

Cells were labeled metabolically with [^{35}S]methionine (50 μCi ml^{-1}, 500 Ci mmole^{-1}) for 12 hours. Lysates of these were immunoprecipitated by monoclonal antibody Y13-259 (kindly provided by Dr. E. Scolnick [Furth et al. 1982]). This antibody is specific for p21 and reacts with p21 from all three *ras* genes (Ha-*ras*, Ki-*ras*, and N-*ras*). The immunoprecipitates were dissolved in electrophoresis sample buffer and electrophoresed in 12% SDS-polyacrylamide gel. The gel was dried and subjected to fluorography.

Molecular cloning and restriction mapping

DNA was cleaved with *Hin*dIII and appropriate areas of the gel containing the band with the first exon were collected, DNA extracted from the agarose by electroelution, purified by chromatography through Elutip (Schleicher and Schüell), and precipitated with ethanol. The DNA fragments were ligated with λ47.1 *Hin*dIII arms at a concentration of 0.5 mg/ml for 48 hours at 15°C. Subsequently, they were packaged according to Maniatis et al. (1982) and plated in BNN45. The efficiencies were around 10^6 recombinant phages/μg of DNA. The phages were screened by standard techniques (Maniatis et al. 1982) using as a probe an *Sst*II–*Xba*I fragment derived from the HiHi 3 plasmid containing the Ki-*ras* sequences. Positive plaques were rescreened, isolated, and grown up in mass culture to obtain phage DNA (Maniatis et al. 1982).

The restriction map was obtained by partial and limit single and double digests of the recombinant insert with different restriction enzymes.

Results

Tumor DNA induces formation of foci in rodent fibroblasts

The criteria for transformation was the formation of foci at 5% serum with cells showing morphological traits of oncogenic transformation (round shape, increased refractility, and disorganized pattern of growth).

All DNAs were tested at least twice with consistent results. As controls, brain DNAs were used from the same animals from which thymomas were tested: There has not been a single focus from these DNAs, so the appearance of transformed foci with thymoma DNAs is statistically highly significant.

We also have used a rat cell line, Rat-2 (Topp 1981), because of its morphologic appearance, growth behavior, and extremely low spontaneous overgrowth rate; these characteristics are very suitable for such studies, although the transformation efficiency of this cell line is lower than that of NIH-3T3. The advantage of using this cell line is that it belongs to a different species. Although very closely related, mouse and rat present differences in the restriction pattern of their genes that can be exploited to demonstrate transformation.

In the NMU-induced thymomas, five out of six tumors were positive in the transformation assay; in the radiation-induced assay, four out of seven activated an oncogene detectable by this protocol. The efficiencies of transformation are similar to those described for the human tumor cell lines, i.e., 0.1–0.2 foci/μg of DNA in the NIH-3T3 cells, with an order of magnitude lower in the Rat-2 cells for the NMU-induced tumors and three to four times less for those induced by radiation.

Transformed foci contain extra copies of c-ras oncogenes

The transformants were tested for the presence of extra bands or for amplification of the endogenous sequences in Southern blots probed with the three ras genes described so far. Figure 2 presents the analysis of three positive NMU-induced tumors with an N-ras probe. The 3T3 transformants display two distinct patterns (Fig. 2a). Some clearly show extra bands, indicating that a new N-ras gene has entered the cell at the time of acquisition of the transformed phenotype (lanes C and G). Others show an evident increase in the endogenous N-ras mouse band (lanes B, D–F) consistent with extra copies of the N-ras gene present in these transformants. All transformations were performed in the presence of a plasmid pAT153 (devoid of poisonous sequences) (Twigg and Sherratt 1980; Lusky and Botchan 1981) as cotransforming agent, all foci contained plasmid sequences indicating transformation (data not shown), and DNAs from all of them induced secondary foci. Southern blots as in Figure 2 probed with Ha-ras or Ki-ras did not have any extra bands or amplification of these genes (data not shown). It appears, therefore, that all positive thymomas analyzed induced by this carcinogen activate the mouse N-ras gene. To confirm that the extra band was transferred with the oncogenic phenotype and to generate rat transformants useful in the study of the properties of this oncogene, DNA from one of the 3T3-transformants (Fig. 2a, lane C) was used to induce foci in Rat-2 cells. The Southern analysis of these rat transformants, shown in Figure 2b, further confirms that the mouse gene homologous to the human N-ras segregates

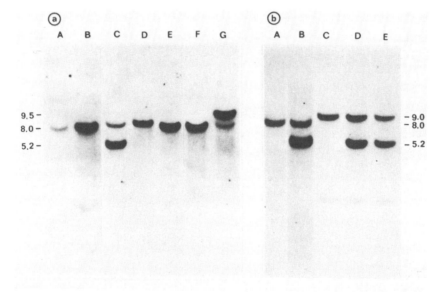

Figure 2 Analysis of the N-ras sequences present in DNA of mouse and rat transformants from carcinogen-induced tumors. Normal and transformant DNAs (20 μg) were digested with restriction endonuclease EcoRI, fractionated by electrophoresis through a 0.8% agarose gel, and transferred to nitrocellulose paper. Filters were incubated with 10^7 cpm of ^{32}P-labeled probe (specific activity >10^8 cpm/μg). The probe was a 1-kb fragment of the human N-ras gene kindly provided by M. Wigler. The exact location of the fragment (R fragment) in the human N-ras gene is in Shimizu et al. (1983a). (a) Analysis of 3T3 primary transformants. (Lane A) NIH-3T3 DNA. Transformants from different tumors are: (lanes B and C) tumor I, (lanes D and E) tumor II, (lanes F and G) tumor III. (b) Analysis of rat secondary transformants. (Lanes A and C) NIH-3T3 DNA and Rat-2 DNA; (lane B) 3T3 transformant from tumor I; (lanes D and E) rat transformants obtained with DNA from lane B.

with the transformed phenotype and must be the activated oncogene in this system. Moreover, it seems to be amplified in all transformants analyzed. Figure 0 presents a similar study with one of the radiation-induced tumors that gave foci in the transformation of NIH-3T3. It shows the Southern blot of normal and transformed DNAs digested with *Hind*III and hybridized with the Ki-*ras* probe from a Kirsten sarcoma virus cDNA clone (Ellis et al. 1981) kindly provided by E. Scolnick (Merck, Sharp, and Dohme). The normal DNA and the transformant induced by the NMU tumor show the same pattern, and the band intensities are similar in both DNAs (lanes A and B). In lane C, the DNA of the transformants obtained from the radiation-induced tumor shows an appreciable increase in the intensity of the two lower bands, indicating that extra copies are present; additionally, in the upper part of the lane there is an extra band, consistent with the idea of a new Ki-*ras* gene being introduced into the cell. The new band might have been generated in the DNA extraction and manipulation or by excision during the transformation process. We already know that the upper band contains the first exon, and presumably the 5′ end of the gene, as will be shown below. The rat cell transformants can clarify this additionally and the blot of such transformants is presented in Figure 3, lanes E–F. The rat endogenous Ki-*ras* sequences give a very different pattern from those of the mouse, as can be observed by comparing lane A with lane D. Due to this useful distinction, it is evident that the DNA from normal rat cells and a rat transformant obtained from DNA originally derived from a carcinogen-induced tumor (Fig. 3, lanes D and E) show the same pattern, confirming once more that the carcinogen-induced tumors do not have an activated Ki-*ras* oncogene. In contrast, lane F shows the profile of a secondary rat transformant from the primary in lane C (from a radiation-induced tumor) and it is clear that a mouse Ki-*ras* pattern is superimposed on that of the endogenous rat. The upper band corresponds to the lower of the doublet in lane C: Everything is consistent with the transfer of a mouse Ki-*ras* gene from the radiation-induced tumor to the NIH-3T3 and subsequently to the rat cells.

We also tested tumor DNA for the presence of gross rearrangements in the activated oncogenes. All tumors examined that were positive or negative in the transformation assay gave the same restriction pattern as normal brain DNA (data not shown).

Transformants obtained with tumor DNA show increased expression of N-*ras* oncogenes

Levels of transcription of these genes in the mouse transformants were also analyzed. In the N-*ras* transformants (by carcinogen), three transcripts of 3.9, 2.4, and 1.5 kb similar to the ones described in humans (Hall et al. 1983) were detected. As shown in Figure 4a, the 3.9-

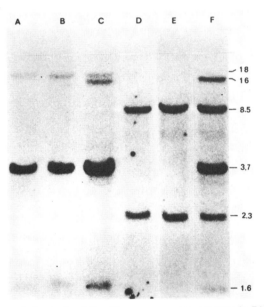

Figure 3 Analysis of the Ki-*ras* sequences present in DNA of mouse and rat transformants from carcinogen- and radiation-induced tumors. The transformant DNAs were digested with *Hind*III and the electrophoresis, transfer, and hybridization were as in Fig. 2, except that the probe used was an *Sst*II–*Xba*I fragment from the HiHi 3 plasmid (Ellis et al. 1981) (kindly provided by E. Scolnick) containing the cloned Ki-*ras* viral cDNA sequences. (Lane *A*) 3T3 DNA; (lane *B*) 3T3 transformant from tumor I (carcinogen); (lane *C*) 3T3 transformant from tumor X (radiation); (lane *D*) Rat-2-DNA; (lane *E*) rat transformant obtained with DNA from lane *B*; (lane *F*) rat transformant obtained with DNA from lane *C*.

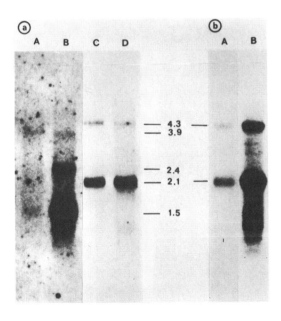

Figure 4 Analysis of the *ras* transcripts in NIH-3T3 transformants obtained from carcinogen- and radiation-induced tumors. The poly (A)⁺ RNAs were electrophoresed in agarose-formaldehyde gels and transferred to nitrocellulose filters (Corces et al. 1981). The hybridization fragments were the same N-*ras* (*a*) (Lanes *A* and *B*) or Ki-*ras* (*b* and *a*) (lanes *C* and *D*) probes described in Figs. 2 and 3. The filters were similarly treated, washed, and autoradiographed. (*a*) (Lanes *A* and *C*) 3T3 RNA; (lanes *B* and *D*) 3T3 transformant from tumor I (carcinogen). (*b*) (Lane *A*) 3T3 RNA; (lane *B*) 3T3 transformant from tumor X (radiation).

kb transcript is at the same level in normal and transformed cells, whereas the two smallest ones show at least 10-fold increase in the transformed cells and are the likely candidates to encode for the transforming protein p21, as will be seen below. Figure 4b shows the same kind of study for the Ki-*ras*-activated oncogene (radiation) and one observes here the presence of two main transcripts that display much greater intensity than in the normal cells. Hybridization of the RNAs, as shown in Figure 4a (lanes A and B), with a Ki-*ras* probe (lanes C and D) shows the same intensity in normal and transformed cells, indicating that the N-*ras* transcripts and their increase are specific.

To obtain a more complete characterization of the system, [35S]methionine-labeled normal and transformed cell extracts were immunoprecipitated with a monoclonal antibody against p21 (Furth et al. 1982), kindly provided by Dr. E. Scolnick.

The results of these experiments are shown in Figure 5. Two different patterns were obtained: In the N-*ras* transformants (activated by carcinogen), there is a marked increase of the p21 protein and moreover the mobility of the polypeptide has been altered (Fig. 5a, lane B; Fig. 5b, lane C) as reported for activated human oncogenes (Reddy et al. 1982; Tabin et al. 1982; Taparowsky et al. 1982). On the other hand, the p21 immunoprecipitated from Ki-*ras*-activated transformants (radiation) shows a clear increase in the transformed cells with respect to the normal parental lines, but in this case no change in mobility is detected.

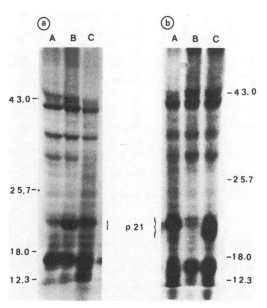

Figure 5 Immunoprecipitation of p21$^{c\text{-}ras}$ from normal and transformed cells. (*a*) Analysis of the normal and transformed mouse cells. (Lane *A*) NIH-3T3; (lane *B*) 3T3 transformant from tumor I (carcinogen); (lane *C*) 3T3 transformant from tumor X (radiation). (*b*) Analysis of the normal and transformed rat cells. (Lane *A*) Rat secondary transformant originally derived from tumor X (radiation); (lane *B*) Rat-2; (lane *C*) rat secondary transformant originally derived from tumor I (carcinogen).

Partial molecular characterization of the mouse Ki-*ras* oncogene

We have cloned a 17-kb *Hind*III fragment from the brain of the mouse that gave tumor X, which showed an activated Ki-*ras* oncogene and the homologous 14-kb piece from a rat transformant derived from tumor X. The rationale behind cloning this particular fragment is that we had identified it as the one containing the first coding exon by using specific probes in genomic blots. Evidence from other laboratories working in the human system indicates that this exon is a likely target for the expected mutation (Capon et al. 1983; Nakano et al. 1984; Shimizu et al. 1983b).

Through a series of double digests, we have obtained a restriction map that is shown in Figure 6. By probing different digests of this recombinant clone with a Ki-*ras* probe (Ellis et al. 1981), we have localized the first coding exon to a 0.65-kb *Eco*RI fragment located to the right of the map (Fig. 6). Comparing the maps obtained from normal mouse DNA and from the transformant, it is noticeable that they differ on the left-hand side, thus indicating that this region is dispensable for transformation, and, therefore, the 5′ portion of the map most likely contains flanking sequences not belonging to the gene. This difference also indicates that the beginning of the gene should be contained within the cloned fragment. As expected, no differences are seen between the two clones (normal and transformant) in the right side of the map (where the gene is supposed to be located) at that level of resolution. The location of the exon in this small *Eco*RI fragment will facilitate the sequencing strategy required to examine this crucial part of the gene.

Discussion

We have shown that DNA extracted directly from tumors obtained in mice by carcinogen (NMU) or radiation induction (Fig. 1) can transform rodent fibroblasts in culture using the foci formation as an assay. There is only one other report in the literature using solid tumors (Pulciani et al. 1982a). The frequency of transformation is very high in NMU-induced tumors (5/6) and a little lower in radiation (4/7). In the tumors analyzed so far, it appears to be activation of a different oncogene depending on the etiological agent: carcinogen, N-*ras*, and radiation, Ki-*ras* (Figs. 2, 3, and 4). Some preliminary results show additional copies of the Ki-*ras* gene in transformants obtained from cell lines derived from radiation-induced thymomas (in collaboration with D. Meruelo, New York University Medical Center), further reaffirming that the radiation-induced tumors contain an activated Ki-*ras* oncogene.

In all transformants analyzed, there is amplification of the transforming oncogene, although this phenomenon is not observed in the tumor DNAs. Gross rearrangements are not detected in these genes.

There is an increased amount of transcripts representing the oncogenes in the 3T3 transformants and this increase is specific for the gene responsible for the transformation (Fig. 4). The increase in the transcripts for the activated genes might be due to the gene am-

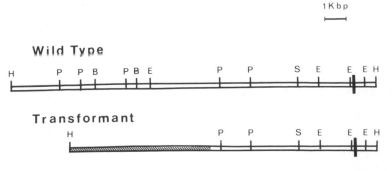

Mouse Ki-ras Exon 1

Figure 6 Restriction maps representing the 5' region of the mouse Ki-*ras* gene from normal and transformant DNA. The recombinant clones were obtained as explained in Methods and the inserts restricted with the enzymes indicated. (E) EcoRI; (B) BglII; (P) PvuII; (S) SstII; (H) HindIII. (□) Mouse Ki-*ras* sequences; (▨) adjacent sequences in the transformant that belong to rat DNA or carrier.

plification present in the transformants, to an enhanced rate of transcription, or to a greater stability of these messages in the transformed cells; due to the large increase, it is likely that a combination of two or more of these mechanisms play a role. The increased expression is also observed at the protein level (Fig. 5) where, besides the elevated levels of p21 in the mouse and rat transformants in the N-*ras*-induced foci, there is a change in the mobility of the protein that might be due to an altered structure of the polypeptide.

Formation of foci does not seem to be due to a retroviral gene but to a cellular one, because in the Southern patterns the newly introduced genes mimic the endogenous ones. Nevertheless, the promoter insertion mechanism of activation is not completely ruled out, because there is increased expression in all transformants analyzed.

The cloning of a portion of the Ki-*ras* gene (from transformant and normal DNA) containing the first exon (Fig. 6) will allow us in the near future to compare the sequences and find out if there is a point mutation in this region; if that is the case, we will subclone a fragment containing the first exon from the transformant into a plasmid containing the last three exons of a normal human Ha-*ras* oncogene and will analyze the ability of this hybrid gene to transform rodent cells. We are also in the process of cloning the second exon from the Ki-*ras* gene and the whole N-*ras* gene from normal and transformant DNAs.

We think that the high incidence of N-*ras* activation with the carcinogen NMU should make this system useful in the study of the genesis of leukemias and for understanding the alterations in preneoplastic stages. For example, precursor cells for thymomas have been reported to be initially in the bone marrow (Haran-Ghera 1973), which, in contrast to many other tissues, can be readily cultured and transplanted, thus providing a powerful tool for dissecting the steps leading to the development of these malignancies.

Acknowledgments

We thank M. Wigler (Cold Spring Harbor Laboratory) for the N-*ras* probe; E. Scolnick (Merck, Sharp, and Dohme) for the monoclonal antibody against p21 and for the Ki-*ras* probe; M. Perucho (State University at Stony Brook, New York) for his ample advice, recipient cells, and constant moral support; P. Calzada and L. Lloyd for excellent technical assistance; and Jon Hart for the preparation of the manuscript. The work has been supported by National Institutes of Health grant CA-16239. A.P. is an Irma Hirschl-Monique Weill-Caulier award recipient.

References

Ball, J.K. and J. A. McCarter. 1971. Repeated demonstration of mouse leukemia virus after treatment with chemical carcinogens. *J. Natl. Cancer Inst.* **46**: 751.

Balmain, A. and I.B. Pragnell. 1983. Mouse skin carcinomas induced *in vivo* by chemical carcinogens have a transforming Harvey-ras oncogene. *Nature.* **303**: 72.

Capon, D.J., P.D. Seeburg, J.P. McGrath, J.S. Hayflick, U. Edman, A.D. Levinson, and D.V. Goeddel. 1983. Activation of Ki-ras 2 gene in human colon and lung carcinomas by two different point mutations. *Nature* **304**: 507.

Cooper, G.M. 1982. Cellular transforming genes. *Science* **218**: 801.

Cooper, G.M. and P. Neiman. 1980. Transforming genes of neoplasms induced by avian lymphoid leukosis viruses. *Nature* **287**: 656.

Cooper, G.M., S. Okenquist, and L. Silverman. 1980. Transforming activity of DNA of chemically transformed and normal cells. *Nature* **284**: 418.

Corces, V., A. Pellicer, R. Axel, and M. Meselson. 1981. Integration, transcription and control of a *Drosophila* heat-shock gene in mouse cells. *Proc. Natl. Acad. Sci.* **78**: 7038.

Duran-Reynals, M.L. and C. Cook. 1974. Resistance to skin tumorigenesis by 3-methylcholanthrene in mice susceptible to leukemia. *J. Natl. Cancer Inst.* **52**: 1001.

Ellis, R.W., D. De Feo, T.Y. Shih, M.A. Gonda, H.A. Young, N. Tsuchida, D.R. Lowy, and E.M. Scolnick. 1981. The p21 src genes of Harvey and Kirsten sarcoma viruses originate from divergent members of a family of normal vertebrate genes. *Nature* **292**: 506.

Furth, M.E., L.J. Davis, B. Fleur de Lys, and E.M. Scolnick. 1982. Monoclonal antibodies to the p21 products of the transforming gene of Harvey murine sarcoma virus and of the cellular ras gene family. *J. Virol.* **43**: 294.

Goldfarb, M., K. Shimizu, M. Perucho, and M. Wigler. 1982. Isolation and preliminary characterization of a human transforming gene from T24 bladder carcinoma cells. *Nature* **296**: 404.

Graham, F.L. and A.J. Van der Eb. 1973. A new technique for the assay of infectivity of human adenovirus 5 DNA. *Virology* **52**: 456.

Hall, A., C.J. Marshall, N.-K. Spurr, and R.A. Weiss. 1983. Identification of a transforming gene in two human sarcoma cell lines as a new member of the ras gene family located on chromosome 1. *Nature* **303:** 396.

Haran-Ghera, N. 1973. Relationship between tumor cells and host in chemical leukemogenesis. *Nat. New Biol.* **246:** 84.

Joshi, V.V. and J.V. Frei. 1970. Effects of dose and schedule of methylnitrosourea on incidence of malignant lymphoma in adult female mice. *J. Natl. Cancer Inst.* **45:** 335.

Kaplan, A.S. 1967. On the natural history of the murine leukemias: Presidential address. *Cancer Res.* **27:** 1325.

Krontiris, T.G. and G.M. Cooper. 1981. Transforming activity of human tumor DNA. *Proc. Natl. Acad. Sci.* **78:** 1181.

Lane, M.-A., A. Sainten, and G.M. Cooper. 1981. Activation of related transforming genes in mouse and human mammary carcinomas. *Proc. Natl. Acad. Sci.* **78:** 5185.

Lusky, M. and M. Botchan. 1981. Inhibition of SV40 replication in simian cells by specific pBR322 DNA sequences. *Nature* **293:** 79.

Maniatis, T., E.F. Fritch, and J. Sambrook, eds. 1982. *Molecular cloning: A laboratory manual.* Cold Spring Harbor Laboratory, Cold Spring Harbor, New York.

Meruelo, D., M. Offer, and N. Flieger. 1981. Genetics of susceptibility to radiation induced leukemia. *J. Exp. Med.* **154:** 1201.

Nakano, H., F. Yamamoto, C. Neville, D. Evans, T. Mizuno, and M. Perucho. 1984. Isolation of transforming sequences of two human lung carcinomas. Structural and functional analysis of the activated c-K-ras oncogene. *Proc. Natl. Acad. Sci.* **81:** 71.

Parada, L.F., C.S. Tabin, C. Shih, and R. Weinberg. 1982. Human EJ bladder carcinoma oncogene is homologue of Harvey sarcoma virus ras gene. *Nature* **297:** 474.

Pellicer, A., D. Robins, B. Wold, R. Sweet, J. Jackson, I. Lowy, J. Roberts, G.-K. Sim, S. Silverstein, and R. Axel. 1980. Altering genotype and phenotype by DNA-mediated gene transfer. *Science* **209:** 1414.

Perucho, M., M. Goldfarb, K. Shimizu, C. Lama, J. Fogh, and M. Wigler. 1981. Human-tumor-derived-cell lines contain common and different transforming genes. *Cell* **27:** 467.

Pulciani, S., E. Santos, A.B. Lauver, L.K. Long, S.A. Aaronson, and M. Barbacid. 1982a. Oncogenes in solid human tumors. *Nature* **300:** 539.

Pulciani, S., E. Santos, A.B. Lauver, L.K. Long, R.C. Robbins, and M. Barbacid. 1982b. Oncogenes in human tumor cell lines: Molecular cloning of a transforming gene from human bladder carcinoma cells. *Proc. Natl. Acad. Sci.* **79:** 2845.

Reddy, E.P., R.K. Reynolds, E. Santos, and M. Barbacid. 1982. A point mutation is responsible for the acquisition of transforming properties by the T24 human bladder carcinoma oncogene. *Nature* **300:** 149.

Santos, E., S.R. Tronick, S.A. Aaronson, S. Pulciani, and M. Barbacid. 1982. T24 human bladder carcinoma oncogene is an activated form of the normal human homologue of BALB- and Harvey-MSV transforming genes. *Nature* **298:** 343.

Shih, C. and R.A. Weinberg. 1982. Isolation of a transforming sequence from a human bladder carcinoma cell line. *Cell* **29:** 161.

Shih, C., C. Padhy, M. Murray, and R.A. Weinberg. 1981. Transforming genes of carcinomas and neuroblastomas introduced into mouse fibroblasts. *Nature* **290:** 261.

Shih, C., B.-Z. Shilo, M.P. Goldfarb, A. Dannenberg, and R.A. Weinberg. 1979. Passage of phenotypes of chemically transformed cells via transfection of DNA and chromatin. *Proc. Natl. Acad. Sci.* **76:** 5714.

Shimizu, K., M. Goldfarb, M. Perucho, and M. Wigler. 1983a. Isolation and preliminary characterization of the transforming gene of a human neuroblastoma cell line. *Proc. Natl. Acad. Sci.* **80:** 383.

Shimizu, K., D. Birnbaum, M.A. Ruley, O. Fasano, Y. Suard, L. Edlund, E. Taparowsky, M. Goldfarb, and M. Wigler. 1983b. Structure of the Ki-ras gene of the human lung carcinoma cell line Calu-1. *Nature* **304:** 497.

Southern, E.M. 1975. Detection of specific sequences among DNA fragments separated by gel electrophoresis. *J. Mol. Biol.* **98:** 503.

Tabin, C.J., S.M. Bradley, C.I. Gargmann, R.A. Weinberg, A.G. Papageorge, E.M. Scolnick, R. Dhar, D.R. Lowy, and E.H. Chang. 1982. Mechanism of activation of a human oncogene. *Nature* **300:** 143.

Taparowsky, E., Y. Suard, O. Fasano, K. Shimizu, M. Goldfarb, and M. Wigler. 1982. Activation of the T24 bladder carcinoma transforming gene is linked to a single amino acid change. *Nature* **300:** 262.

Topp, W. 1981. Normal rat cell lines deficient in nuclear thymidine kinase. *Virology* **113:** 408.

Twigg, A.J. and D. Sherratt. 1980. Trans-complementable copy-number mutant of plasmid ColE1. *Nature* **283:** 216.

Wigler, M., A. Pellicer, S. Silverstein, and R. Axel. 1978. Biochemical transfer of single-copy eucaryotic genes using total cellular DNA as donor. *Cell* **14:** 725.

Study of Possible Relationships among Retroviral Oncogenes Using Flat Revertants Isolated from Kirsten Sarcoma Virus-transformed Cells

R.H. Bassin and M. Noda

Laboratory of Tumor Immunology and Biology, National Cancer Institute, Bethesda, Maryland 20205

E.M. Scolnick

Virology Division, Merck, Sharp and Dohme, West Point, Pennsylvania 19486

Z.S. Selinger

Division of Life Sciences, Hebrew University, Jerusalem, Israel 91904

The nucleotide sequences of many retroviral oncogenes, as well as the primary structures of the polypeptides that they encode, have recently been reported. Various activities have been assigned to retroviral oncogene products. In particular, protein kinase activities have been associated with the products of *src, yes, fps, fes,* and *abl,* whereas GDP-binding and autophosphorylating activities have been reported for p21, the peptide specified by the *ras* family of oncogenes (for review, see Bishop and Varmus 1982). Studies with temperature-sensitive mutants and with mutants constructed in vitro have indicated that at least some of these enzyme activities are linked to the ability of oncogenes to transform cells in culture. In addition, there appears to be an association between the production by cells of low-molecular-weight peptide growth factors (TGFs) and transformation by retroviruses (DeLarco and Todaro 1978; Ozanne et al. 1980). Recently, the gene product p28 of the retroviral oncogene *sis* has been shown to bear close structural homology to a cellular peptide, platelet-derived growth factor (PDGF) (Doolittle et al. 1983; Waterfield et al. 1983). In spite of these observations, the fundamental mechanisms responsible for cell transformation have yet to be elucidated.

The isolation of mutant cells that contain alterations in one or more of the cellular "target" molecules directly involved in transformation by retroviral oncogenes could be of immense value in this area, but such studies have met with very limited success to date (Stephenson et al. 1973; Morris et al. 1980; Inoue et al. 1983; for review, see Ozer and Jha 1977). Such cells are usually isolated as flat revertants from populations of retrovirus-transformed cells. A frequent problem in the isolation of revertants resulting from changes in cellular target molecule(s) (i.e., cellular revertants) is the apparent abundance of flat revertants that have defective or missing retroviral oncogenes (viral revertants) and are of little value in studies on cellular aspects of transformation.

In this paper, two new methods are presented for enriching, in mixed cell populations, the proportion of cellular revertants apparently resulting from changes in host cell genomes. Further characteristics of two revertants, C-11 and F-2, which have been isolated from Kirsten murine sarcoma virus (Ki-MSV)-transformed NIH-3T3 cells are also given.

Experimental Procedures

Cells and viruses

The origins of the following cell lines have been described previously (Noda et al. 1983): NIH-3T3, DT, TK⁻NIH, Ki/Tk⁻NIH, and revertants C-11, C-11 Oua^R, F-2, and F-2 Oua^R. C-11 Neo^R cells were derived from C-11 cells by transfecting pSV2-*neo* plasmid DNA followed by selection with 400 μg/ml of G-418 (Southern and Berg 1982). Cell culture and somatic cell hybridization experiments were performed as described (Noda et al. 1983).

Techniques for rescuing transforming viruses from nonproducer cells (Bassin et al. 1970), infectious center procedures (Duran-Troise et al. 1977), and assays for infectious murine leukemia and sarcoma viruses (Bassin et al. 1971) have also been described.

Ouabain selection

Cells were plated at densities of 10^2–10^5 per 60-mm dish in growth medium. After overnight incubation at 37°C, cells were rinsed twice with K⁺-free growth medium and refed with K⁺-free medium containing 10% fetal calf serum and 1 mM ouabain. After incubation for 1–7 days, the medium on the plates was replaced with growth medium, and incubation was continued until sufficiently large colonies were observed.

Blot hybridization

High-molecular-weight DNA of actively growing cells in culture was extracted by the method of Gross-Bellard et al. (1973), digested with *Eco*RI (New England Biolabs), and resolved by electrophoresis in 0.6% agarose. Blot hybridization analysis was carried out by the method of Southern (1975) using a ^{32}P-labeled fragment of cloned *c*-Ki-*ras* (human) DNA as a probe (Chang et al. 1982).

Tumorigenicity testing

Cultured cells were trypsinized, rinsed, diluted, and injected subcutaneously into 8–10-week-old NIH Swiss nu/nu mice. Mice were examined periodically for evidence of tumors until the experiment was terminated after 58 days. Several cell concentrations were tested from each cell line, and the activities are expressed as the cumulative number of mice with tumors and as the median latent period to tumor formation.

DNA transfection

Transfection of plasmid DNAs and high-molecular-weight DNAs was carried out by the method of Graham and Van der Eb (1973), as modified by Lowy et al. (1978).

Results

Selection of revertant cells with ouabain

Because the existing methods for enriching the proportion of nontransformed cells in mixed populations seemed less than ideal (Vogel and Pollack 1974), we tested novel selective procedures for their value in the isolation of flat cellular revertants. Morphological transformation of cultured cells is accompanied by a variety of changes involving alterations at the cell surface (Hynes 1979). Therefore, it was not surprising to find a difference in the apparent toxicity for transformed and nontransformed NIH-3T3 cells following treatment with the cardiac glycoside ouabain, a drug whose specific target, Na⁺-K⁺ ATPase, is a cell-surface-associated enzyme (Schwartz et al. 1975).

Figure 1 shows the results of a dose-response ex-

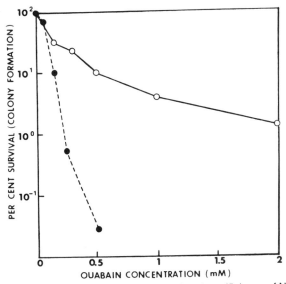

Figure 1 Effect of ouabain on colony-forming efficiency of NIH-3T3 and DT cells—dose-response curve. Per cent survival is the number of cells able to give rise to colonies after ouabain treatment divided by the number of colonies observed in cultures without ouabain treatment. (o) NIH-3T3 cells; (●) DT cells.

periment in which the colony-forming ability of the DT cell line, a 6-thioguanine(TG)-resistant, Ki-MSV-transformed derivative of the NIH-3T3 cell line (Noda et al. 1983) is compared with that of control NIH-3T3 cells following 24 hours of treatment with increasing doses of ouabain. The transformed DT cell line is much more sensitive to treatment with ouabain than is the parental NIH-3T3 cell line itself.

The value of ouabain treatment for the selection of flat cells from mixed populations containing a much larger number of transformed cells (as might be encountered in attempts to isolate revertants) was confirmed in a reconstruction experiment. The transformed DT cell line can readily be distinguished from wild-type cell lines, such as NIH-3T3, by its inability to survive in medium containing HAT (Littlefield 1964). Mixtures containing NIH-3T3 cells together with either a 100-fold or a 1000-fold excess of DT cells were plated at several dilutions in growth medium. The following day, half of the plates were treated with 1 mM ouabain for 24 hours and half were kept as mock-treated controls. After an additional 24 hours of incubation, ouabain was removed and the proportion of viable NIH-3T3 cells in each of the two groups was estimated by measuring colony-forming activity in both regular growth medium and in growth medium containing HAT. The results (Table 1) show that treatment of the mixed cell populations with ouabain resulted in a differential toxicity such that the proportion of HAT-resistant normal NIH-3T3 cells was increased by as much as 160-fold. The experiments described above indicate that ouabain treatment may be of use in the selection of untransformed cells in mixed populations. Varmus et al. (1981) have reported a similar selection of flat revertant cells from mixtures with *src*-transformed chicken cells using hydroxyurea.

Use of doubly transformed cells to reduce numbers of revertants with altered or missing viral oncogenes

Our strategy for the isolation of new classes of flat cellular revertants also involved the use of virus-transformed cells that contain more than one copy of the oncogene responsible for transformation. Such doubly transformed (DT) cells should rarely give rise to revertants in which both copies of the viral oncogene have been lost or inactivated. As a result, the relative frequency of revertants resulting from changes in cellular factors involved in the transformation process should be correspondingly increased. The DT cells employed in these experiments were NIH-3T3 cells that had been infected on two separate occasions with Ki-MSV. The presence of two copies of *v*-Ki-*ras* sequences in these cells was demonstrated in a blot hybridization experiment (Fig. 2, lane 8). As expected, two copies of the cellular proto-oncogene *c*-Ki-*ras* were also present in the DT cell line as well as in control NIH-3T3 cells (Fig. 2, lanes 1 and 8) (Ellis et al. 1981).

Characterization of revertants C-11 and F-2

The ouabain selection procedure described above has been used successfully to isolate two flat revertants, C-

Table 1 Selection of Flat Cells with Ouabain: Reconstruction Experiment[a]

| Initial ratio (NIH-3T3:DT) | Cloning efficiency (%) | | | | | |
| | control | | | ouabain selected | | |
	HAT[Rb]	total	MAT[R]/total	HAT[R]	total	HAT[R]/total
1:1000 (0.1%)	0.05	90	(0.055%)	0.021	0.13	(16%)
1:100 (1%)	0.42	93	(0.45%)	0.083	0.13	(64%)
NIH-3T3 contol	21	20	(105%)	5.5	5.8	(95%)
DT control	<0.001	95	(<0.001%)	<0.001	0.043	(<2.3%)

[a]Mixtures containing the indicated ratios of wild-type NIH-3T3 cells and DT cells were plated in 60-mm dishes at several concentrations. The following day, 1 mM ouabain was added to the ouabain-selected dishes, while the control dishes were mock-treated. Ouabain was removed 16 hr later, at which time half of the plates in each group were treated with HAT medium for 48 hr. All dishes were incubated for an additional 5 days and the resulting colonies of growing cells were counted under a microscope.

[b]HAT[R] = Cells able to form colonies following 48 hr exposure to medium containing HAT.

11 and F-2, from the Ki-MSV-transformed DT cell line (Noda et al. 1983). Our initial studies showed that the C-11 and F-2 revertants have a nontransformed appearance when grown as monolayers and fail to grow in agar suspension cultures. However, the revertants retain several characteristics of their transformed progenitor line, including elevated levels of the v-Ki-ras gene product p21 as well as an ability to grow in medium with 1% serum (Noda et al. 1983). Additional properties of the C-11 and F-2 revertants are presented below.

The ability of the revertant lines to produce tumors in nude mice is shown in Table 2. C-11 cells are less than

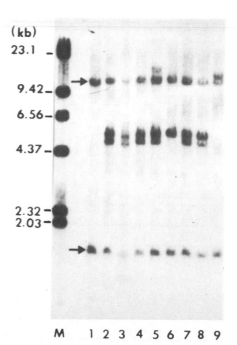

Figure 2 Southern blot experiment. Cellular DNAs were digested with EcoRI and probed with a ^{32}P-labeled c-Ki-ras (human) DNA (1.2 kb BglII–HindIII). (Lane M) Size marker (λ DNA digested with HindIII); (lane 1) NIH-3T3; (lane 2) C-11; (lane 3) F-2; (lane 4) C-11 Oua[R]; (lane 5) F-2 Oua[R]; (lane 6) DO-4 (a third clone which was isolated but which has apparently lost one copy of v-Ki-ras); (lane 7) ZS-156 (another flat revertant with two copies of v-Ki-ras); (lane 8) DT; (lane 9) Ki/TK⁻NIH. Arrows indicate the two endogenous c-Ki-ras sequences.

1/100 as tumorigenic as the parental DT cell line, whereas F-2 cells and control NIH-3T3 cells exhibit almost no tumorigenic activity at the highest concentration of inoculated cells, 1 × 10[7] per mouse, and are apparently less than 1/2000 as tumorigenic as the transformed DT cell line. Thus, tumorigenicity in nude mice appears to be one of the transformation-specific properties not expressed in the revertant cells. The low level of tumors induced by the C-11 revertant line may be the result of occasional rerevertants present in the cell population (R.H. Bassin et al., in prep.).

Southern blot analysis (Fig. 2, lanes 2–5) indicated that both the C-11 and F-2 revertants retain two copies of the v-Ki-ras gene with no apparent structural alterations. In addition, each of the revertants appears to contain elevated levels of p21 (Noda et al. 1983). These results do not exclude the possibility that the p21 present in the revertants is inactive as a result of some minor alteration in the v-Ki-ras sequence(s).

A series of experiments designed to characterize the activity of the v-Ki-ras genes present in the revertants was undertaken. Revertant cell lines were examined for the presence of potentially functional v-Ki-ras genes in a rescue experiment. Cells were superinfected with murine leukemia helper virus, and the proportion of cells able to register as infectious centers for transforming virus was determined by plating the infected cells on a monolayer of lawn cells, in this case untransformed NIH-3T3 cells. As shown in Table 3, infection of the C-11 or F-2 revertant cell lines with either of two murine leukemia viruses induced the production of transforming Ki-MSV with frequencies similar to those observed following infection of the DT cell line.

The functional integrity of Ki-MSV proviral sequences in the revertant cell lines was also tested directly by transfection of focus-forming activity to susceptible NIH-3T3 cells using purified DNA from the revertant cell lines. The data shown in Table 4 are the results of a preliminary transfection experiment and show that a low level of focus-forming activity, comparable with that seen with DNA from a line of Ki-MSV-transformed NIH cells, is associated with DNA recovered from each of the revertants. Thus, the Ki-MSV provirus and the p21 trans-

Table 2 Tumorigenicity of Revertants C-11 and F-2 in Nude Mice[a]

Cell line	Number of cells inoculated	Positive/total	Average latent period[b]
DT	5×10^6	10/10	<8 days
DT	5×10^5	9/10	9
DT	5×10^4	7/10	20
DT	5×10^3	3/10	—
C-11	1×10^7	8/8	46
C-11	5×10^6	1/7	—
C-11	1×10^6	0/8	—
F-2	1×10^7	0/10	—
F-2	1×10^6	0/8	—
NIH-3T3	1×10^7	2/8	—
NIH-3T3	1×10^6	1/8	—

[a]Nude mice were inoculated subcutaneously in the interscapular region with trypsinized cell suspensions from each cell line. They were examined periodically for signs of tumor formation near the area inoculated until the experiment was terminated at 58 days. In all cases tumors grew progressively until the animals were sacrificed. Data from two experiments are combined.

[b]Average latent period, time in days required for 50% of inoculated animals to exhibit tumor formation. Estimated graphically.

forming protein present in the revertant cell lines are functional when transferred to normal host cells, and their action is blocked in the revertant cells.

Retransformation of revertants

If the revertant cell lines contain active *v-Ki-ras* genes, and if, as stated above, the revertant lines represent cellular variants resistant to the action of functional p21, it follows that the revertant cell lines should be resistant to challenge with additional Ki-MSV. We have chosen two procedures to introduce new copies of functioning Ki-MSV DNA into the revertant cell lines—hybridization of revertant cells to Ki-MSV-transformed cells and direct infection with Ki-MSV pseudotypes.

Before attempting to determine the behavior of selected retroviral oncogenes in hybrid cells, we carried out two sets of control experiments. Fusion of TG-resistant DT cells to BrdUrd-resistant NIH cells (TK⁻NIH) followed by selection in HAT medium (Littlefield 1964) resulted in hybrid colonies, 85% of which appeared to be composed of transformed cells in the liquid medium assay and 52% of which formed colonies in semisolid medium (Table 5). A similar experiment in which ouabain-resistant, Ki-MSV-transformed TK⁻NIH cells (Ki/TK⁻NIHOua^R) and wild-type NIH-3T3 cells were fused together gave essentially the same results (Table 5). These data indicate that the transformed phenotype is dominant in crosses between *v-Ki-ras*-transformed cells and normal NIH cells.

Fusion of either the C-11 or the F-2 revertant cell line to nontransformed TK⁻NIH cells using the same HAT selection system resulted in hybrid cells that almost al-

Table 3 Rescue of Ki-MSV from Revertants—Infectious Center Assay

"Helper" virus	moi[a]	Cell line			
		NIH-3T3	DT	C-11Oua^R	F-2Oua^R
Ampho[b]	1	0	0.60	0.11	0.10
	0.01	0	0.01	0.01	0.02
Eco[c]	1	0	0.31	0.79	0.61
	0.01	0	0.04	0.08	0.18
None[d]	—	0	0	0	0

Cells (500,000) of each type were seeded in replicate flasks. The following day, cells were infected with the indicated moi of either amphotropic MLV or ecotropic MLV at the moi indicated. Approximately 16 hr after infection, cells were treated with 20 μg/ml of Mitomycin C for 2 hr, rinsed, and trypsinized. The number of Ki-MSV-producing cells was determined by plating the test cells on a previously seeded "lawn" of NIH-3T3 cells and scoring foci of transformed cells 12 days later.

[a]moi, multiplicity of infection.
[b]Amphotropic MLV.
[c]Ecotropic MLV.
[d]Mock-infected with growth medium.

Table 4 Transforming Activities of Revertant DNAs

Cell line	Foci per μg DNA
NIH-3T3	0
C-11 Oua^R	0.27
F-2 Oua^R	0.20
Ki/TK$^-$ NIH	0.07

NIH-3T3 cells were plated at 3×10^5/ 35-mm dish. On the following day, 20 μg of high-molecular-weight DNA from each cell line was transfected by the method of Lowy et al. (1978). Transfected cells were trypsinized the following day and replated into four 60-mm dishes per original 35-mm dish. Foci of transformed cells were counted approximately 10 days later.

mycin-resistant cells (Southern and Berg 1982). Finally, a preliminary experiment (Table 5) indicated that SH1-1, an NIH-3T3 cell line transfected with DNA from human neuroblastoma cells (Perucho et al. 1981), produced flat hybrids following fusion with C-11 Neo^R cells, in agreement with the identification of a ras-related gene (N-ras) as the transforming agent in this system. The reader is referred to a previous publication for a description of additional cell hybridization studies involving the C-11 and F-2 revertants (Noda et al. 1983).

In addition to the cell hybridization experiments described above, we attempted to measure the susceptibility of the revertant cell lines to retransformation by v-Ki-ras sequences by superinfecting revertant cells with infectious virus. Revertant C-11 cells were seeded sparsely in Petri dishes and were infected the following day with ecotropic pseudotypes of several defective retroviruses known to transform NIH-3T3 cells. Infected cultures were examined periodically for evidence of transformation as determined by alterations in cell morphology, refractility, and an enhanced ability to grow in multilayers. As shown in Figure 3, C-11 cells appear to be resistant to challenge with either Kirsten or Harvey sarcoma viruses following infection with moderate amounts (moi = 0.1) of these agents. Comparison of infected cultures indicated that the revertants were approximately 1000-fold less sensitive to either Ki-MSV or Ha-MSV than were control NIH-3T3 cells. In contrast, relatively small amounts of Moloney (Mo)-MSV are capable of retransforming the C-11 cell line (Fig. 3), although the C-11 revertant appears to be about 10-fold less susceptible than NIH-3T3 cells to retransformation by Mo-MSV. Thus, the revertant C-11 is significantly more resistant to retransformation by the ras oncogene than by the mos oncogene. Studies on superinfection of revertants with other transforming viruses are in progress.

It was noted during the course of these experiments that infection of either revertant with high moi values (>1) of Ki-MSV caused visible transformation in C-11

ways gave rise to flat colonies in liquid medium and failed to grow in semisolid medium (Table 5). This important control experiment indicates that the revertant phenotype in the C-11 and F-2 cell lines does not result from the absence of some cellular component necessary for the transformation process. The results of these two control experiments indicated that the introduction of additional v-Ki-ras sequences into revertant cells following hybridization can be used to assess their resistance to retransformation. Therefore, C-11 and F-2 cells were each fused to Ki/TK$^-$NIH cells, and the resulting hybrids were plated in both liquid medium and in semisolid agar. The results (Table 5) indicate that the vast majority of such hybrids exhibit a nontransformed phenotype when grown in liquid medium and do not form colonies in semisolid agar. Thus, the revertants appear to be resistant to retransformation by v-Ki-ras. Essentially, the same result was obtained following fusion of a neomycin-resistant derivative of C-11 cells to Ki/TK$^-$NIH cells followed by selection in medium containing HAT and G-418, a drug which may be used as a selective agent for neo-

Table 5 Frequency of Transformed Colonies after Plating Cell Hybrids in Liquid or Agar Suspension Cultures

Hybrid	Frequency of transformed colonies			
	liquid medium[a]	(%)	semisolid medium[b]	(%)
DT × TK$^-$NIH[c]	76/89	(85)	846/1620	(52)
Ki/TK$^-$NIH × NIH-3T3[d]	130/162	(80)	297/810	(36)
C-11 × TK$^-$NIH[d]	0/17	(<6)	0/170	(<.6)
F-2 × TK$^-$NIH[d]	0/7	(<14)	1/70	(1.4)
C-11 × Ki/TK$^-$NIH[d]	3/96	(3.1)	3/410	(0.7)
F-2 × Ki/TK$^-$NIH[d]	5/60	(8.3)	5/480	(1.0)
C-11 Neo^R × Ki/TK$^-$NIH[e]	10/62	(16)	N.T.	—
C-11 Neo^R × SH1-1[e]	1/19	(5.3)	N.T.	—

[a]Number of colonies with transformed morphology/total number of colonies after fusion and growth for about 2 weeks in selective medium.
[b]Number of colonies in semisolid medium/total number of viable cells plated after fusion and growth for 2–3 weeks in selective medium.
[c]Selective medium contained HAT only.
[d]Selective medium contained HAT and 1 mM ouabain.
[e]Selective medium contained HAT and 400 μg/ml G-418.

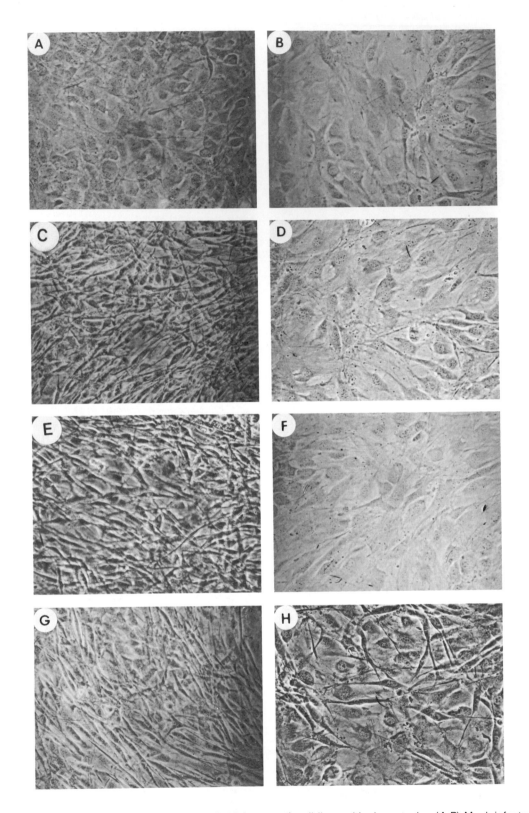

Figure 3 Superinfection of NIH-3T3 (control) and C-11 (revertant) cell lines with virus stocks. (*A,B*) Mock-infected NIH-3T3 and C-11 cells, respectively; (*C,D*) NIH-3T3 and C-11 cells, respectively, infected with Ha-MSV; (*E,F*) NIH and C-11 cells, respectively, infected with Ki-MSV; (*G,H*) NIH and C-11 cells, respectively, infected with Mo-MSV. All viruses were diluted to give an moi of 0.1. Cells were photographed 7 days after infection.

cells. Since the transforming virus is presumably able to replicate in the revertant cells, the actual multiplicity of infection cannot be determined, and the significance of this observation is not clear at present.

Discussion

A small proportion of the cells in a population transformed by retroviruses exhibits a tendency to revert, exhibiting a more or less flat or nontransformed phenotype. The frequency of reversion is low and depends on the particular experimental conditions employed. Either of two general mechanisms may be responsible for reversion: (1) the retroviral oncogene causing transformation may become damaged or entirely lost (giving rise to a viral revertant); or (2) a modification in the cellular genome may result in cellular revertants, which inhibit the expression of the oncogene or are resistant to its action because of an alteration in one of the cell components involved in the transformation process. These two classes of revertants can, in theory, be readily distinguished from one another: Viral revertants should not contain rescuable transforming virus and should be susceptible to retransformation by the same or closely related oncogenes, whereas cellular revertants should display the opposite properties.

Attempts to isolate revertants from cells transformed by any of several oncogenes have often resulted in the isolation of flat cells which, after study, have proven to be viral revertants lacking functional retroviral oncogenes. On the other hand, cellular revertants have been described only rarely. It was apparent, therefore, that new methods would be required for the isolation of cellular revertants. Two such methods are described in this study: (1) the use of ouabain to kill selectively Ki-MSV-transformed cells, thereby greatly increasing the frequency of revertants in mixed populations; and (2) the use of cells containing more than a single copy of an integrated retroviral oncogene to reduce the occurrence of revertants resulting from changes in the oncogene itself.

Treatment of Ki-MSV-transformed DT cells and control NIH-3T3 cells with ouabain appears to be an effective technique for enriching the proportion of flat cells in mixed populations by as much as 1000-fold (Fig. 1; Table 1). The fact that ouabain is more active in killing DT cells than NIH-3T3 cells may have some implications for the mechanism of transformation. Ouabain is an inhibitor of Na^+-K^+ ATPase, and its differential effect on normal and transformed cells may indicate fundamental differences in ion transport mechanisms in the revertant cells. Additional Ki-MSV-transformed NIH-3T3 cell lines have been examined and appear to vary in their sensitivity to ouabain, so that no general conclusions regarding the relationship between ouabain sensitivity and transformation can be drawn at this time. Nevertheless, there is a good deal of evidence that these two properties are linked in DT cells based on the data shown here and on results with cell hybrids between DT cells and NIH-3T3 cells in which transformation and ouabain sensitivity appear to be closely correlated (R.H. Bassin et al., in prep.). In addition, our preliminary studies have shown that NIH-3T3 cells are more sensitive than are DT cells to bumetanide, a second drug that affects a different Na^+ and K^+ transport pathway.

A second method for increasing the proportion of cellular revertants in mixed populations involves the use of transformed cells that contain two copies of a transforming viral oncogene. The DT cell line used in this study had been infected on two separate occasions with Ki-MSV and contained two copies of the v-Ki-ras gene as confirmed by Southern blot hybridization (Fig. 2). Although it was not possible to confirm that both copies of v-Ki-ras were transcriptionally active, the fact that neither of the flat cell lines isolated in this study appeared to be viral revertants (see below) is consistent with the presence of more than one active transforming gene in the DT cell line.

The C-11 and F-2 revertants, which were isolated using the techniques described above, appear to demonstrate several properties which indicate that they are cellular revertants and are not the result of changes in the genome of the original transforming virus, Ki-MSV. The revertants contain two apparently unaltered copies of v-Ki-ras (Fig. 2), a rescuable (and transfectable) provirus capable of transforming control NIH-3T3 cells (Tables 3 and 4), and elevated levels of the ras gene product p21 (Noda et al. 1983). Furthermore, the revertants exhibit certain characteristics associated with transformation by the ras oncogene, including an ability to grow in medium with 1% serum (Noda et al. 1983) as well as the production of a growth-stimulating factor (D. Salomon et al., in prep.).

For an additional indication of the mechanism responsible for reversion in the C-11 and F-2 cell lines, we attempted to retransform these cells with Ki-MSV. As stated previously, cellular revertants, which are the result of changes in cellular components involved in the transformation process, should resist retransformation by the original transforming agent, whereas viral revertants, which arise as a result of a loss or change in the viral ras gene or in its product p21, should be permissive to retransformation. We have attempted to assess the susceptibility of the C-11 and F-2 revertants to retransformation by two different methods: (1) hybridization of the revertants to cell lines transformed by various retroviral oncogenes; and (2) direct superinfection of the revertants with a variety of retroviruses. Cell hybridization between transformed and nontransformed cells is known to give rise to hybrids with the phenotype of either the transformed or the nontransformed parent, depending on the particular system employed (Ozer and Jha 1977). For example, Rous sarcoma virus-transformed mouse cells are known to give rise to flat hybrid colonies following fusion to normal mouse cells (Marshall 1980; Dyson et al. 1982). It was necessary, therefore, to establish the phenotype of hybrids between normal NIH-3T3 cells and Ki-MSV cells before attempting to assess the behavior of the revertant cells by this method. The data presented here (Table 5) indicate that two different combinations of nontransformed and *ras*-transformed NIH cells give hybrids that are transformed as measured in liquid or agar suspension cultures. Additional experiments using other *ras*-transformed cell lines have given identical results (Noda et al. 1983). In a more complete study, it was found that both the C-11 and F-2 revertants gave phenotypically flat hybrids when fused to cells transformed not only by *ras*, but also when fused to cells transformed by *fes* and *src*. Fusion of either revertant to cell transformed by *mos*, *fms*, and *sis*, however, resulted in hybrid colonies that were transformed (Noda et al. 1983).

The second method of testing the susceptibility of the revertants to retransformation involved superinfection of the C-11 revertant with transforming Ki-MSV (Fig. 3). The results of this experiment showed that retransformation by Ki-MSV was severely inhibited (1000-fold) in the C-11 revertant whereas retransformation by Mo-MSV was only slightly inhibited (about 10-fold). These results agree with the cell hybridization studies, and again indicate that revertants are resistant to retransformation by certain oncogenes but are susceptible to retransformation by others.

It seems likely from the data presented here that the C-11 and F-2 revertants have acquired some cellular change that confers upon them resistance to transformation by certain viral oncogenes but not by others. Although the basis for this discrimination is not at all clear at present, members of the inhibited group of retroviral oncogenes (*ras*, *fes*, and *src*) do not appear to be structurally related to one another nor to members of the uninhibited group (*mos*, *fms*, and *sis*). It seems a likely possibility, therefore, that the oncogenes in the first group must bear some unknown functional similarity. The similarity in the restricted group of oncogenes may represent a common site of action, such as a need to interact with the cell membrane. On the other hand, there may be a common requirement for a cellular substrate by the *ras*, *fes*, and *src* gene products. In contrast, the inhibited group of oncogenes may be able to transform cells without a requirement for this particular function. The fact that oncogenes from human tumors may also be inhibited by the C-11 and F-2 revertants (Table 5; Noda et al. 1983) indicates that an understanding of the mechanism of reversion should be of value in the future.

Acknowledgments

It is a pleasure to acknowledge the technical assistance of B. Wallace, A. Brown, and M. Thistlethwaite. P. Minor, Meloy Laboratories, Springfield, Virginia, conducted the nude mouse study. We thank L. Benade, American Type Culture Collection, Rockville, Maryland, for critically evaluating the manuscript. We also thank M. Furth, Sloan Kettering Memorial Cancer Institute, New York, for advice with the cell fusion studies and E. Chang, Uniformed Services University, Bethesda, Maryland, for advice and assistance with the Southern blotting. M.N. is a Visiting Fellow on leave from Keio University, Tokyo.

References

Bassin, R.H., N. Tuttle, and P.J. Fischinger. 1970. Isolation of murine sarcoma virus-transformed mouse cells which are negative for leukemia virus from agar suspension cultures. *Int. J. Cancer* **6**: 95.

———. 1971. Rapid cell culture assay technique for murine leukaemia viruses. *Nature* **229**: 564.

Bishop, J.M. and H. Varmus. 1982. Functions and origins of retroviral transforming genes. In *Molecular biology of tumor viruses*, 2nd edition: *RNA tumor viruses* (ed. R. Weiss et al.), p. 999. Cold Spring Harbor Laboratory, New York.

Chang, E.H., M.A. Gonda, R.W. Ellis, E.M. Scolnick, and D.R. Lowy. 1982. Human genome contains four genes homologous to transforming genes of Harvey and Kirsten murine sarcoma viruses. *Proc. Natl. Acad. Sci.* **79**: 4848.

DeLarco, J.E. and G.J. Todaro. 1978. Growth factors from murine sarcoma virus transformed cells. *Proc. Natl. Acad. Sci.* **75**: 4001.

Doolittle, R.F., M.W. Hunkapiller, L.E. Hood, S.G. Devare, K.C. Robbins, S.A. Aaronson, and H.N. Antoniades. 1983. Simian sarcoma virus *onc* gene, v-*sis*, is derived from the gene (or genes) encoding a platelet-derived growth factor. *Science* **221**: 275.

Duran-Troise, G., R.H. Bassin, A. Rein, and B.I. Gerwin. 1977. Loss of Fv-1 restriction in BALB/3T3 cells following infection with a single N-tropic murine leukemia virus particle. *Cell* **10**: 479.

Dyson, P.J., K. Quade, and J.A. Wyke. 1982. Expression of the ASV *src* gene in hybrids between normal and virally transformed cells: Specific suppression occurs in some hybrids but not others. *Cell* **30**: 491.

Ellis, R.W., D. DeFeo, T.Y. Shih, M.A. Gonda, H.A. Young, N. Tsuchida, D.R. Lowy, and E.M. Scolnick. 1981. The p21 *src* gene of Harvey and Kirsten sarcoma viruses originate from divergent members of a family of normal vertebrate genes. *Nature* **289**: 127.

Graham, R. and A. Van der Eb. 1973. A new technique for the assay of infectivity of human adenovirus 5 DNA. *Virology* **52**: 456.

Gross-Bellard, M., P. Oudet, and P. Chambon. 1973. Isolation of high-molecular weight DNA from mammalian cells. *Eur. J. Biochem.* **36**: 32.

Hynes, R.O., ed. 1979. *Surfaces of normal and malignant cells.* Wiley, New York.

Inoue, H., M. Yutsudo, and A. Hakura. 1983. Rat mutant cells showing temperature sensitivity for transformation by wildtype Moloney murine sarcoma virus. *Virology* **125**: 242.

Littlefield, J.W. 1964. Selection of hybrids from matings of fibroblasts in vitro and their presumed recombinants. *Science* **145**: 709.

Lowy, D.R., E. Rands, and E.M. Scolnick. 1978. Helper-independent transformation by unintegrated Harvey sarcoma virus DNA. *J. Virol.* **26**: 291.

Marshall, C.J. 1980. Suppression of the transformed phenotype with retention of the viral 'src' gene in cell hybrids between Rous sarcoma virus-transformed rat cells and untransformed mouse cells. *Exp. Cell Res.* **127**: 373.

Morris, A., C. Clegg, J. Jones, B. Rodgers, and R.J. Avery. 1980. The isolation and characterization of a clonally related series of murine retrovirus-infected mouse cells. *J. Gen. Virol.* **49**: 105.

Noda, M., Z. Selinger, E.M. Scolnick, and R.H. Bassin. 1983. Flat revertants isolated from Kirsten sarcoma virus-transformed cells are resistant to the action of specific oncogenes. *Proc. Natl. Acad. Sci.* **80**: 5602.

Ozanne, B., R.J. Fulton, and P.L. Kaplan. 1980. Kirsten murine sarcoma virus transformed cell lines and a spontaneously transformed rat cell line produce transforming factors. *J. Cell. Physiol.* **105**: 163.

Ozer, H.L. and K.K. Jha. 1979. Malignancy and transformation: Expression in somatic cell hybrids and variants. *Adv. Cancer Res.* **25**: 53.

Perucho, M., M. Goldfarb, K. Shimizu, C. Lama, J. Fogh, and M. Wigler. 1981. Human-tumor-derived cell lines contain common and different transforming genes. *Cell* **27**: 467.

Schwartz, A., G.E. Lindenmayer, and J.C. Allen. 1975. The sodium-potassium adenosine triphosphatase: Pharmacological, physiological and biochemical aspects. *Pharmacol. Rev.* **27**: 3.

Southern, E.M. 1975. Detection of specific sequences among DNA fragments separated by gel electrophoresis. *J. Mol. Biol.* **98**: 503.

Southern, P.J. and P. Berg. 1982. Transformation of mammalian cells to antibiotic resistance with a bacterial gene under control of the SV40 early region promoter. *J. Mol. Appl. Genet.* **1**: 327.

Stephenson, J.R., R.K. Reynolds, and S.A. Aaronson. 1973. Characterization of morphologic revertants of murine and avian sarcoma virus-transformed cells. *J. Virol.* **11**: 218.

Varmus, H.E., N. Quintrell, and S. Ortiz. 1981. Retroviruses as mutagens: Insertion and excision of a nontransforming provirus alter expression of a resident transforming provirus. *Cell* **25**: 23.

Vogel, H.L. and R. Pollack. 1974. Methods for obtaining revertants of transformed cells. *Methods Cell Biol.* **8**: 75.

Waterfield, M.D., G.T. Scrace, N. Whittle, P. Stroobant, A. Johnsson, A. Wasteson, B. Westermark, C.-H. Heldin, J.S. Huang, and T.F. Deuel. 1983. Platelet-derived growth factor is structurally related to the putative transforming protein p28^{sis} of simian sarcoma virus. *Nature* **304**: 35.

Cellular and Viral Oncogenes Cooperate to Achieve Tumorigenic Conversion of Rat Embryo Fibroblasts

H. Land, L.F. Parada, and R.A. Weinberg

Center for Cancer Research and Department of Biology, Massachusetts Institute of Technology and The Whitehead Institute for Biomedical Research, Cambridge, Massachusetts 02139

Gene transfer experiments have shown that certain types of chemically transformed cells as well as a large number of human tumor cell lines and tumor biopsies carry oncogenic sequences in their DNAs (Shih et al. 1979; Cooper 1982; Weinberg 1982).

Several of the active tumor oncogenes have been isolated by molecular cloning. These include the oncogene of the T24/EJ human bladder carcinoma cell line (EJ c-Ha-ras-1; Goldfarb et al. 1982; Pulciani et al. 1982; Shih and Weinberg 1982), the Blym oncogene of a chicken lymphoma (Goubin et al. 1983), an oncogene of a human lung carcinoma (c-Ki-ras-2; Capon et al. 1983; Shimizu et al. 1983b), and one isolated from a neuroblastoma, a sarcoma, and a leukemia (N-ras; Hall et al. 1983; Murray et al. 1983; Shimizu et al. 1983a).

The initial detection of these oncogenes depended in all cases on the use of the mouse fibroblast cell line NIH-3T3 as the source for the recipient cells in the transfection-focus assay. These cells were chosen because they grow as monolayers and were found to be particularly efficient at taking up and fixing exogenous, transfected DNAs (Smotkin et al. 1975). However, although the NIH-3T3 cells have proven to be a useful tool in the isolation of active oncogenes from cellular DNA, they seemed not to be an appropriate system to investigate the possible role of these particular oncogenes within the multiple and distinct stages of tumorigenesis. Because these cells have been established and passaged in vitro for several years, they may deviate substantially from normal target cells that are altered by the activity of oncogenes in vivo. The immortalized state of these NIH-3T3 cells might be sufficient to predispose these cells to tumorigenic conversion by a single event such as acquisition of an oncogene. This contrasts with the often repeated observation that experimental induction of a tumor requires two or more distant stimuli, such as initiators and promoters (for review, see Farber and Cameron 1980).

Recent work has shown that DNA tumor viruses such as polyoma and adenovirus carry at least two genes encoding distinct functions, both of which must be expressed to induce the tumor cell phenotype in primary cultures of rodent cells (Houweling et al. 1980; Rassoulzadegan et al. 1982, 1983; van den Elsen et al. 1982). These data suggest that multistep tumorigenesis might have an explanation at the genetic level: each step may require the activation of a distinct gene, and the final phenotype may require the concomitant expression of many of the previously activated genes.

More support for this model comes from the observation that the induction of bursal lymphomas by avian leukosis virus appears to require the activation of two different oncogenes during lymphomagenesis. The myc gene becomes activated via adjacent integration of a proviral promoter-enhancer element (Hayward et al. 1981; Payne et al. 1982), while the Blym gene (Cooper and Neiman 1981) can be detected as a focus-inducing oncogene on NIH-3T3 fibroblasts. Studies of a promyelocytic leukemia and an American Burkitt's lymphoma revealed that in each case the cells carry altered myc genes as well as activated forms of the N-ras oncogene (Murray et al. 1983).

We undertook experiments that were designed to reconcile these two conflicting results—single-hit transformation by transfection and multi-hit carcinogenesis in vivo. We utilized secondary embryo fibroblasts as recipients in transfections, reasoning that these cells, more than NIH-3T3 cells, resembled the targets of carcinogenesis in vivo. We could show that after transfecting the EJ c-Ha-ras-1 (EJ ras) gene into rat embryo fibroblasts, the cells did not undergo tumorigenic conversion unless they were established and immortalized before transfection. Secondary embryo fibroblasts become tumorigenic, however, if a second oncogene such as the viral or cellular myc gene, the gene for the polyoma large T antigen, or the adenovirus early region 1A was introduced together with the EJ ras gene (Land et al. 1983).

Materials and Methods

Transfection of secondary rat embryo fibroblasts and Rat-1 cells

Primary cultures of rat embryo fibroblasts (REF) were prepared as described by Pollack et al. (1974) from 12–14-day-old Fisher rat embryos. Three to four days later, the cells were passaged and 1.2×10^6 cells were seeded onto 100-mm Petri dishes in Dulbecco's modified Eagle's medium (DMEM) supplemented with 10% fetal bovine serum (Hyclone) (normal medium). Parallel cultures of the Rat-1 cell line (Freeman et al. 1973) were seeded at a density of 5×10^5 cells (normal medium) so that 18–24 hours later both types of culture plated at similar cell densities (8×10^5 to 1.2×10^6 cells/dish). Transfections were carried out as previously described (Graham and van der Eb 1973; Andersson et al. 1979) with 75 μg REF carrier DNA, 10 μg each of the oncogene-carrying plasmid DNAs, and 2 μg of pSV2-gpt DNA per 2×10^6 cells (two dishes). After 24 hours, the transfected cells were pooled. The REFs were split in a ratio of 1:3 and the Rat-1 cells in a ratio of 1:10. One day later, half of the cultures were put under mycophenolic acid selection (Mulligan and Berg 1981). Cultures were refed every 4 days. For plating in soft agar, 10^6 cells were seeded 36 hours after transfection into normal medium containing 0.3% low-melting agarose (Sea Plaque). Foci or colonies were counted 14–16 days after transfection.

Assay for tumorigenicity

To test for in vivo growth potential, the transfected cells were collected 16–18 days after transfection, washed with phosphate-buffered saline (without Ca^{++}), and injected subcutaneously into 30–40-day-old nude mice. The mice had been irradiated with 500 rads 24 hours prior to injection to eliminate natural killer cells. The contents of a single culture dish (5×10^6 cells) were used as one inoculum. Cells that had previously been under mycophenolic acid selection were adjusted to normal culture conditions 2–3 days before they were injected. This was done by refeeding with mycophenolic acid selection medium (Mulligan and Berg 1981) not containing mycophenolic acid and aminopterin. Finally, cells from one of these dishes were mixed with 5×10^6 untransfected secondary (2°) REFs and used for a single injection. The animals were observed for tumor formation on a weekly basis over a period of 4 weeks. Tumors appeared between 7 and 10 days after injection.

Construction of plasmids containing active viral and cellular *myc* genes

p-v-*myc* (a kind gift from J.M. Bishop, University of California, San Francisco) contains a permuted copy of the avian MC29 provirus DNA (5.5 kb; Vennstrom et al. 1981). To provide a polyadenylation signal, the circularly permuted provirus clone was completed by duplication of the 5′ proximal 1.1-kb *Eco*RI–*Kpn*I restriction fragment at the 3′ proximal end of the provirus. To achieve this, the *Eco*RI–*Kpn*I fragment, which contains the two long terminal repeats (LTRs), was subcloned into the *Eco*RI and *Kpn*I sites of pSV2-*gpt* (Mulligan and Berg 1981). In a second step, the *Eco*RI fragment containing the entire permuted proviral DNA was ligated into the modified vector. In the resulting plasmid, termed pSV*v-myc*, the SV40 early promoter (PE) has the opposite polarity compared with the direction of transcription of the proviral DNA. The pSV*v-myc* del plasmid, a further modification of the above described pSV*v-myc*, had a 1.6-kb *Sac*I fragment deleted by cleavage with this enzyme and recircularization by ligation. This deletion removes a large portion of the sequences that encode the *gag-myc* fusion protein. pc-*myc* (a kind gift from M. Cole) contains the second and third exons of the cellular mouse *myc* gene within a 5.6-kb *Bam*HI fragment. It originated from DNA of the mouse plasmacytoma MOPC-315, in which this *myc* gene had been translocated into the immunoglobulin C_α-locus (Shen-Ong et al. 1982). These immunoglobulin sequences were removed during construction of the pc-*myc* plasmid. To express the mouse

cellular *myc* gene of the pc-*myc* plasmid, we created a plasmid termed pSV*c-myc*-1, in which transcription of the *myc* gene is driven by the SV40 early promoter (PE). By linker litigation, an *Xba*I site was added to the *Hind*III site of pSV2-*gpt* (Mulligan and Berg 1981). Following that, the 4.8-kb *Xba*I–*Bam*HI fragment of the pc-*myc* insert was cloned into this vector, putting transcriptional start and AUG 40 nucleotides apart. pSV*c-myc*-2 contains the *Bam*HI insert of pc-*myc* in pSV2-*gpt* in opposite transcriptional orientation relative to the SV40 early promoter-enhancer sequences (see also Fig. 1).

Results

Limited transformation capacity of the *ras* oncogene

The oncogene of the human EJ bladder carcinoma line (Shih and Weinberg 1982) is a variant of the human c-Ha-*ras*-1 proto-oncogene (Der et al. 1982; Parada et al. 1982; Santos et al. 1982). This EJ *ras* gene is a member of the *ras* gene family and is thereby closely related to the Ki-*ras* and N-*ras* oncogenes. When a clone of this oncogene, termed pEJ6.6, was introduced into 2°REFS, no foci of morphologically altered cells were observed 14–21 days after transfection. To prove that these 2°REFs are able to take up and express exogenous DNA, we transfected the cells with pSV2-*gpt* (Mulligan and Berg 1981). This plasmid carries the *Ecogpt* gene that serves as a dominant marker conferring resistance to growth inhibition by mycophenolic acid. Transfected cultures of 10^6 REFs formed 150 mycophenolic acid-resistant colonies that were observable 16–21 days after transfection.

To detect the REFs that had received the EJ *ras* oncogene, we cotransfected the oncogene together with the *Ecogpt* marker. As had been shown previously by others, cotransfected markers are efficiently incorporated by those cells in the culture that are transfection-competent (Perucho et al. 1980). Indeed, the resulting mycophenolic acid-resistant colonies were found to include a high percentage (80%) of morphologically altered cells (Table 1). This alteration of the cell phenotype that is exerted by the EJ *ras* oncogene could only be observed under conditions of mycophenolic acid selection in which nontransfected cells were prevented from growing. The presence of the EJ *ras* could also be detected in another way. If the REF cultures were seeded into soft agar 36 hours after transfection, then colonies of transformants grew out. No colonies could be observed in soft agar cultures of REF transfected with carrier DNA. This indicated that the transformation phenotype of anchorage independence could indeed be induced by the EJ *ras* oncogene (not shown).

We also used as recipients cells of the Rat-1 cell line, which had been derived originally from Fisher rat embryo fibroblasts (Freeman et al. 1973). These cells yielded up to 2×10^3 to 3×10^3 foci/10^6 cells when transfected with the EJ *ras* gene. The Rat-1 cells behaved in this respect like cells of the established NIH-3T3 line. Contrasting with the behavior of REFs, the formation of foci

Table 1 Complementation of Transformation by Cotransfection of Different Oncogenes into REFs

Transfected oncogene clones	Normal medium (foci/10^6 cells)	*Ecogpt* selection medium		Tumorigenicity in nude mice (number of tumors/ number injections)
		number of colonies/ 10^6 cells	percent of colonies with morphologically transformed cells	
pSV2-*gpt* (alone)	0	150	0	0/10
pEJ6.6	0	200	80	0/11
pPyMT1	0–10	75	15	0/6
pLT214	0	150	0	0/5
pEJ6.6 + pPyMT1	0–10	70	10	0/5
pEJ6.6 + pLT214	200	200	80	6/6
pE1a	0	150	80[b]	0/5
pE1a + pEJ6.6	80	150	80	5/5
pE1a + pPyMT	80	60	20	0/6
pSV*v-myc*	0	100	0	0/7
pSV*c-myc*-1	0	120	0	0/6
pEJ6.6 + pSV*v-myc*	200	200	80	10/10
pEJ6.6 + pSV*v-myc* del *SacI*	0	200	80	0/9
pEJ6.6 + p*v-myc*	80	200	80	7/7
pEJ6.6 + p*c-myc*	0	200	80	0/11
pEJ6.6 + pSV*c-myc*-1	220	220	80	9/9
pEJ6.6 + pSV*c-myc*-2	25	200	80	6/6
pEC6.6	0	100	0	0/3
pEC6.6 + pSV*v-myc*	0	100	0	0/3
pHu-*c-myc*	0	100	0	0/3
pHu-*c-myc* + pEJ6.6	0	200	80	0/3
N-*ras*[a]	0	140	15	0.5
N-*ras*[a] + pSV*v-myc*	25	140	20	5/5
pPyMT1 + pSV*v-myc*	60	100	15	2/5
pLT214 + pSV*v-myc*	0	100	0	0/4
pE1a + pSV*v-myc*	0	150	80[b]	0/5
pSV12	0	30	0	0/4
pSV12 + pEJ6.6	30	200	80	4/4

Cultures of 2°REFs were transfected by combinations of different cloned oncogenes as indicated. In each transfection, 1 μg of pSV2-*gpt* per 2 × 10^6 cells was transfected together with 10 μg of each oncogene-carrying plasmid. Focus, colony, and tumorigenicity assays are described in detail in Materials and Methods. The data represent a summation of several experiments for each test.
[a]2 μg of phage DNA were used.
[b]E1A-specific morphological alteration.

was not dependent on a cotransfection-selection protocol. More importantly, while transformed Rat-1 cells yielded rapidly growing cell lines upon cloning, colonies of transformed REFs entered cell crisis after replating, reaching sizes of only 500–5000 cells.

To test for tumorigenicity, we inoculated various transfected cultures into nude mice. Cultures of REFs were cotransfected with the EJ *ras* and *Ecogpt* clones and were placed under mycophenolic acid selection thereafter. About 80 colonies per dish grew out containing approximately 5 × 10^4 morphologically transformed cells in total. The cells of each dish were harvested, mixed with 5 × 10^6 untransfected 3°REFs, and injected into a single site. Three weeks after inoculation, the cells had developed into small subcutaneous, cartilaginous nodules (average size: 3 mm in diameter). However, when 5 × 10^4 EJ *ras*-carrying Rat-1 cells plus 2 × 10^6 untransfected Rat-1 cells were inoculated into one site of a nude mouse, rapidly growing fibrosarcomas grew

out that were readily detectable after 1 week and reached sizes of 3 cm in diameter after 3 weeks.

These data clearly show that the EJ *ras* oncogene has only a limited ability to transform REFs. It was not able to induce foci in dense monolayers; the transfected cells had a limited lifespan and they were not tumorigenic in nude mice. However, intrinsic functions of the Rat-1 cells could supply activities lacked by the oncogene. We suppose that these functions which can cooperate with the *ras* oncogenes to focus a tumorigenic cell were acquired during the process of in vitro establishment. A similar conclusion has been reached by Newbold and Overell (1983).

Cooperation between *ras* and viral oncogenes

We have mentioned above that certain DNA tumor viruses contain genes that are able to induce continuous growth of primary cells in tissue culture (Houweling et al. 1980; Rassoulzadegan et al. 1982, 1983; van den

Elsen et al. 1982) and thus mimic the process of in vitro establishment of these cells.

The "early" replicative region of the polyoma viral genome, which is also expressed in virus-transformed cells, encodes for three separate proteins, the small, middle, and large T antigens. These genes have been isolated as separate molecular clones (Treisman et al. 1981; Tyndall et al. 1981). As reported by Rassoulzadegan et al. (1982, 1983), these genes confer distinct and separable phenotypes on rat cells. The middle T antigen induces morphologic alteration and anchorage independence, whereas the large T antigen affects serum dependency and cell immortalization. Perhaps the phenotypes of establishment/immortalization that rendered cells reactive to the EJ *ras* oncogene could be elicited as well by one or another of these viral oncogenes. Initial transfections with the large T antigen clone showed that it strongly inhibited the formation of mycophenolic acid-resistant colonies. This cytopathic effect is probably due to large amounts of large T protein shortly after transfection, which might have led to abortive rounds of virus replication. To circumvent this problem, we used a clone, termed pLT214, given by R. Kamen. This clone encodes a truncated large T molecule which represents its aminoproximal half. This part of the large T molecule appears to be sufficient for its capacities in alteration of serum dependency and immortalization (Rassoulzadegan et al. 1982), whereas the lacking carboxyterminal part is required for mediating viral replication.

No change in morphology of 3°REF monolayer cultures was observed after transfection of pLT214 alone. However, cotransfection of the truncated large T clone with the EJ *ras* oncogene resulted in the appearance of dense foci within 10 days. When these cultures were injected into nude mice, rapidly growing tumors were observed in all cases. After 3 weeks, the tumors reached average diameters of 3–4 cm.

Whereas the EJ *ras* oncogene alone behaved like an incomplete oncogene, now it was clear that the EJ *ras* gene and the polyoma large T antigen gene acting cooperatively could convert the normal REFs into tumorigenic cells. Transfection of the middle T clone pPyMT1 alone or cotransfection of this clone with pEJ6.6 neither induced foci in dense monolayer culture nor yielded tumorigenic cells (see also Table 1).

Concurrent with our work, H.E. Ruley (1983) was performing experiments to examine the cooperation of the *ras* oncogene with the E1A early gene of adenovirus. Experiments in our laboratory confirmed Ruley's finding that the E1A gene can replace the function provided by the polyoma large T antigen in a cotransfection with the *ras* oncogene. Cotransfection of pE1A (contains the leftmost 1632 nucleotides of adenovirus 5; a gift from Tom Shenk, State University of New York, Stony Brook) with pPyMT1 led to focus formation in normal culture medium but repeated tests for tumorigenicity of the transfectants remained negative. As we learned from M. Rassoulzadegan (pers. comm.), the small T antigen clone has to be present in the cotransfections of pPyMT1 and pPyLT1 to achieve the reconstitution of the transforming capacity

of polyoma wild-type DNA. It might be possible that in the cotransfection of pE1a and pPyMT1 a third factor is required to achieve a fully transformed phenotype. However, at least two distinct genes, one cellular and one viral, acting in a cooperative fashion are sufficient for tumorigenic conversion.

Cooperation between *ras* and *myc*

We next wanted to examine the possibility of a cellular rather than a viral gene cooperating with the EJ *ras* gene to create a tumor cell. The cellular *myc* gene presented itself as the most likely candidate because altered versions of this gene were found to exist in a variety of tumor cell lines, which in addition carry a second oncogene that is able to transform NIH-3T3 cells (Goubin et al. 1983; Murray et al. 1983). To test the activities of the *myc* gene, we first chose to utilize the oncogene carried by the avian myelocytomatosis virus MC29. A proviral clone termed p*v-myc* (Fig. 1, Vennstrom et al. 1981) was kindly provided by J.M. Bishop. The circularly permuted provirus clone was reconstructed to carry a complete provirus by attaching an additional proviral fragment to its 3' proviral end (pSV*v-myc*; Fig. 1). When this clone was applied to NIH-3T3 cells, Rat-1 cells, or 2°REFs, either alone or together with DNA of the *Ecogpt* clone, no obvious effect was observed on these transfected cultures. However, transfection of either p*v-myc* or pSV*c-myc*-1 (see below and Fig. 1) together with the *Ecogpt* clone followed by mycophenolic acid selection resulted in detection of drug-resistant colonies with a longer lifespan than colonies carrying only the *Ecogpt* clone.

When the EJ *ras* and the *myc* clone (pSV*v-myc*) were transfected together into 2°REFs, both genes caused a dramatic alteration of the cell phenotype under conditions in which neither *ras* nor *myc* alone had any obvious effect on the monolayer cultures. Foci of refractile cells became apparent within 8 days of transfection. These foci could expand into the surrounding monolayer, under all described conditions of culture. In contrast to REFs carrying only the EJ *ras* gene, the EJ *ras/myc* cotransfectant grew rapidly (doubling time <24 hr) into mass cultures of morphologically transformed cells. When the cotransfected cells were tested in the tumorigenicity assay (as described in Materials and Methods), they were found to yield tumors in nude mice or in young Fisher rats that grew to a size of 1 cm within 2 weeks after injection. Southern blot analysis of the DNAs from five of these lines confirmed the presence of multiple copies of both the transfected EJ *ras* and *v-myc* segments in these DNAs (not shown).

Since the pSV*v-myc* construct contained two pairs of viral LTRs as well as an SV40 early promoter-enhancer element, it was possible that these *cis*-acting control elements alone would be responsible for the observed activity of the clone. Therefore, we deleted a 1.6-kb *Sac*I fragment from pSV*v-myc* that contains parts of the protein-encoding sequences of the *gag-myc* viral oncogene (Fig. 1). When cotransfected with the *ras* oncogene

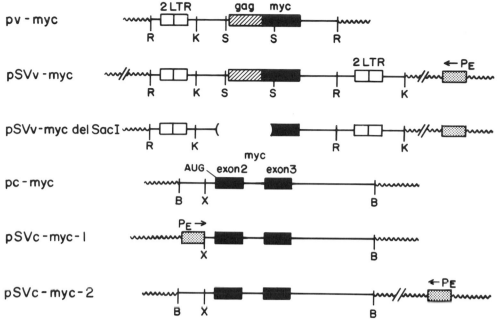

Figure 1 Schematic representation of the viral and mouse cellular *myc* genes used in cotransfection experiments. Details are given in Materials and Methods. (Reprinted, with permission, from Land et al. 1983.)

DNA, this modified provirus induced no detectable phenotype. Thus, activity of the *myc* clone depends upon synthesis of part or all of the *gag-myc* protein and not simply upon action of regulatory sequences.

We then tested a cellular rodent *myc* gene for its ability to cooperate with the EJ *ras* gene. A mouse *myc* clone, was obtained from M. Cole (Shen-Ong et al. 1982), originally isolated from the DNA of the mouse plasmacytoma MOPC-315. In this DNA, the *c-myc* gene had been rearranged by a chromosomal translocation and was found to be juxtaposed to the immunoglobulin C_α locus. The clone was modified by removing all immunoglobulin sequences and placing the two translated exons under control of the SV40 early region promoter present in the pSV2-*gpt* vector (Mulligan and Berg 1981). The promoter was located approximately 40 nucleotides upstream from the translational start codon (pSV*c-myc*-1; Fig. 1). This construct was effective in cooperating with EJ *ras* when tested in the cotransfection assay, and by that measure it was indistinguishable from the MC29 proviral *myc* gene (Table 1). A 10-fold lower focus-forming activity in this assay was yielded by an alternative *c-myc* clone. This construction harbored the SV40 promoter-enhancer fragment downstream of the gene and in opposite transcriptional polarity (pSV*c-myc*-2; Fig. 1; Table 1). Lacking any promoter-enhancer element, the *c-myc* clone (p*c-myc*; Fig. 1) did not show any biological activity in the cotransfection assay (Table 1).

Cotransfection of the normal human *c-Ha-ras*-1 gene carried by the plasmid pEC6.6 together with pSV*v-myc* did not yield any foci of transformed cells. Furthermore, we did not find cooperative effects between a human *c-myc* clone (Dalla Favera et al. 1982) and the EJ *ras* clone (Table 1). This *myc* clone (pHu-*c-myc*) contains all of the three exons and no foreign regulator sequences (a kind

gift from R. Dalla Favera). These data indicate that to achieve cooperative effects on transformation of 2°REFs, both of the transfected oncogenes have to be in an activated configuration.

Complementation groups of viral and cellular oncogenes

The ability of the EJ *ras* gene to cooperate with *myc* genes, polyoma large T, and adenovirus E1A genes suggested that the genes could be placed into complementation groups, meaning that differently acting genes should be able to cooperate in converting REFs into tumor cells, but similarly acting genes should not. In addition, other genes could be placed into the groups by their particular ability in cooperating either with EJ *ras* or *myc* in the focus assay.

In this type of assay, the N-*ras* oncogene behaved like the previously tested EJ *ras* clone in its ability to cooperate with *myc* (Table 1). The two *ras* genes therefore were placed into the same complementation group. When the polyoma MT clone was cotransfected with *myc* sequences, some foci grew out which in turn only rarely led to formation of tumors after inoculation into the nude mouse. Polyoma large T, *v-myc* and adenovirus E1A do not cooperate with one another (Table 1).

Based on these results, we would place Ha-*ras* and N-*ras* into one complementation group. The polyoma middle T antigen gene cannot be easily placed into this group, because establishment of this transforming function in the cell might need the presence of a third factor, such as the small T antigen gene (see above). Polyoma large T, the *myc* genes, adenovirus E1A, and the function of "in vitro establishment" can be ordered together into another group of genes serving a prolongation of the lifespan or immortalization of cells in vitro.

Discussion

The present results show that the EJ *ras* oncogene, while able to convert established cell lines into tumorigenic cells, has only a limited ability to transform 2°REFs. In monolayer cultures in which the nontransfected cells are suppressed from growing, it can be shown that the EJ *ras* gene is able to alter the morphology of REFs. In addition, EJ *ras*-carrying REFs are able to form colonies in soft agar. However, the EJ *ras* oncogene is neither able to induce foci in cultures of densely growing normal cells nor does it permit unlimited proliferation of the transfectants, which limits their tumorigenic potential. Observations describing the tumorigenic abilities of Harvey and Kirsten sarcoma viruses that have acquired very related *ras* genes (Gross 1970) might seem to contrast with the data described here. However, while tumor induction by these viruses might be interpreted as single-hit events, we would like to point out that viral tumorigenesis in vivo is still poorly understood and that other cell-specific factors might be required for tumor development.

The *myc* oncogene, when cotransfected with the *Ecogpt* gene, seems to prolong the lifespan of REFs. However, we are unable to confirm other reports concerning transformation of rodent fibroblasts by the avian *myc* oncogene (Quade 1979; Copeland and Cooper 1980). It is possible that such v-*myc* transformations resulted from rare events involving secondary alterations.

Our results clearly show that *ras* and *myc* genes exert qualitatively different functions. Alone they induce limited but distinct changes of the cell phenotype that might involve different cellular targets. In combination, however, they induce a tumorigenic phenotype that neither gene is able to achieve on its own.

The ability of the *myc* gene to cooperate with the EJ *ras* oncogene is at least in part comparable with the effect of in vitro "establishment" on *ras* transformation. This does not indicate that both functions lead to the same changes in the cellular phenotype. Indeed, we do not have any evidence that the *myc* gene is able to immortalize REFs, and we do not know whether the *myc* gene is necessarily involved in the process of cellular immortalization. However, both *myc* and in vitro "establishment" interact with *ras* in a similar way. This led us to postulate a complementation group in which, in addition to *myc* and "establishment," we placed the large T antigen gene of polyoma virus and the early 1A region of adenovirus, the latter of which had been shown earlier to be able to immortalize primary rat cells in culture (Houweling et al. 1980; Rassoulzadegan et al. 1982, 1983).

Another complementation group of transforming genes is comprised by Ha-*ras*, N-*ras*, and tentatively the polyoma middle T. This second class, which induces morphological alteration and anchorage independence, represents gene products that have been localized to the inner surface of the plasma membrane (Ito 1979; Willingham et al. 1981; Schaffhausen et al. 1982). In contrast, the genes of the previously described class specify proteins that are located within nuclear structures (Ito et al. 1977; Abrams et al. 1982; Donner et al. 1982, Feldman and Nevins 1983). The common site of cellular localization of the members of these groups may reflect molecular mechanisms, particularly involving interactions with common cellular targets.

It is not clear so far that the two described steps will be sufficient to convert a normal cell into a fully competent neoplastic cell. Although *myc* and *ras* together will induce a tumorigenic phenotype in REFs, the respective tumors grow to a large but static size. In contrast, *ras*-transformed cells that have undergone in vitro establishment or are cotransfected with the large T antigen gene seed tumors with unlimited growth capacity. This suggests that a third distinct gene together with *ras* and *myc* may be required to create a nonstatic tumor phenotype. However, the number of distinct genetic alterations required for tumorigenesis seems to be limited. This is promising, in that our understanding of the basis of this process may soon focus on a small number of molecular events.

Acknowledgments

We thank R. Kamen for his very useful discussions and for his generosity in providing T antigen clones. J. M. Bishop, M. Cole, and R. Dalla Favera are thanked for their gifts of *myc* clones, as well as T. Shenk for his gift of an E1A clone. We also thank W.R. Fields of the Lilly Research Laboratories for his kind gift of mycophenolic acid. H. Beug provided especially useful suggestions. The excellent technical assistance of J. Clark and A. Chen is gratefully acknowledged. H.L. is supported by the Deutsche Forschungsgemeinschaft. This work was supported by grants CA26717 and CA14051 of the U.S. National Cancer Institute.

References

Abrams, H.D., L.R. Rohrschneider, and R.N. Eisenman. 1982. Nuclear location of the putative transforming protein of avian myelocytomatosis virus. *Cell* **29:** 427.

Andersson, P., M. Goldfarb, and R.A. Weinberg. 1979. A defined subgenomic fragment of in vitro synthesized Moloney sarcoma virus DNA can induce cell transformation upon transfection. *Cell* **16:** 63.

Capon, D.J., P.H. Seeburg, J.P. McGrath, J.S. Hayflick, U. Edman, A.L. Levinson, and D.V. Goeddel. 1983. Activation of Ki-*ras*2 gene in human colon and lung carcinomas by two different point mutations. *Nature* **304:** 507.

Cooper, G. 1982. Cellular transforming genes. *Science* **218:** 801.

Cooper, G. and P.E. Neiman. 1981. Two distinct candidate transforming genes of lymphoid leukosis virus-induced neoplasms. *Nature* **292:** 857.

Copeland, N.G. and G.M. Cooper. 1980. Transfection by DNAs of avian erythroblastosis virus: An avian myelocytomatosis virus strain MC29. *J. Virol.* **33:** 1199.

Dalla Favera, R., E.P. Gelman, S. Martinotti, G. Franchini, T.S. Papas, R.C. Gallo, and F. Wong-Staal. 1982. Cloning and characterization of different human sequences related to the onc gene (v-*myc*) of avian myelocytomatosis virus (MC29). *Proc. Natl. Acad. Sci.* **79:** 6497.

Der, C.J., T.G. Krontiris, and G.M. Cooper. 1982. Transforming genes of human bladder and lung carcinoma lines are homologs to the *ras* genes of Harvey and Kirsten sarcoma viruses. *Proc. Natl. Acad. Sci.* **79:** 3637.

Donner, P., I. Greiser-Wilke, and K. Moelling. 1982. Nuclear localization and DNA binding of the transforming gene product of avian myelocytomatosis virus. *Nature* **296:** 262.

Farber, E. and R. Cameron. 1980. The sequential analysis of cancer development. *Adv. Cancer Res.* **31:** 125.

Feldman, L.T. and J.R. Nevins. 1983. Localization of the adenovirus E1a protein, a positive-acting transcriptional factor in infected cells. *Mol. Cell. Biol.* **3:** 829.

Freeman, A.E., R.V. Gilder, M.L. Vernon, R.G. Wolford, P.E. Hugunin, and R.J. Huebner. 1973. 5-Bromo-2'-deoxyuridine potentiation of transformation of rat embryo cells induced *in vitro* by 3-methylcholanthrene: Induction of rat leukemia virus gs antigen in transformed cells. *Proc. Natl. Acad. Sci.* **70:** 2415.

Goldfarb, M., K. Shimizu, M. Perucho, and M. Wigler. 1982. Isolation and preliminary characterization of a human transforming gene from T24 bladder carcinoma cells. *Nature* **296:** 404.

Goubin, G., D.S. Goldman, J. Luce, P.E. Neiman, and G.M. Cooper. 1983. Molecular cloning and nucleotide sequence of a transforming gene detected by transfection of chicken B-cell lymphoma DNA. *Nature* **302:** 114.

Graham, F.L. and A.J. van der Eb. 1973. A new technique for the assay of infectivity of human adenovirus 5 DNA. *Virology* **52:** 456.

Gross, L. 1970. *Oncogenic viruses*, 2nd ed., p. 931. Pergamon Press, Oxford.

Hall, A., C.J. Marshall, N.K. Spurr, and R.A. Weiss. 1983. Identification and transforming gene in two sarcoma cell lines as a new member of the *ras* gene family located on chromosome 1. *Nature* **303:** 396.

Hayward, W.S., B.G. Neel, and S.M. Astrin. 1981. Activation of a cellular *onc* gene by promoter insertion in ALV-induced lymphoid leukosis. *Nature* **290:** 475.

Houweling, A., P.J. van der Elsen, and A. van der Eb. 1980. Partial transformation of primary rat cells by the leftmost 4.5% fragment of adenovirus 5 DNA. *Virology* **105:** 537.

Ito, Y. 1979. Polyoma virus-specific 55K protein isolated from plasma membrane of productively infected cells is virus-coded and important for cell transformation. *Virology* **98:** 261.

Ito, Y., N. Spurr, and R. Dulbecco. 1977. Characterization of polyoma virus T antigen. *Proc. Natl. Acad. Sci.* **74:** 1259.

Land, H., L.F. Parada, and R.A. Weinberg. 1983. Tumorigenic conversion of primary embryo fibroblasts requires at least two cooperating oncogenes. *Nature* **304:** 596.

Mulligan, R. and P. Berg. 1981. Selection for animal cells that express the *E. coli* gene coding for xanthine-guanine phosphoribosyltransferase. *Proc. Natl. Acad. Sci.* **78:** 2072.

Murray, M., J. Cunningham, L.F. Parada, F. Dautry, P. Lebowitz, and R.A. Weinberg. 1983. The HL-60 transforming sequence: A *ras* oncogene coexisting with altered *myc* genes in hematopoietic tumors. *Cell* **33:** 749.

Newbold, R.F. and R.W. Overell. 1983. Fibroblast immortality is a prerequisite for transformation by EJ c-Ha-*ras* oncogene. *Nature* **304:** 648.

Parada, L.F., C.J. Tabin, C. Shih, and R.A. Weinberg. 1982. Human EJ bladder carcinoma oncogene is homologue of Harvey sarcoma virus *ras* gene. *Nature* **297:** 474.

Payne, G.S., J.M. Bishop, and H.E. Varmus. 1982. Multiple arrangements of viral DNA and an activated host oncogene in bursal lymphomas. *Nature* **295:** 209.

Perucho, M., D. Hanahan, and M. Wigler. 1980. Genetic and physical linkage of exogenous sequences in transformed cells. *Cell* **22:** 309.

Pollack, R., R. Risser, S. Coulon, and D. Rifkin. 1974. Plasminogen activator production accompanies loss of anchorage regulation in transformation of primary rat embryo cells by simian virus 40. *Proc. Natl. Acad. Sci.* **71:** 4792.

Pulciani, S., E. Santos, A.V. Lauver, L.K. Long, K.C. Robbins,

and M. Barbacid. 1982. Oncogenes in human tumor cell lines: Molecular cloning of a transforming gene from human bladder carcinoma cells. *Proc. Natl. Acad. Sci.* **79:** 2845.

Quade, K. 1979. Transformation of mammalian cells by avian myelocytomatosis virus and avian erythroblastosis virus. *Virology* **98:** 461.

Rassoulzadegan, M., A. Cowie, A. Carr, N. Glaichenhaus, R. Kamen, and F. Cuzin. 1982. The roles of individual polyoma virus early proteins in oncogenic transformation. *Nature* **300:** 713.

Rassoulzadegan, M., Z. Naghashfar, A. Cowie, A. Carr, M. Grisoni, R. Kamen, and F. Cuzin. 1983. Expression of the large T protein of polyoma virus promotes the establishment in culture of "normal" rodent fibroblast cell lines. *Proc. Natl. Acad. Sci.* **80:** 4354.

Ruley, H.E. 1983. Adenovirus early region 1A enables viral and cellular transforming genes to transform primary cells in culture. *Nature* **304:** 602.

Santos, E., S. Tronick, S.A. Aaronson, S. Pulciani, and M. Barbacid. 1982. The T24 human bladder carcinoma oncogene is an activated form of the normal human homologue of Balb- and Harvey-MSV-transforming genes. *Nature* **298:** 343.

Schaffhausen, B.S., J. Dorai, G. Arakere, and T.L. Benjamin. 1982. Polyoma virus middle T antigen: Relationship to cell membrane and apparent lack of ATP-binding activity. *Mol. Cell. Biol.* **2:** 1187.

Shen-Ong, G.L.C., E.J. Keath, S.P. Piccoli, and M.D. Cole. 1982. Novel *myc* oncogene RNA from abortive immunoglobulin-gene recombination in mouse plasmacytoma. *Cell* **31:** 443.

Shih, C. and R.A. Weinberg. 1982. Isolation of a transforming sequence from a human bladder carcinoma cell line. *Cell* **29:** 161.

Shih, C., B.-Z. Shilo, M. Goldfarb, A. Dannenberg, and R.A. Weinberg. 1979. Passage of phenotypes of chemically transformed cells via transfection of DNA and chromatin. *Proc. Natl. Acad. Sci.* **76:** 5714.

Shimizu, K., M. Goldfarb, M. Perucho, and M. Wigler. 1983a. Isolation and preliminary characterization of the transforming gene of a human neuroblastoma cell line. *Proc. Natl. Acad. Sci.* **80:** 383.

Shimizu, K., D. Birnbaum, M.A. Ruley, O. Fasano, Y. Sciard, L. Edlund, E. Taparowsky, M. Goldfarb, and M. Wigler. 1983b. Structure of the Ki-*ras* gene of the human lung carcinoma cell line Calu-1. *Nature* **304:** 497.

Smotkin, D., A.M. Gianni, S. Rozenblatt, and R.A. Weinberg. 1975. Infectious viral DNA of murine leukemia virus. *Proc. Natl. Acad. Sci.* **72:** 569.

Treisman, R., U. Novak, J. Favaloro, and R. Kamen. 1981. Transformation of rat cells by an altered polyoma virus genome expressing only the middle T protein. *Nature* **292:** 595.

Tyndall, C., G. LaMantia, C.M. Thacker, J. Favaloro, and R. Kamen. 1981. A region of the polyoma virus genome between the replication origin and late protein coding sequences is required in *cis* for both early gene expression and viral DNA replication. *Nucleic Acids Res.* **9:** 6231.

van den Elsen, P.J., S. de Pater, A. Houweling, J. van der Veer, and A. van der Eb. 1982. The relationship between region E11 and E1b of human adenoviruses in cell transformation. *Gene* **18:** 175.

Vennstrom, B., C. Moscovici, H.M. Goodman, and J.M. Bishop. 1981. Molecular cloning of the avian myelocytomatosis virus genome and recovery of infectious virus by transfection of chicken cells. *J. Virol.* **39:** 625.

Weinberg, R.A. 1982. Oncogenes of spontaneous and chemically induced tumors. *Adv. Cancer Res.* **36:** 149.

Willingham, M.C., I. Pastan, T.Y. Shih, and E.M. Scolnick. 1981. Localization of the *src* gene product of the Harvey strain of MSV to plasmid membrane of transformed cells by electron microscope immunocytochemistry. *Cell* **19:** 1005.

Avian Myelocytomatosis Virus *myc* and Adenovirus Early Region 1A Promote the In Vitro Establishment of Cultured Primary Cells

H.E. Ruley, J.F. Moomaw, and K. Maruyama
Cold Spring Harbor Laboratory, Cold Spring Harbor, New York 11724

Previous experiments have demonstrated that the T24 Ha-*ras*-1 and the polyoma virus middle T antigen genes individually are unable to transform primary baby rat kidney (BRK) cells following DNA-mediated gene transfer. However, early region 1A of adenovirus type 2 (Ad2) is able to provide functions required by these genes to transform primary cells in culture (Ruley 1983). The activity of E1A that enables these genes to transform primary BRK cells is presently unknown; however, the E1A functions important in transformation appear to be linked to activities present in continuous cell lines following in vitro establishment. Thus, cells from several previously established cell lines are readily transformed by the polyoma middle T antigen and activated *ras* genes (Triesman et al. 1981; Goldfarb et al. 1982; Capon et al. 1983), whereas primary cells are not transformed by these genes acting alone (Rassoulzadegan et al. 1982; Land et al. 1983, Newbold and Overell 1983, Ruley 1983). In addition, E1A itself expresses functions that facilitate the in vitro establishment of primary cells (van der Eb et al. 1980).

The linkage between in vitro establishment and functions required by *ras* and the polyoma middle T antigen genes to transform primary cells is further demonstrated by the fact that a portion of the polyoma large T antigen facilitates establishment of primary cells (Rassoulzadegan et al. 1983) and enables activated *ras* genes to transform secondary rat embryo fibroblasts (2° REF) (Land et al. 1983). Thus, it appears that transformation of primary cells in culture by certain oncogenes requires separate establishment and transforming functions.

As E1A and the polyoma virus middle T are viral genes, the question arises as to whether there are cellular genes expressing analogous activities that might be important in establishment and malignant transformation. A potential candidate for such a gene is *myc*, since *myc* is activated in a variety of tumor cells (Perry 1983) and yet *myc* apparently does not transform NIH-3T3 cells. Moreover, recent studies (Land et al. 1983) have shown that both *c-myc* and *v-myc* can cooperate with activated *ras* genes to transform 2° REF. However, attempts to demonstrate that *myc* could directly facilitate the establishment of 2° REF were unsuccessful, and as a result, the linkage between establishment functions and activities enabling activated *ras* genes to transform primary cells is less clear.

In the present report, the function of the *v-myc* oncogene of MC29 virus in transformation was examined by testing for its ability (1) to provide functions required by the T24 Ha-*ras*-1 gene to transform primary BRK cells and (2) to facilitate the establishment of primary BRK cells in culture. We find that *v-myc* expresses both activities, indicating that the functions required by activated *ras* genes to transform primary cells in culture are tightly linked to functions promoting in vitro establishment.

Methods

Plasmid DNAs
The following plasmids were tested individually and in combination to look for potential interactions leading to oncogenic transformation: pv-*myc*, a portion of the MC29 avian myelocytomatosis virus genome containing the coding sequences for $p110^{gag-myc}$ and the 5′ long terminal repeat (LTR) (Vennstrom et al. 1981); pT24, an activated *ras* transforming gene, T24 Ha-*ras*-1, isolated from T24 human bladder carcinoma cells (Goldfarb et al. 1982); pN-*ras*, an activated *ras* transforming gene isolated from SK-N-SH human neuroblastoma cells (Shimizu et al. 1983); and p1A, early region 1A from adenovirus type 5 (Ad5), extending from nucleotides 1 to 1834.

Transfection of primary baby rat kidney cells
Cultures of primary BRK were prepared and transfected by the DNA-calcium phosphate coprecipitation method as described previously (Ruley 1983). Primary BRK cells prepared in this manner consisted largely of epithelial cells, with fibroblasts accounting for a few percent of the total. Aliquots (0.5 ml) of DNA-calcium phosphate precipitate containing 250 ng of each plasmid and 10 μg rat carrier DNA were added to four 00-mm dishes of primary BRK cells. Cells were fixed with methanol:acetone (1:1) and stained 3–8 weeks posttransfection.

Isolation of established cells
Transfection of E1A and *v-myc* plasmids resulted in colonies of cells with extended growth potential in culture. Initial attempts to isolate cell lines derived from such colonies using cloning cylinders proved unsuccessful. Established cell lines derived from cells transfected by *v-myc* plasmids were isolated by challenging the cells to form colonies in dilute culture. Cultures were trypsinized 3 weeks after DNA transfection and plated at 10^5, 10^4, and 10^3 cells/60-mm dish. Cells from well-isolated colonies were trypsinized within cloning cylinders, seeded

in 2-cm² cloning wells, and subsequently expanded to mass culture.

Isolation of a mixed population of cells established by Ad5 E1A was accomplished by passaging transfected cultures containing several colonies to a second 60-mm dish 4 weeks posttransfection. This dish was nearly confluent within 4 weeks, at which time, cells were expanded to a 10-cm dish and subsequently passaged 1:2 at twice-weekly intervals. After four passages, cells were seeded at low cell densities for single-cell cloning. Well-separated colonies were picked using cloning cylinders and seeded into 2-cm² culture wells and expanded to mass culture.

Results

The ability of viral and cellular genes to transform primary BRK cells was tested following DNA-calcium phosphate cotransfection. Transformation was monitored by the appearance of dense foci of cells 2–4 weeks posttransfection. Cultures without foci were maintained for an additional 4 weeks to screen for slowly replicating clones of cells. Plasmids containing the following DNA sequences were tested individually and in combinations: Ad5 early region 1A, v-myc, cellular oncogenes (T24 Ha-ras-1 and N-ras) isolated from T24 bladder carcinoma and SK-N-SH neuroblastoma cells, and a modified polyoma virus genome encoding the polyoma virus middle T antigen species.

The results of several transformation experiments are listed in Table 1. As previously, shown, plasmids containing the polyoma virus middle T antigen and ras transforming genes were individually unable to transform primary BRK cells. In addition, plasmids containing the activated N-ras gene were also nontransforming. The failure of these genes to transform primary NRK cells is particularly interesting in view of the fact that all three genes readily transform a variety of established cell lines.

Early region 1A of Ad2 was previously shown to express functions that enable both the T24 Ha-ras-1 and polyoma virus middle T antigen genes to transform primary BRK cells (Ruley 1983). Similar results were ob-

tained in the present study with the early region 1A of Ad5. In addition, the N-ras gene was similarly dependent on E1A for transformation. The N-ras gene is related to both the Ha-ras and Ki-ras genes, having a similar nucleotide sequence. A single amino acid change at position 61 is responsible for the transforming properties of the N-ras gene (Taparowsky et al. 1983). These results suggest that although ras genes can be activated by amino acid changes at several positions, none of these is sufficient for the transformation of primary BRK cells.

Table 1 also indicates that the v-myc gene of MC29 virus can also provide functions required by the T24 Ha-ras-1 gene for transformation of primary BRK cells. However, the efficiency of transformation by cotransfer of v-myc and T24 Ha-ras-1 was 20-to 50-fold lower than the frequency obtained following cotransfer of Ad5 E1A and T24 Ha-ras-1. The low transformation frequency is nevertheless significant since the background in these experiments is exceedingly low. Indeed, transfection of several hundred plates with the T24 Ha-ras plasmid alone has failed to produce even a single focus resembling those obtained following cotransfer of v-myc or E1A (data not shown).

Transfection of Ad5 E1A or v-myc plasmids alone did not produce transformed foci. However, both E1A and v-myc gave rise to cell colonies with extended growth potential in culture. In the case of v-myc, isolation of established cell cultures proved to be straightforward. As shown in Figure 1, the ability of v-myc to establish primary BRK cells was demonstrated by the ability of the transfected cells to form colonies in dilute culture. The colonies in turn were trypsinized within cloning cylinders, plated into 2-cm² culture wells and subsequently passaged to larger culture vessels.

Initial efforts using cloning cylinders to isolate colonies of cells established by E1A were unsuccessful. Presumably these failures resulted because of a requirement for a high density of feeder cells for cell growth. Cells established by E1A-containing plasmids were isolated by passaging transfected cultures into dishes of similar surface area to maintain high cell densities.

Cells established by both E1A and v-myc have been cultured continuously for several months without crisis. In both cases, the cells retain and express sequences homologous to the transfected plasmids as judged by DNA and RNA blot hybridization (data not shown). These results suggest that E1A and v-myc have directly altered the growth potential of primary BRK cells following DNA-mediated gene transfer. However, it is presently not clear whether v-myc and E1A induce an immortal phenotype directly or give rise to a population of cells with extended growth potential from which immortal variants arise.

Cells established by E1A and v-myc are shown in Figure 2. The cells are flat and fail to overgrow a monolayer. In short, their morphological and growth properties are characteristic of nontransformed established cell lines. In contrast, cells transformed with E1A or v-myc and T24 Ha-ras-1 possess properties characteristic of oncogenically transformed cells: They overgrow a monolayer,

Table 1 Transfection of Primary Baby Rat Kidney Cells

	Experiment	
Plasmid	I	II
None (carrier only)	0	0
p1A	(8)	(14)
p1A + T24 Ha-ras-1	25	38
p1A + N-ras	17	26
pv-myc	(0)	(0)
pv-myc + T24 Ha-ras-1	1	1
T24 Ha-ras-1	0	0
N-ras	0	0

The total number of transformed foci in each experiment is indicated. Cells transfected with p1A did not produce transformed foci but formed colonies that could be stained; these are indicated in parenthesis. Cells transfected with v-myc formed neither foci nor colonies, as revealed by staining.

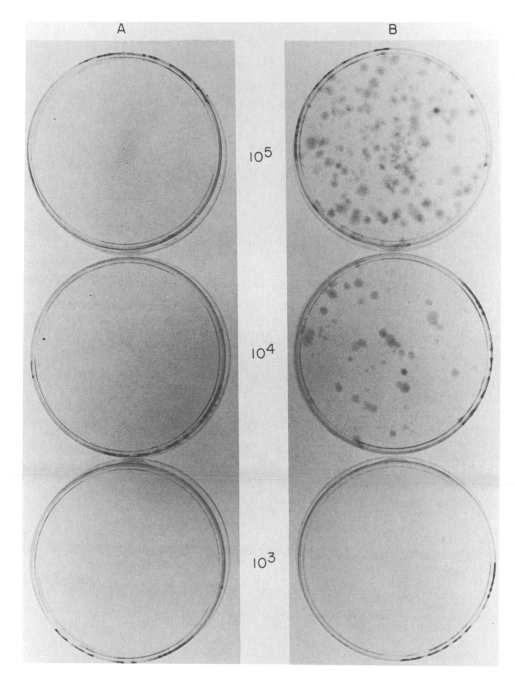

Figure 1 Establishment of primary BRK cells by the *v-myc* oncogene of MC29 virus. The ability of the *v-myc* oncogene to promote establishment was demonstrated by the outgrowth of colonies after transfected cells were plated in dilute culture. Cell cultures transfected with rat carrier DNA (*A*) or carrier plus pv-*myc* plasmid DNA (*B*) were trypsinized 3 weeks posttransfection and replated at 10^5, 10^4, and 10^3 cells per 60-mm dish. The plates were fixed with methanol:acetone (1:1) and stained with Giemsa after 3 weeks.

they are capable of anchorage-independent growth, and cells transformed by E1A and *ras* form tumors when injected into syngeneic animals. We are currently testing whether cells transformed by *v-myc* and T24 Ha-*ras*-1 are tumorigenic. A more detailed description of the properties of established and transformed BRK cells will be published elsewhere.

Discussion

Several genes, including the polyoma middle T antigen gene and activated *ras*-related transforming genes, are unable to transform primary BRK cells following DNA-mediated gene transfer. Functions provided by adenovirus early region 1A or the *v-myc* gene of MC29 virus enable these genes to transform. Both E1A and *v-myc* express functions that lead to the ability of primary BRK cells to grow for extended periods in culture. Indeed, cells transfected with E1A or *v-myc* have been passaged for over 6 months in culture with no indication of crisis. By contrast, BRK cells transfected with carrier DNA alone fail to establish beyond the first passaging except for rare variants that require months to establish and

EIA   EIA + Ha−<u>ras</u>

v−<u>myc</u>   v−<u>myc</u> + Ha−ras

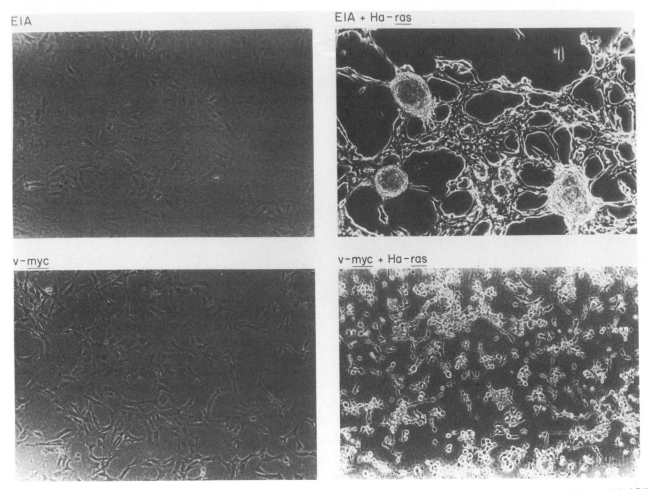

Figure 2 Phase-contrast photomicrographs of established and transformed BRK cells. Clones of BRK cells established with AD5 early region 1A or the *v-myc* oncogene of MC29 virus and transformed by a combination of Ad5 E1A or *v-myc* and the T24 Ha-*ras*-1 oncogene are pictured.

grow into mass culture. These results provide further evidence that separate establishment and transforming functions are required to transform primary cells in culture.

The activities of *v-myc* and E1A that lead to in vitro establishment correspondingly have been designated establishment functions. We prefer the term establishment over immortalization since it is not possible to demonstrate that *v-myc* and E1A directly confer the ability of indefinite growth in culture. Thus, it is possible that *v-myc* and E1A only extend the growth potential of primary BRK cells, and variants capable of indefinite growth arise subsequently. However, the use of the term "establishment" in this manner should not be confused with an earlier literature in which functions required to initiate (establish) transformation are distinguished from those required to maintain the transformed phenotype.

A recent report (Land et al. 1983) has shown that *myc* genes can cooperate with activated *ras* genes and the polyoma virus middle T antigen gene for transformation of 2° REF. However efforts to detect establishment functions following transfection of either *v-myc* or *c-myc* were unsuccessful. The reason for the difference between the study of Land et al. and this one is not clear. One pos-

sibility is that the different cell types used—2° REF as opposed to kidney epithelial cells—respond differently to the establishment functions of *myc*. Alternatively, Land et al. routinely selected transfected cells for mycophenolic acid resistance as well as establishment following cotransfection of *myc* and *Ecogpt* plasmids. It is possible that factors attending *Ecogpt* selection interfere with the outgrowth of established cell clones.

A third gene, encoding the polyoma large T antigen, is also able to provide functions required by transforming genes to transform 2° REF (Land et al. 1983). Moreover the large T antigen alone expresses an establishment function when introduced into primary cells (Rassoulzadegan et al. 1983). Thus, the functions required by transforming genes for transformation of primary cells are tightly linked to activities that lead to in vitro establishment.

The question arises whether the requirement for separate establishment and transforming functions in primary cell transformation is important in oncogenesis in vivo or simply reflects a peculiarity of in vitro transformation assays. Clearly, cultured cells must be able to grow in order to be transformed.

There are several reasons for believing that establishment functions are important in malignant transformation in vivo at least as far as activated *ras* genes are concerned. First, cells transfected by *ras* alone are not tumorigenic when transplanted into nude mice (Land et al. 1983). This suggests that the failure of *ras* to transform primary cells in culture is not due to the absence of growth factors that might be present in vivo. Second, several human tumor cell lines contain activated *myc* oncogenes in addition to activated oncogenes capable of transforming NIH-3T3 cells (Diamond et al. 1983; Murray et al. 1983). Third, it seems unlikely that the single-base changes responsible for the transforming properties of the activated *ras* genes are sufficient for malignant transformation, given the clinical and epidemiological evidence indicating that carcinogenesis is a progressive, multistep process. Finally, cell transfer experiments suggest that primary cells also have a limited proliferative potential in vivo as well as in vitro (Cudkowicz et al. 1964; Williamson and Askonas 1972; Daniel et al. 1975). In contrast, certain premalignant cells have an apparently unlimited proliferative potential in vivo (Daniel et al. 1975), suggesting that establishment functions may be associated with an enhanced proliferative potential in vivo as well as in vitro.

Establishment genes appear to enable primary cells (1) to respond to serum growth factors, allowing the cell to be cultured indefinitely and (2) to respond to the activities of transforming genes. A very simple model focusing on the relationship between establishment and transforming functions is shown in Figure 3. This model supposes that a cell can be in one of two metabolic states in regard to the potential of the cell to replicate. State I is characteristic of established cells. Such cells will respond to growth factors present in serum and can grow indefinitely in tissue culture. These cells can also be transformed by activated *ras* or the polyoma middle T antigen genes. State II is characteristic of primary cells on the road to senescence. These cells have a limited proliferative potential and eventually die. The limitation

is not overcome by serum growth factors or by the introduction of transforming genes. In contrast, establishment functions have the appearance of moving cells into state I (or of blocking entry into state II), thus enabling primary cells to respond to serum growth factors and leading directly or indirectly to in vitro establishment.

Given the association between establishment functions and proliferation in vitro, the question arises whether establishment functions, such as those expressed by *myc*, have a role in cell proliferation in vivo. If such is the case, proliferating stem cells in vivo may also occupy state I, whereas differentiated cells, which have a greatly reduced proliferative potential, would fall into state II. This model leads to the prediction that cellular genes expressing establishment functions should be repressed during differentiation. Although this an easily tested hypothesis, there is at least one example in which *myc* appears to be repressed following differentiation (Westin et al. 1982). Additional experiments will be required to demonstrate whether reduced *myc* expression directly influences the loss of proliferative potential characteristic of differentiation or is merely one of the many consequences of differentiation.

Although little is known about the metabolic functions of establishment and transforming proteins, it is interesting that the proteins of each group reside in similar cellular locations. Thus, proteins that express establishment functions are located within the nucleus (Ito et al. 1977; Abrams et al. 1982; Donner et al. 1982; Feldman and Nevins 1983), whereas *ras*-encoded p21 proteins and the polyoma middle T antigen are associated with the cytoplasmic membrane (Ito 1979; Willingham et al. 1980). Moreover, a sequence homology between E1A and *myc* proteins has recently been noted (R. Ralston and M. Bishop, in prep.). These structural and functional similarities encourage the hope that the establishment and transforming proteins each have similar metabolic functions and interact with similar targets within the cell. It remains to be seen whether this will prove to be true.

Acknowledgments

This work was supported by National Cancer Institute grant CA13106. K.M. is supported by the Robertson Research Fund.

References

Abrams, H.D., L.R. Rohrschneider, and R.N. Eisenman. 1982. Nuclear location of the putative transforming protein of avian myelocytomatosis virus. *Cell* **29:** 427.

Capon, D.J., E.Y. Chen, A.D. Levinson, P.H. Seeburg, and D.V. Goeddel. 1983. Complete nucleotide sequences of the T24 human bladder carcinoma oncogene and its normal homologue. *Nature* **302:** 33.

Cudkowicz, G., A.C. Upton, G.M. Shearer, and W.L. Hughes. 1964. Lymphocyte content and proliferative capacity of serially transplanted mouse bone marrow. *Nature* **201:** 165.

Daniel, C.W., B.D. Aidells, D. Medina, and L.J. Faulkin. 1975. Unlimited division potential of precancerous mouse mammary cells after spontaneous or carcinogen-induced transformation. *Fed. Proc.* **34:** 64.

Diamond, A., G.M. Cooper, J. Ritz, and M. Lane. 1983. Iden-

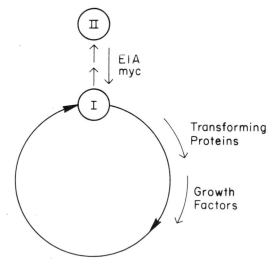

Figure 3 A model illustrating the relationship between establishment functions and cell proliferation. See text for details.

tification and molecular cloning of the human Blym transforming gene activated in Burkitt's lymphomas. *Nature* **305**: 112.

Donner, P., I. Greiner-Willke, and K. Moelling. 1982. Nuclear localization and DNA binding of the transforming gene product of avian myelocytomatosis virus. *Nature* **296**: 262.

Feldman, L.T. and J.R. Nevins. 1983. Localization of the adenovirus E1a protein, a positive-acting transcriptional factor, in infected cells. *Mol. Cell. Biol* **3**: 829.

Goldfarb, M., K. Shimizu, M. Perucho, and M. Wigler. 1982. Isolation and preliminary characterization of a human transforming gene from T24 bladder carcinoma cells. *Nature* **296**: 404.

Ito, Y. 1979. Polyoma virus-specific 55K protein isolated from plasma membrane of productively infected cells is virus-coded and important for cell transformation. *Virology* **98**: 261.

Ito, Y., N. Spurr, and R. Dulbecco. 1977. Characterization of polyoma virus T antigen. *Proc. Natl. Acad. Sci.* **74**: 1259.

Land, H., L.F. Parada, and R.A. Weinberg. 1983. Tumorigenic conversion of primary embryo fibroblasts requires at least two cooperating oncogenes. *Nature* **304**: 596.

Murray, M.J., J.M. Cunningham, L.F. Parada, F. Dautry, P. Lebowitz, and R.A. Weinberg. 1983. The HL-60 transforming sequence: A *ras* oncogene coexisting with altered *myc* genes in hematopoietic tumors. *Cell* **33**: 749.

Newbold, R.F. and R.W. Overell. 1983. Fibroblast immortality is a prerequisite for transformation by EJ c-Ha-*ras* oncogene. *Nature* **304**: 648.

Perry, R.P. 1983. Consequences of *myc* invasion of immunoglobin loci: Facts and speculation. *Cell* **33**: 647.

Rassoulzadegan, M., A. Cowie, A. Carr, N. Glaichenhaus, R. Kamen, and F. Cuzin. 1982. The roles of individual polyoma virus early proteins in oncogenic transformation. *Nature* **300**: 713.

Rassoulzadegan, M., Z. Naghashfar, A. Cowie, A. Carr, M. Grisoni, R. Kamen, and F. Cuzin. 1983. Expression of the large T protein of polyoma virus promotes the establishment in culture of "normal" rodent fibroblast cell lines. *Proc. Natl. Acad. Sci.* **90**: 1054.

Ruley, H.E. 1983. Adenovirus early region 1A enables viral and cellular transforming genes to transform primary cells in culture. *Nature* **304**: 602.

Shimizu, K., M. Goldfarb, M. Perucho, and M. Wigler. 1983. Isolation and preliminary characterization of the transforming gene of a human neuroblastoma cell line. *Proc. Natl. Acad. Sci.* **80**: 383.

Taparowsky, E., K. Shimizu, M. Goldfarb, and M. Wigler. 1983. Structure and activation of the human N-*ras* gene. *Cell* **34**: 581.

Treisman, R., U. Novak, J. Favaloro, and R. Kamen. 1981. Transformation of rat cells by an altered polyoma virus genome expressing only the middle-T protein. *Nature* **292**: 595.

van der Eb, A.J., H. van Ormondt, P.I. Schrier, J.H. Lupker, H. Jochemsen, P.J. van den Elsen, R.J. DeLeys, J. Maat, C.P. van Beveren, R. Dijkema, and A. de Waard. 1980. Structure and function of the transforming genes of human adenoviruses and SV40. *Cold Spring Harbor Symp. Quant. Biol.* **44**: 383.

Vennstrom, B., C. Moscovici, H.M. Goodman, and J.M. Bishop. 1981. Molecular cloning of the avian myelocytomatosis virus genome and recovery of infectious virus by transfection of chicken cells. *J. Virol.* **39**: 625.

Westin, E.H., F. Wong-Staal, E.P. Gelmann, R. Dalla-Favera, T.S. Papas, J.A. Lautenberger, A. Eva, E.P. Reddy, S.P. Tronick, S.A. Aaronson, and R.C. Gallo. 1982. Expression of cellular homologues of retroviral onc genes in human hematopoietic cells. *Proc. Natl. Acad. Sci.* **79**: 2490.

Williamson. A.R. and B.A. Askonas. 1972. Senescence of an antibody-forming cell clone. *Nature* **238**: 337.

Willingham, M.C., I. Pastan, T.Y. Shih, and E.M. Scolnick. 1980. Localization of the *src* gene product of the Harvey strain of MSV to plasma membrane of transformed cells by electron microscopic immunocytochemistry. *Cell* **19**: 1005.

Resistance of Human Cells to Oncogenic Transformation

R. Sager

Division of Cancer Genetics, Dana-Farber Cancer Institute and Department of Microbiology and
Molecular Genetics, Harvard Medical School, Boston, Massachusetts 02115

The view of oncogenesis as a one-step process and of oncogenes as total determinants of tumor formation has been widely held, especially after transforming genes were identified in retroviruses (for review, see Klein 1982). This view was further strengthened by the identification of genes (proto-oncogenes) in normal cells related to the transforming genes of retroviruses, and by the discovery of retroviral DNA integrated near the c-myc proto-oncogene in chicken lymphomas induced by weakly oncogenic viruses (Hayward et al. 1981). Above all, the discovery that DNA sequences from some human tumors could transform NIH-3T3 cells (for review, see Cooper 1982) led to the assumption that the DNA effective in 3T3 transformation must also have been responsible for the human tumors, despite the overwhelming evidence that the 3T3 cells were already partially transformed, and the absence of evidence that the cloned DNA sequences could transform human cells in culture.

This simplistic view of oncogenesis has now been criticized cogently by virologists examining the detailed experimental record (Duesberg 1983; Temin 1983). More generally, the concept of neoplasia as a complex multistep process is supported by a huge literature, both experimental and clinical, documenting tumor formation as a slow, uncertain, multistage process (e.g., Foulds 1975; Owens et al. 1982). The one-step view of tumorigenesis has finally been shattered even for its strongest protagonists by the discovery that the mutant c-Ha-ras oncogene cloned from human bladder carcinoma cell line EJ could only partially transform early-passage rat embryo fibroblasts (Land et al. 1983).

The new findings (Land et al. 1983; Newbold and Overell 1983; Ruley 1983) have led to the proposal that two oncogenes rather than one are necessary and sufficient for oncogenesis, but this view is basically inadequate. In terms of the experiments, we may ask for evidence that no additional genetic changes occurred in the transformed recipient cells beyond the addition of two oncogenes. This question is based on the fact that tumor cells characteristically contain abnormal genomes with rearranged chromosomes, and undergo further rearrangements during growth in culture or in vivo. The oncogene hypothesis does not consider chromosomal abnormalities as an intrinsic feature of the process of oncogenesis. The presence of chromosomal changes in the focus cells derived from treatment with two oncogenes would signal the presence of unidentified genetic changes, although inability to detect abnormalities by current methods does not preclude their existence at a submicroscopic level. Also, the occurrence needs to be examined in these experiments of "hit and run" transformation (Paraskeva et al. 1982; Galloway and McDougall 1983; C.C. Lau and R. Sager, in prep.) in which transformed cells no longer contain the inducing viral DNA.

The current state of our knowledge leads to two fundamental questions. Is oncogenesis the result solely of mutation, activation, or inactivation of the same short list of genes, such that if one could introduce those genes into normal cells without perturbing the genome, the cells would then be tumor cells? Second, what is the significance of the chromosomal rearrangements that are seen characteristically in tumor cells? A suggested answer is that chromosomal rearrangements provide the driving force for the multiple genetic changes required during oncogenesis. It is evident from clinical and epidemiological evidence that fully neoplastic cells arise in a step-wise fashion, but estimates of the number of steps vary widely (Peto 1977). If ongoing chromosomal rearrangements were responsible for the genetic changes underlying oncogenesis, the difficulty in assessing the number of such steps would be understandable. The importance of using early precrisis cells in the genetic analysis of tumorigenesis is now abundantly clear, but most rodent species are unsuitable because of the rapidity and heterogeneity with which they become genetically unstable in culture.

Human cells differ dramatically from rodent cells in their ability to remain stably diploid under conventional culture conditions for about 50 population doublings before they senesce (Hayflick 1965). With improved media, the number of presenescent doublings may be extensively increased. Thus, human embryo or foreskin cells would appear to provide the very best experimental material for studies of oncogenesis. However, normal human cells in culture are remarkably resistant to transformation, both spontaneous and induced, in comparison with rodent cells (Kakunaga 1980; DiPaolo 1983). Indeed, the difficulties encountered by many investigators in transforming human cells in culture (see Discussion) have led us to propose that the resistance to transformation of human cells may be in large part determined by their genomic stability.

We have begun to test this proposal experimentally by introducing known oncogenes into human cells to determine whether they are more resistant than rodent cells to transformation by these agents, and if so, to investigate the molecular basis of this resistance.

This paper summarizes preliminary studies (Sager et

al. 1983; R. Sager and L. Stephens, in prep.) of the responses of normal human cells of foreskin origin to transfection with SV40 DNA (deleted in the late region) and with the cloned EJ gene, a mutant form of the human *c*-Ha-*ras* gene, derived from a human bladder carcinoma cell line (Shih and Weinberg 1982). Transfection with SV40 DNA was of particular interest in view of the clinical record that demonstrates unequivocally the nontumorigenicity of SV40 viral infection in the human population (Fraumeni et al. 1963; Mortimer et al. 1981). The EJ gene was chosen for these experiments because its role in human cancer has been inferred indirectly from its effectiveness in transforming NIH-3T3 cells, although no direct evidence has been reported showing that the mutant gene has a transforming effect on normal human cells.

The results to be described here demonstrate that transfection of normal human cells with SV40 DNA leads to morphological transformation and expression of T antigen, but not to the acquisition of tumor-forming ability. Transfection with the EJ gene, however, leads neither to morphological transformation nor to tumorigenicity, despite the presence of the intact gene as shown by restriction site mapping, and overexpression of the Ha-*ras*-coded p21 protein. This result is in contrast with the findings with rat embryo fibroblasts reported by Land et al. (1983), in which precrisis rodent cells did exhibit morphological changes and increased ability to grow in soft agar following transfection with the same plasmid that we have used.

Methods of Experimental Procedures

Cells and media

FS-2 fibroblasts were derived from a human foreskin cultured in NCTC 135 medium plus 15% fetal calf serum (FCS). The minced FS-2 sample was distributed into six 35-mm dishes, and large outgrowths of fibroblasts appeared within 10 days. The cultures were trypsinized 2 weeks after seeding, and the pooled suspensions containing a total of 3×10^6 cells were reseeded as passage 1. A stock of 24 vials was frozen and maintained in liquid nitrogen at passage 4. The number of doublings to senescence has not yet been determined, but cells have grown at an average rate of three population doublings per week for more than 30 doublings. FS-2 cells do not form colonies in methylcellulose, although some cells undergo a few doublings. No tumors have formed in nude mice injected with 10^7 cells per site. Cells were grown in Dulbecco's modified Eagle's medium (DME) (Flow Laboratory) with 10% FCS (Gibco) in the experiments reported here. To test for anchorage independence, plates were coated with 0.6% agar bases, and cells were added in suspension in 1.3% methylcellulose (Fisher) as previously described (Sager and Kovac 1978).

Vectors

Transforming DNAs were introduced in the following vectors: (1) λSV-9 is a cloned fragment in λgtWes from the SV40-transformed mouse cell line SVT2 containing an integrated copy of SV40 DNA deleted in the late region (Sager et al. 1981); (2) pEJ contains the EJ gene as the 6.6-kb *Bam*HI fragment in plasmid pBR322 (Shih and Weinberg 1982); (3) pSV-*gpt*EJ, and (4) pSV-*neo*EJ (Bethesda Research Laboratory) are two similar shuttle vectors developed by Mulligan and Berg (1981) into which we introduced the 6.6-kb *Bam*HI fragment containing the EJ gene (Sager et al. 1983). After transfection, cells containing λSV-9 or pEJ were selected on the basis of focus formation, whereas transfectants containing one of the shuttle vectors were selected either with 25 μg/ml mycophenolic acid (*gpt* selection) or with 400 μg/ml of the drug G418 (Gibco) (*neo* selection). Subsequently, drug-resistant cells were grown continuously in the presence of the selective drug.

Transfection

FS-2 cells were transfected as described (Smith et al. 1982) except that DMSO treatment was omitted and 15% glycerol was added for 4 minutes about 18 hours after DNA addition. The cells were then washed with DME salts and refed. Three days later, cells were trypsinized and replated at 5×10^5 cells per 100-mm dish in medium containing selective drugs when specified.

Restriction site analysis

See Sager et al. (1981).

Identification of p21

Metabolic labeling of cells and p21 immunoprecipitations were carried out essentially as described (Der and Cooper 1983) with minor modifications. Immunoprecipitation was performed with 10^7 trichloracetic acid-precipitable cpm per sample, and immunoprecipitates were subjected to electrophoresis in 5–15% linear gradient polyacrylamide slab gels. For immunoprecipitation, the rat monoclonal antibody preparation #238 that reacts specifically with the Ha-*ras* p21 was used (Furth et al. 1982).

Results

Evidence of transformation of fibroblasts in culture is conventionally based upon a number of criteria of which the following appear to be the most reliable: morphological transformation, focus formation, growth in semisolid medium as evidence of anchorage independence, growth in low serum as evidence of loss of growth factor requirements, and tumor formation either in the nude mouse or in a syngeneic host. In transfection experiments with genomic DNA or cloned oncogenes, focus formation has been used often coupled with morphological transformation as the principal criterion both for selection and for quantitation. A few foci have then been chosen for tests with other criteria. In transformation studies with chemical and physical agents, growth in semisolid media has frequently been used as the primary criterion for selection and quantitation. Focus formation, morphological change, and growth in semisolid media are all empirical criteria that measure different parameters of transformation. In Chinese hamster CHEF cells,

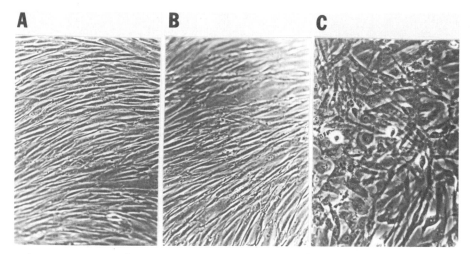

Figure 1 Morphology of normal and transfected FS-2 cells. (*A*) Confluent monolayer of FS-2 cells showing typical spindle shape and parallel orientation of fibroblasts in culture. (*B*) Confluent monolayer of gEF4 cells containing integrated EJ gene. Morphology resembles FS-2. (*C*) Confluent SV-46 cells containing integrated defective SV40 DNA. Rounded cell morphology and criss-cross orientation is typical of transformed cells. (Reprinted, with permission, from Sager et al. 1983.)

we have found at least two complementation groups that regulate anchorage independence and segregate independently in somatic cell hybrids (Marshall and Sager 1981). One anchorage gene affects morphology and tumorigenicity whereas the other does not. Furthermore, anchorage-independence and tumorigenicity are genetically separable in CHEF cells; many mutants have been recovered that are anchorage independent, but nontumorigenic, as well as tumor-derived cells that are anchorage-dependent (Smith and Sager 1982). In addition, anchorage independence varies greatly with the serum batch and concentration (Peehl and Stanbridge 1981) and is a difficult end point for quantitation because of the heterogeneous size of colonies.

Transformation of FS-2 cells by cloned SV40 DNA

As previously reported (Sager et al. 1983), FS-2 cells were transfected with phage λSV-9 DNA. This DNA effectively transforms CHEF/18 cells (Smith et al. 1982) and induces tumorigenicity. In transfection experiments with FS-2 cells, yields were about 15 foci/10^6 cells per microgram of vector DNA in one set of experiments, and about 3 foci/10^6 cells in a second set. The cells were morphologically transformed (Fig. 1). A sample set of foci chosen from these experiments contained SV40 DNA, produced T antigen, and was nontumorigenic in nude mice (Table 1). Plating efficiencies in methylcellulose were low, varied independently of T antigen pro-

duction, and did not correlate with the extent of SV40 DNA incorporation into the genome. T antigen was detected by indirect immunofluorescence of cells treated with fluorescein-conjugated anti-T antiserum.

These results are consistent with previous reports that SV40 virus-transformed human cells are not tumorigenic in the nude mouse assay (Stiles et al. 1975), and with the clinical evidence that inoculation with SV40 virus does not lead to cancer in humans (Fraumeni et al. 1963; Mortimer et al. 1981). The results demonstrate that one mechanism of resistance to oncogenesis by SV40 DNA lies at the cellular level, rather than in immune surveillance.

Transfection of the EJ gene into FS-2 cells

Availability of the cloned EJ gene (Shih and Weinberg 1982) made possible a direct test of its ability to transform FS-2 cells. Successful transfection of these cells with cloned SV40 DNA demonstrated that the cells were transfectable with a reasonable yield and that focus formation was an excellent criterion for selection of transformants. When FS-2 cells were transfected with pEJ, however, no foci were recovered in several attempts (Sager et al. 1983). Therefore it became necessary to establish whether or not the EJ DNA was integrated into the FS-2 genome. For this purpose, the selectable shuttle vectors pSV-*gpt* and pSV-*neo* (Mulligan and Berg 1981) were utilized. The cloned EJ gene was introduced

Table 1 Properties of SV40-transformed FS-2 cells

Cell line	SV40 DNA	T-antigen	Plating efficiency (%)		Tumor formation
			plastic	methocel	
FS-SV 32	single copy	+	15.5	0.1	0/4
FS-SV 35	many copies	+	12.1	0.2	0/4
FS-SV 39	single copy	+	10.0	0.02	0/4
FS-SV 46	many copies	+	26.0	0	0/4
FS-2	—	—	27.0	0.003	0/4

Vector λSV-9 contains DNA defective in the late region inserted into λgtWes.

into each vector at the *Eco*RI site and conditions were established for drug selection: 5–25 µg/ml of mycophenolic acid for *gpt* selection, and 400 µg/ml for *neo* selection. The results of these experiments are summarized in Table 2.

Excellent yields of permanently drug-resistant colonies were obtained, but the cells were not morphologically transformed (Fig. 1) in contrast to the SV40-transformed FS-2 cells. As previously reported, 30 mycophenolic acid-resistant colonies were picked and examined for the presence of EJ-DNA by Southern blot analysis (Sager et al. 1983). DNAs from eight of these clones, containing restriction fragments in the expected size range, were examined in detail using restriction enzymes that cut large fragments consisting of both the EJ gene and the adjacent *gpt* gene. An example from this study is shown in Figure 2. Fragments corresponding to the expected 6.8-kb *Sph*I fragment were present in five of the eight gEF cell DNAs tested: gEF 4, 22, 24, 25, and 29. In the other three gEF DNAs, fragments were present that hybridized with the 6.6-kb EJ probe, but their sizes were off. In gEF 23, the fragment was slightly smaller than 6.8 kb, whereas in gEF 20 and 27, only larger fragments were present.

The eight clones of gEF cells were examined for tumorigenicity in the nude mouse assay. No tumors developed in 4–6 months at a total of 25 sites, each injected with 5 × 10⁶ to 10 × 10⁶ cells (3–4 sites per gEF clone).

Presence of p21 protein in gEF cells

The *ras* gene family codes for a set of closely related proteins of about 21-kD molecular weight, the p21 proteins. Availability of anti-p21 monoclonal antibodies (Furth et al. 1982) has made it possible to immunoprecipitate these proteins, and it has been shown by immunoprecipitation and gel electrophoresis that the EJ gene product migrates slightly slower than the related protein coded by the normal *c*-Ha-*ras* gene (Tabin et al. 1982). This distinction in electrophoretic mobility between normal and mutant gene products, which is barely

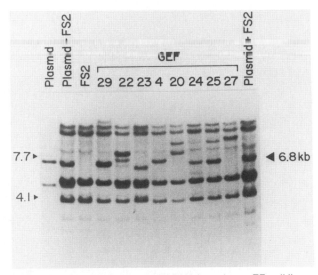

Figure 2 Integrated copies of EJ DNA in various gEF cell lines. Restriction fragments of genomic DNAs from gEF cell lines were cleaved by *Sph*I digestion, electrophoresed on a 0.8% agarose gel, transferred to nitrocellulose, and hybridized with a nick-translated, ³²P-labeled 6.6-kb *Bam*HI fragment of pEJ as described. (Reprinted, with permission, from Sager et al. 1983.)

detectable in mouse cells containing transfected copies of the human Ha-*ras* genes, is even more difficult on the background of human cell proteins.

We have examined proteins recovered from the eight gEF clones, in comparison with proteins from normal FS-2 and from the EJ cell line, using two different rat monoclonals against p21 (Furth et al. 1982). With monoclonal antibody #259, which detects mainly Ki-*ras*-coded p21 (M.E. Furth, pers. comm.), we did not find a consistent difference between FS-2, EJ, and gEF-derived proteins although gEF 25 may have a significantly higher amount of p21 than any of the others. With monoclonal antibody #238, which recognizes primarily Ha-*ras*-coded p21, however, the FS-2- and EJ-derived proteins gave distinctly different gel patterns, and all of the gEF-derived proteins except gEF 22, resembled the EJ pattern (R. Sager and L. Stephens, in prep.), as shown in Figure 3.

These results demonstrate that the transfected human cells are producing the EJ-coded p21 protein, but that it is inactive in altering their phenotype. Thus, resistance of human cells to transformation by the EJ gene is not at the level of transcription or translation. As with SV40 transformation, the resistance is evidently post-translational.

Discussion

The experiments described here are the first to examine directly the response of normal human cells to the introduction of cloned oncogenic DNA. Underlying these studies, which have just begun, is the extensive evidence that human cells are more resistant to transformation than are rodent cells of similar tissue origin. For clarification, this evidence will be briefly summarized here.

Table 2 Drug-resistant Colony Formation after Transfection of FS-2 Cells with pSV-*gpt*EJ or pSV-*neo*EJ

DNA	Colonies/pmole EJ DNA[a]
pSV-*gpt*EJ	
circular	36
linear	172
pSV-*neo*EJ	
circular	64
linear	133
Salmon sperm	0

Reprinted, with permission, from Sager et al. (1983).

[a]Two or more experiments, each with five or more dishes containing 5 or 10 × 10⁵ cells treated with 1 µg vector DNA plus 20 µg salmon sperm DNA and five dishes with 20 µg salmon sperm DNA alone.

a b c d e f g h i j k l m n o p

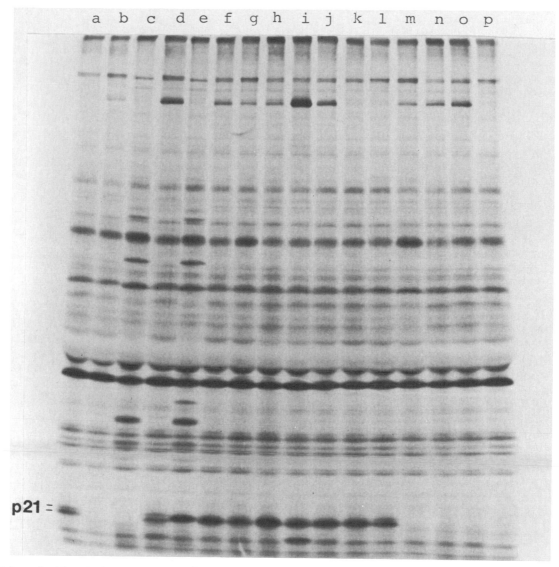

p21 =

Figure 3 Polyacrylamide gel electrophoresis of ^{35}S-labeled cell proteins immunoprecipitated with anti-p21 monoclonal antibody (lanes *a, d–l*) or normal rat serum (lanes *b, c, m–p*). Lanes are (*a*) gEF22, (*b*) FS-2 control, (*c*) EJ control, (*d*) FS-2, (*e*) EJ, (*f*) gEF4, (*g*) gEF20, (*h*) gEF23, (*i*) gEF24, (*j*) gEF 25, (*k*) gEF27, (*l*) gEF29, (*m*) gEF20 control, (*n*) gEF23 control, (*o*) gEF25 control, and (*p*) gEF29 control. Position of p21 determined by migration in relation to molecular weight standards.

Resistance of human cells to transformation

Only early passages of precrisis cells will be considered, since cells that survive crisis or senescence to become established cell lines have undergone genetic changes with unknown and variable consequences. Normal diploid populations of fibroblasts from embryonic or neonatal humans and from rodents differ dramatically during growth in culture. Human fibroblasts can be maintained as diploids with a constant doubling rate for about 50 doublings before senescence and death (Hayflick 1965). No spontaneous transformants have ever been reported in such cultures, nor have clones of spontaneous immortalized cells been found (Kakunaga 1980; DiPaolo 1983). In sharp contrast, rodent fibroblasts begin to undergo genomic rearrangements in very early passages, and spontaneous transformants arise as cell populations become increasingly heterogeneous in

karyotype and phenotype. The rapidity of these changes varies with the species, faster with mouse cells than with cells from Syrian or Chinese hamsters (DiPaolo 1983). Regardless of the species, however, spontaneous transformations occur characteristically during culture of freshly excised rodent fibroblasts but not in comparable cultures of human cells.

Human and rodent early passage cells also differ dramatically in their response to chemical and physical transforming agents. Whereas rodent cells are readily transformed by chemical carcinogens and UV and ionizing radiation, the many efforts to transform human cells were almost totally unsuccessful until complex new protocols were introduced (Milo and DiPaolo 1978) and applied (Borek 1980; Silinskas et al. 1981; Zimmerman and Little 1983). The essential common feature of these protocols is synchronization at the G_1/S boundary by starvation, using either amino acid-depleted medium or low serum concentrations. The cells are then released into rich media and mutagenized during early S phase. The requirement for synchronization is remarkable because no transformants whatsoever are recovered without it, despite the fact that about one-third of the cells in exponentially growing cultures are in the S phase. Although no explanation of the synchrony requirement has been generally accepted, it is likely that the prolonged starvation in these protocols leads to chromosome breakage, and thereby potentiates further genetic changes. Because of the special protocols required for human cells, it is difficult to compare their responses quantitatively with those of rodent cells. In an attempt to do so, Borek (Borek and Andrews 1983) has reported about a 100-fold difference in transformation frequency, assayed as colony formation in soft agar, between synchronized human and unsynchronized hamster cells exposed to 400 rads of x-irradiation.

Human cells are also much more resistant than rodent cells to virally induced transformation, as shown by the minor and indirect role that tumor viruses play in human cancer compared with that seen in rodent and chickens (Weiss et al. 1982). An impressive example comes from the inadvertant inoculation of 5,000–10,000 individuals with SV40 virus present as a contaminant in early polio vaccines (Fraumeni et al. 1963). Not a single instance of cancer has been reported from this exposure over the intervening 20-year period (Mortimer et al. 1981). Thus, the resistance of human cells to tumorigenesis must take into account viral as well as chemical and physical transforming agents.

Mechanisms of resistance to oncogenic transformation

To cope realistically with the question of resistance mechanisms, one needs to reach a pro tem decision about the number of genetic events involved in transformation. If a very few mutations, say two or three, are sufficient, the problem is a simple one of iterating mutation rates and determining whether mutation rates to ordinary genes are significantly lower in human cells than in rodents. From existing evidence, mutation rates in human diploids and in established cell lines of rodents are quite comparable. This evidence already suggests that there is something special about oncogenesis, not obviously comparable with single gene mutations.

One possibility is that quite a lot of mutations are required, and therefore that the iterated frequency of spontaneous mutation rates for a set of individual genes will be too slow. This ad hoc reasoning leads to the need for accelerated mutation rates to create neoplastic cells, and one known mechanism for achieving this is by turning on transposition (McClintock 1965, 1978). As discovered and analyzed by McClintock, transposition rates can be tremendously elevated following initiation by chromosome breakage. The consequences of transposition, including deletions, duplications, and translocations are hallmarks of the karyotypic chaos seen in malignant tumor cells.

On this hypothesis, evolution is greatly accelerated during tumorigenesis, with transposition as the driving force. As a consequence, changes arise in the coding sequences and in the regulation of many genes, leading to the phenotypic diversity acted on by natural selection, and resulting in the origin and heterogeneity of tumor cells (Owens et al. 1982). One would then propose that human cells are genomically stabler than rodent cells, and thereby less susceptible to transpositionally induced phenotypic changes.

An alternative explanation for the relative resistance to transformation of human cells could be that they require additional genetic steps, that is, additional oncogenic mutations beyond those required by rodent cells, but few enough to accumulate within the human lifetime. The two hypotheses are not mutually exclusive, and both may contribute to the resistance of human cells and survival of the species. Both suggested mechanisms are consistent with the evidence of cancer as a disease primarily of old age. Since we live about 50 times as long as mice, we need protection against the tumors they acquire in 1–2 years.

If chromosome stability is the key to cancer resistance, then new approaches to chemotherapy and prevention could be based on the elimination of cells with unstable genomes (Kakunaga 1975; Lau and Pardee 1982).

Acknowledgment

Most of the research was previously published and acknowledged. I thank Laurie Stephens for new experiments published here and Stephanie James for preparing the manuscript.

References

Borek, C. 1980. X-ray induced *in vitro* neoplastic transformation of human diploid cells. *Nature* **283**: 776.

Borek, C. and A.D. Andrews. 1983. Oncogenic transformation of normal XP and Bloom syndrome cells by X rays and ultraviolet B irradiation. In *Human carcinogenesis* (ed. H. Antrup and C.C. Harris), p. 519. Academic Press, New York.

Cooper, G.M. 1982. Cellular transforming genes. *Science* **218**: 801.

Der, C.J. and G.M. Cooper. 1983. Altered gene products are associated with activation of cellular *ras* genes in human lung and colon carcinomas. *Cell* **32**: 201.

DiPaolo, J.A. 1983. Relative difficulties in transforming human and animal cells in vitro. *J. Natl. Cancer Inst.* **70**: 3.

Duesberg, P.H. 1983. Retroviral transforming genes in normal cells? *Nature* **304**: 219.

Foulds, L. 1975. *Neoplastic development*, vol. 2. Academic Press, New York.

Fraumeni, J.F., Jr., F. Ederer, and R.W. Miller. 1963. An evaluation of the carcinogenicity of simian virus 40 in man. *J. Am. Med. Assoc.* **185**: 713.

Furth, M.E., L.J. Davis, B. Fleurdelys, and E.M. Scolnick. 1982. Monoclonal antibodies to the p21 products of the transforming gene or Harvey murine sarcoma virus and of the cellular *ras* gene family. *J. Virol.* **43**: 294.

Galloway, D.A. and J.K. McDougall. 1983. The oncogenic potential of herpes simplex viruses: Evidence for a 'hit-and-run' mechanism. *Nature* **302**: 21.

Hayflick, L. 1965. The limited *in vitro* lifetime of human diploid cell strains. *Exp. Cell Res.* **37**: 614.

Hayward, W.S., B.G. Neel, and S.M. Astrin. 1981. Activation of a cellular *onc* gene by promoter insertion in ALV-induced lymphoid leukosis. *Nature* **290:** 475.

Kakunaga, T. 1975. Caffeine inhibits cell transformation by 4-nitroquinoline-1-oxide. *Nature* **258:** 248.

———. 1980. Approaches toward developing a human transformation assay system. In *Advances in modern environmental toxicology* (ed. N. Mishra et al.), vol. 1, p. 355. Senate Press, New Jersey.

Klein, G., ed. 1982. *Advances in viral oncology*, vol. 1. Raven Press, New York.

Land, H., L.F. Parada, and R.A. Weinberg. 1983. Tumorigenic conversion of primary embryo fibroblasts requires at least two cooperating oncogenes. *Nature* **304:** 596.

Lau, C.C. and A.B. Pardee. 1982. Mechanism by which caffeine enhances lethality of nitrogen mustard. *Proc. Natl. Acad. Sci.* **79:** 2942.

Marshall, C.J. and R. Sager. 1981. Genetic analysis of tumorigenesis: IX. Suppression of anchorage independence in hybrids between transformed hamster cell lines. *Somatic Cell Genet.* **7:** 713.

McClintock, B. 1965. The control of gene action in maize. *Brookhaven Symp. Biol.* **18:** 162.

———. 1978. Mechanisms that rapidly reorganize the genome. *Stadler Genet. Symp.* **10:** 25.

Milo, G.E., Jr. and J.A. DiPaolo. 1978. Neoplastic transformation of human diploid cells *in vitro* after chemical carcinogen treatment. *Nature* **275:** 130.

Mortimer, E.A., Jr., M.L. Lepow, E. Gold, F.C. Robbins, G.J. Burton, and J.F. Fraumeni. 1981. Long-term follow-up of persons inadvertently innoculated with SV40 as neonates. *New Engl. J. Med.* **305:** 1517.

Mulligan, R.C. and P. Berg. 1981. Selection for animal cells that express the *Escherichia coli* gene coding for xanthine guanine phosphoribosyltransferase. *Proc. Natl. Acad. Sci.* **78:** 2072.

Newbold, R.F. and R.W. Overell. 1983. Fibroblast immortality is a prerequisite for transformation by EJ *c-Ha-ras* oncogene. *Nature* **304:** 648.

Owens, A.H., S.B. Baylin, and D.S. Coffey, eds. 1982. *Tumor cell heterogeneity: Origins and implications.* Academic Press, New York.

Paraskeva, C., K.W. Brown, A.R. Dunn, and P.H. Gallimore. 1982. Adenovirus type 12-transformed rat embryo brain and rat liver epithelial cell lines: Adenovirus type 12 genome content and viral protein expression. *J. Virol.* **44:** 759.

Peehl, D.M. and E.J. Stanbridge. 1981. Anchorage-independent growth of normal human fibroblasts. *Proc. Natl. Acad. Sci.* **78:** 3053.

Peto, R. 1977. Epidemiology, multistage models, and short-term mutagenicity tests. In *Origins of human cancer* (ed. H.H. Hiatt et al.), p. 1403. Cold Spring Harbor Laboratory, Cold Spring Harbor, New York.

Ruley, H.E. 1983. Adenovirus early region 1A enables viral and cellular transforming genes to transform primary cells in culture. *Nature* **304:** 602.

Sager, R. and P. Kovac. 1978. Genetic analysis of tumorigenesis: I. Properties of a pair of tumorigenic and non-tumorigenic hamster cell lines. *Somatic Cell Genet.* **4:** 375.

Sager, R., A. Anisowicz, and N. Howell. 1981. Genomic rearrangements in a mouse cell line containing integrated SV40 DNA. *Cell* **23:** 41.

Sager, R., K. Tanaka, C.C. Lau, Y. Ebina, and A. Anisowicz. 1983. Resistance of human cells to tumorigenesis induced by cloned transforming genes. *Proc. Natl. Acad. Sci.* **80:** 7601.

Shih, C. and R.A. Weinberg. 1982. Isolation of a transforming sequence from a human bladder carcinoma cell line. *Cell* **29:** 161.

Silinskas, K.C., S.A. Kately, J.E. Tower, V.M. Maher, and J.J. McCormick. 1981. Induction of anchorage-independent growth in human fibroblasts by propane sultone. *Cancer Res.* **41:** 1620.

Smith, B.L. and R. Sager. 1982. Multistep origin of tumor forming ability in Chinese hamster embryo fibroblast cells. *Cancer Res.* **42:** 389.

Smith, B.L., A. Anisowicz, L.A. Chodosh, and R. Sager. 1982. DNA transfer of focus- and tumor-forming ability into non-tumorigenic CHEF cells. *Proc. Natl. Acad. Sci.* **79:** 1964.

Stiles, C.D., W. Desmond, Jr., G. Sato, and M.H. Saier, Jr. 1975. Failure of human cells transformed by simian virus 40 to form tumors in athymic nude mice. *Proc. Natl. Acad. Sci.* **72:** 4971.

Tabin, C.J., S.M. Bradley, C.I. Bergmann, R.A. Weinberg, A.G. Papageorge, E.M. Scolnick, R. Dhar, D.R. Lowy, and E.H. Chang. 1982. Mechanism of activation of human oncogene. *Nature* **300:** 143.

Temin, H. 1983. We still don't understand cancer. *Nature* **302:** 656.

Weiss, R., N. Teich, H. Varmus, and J. Coffin, eds. 1982. *Molecular biology of tumor viruses*, 2nd edition: *RNA tumor viruses.* Cold Spring Harbor Laboratory, Cold Spring Harbor, New York.

Zimmerman, R.J. and J.B. Little. 1983. Characterization of a quantitative assay for the *in vitro* transformation of normal human diploid fibroblasts to anchorage independence by chemical carcinogenes. *Cancer Res.* **43:** 2176.

Tumorigenic Conversion of Early-passage Rodent Cells Can Be Achieved with a Single Activated Human Oncogene

D.A. Spandidos* and N.M. Wilkie

Beatson Institute for Cancer Research, Glasgow G61 1BD, Scotland

It is generally acknowledged that carcinogenesis is a multistep process (Armitage and Doll 1957; Peto et al. 1975; Knudson 1983; Spandidos 1983), although the nature and number of steps are still only poorly understood. On the basis of genetic analyses of hereditary cancers and the age distribution of other cancers, it has been proposed that the process in all cancers may occur in two stages—an initiating stage and a completing stage (Armitage and Doll 1957; Knudson 1971; Moolgavkar and Knudson 1981). Recently, some 16 cellular genes (or groups of genes) have been identified that are closely related to the active transforming genes of highly oncogenic retroviruses (for review, see Duesberg 1983) and may play a direct role in spontaneous cancer. One major question of interest is whether such genes are active in the primary or secondary stages of the carcinogenic process. Several in vitro systems have been described that have been used to mimic some steps in in vivo carcinogenesis. The malignant transformation of primary cultures of rodent cells is a commonly used model. In this system, the process has been divided into two conceptual stages: (1)"rescue from senescence" or "immortalization" and (2) "progression" or acquisition of a malignant phenotype (Spandidos and Siminovitch 1977a,b; Spandidos and Siminovitch 1978a,b; Barrett and Ts'o 1978). A major unanswered question is how these two stages of in vitro transformation are related to the proposed two-stage model of in vivo carcinogenesis. Recently, NIH-3T3 cells have been successfully used as recipients in gene transfer in vitro transformation experiments which have identified activated forms of cellular proto-oncogenes in human, rodent, and avian cancers (Cooper 1982; Goldfarb et al. 1982; Parada et al. 1982; Santos et al. 1982; Capon et al. 1983; Diamond et al. 1983; Goubin et al. 1983; Hall et al. 1983; Shimizu et al. 1983). Since NIH-3T3, cells are considered to be already partially transformed, it has been argued that this assay identifies only late-stage dominantly acting transforming genes (Littlefield 1982; Pollack 1982). More recently, it has been argued that one such gene, the Ha-ras-1 gene from the T24 bladder carcinoma line will only induce transformation of early-passage rodent cells only in combination with other genes or mutational events, which "rescue" the cells from senescence (Land et al. 1983; Newbold and Overell 1983; Ruley 1983). In this study, we show that this is not necessary, and that the introduction of the single T24 oncogene, in the appropriate vector, is sufficient to trigger the complete malignant transformation of early-passage Chinese hamster lung (CHL) cells.

Methods of Experimental Procedures

Cells and growth medium

CHL cells were derived from explants of female hamsters and were grown in Ham's modified SF12 medium (Flow Laboratories) containing 15% Hyclone serum (Sterile Systems Inc.)

Recombinant plasmids

The recombinant plasmids used in this study are shown in Figure 1. Plasmid pAG60 (Colbere-Garapin et al. 1981) contains the bacterial Tn5-coded aminoglycoside phosphotransferase (aph) gene under the transcriptional control of the herpes simplex virus thymidine kinase gene (HSV-1 tk) 5' and 3' signals. Plasmids pAGT1 and pAGT2 were obtained by insertion into the BamHI site of pAG60 of a 6.6-kb BamHI fragment containing the human T24 bladder carcinoma Ha-ras-1 oncogene (Santos et al. 1982). Plasmid pAGT1 contains the T24 gene in the same orientation as the aph gene and plasmid pAGT2 in the opposite orientation. Homer 6 was derived from the cosmid vector Homer 5 by Jonathan Wolf (Imperial College, London). Homer 6 contains the aph gene under the 5' transcriptional control of the Moloney murine sarcoma virus (Mo-MSV) long terminal repeat (LTR) promoter and enhancer regions (Lang et al. 1983) and the 3' polyadenylation signal derived from the HSV-1 tk gene. Homer 6 also contains the 430-bp HpaII–HindIII fragment of SV40 spanning the origin of replication and carrying the "enhancer" region, and the packaging signal of phage λ (λ COS). Plasmids pH06T1 and pH06T2 were obtained by inserting the 6.6-kb T24 Ha-ras-1 oncogene fragment into the BamHI site of Homer 6. Plasmid pH06T2 contains the T24 gene in the same orientation as aph and pH06T1 in the opposite orientation.

Cell transformation assays

Transfections of third-passage Chinese hamster lung CHL(F3) cells and second-passage rat embryo or baby rat skin, muscle, lung, or kidney cells were carried out using the calcium phosphate technique (Graham and Van der Eb 1973) with the following modifications. The

---

*Permanent address: Hellenic Anticancer Institute, Athens, Greece.

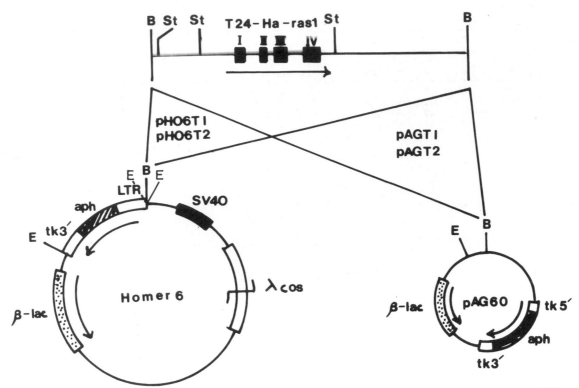

Figure 1 Schematic representation of pAG60 (8.2 kb), Homer 6 (7.7 kb), pH06T1, and derivative plasmids pAGT1, pAGT2, pH06T1, and pH06T2. The *Bam*HI fragment containing the T24 Ha-*ras*-1 oncogene is 6.6 kb. Details of their constructions are described in Methods of Experimental Procedures. The following designated sequences are defined in Methods: (*aph*) aminoglycoside phosphotransferase; (*tk*) HSV thymidine kinase; (LTR) Mo-MSV long terminal repeat; (SV40) simian virus 40; (λ COS) packaging signal of phage λ; (β-lac) β-lactamase sequences; (B) *Bam*HI; (E) *Eco*RI; (St) *Sst*I. The maps are not drawn to scale. (I–IV) Exons of the human T24 Ha-*ras*-1 (T24-Ha-*ras*-1) oncogene.

DNA-calcium phosphate coprecipitate was added to the culture medium at a ratio of 1.0 ml coprecipitate/10 ml medium · 1 × 10^5 to 2 × 10^5 exponentially growing recipient cells/25 cm^2 flask. After 20 hours, the medium was replaced with fresh nonselective medium (SF12 containing 15% Hyclone serum) for an additional 24 hours before selective medium (SF12 containing 15% Hyclone serum and 200 μg/ml geneticin-Gibco) was applied. The medium was changed every 2–3 days for up to 10 days before colonies were counted. Colonies were scored for morphological transformation with phase-contrast microscopy. Normal untransformed colonies display an organized parallel arrangement of cells with very little piling up. Morphologically transformed colonies exhibit a random orientation growth pattern with increased number of multinucleated giant cells and extensive piling up. Colonies were picked using sterile stainless steel cloning rings or the cells were fixed with 100% methanol for 10 minutes and stained with 10% Giemsa in H$_2$O. The methocel assay has been described in detail elsewhere (Spandidos et al. 1982).

Tumorigenicity studies
Cultures were trypsinized and suspended in SF12 medium of varying concentrations of cells and 0.1 ml were subcutaneously injected into male nude mice (30 days old). All animals were checked every day for the appearance of tumors.

Karyological analysis
Forty metaphases from each cell line were counted for the modal chromosome number. Fifteen G-banded late prophase or prometaphase cells were photographed to prepare the karyotypes.

Isolation of RNA and DNA and filter hybridizations
Extraction of RNA and DNA from cells and blotting onto nitrocellulose was carried out as described previously (Spandidos and Paul 1982). DNA from recipient and transformed cells was obtained from CsCl gradients, which were also used to isolate the RNA, and further treated with proteinase K, phenol, and chloroform before ethanol precipitation. Filter hybridizations were performed in 5× SSC, 50% formamide for 24 hours at 42°C with 10 ng/ml denatured, nick-translated ^{32}P-labeled DNA, specific activity 1 × 10^8 to 3 × 10^8 cpm/μg; using 2× Denhardt's solution. The nitrocellulose sheets were washed in 0.5× SSC at 60°C and exposed to X-ray films at −70°C.

Results
Transformation of Chinese hamster lung cells
Recombinant plasmids pAG60, pAGT1, Homer 6, pH06T1, and pH06T2 described in Methods and Experimental Procedures and in Figure 1, were used to transfect passage-3 Chinese hamster lung cells

Table 1 Transformation of Chinese Hamster Lung CHL(F3) Cells with *aph* Recombinants

| Donor DNA[a,b] | Colonies/25 cm² flask in liquid medium[c] | | Colonies/10-cm plate Methocel medium[d] (average) |
	morphologically normal (average)	morphologically transformed (average)	
pAG60	3, 5, 8, 10 (6.5)	0, 0, 0, 0 (0)	0, 0, 0, 0 (0)
pAGT1	17,12,23,10 (16)	0, 0, 0, 0 (0)	0, 0, 0, 0 (0)
Homer 6	32,47,65,54 (50)	0, 0, 0, 0 (0)	0, 0, 0, 0 (0)
pH06T1	78,111,96,105 (98)	75,106,90,101 (93)	250,196,210,215 (218)
pH06T2	56, 72, 83, 97 (77)	56, 69,78, 92 (74)	182,195,173,224 (194)
Salmon	0, 0, 0, 0 (0)	0, 0, 0, 0 (0)	0, 0, 0, 0 (0)

[a]All selective media contained 200 μg/ml geneticin.
[b]Use 10 μg supercoiled donor DNA per flask or plate, in the absence of carrier DNA.
[c]1×10^5 cells plated per 25-cm² flask.
[d]2×10^5 cells plated per 10-cm² flask.

CHL(F3) using the calcium phosphate technique (Graham and Van der Eb 1973). After the addition of 200 μg/ml geneticin in the selective medium, background cells died within 3–5 days, and within 7–10 days geneticin-resistant colonies became apparent. The colonies were counted at day 10 and the results are given in Table 1. Geneticin-resistant colonies were obtained after transfection with all of the recombinants tested, but at widely different frequencies. No colonies were obtained when salmon sperm DNA was used as donor. Homer 6 gave approximately seven to eight times more colonies than pAG60. We assume that this is due to the presence of the Mo-MSV LTR and SV40 "enhancers" in the former plasmid (Blair et al. 1980; Banerji et al. 1981; Gruss et al. 1981; Moreau et al. 1981; Spandidos and Wilkie 1983). In each case, the presence of the T24 oncogene resulted in significantly increased numbers of geneticin-resistant colonies. The reasons for this are not yet known. Perhaps the presence of an activated *ras* gene improves the ability of cells to survive at low cell densities without necessarily displaying morphological changes. Alternatively, the *ras* gene sequence may itself contain an "enhancer" that additionally affects expression of the *aph* gene.

The geneticin-resistant colonies were scored for evidence of morphological transformation and the results are given in Table 1. No morphologically altered colonies were obtained with plasmid pAG60, pAGT1, or Homer 6, whereas more than 90% of the geneticin-resistant colonies obtained with pH06T1 and pH06T2 were morphologically altered by the criteria described in Methods and Experimental Procedures and as shown in Figure 2. Transfection of CHL(F3) cells with pH06T1 or pH06T2 also resulted in the appearance of geneticin-resistant colonies with an anchorage-independent phenotype. This was assayed by direct simultaneous selection in semisolid medium containing geneticin (Table 1). Morphologically altered cells from liquid cultures, when picked and subcultured, also grow in semisolid medium. On subsequent subculture in liquid medium, colonies isolated from both semisolid medium and liquid culture have a higher plating efficiency than CHL(F3) cells (80–90% vs. 10–20%), a lower doubling time (7–10 hr vs. 24–30 hr), and grow to a higher density. Morphologically altered cells have abnormal karyotypes (marker chromosomes; aneuploidy; deletions and translocations) and produce tumors in nude mice 5–7 days after the subcutaneous inoculation of 10⁶ cells. (CHL[F3]) cells do not produce tumors.)

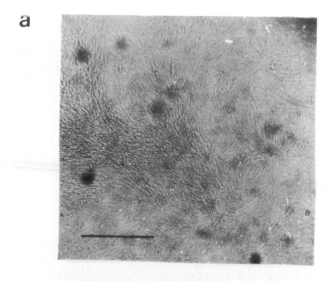

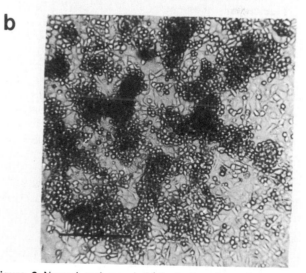

Figure 2 Normal and morphologically transformed cells. (*a*) Geneticin-resistant CHL(F3) cells transformed with recombinant pAG60. (*b*) Geneticin-resistant CHL(F3) cells transformed with recombinant pH06T1. Bar, 0.5 mm.

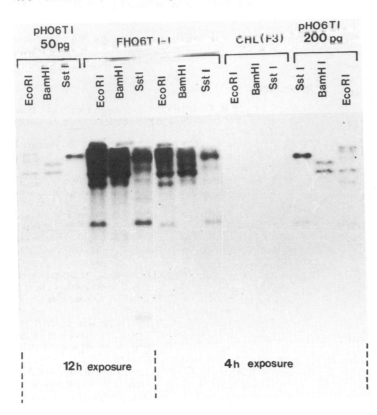

12h exposure   4h exposure

Figure 3 An autoradiograph showing a Southern blot hybridization analysis of recipient CHL(F3) and transformed FH06T1-1 cells containing multiple copies of the pH06T1 recombinant. ^{32}P-labeled, nick-translated pH06T1 plasmid was used as probe. pH06T1 DNA (50 and 200 pg) cut with *Eco*RI, *Bam*HI, or *Sst*I were used as a marker.

Analyses of DNA and RNA

Several morphologically transformed cell lines were analyzed for the presence and state of donor plasmid DNA. The data for cell line FH06T1-1, derived after transfection with plasmid pH06T1, is shown in Figure 3, with control lanes for the original CHL(F3) cells and pH06T1 plasmid DNA. Analysis with restriction enzymes *Eco*RI, *Bam*HI, and *Sst*I shows the presence of three to five copies of full-length pH06T1 DNA, presumably present as head-to-tail tandem duplications. Additional DNA fragments not observed with control pH06T1 plasmid DNA may be due to partial digestion with the restriction endonucleases or fragments representing junctions between pH06T1 DNA and cell DNA. In other cell lines, no full-length copies were detected, indicating integration of donor DNA into recipient DNA.

Figure 4 shows the analysis of T24 gene-related transcripts in several morphologically altered cell lines obtained after transformation with pH06T1 or pH06T2, in comparison to recipient CHL(F3) cells and the original human T24 bladder carcinoma cell line. We could detect very little Ha-*ras*-1-related RNA in CHL(F3) cells. In contrast, the T24 line and the morphologically altered transformed hamster cells had abundant 1.2-kb Ha-*ras*-1-related transcripts, the expected size for the T24 gene (Santos et al. 1982; Goldfarb et al. 1982; Parada et al. 1982). The most abundant RNA was found in the morphologically altered hamster cells transformed with pH06T1 or pH06T2 DNAs.

Discussion

Our data clearly shows that transfer of a single activated human oncogene (Ha-*ras*-1) is sufficient to trigger the

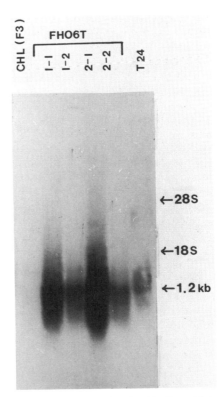

←28S

←18S

←1.2 kb

Figure 4 An autoradiograph showing Northern blot hybridization analysis of Ha-*ras*-1 RNA in recipient CHL(F3), cells morphologically transformed with pH06T1 (FH06T1-1, FH06T1-2) or pH06T2 (FH06T2-1, FH06T2-2) and the human T24 bladder carcinoma cell line. Total cell RNAs (20 μg) from cells indicated on the figure were fractionated at 1% agarose-formaldehyde-containing gels, blotted onto nitrocellulose, and probed with ^{32}P-labeled pT24C3 (Santos et al. 1982) DNA.

process of full conversion to malignant phenotype of primary Chinese hamster cells. The result is not confined to Chinese hamster cells, since we have obtained equivalent results with cells explanted from the tissues of both embryonic and newborn rats (D.A. Spandidos and N.M. Wilkie, in prep.).

These results contrast with recent reports that the T24 oncogene only transforms primary rodent cells only when they have been treated with chemical carcinogens, or other transforming viral genes (Land et al. 1983; Newbold and Overell 1983; Ruley 1983). We interpret our results to mean that if sufficient transcriptional activation is obtained, the T24 gene alone can trigger the conversion of a fully malignant phenotype. In agreement with the previous workers, we could find no morphological transformation when the T24 gene was introduced into the recipient cells in a vector lacking "enhancer" sequences. Our results are also consistent with previous studies which show that either ras gene mutation (Reddy et al. 1982; Tabin et al. 1982; Taparowsky et al. 1982) or increased levels of wt ras-gene transcripts (Chang et al. 1982) can result in tumorigenic conversion of 3T3 cells: in the present study, the T24 gene active in the malignant conversion of primary cells contains the previously described mutation at amino acid position 12 (Reddy et al. 1982) and is also transcriptionally activated. Our recombinants, which carry the mutated ras gene, and also strong transcriptional "enhancers," may be compared with some of the acute transforming retroviruses. Indeed, it is long established that some of these viruses can directly transform cells in vitro to a fully malignant phenotype (for reviews, see Weiss et al. 1982 and Duesberg 1983). For example, Rous sarcoma virus, which contains a mutationally altered homolog of the cellular src gene, transforms avian fibroblasts with single-hit kinetics (Temin and Rubin 1958). In these cases, it seems likely that both mutation of amino acid-coding sequences and transcriptional activation contribute to the highly transforming phenotype.

To date, the models proposed for ras gene activation during in vitro carcinogenesis have concentrated on mutational events that alter the primary coding potential (Reddy et al. 1982; Tabin et al. 1982; Taparowsky et al. 1982; Capon et al. 1983; Yuasa et al. 1983). However, recently we have detected highly elevated levels of ras gene transcripts in premalignant tissues of the human colon (D.A. Spandidos and I.B. Kerr, in prep.). Taken together with the present report, these results suggest that altered ras genes may play an early role in the carcinogenic process. Perhaps multistep events, acting at only a single locus, or only a small number of loci, are sufficient to trigger the processes that inevitably lead to a malignant phenotype.

Acknowledgments

We would like to thank M. Freshney and R. Balfour for excellent technical assistance and J. Neil for critical reading of the manuscript.

We are most grateful to M. Barbacid for plasmid pT24C3 containing the T24, Ha-ras-1 gene, to J. Wolfe and P. Rigby for the Homer 6 vector, and to A.C. Garapin for pAG60. We gratefully acknowledge the continuing support of the Cancer Research Campaign of Great Britain.

References

Armitage, P. and R. Doll. 1957. A two stage theory of carcinogenesis in relation to the age distribution of human cancer. *Br. J. Cancer* **11**: 161.

Banerji, J., S. Rusconi, and W. Schaffner. 1981. Expression of β-globin gene is enhanced by remote SV40 DNA sequences. *Cell* **27**: 299.

Barrett, J.C. and P.O.P. Ts'o. 1978. Evidence for the progressive nature of neoplastic transformation in vitro. *Proc. Natl. Acad. Sci.* **75**: 3761.

Blair, D.G., W.L. McClements, M.K. Oskarsson, P.J. Fischinger, and G.F. Vande Woude. 1980. Biological activity of cloned Moloney sarcoma virus DNA: Terminally redundant sequence may enhance transformation efficiency. *Proc. Natl. Acad. Sci.* **77**: 3504.

Capon, D.J., P.H. Seeburg, J.P. McGrath, J.S. Hayflick, U. Edman, A.D. Levinson, and D.V. Goeddel. 1983. Activation of Ki-ras2 gene in human colon and lung carcinomas by two different point mutations. *Nature* **304**: 507.

Chang, E.J., M.F. Furth, E.M. Scolnick, and D.R. Lowy. 1982. Tumorigenic transformation of mammalian cells induced by a normal human gene homologous to the oncogene of Harvey murine sarcoma virus. *Nature* **297**: 479.

Colbere-Garapin, F., F. Horodniceanu, P. Kourilsky, and A.C. Garapin. 1981. A new dominant hybrid selective marker for higher eukaryotic cells. *J. Mol. Biol.* **150**: 1.

Cooper, G.M. 1982. Cellular transforming genes. *Science* **218**: 801.

Diamond, A., G.M. Cooper, J. Ritz, and M.A. Lane. 1983. Identification and molecular cloning of the human Blym transforming gene activated in Burkitt's lymphomas. *Nature* **305**: 112.

Duesberg, P.H. 1983. Retroviral transforming genes in normal cells? *Nature* **304**: 210.

Goldfarb, M., K. Shimizu, M. Perucho, and M. Wigler. 1982. Isolation and preliminary characterization of a human transforming gene from T24 bladder carcinoma cells. *Nature* **296**: 404.

Goubin, G., D.S. Goldman, J. Luce, P.E. Neiman, and G.M. Cooper. 1983. Molecular cloning and nucleotide sequence of a transforming gene detected by transfection of chicken B-cell lymphoma DNA. *Nature* **302**: 114.

Graham, F.L. and A.J. Van der Eb. 1973. A new technique for the assay of infectivity of human adenovirus DNA. *Virology* **52**: 456.

Gruss, P., R. Dhar, and G. Khoury. 1981. Simian virus 40 tandem repeated sequences as an element of the early promoter. *Proc. Natl. Acad. Sci.* **78**: 943.

Hall, A., C.J. Marshall, N.K. Spurr, and R.A. Weiss. 1983. Identification of transforming gene in two human sarcoma cell lines as a new member of the ras gene family located on chromosome 1. *Nature* **303**: 396.

Knudson, A.G. 1971. Mutation and cancer: Statistical analysis of retinoblastoma. *Proc. Natl. Acad. Sci.* **68**: 820.

———. 1983. Hereditary cancers of man. *Cancer Invest.* **1**: 187.

Land, H., L.F. Parada, and R.A. Weinberg. 1983. Tumorigenic conversion of primary embryo fibroblasts requires at least two co-operating oncogenes. *Nature* **304**: 596.

Lang, J.C., N.M. Wilkie, and D.A. Spandidos. 1983. Characterization of eukaryotic transcriptional control signals by assay of herpes simplex virus type 1 thymidine kinase. *J. Gen. Virol.* **64**: 2679.

Littlefield, J.W. 1982. NIH 3T3 cell line. *Science* **218**: 214.

Moolgavkar, S.H. and A.G. Knudson. 1981. Mutation and cancer: A model for human carcinogenesis. *J. Natl. Cancer Inst.* **66**: 1037.

Moreau, P., R. Hen, B. Wasylyk, R. Everett, M.P. Gaub, and P. Chambon. 1981. The SV40 72 base pair repeat has a striking effect on gene expression both in SV40 and other chimeric recombinants. *Nucleic Acids Res.* **9**: 6047.

Newbold, R.F. and R.W. Overell. 1983. Fibroblast immortality is a prerequisite for transformation by EJ c-Ha-ras oncogene. *Nature* **304**: 040.

Parada, L.F., C.J. Tabin, C. Shih, and R.A. Weinberg. 1982. Human EJ bladder carcinoma oncogene is homologue of Harvey sarcoma virus *ras* gene. *Nature* **297**: 474.

Peto, R., F.J.C. Roe, P.N. Lee, L. Levy, and J. Clack. 1975. Cancer and ageing in mice and men. *Br. J. Cancer* **32**: 411.

Pollack, R.E. 1982. Oncogenes. *Science* **218**: 1069.

Reddy, E.P., R.K. Reynolds, E. Santos, and M. Barbacid. 1982. A point mutation is responsible for the acquisition of transforming properties by the T24 human bladder carcinoma oncogene. *Nature* **300**: 149.

Ruley, H.E. 1983. Adenovirus early region 1A enables viral and cellular transforming genes to transform primary cells in culture. *Nature* **304**: 602.

Santos, E., S.R. Tronick, S.A. Aaronson, S. Pulciani, and M. Barbacid. 1982. T24 human bladder carcinoma oncogene is an activated form of the normal human homologue of BALB- and Harvey-MSV transforming genes. *Nature* **298**: 343.

Shimizu, K., D. Birnboim, M.A. Ruley, O. Fasano, Y. Suard, L. Edlund, E. Taparowsky, M. Goldfarb, and M. Wigler. 1983. Structure of the Ki-*ras* gene of the human lung carcinoma cell line Calu-1. *Nature* **304**: 497.

Spandidos, D.A. 1983. Cellular oncogenes, mutations and cancer. *Anticancer Res.* **3**: 121.

Spandidos, D.A. and J. Paul. 1982. Transfer of human globin genes to erythroleukaemic mouse cells. *EMBO J.* **1**: 15.

Spandidos, D.A. and L. Siminovitch. 1977a. Transfer of anchorage independence by isolated metaphase chromosomes in hamster cells. *Cell.* **12**: 675.

———. 1977b. Genetic analysis of chromosome mediated gene transfer in hamster cells. *Brookhaven Symp. Biol.* **29**: 127.

———. 1978a. Transfer of the marker for the morphologically transformed phenotype by isolated metaphase chromosomes in hamster cells. *Nature* **271**: 259.

———. 1978b. The relationship between transformation and somatic mutation in human and Chinese hamster cells. *Cell* **13**: 651.

Spandidos, D.A. and N.M. Wilkie. 1983. Host specificities of papillomavirus, Moloney murine sarcoma virus and simian virus 40 enhancer sequences. *EMBO J.* **2**: 1193.

Spandidos, D.A., P.R. Harrison, and J. Paul. 1982. Replication and amplification of recombinant plasmid molecules as extrachromosomal elements in transformed mammalian cells. *Exp. Cell Res.* **141**: 149.

Tabin, C.J., S.M. Bradley, C.I. Bargmann, R.A. Weinberg, A.G. Papageorge, E.M. Scolnick, R. Dhar, D.R. Lowy, and E.H. Chang. 1982. Mechanism of activation of a human oncogene. *Nature* **300**: 143.

Taparowsky, E., Y. Suaro, O. Fasano, K. Shimizu, M. Goldfarb, and M. Wigler. 1982. Activation of the T24 bladder carcinoma transforming gene is linked to a single amino acid change. *Nature* **300**: 762.

Temin, H.M. and H. Rubin. 1958. Characteristics of an assay for Rous sarcoma virus and Rous sarcoma cells in tissue culture. *Virology* **6**: 669.

Weiss, R.A., N.M. Teich, H. Varmus, and J.M. Coffin, eds. 1982. *The molecular biology of tumor viruses*, 2nd edition: *RNA tumor viruses*. Cold Spring Harbor Laboratory, Cold Spring Harbor, New York.

Yuasa, Y., S.K. Srivastava, C.Y. Dunn, J.S. Rhim, E.P. Reddy, and S.A. Aaronson. 1983. Acquisition of transforming properties by alternative point mutations with c-*bas/has* human proto-oncogene. *Nature* **303**: 775.

Altered Expression of Cellular Genes in Adenovirus-transformed Cells

A.J. van der Eb, R. Bernards, P.I. Schrier, J.L. Bos, R.T.M.J. Vaessen, A.G. Jochemsen, and C.J.M. Melief†

Department of Medical Biochemistry, Sylvius Laboratories, 2333 AL Leiden, The Netherlands; †Department of Tumor Immunology, Central Laboratory of the Netherlands Red Cross Blood Transfusion Service, 1066 CX Amsterdam, The Netherlands

Human adenoviruses provide unique model systems for studies on basic mechanisms of carcinogenesis. An important advantage of this group of viruses is that both oncogenic and nononcogenic species are found within the same virus group. Although only the members of the subgenera A and B (e.g., Ad12 and Ad7, respectively) can cause tumors in newborn hamsters and some other rodents (Huebner 1967), all human adenoviruses studied so far are capable of transforming cells in vitro. In this article, we summarize a number of experiments designed to obtain some understanding of the role of the transforming genes of oncogenic Ad12 and nononcogenic Ad5 in oncogenesis and transformation.

The transforming activity of all human adenoviruses studied so far is associated with early region 1 (E1), which consists of two transcriptional units, E1A and E1B. In transformed cells, region E1A codes for two coterminal RNAs (12S and 13S) that differ only in the amount of RNA removed internally by splicing. The RNAs code for two polypeptides (of about 26 kD and 32 kD) that are structurally related. Region E1B codes for one major RNA species (in transformed cells) of 22S, which specifies two polypeptides of about 20 kD and 55 kD. These two proteins are translated in different reading frames and, hence, are not related (references in Pettersson and Akusjärvi 1983; van der Eb and Bernards 1983).

Rat cells transformed by region E1 of Ad5 or Ad12 are indistinguishable from cells transformed by intact DNA or virions, indicating that all transforming functions are located in region E1. DNA fragments comprising certain parts of region E1 may still contain transforming activity, although the resulting transformed cells show abnormal phenotypes. The smallest segment containing transforming activity is region E1A (0–4.5%). Cells transformed by E1A only exhibit a semitransformed phenotype and grow to low saturation densities. Ad5 E1A-transformed baby rat kidney (BRK) cells mainly differ from the untransformed primary cells in that they are immortalized (Houweling et al. 1980). Cells transformed by region E1A plus the adjoining 50% of region E1B appear almost completely transformed, but they differ from E1-transformed cells in that they have lost their oncogenicity in nude mice (Jochemsen et al. 1982). Region E1B alone has no detectable transforming activity, even under conditions where it is fully expressed (van den Elsen et al. 1983). These results indicate that region E1A has an initiating (and perhaps major) role in transformation (cf. van der Eb and Bernards 1984).

Several lines of evidence suggest that region E1B must have an important function in oncogenesis. First, introduction of a mutation in one of the two Ad12 E1B proteins results in a loss of oncogenicity, even in nude mice (Jochemsen et al. 1982; Bernards et al. 1983a). Second, transplantation studies using cells transformed by Ad5/Ad12 hybrid E1 regions, consisting of region E1A of nononcogenic Ad5 and E1B of oncogenic Ad12, and vice versa, have shown that the high oncogenic potential of Ad12-transformed cells in nude mice is determined by region E1B (Bernards et al. 1982), and specifically by the 54-kD E1B protein (Bernards et al. 1983a).

In the present study we report a major contribution of Ad12 region E1A in oncogenicity. We have found that expression of this region in transformed rat cells causes suppression of the production of class-I transplantation antigens and of a 32-kD cellular protein, resulting in a considerable reduction in susceptibility of the transformed cells to the cellular immune defense. This resistence to the host immune defense presumably causes the cells to be tumorigenic, even in immunocompetent animals.

Methods of Experimental Procedures

Transformed cells

All adenovirus-transformed cells discussed in this paper were obtained by transforming primary cultures of BRK cells (from 6-day-old Wag Rij rats) with recombinant plasmids containing the viral DNA inserts. The transformations were carried out by use of the calcium technique (Graham and van der Eb 1973; van der Eb and Graham 1980). BRK cells transformed by the following recombinant plasmids were used:

pAd5XhoC (Ad5 region E1 of Ad5; Bernards et al. 1982)
pAd5HindIIIG (Ad5 region E1A + 19-kD E1B gene; Bernards et al. 1983a)
pAd5d1Sac (Ad5 region E1A + 55-kD E1B gene; Bernards et al. 1983a)
pAd5HpaIE (Ad5 region E1A; Bernards et al. 1982)
pAd12RIC (Ad12 region E1; Bos et al. 1981)
pAd12HindIIIG (Ad12 region E1A + 19-kD E1B gene; Jochemsen et al. 1982)

pAd12d1Acc (Ad12 region E1A + 54-kD F1R gene; Bernards et al. 1983a)

pAdb12 (Ad5 E1A + Ad12 E1B; Bernards et al. 1982)

pAd125 (Ad12 E1A + Ad5 E1B; Bernards et al. 1982)

pAd512pm975 (Ad12 region E1 + Ad5 region E1A 13S product; Bernards et al. 1983b)

pAd512HL1007 (Ad12 region E1 + Ad5 E1A 12S product; Bernards et al. 1983b)

pAd51212 (Ad12 region E1 + Ad5 E1A; Bernards et al. 1983b)

pSVR7 (Ad12 region E1, but lacking 13S E1A product + SV40 enhancer; Bos et al. 1983)

pSVR11 (AD12 region E1, lacking 12S and 13S E1A products + SV40 enhancer; Bos et al. 1983)

pST12 (Ad5 + Ad12 region E1A + 19-kD Ad12 and 58-kD Ad5; Bernards et al. 1983a)

pLT12 (Ad5 + Ad12 region E1A + 19-kD Ad5 and 54-kD Ad12; Bernards et al. 1983a)

Assay for oncogenicity

Transformed cells (10^7) were injected subcutaneously into 4-day-old Wag-Rij rats or into adult athymic nude mice or nude Wag-Rij rats.

CTL reactions

Anti-RT1^u allogeneic cytotoxic T lymphocytes (CTL) were generated in a 6-day primary mixed lymphocyte culture: 10^7 spleen cells from an ACI rat were cultured with 3×10^6 x-irradiated spleen cells derived from Wag-Rij rats. Target cells were labeled in 100 μl of PBS containing 100 μCi of [^{51}Cr]sodium chromate for 30 minutes at 37°C. Lysis was measured in microtiter dishes during 4 hours at 37°C using 10^4 target cells per well. The specific lysis was calculated according to $(E-C)/(M-C) \times 100\%$, where E = counts released from target in the presence of CTL; C = counts released in the absence of CTL; and M = counts released from targets in the presence of 5% Triton X-100.

Sera and immunoprecipitation technique

Antisera against primary BRK cells were prepared by immunizing 10-week-old BALB/c mice with 10^7 BRK cells (derived from 6-day-old Wag-Rij rats, a highly inbred rat strain). Three intraperitoneal injections were given, with 10-day intervals, the first with complete Freund's adjuvant. Serum was collected 2 weeks after the last injection. Immunoprecipitations were carried out as described (Bernards et al. 1982). ^{125}I-labeling was carried out according to Markwell and Fox (1978).

Results

Region E1A has a major role in oncogenicity

In previous experiments, we had established a series of BRK lines transformed by Ad5 region E1, Ad12 region E1, Ad5 E1A + Ad12 E1B, and Ad12 E1A + Ad5 E1B. All four types of transformed cells were found to be oncogenic in athymic nude mice (Bernards et al. 1982). However, when the oncogenicity of the transformed cells was tested in immunocompetent syngeneic rats, a surprising result was obtained.

BRK cells transformed by intact region E1 of Ad5 were weakly oncogenic in nude mice and nononcogenic in immunocompetent rats, whereas cells transformed by region E1 of Ad12 were highly oncogenic in both types of animals. Cells transformed by Ad5 E1A and Ad12 E1B were highly oncogenic in nude mice but, surprisingly, completely nononcogenic in normal rats. Cells transformed by Ad12 E1A plus Ad5 E1B were weakly oncogenic, not only in nude mice but, to the same extent, also in normal rats (Table 1). These results indicated that region E1A determines whether or not a transformed cell is rejected in an immunocompetent animal: when E1A is derived from Ad12, the transformed cells apparently are sufficiently resistant to the host immune defense to be able to form a tumor, whereas when E1A is derived from Ad5, the transformed cells are always rejected, even when they are intrinsically highly tumorigenic in nude mice. This suggested that the oncogenic potential of transformed cells in immunocompetent animals is dependent on whether or not the cells can escape the immune surveillance of the host. Two alternative explanations might account for the observed differences in oncogenicity: (1) transformed cells that are oncogenic in immunocompetent rats are less immunogenic to the host than nononcogenic transformed cells or (2) oncogenic cells are resistant to the immune defense whereas nononcogenic cells are susceptible.

Table 1 Oncogenicity of Adenovirus-transformed Cells in Nude Mice, Syngeneic Rats, and Nude Rats

Plasmids used for transformation	Expression in transformed cell		Oncogenicity of transformed cells in:		
	E1A	E1B	nude mice	syngeneic rats	nude rats
pAd5XhoC	5	5	50% (15/31)	0% (0/51)	n.d.[c]
pAd12RIC	12	12	100% (23/23)	100% (18/18)[a]	n.d.
pAd512	5	12	100% (18/18)	0% (0/26)	100% (6/6)[d]
pAd125	12	5	10% (2/19)	10% (6/60)[b]	n.d.
p51212	5 + 12	12	100% (12/12)	0% (0/18)	n.d.

For each type of of transformed cells, at least three independently isolated cell lines were used. The numbers between brackets indicate the total number of animals with tumors/total number of animals injected.

[a]Average latent period, 6 weeks.
[b]Average latent period, 4 months.
[c]n.d., not done.
[d]Average latent period, 3 months.

The interactions between transformed cells and the immune system of the host will be either mediated by viral T antigens, by cellular proteins which are modulated by the viral transforming genes, or by both. To investigate whether specific cellular proteins play a role in determining whether or not a transformed rat cell is capable of inducing a tumor in immunocompetent oncogenic rats, we have prepared antisera against untransformed BRK cells in BALB/c mice. To screen for differences in cellular gene expression, the sera were used to analyze a panel of transformed cells, using the immunoprecipitation procedure.

Ad12 region E1A suppresses the synthesis of a cellular 32-kD protein

BALB/c mice were immunized with untransformed primary BRK cells derived from 6-day-old Wag-Rij rats. Preliminary experiments showed that the sera precipitated a rather limited set of proteins from the rat cells and that differences in protein content could be detected between untransformed and Ad12-transformed cells. The clearest differences were found for 38-kD and 32-kD proteins, which were both present in untransformed BRK cells but absent in Ad12-transformed cells. Sur-

prisingly, the 32-kD protein was present in normal amounts in Ad5-transformed cells but the 38-kD protein was not detectable in this line. To study the occurrence of these proteins in more detail, a pool of several mouse sera was used to immunoprecipitate a panel of Ad-transformed cells including cell lines transformed by hybrid plasmids consisting of Ad5 E1A and Ad12 E1B (pAd512), or Ad12 E1A and Ad5 E1B (pAd125).

The results presented in Figure 1 show that the 32-kD protein is present in primary BRK cells and in all Ad5-transformed cell lines that contain Ad5 region E1A, irrespective of whether one of the E1B proteins is mutated, or even both are absent. The protein is absent in all cells expressing Ad12 E1A, again independent of the presence of mutations in one of the E1B proteins. The 38-kD protein is absent in all cell lines harboring Ad12 E1A and is present in some, but not all, lines containing Ad5 E1A. When the immunoprecipitation results are considered in relation to the oncogenicity data, it is obvious that a strict correlation exists between presence of region E1A of Ad12, the lack of the 32-kD protein, and oncogenicity in immunocompetent syngeneic rats. It appeared to be of interest, therefore, to investigate whether the 32-kD protein is a membrane protein ex-

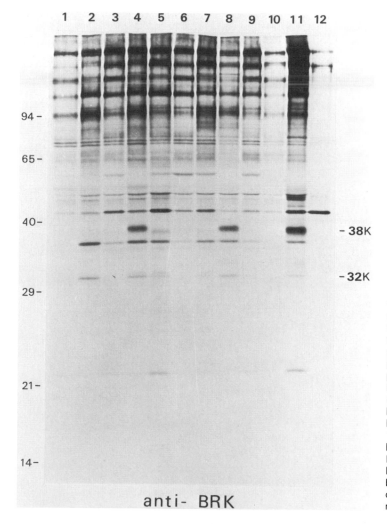

anti- BRK

Figure 1 Proteins immunoprecipitated from extracts of [^{35}S]methionine-labeled adenovirus-transformed rat cells with pooled serum from BALB/c mice immunized with primary baby rat kidney (BRK) cells. The rat cells were transformed by the following plasmids: (lane 1) pAd12RIC (containing Ad12 region E1); (lane 2) pAd5XhoC (containing Ad5 region E1); (lane 3) pAd12HindIIIG (containing Ad12 region E1A + part of E1B; lacks the 54-kD protein); (lane 4) pAd5HindIIIG (containing Ad5 region E1A + part of E1B; lacks the 58-kD protein); (lane 5) pAd5HpaIE (containing Ad5 region E1A); (lane 6) pAd12d1Acc (Ad12 region E1, lacking the 19-kD E1B protein); (lane 7) pAd5dlSac (Ad5 region E1, lacking the 19-kD E1B protein); (lane 8) pAd512 (Ad5 E1A + Ad12E1B); (lane 9) pAd125 (Ad12 E1A + Ad5 E1B); (lane 10) cell line derived from a tumor induced by pAd125-transformed cells; (lane 11) primary BRK cells; (lane 12) primary BRK cells precipitated with normal mouse serum.

posed on the outside of the cell membrane, where immune recognition is expected to occur.

To this end, primary BRK cells and Ad12-transformed BRK cells were labeled with ^{125}I and immunoprecipitated with the pooled BALB/c anti-BRK serum. No radioactive 32-kD protein could be precipitated, suggesting that it is not a membrane component, or at least is not exposed on the outer surface. However, prominent 38-kD and 12-kD proteins were precipitated from the primary cells which were absent in the Ad12-transformed cells (Fig. 2, lanes 1b and 2b). The 38-kD protein comigrated with the [^{35}S]methionine-labeled 38-kD protein precipitated by the same serum.

The coprecipitation of the 38-kD protein with a 12-kD component suggested that the two polypeptides might belong to the class-I major histocompatibility complex (MHC), which is known to consist of a heavy chain in the 40–45-kD molecular-weight range, associated with β_2-microglobulin (β_2-m; 12-kD molecular weight). Therefore, the ^{125}I-labeled extracts were immunoprecipitated with an antiserum directed against human β_2-m, which cross-reacts with rat β_2-m. A considerable amount of 12-kD β_2-m was precipitated from untransformed BRK cells, but only very small amounts of this protein were found in the extract of Ad12-transformed cells (Fig.2, lanes 3d and 5d). No heavy-chain molecules were co-

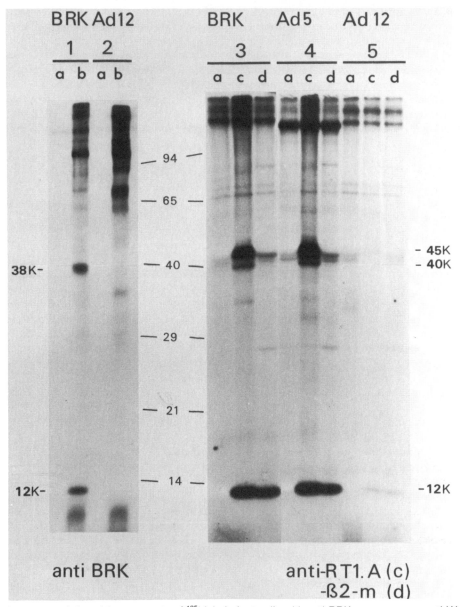

Figure 2 Proteins immunoprecipitated from extracts of ^{125}I-labeled rat cells with anti-BRK mouse serum, anti-Wag-Rij alloantiserum, and an antiserum against human β_2-m. Extracts of the following cells were used for immunoprecipitation: (lanes *1* and *3*) primary BRK cells; (lanes *2* and *5*) pAd12RIC-transformed BRK cells; (lane *4*) pAd5XhoC-transformed BRK cells. The following sera were used: normal mouse serum (lanes *a*); mouse anti-BRK serum (lanes *b*); Lewis anti-Wag-Rij hyperimmune alloantiserum (lanes *c*); and anti-human β_2-m serum (lanes *d*).

precipitated, probably due to the fact that the heterologous antiserum does not precipitate β_2-m when it is complexed to the heavy chain. In later experiments, an antiserum against rat β_2-m was used that did coprecipitate 45-kD heavy-chain molecules. The finding that Ad12-transformed cells contain minimal amounts of β_2-m molecules at the cell surface directly suggested to us that the amount of class-I heavy-chain molecules, to which the β_2-m molecules are normally complexed, would also be reduced.

Expression of RT1.A class-I genes is greatly reduced in cells harboring Ad12 region E1

The expression of class-I MHC antigens in adenovirus-transformed cells was further investigated with specific rat alloantisera. The rat cells used for the transformation assays originated from Wag-Rij rats, a highly inbred strain carrying the RT1^u haplotype. (The RT1 complex of the rat comprises five loci, two of which, RT1.A and RT1.E, code for the serologically detectable class-I antigens.) Figure 2, lane 3c, shows that these alloantisera precipitated predominantly a 45-kD and a 12-kD protein from ^{125}I-labeled untransformed BRK cells, representing the class-I heavy-chain molecules and β_2-m, respectively. These two proteins were also precipitated from cells expressing Ad5 E1 (Fig. 2, lane 4c), but they were absent, or present in greatly reduced amounts, in the lines expressing Ad12 E1 (Fig.2, lane 5c). Basically similar results were obtained with ^{125}I-labeled and ^{35}S metabolically labeled extracts. Further experiments showed that expression of the class-I heavy-chain molecules exactly paralleled that of the 32-kD protein detected by the BALB/c sera: Expression of 32-kD protein is greatly reduced in the presence of Ad12 E1A but normal with Ad5 E1A (Table 2). This suggests that expression of class-I protein and of 32-kD protein is controlled in a similar way by Ad12 E1A.

Expression of class-I genes is suppressed at the level of mRNA accumulation

The almost complete absence of class-I molecules on the surface of Ad12-transformed BRK cells can have several causes, for example, inhibition of transcription of class-I genes, reduced stability of class-I mRNAs, or absence of β_2-m. To test the latter possibility, transformed cells were metabolically labeled with [^{35}S]methionine and subsequently precipitated with antiserum against human β_2-m. It was found that Ad12-transformed cells, which lack 45-kD heavy chains, contain normal amounts of ^{35}S-labeled β_2-m as compared with Ad5-transformed cells. To investigate whether reduced expression of heavy-chain molecules is caused by the absence of mRNA transcripts, a number of transformed cell lines were studied by Northern blot analysis, using a DNA probe containing conserved sequences of the human HLA B7 gene. The probe was found to hybridize to a 1.7-kb RNA, which most likely represents the mRNA coding for the RT1.A heavy chain. This RNA band was present in untransformed BRK cells and in cells containing Ad5 E1A, but it was almost completely lacking in cells expressing Ad12 E1A (Fig. 3). This demonstrates that the absence of heavy-chain molecules is caused by a greatly reduced concentration of mRNA transcripts. Since the HLA B7 probe will react with all RT1.A gene transcripts, this result also shows that no other (alien) class-I alloantigens are expressed instead of the RT1.A^u heavy chains.

Reduced expression of 32-kD and 45-kD proteins is a function of the Ad12 13S mRNA product

In transformed cells, the E1A region of human adenoviruses is transcribed into two coterminal mRNAs of 12S and 13S, which only differ in the amount of RNA removed internally by splicing. To investigate which of these RNAs, if not both, is responsible for suppression of 32-kD protein production, we investigated the presence of this protein in rat cells transformed by an Ad12-region E1 plasmid carrying a mutation affecting the 13S mRNA product only (pSVR7; Bos et al. 1983). Figure 4, lane 8B, shows that cells transformed by pSVR7 have normal expression of the 32-kD protein. Similar results were obtained with cells transformed by pSV11, which carries a mutation affecting both E1A gene products (Fig. 4, lane 9B), indicating that the 13S mRNA product must be responsible for turning-off 32-kD gene expression. Similar results were obtained for expression of class-I genes (Bernards et al. 1983b; Table 2).

Ad5 E1A prevents Ad12 E1A from inhibiting expression of 32-kD and 45-kD proteins

Expression of the 32-kD protein was also studied in three cell lines containing the E1A regions of both Ad5 and Ad12. S1 nuclease analysis had shown that the two E1A regions were transcribed to the same extent (Bernards et al. 1983a,b). Analysis by immunoprecipitation with anti-BRK serum showed that all three cell lines expressed normal levels of 32-kD proteins, which indicates that the E1A region of Ad5 blocks the inactivating activity of Ad12 E1A (Fig.4, lanes 5, 6, and 7). To investigate which Ad5 E1A product is responsible for the dominant effect, 32-kD protein expression was determined in transformed cells carrying region E1 of Ad12 as well as a mutant E1A region of Ad5. Two plasmids were tested, one allowing expression of Ad12 E1 plus Ad5 13S E1A RNA (pAd512 pm975), the other of Ad12 E1 plus Ad5 12S E1A RNA (pAd512 HL1007) (Bernards et al. 1983b). It was found that coexpression of the Ad5 13S E1A mRNA product and Ad12 region E1 resulted in normal production of the 32-kD protein, whereas coexpression of the Ad5 12S E1A mRNA product and Ad12 region E1 gave rise to suppression of this protein (Fig. 4, lanes 3 and 4). Thus, the dominant effect exerted by Ad5 E1A on Ad12 E1A is also a function of the 13S mRNA. Again, the expression of class-I heavy-chain molecules paralleled that of the 32-kD protein in the above-mentioned cell lines. Thus, rat cells coexpressing all transforming genes of Ad12 as well as region E1A of Ad5 had normal levels of class-I genes (not shown). These cells were nononcogenic in immunocompetent rats, in spite of their high oncogenicity in nude mice (Table 1). This suggests

Table 2 Cellular Proteins Present in a Series of Adenovirus-transformed Cell Lines with Different Oncogenic Potential

transformed by[a]	Expression of Ad5 or Ad12 region		Proteins detected in transformed cells[b]			Oncogenicity	
	E1A	E1B	32 kD	(45 kD)	(12 kD)	mice	rats
BRK (untransformed)	—		+	+	+	—	—
pAd5XhoC	5	5	+	+	+	+/−	—
pAd5HindIIIG	5	5 (only 19 kD)[c]	+	+	+	—	n.d.
pAd5d1Sac	5	5 (only 58 kD)[c]	+	+	+	—	n.d.
pAd5HpaIE	5	—	+	+	+	—	n.d.
pAd12RIC	12	12	−	−	+	+	+
pAd12HindIIIG	12	12 (only 19 kD)[c]	−	−	+	−	−
pAd12dlAcc	12	12 (only 54 kD)[c]	−	−	+	−	−
pAd512	5	12	+	+	+	+/−	−
pAd125	12	5	−	−	+	+/−	+/−
pAd51212	12	12	+	+	+	+	−
pST12	5 + 12	Ad12 19 kD + Ad5 58 kD	+	+	+	+/−	−
pLT12	5 + 12	Ad5 19 kD + Ad12 54 kD	+	+	+	+	—
pAd512pm975	12 + 5 (only 13S product)[c]	12	+	+	+	n.d.	n.d.
pAd512HL1007	12 + 5 (only 12S product)[c]	12	−	−	+	n.d.	n.d.
pSVR7	12 (only 12S product)[c]	12	+	+	+	+	n.d.
pSVR11	12 (no 12S product)[c] (no 13S product)	12	+	+	+	+	n.d.

[a]The composition of the various recombinant plasmids is given in Methods of Experimental Procedures.
[b]+, Highly oncogenic; +/−, weakly oncogenic; −, nononcogenic; n.d., not done.
[c]Truncated products from mutated genes can still be present.

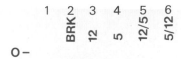
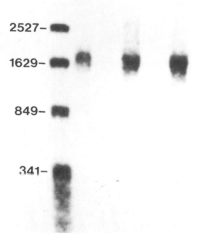

Figure 3 Northern blot analysis of RNA extracted from primary and adenovirus-transformed BRK cells, using a nick-translated human HLA B7 cDNA clone as described by Schrier et al. (1983). (Lane *1*) HaeIII-digested M13mp8 marker DNA; (lane *2*) RNA isolated from primary BRK cells; (lane *3*) RNA from cells transformed by pAd12RIC; (lane *4*) DNA from cells transformed by pAd5XhoC; (lane *5*) RNA from cells transformed by pAd125; (lane *6*) RNA from cells transformed by pAd512.

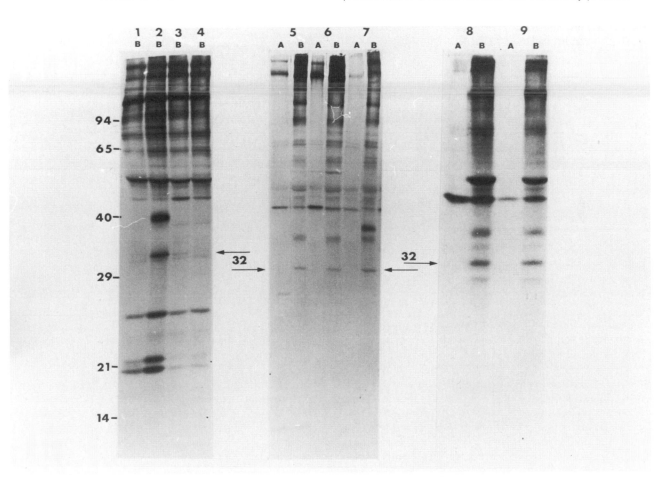

Figure 4 Proteins immunoprecipitated from extracts of [^{35}S]methionine-labeled transformed cells using an anti-BRK serum (lanes *B*) or nonimmune serum (lanes *A*). (Lane *1*) pAd12RIC; (lane *2*) pAd5HindIIIG; (lane *3*) p512 pm975; (lane *4*) p512HL1007; (lane *5*) p51212; (lane *6*) pLT12; (lane *7*) pST12; (lane *8*) pSVR7; (lane *9*) pSVR11. For details on plasmids, see Methods section.

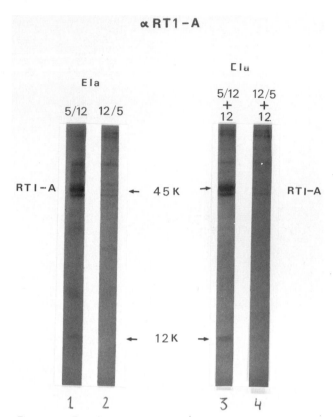

Figure 5 Proteins immunoprecipitated from extracts of [^{35}S]methionine-labeled adenovirus-transformed BRK cells, using a specific anti-RT1.A^u alloantiserum. Extracts were obtained from cells transformed by the following adenoviral DNAs. (*Left panels*) Cells transformed by Ad2 E1B plus either a hybrid E1 region in which the first exon is derived from Ad5 and the second from Ad12 (lane *1*), or a hybrid E1A region with the first exon of Ad12 and the second of Ad5 (lane *2*). (*Right panels*). Cells transformed by complete region E1 of Ad12 plus either a hybrid E1A region with the first exon of Ad5 and the second of Ad12 (lane *3*), or a hybrid E1A region with the first exon of Ad12 and the second of Ad5 (lane *4*).

that the property of Ad12 E1A to suppress class-I antigen synthesis is the basis of the highly oncogenic phenotype of Ad12-transformed cells in immunocompetent animals.

Inhibitions of class-I gene expression is a function of the first exon of Ad12 E1A mRNA

To investigate whether the suppressing activity of Ad12 E1A can be assigned to a particular domain of the gene product, plasmids were constructed containing hybrid Ad5/Ad12 E1A regions. For the construction of these recombinants, use was made of an *Ava*II site occurring at corresponding positions in the Ad5 and Ad12 E1A regions, at the splice-acceptor site of both E1A mRNAs. Cells transformed by these hybrid E1A regions plus Ad12 E1B were tested for the presence of class-I antigens. It was found that class-I proteins were virtually absent in cells transformed by a hybrid E1A region in

which the first exon was derived from Ad12 and the second from Ad5, while these proteins were normally present with an E1A region in which the first exon is derived from Ad5 and the second from Ad12 (Fig. 5). Thus, inhibition of class-I gene expression is an activity associated with the first "domain" of the 13S mRNA product of Ad12. Since the 12S mRNA product(s) apparently do not influence MHC gene expression, the segment that is unique to 13S mRNA must have an important role in this activity. Further studies showed that the dominant activity of Ad5 E1A over Ad12 E1A in suppressing class-I gene expression is also encoded by the first exon of the Ad5 13S mRNA (Fig. 5). This indicates that these opposite activities of Ad5 and Ad12 E1A are functions of the same protein domains, and hence might be based on similar pathways or mechanisms.

Evidence has recently been presented that the Ad5 DNA region in front of the E1A major cap site has an enhancer activity. To investigate the possibility that the effect of Ad12 E1A on class-I gene expression is caused by an activity of this upstream DNA sequence, we have studied cell lines transformed by an Ad12 E1 region in which this enhancer region is replaced by the corresponding segment of Ad5. It was found that in these lines class-I gene production was as strongly suppressed as in control Ad12-transformed cells, showing that this effect is not a function of the Ad12 DNA segment in front of the E1A cap site (results not shown).

Cells expressing Ad12 E1A are less susceptible to cytotoxic T cells than those expressing Ad5 E1A

Cells of a particular animal expressing foreign antigens, such as viral tumor antigens, will only be recognized by the animal's cytotoxic T cells (CTL) if the neoantigens are presented on the cell surface together with the class-I MHC molecules. Cells having reduced expression of class-I antigens, such as Ad12-transformed BRK cells, would therefore be able to escape from lysis by CTL, even when they express viral T antigens on the plasma membrane. If this assumption were correct, it would explain why cells expressing Ad12 E1A are oncogenic in immunocompetent animals. To investigate whether reduced expression of class-I molecules indeed results in lower susceptibility to CTL, we have measured the lysis of a panel of Ad5- and Ad12-transformed cells by allogeneic cytotoxic T lymphocytes generated in a primary mixed lymphocyte culture. Such CTLs are mainly directed against the allogeneic class-I MHC molecules (Bevan 1977). Absence of class-I molecules would therefore prevent killing by cytotoxic T cells. Figure 6 shows that the allogeneic CTLs exhibited a strong lytic response against Ad5 E1- and pAd512-transformed cells (both containing E1A of Ad5), but that the spleen cells reacted only weakly with Ad12 E1- and pAd125-transformed cells (both containing E1A of Ad12). This result is in agreement with the model that cells expressing Ad12 E1A are oncogenic in immunocompetent syngeneic hosts because they can escape from the T-cell-mediated immune response. That the phenomenon is not restricted to rat cells of a particular haplotype was shown by an experiment in which the CTLs were derived from

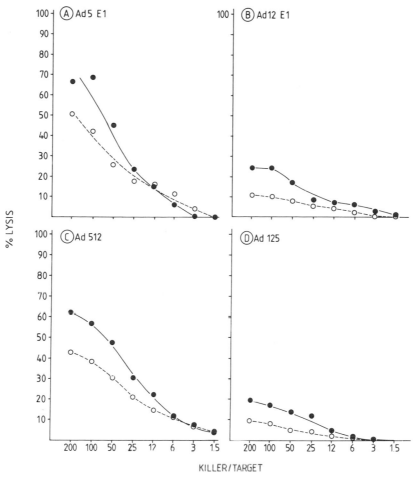

Figure 6 Susceptibility of adenovirus-transformed Wag-Rij cells to allogeneic CTL. In each of the four panels, percentage of cell lysis by allogeneic CTLs is shown for two independently derived transformed cell lines. Cell killing is plotted against different ratios of killer lymphocytes versus target adenovirus-transformed cells. (A) Cells transformed by Ad5 region E1 (pAd5XhoC); (B) cells transformed by Ad12 region E1 (pAd12RIC); (C) cells transformed by a plasmid containing Ad5 E1A plus Ad12 E1B (pAd512); (D) cells transformed by a plasmid containing Ad12 E1A plus Ad5 E1B (pAd125).

Wag-Rij rats and the stimulator lymphocytes and target cells from Brown Norway (BN) rats (RT1^n haplotype). Again, a similar difference in susceptibility to allogeneic CTLs was found between Ad5- and Ad12-transformed BN cells.

To further confirm the model, the reactivity of virus-specific syngeneic T cells was measured against Ad-transformed cells of the same haplotype as the T cells, in a secondary syngeneic CTL reaction. The T killer cells were now specifically directed against the viral antigens. It was found that Ad5-transformed cells were efficiently killed by Ad5-stimulated CTLs whereas Ad12-transformed cells were only poorly lysed by Ad12-stimulated CTLs (results not shown). Thus, basically similar results were obtained with virus-specific syngeneic CTLs as with allogeneic primary CTLs.

Discussion

The study reported in this paper was undertaken to search for differences at the protein level between oncogenic and nononcogenic adenovirus-transformed rat

cells. Two proteins were identified, of 32 kD and 45 kD, that were absent in Ad12-transformed cells (or present in greatly reduced amounts), but present in normal concentrations in Ad5-transformed and untransformed cells. The 45-kD protein was identified as the heavy chain of the class-I MHC antigens, RT1.A, of the rat. Suppression of heavy-chain production was shown to occur at the level of mRNA accumulation, whereas synthesis of the light chain, β_2-m was unaffected. The suppressing activity of Ad12 region E1 was shown to be a function of the 13S mRNA (probably its product) encoded by region E1A, and specifically of the first exon. We have recently shown that the same Ad12 13S mRNA product is also required for activation of the E1B promoter (Bos and Ten Wolde-Kraamwinkel 1983). A similar property has been described for the Ad5 13S E1A mRNA, not only for activation of region E1B but also of the other adenoviral early regions, as well as for activation of a cellular gene coding for a heat-shock protein (Nevins 1982). Thus, the E1A regions of both Ad5 and Ad12 are capable of activating their own early genes and cellular heat-shock genes (shown for Ad5 only), whereas Ad12 E1A, but not Ad5 E1A, can suppress the activity of at least two different cellular genes, the 45-kD class-I MHC genes and a gene coding for a 32-kD protein. The suppressing activity of Ad12 E1A is counteracted by Ad5 E1A, if both regions are present within the same rat cell. Since the suppressing activity of Ad12 E1A on class-I gene expression and the Ad5 activity in preventing this suppression by Ad12 E1A are both associated with the first exon of the respective 13S mRNAs, a reasonable working hypothesis would be that the two viral polypeptides compete for the same cellular binding or effector site. The Ad5 product would then have a higher affinity than the Ad12 product. More difficult to explain is how the Ad12 product would cause inhibition of class-I gene expression while the Ad5 product does not affect expression of these genes, although the E1A products of the two viruses are otherwise homologous in function and can complement each other in transformation.

So far, we have assumed that the strongly reduced expression of the 45-kD and 32-kD proteins is caused by an inhibition of mRNA transcription or a reduction of mRNA stability. It cannot be excluded, however, that Ad12 region E1, and more specifically region E1A, can only transform cells that have no, or reduced, expression of these two proteins. This possibility is supported by the observation that Ad12 usually transforms with an at least 10-fold lower efficiency than Ad5. On the other hand, preliminary experiments have shown that the level of expression of Ad12 region E1A is inversely correlated with that of class-I genes. An Ad12-transformed hamster line, derived from an Ad12 DNA-induced tumor, and a subclone of this line, were found to differ in viral T antigen expression, one containing high levels of T antigens, the other low levels. Northern blotting analysis showed that the line with high T antigen concentration had a very low expression level of class-I antigens, and vice versa. This result suggests that the Ad12 products can indeed switch-off expression of class-I genes. Further experiments to distinguish between the alternative possibilities are in progress.

The results presented in the last paragraph show that transformed BRK cells containing Ad12 E1A are much less susceptible to allogeneic CTLs than cells containing Ad5 E1A. Whether this observation can be extrapolated to an in vivo situation is not certain, but is strongly suggested by the finding that cells expressing Ad12 E1A can form tumors in immunocompetent rats whereas cells expressing Ad5 E1A cannot. Thus, as a result of the decreased susceptibility to CTL, a sufficient number of Ad12-transformed cells will escape the immune surveillance so that a tumor can be formed, while transformed cells expressing Ad5 E1A will be eliminated and hence will only be able to form tumors when they are introduced into immunodeficient animals, such as nude mice.

Preliminary experiments with a viable Ad5 recombinant virus containing a genome in which the E1 region is replaced by the corresponding E1 region of Ad12, have shown that this virus may be nononcogenic in hamsters. If this is correct, it would indicate that other regions of the viral genome can also influence oncogenicity of intact virions.

Acknowledgments

The authors thank Drs. L.C. Paul (Leiden) and I. Vaessen (Rotterdam) for providing the rat alloantisera, Dr. S.M. Weissman (Yale) for the cDNA probe of HLA B7, and Dr. A.J. Berk for the gift of pEKpm975.

This work was supported in part by the Netherlands Organization for the Advancement of Pure Research (ZWO) through the foundation for Fundamental Medical Research.

References

Bernards, R., A. Houweling, P.I. Schrier, J.L. Bos, and A.J. van der Eb. 1982. Characterization of cells transformed by Ad5/Ad12 hybrid early region 1 plasmids. *Virology* **120**: 422.

Bernards, R., P.I. Schrier, J.L. Bos, and A.J. van der Eb. 1983a. Role of adenovirus types 5 and 12 early region 1b tumor antigens in oncogenic transformation. *Virology* **127**: 45.

Bernards, R., P.I. Schrier, A. Houweling, J.L. Bos, A.J. van der Eb, M. Zijlstra, and C.J.M. Melief. 1983b. Tumorigenicity of cells transformed by adenovirus type 12 by evasion of T-cell immunity. *Nature* **305**: 776.

Bevan, M.J. 1977. Killer cells reactive to altered-self antigens can also be alloreactive. *Proc. Natl. Acad. Sci.* **74**: 2094.

Bos, J.L. and H.C. Ten Wolde-Kraamwinkel. 1983. The E1b promoter of Ad12 in mouse L tk⁻ cells is activated by adenovirus region E1a *Embo J.* **2**: 73.

Bos, J.L., A.G. Jochemsen, R. Bernards, P.I. Shrier, H. van Ormondt, and A.J. van der Eb. 1983. Deletion mutants of region E1a of Ad12 E1 plasmids: Effect on oncogenic transformation. *Virology* **129**: 393.

Bos, J.L., L.J. Polder, R. Bernards, P.I. Schrier, P.J. van den Elsen, A.J. van der Eb, and H. van Ormondt. 1981. The 2.2 kb E1b mRNA of human Ad12 and Ad5 codes for two tumor antigens starting at different AUG triplets. *Cell* **27**: 121.

Graham, F.L. and A.J. van der Eb. 1973. A new technique for the assay of infectivity of human adenovirus DNA. *Virology* **52**: 456.

Houweling, A., P.J. van den Elsen, and A.J. van der Eb. 1980. Partial transformation of primary rat cells by the leftmost 4.5% fragment of adenovirus 5 DNA. *Virology* **105**: 537.

Huebner, R.J. 1967. Adenovirus-directed tumor and T antigens. *Perspect. Virol.* **5**: 147.

Jochemsen, H., G.S.G. Daniëls, J.J.L. Hertoghs, P.I. Schrier, P.J. van den Elsen, and A.J. van der Eb. 1982. Identification of adenovirus type 12 gene products involved in transformation and oncogenesis. *Virology* **122**: 15.

Markwell, M.A.K. and G.F. Fox. 1978. Surface specific iodenation of membrane proteins of viruses and eucaryotic cells using 1,3,4,6-tetra-chloro-3α, 6α-diphenylglycoluril. *Biochemistry* **173**: 4807.

Nevins, J.R. 1982. Induction of the synthesis of a 70.000 dalton mammalian heat shock protein by the adenovirus E1a gene product. *Cell* **29**: 913.

Pettersson, U. and G. Akusjärvi. 1983. Molecular biology of adenovirus transformation. *Adv. Viral Oncol.* **3**: 83.

Schrier, P.I., R. Bernards, R.T.M.J. Vaessen, A. Houweling, and A.J. van der Eb. 1983. Expression of class I major histocompatability antigens switched off by highly oncogenic adenovirus 12 in transformed rat cells. *Nature* **305**: 771.

van den Elsen, P.J., A. Houweling, and A.J. van der Eb. 1983. Expression of region E1b of human adenoviruses in the absence of region E1a is not sufficient for complete transformation. *Virology* **128**: 377.

van der Eb, A.J. and R. Bernards. 1984. Transformation and oncogenicity by adenoviruses. *Curr. Top. Microbiol. Immunol.* **110**: (in press).

van der Eb, A.J. and F.L. Graham. 1980. Assay of transforming activity of tumor virus DNA. *Methods Enzymol.* **65**: 826.

Adenovirus-2 *lp*⁺ Locus and Cell Transformation

G. Chinnadurai

Institute for Molecular Virology, St. Louis University Medical Center, St. Louis, Missouri 63110

The transforming genes of human adenovirus have been localized within the left 12% of the viral genome by analysis of viral sequences that are expressed in adenovirus-transformed cell lines (Gallimore et al. 1974; Flint et al. 1976) and by in vitro transformation experiments using transfection with restriction fragments of the viral DNA (Graham et al. 1974). The transforming region (F1) of adenovirus type 2 (Ad2) (and closely related adenovirus type 5 [Ad5]) is comprised of two transcriptional units, E1A and E1B. E1A maps between map positions 1.3 and 4.4 and E1B between map positions 4.5 and 11.2 (reviewed in Tooze 1980).

DNA transfection studies have shown that the E1A-coding sequences (left 4.5% of the Ad5 genome) can transform rat embryo cells in vitro to a "partially transformed" state (Houweling et al. 1980) but at a lower frequency compared with the leftmost 8% (HindIII-G fragment) of the viral genome (van der Eb et al. 1977). Similarly with the Ad12 system, a DNA fragment (AccI-H fragment) representing the left 4.5% of the viral genome has been shown to induce partial transformation (Shiroki et al. 1979), whereas the left 6.8% (HindIII-G fragment) induced complete transformation (Shiroki et al. 1977). These results indicate that the DNA sequences containing E1A and the portion of E1B that contains the complete sequences coding for the E1B 19-kD tumor antigen and the amino terminus of the E1B 53-kD tumor antigen is sufficient to induce a fully transformed phenotype.

A number of viral mutants with lesions in E1 have been isolated and characterized with regard to cellular transformation. Two complementation groups (hrI and hrII) of Ad5 host-range mutants defective in cell transformation have been isolated (Harrison et al. 1977; Ho et al. 1982). Mutants in hrI and hrII groups have been mapped within E1A and E1B, respectively (Galos et al. 1980; Ho et al. 1982). The hrI-E1A mutants (i.e., hr1–5) induce abortive transformation, in that these mutants induce small transformed foci from which permanent cell lines could not be easily established (Graham et al. 1978). The hrI cold-sensitive (cs) mutants have been shown to possess a cs transformation phenotype and the temperature-shift experiments indicate that E1A function is required, either indirectly or directly, for maintenance of transformation (Ho et al. 1982). One of the Ad5 deletion mutants isolated by Jones and Shenk (1979a) that maps entirely within E1A (dl312) has also been shown to be transformation defective. It is difficult to judge fully the effect of hrI and dl312 on transformation because these mutants are defective in the normal expression of E1B (Berk et

al. 1979; Jones and Shenk 1979b). However, an Ad2 E1A mutant, hr440 that expresses normal amounts of E1B has been shown to be transformation defective (Solnick and Anderson 1982), indicating that E1A gene products are indeed needed for transformation. All the available E1B mutants fall under the complementation group hrII. Members of the hrII group have been shown to be defective in the E1B 53-kD tumor antigen (Lassam et al. 1979). It has been shown that these mutants are transformation defective when used as viral particles (Graham et al. 1978; Ho et al. 1982) but can transform as does wild-type virus when viral DNA is used in the transfection assay (Rowe and Graham 1983). These results in conjunction with the observation that the left 8% of the viral genome can induce "fully-transformed" phenotype (Graham et al. 1974; van der Eb et al. 1977) indicate that the E1B 53-kD tumor antigen may not play an essential role in DNA-mediated cell transformation.

We have isolated a set of Ad2 mutants that produce clear large plaques (lp) on human KB cells. These mutants are defective in cell transformation and have been mapped within the 19-kD tumor antigen-coding region of E1B. Our results indicate that the 19-kD tumor antigen plays an essential role in cell transformation.

Results

Isolation and mapping of Ad2 lp mutants

We have isolated four lp mutants (lp1–4) by mutagenesis of Ad2 viral particles with hydroxylamine (Chinnadurai et al. 1979). The plaque morphology of mutant lp3 is shown in Figure 1. Mutant lp3 was mapped within the left 42% of the Ad2 genome by dissection of viral DNA from Ad2 (lp3)-Ad5 intertypic recombinants according to a method developed by Sambrook et al. (1975). The intertypic recombinants between Ad2 lp3 and Ad5 were constructed by the overlap recombination method that we have developed (Chinnadurai et al. 1979) and are illustrated schematically in Figure 2. From the overlap recombination assay, 10 plaques were isolated and the viral DNA was analyzed using restriction endonucleases BamHI and EcoRI.

All 10 isolates were found to be true recombinants and to exhibit the lp phenotype. Two types of recombinants were seen. Eight isolates (type I) had BamHI cleavage patterns identical to Ad2 and EcoRI cleavage patterns identical to Ad5. Two isolates (type II), after cleavage with BamHI, yielded one fragment similar in size to the Ad5 B or Ad2 A fragment and two other fragments similar in size to Ad2 B fragment. Cleavage

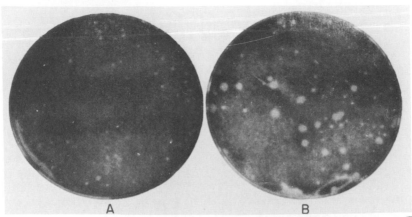

Figure 1 Plaque morphology of Ad2 *wt* and *lp*3 on KB cells. Infected cells were maintained at 33°C, stained with Neutral Red, and photographed with Polaroid type-55 film on day 12. (Reprinted, with permission, from Chinnadurai et al. 1979.)

of DNA from type-II recombinants with *Eco*RI yielded three fragments identical to Ad5 *Eco*RI fragments. These results indicate that all the recombinants might have been generated by recombination between *Eco*RI-A of Ad2 *lp*3 DNA and *Sal*I-A or *Sal*I-A to *Sal*I-C (see below) of Ad5 DNA. The points of crossover for type-I recombinants may be located within map positions 42–59 (Fig. 2) since the DNAs of these recombinants contain the Ad2 *Bam*HI cleavage sites located at map positions 30–42. On the other hand, sites of crossover for type-II recombinants may be located within map positions 30–42 because the Ad2 *Bam*HI cleavage site at map position 42 (Fig. 2) is absent in the recombinant DNA, but the cleavage site at map position 30 is present. The simplest mode by which these recombinants may have arisen is by a single recombination event between *Eco*RI-A of Ad2 *lp*3 DNA and small portions of Ad5 DNA consisting of *Sal*I-A to *Sal*I-C molecules that may have been produced by incomplete digestion with *Sal*I. All 10 recombinants selected were of the *lp* phenotype, indicating that *lp* mutation of Ad2 is located anywhere between map positons 0–42.

Subsequently, we isolated three other *lp* mutants by local mutagenesis of the left 15% of the viral genome. The scheme for isolation of these mutants is shown in Figure 3A. The left 15% (*Xho*I-C fragment) of the Ad2 genome was cloned using plasmid vector pBR322. The

cloned DNA was mutagenized with hydroxylamine (Chu et al. 1979) and cotransfected with a terminal DNA-protein complex from an Ad2 E1A-E1B host-range deletion mutant *dl*201.2 (Brusca and Chinnadurai 1981) in human KB cells. KB cells are nonpermissive for *dl*201.2 and therefore only viable recombinants between the mutagenized DNA and the genome of *dl*201.2 will yield plaques. Three *lp* mutants were isolated from about 200 plaques examined. These results indicated to us that the *lp* mutation is located within the left 15% of the viral genome.

Since mutagenesis of the left 15% of the viral genome produced *lp* mutants, we assumed that the likely candidate region for the mutation would be the early gene block E1 that encompasses the left 11.2% of the genome. Consistent with this expectation, in pilot studies cotransfection of the left 9.4% (*Bgl*II-E fragment) of mutant *lp*5 DNA with *dl*201.2 DNA protein complex was found to generate *lp* progeny viruses. To map precisely the *lp* mutation within the E1 region, we constructed recombinant plasmids in which segments of *wt* sequences were fused with *lp* sequences. This reconstruction results in sequences with overlapping homology with the sequences present on both sides of the deleted region (map positions ~2.0–7.0) in the *dl*201.2 genome. These overlapping sequences are essential for marker rescue of *dl*201.2 by homologous in vivo recombination

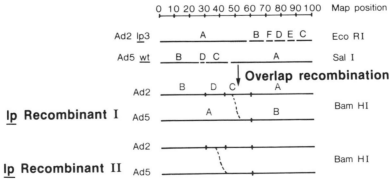

Figure 2 Mapping of Ad2 *lp*3 by overlap recombination. Ad5-Ad2 *lp*3 recombinants were constructed and analyzed as described by Chinnadurai et al. (1979).

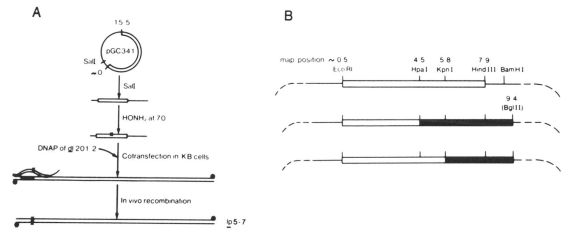

Figure 3 (*A*) Scheme for isolation of Ad2 *lp* mutants by local mutagenesis. About 5 μg of plasmid DNA (pGC341) was linearized with restriction endonuclease *Sal*I and mutagenized with 0.05 M hydroxlyamine at 70°C for 13 min (Chu et al. 1979). The plasmid DNA was then cotransfected into human KB cells along with 1 μg of DNA-terminal protein complex (Chinnadurai et al. 1978) from *dl*201.2 and 4 μg of carrier salmon sperm DNA. Progeny virus was collected after 4–6 days and plaque-assayed on KB cells. (*B*) Structure of Ad2 *wt-lp* DNA constructs used for marker rescue of *dl*201.2. The map positions of the cleavage sites on the viral DNAs are shown above the restriction enzymes. The *wt* sequences are shown with the open bars and the *lp* sequences are shown with the filled bars. For construct I, pGC212 DNA (in which the left 7.9% of the viral genome, i.e., the *Hind*III-G fragment, has been cloned between the *Eco*RI and *Hind*III sites of pBR322) was cleaved with *Hpa*I and *Bam*HI. The excised DNA segment containing viral DNA and vector DNA was replaced with a viral DNA fragment from map position 4.5 (*Hpa*I site) to map position 9.4 (*Bgl*II site) of DNAs from *lp*3 or *lp*5. In construct II, pGC212 DNA was cleaved with *Kpn*I and *Bam*HI and the *wt* DNA from map position 5.8 (*Kpn*I site) to map position 7.9 and part of the vector DNA was replaced with an *lp*3 or *lp*5 DNA fragment from map positions 5.8 to 9.4. (Reprinted, with permission, from Chinnadurai 1983.)

as illustrated in Figure 1A. In these constructs, we used DNAs from both *lp*3 (isolated by mutagenesis of viral particles) and *lp*5 (isolated by local mutagenesis). The structures of the constructs are shown in Figure 3B.

When construct I containing *wt* DNA from map positions ~0.5–4.5 and *lp*3 or *lp*5 DNA from map positions 4.5–9.4 was used for marker rescue of *dl*201.2, all the progeny virus were of *lp* phenotype indicating that the *lp* mutation is located within the E1B region (i.e., between map positions 4.5 and 9.4). When construct II containing *lp*3 or *lp*5 DNA was used in marker rescue of *dl*201.2, all the progeny virus were of *wt* phenotype. These results indicated that the mutations causing the *lp* phenotype in *lp*3 and *lp*5 are located between map positions 4.5 and 5.8.

DNA sequence analysis of *lp* mutants

Guided by the marker-rescue studies, we focused our DNA sequence analysis between map positions 4.5 and 6.5 using the construct I *wt-lp* plasmid DNAs. The DNA sequence analysis of Ad5 and Ad2 carried out by Bos et al. (1981) and Gingeras et al. (1982) and the aminoterminal amino acid analysis of the 19-kD polypeptide (Anderson and Lewis 1980) have indicated that this region contains the coding sequences for E1B 19-kD tumor antigen and the aminoterminus of E1B 53-kD tumor antigen. We sequenced about 680 bp from positions 1568 to 2250 of *wt*, *lp*3, and *lp*5 DNA by the method of Maxam and Gilbert (1980). The effect of the mutations on the 19-kD polypeptide is illustrated diagramatically in Figure 4. The *wt* sequence of this region was found to be entirely in accordance with the Ad2 sequence pub-

lished by Gingeras et al. (1982). In the sequenced region, *lp*3 revealed a single base pair change at position 1718 where there is a C → T transition. In the case of *lp*5, alterations at two sites were observed. There is a G → T transversion at position 1954. The second change is located at position 2237, where there is also a G → T transversion. In both *lp*3 and *lp*5, the observed mutational change is located within the 19-kD tumor antigen-coding sequence. The G → T transversion of *lp*5 at position 2237 is located in the aminoterminal region of the 53-kD tumor antigen, where it causes an amino acid substitution from methionine to isoleucine. In *lp*3, the single base pair mutational change results in the substitution of valine for alanine at the aminoterminus of the 19-kD polypeptide. In the case of *lp*5, the first mutational change results in the substitution of tyrosine for aspartic acid. The second mutation changes the normal termination codon of the 19-kD polypeptide into a leucine codon.

Published results (Bos et al. 1981; Gingeras et al. 1982) indicate that the 19-kD polypeptide could be coded by both a 13S and a 22S mRNA (Fig. 4). Thus, the loss of normal termination of the 19-kD polypeptide of *lp*5 would result in two 19-kD-related polypeptides of higher molecular weight. When translation is initiated on the 22S mRNA, the altered 19-kD polypeptide would terminate at position 2272 resulting in 12 extra amino acids. When translation is initiated on the 13S mRNA in which nucleotide 2249 is juxtaposed next to nucleotide 3589 by splicing (Perricaudet et al. 1980), the translation would terminate at position 3617 resulting in 14 extra amino acids.

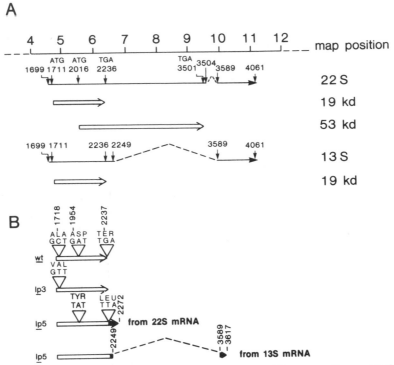

Figure 4 Organization of the Ad2 E1B sequences coding for the 53-kD and 19-kD tumor antigens. (*A*) Organization of E1B coding for the two tumor antigens. This is drawn according to the data of Gingeras et al. (1982). (*B*) Structure of 19-kD tumor antigen coded by *wt* and *lp* mutants. The sites of the mutations in the 19-kD polypeptide of the *lp* mutants and the corresponding region on the *wt* sequences are denoted by triangles. The triplets and amino acid sequence of the *wt* and mutant 19-kD polypeptide are also shown. The extra amino acids on the altered 19-kD polypeptide coded by *lp*5 are indicated by the filled bar or by the bar with slanted lines. (Reprinted, with permission, from Chinnadurai 1983.)

Analysis of E1B proteins coded by the *lp* mutants

It has been established by other investigators that the E1B region codes for a 53-kD and a 19-kD tumor antigen by in vitro translation (Halbert et al. 1979; Esche et al. 1980). In addition to these polypeptides, an E1B 20-kD polypeptide has also been identified both by analysis of in vivo synthesized proteins by immunoprecipitation and by in vitro translation (Green et al. 1982). We have analyzed the E1B proteins coded by Ad2 *wt*, *lp*3, and *lp*5 by immunoprecipitation of in vivo-synthesized proteins using antiserum prepared against the Ad2-transformed cell line F17 (Fig. 5).

The F17-antiserum has been extensively characterized by Green, Wold, and co-workers and has been shown to contain antibodies to E1B proteins (Gilead et al. 1976; Wold and Green 1979). In cells infected with *wt* virus, we could detect three major polypeptides that are specific for infected cells. The sizes of these three polypeptides are 53 kD, 20 kD, and 19 kD. It has been shown that the 53-kD and the 20-kD polypeptides are related to one another and the 19-kD polypeptide is distinct from them. These three polypeptides have been described in detail by Green et al. (1982). Cells infected with *lp*3 also synthesized the three polypeptides similar to those observed in *wt*-infected cells. In cells infected with *lp*5, the 53-kD and the 20-kD polypeptides were similar to those observed in *wt*-infected cells. As expected, the 19-kD polypeptide was absent and instead low amounts of the

19-kD-related 21-kd polypeptide were observed. The relatedness of the *lp*5-coded 21-kD polypeptide and *wt* 19-kD polypeptide has also been established by immunoprecipitation with sera raised against synthetic pep-

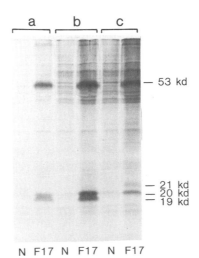

Figure 5 SDS-PAGE analysis of E1B polypeptides synthesized in KB cells infected with Ad2 *wt* and *lp* mutants. Immunoprecipitation was with normal rat serum (N) or F17 antiserum (F17). (Lanes *a*) *wt*-infected cells; (lanes *b*) *lp*3-infected cells; (lanes *c*) *lp*5-infected cells. (Reprinted, with permission, from Chinnadurai 1983.)

tides predicted from the 19-kD polypeptide coding region (M.Green, pers. comm.).

Transformation of rat 3Y1 cells by *lp* mutants

Since we have localized the *lp* mutation within the E1B 19-kD tumor antigen-coding region, we wanted to examine the role of this protein in inducing cell transformation of the established rat embryo fibroblast cell line, 3Y1 (Kimura et al. 1975). This cell line has been shown to be very sensitive to transformation by human adenoviruses (Shiroki et al. 1977).

As seen in Table 1, when 3Y1 cells were infected with different Ad2 *lp* mutants, *lp*5 was found to be completely transformation defective, *lp*3 and *lp*4 showed greatly reduced transformation efficiency (i.e., about 10-fold lower than *wt*), and *lp*1 and *lp*2 were partially transformation defective (about two-fold lower than *wt*). In addition, transfection with the DNAs of the transformation-defective mutants *lp*3 or *lp*5 did not result in significant transformation. These results indicate that the E1B 19-kD tumor antigen coded by the *lp*⁺ locus plays an essential

Table 1 Transformation of Rat 3Y1 Cells with Ad2 *wt* and *lp* Mutants

	Virus [a]	Viral DNA [b]
	foci per flask	
wt	42	15
*lp*1	15	n.d. [c]
*lp*2	18	n.d.
*lp*3	4	3
*lp*4	4	n.d.
*lp*5	0	1
No virus or viral DNA	0	1

Confluent cultures of 3Y1 cells were trypsinized (1 or 2 days after confluency) and about 10⁵ cells were plated per 25-cm² bottle. After 2 hr, cells were infected with Ad2 *wt* or *lp* mutants at an input multiplicity of 10–20 pfu/cell. Infected cells were maintained in Ca⁺⁺-free-Dulbecco's modified Eagle's media containing 10% fetal calf serum for about 1 week. Subsequently, the liquid media was replaced with 10 ml of semisolid media containing 0.3% agarose. The cells were fed with another 5 ml of agarose overlay media on the third week. After 4–5 weeks, agarose overlays were removed and the transformed foci were counted by staining with Giemsa. Transformation assays using viral DNAs were carried out essentially as described above. Flasks (25 cm²) containing about 5 × 10⁵ cells were transfected with 1 μg of viral DNA along with 9 μg of carrier salmon sperm DNA. DNA transfections were carried out by the calcium method of Graham and van der Eb (1973). (Reprinted, with permission, from Chinnandurai 1983.)
[a] Cells were infected with Ad2 *wt* or *lp* mutants at 10–20 pfu cell.
[b] One μg of viral DNA was transfected on 5 × 10⁵ cells contained in a 25-cm² flask.
[c] n.d., not determined.

role in cell transformation. The observed effect on cell transformation is not due to excessive cell killing by the *lp* mutants since the cloning efficiencies of *wt* and mutant-infected cells are the same (results not shown).

Discussion

We have identified a class of Ad2 mutants that is defective in inducing cell transformation. These viable mutants produce large clear plaques on human KB cells and are therefore designated *lp* (large plaque) mutants. These mutants resemble the cytocidal (*cyt*) mutants of Ad12 isolated by Takemori and co-workers (Takemori et al. 1968). Ad12 *cyt* mutants produce large plaques on human embryonic kidney cells. These mutants are also defective in cell transformation and are poorly (or non-) oncogenic in newborn hamsters. We have localized the Ad2 *lp* mutation within the section of early-region E1B coding for a 19-kD tumor antigen by marker-transfer, by DNA sequence analysis, and by analysis of viral proteins. Comparable data for Ad12 *cyt* mutants are not yet available. Mapping studies of Ad12 *cyt* mutants should reveal whether the *lp*⁺ locus of Ad2 and the *cyt*⁺ of locus of Ad12 are similar.

Our results demonstrate that the E1B 19-kD tumor antigen plays an essential role in inducing cell transformation. It is noteworthy that the Ad2 19-kD tumor antigen is associated with plasma membrane (Persson et al. 1982) as are other transformation proteins such as polyoma middle T antigen (Ito 1979) and avian sarcoma virus-coded pp60ˢʳᶜ (Willingham et al. 1979; Levinson et al. 1980). It remains to be determined whether the adenovirus 19-kD tumor antigen is an analog of these transforming proteins. We do not know the role of this polypeptide during productive infection. Since 19-kD polypeptide is synthesized in higher abundance during late stages of viral infection (Esche et al. 1980), it may play a role in viral DNA replication or in late gene expression.

Conclusions that can be inferred from DNA transfection studies complement our results on cell transformation. Immunoprecipitation studies (Schrier et al. 1979) have revealed that cells "fully transformed" by the Ad5 *Hind*III-G fragment (map positions 0–7.9) do not synthesize the Ad5 E1B 53 kD (also referred to as 65 kD) tumor antigen but express E1B 19-kD tumor antigen. Ad5 *Hpa*I-E fragment- (map positions 0–4.5) transformed cells (partially transformed) do not express E1B 19-kD tumor antigen, and, therefore, the partially transformed state of the *Hpa*I-E-transformed cells may be due to the absence of the 19-kD tumor antigen. Recently, by transfection of cloned E1 DNA with random insertional mutations generated by the bacterial transposon Tn*5*, McKinnon et al. (1982) have shown that the aminoterminal region of E1B plays an essential role in transformation. These results are also consistent with the observation that all Ad2- or Ad5-transformed cell lines examined express the 19-kD tumor antigen (Matsuo et al. 1982).

The functional domains of the 19-kD tumor antigen that

may be essential for inducing cell transformation can be inferred from the DNA sequence analysis data of Ad2 (Gingeras et al. 1982) and Ad5 (Bos et al. 1981) and our analysis of Ad2 *lp* mutants. Comparison of the sequences of Ad2 and Ad5 19-kD tumor antigen-coding regions reveals that the carboxyterminal region exhibits variations leading to amino acid substitutions but the amino terminus is highly conserved between the two serotypes. This suggests that the amino terminus of the 19-kD tumor antigen contains important functional information. This view is strengthened by the observation that *lp3* DNA contains a single base pair change resulting in a single amino acid substitution at the amino terminus that greatly reduces the transforming potential of this mutant.

It has also been observed that adenoviral genes that lie outside the E1 region play a role in the transformation process when infection is performed with viral particles. Ad5 *ts* mutants that map at map positions 18.0–22.5 have been shown to be defective in the initiation of transformation (Williams et al. 1974). On the other hand, Ad5 *ts125*, which is defective in the 72-kD single-stranded DNA-binding protein encoded by the E2A region, enhances transformation (Ginsberg et al. 1974). Possible interactions between these proteins and the 19-kD tumor antigen remain to be investigated.

Acknowledgment

This work was supported by a research grant from the National Cancer Institute (CA-33616). The author is an Established Investigator of the American Heart Association.

References

Anderson, C.W. and J.B. Lewis. 1980. Amino-terminal sequence of adenovirus type 2 proteins: Hexon, fiber, component IX and early protein 1B-15K. *Virology* **104:** 27.

Berk, A.J., F. Lee, T. Harrison, J. Williams, and P. Sharp. 1979. Pre-early adenovirus 5 gene product regulates synthesis of early viral messenger RNAs. *Cell* **17:** 935.

Bos, L., L.J. Polder, S.R. Bernards, P.I. Schrier, P.J. van den Elsen, A.J. van der Eb, and H. van Ormondt. 1981. The 2.2 kb E1B mRNA of human Ad12 and Ad5 codes for two tumor antigens starting at different AUG triplets. *Cell* **27:** 121.

Brusca, J.S. and G. Chinnadurai. 1981. Transforming genes among three different oncogenic subgroups of human adenoviruses have similar replicative functions. *J. Virol.* **39:** 300.

Chinnandurai, G. 1983. Adenovirus 2 *lp⁺* locus codes for a 19 kd tumor antigen that plays an essential role in cell transformation. *Cell* **33:** 759.

Chinnadurai, G., S. Chinnadurai, and J. Brusca. 1979. Physical mapping of a large plaque mutation of adenovirus type 2. *J. Virol.* **32:** 623.

Chinnaduai, G., S. Chinnadurai, and M. Green. 1978. Enhanced infectivity of adenovirus type 2 DNA and a DNA-protein complex. *J. Virol.* **26:** 195.

Chu, C.-T, D.S. Parris, R.A.F. Dixon, F.E. Farber, and P.A. Schaffer. 1979. Hydroxylamine mutagenesis of HSV DNA and DNA fragments: Introduction of mutations into selected regions of the viral genome. *Virology* **98:** 168.

Esche, H., M.B. Mathews, and J.B. Lewis. 1980. Proteins and messenger RNAs of the transforming region of wild-type and mutant adenoviruses. *J. Mol. Biol.* **142:** 399.

Flint, S.J., J. Sambrook, J.E. Williams, and P. Sharp. 1976. Viral nucleic acid sequences in transformed cells, IV. A study of the sequences of adenovirus 5 DNA and RNA in four lines of adenovirus-transformed rodent cells using specific fragments of the viral genome. *Virology* **72:** 456.

Gallimore, P.H., P.A. Sharp, and J. Sambrook. 1974. Viral DNA in transformed cells, II. A study of the sequences of adenovirus 2 DNA in nine lines of transformed rat cells using specific fragments of the viral genome. *J. Mol. Biol.* **89:** 49.

Galos, R., J. Williams, T. Shenk, and N. Jones. 1980. Physical location of host-range mutants of adenovirus type 5; deletion and marker-rescue mapping. *Virology* **104:** 510.

Gilead, Z., Y. Jeng, W.S.M. Wold, K. Sugawara, H.M. Rho, M.L. Harter, and M. Green. 1976. Immunological identification of two adenovirus 2-induced early proteins possibly involved in cell transformation. *Nature* **264:** 263.

Gingeras, T.R., D. Sciaky, R.E. Gelinas, J. Bing-Dong, C. Yen, M. Kelly, P. Bullock, B. Parsons, K. O'Neil, and R.J. Roberts. 1982. Nucleotide sequences from the adenovirus-2 genome. *J. Biol. Chem.* **257:** 13475.

Ginsberg, H.S., M.G. Ensinger, R.S. Kauffman, A.J. Mayer, and U. Lundholm. 1974. Cell transformation: A study of regulation with type 5 and adenovirus temperature sensitive mutants. *Cold Spring Harbor Symp. Quant. Biol.* **39:** 419.

Graham, F.L. and A.J. van der Eb. 1973. A new technique for the assay of infectivity of human adenovirus type 5 DNA. *Virology* **52:** 456.

Graham, F.L., T. Harrison, and J. Williams. 1978. Defective transforming capacity of adenovirus type 5 host-range mutants. *Virology* **86:** 10.

Graham, F.L., P.J. Abrahams, C. Mulder, H.L. Heijneker, S.O. Warnaar, F.A.J. DeVries, W. Fiers, and A.J. van der Eb. 1974. Studies on in vitro transformation by DNA and DNA fragments of human adenoviruses and SV40. *Cold Spring Harbor Symp. Quant. Biol.* **39:** 637.

Green, M., K.H. Brackmann, M.A. Cartas, and T. Matusuo. 1982. Identification and purification of a protein coded by the human adenovirus type 2 transforming region. *J. Virol.* **42:** 30.

Halbert, D., D. Spector, and H.J. Raskas. 1979. In vitro translation products specified by the transforming region of adenovirus type 2. *J. Virol.* **31:** 621.

Harrison, T., F.L. Graham, and J. Williams. 1977. Host range mutants of adenovirus type 5 defective for growth in HeLa cells. *Virology* **77:** 319.

Ho, Y.-S., R. Galso, and J. Williams. 1982. Isolation of type 5 adenovirus mutants with a cold-sensitive host range phenotype: Genetic evidence for an adenovirus transformation maintenance function. *Virology* **122:** 109.

Houweling, A., P.J. van den Elsen, and A.J. van der Eb. 1980. Partial transformation of primary rat cells by the leftmost 4.5% fragment of adenovirus 5 DNA. *Virology* **105:** 537.

Ito, Y. 1979. Polyoma virus-specific 55K protein isolated from plasma membrane of productively infected cell is virus-coded and important for cell transformation. *Virology* **98:** 261.

Jones, N. and T. Shenk. 1979a. Isolation of adenovirus type 5 host range deletion mutants defective for transformation of rat embryo cells. *Cell* **17:** 683.

———. 1979b. An adenovirus type 5 early gene function regulates expression of other early viral genes. *Proc. Natl. Acad. Sci.* **76:** 3665.

Kimura, G., S. Itagaki, and J. Summers. 1975. Rat cell line 3Y1 and its virogenic polyoma and SV40 transformed derivatives. *Int. J. Cancer* **15:** 694.

Lassam, N.J., S.T. Bayley, and F.L. Graham. 1979. Tumor antigens of human Ad5 in transformed cells and in cells infected with transformation-defective host-range mutants. *Cell* **18:** 781.

Levinson, A.D., S.A. Courtneidge, and J.M. Bishop. 1980. Structural and functional domains of the Rous Sarcoma Virus transforming protein (pp60*src*). *Proc. Natl. Acad. Sci.* **78:** 1624.

Matsuo, T., W.S.M. Wold, S. Hashimoto, A. Rankin, J. Symington, and M. Green. 1982. Polypeptides encoded by transforming region E1b of human adenovirus 2: Immunoprecipitation from transformed and infected cells and cell-free translation of E1b-specific mRNA. *Virology* **118:** 456.

Maxam, A. and W. Gilbert. 1980. Sequencing end-labeled DNA with base-specific chemical cleavages. *Methods Enzymol.* **65:** 499.

McKinnon, R.D., S. Bacchetti, and F.L. Graham. 1982. Tn5 mutagenesis of the transforming genes of human adenovirus type 5. *Gene* **19:** 33.

Perricaudet, M., J.M. LeMoullec, and U. Petterson. 1980. The predicted structure of two adenovirus T antigens. *Proc. Natl. Acad. Sci.* **77:** 3778.

Persson, H., M.G. Katze, and L. Philipson. 1982. Purification of a native membrane-associated adenovirus tumor antigen. *J. Virol.* **42:** 905.

Rowe, D.T. and F.L. Graham. 1983. Transformation of rodent cells by DNA extracted from transformation defective adenovirus mutants. *J. Virol.* **46:** 1039.

Sambrook, J., J. Williams, P.A. Sharp, and T. Grodzicker. 1975. Physical mapping of temperature sensitive mutations of adenoviruses. *J. Mol. Biol.* **97:** 369.

Schrier, P.I., P.J. van den Elsen, J.J.L. Hertoghs, and A.J. van der Eb. 1979. Characterization of tumor antigens in cells transformed by fragments of adenovirus type 5 DNA. *Virology* **99:** 372.

Shiroki, K., H. Shimojo, Y. Sawada, Y. Uemizu, and K. Fujinaga. 1979. Incomplete transformation of rat cells by a small fragment of adenovirus 12 DNA. *Virology* **95:** 127.

Shiroki, K., H. Handa, H. Shimojo, S. Yano, S. Ojima, and K.

Fujinaga. 1977. Establishment and characterization of rat cell lines transformed by restriction endonuclease fragments of adenovirus 12 DNA. *Virology* **82:** 462.

Solnick, D. and M.A. Anderson. 1982. Transformation-deficient adenovirus defective in expression of region IA and not region IB. *J. Virol.* **42:** 106.

Takemori, N., J.L. Riggs, and C.D. Aldrick. 1968. Genetic studies with tumorigenic adenovirus I. Isolation of cytocidal (*cyt*) mutants of adenovirus type 12. *Virology* **36:** 575.

Tooze, J., ed. 1980. *Molecular biology of tumor viruses*, 2nd edition: *DNA tumor viruses*. Cold Spring Harbor Laboratory, Cold Spring Harbor, New York.

van der Eb, A.J., C. Mulder, F.L. Graham, and A. Houweling. 1977. Transformation with specific fragments of adenovirus DNAs, I. Isolation of specific fragments with transforming activity of adenovirus 2 and 5 DNA. *Gene* **2:** 115.

Williams, J.F., H. Young, and P. Austin. 1974. Genetic analysis of adenovirus type 5 in permissive and nonpermissive cells. *Cold Spring Harbor Symp. Quant. Biol.* **39:** 427.

Willingham, M.D., G. Jay, and I. Pastan. 1979. Localization of the ASV src gene product to the plasma membrane of transformed cells by electron microscopic immunocytochemistry. *Cell* **18:** 125.

Wold, W.S.M. and M. Green. 1979. Adenovirus type 2 early polypeptides immunoprecipitated by antisera to five lines of adenovirus-transformed rat cells. *J. Virol.* **30:** 297.

An Examination of the Transforming and Tumor-inducing Capacity of a Number of Adenovirus Type 12 Early-region 1, Host-range Mutants and Cells Transformed by Subgenomic Fragments of Ad12 E1 Region

P. Gallimore, P. Byrd, R. Grand, and J. Whittaker

Department of Cancer Studies, Cancer Research Campaign Laboratories, University of Birmingham Medical School, Birmingham, B15 2TJ, England

D. Breiding and J. Williams

Department of Biological Sciences, Carnegie-Mellon University, Pittsburgh, Pennsylvania 15213

It is extremely appropriate that we should be considering adenovirus 12 (Ad12) oncogenesis at this meeting because it is 21 years since Trentin et al. (1962) first reported that this human virus induced tumors in hamsters. Since that original observation, the oncogenic host range of Ad12 has been extended from a number of different rodent species, including the rat (Huebner et al. 1963), mouse (Yabe et al. 1964), and mastomys (Rabson and Kirschstein 1964) to the baboon (Mukai et al. 1980). This has encouraged research funding agencies to support experimentation designed to determine how adenoviral protein(s) switch cell growth control from a normal to a malignant mode. Two initial approaches were made to this problem. First, restriction endonucleases were used to map the adenoviral genetic information retained and expressed in transformed cells (Gallimore et al. 1974; Sambrook et al. 1974; Sharp et al. 1974) and, second, DNA transfection was used to examine which region of the adenoviral genome is responsible for transformation in vitro (Graham et al. 1974; Shiroki et al. 1979; van der Eb et al. 1979). The results from these studies showed that the left-hand 12% of the adenoviral genome, now referred to as the early region 1 (E1), contained the genetic information responsible for morphological transformation. These findings provided the basis for more refined molecular (Jones and Shenk 1979a) and genetic (Harrison et al. 1977; Graham et al. 1978) investigations. The results of these studies together with transcription mapping data (Berk and Sharp 1978) showed that the E1 region comprises two gene blocks (E1A and E1B). Recently, the DNA nucleotide sequence for both AD12 E1A (Sugisaki et al. 1980) and E1B (Bos et al. 1981; Kimura et al. 1981) have been reported. The biological activities of the proteins expressed from E1 remain elusive, but it is clear from genetic and transformation studies that expression of the E1B region is under the control of E1A (Berk et al. 1979; Jones and Shenk 1979b; Bos and ten Wolde-Kraamwinkel 1983) and that E1B alone cannot transform rodent cells (van den Elsen et al. 1982). It is questionable if these elegant studies carried out in tissue culture reflect the virus-cell interactions occurring during Ad12 oncogenesis in vivo.

This paper describes a collaborative study aimed at resolving this by a genetic approach with the development of AD12 E1 mutant viruses that can be examined for tumorigenicity, morphological transformation in vitro, and for the induction of tumor-specific transplantation immunity.

Initially, we describe the use of Ad12 E1 recombinant plasmids in transformation experiments carried out on nonpermissive baby rat kidney (BRK) and permissive human embryo retinal (HER) cell cultures that provided evidence of the biological activity of the plasmids; these studies have allowed us to develop human cell lines carrying and expressing Ad12 E1 proteins. We then present data on the malignant phenotype of these transformed cell lines and finally describe the isolation and properties of Ad12 E1 mutant viruses developed by classical mutagenesis and molecular genetic techniques.

Methods

Ad12 recombinant plasmids

The isolation, growth, and restriction endonuclease maps for the Ad12 recombinant plasmids used in this study have been previously reported (Byrd et al. 1982b). The plasmids contain the following AD12 DNA, pAsc 2, the EcoRI-C fragment (0–16.5 map units); pAsc 10.3 the SalI-C fragment (0–10.3 map units); pAsc 6.8, the HindIII-G fragment (0–6.8 map units); and pAsc 4.7, the AccI-H fragment (0–4.7 map units).

Transformation assays

Transformation experiments using Hooded Lister baby rat kidney cells (HLBRK) and plasmid DNA were carried out as described by Byrd et al. (1982b) with the exception that no carrier DNA was used. BALB/c mouse embryo and baby mouse kidney cell cultures were used for the studies with Ad12 hr mutants. Both cell types were infected with 10 pfu/cell, the kidney cells being passaged immediately after infection (5 × 10⁵ cells/dish) whereas the embryo cells were passaged 24 hours after infection (9.0×10^5 cells/dish). Transformed colonies were counted at 4 weeks postinfection (kidney cells) and 6 weeks postinfection (embryo cells).

Development of mutant viruses

Ad12 strain Huie was obtained from the ATCC, plaque purified, and grown on A549 cells (Giard et al. 1973; ATCC#CCL 185) or human embryo kidney (HEK) cells to provide high-titer working stocks. Mutagenesis of whole virus was carried out as previously described (Williams et al. 1971), using nitrous acid (0.7 M) as the mutagen. Mutagenized virus was plated on Ad12 HER3 cells (established as described by Byrd et al. 1982a) at 37°C; well-isolated plaques were picked and these were tested for growth on A594 cells by "rapid assay" (Harrison et al. 1977). Putative mutants were plaque purified on AD12 HER3 cells and propagated upon these cells to provide high-titer working stocks.

A second approach was to develop a system for isolating site-directed E1 mutants. Initially, this involved the isolation of an Ad12 variant with one SalI restriction site (wild-type virus has two SalI sites) at 10.3 map units. Plaque-purified virus was passaged at high input multiplicity for five passages. Ad12 DNA with terminal protein complex was then prepared, cut with SalI, religated with T4 DNA ligase, and plaqued on HEK cells using the DNA transfection technique (Graham and van der Eb 1973). Four variants that had lost the SalI site at 48.8 map units were isolated and one of these (Ad12 Salt7) was grown to high-titer stocks on HEK cells. The recombinant plasmid pAsc 6.8 which contains the Ad12 HindIII-G fragment was manipulated by the insertion of an 8-bp BclI linker d(CTGATCAG) at the RsaI site at nucleotide 1004. This insertion places a stop codon at nucleotide 1022 in frame within the coding sequences of the Ad12 E1A 13S mRNA, leaving the 12S E1A mRNA unaltered. The purified, mutated Ad12 HindIII-G fragment was then ligated with the large EcoRI–HindIII fragment of pAsc 10.3 and the reconstructed SalI-C fragment was then rescued on Ad12 HER 3 cells using a SalI-cleaved Ad12 Salt7 DNA terminal protein complex. This mutant is referred to as H12 *in*600.

Detection of Ad12 E1 proteins

These proteins were detected by two techniques (1) immunoprecipitation (see Paraskeva et al. 1982) and (2) a modification of the Western blotting technique previously described by Towbin et al. (1979). Cells were solubilized (2×10^7/ml) in 8 M urea, 50 mM Tris-HCl (pH 7.6), 150 mM β-mercaptoethanol, 1% SDS. Aliquots (15 μl) were electrophoresed on 13% polyacrylamide gels and the proteins were electrophoretically transferred to cellulose nitrate filters. After exposure to Tris/saline (pH 7.4) containing 3% BSA (Buffer A) for 1 hour at 40°C, the filters were incubated in Ad12 rat tumor bearer serum (TBS) appropriately diluted (1 in 200) in Buffer A. After 2 hours at 30°C, the filters were washed extensively and then incubated in Buffer A containing ^{125}I-labeled sheep anti-rat antibody ($\sim 5 \times 10^4$ cpm cm^{-2}

of filter). After a further 2 hours, unbound radioactivity was removed by exhaustive washing with Tris/saline containing 0.1% SDS and 0.5% Triton X-100; the filters were dried and autoradiographed for 1–2 days. Two Ad12 TBS were used in these studies: Ad12/100-1 TBS (Paraskeva et al. 1982) identified 18K and 52K E1B proteins and the Ad12 ECO.C1 TBS identified the 41K E1A protein and the 52K E1B protein.

Tumorigenicity and transplantation immunity

One-day-old HL rats were inoculated intraperitoneally (i.p.) with either Ad12 wild-type (wt) or mutant virus at 1×10^8 pfu per rat. For the Ad12 wt, this is equivalent to 100 tumor-producing dose (TPD$_{50}$). Animals were examined for tumor development weekly, for a year.

Ad12 tumor-specific transplantation immunity was measured by the ability of Ad12 mutant viruses to protect rats inoculated at 1 day old with 100 TPD$_{50}$ of Ad12 wt virus. Animals 14 and 21 days old were immunized with either Ad-12 wt (positive control) or mutant viruses (1×10^7 pfu given i.p. per rat at each immunization).

Results

The relative transforming activities of the Ad12 recombinant plasmids in HLBRK cells were calculated from three experiments in which pAsc 2 (29 dishes), pAsc 6.8 (45 dishes), and pAsc 4.7 (45 dishes) were compared directly and two experiments in which pAsc 10.3 was also included. All four plasmids transformed these rat cells and the mean transformants per microgram genome equivalent were 0.152, 0.0442, 0.0186, and 0.0057 for pAsc 2, pAsc 10.3, pAsc 6.8, and pAsc 4.7, respectively. Expressed more simply, the transforming activities of pAsc 2, pAsc 10.3, and pAsc 6.8 were 31.23, 14.31, and 4.26 times higher than that of pAsc 4.7, respectively.

When transformed foci were picked with the aim of developing cell lines, immortal cell lines were established directly from foci induced by either pAsc 2 or pAsc 10.3. These cell lines were phenotypically indistinguishable from Ad12 virion-induced BRK cell lines. pAsc 6.8 transformants grew slowly after initial isolation, mainly due to a high proportion of cells flattening, stretching, and finally falling off the plastic. The cells that remained attached continued to divide and all six of the foci picked developed into cell lines. More growth problems were encountered with pAsc 4.7-induced foci. Six out of seven that were picked failed to develop into cell lines at the first and second isolation attempts. Between isolation procedures, the transformed foci were allowed to reform on the original dishes and at the third attempt all of these six foci slowly developed into cell lines. Following isolation, the growth pattern of the seventh pAsc 4.7 focus was the same as the pAsc 6.8 foci described above. Representative phase-contrast photomicrographs of Ad12 plasmid-transformed BRK cell lines are shown in Figure 1. All the cell lines had an overall epithelioid morphology. pAsc 2 and pAsc 10.3 transformants grew as tightly packed colonies whereas pAsc 6.8 and 4.7 trans-

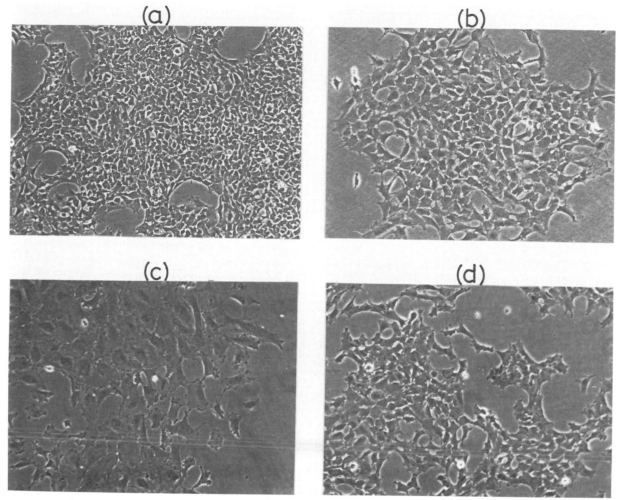

Figure 1 Phase-contrast photomicrographs of Ad12 recombinant plasmid-transformed HLBRK cell lines. (*a*) pAsc 2 transformant ECO.C1; (*b*) pAsc 6.8 transformant HIN.G1; (*c*) pAsc 4.7 transformant ACC.H1; and (*d*) pAsc 4.7 transformant ACC.H2.

formed lines showed loose contact between cells and the borders of individual cells were highly ruffled.

The results of tumorigenicity experiments carried out in 1-day-old syngeneic rats are shown in Table 1. A clear distinction in both tumor latent period and time of death was noted for pAsc 2- and pAsc 10.3-transformed lines, compared with pAsc 6.8- and pAsc 4.7-transformed lines, in that these were three times longer for the latter cell lines. One pAsc 6.8 cell line and three pAsc 4.7 cell lines were nontumorigenic at a standard inoculum of 2×10^6 cells per rat. Immunoprecipitation and Western

blotting experiments revealed that all of the plasmid-transformed cell lines expressed the 41K (E1A) protein and three of the six pAsc 6.8 transformants also expressed the E1B 18K protein, whereas all of the pAsc 10.3 and pAsc 2 transformants produced the E1B 52K protein in addition to the proteins just mentioned (Table 1).

We have previously described a human cell system in which pAsc 2 reliably induced morphological transformation (Byrd et al. 1982a). A number of experiments have been carried out using the HER cell system with

Table 1 Ad12 Protein Content and Tumorigenicity of Ad12 DNA-Transformed Baby Rat Kidney Cells

Ad12 plasmid used to produce BRK cell lines (Ad12 map units)	Tumor-positive lines/ number of cell lines examined	Tumor-positive rats/ number inoculated (%)	Mean tumor latent period	Mean time of death	Ad12 proteins identified
pAsc 2 (0–16.5)	7/7	88/88 (100)	34 days	70 days	41K, 52K, 18K
pAsc 10.3 (0–10.3)	3/3	23/23 (100)	40 days	77 days	41K, 52K, 18K
pAsc 6.8 (0–6.8)	5/6	45/56 (80.4)	129 days	219 days	41K, 18K +/−
pAsc 4.7 (0–4.7)	4/7	42/75 (56)	118 days	209 days	41K

2×10^6 cells inoculated subcutaneously into 1-day-old syngeneic rats.

both pAsc 2 and pAsc 6.8 DNA as the transfected molecules. pAsc 2 was found to tranform HER cells 10- to 20-fold less efficiently than HLBRK cells. In contrast, pAsc 6.8 induced rare transformants in HER cultures at a frequency of at least an order of magnitude lower than pAsc 2. Nineteen out of nineteen picked pAsc 2-transformed HER foci developed into cells lines, whereas all seven pAsc 6.8 HER-transformed foci that were picked aborted in primary culture. Fifteen pAsc 2-transformed HER cell lines have been inoculated intracerebrally (i.c.) into 2-week-old congenitally athymic nude mice (1 × 10^5 cells per mouse) and all lines produced lethal neoplasms within 90 days (P.H. Gallimore and P. Byrd, unpubl.).

Figure 2 illustrates the morphology and monolayer

characteristic of one pAsc 2-transformed HER cell line, namely Ad-12 HER3. These cells express the Ad12 E1A and E1B proteins, contain only three or four copies of the Ad12 sequences (Byrd 1983), and give Ad12 virus yields and plaque-forming units in the same range as normal HEK cells (the best permissive cell type for Ad12). Consequently, this cell line was chosen as the permissive cell type for the isolation of Ad12 E1 mutants and for the growth of high-titer stocks of such mutants.

Properties of Ad12 E1 mutant viruses

To date, roughly 2% of plaques isolated from nitrous acid-treated virus stocks were shown to be *hr* mutants, i.e., they grew less well on A549 cells than on Ad12 HER3 cells. A comparison of the ratios of plaque-forming

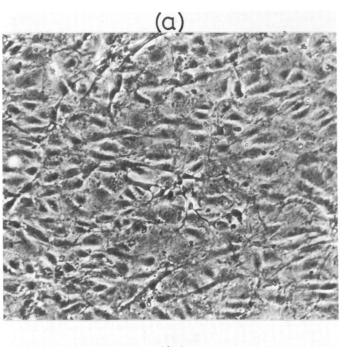

(a)

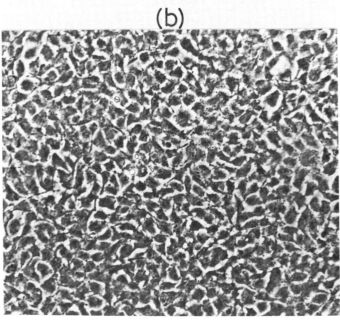

(b)

Figure 2 Phase-contrast photomicrographs of normal human embryo retinoblasts and the Ad12 HER3 cell line. (*a*) Normal HER cells after 6 weeks in tissue culture; (*b*) Ad12 HER3 cells left confluent for 10 days (note retention of monolayer).

units for four *hr* mutants measured on Ad12 HER3 cells and A549 were as follows: H12 *hr*700, 8.1×10^3; H12 *hr*702, 2.5×10^3; H12 *hr*703, 1.0×10^5; and H12*hr* 704, 2.3×10^4. The ratio for Ad12 wt was 2.4. None of these *hr* mutants demonstrates any temperature sensitivity. Table 2 shows the data obtained from experiments in which the same *hr* mutants were used to infect both A549 and Ad12 HER3 cells at 10 pfu per cell and the virus yields obtained at 46 hours determined on Ad12 HER3 cells. At the higher multiplicity used in this type of experiment, one of these mutants (H12 *hr*700) was considerably leakier on A549 cells than the other mutants studied. The leaky phenotype of H12 *hr*700 was even more pronounced on normal HEK cells (data not shown). Because this mutant and a few more recent isolates are quite leaky on A549 cells, we have also measured their growth upon HeLa cells. The *hr* phenotype of all mutants tested (see Table 3) was found to be considerably tighter on HeLa cells, making these cells more suitable for complementation analysis. For complementation, HeLa cells were infected at an input multiplicity of 10 pfu/cell in single infection with each mutant, and at 5 pfu/cell with each mutant in double infection. Infected cells were incubated at either 37°C (46–48 hr), or 38.5°C (42–44 hr). As is clear from Table 3, six mutants that were tested were found to fall into two groups, one comprising H12 *hr*700 and H12 *hr*701, and the other consisting of H12 *hr* mutants 702, 703, 704, and 705. Recent complementation tests of some of these mutants with E1A and E1B *hr* and *dl* mutants of Ad5 suggest that H12 *hr*700 and H12 *hr*701 are E1A mutants, whereas the other four are E1B mutants (data not shown). In addition, preliminary marker rescue of *hr*703 and *hr*704 DNA complex with DNA fragments derived from Ad12 E1 plasmids and deletion plasmids places these mutations within the E1B 52K reading frame (D. Breiding, unpubl.). This observation was supported by immunoprecipitation and Western blotting experiments carried out on mutant virus-infected normal HEK cells, in that the E1B 52K protein was not produced by either of these mutants in this cell type (Table 4).

Transformation experiments carried out on primary mouse cells revealed that Ad12 transformed these cells 50–100 times more efficiently than Ad5 (J. Williams, unpubl.). In transformation experiments carried out at 37°C on both BALB/c mouse embryo and mouse kidney cells with all the mutants described in Table 3, only H12 *hr*700

Table 2 Yields of Type-12 Human Adenovirus *hr* Mutants Grown in HER3 and A549 Cells at 37°C

Virus	Yield at 46 hr[a]		Ratio HER3/ A549
	HER3	A549	
Wild type	1.7×10^{9b}	4.5×10^9	0.37
H12 *hr*700	1.8×10^9	9.0×10^7	20
H12 *hr*702	2.2×10^9	7.0×10^6	3.1×10^2
H12 *hr*703	2.6×10^9	1.2×10^5	2.2×10^4
H12 *hr*704	3.4×10^9	2.4×10^5	1.4×10^4

[a]Monolayers infected at an input multiplicity of 10 pfu/cell, and harvested at 46 hr postinfection.
[b]Yield, pfu/dish, measured on HER3 cells at 37°C.

and 701 produced transformed foci (input multiplicity 10 pfu/cell). Comparison of the transforming frequencies of these mutant viruses with Ad12 wild-type virus showed them to be at least an order of magnitude lower. Transformation experiments were also carried out at 32.5°C and 38.5°C and it was found that none of the mutants reported here showed a temperature-sensitive phenotype. Table 4 contains the summary data for both tumorigenicity and Ad12 tumor-specific transplantation immunity induction in HL rats. Of the four *hr* mutants tested, only H12 *hr*700 produced tumors (2 out of 10 rats injected) at an inoculation dose (1×10^8 pfu/rat) equivalent to 100 TPD_{50} of Ad12 wt. H12 *hr*703 and 704 both failed to produce tumors in two experiments. However, in a single transplantation immunity experiment, both of these *hr* mutants gave 100% protection to rats inoculated at birth with 100 TPD_{50} of Ad12 wt virus. In the same experiment, H12 *hr*700 was shown to induce a low level of tumor transplantation immunity because half of the rats, immunized with this virus, succumbed to Ad12 tumors.

The single site-directed mutant virus described in this study, H12 *in*600, was found to be a "tight" host-range mutant. A cesium chloride gradient-purified virus stock gave titers of 1.3×10^{10} pfu/ml on Ad12 HER3 cells and 2.3×10^5 pfu/ml on primary HEK cells. In preliminary transformation experiments carried out on HLBRK cells, H12 *in*600 failed to transform these cells at the three temperatures tested (32.5°C, 37°C, and 38.5°C). In these experiments, both Ad12 wt and Ad12 Salt7 (the virus used to rescue the site-directed mutated recom-

Table 3 Complementation between Type-12 *hr* Mutants on HeLa Cells at 37°C

Mutant	700	701	702	703	704	705
H12 *hr*700	1.8×10^{6a}	0.5^b	9.0	40	94	—
H12 *hr*701	—	2.2×10^6	26	31	146	161
H12 *hr*702	—	—	3.4×10^5	0.7	1.3	—
H12 *hr*703	—	—	—	2.1×10^4	1.4	2.6
H12 *hr*704	—	—	—	—	2.8×10^4	2.3
H12 *hr*705	—	—	—	—	—	3.1×10^4

[a]Infectivity of single infection yields (pfu/ml) measured on HER3 cells at 37°C.
[b]Complementation index: ratio of double infection yield/higher of two single infection yields.

Table 4 A Summary of the Biological Properties of Five AD12 E1 Mutant Viruses

Viruses	Transformation of rodent cells[a]	Tumorigenicity[b] in 1-day-old rats (% positive)	Induction of Ad12 tumor-specific transplantation immunity	Ad12 E1 proteins[c] expressed in infected normal HEK cells
Ad12 Huie (wt)	positive (M and R)	tumorigenic (100)	positive	41K, 52K & 18K
H12 hr700	weakly positive (M)	weakly tumorigenic (20)	weakly positive	41K, 52K & 18K (leaky)
H12 hr702	negative (M)	nontumorigenic	N.D.	41K, 52K (very low)
H12 hr703	negative (M)	nontumorigenic	positive	41K, 18K (low)
H12 hr704	negative (M)	nontumorigenic	positive	41K, 18K (low)
H12 in600	negative (R)	N.D.[d]	N.D.	41K, 30K,[e] 52K (low), and 18K (low)

[a]M, Mouse kidney and mouse embryo cells; R, rat kidney cells.
[b]1×10^8 pfu/rat intraperitoneally ($=$ 100 tumor-producing dose$_{50}$ for weight).
[c]By immunoprecipitation and Western blotting.
[d]N.D., Not done.
[e]Truncated E1A protein, not found to be equimolar with 41K.

binant plasmid) transformed HLBRK cells at all three temperatures. Using an Ad12 tumor-bearer serum that only reacts with E1A 41K protein from Ad12-infected and Ad12-transformed cells (derived from a rat bearing a tumor induced by one of the pAsc 4.7 HLBRK cell lines), H12 in600 was found to produce Ad12 proteins of approximately 40K and 30K in infected normal HEK cells, 28 hours postinfection (20 pfu/cell).

Discussion

Two approaches to the study of the Ad12 gene(s) involved in oncogenesis are described here, namely DNA transformation studies on normal rat and human cells and the development of Ad12 E1 mutant viruses. In respect to morphological transformation and tumorigenicity, our findings strongly implicate the E1B 52K protein. In the absence of this protein, transformation of BRK and HER cells is significantly reduced. Problems are encountered after picking transformed foci during the development of cell lines, and the overall behavior of the 52K negative lines in vivo is clearly distinguishable from those lines expressing this protein (Table 1). Our study is the first to report the establishment of Ad12 E1A-transformed normal rat cells. These seven pAsc 4.7-transformed BRK cell lines are anchorage dependent (data not shown) and fail to produce tumors in congenitally athymic nude mice (data not shown), but four were found to produce invasive tumors in syngeneic rats (Table 1). The discrepancy between the nude mouse and rat results could be explained by the long tumor latent periods observed in the rats. In the nude mouse, only two out of the six pAsc 6.8 transformants produced tumors compared with five out of six in the syngeneic host (Table 1). Our findings are different from those reported by Jochemsen et al. (1982) in that none of their six Ad12

HindIII-G-transformed BRK cell lines were tumorigenic in the nude mouse.

In agreement with our findings, Rowe and Graham (1983) have recently reported that hamster cells expressing only Ad5 E1A proteins can produce tumors when inoculated into hamsters. What is unclear at present from our study is what effect in vitro selection had on our E1A transformants during the "crisis growth phase," whether the presence of the E1B promoter in the pAsc 4.7 plasmid is functional on integration, and whether the recovery from crisis signals a change in cellular gene expression.

The development of Ad12 E1 mutant viruses allowed us to carry out in vitro transformation and in vivo tumorigenicity and transplantation immunity studies. From the results obtained so far, we can conclude that the E1B 52K protein is required for Ad12 oncogenesis and transformation, but is not required for tumor-specific transplantation immunity (see data for H12 hr703 and 704 in Table 4). The most likely protein to be involved in transplantation immunity is the E1B 18K protein, which, like the Ad2 E1B 15K protein (Persson et al. 1982), is almost exclusively found in the cell membrane (R.J.A. Grand and P.H. Gallimore, unpubl. observ.). The in vivo and in vitro findings for the E1A mutant H12 hr700 coupled with the failure of H12 in600 to transform BRK cells clearly also implicates E1A in both Ad12 transformation and tumorigenesis. It would be premature to assign specific role(s) for the Ad12 E1 proteins, but we can tentatively hypothesize that E1A has a role in the induction of transformation and that the 52K E1B protein enhances or stabilizes the effect of E1A. It should be borne in mind that a product of E1A controls the expression of the E1B gene region (Berk et al. 1979; Jones and Shenk 1979b), and recently Bos and ten Wolde-Kraamwinkel (1983) have provided data that the Ad12 E1B promoter is activated by the E1A gene region. The transformation of BRK cells described in this study suggests that E1A is not simply functioning as an activator of E1B.

Finally, the recent finding that the Ad12 but not the Ad5 E1A gene region depresses the level of expression of class-1 major histocompatibility (MHC) antigens (A.J. van der Eb, pers. comm.) may provide an explanation for the oncogenic phenotype or subgroup-A adenoviruses (which includes Ad12). Similarly, K. Raska (pers. comm.) has examined MHC class-1 expression on a number of the HLBRK-transformed cell lines described in this report and has found that the level of expression of the Ag-B5 (H − 1^c) MHC antigen is reduced by 55–90%. Two notes of caution should be added to these observations: (1) Ad12 virus only produces tumors when inoculated into immunologically immature rodents and (2) animals immunized with Ad12 virus are protected from Ad12 oncogenesis and tumor induction by Ad12-transformed cell lines.

In spite of the time that has elapsed since Trentin et al. (1962) discovered Ad12 oncogenesis, we have so far been unable to discover the biological property (or properties) of the products of the adenoviral E1 gene region. The development of molecular biology techniques has enabled us to produce a permissive cell system for the detection and the isolation of Ad12 E1 mutants. It is hoped that a study of the effect of these mutants on cell physiology and gene expression will lead to a better understanding of how Ad12 changes a normal cell into a cancer cell.

Acknowledgments

The following technicians are thanked for their considerable contributions to this study: A. Maguire, V. Nash, P. Reeve, C. Roberts, M. Williams, and L. Withington. The secretarial skills of J. Meers and D. Williams were very much appreciated.

This study was jointly funded by the Cancer Research Campaign, England, and by the National Cancer Institute (Grant CA-21375).

References

Berk, A.J. and P.A. Sharp. 1978. Structure of the adenovirus 2 early m-RNAs. *Cell* **14:** 695.

Berk, A.J., F. Lee, T. Harrison, J. Williams, and P.A. Sharp. 1979. Pre-early adenovirus 5 gene product regulates synthesis of early viral messenger RNAs. *Cell* **17:** 935.

Bos, J.L. and H.C. ten Wolde-Kraamwinkel. 1983. The E1b promoter of Ad-12 in mouse L tK⁻ cells is activated by adenovirus region E1a. *EMBO J.* **2:** 73.

Bos, J.L., L.J. Polder, R. Bernards, P.I. Schrier, P.J. van den Elsen, A.J. van der Eb, and H. van Ormondt. 1981. The 2.2 Kb E1b m-RNA of human Ad-12 and Ad-5 codes for two tumour antigens at different AUG triplets. *Cell* **27:** 121.

Byrd, P.J. 1983. "Transformation of mammalian cells by human adenovirus DNA." Ph. D. thesis, University of Birmingham, England.

Byrd, P.J., K.W. Brown, and P.H. Gallimore. 1982a. Malignant transformation of human embryo retinoblasts by cloned adenovirus 12 DNA. *Nature* **298:** 69.

Byrd, P.J., W. Chia, P.W.J. Rigby, and P.H. Gallimore. 1982b. Cloning of DNA fragments from the left end of the adenovirus

type 12 genome: Transformation by cloned early region 1. *J. Gen. Virol.* **60:** 279.

Gallimore, P.H., P.A. Sharp, and J. Sambrook. 1974. Viral DNA in transformed cells. III. A study of the sequences of adenovirus 2 DNA in nine lines of transformed rat cells using specific fragments of the viral genome. *J. Mol. Biol.* **89:** 49.

Giard, R.J., S.A. Aaronson, G.J. Todaro, P. Arnstein, J.H. Kersey, H. Posik, and W.P. Parks. 1973. In vitro cultivation of human tumours: Establishment of cell lines derived from a series of solid tumors. *J. Natl. Cancer Inst.* **51:** 1417.

Graham, F.L. and A.J. van der Eb. 1973. A new technique for the assay of infectivity of human adenovirus 5 DNA. *Virology* **52:** 456.

Graham, F.L., T. Harrison, and J. Williams. 1978. Defective transforming capacity of adenovirus type 5 host-range mutants. *Virology* **86:** 10.

Graham, F.L., P.J. Abrahams, C. Mulder, H.L. Heijneker, S.O. Warnaar, F.A.J. de Vries, W. Friers, and A.J. van der Eb. 1974. Studies on the in vitro transformation by DNA and DNA fragments of human adenoviruses and simian virus 40. *Cold Spring Harbor Symp. Quant. Biol.* **39:** 637.

Harrison, T., F. Graham, and J. Williams. 1977. Host-range mutants of adenovirus type 5 defective for growth in Hela cells. *Virology* **77:** 319.

Huebner, R.J., W.P. Rowe, H.C. Turner, and W.T. Lane. 1963. Specific adenovirus complement-fixing antigens in virus free hamster and rat tumours. *Proc. Natl. Acad. Sci.* **50:** 379.

Jochemsen, H., G.S.G. Daniels, J.J.L. Hertoghs, P.I. Schrier, P.J. van den Elsen, and A.J. van der Eb. 1982. Identification of adenovirus-type 12 gene products involved in transformation and oncogenesis. *Virology* **122:** 15.

Jones, N. and T. Shenk. 1979a. Isolation of adenovirus type 5 host range deletion mutants defective for transformation of rat embryo cells. *Cell* **17:** 683.

———. 1979b. An adenovirus type 5 early gene function regulates expression of the other early viral genes. *Proc. Natl. Acad. Sci.* **76:** 3665.

Kimura, T., Y. Sawada, M. Shinagawa, Y. Shimizu, K. Shiroki, H. Shimojo, H. Sugisaki, M. Takanami, Y. Uemiza, and K. Fujinaga. 1981. Nucleotide sequence of the transforming early region E1b of adenovirus type 12 DNA; structure and gene organisation, and comparison with those of adenovirus type 5 DNA. *Nucleic Acids Res.* **9:** 6571.

Mukai, N., S.S. Kalter, L.B. Cummins, V.A. Matthews, T. Nishida, and T. Nakajima. 1980. Retinal tumour induced in the baboon by human adenovirus 12. *Science* **210:** 1023.

Paraskeva, C., K.W. Brown, A.R. Dunn, and P.H. Gallimore. 1982. Adenovirus type 12 transformed rat embryo brain and rat liver epithelial cell lines: Adenovirus type 12 genome content and viral protein expression. *J. Virol.* **44:** 759.

Persson, H., M.G. Katze, and L. Philipson. 1982. Purification of a native membrane-associated adenovirus tumour antigen. *J. Virol.* **42:** 905.

Rabson, A.S. and R.L. Kirschstein. 1964. Tumours produced by adenovirus 12 in mastomys and mice. *J. Natl. Cancer Inst.* **32:** 77.

Rowe, D.T. and F.L. Graham. 1983. Transformation of rodent cells by DNA extracted from transformation-defective adenovirus mutants. *J. Virol.* **46:** 1039.

Sambrook, J., M. Botchan, P. Gallimore, B. Ozanne, U. Pettersson, J. Williams, and P.A. Sharp. 1974. Viral DNA sequences in cells transformed by simian virus 40, adenovirus type 2 and adenovirus type 5. *Cold Spring Harbor Symp. Quant. Biol.* **39:** 615.

Sharp, P.A., P.H. Gallimore, and S.J. Flint. 1974. Mapping of adenovirus 2 RNA sequences in lytically infected cells and transformed cell lines. *Cold Spring Harbor Symp. Quant. Biol.* **39:** 457.

Shiroki, K., K. Segawa, I. Saito, H. Shimojo, and K. Fujinaga. 1979. Products of the adenovirus 12 transforming genes and their functions. *Cold Spring Harbor Symp. Quant. Biol.* **44:** 533.

Sugiska, H., K. Sugimoto, M. Takamani, K. Shiroki, I. Saito, H.

Shimojo, Y. Sawada, Y, Uemizu, S. I. Uesugi, and K. Fujinaga. 1980. Structure and gene organization in the transforming *Hin*dIII-G fragment of Ad-12. *Cell* **20:** 777.

Towbin, H., T. Staehelin, and J. Gordon. 1979. Electrophoretic transfer of proteins from polyacrylamide gels to nitrocellulose sheets: Procedure and some applications. *Proc. Natl. Acad. Sci.* **76:** 4350.

Trentin, J.J., Y. Yabe, and G. Taylor. 1962. The quest for human cancer viruses. *Science* **137:** 835.

van den Elsen, P., S. de Pater, A. Houweling, J. van der Veer, and A.J. van der Eb. 1982. The relationship between E1a and E1b of human adenoviruses in cell transformation. *Gene* **18:** 175.

van der Eb, A.J., H. van Ormondt, P.I. Schrier, J.H. Lupker, H. Jochemsen, P.J. van den Elsen, R.J. DeLeys, J. Maat, C.P. van Beveren, R. Dijkema, and A. de Waard. 1979. Structure and function of the transforming genes of human adenoviruses and SV40. *Cold Spring Harbor Symp. Quant. Biol.* **44:** 383.

Williams, J.F., M. Gharpure, S. Ustacelebi, and S. McDonald. 1971. Isolation of temperature-sensitive mutants of adenovirus type 5. *J. Gen. Virol.* **11:** 95.

Yabe, Y., L. Samper, E. Bryan, G. Taylor, and J.J. Trentin. 1964. Oncogenic effect of human adenovirus type 12 in mice. *Science* **143:** 46.

Functional Analysis of Adenovirus Type-5 Early Region 1B

J. Logan, S. Pilder, and T. Shenk

Department of Microbiology, Health Sciences Center, State University of New York, Stony Brook, New York 11794

The information necessary and sufficient for transformation of rodent cells by adenoviruses is contained in the E1A and E1B transcription units (Gallimore et al. 1974; Graham et al. 1974, 1978; Sambrook et al. 1974; Flint et al. 1975; Harrison et al. 1977; van der Eb et al. 1977; Jones and Shenk 1979a). The E1A transcription unit lies at the extreme left end of the viral chromosome. Early after infection, it gives rise to two mRNAs (12S and 13S) that have common 5′ and 3′ ends but differ in their splicing patterns (see Fig. 1). The 12S and 13S mRNAs contain coding regions that specify 26.5-kD and 31.9-kD polypeptides, respectively (Maat and Van Ormondt 1979; Gingeras et al. 1982). These two RNAs encode a family of four to six polypeptides in vivo with apparent molecular weights of 40,000–60,000 (e.g., Smart et al. 1981) that are localized in both the nucleus and cytoplasm of the infected cell (Feldman and Nevins 1983; Yee et al. 1983). An E1A gene product is required for efficient expression of all remaining viral transcription units (Berk et al. 1979; Jones and Shenk 1979b). The E1B unit lies directly to the 3′ end of the E1A unit (see Fig. 1). It also encodes two mRNAs (13S and 22S) early after infection. The 22S mRNA can code both a 21K and 55K polypeptide, whereas the 13S mRNA codes only the 21K species (Bos et al. 1981). The 21K coding region begins just 13 nucleotides downstream of the mRNA 5′ end. The 55K coding region overlaps the carboxyterminal portion of the 21K region in a second reading frame. The 55K polypeptide is located in the nucleus and cytoplasm (Yee et al. 1983), whereas the 21K moiety is found in the plasma membrane of infected cells (Persson et al. 1982).

Here we describe mutants designed to probe the function of E1B polypeptides in both the lytic and transforming cycles of adenovirus type 5 (Ad5). To determine whether E1B gene products can transform rat cells in the absence of E1A products, dl349 was constructed. This mutant lacks the E1A coding region and its E1B coding sequences are fused to the E1A 5′-flanking sequences. As a result, dl349 carries no E1A function but efficiently expresses its E1B gene. It fails to transform primary rat embryo cells, demonstrating that the E1B region cannot transform in the absence of E1A products. To probe the function of the E1B 21K and 55K polypeptides, deletion mutants (dl337 and dl338) were constructed which carry lesions in one or the other of these coding regions. Their phenotypes suggest that both E1B polypeptides are required for optimal virus production during the lytic cycle, but deletion of the 55K species has a much greater effect on virus yield than deletion of the 21K species. The 55K species is required for normal expression of the major late transcription unit. Both E1B polypeptides are also required for efficient transformation.

Methods of Experimental Procedures

Plasmids, viruses, and cells

Mutations were originally constructed in a recombinant plasmid (pA5-XhoIC, 0–15 Ad5 map units) by dropping segments between conveniently located restriction endonuclease cleavage sites. Mutated plasmid sequences were rebuilt into intact viral chromosomes by overlap recombination (Chinnadurai et al. 1979; Ho et al. 1982).

H5dl309 was selected as an Ad5 variant that contained only one XbaI endonuclease cleavage site (1339 bp from the left end of the chromosome) (Jones and Shenk 1978), and it served as the parent for the viral mutants described in this report (dl337, 338, 339, and 349).

The 293 cell line (a human embryonic kidney cell line transformed with a DNA fragment carrying the left 11% of the Ad5 genome) was obtained from H. Young and has been described by Graham et al. (1977). HeLa cells were from the American Type Culture Collection and primary rat embryo cells were from 15-day Fisher rat embryos.

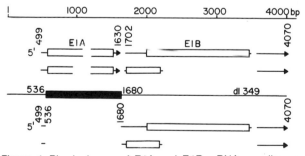

Figure 1 Physical map of E1A and E1B mRNAs, coding regions, and the dl349 mutation. The top of the figure positions the map in terms of nucleotide sequence position relative to the left end of the viral chromosome (Maat and Van Ormondt 1979; Bos et al. 1981; Gingeras et al. 1982). mRNAs are designated by lines, intervening sequences by spaces, and polypeptide coding regions by open boxes. The 349 deletion is represented by a closed box, and the first and last base pairs that are present bracketing the deletion are indicated. Wild-type mRNAs are diagrammed above the deletion and the novel E1B mRNAs predicted by the position of the 349 lesion are drawn below the deletion.

Analysis of mutant phenotypes

For Northern-type analysis, cytoplasmic poly(A)$^+$ RNA was isolated by the procedure of McGrogan et al. (1979). A 200-ng portion of the RNA was subjected to electrophoresis in an agarose gel (1%) containing formaldehyde (3%) using the conditions described by Rave et al. (1979). The probes were cloned viral sequences that were ^{32}P-labeled by nick-translation according to the procedure of Rigby et al. (1977). For analysis of polypeptides, infected cells were labeled with [^{35}S]methionine (1100 Ci/mmole, 50 μCi/ml). Preparation of cellular extracts, immunoprecipitations, and SDS-polyacrylamide gel electrophoresis were carried out as described by Sarnow et al. (1982). Transformation of primary rat embryo cells was as described by Logan et al. (1981).

Results

The E1B gene alone is not sufficient to transform primary rat embryo cells

To determine whether E1B gene products can induce transformation in the absence of E1A products, *dl*349 was constructed (Fig. 1). This variant is defective for growth in HeLa cells but can be propagated in 293 cells that provide E1A function (Table 1). It lacks the entire E1A coding region and E1B 5′-flanking region. The E1A transcriptional control sequences are fused to the E1B coding region, controlling E1B transcription. Although the E1B unit normally requires an E1A gene product for its transcription, the *dl*349 unit does not. Thus, *dl*349 should produce E1B gene products and transform cells unless the E1A gene plays a role in the transformation process beyond simply turning on E1B expression.

The experiment depicted in Figure 2 demonstrates that *dl*349 does efficiently express the E1B-55K polypeptide. In fact, it produces the polypeptide at near wild-type levels. The same is true for the E1B-21K species (data not shown).

In spite of the fact that *dl*349 produces the E1B gene products, it is unable to transform primary rat embryo cells, even at very high multiplicities of infection (Fig. 3). The *dl*349 E1B gene is potentially functional since *dl*349 DNA plus a cloned E1A segment can transform rat embryo cells (data not shown). We conclude that the Ad5 E1B-55K and 21K polypeptides cannot induce transformation of primary rat embryo cells in the absence of E1A products.

Table 1 Host-range Characteristics of *dl*349

Virus	pfu/ml	
	293	HeLa
*dl*309	2×10^9	1×10^9
*dl*349	1×10^9	5×10^4

Stocks of the parental (*dl*309) and mutant (*dl*349) viruses were titered by plaque assay on 293 and HeLa cells.

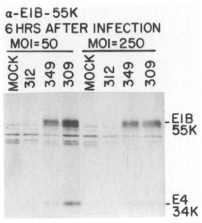

α-E1B-55K
6 HRS AFTER INFECTION
MOI=50   MOI=250

Figure 2 Electrophoretic analysis of the E1B-55K polypeptide synthesized in HeLa cells after infection with *dl*349 or its wild-type parent, *dl*309. ^{35}S-labeled extracts were prepared at 5 hr after infection and subjected to immunoprecipitation using a monoclonal antibody (2A6; gift from A. Levine) specific for the E1B-55K polypeptide. *dl*349 expresses E4 mRNAs and polypeptides, and the E4-34K polypeptides designated on the autoradiogram coprecipitates with the E1B-55K moiety.

Role of the E1B-coded polypeptides during lytic growth

To study the function of E1B polypeptides, several deletion mutants were constructed that lack portions of the E1B coding regions (Fig. 4). *dl*337 lacks a 146-bp segment (between sequence positions 1770–1916) located exclusively within the E1B-21K coding region, whereas *dl*338 carries a 521-bp deletion (between sequence positions 2808–3329) which disrupts only the 55K coding region. *dl*339 contains both the 21K and 55K deletions.

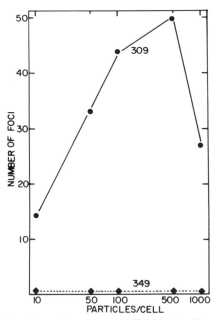

Figure 3 Transformation of primary Fisher rat embryo cells using *dl*349 or its wild-type parent, *dl*309. Transformations were carried out using gradient-purified virions. Colonies were counted 6 weeks after infection. (●) *dl*309; (♦) *dl*349.

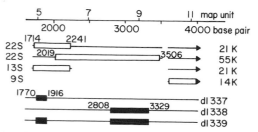

Figure 4 Physical map of E1B mRNAs, coding regions, and mutations that alter specific E1B coding regions. The symbols and designations are as described in the legend to Fig. 1.

Table 2 Host-range Characteristics of E1B Deletion Mutants

Virus	pfu/ml	
	293	HeLa
*dl*309	7×10^8	6×10^8
*dl*337	7×10^8	5×10^7
*dl*338	6×10^8	5×10^6
*dl*339	6×10^8	3×10^7

Virus stocks were titered by plaque assay on 293 and HeLa cells. *dl*338 produces very tiny plaques on HeLa cells whereas *dl*337 and 339 produce a mixture of wild-type and extra-large plaques.

*dl*338 is quite defective for lytic growth in HeLa cells as compared with 293 cells which provide E1B function (Table 2); its yield is reduced 100-fold and the plaques are much smaller than those produced by wild-type virus. In contrast, *dl*337 is only reduced 10-fold in plaque-forming ability on HeLa as compared with 293 cells. Its plaques are a mixture of wild-type and extra-large size. Interestingly, the double mutant, *dl*339 displays the 337 plaque morphology, indicating that the 21K lesion's phenotype is dominant over the 55K defect in this respect. The E1B polypeptides produced by these viruses were analyzed by immunoprecipitation. As expected, *dl*337 produced the E1B-55K but not 21K polypeptide, *dl*338 produced the E1B-21K but not 55K species, and *dl*339 failed to produce either polypeptide (data not shown).

Since the 55K-minus virus (*dl*338) grew quite poorly in HeLa cells, its physiological defect was examined. The mutant expressed all of its early genes and replicated its DNA normally. Late after infection, two perturbations in gene expression were observed. First, the E2A-coded

DNA-binding protein was produced in about three-fold excess as compared with the wild-type (data not shown). Second, all of the families of late mRNAs produced from the major late transcription unit were present at three- to fivefold reduced levels as compared with a wild-type infection (Fig. 5A). The reduction in late mRNA levels was clearly mimicked at the protein level for some late polypeptides (e.g., polypeptides II, IV, and pVI, Fig. 5B), but, curiously, other species were not reduced (e.g., 100K and III, Fig. 5B). Thus, the 55K-minus mutant appears to carry out its early functions normally, but it produces altered levels of late mRNAs and may also translate some mRNAs more efficiently than others late after infection.

As yet, the physiological consequences of the E1B-21K mutation (*dl*337) have not been evaluated. We have observed, however, that the virus replicates its DNA normally.

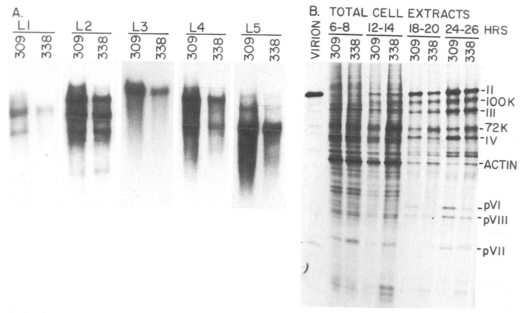

Figure 5 Analysis of major late transcription unit mRNAs and proteins made by *dl*309. (*A*) Northern-type analysis of viral mRNAs. RNAs were prepared 24 hr after infection at a multiplicity of 20 pfu/cell. Plasmid DNA probes were utilized that were specific for the indicated late families of mRNAs. (*B*) Electrophoretic analysis of polypeptides synthesized in HeLa cells after infection at a multiplicity of 20 pfu/cell. Labeled virion proteins were included as size markers.

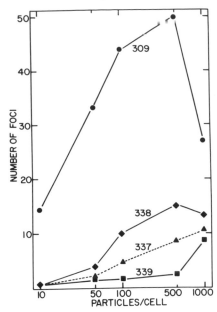

Figure 6 Transformation of primary Fisher rat embryo cells using E1B mutants or their wild-type parent, *dl*309. Details were described in the legend to Fig. 3. (●) *dl*309g; (▲) *dl*337; (♦) *dl*338; (■) *dl*339.

Both E1B-coded polypeptides are required for efficient transformation

All of the mutants were reduced in their ability to transform primary rat embryo cells (Fig. 6). The 55K-minus variant (*dl*338) was reduced four- to fivefold, the 21K-minus virus (*dl*337) about 10-fold, and the double mutant (*dl*339) only transformed at the very highest multiplicities of infection. The phenotypes of mutant as compared with wild-type-transformed cell lines are presently under evaluation.

Discussion

The viral mutants described in this report were produced to address two questions. First, can the E1B gene products induce the transformed phenotype in the absence of E1A products, and second, what are the roles of E1B products during the lytic and transforming cycles of the virus? It seems clear that E1B products alone cannot induce transformation of primary rat embryo cells. E1A products must play a role in this process beyond simply facilitating expression of the E1B transcription unit. This conclusion is consistent with other mutant studies performed by Carlock and Jones (1981) and Solnick and Anderson (1982). We are presently testing the possibility that *dl*349 might transform established rat cell lines. Conceivably, the requirement for E1A function might be reduced in an established line as compared with primary cells.

Neither E1B gene product appears to be required for DNA replication during the Ad5 lytic growth cycle. The E1B-55K mutant phenotype appears complex. Alterations are evident in the levels of late mRNAs. The E2A-coded, DNA-binding protein mRNA is increased and

other late mRNAs are decreased. Curiously, none of the effects observed so far (three- to fivefold differences between mutant and wild-type) obviously account for the 100-fold decrease in yield displayed by *dl*338. However, it is difficult to evaluate what effect a series of modest alterations might have on the overall dynamics of viral replication. Further, it is possible that some minor viral gene products are more severely affected than those we have monitored.

It is not clear which aspects of the *dl*338 phenotype are primary effects of its inability to express the 55K polypeptide and which are indirect. The levels of DNA-binding proteins are increased in *dl*338-infected HeLa cells and it is known that this protein influences expression and levels of other viral mRNAs (Nevins and Winkler 1980; Babich and Nevins 1981). Therefore, the alterations in *dl*338-coded late mRNA and protein levels could be due at least in part to increased levels of the DNA-binding protein.

As yet, the effects of the *dl*337 (E1B-21K) mutation during the lytic cycle have not been evaluated. Its large-plaque phenotype is similar to that of the Ad12 *cyt* mutants (Takemori et al. 1968), which are believed to map in the E1B region (Lai Fatt and Mak 1982). Possibly then, the *cyt* mutations lie within the E1B-21K coding regions. Chinnadurai (1983) has also reported a large-plaque phenotype for Ad2 mutants that carry substitution mutations within the E1B-21K coding region.

All E1B mutants were reduced in the efficiency with which they transform primary rat embryo cells. Three groups of Ad2 and Ad5 E1B mutants have previously been reported to be transformation defective: host-range point mutations (e.g, *hr*6 and *hr*cs13, Harrison et al. 1977; Graham et al. 1978; Ho et al. 1982), host-range deletion mutations (e.g., *dl*313, Jones and Shenk 1979a), and large-plaque mutations (e.g., *lp*3, Chinnadurai 1983). The *hr*6 and *hr*cs13 mutants fail to produce detectable E1B-55K polypeptide and appear considerably more impaired in their transforming ability than *dl*338, which is also 55K minus. The difference in *hr*6 and *hr*13 as compared with the *dl*338 phenotype might be explained if the *hr* lesions alter both 21K and 55K moieties whose coding regions partially overlap. The precise positions of the *hr* lesions have not been reported. In fact, there is a third reading frame on the opposite strand (of unknown function) which could also be altered by *hr*6 and *hr*13 but not by the 338 deletion (see Bos et al. 1981; Gingeras et al. 1982). If the *hr* mutations alter multiple polypeptides, their relatively severe transformation defects could be explained. Alternatively, *dl*338 might produce an unstable but biologically active aminoterminal fragment of the E1B 55K polypeptide, alleviating its transformation defect. Additional mutations in the E1B region are being constructed to distinguish between these various possibilities.

The *lp* mutants described by Chinnadurai (1983) alter the 21K polypeptide and were reported to be defective for transformation. The 21K mutant reported here, *dl*337, appears similar to the *lp* mutants in its transformation phenotype.

Finally, it is interesting to note that the lytic cycle phenotype of *dl*338 (55K-minus), appears identical to that of *dl*355, a mutant that carries a small deletion in the E4-34K coding region (D. Halbert et al., unpubl.). This makes sense because the E1B-55K and E4-34K polypeptides are physically associated, existing as a complex in infected cells (Sarnow et al. 1984). In contrast to the lytic cycle, *dl*338 and 355 differ dramatically in their ability to transform primary rat embryo cells. *dl*338 transforms less efficiently whereas *dl*355 transforms at least fivefold more efficiently than wild-type virus. There are several ways to explain this phenomenon. It is tempting to speculate that the absence of the E4-34K species allows the *dl*355 E1B-55K polypeptide to enter more efficiently into a complex with the p53 cellular tumor antigen (DeLeo et al. 1979; Lane and Crawford 1979; Linzer and Levine 1979). An E1B-55K/p53 complex has been identified by Sarnow et al. (1984). This complex might be important for the transforming function of the E1B-55K polypeptide.

Acknowledgments

We acknowledge the competent technical assistance of Ms. Martha Marlow. This work was supported by grants from the American Cancer Society (MV-45) and the National Cancer Insitute (CA 28146).

References

Alwine, J.C., S.I. Reed, and G.R. Stark. 1977. Characterization of the autoregulation of SV40 gene A. *J. Virol.* **24:** 22.

Babich, A. and J.R. Nevins. 1981. The stability of early adenovirus mRNA is controlled by the viral 72kd DNA-binding protein. *Cell* **26:** 371.

Berk, A.J., F. Lee, T. Harrison, J. Williams, and P.A. Sharp. 1979. Pre-early Ad5 gene product regulates synthesis of early viral mRNAs. *Cell* **17:** 935.

Bos, J.L., L.J. Polder, R. Bernards, P.I. Schrier, P.J. van den Elsen, A.J. van der Eb, and H. van Ormondt. 1981. The 2.2 kb E1B mRNA of human Ad12 and Ad5 codes for two tumor antigens starting at different AUG triplets. *Cell* **27:** 121.

Carlock, L.R. and N.C. Jones. 1981. Transformation-defective mutant of adenovirus type 5 containing a single-altered E1A mRNA species. *J. Virol.* **40:** 657.

Chinnadurai, G. 1983. Adenovirus 2 *lp+* locus codes for a 19kd tumor antigen that plays an essential role in cell transformation. *Cell* **33:** 759.

Chinnadurai, G., S. Chinnadurai, and J. Brusca. 1979. Physical mapping of a large plaque mutation of adenovirus type 2. *J. Virol.* **32:** 623.

DeLeo, A.B., G. Jay, E. Apella, G.C. Dubois, L.W. Law, and L.J. Old. 1979. Detection of a transformation-related antigen in chemically induced sarcomas and other transformed cells of the mouse. *Proc. Natl. Acad. Sci.* **76:** 2420.

Feldman, L.T. and J.R. Nevins. 1983. Localization of the adenovirus E1A a protein, a positive acting transcription factor, in infected cells. *Mol. Cell. Biol.* **3:** 829.

Flint, S.J., P.H. Gallimore, and P.A. Sharp. 1975. Comparison of viral RNA sequences in adenovirus 2-transformed and lytically infected cells. *J. Mol. Biol.* **96:** 47.

Gallimore, P.H., P.A. Sharp, and J. Sambrook. 1974. Viral DNA in transformed cells. II. A study of the sequences of adenovirus 2 DNA in nine lines of transformed rat cells using specific fragments of the viral genome. *J. Mol. Biol.* **89:** 49.

Gingeras, T.R., D. Sciaky, R.E. Gelinas, J. Bing-Dong, C.E. Yen, M.M. Kelly, P.A. Bullock, B.L. Parsons, K.E. O'Neill, and R.J. Roberts. 1982. Nucleotide sequences from the adenovirus 2 genome. *J. Biol. Chem.* **257:** 13475.

Graham, F.L., T. Harrison, and J. Williams. 1978. Defective transforming capacity of adenovirus type 5 host-range mutants. *Virology* **86:** 10.

Graham, F.L., J. Smiley, W.C. Russell, and R. Nairu. 1977. Characteristics of a human cell line transformed by DNA from human adenovirus type 5. *J. Gen. Virol.* **36:** 59.

Graham, F.L., P.J. Abrahams, C. Mulder, H.L. Heijneker, S.O. Warnaar, F.A.J. De Vries, W. Fiers, and A.J. van der Eb. 1974. Studies on *in vitro* transformation by DNA and DNA fragments of human adenovirus and simian virus 40. *Cold Spring Harbor Symp. Quant. Biol.* **39:** 637.

Harrison, T., F. Graham, and J. Williams. 1977. Host-range mutants of adenovirus type 5 defective for growth in HeLa cells. *Virology* **77:** 319.

Ho, Y.-S., R. Galos, and J. Williams. 1982. Isolation of type 5 adenovirus mutants with a cold-sensitive host-range phenotype: Genetic evidence of an adenovirus transformation maintenance function. *Virology* **122:** 109.

Jones, N. and T. Shenk. 1978. Isolation of deletion and substitution mutants of adenovirus type 5. *Cell* **13:** 181.

———. 1979a. Isolation of Ad5 host range deletion mutants defective for transformation of rat embryo cells. *Cell* **17:** 683.

———. 1979b. An adenovirus type 5 early gene function regulates expression of other early viral genes. *Proc. Natl. Acad. Sci.* **76:** 3665.

Lai Fatt, R.B. and S. Mak. 1982. Mapping of an adenovirus function involved in the inhibition of DNA degradation. *J. Virol.* **42:** 969.

Lane, D.P. and L.V. Crawford. 1979. T antigen is bound to a host protein in SV40 transformed cells. *Nature* **278:** 261.

Linzer, D.I. and A.J. Levine. 1979. Characterization of a 54K dalton cellular SV40 tumor antigen present in SV40-transformed cells and uninfected embryonal carcinoma cells. *Cell* **17:** 43.

Logan, J., J.C. Nicolas, W.C. Topp, M. Girard, T. Shenk, and A.J. Levine. 1981. Transformation by adenovirus early region 2A temperature-sensitive mutants and their revertants. *Virology* **115:** 419.

Maat, J. and H. Van Ormondt. 1979. The nucleotide sequence of the transforming HindIII-G fragment of Ad5: The region between map positions 4.5(Hpal site) and 8.0 (*Hind*III site). *Gene* **6:** 75.

McGrogan, M., D.J. Spector, C. Goldenberg, D.N. Halbert, and H.J. Raskas. 1979. Purification of specific adenovirus 2 RNAs by preparative hybridization and selective thermal elution. *Nucleic Acids Res.* **6:** 593.

Nevins, J.R. and J.J. Winkler. 1980. Regulation of early adenovirus transcription: A protein product of early region 2 specifically represses region 4 transcription. *Proc. Natl. Acad. Sci.* **77:** 1893.

Persson, H., M.G. Katze, and L. Philipson. 1982. Purification of a native membrane-associated tumor antigen. *J. Virol.* **42:** 905.

Rave, N., R. Crkenjakov, and H. Boedtker. 1979. Identification of procollagen mRNAs transferred to diazobenzylomethyl paper from formaldehyde agarose gels. *Nucleic Acids Res.* **6:** 3559.

Rigby, P.W.J., M. Dieckmann, C. Rhodes, and P. Berg. 1977. Labeling DNA to high specific activity *in vitro* by nick translation with DNA polymerase I. *J. Mol. Biol.* **113:** 237.

Sambrook, J., M. Botchan, P. Gallimore, B. Ozanne, U. Pettersson, J.F. Williams, and P.A. Sharp. 1974. Viral DNA sequences in cells transformed by simian virus 40, adenovirus type 2 and adenovirus type 5. *Cold Spring Harbor Symp. Quant. Biol.* **39:** 615.

Sarnow, P., Y.S. Ho, J. Williams, and A.J. Levine. 1982. Adenovirus E1B tumor antigen and SV40 large tumor antigen are physically associated with the same 54kd cellular protein in transformed cells. *Cell* **28:** 387.

Sarnow, P., P. Hearing, C.W. Anderson, D.N. Halbert, T. Shenk, and A.J. Levine. 1984. Adenovirus early region 1B 58,000-dalton tumor antigen is physically associated with an early region 4 25,000-dalton protein in productively infected cells. *J. Virol.* **49:** (in press).

Smart, J.E., J.B. Lewis, M.B. Mathews, M.L. Harter, and C.W. Anderson. 1981. Adenovirus type 2 early proteins: Assignment of the early region 1A proteins synthesized *in vivo* and *in vitro* to specific mRNAs. *Virology* **112:** 703.

Solnick, D. and M.A. Anderson. 1982. Transformation deficient adenovirus mutant defective in expression of region 1A but not region 1B. *J. Virol.* **42:** 106.

Takemori, N., J.L. Riggs, and C. Aldrich. 1968. Genetic studies with tumorigenic adenoviruses. I. Isolation of cytocidal (cyt) mutants of adenovirus type 12. *Virology* **36:** 575.

van der Eb, A.J., C. Mulder, F.L. Grahams, and A. Houweling. 1077. Transformation with specific fragments of adenovirus DNAs. *Gene* **2:** 115.

Yee, S.-P., D.T. Rowe, M.L. Tremblay, M. McDermott, and P.E. Branton. 1983. Identification of human adenovirus early region 1 products by using antisera against synthetic peptides corresponding to the predicted carboxy terminal. *J. Virol.* **46:** 1003.

Role of the Adenoviral E1A Gene Product in Transcriptional Activation

J.R. Nevins, M.J. Imperiale, H.-T. Kao, and L.T. Feldman*

The Rockefeller University, New York, New York 10021

The control of transcriptional initiation is clearly a key event in determining the ultimate phenotype of a given cell, whether in relation to a state of differentiation, a response to a hormone stimulus, or the expression of a malignant phenotype. Of central importance to the study of transcriptional control are the factors that mediate the process, including positive-acting regulatory proteins. One such protein is the product of the adenoviral E1A gene. This particular protein is responsible for the activation of transcription of five other viral transcriptional units during an early lytic infection (Berk et al. 1979; Jones and Shenk 1979; Nevins 1981). Thus, the expression of the adenoviral genome during an early lytic infection presents a system of coordinate regulation of transcription mediated by a known protein. Of added significance is the fact that the adenoviral E1A gene is an active participant, along with the E1B gene, in adenoviral transformation of cells in culture (Flint 1981). In fact, the E1A gene working alone, independent of the E1B gene, possesses the ability to immortalize a primary cell line that otherwise would cease to grow in culture (Houweling et al. 1980). In this paper, we will present evidence that deals with the question of E1A-mediated transcriptional control as it concerns the activation of the early viral genes as well as the activation of certain cellular genes.

Methods of Experimental Procedures

All procedures have been detailed in previous publications (Nevins 1980, 1981; Feldman et al. 1982; Kao and Nevins 1983; Imperiale et al. 1983). The plasmids pGC212 (an E1A-containing plasmid) and pIE (a plasmid containing the pseudorabies virus immediate early gene) were kind gifts of G. Chinnadurai (St. Louis University) and T. Ben-Porat (Vanderbilt University), respectively.

Results

Experiments carried out over the past few years have established the fact that the adenoviral E1A gene product is required for early viral transcription during lytic infection (Berk et al. 1979; Jones and Shenk 1979; Nevins 1981) as well as for processing of early viral RNA (Katze et al. 1981). Some of these experiments also hinted at a possible mechanism for the activation. In certain instances, the E1A gene product was found to

be nonessential for early transcription. For instance, using a high multiplicity of infection with the E1A mutant dl312, one can overcome the need for the E1A function (Nevins 1981; Shenk et al. 1979) (Fig. 1). The same result can be obtained through the inhibition of protein synthesis during a dl312 infection (Katze et al. 1981; Nevins 1981). On the basis of these results, the suggestion was made that the E1A protein counteracted a cellular regulatory factor so as to achieve both transcriptional (Nevins 1981) as well as posttranscriptional (Katze et al. 1981) activation. This finding led to the notion that if there were a cellular regulator of transcription that was the target of the E1A protein, it likely did not have the sole function of controlling the viral genes, but instead was surely involved in the control of certain cellular genes. One would thus predict that such cellular genes would be activated as a result of the action of the E1A gene product. We have been interested in defining such a system of cellular gene control and began with a search for a cellular gene subject to E1A activation. Such an induction was found in the form of a cellular 70-kD protein that was induced during an early lytic in-

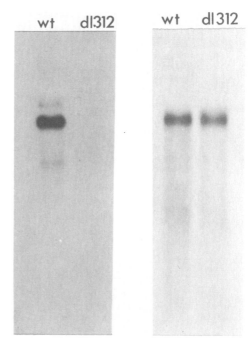

Figure 1 Production of E1B mRNA in a wild-type Ad5 and dl312 infection of HeLa cells. (*Left*) Multiplicity of infection of 100 particles per cell. (*Right*) Multiplicity of infection of 10,000 particles per cell.

*Present address: Department of Microbiology, UCLA School of Medicine, Los Angeles, California 90024.

fection by Ad5 (Nevins 1982). The identity of this protein became clear when it was found that a heat shock of HeLa cells also induced the same protein (Nevins 1982). This 70-kD heat-shock protein of HeLa cells appears to be analogous to the well-studied major hsp70 gene product of *Drosophila* (Ashburner and Bonner 1979).

E1A-mediated induction of the human 70-kD heat-shock gene

To extend these initial observations, we proceeded to isolate a cDNA clone for the human heat-shock mRNA. Such a clone was obtained and subsequently employed as a probe for the expression of the heat-shock gene during an adenoviral infection. As shown in Figure 2, left, the heat-shock mRNA is dramatically induced between about 5 and 8 hours of adenoviral lytic infection. Surprisingly, the abundance of the mRNA then fell back to preinduced levels. In contrast, the concentration of a distinct HeLa mRNA did not change during this period, indicating that the induction was indeed specific. That the induction was the result of the E1A gene product is shown by the experiment depicted in Figure 2, right. In this case, the abundance of the heat-shock mRNA was assayed in a wild-type and a *dl*312 infection. The wild-type infection was at a multiplicity of 100 viral particles per cell, whereas the *dl*312 infection was at a multiplicity of 10,000 particles per cell. Under these conditions, the *dl*312 infection is equivalent to the wild-type infection in terms of early gene expression with the exception that there is no E1A gene expression (Kao and Nevins 1983). Thus, from the results of Figure 2, right, it is clear that in the absence of E1A function, and despite the fact that

there is a full viral infection proceeding that equals a wild-type infection in yields of virus (Shenk et al. 1979), there is no induction of the heat-shock gene.

Similar experiments employing wild-type and *dl*312 infections but measuring the nuclear transcription rate of the heat-shock gene demonstrate that the increase in mRNA abundance is due to an activation of the transcription of the gene (Fig. 3). Furthermore, the decline in mRNA abundance in the cytoplasm is a reflection of a decline in transcription rate of the gene in the nucleus. This result suggests two phenomena: (1) a control of transcription that is only transient during the lytic infection and (2) a short mRNA half-life in the cytoplasm. In fact, from the data shown, the half life of the RNA must be no more than 30 minutes.

What is responsible for the control of the transcription of the heat-shock gene with respect to the decline after the maximum is reached? We believe the transcription rate reflects the presence of the inducer, the E1A protein. Recently, we have used an antiserum specific to the 13S E1A product (Feldman and Nevins 1983) to measure the concentration of E1A protein within the cell during the course of a normal lytic infection. The results indicate that the E1A protein is only present transiently during the early lytic infection with a peak abundance at about 8 hours (L. Feldman and J. Nevins, unpubl.). By 15 hours postinfection, the level of E1A protein has dropped to about 10% of its maximal level and by 24 hours it has completely disappeared. The transcription of the heat-shock gene exactly parallels the presence of the E1A protein in the cell, suggesting that the continual presence of the protein is required for transcription.

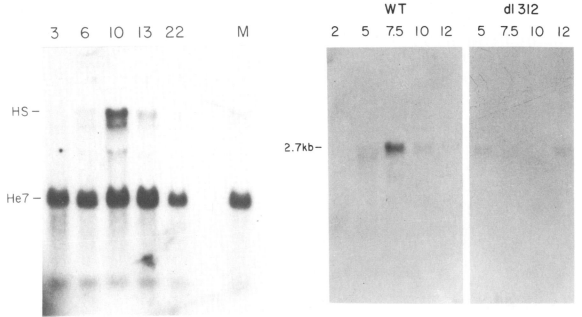

Figure 2 Induction of the human heat-shock mRNA during an adenovirus infection. (*Left*) Northern blot analysis of RNA from various times after a wild-type Ad5 infection of HeLa cells and probed with a heat-shock cDNA probe (HS) and a cDNA probe for an abundant HeLa mRNA (He7). (*Right*) Northern blot analysis of RNA from various times after a wild-type Ad5 infection (100 particles per cell) or a *dl*312 infection (10,000 particles per cell) and probed with the heat-shock cDNA. (Reprinted, with permission, from Kao and Nevins 1983.)

NUCLEAR TRANSCRIPTION RATE

CYTOPLASMIC mRNA

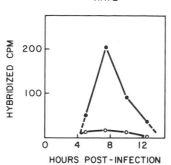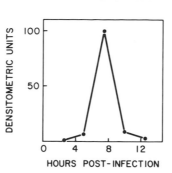

Figure 3 Transcriptional rate of heat-shock gene during adenovirus infection. HeLa cells were infected with wild-type Ad5 (●) at 100 particles per cell or with dl312 (○) at 10,000 particles per cell. Nuclei were prepared at the indicated times and labeled in vitro. Nuclear RNA was hybridized to filters bearing the heat-shock cDNA clone and RNase-resistant cpm were scored. The cytoplasmic RNA abundance was determined by densitometric scanning of the autoradiogram depicted in Fig. 2B. (Reprinted, with permission, from Kao and Nevins 1983.)

Cell-specific control of heat-shock gene expression reflecting an E1A-like activity

The preceding description indicates that the same cellular mechanisms affect the expression of both the adenoviral early genes and the heat-shock gene. This observation has led us to ask if the expression of the heat-shock gene can serve as an indicator of regulation in the cell that would also affect transcription of the early adenoviral genes. That is, if the action of the E1A protein is to alter transcriptional control in the cell so as to enhance viral transcription, then cells that are already partially altered, as reflected by a high level of expression of the heat-shock gene, should allow expression of early viral genes in the absence of the normally required inducer of early viral transcription, the E1A gene product. We have therefore measured the uninduced rate of expression of the heat-shock gene in various human cell lines, both by measuring heat-shock protein levels with a specific antiserum as well as by measuring RNA levels with the heat-shock cDNA clone. The results indicate that there is indeed expression of the heat-shock gene in the absence of heat induction and that the level of expression is very dependent on the particular cell type. Specifically, there is a reasonably high level of expres-

sion in HeLa cells as compared with 143B cells (a human osteogenic line transformed by Kirsten sarcoma virus), WI38 cells, or HEK cells. On the basis of our previous findings, we would then predict that there would be less of an E1A requirement in the HeLa cells than in the other cells. This is, in fact, true. The E1A mutant dl312, when introduced into HeLa cells at a high multiplicity, expressed early genes. However, no matter what the multiplicity of infection, there was no expression of the early viral genes during a dl312 infection of 143B, WI38, or HEK. That is, there is a strict requirement for the E1A function in these cells where there is also tight control of the heat-shock gene. Various other cells have been tested with the conclusion that every cell line derived from a human tumor source that has been tested behaves similarly to the HeLa cells. We would conclude that these cells that allow E1A independent early gene expression as well as uninduced heat-shock gene transcription likely express a function analogous to the E1A function.

The herpesvirus immediate early gene stimulates adenoviral transcription

Given the fact that there appeared to be a function in certain cells that could provide E1A function, we have asked if there were any other such activities, possibly in a form more amenable to study, that could be identified. We have turned to the herpesviruses for such a possibility. Adenovirus and herpesvirus have in common the fact that they both replicate in the nucleus and utilize host enzymes. Both viruses also progress through a temporally regulated pattern of gene expression (Spear and Roizman 1981). Furthermore, the herpesviruses possess a gene that is expressed immediately after infection and that is required for the activation of the remaining genes (Preston 1979; Dixon and Schaffer 1980; Watson and Clements 1980), thus analogous to E1A. Therefore, we have questioned whether the herpesvirus immediate early gene could substitute for the E1A gene in the activation of the adenoviral genes. As shown in Figure 4, cells infected with dl312 at a low multiplicity of infection did not express the adenoviral E2 gene; however, coinfection with pseudorabies virus (a herpesvirus) resulted in high levels of E2 expression, indeed even higher than that attained in a wild-type adenovirus infection. To demonstrate that the herpesvirus-mediated activation was due to the action of the immediate early gene, we have

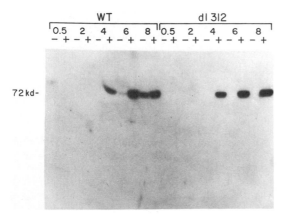

Figure 4 Synthesis of the adenoviral E2 gene product (72-kD protein) during pseudorabies virus coinfection of HeLa cells with wild-type adenovirus (WT) or dl312. Samples were taken at the indicated times postinfection and assayed for formation of the 72-kD E2 gene product by Western blot analysis. The (−) and (+) refer to the absence or presence of pseudorabies virus. (Reprinted, with permission, from Feldman et al. 1982.)

utilized transient DNA transfection assays. A plasmid containing the E2 gene was inactive when assayed after transfection into mouse L cells (Fig. 5). Cotransfection with an E1A plasmid increased E2 expression approximately three- to fivefold. Cotransfection with a plasmid containing the pseudorabies immediate early gene increased E2 expression 20–50-fold. Thus, the herpesvirus immediate early gene can stimulate transcription of the adenoviral E2 gene and apparently much more efficiently than the homologous E1A-mediated stimulation.

This result strongly suggests that there is something common about the induction mediated by the E1A protein and the immediate early (IE) protein. It seems likely that direct sequence recognition by these proteins is ruled out as these two viruses are not genetically related. Furthermore, the fact that the heterologous activation (E2 induction by herpes IE) is more efficient than the homologous activation argues against a sequence recognition. Rather, the results would suggest that the action of these proteins is indirect, possibly involving a common target in the host cell.

Discussion

The product of the adenoviral 13S E1A mRNA mediates transcriptional induction of viral genes as well as at least one cellular gene. Those facts are reasonably clear. What is not clear at the present time is the mechanism of this activation and what role this function plays in cell growth and transformation. The activation mechanism appears to be rather nonspecific based on the following: The herpesvirus immediate early gene can efficiently activate adenoviral genes; the E1A gene can stimulate transcription of the heat-shock gene; and the E1A gene can stimulate expression of the human β-globin gene upon transfection into HeLa cells (Green et al. 1983). These results argue against a direct role for the E1A protein or the IE protein in transcription induction. That is, it does not seem likely that the E1A protein recognizes and binds promoter sequences so as to stimulate transcription. Instead, it would appear that the protein works indirectly so as to effect a stimulation of transcription. How might this take place? It seems certain that there must be positive-acting transcriptional factors that interact with promoters to achieve efficient transcription of the gene. Certainly the results of Dynan and Tjian (1983) indicate the presence of such factors and moreover that there is some specificity. These results also suggest that the viral promoters can utilize cellular factors for transcription, factors that must be present in the cell normally for the use by certain cellular promoters. Similar but distinct factors are likely utilized by the early adenovirus promoters. If such factors were limiting in the cell, then a role for the E1A protein could be in mediating an increase in the availability of such factors. On the basis of the results described in this paper, we would suggest that the differences observed in the various cell lines, with respect to allowing heat shock and early adenoviral gene expression, represented differences in the levels of transcription factors available for these promoters. How then

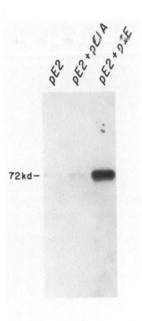

Figure 5 *Trans*-induction of E2 expression by E1A and IE genes in transient transfections. Mouse L cells were transfected with a plasmid containing the Ad5 E2 gene (pE2) or were transfected with a mixture of pE2 and pGC212 (E1A plasmid) or with a mixture of pE2 and pIE (immediate early gene plasmid). Production of the 72-kD protein (E2 gene product) was scored by Western blot analysis. (Reprinted, with permission, from Imperiale et al. 1983.)

is the E1A transcription unit utilized at the beginning of infection at a time when the other viral promoters are not active? We and others have shown that the region upstream from the E1A transcriptional start site possesses enhancer activity (Hearing and Shenk 1983; Imperiale et al. 1983; P. Sassone-Corsi, pers. comm.). We would suggest that the E1A promoter, like the early SV40 promoter and any promoter possessing an enhancer element, had a higher affinity for the factors and thus under limiting conditions was able to out-compete the other early promoters. An alternative explanation would be that enhancer elements utilized transcriptional factors not used by the inducible promoters and that these factors were nonlimiting.

Finally, how do these results bear on the role of the E1A gene product in the alteration of cell growth during transformation. Perhaps the E1A protein alters the growth potential of cells in culture by providing a general stimulus of transcription, possibly in the form of increasing transcriptional factors as discussed above. The specificity of E1A-mediated induction appears to be broad, as detailed before. There is some specificity since the E1A gene product does not activate transcription of the herpesvirus *tk* gene whereas the IE gene product does (M.J. Imperiale and J.R. Nevins, unpubl.). There also must be specificity dependent upon the chromatin structure of the gene since the β-globin gene can be stimulated upon transfection but the endogenous gene is silent. Thus, E1A might stimulate a certain group of genes in the cell that were structurally activated in the chromosome possibly dependent upon the differentiated nature of the cell.

It has recently been shown that E1A and the cellular oncogene *myc* can alter primary cells so as to allow transformation by the *ras* oncogene (Land et al. 1983; Ruley 1983). Although the role of E1A or *myc* in such transformation is far from clear, one obvious possibility is in the stimulation of expression of various cellular genes, one or more of which is a substrate for the action of *ras*. In combination, E1A or *myc* may also stimulate the expression of the *ras* gene to sufficient levels to allow function. In addition, these results that suggest a functional equivalence between E1A and *myc* pose the possibility that the E1A-like function that we observe in certain cells (those that express heat shock and early adenoviral genes and happen to be rapidly growing cells of a tumor origin), might be the *myc* gene.

Acknowledgments

We thank H. Ali and S. Willis for their excellent technical assistance. M.J.I. is a Damon Runyon-Walter Winchell postdoctoral fellow; L.T.F. holds a National Institutes of Health postdoctoral fellowship; J.R.N. is the recipient of a Research Career Development Award (CA00666). The work was supported by grants from the American Cancer Society (MV141) and the National Institutes of Health (GM26765-05).

References

Ashburner, M. and J.J. Bonner. 1979. The induction of gene activity in *Drosophila* by heat shock. *Cell* **17**: 241.

Berk, A.J., F. Lee, T. Harrison, J. Williams, and P.A. Sharp. 1979. Pre-early adenovirus 5 gene product regulates synthesis of early viral messenger RNAs. *Cell* **17**: 935.

Dixon, R.A.F. and P.A. Schaffer. 1980. Fine structure mapping and functional analysis of temperature sensitive mutants in the gene encoding the herpes simplex virus type 1 immediate early protein VP175. *J. Virol.* **36**: 189.

Dynan, W.S. and R. Tjian. 1983. Isolation of transcription factors that discriminate between different promoters recognized by RNA polymerase II. *Cell* **32**: 669.

Feldman, L.T. and J.R. Nevins. 1983. Localization of the adenovirus E1Aa protein, a positive acting transcriptional factor, in infected cells. *Mol. Cell. Biol.* **3**: 829.

Feldman, L.T., M.J. Imperiale, and J.R. Nevins. 1982. Activation of early adenovirus transcription by the herpesvirus immediate early gene: Evidence for a common cellular control factor. *Proc. Natl. Acad. Sci.* **79**: 4952.

Flint, S.J. 1981. Transformation by adenoviruses. In *Molecular biology of tumor viruses*, 2nd edition, revised: *DNA tumor viruses* (ed. J. Tooze), p. 547. Cold Spring Harbor Laboratory, Cold Spring Harbor, New York.

Green, M.R., R. Treisman, and T. Maniatis. 1983. Transcriptional activation of cloned human β-globin genes by viral immediate-early gene products. *Cell* **35**: 137.

Hearing, P. and T. Shenk. 1983. The adenovirus type 5 E1A transcriptional control region contains a duplicated enhancer element. *Cell* **33**: 695.

Houweling, A., P. van den Elsen, and A.J. van der Eb. 1980. Partial transformation of primary rat cells by the leftmost 4.5% fragment of adenovirus 5 DNA. *Virology* **105**: 537.

Imperiale, M.J., L.T. Feldman, and J.R. Nevins. 1983. Activation of gene expression by adenovirus and herpesvirus regulatory genes acting in trans and by a cis acting adenovirus enhancer element. *Cell* **35**: 127.

Jones, N. and T. Shenk. 1979. An adenovirus type 5 early gene function regulates expression of other early viral genes. *Proc. Natl. Acad. Sci.* **76**: 3665.

Kao, H.-T. and J.R. Nevins. 1983. Transcriptional activation and subsequent control of the human heat shock gene during adenovirus infection. *Mol. Cell. Biol.* **3**: 2058.

Katze, M.G., H. Perrson, and L. Philipson. 1981. Control of adenovirus early gene expression: Posttranscriptional control mediated by both viral and cellular gene products. *Mol. Cell. Biol.* **1**: 807.

Land, H., L.F. Parada, and R.A. Weinberg. 1983. Tumorigenic conversion of primary embryo fibroblasts requires at least two cooperating oncogenes. *Nature* **304**: 596.

Nevins, J.R. 1980. Definition and mapping of adenovirus 2 nuclear transcription. *Methods Enzymol.* **65**: 768.

———. 1981. Mechanism of activation of early viral transcription by the adenovirus E1A gene product. *Cell* **26**: 213.

———. 1982. Induction of the synthesis of a 70,000 dalton mammalian heat shock protein by the adenovirus E1A gene product. *Cell* **29**: 913.

Preston, C.M. 1979. Control of herpes simplex virus type 1 mRNA synthesis in cells infected with wild type virus or the temperature sensitive mutant tsK. *J. Virol.* **29**: 275.

Ruley, H.E. 1983. Adenovirus early region 1A enables viral and cellular transforming genes to transform primary cells in culture. *Nature* **304**: 602.

Shenk, T., N. Jones, W. Colby, and D. Fowlkes. 1979. Functional analysis of adenovirus type 5 host range deletion mutants defective for transformation of rat embryo cells. *Cold Spring Harbor Symp. Quant. Biol.* **44**: 367.

Spear, P.G. and B. Roizman. 1981. Herpes simplex viruses. In *Molecular biology of tumor viruses*, 2nd edition, revised: *DNA tumor viruses* (ed. J. Tooze), p. 615. Cold Spring Harbor Laboratory, Cold Spring Harbor, New York.

Watson, R.J. and J.B. Clements. 1980. A herpes simplex virus type 1 function required for early and late virus RNA synthesis. *Nature* **285**: 329.

Regulation of Gene Expression by the Adenoviral E1A Region and by *c-myc*

R.E. Kingston and P.A. Sharp
Center for Cancer Research and Department of Biology, Massachusetts Institute of Technology, Cambridge, Massachusetts 02139

R.J. Kaufman
Genetics Institute, Boston, Massachusetts 02115

The E1A region of adenovirus specifies a 13S mRNA that encodes a protein of 289 amino acids (Halbert et al. 1979; Perricaudet et al. 1979). This protein stimulates transcription of other viral promoters during the early stage of infection (Berk et al. 1979; Jones and Shenk 1979; Nevins 1981; Montell et al. 1982). A group of host-range mutants (Ad5 *hr*) that have either frameshift or deletion mutations in sequences coding for this protein fail to accumulate mRNAs at early times. However, the E1A-289 protein is not absolutely required for transcription of any viral promoter since infection with host-range deletion mutants at high multiplicities results in synthesis of most viral mRNAs. Transcription of the E1A-289 gene is dependent upon the presence of enhancer sequences (Hearing and Shenk 1983). Most interestingly, enhancer elements have not been identified in the adenoviral genome outside the E1A region.

Adenovirus infection of resting monolayers stimulates the synthesis of many cellular activities; among these are thymidine kinase, deoxycytidine kinase, and galactose kinase (McDougall et al. 1974). In the case of adenovirus 12 (Ad12), chromosomal breaks, perhaps due to puffing, can develop at positions of thymidine and galactose kinase genes. More recently, it has been shown that adenovirus infection induces the synthesis of a cellular heat-shock protein with a molecular weight of 70,000 (Nevins 1982). This induction is at the level of mRNA and does not occur when cells are infected with a mutant deleted in the E1A gene. The activities of the cellular heat-shock proteins are not known but their strong conservation in amino acid and DNA sequence in widely divergent species suggests a critical function. Induction of these proteins occurs following many different types of cellular stress, including heat shock.

The oncogenes of adenovirus are encoded in the E1A and E1B regions (Houweling et al. 1980; van den Elsen et al. 1982). Expression of three different viral proteins is thought to be essential for complete oncogenic transformation of cells. However, transfection of cells with only one or two of the viral oncogenes results in alterations of cell growth. Sequences encoding the E1A-289 protein can confer immortalization to primary cells (Houweling et al. 1980). Segments encoding the 19K and 55K proteins from the E1B region can alter the phenotype of established mouse lines (P. Jat and C. Cepko, pers. comm.). Some of the previously mentioned host-range mutants of adenovirus 5 (Ad5) are cold sensitive

for phenotypes associated with transformation. For example, a mutant with a frameshift mutation in the E1A-289 gene, fails to form colonies in agar at low temperatures but does so readily at high temperatures (Ho et al. 1982). These data and similar data for the host-range mutants in the E1B region suggest that continuous expression of several viral genes is necessary for maintenance of transformation.

As mentioned above, the E1A-289 protein can induce immortalization of primary cells. Such an activity has also been associated with the large T antigen of polyoma virus (Rassoulzadegan et al. 1983). It has recently been recognized that a number of cellular (EJ-*ras*, Ki-*ras*, and N-*ras*) and viral (polyoma middle T) genes can transform established cells but cannot transform primary cells (Parada et al. 1982; Rassoulzadegan et al. 1982; Taparowsky et al. 1982; Murray et al. 1983). Transformation occurs when oncogenes capable of immortalization are cotransfected into primary cells with a representative of the latter set (Land et al. 1983; Ruley 1983). Somewhat surprisingly, the c-*myc* oncogene also complements both *ras* and polyoma middle T genes in transformation of primary cells. Whether this complementation reflects an immortalization function conferred by *myc* is not clear; direct evidence that *myc* possesses this potential has not been reported. Alterations in *myc* gene activity are also certainly involved in a range of tumors associated with hematopoietic diseases. At present, no cellular activity has been assigned to the protein encoded by the *myc* gene.

Methods of Experimental Procedure

Recombinant DNA

All dihydrofolate reductase (DHFR)-encoding vectors are derivatives of pAdD26SV(A) (Kaufman and Sharp 1982a). Details of the constructions will be described separately. The promoter regions contained in each plasmid are described in Figure 1. Plasmids were grown in *Escherichia coli* HB101, and were purified by banding twice in cesium chloride.

Stable transfection assay

DHFR-deficient cells were plated at 7% confluence (approximately 7×10^5 cells per 10-cm dish) 1 day prior to transfection. DNA was transfected by a modification

pEII-DHFR

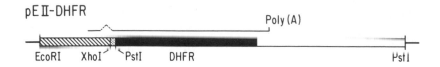

pHS-DHFR

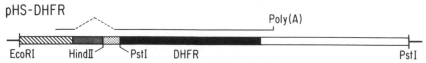

Figure 1 The promoter and DHFR cDNA regions of vectors used are shown. The hatched area of pEII-DHFR contains sequences from −284 (EcoRI) to +119 (XhoI) of the Ad2 EII early promoter, where +1 is the in vivo transcription initiation site. The hatched area in pHS-DHFR contains from −194 (at EcoRI) to +86 of the hsp70 promoter of Drosophila (Karch et al. 1981). Plasmid p72HS-DHFR contains bases 5107–493 of SV40. Base 493 is fused to the EcoRI site. pHSD26 contains 1.1 kb of flanking Drosophila sequence upstream of −194 (the site at −194 in pHSD26 is an XhoI site). The solid area and the stipled regions of both plasmids are the DHFR cDNA-containing fragment and a 3′ splice site of pAdD26SV(A) (Kaufman and Sharp 1982a). The lightly shaded region of pHS-DHFR encodes the 5′ splice site of the adenovirus major late promoter. The open areas of both constructions are the BclI–PstI fragment of SV40.

of the calcium phosphate procedure of Graham and Van der Eb (1973; see Kaufman and Sharp 1982b). Two days after transfection, cells were split 1/15 to selective media (α⁻ with 10% dialyzed fetal calf serum) containing either 0, 0.005 μM, or 0.02 μM methotrexate. Cells were fed once, and colonies were stained and counted 12 days after transfection. Colonies contained at least 40 cells.

Results

Previous studies have shown that the E1A-289 protein stimulates the transcription of a number of viral promoters. A biological assay has been developed to study the nature of the specificity of stimulation by E1A. We have constructed plasmid vectors in which a cDNA of the *dhfr* gene is transcribed from a specified promoter (Kaufman and Sharp 1982a). We have used two such vectors, one containing the adenoviral EII promoter and one containing the *Drosophila* heat-shock protein 70 (hsp70) promoter, to study the regulatory effects of the adenoviral E1A region. When either of these vectors is transfected into a DHFR-deficient Chinese hamster ovary (CHO) cell line (Urlaub et al. 1983), they are capable of transforming a certain fraction of the cells to a DHFR⁺ phenotype (see Fig. 2). The number of transformants decreases as the selectivity of the media is increased by adding methotrexate, a potent inhibitor of DHFR. A characteristic number of such transformants is obtained at each methotrexate level from transfection of 1 μg of any specified vector. These values reflect the ability of the vector to express the contained *dhfr* gene.

Response of pEII-DHFR in a stable contransfection assay

The E1A gene product is capable of stimulating expression of the adenoviral EII promoter in *trans* when both the promoter and the E1A region are stably integrated in chromosomal DNA (R. Kingston, unpubl.). This prop-

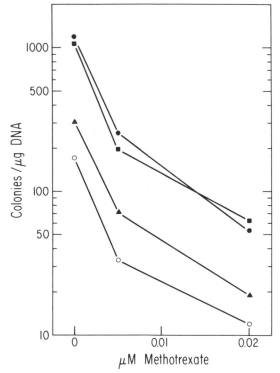

Figure 2 The effect of various E1A mutants on pEII-DHFR. Plasmid pEII-DHFR (1 μg) was transfected either with pBR322 DNA (5 μg) (○); pHindIIIG DNA (5 μg) (■); pEKpm975 DNA (5 μg) (●); or pGhr1 DNA (5 μg) (▲) into DHFR-deficient CHO cells (Urlaub et al. 1983). The values are plotted as a function of colonies per microgram of DHFR containing DNA against the concentration of methotrexate in the selective media. pHindIIIG was constructed by Dr. K. Berkner and contains map units 0–7.9 of Ad5 in pBR322. pEKpm975 (Montell et al. 1982) contains a point mutant that eliminates a splice junction necessary to make the E1A 12S message. pEKpm975 contains from 0–5.8% of Ad5. pGhr1 contains the *hr1* mutant of Ad5 in a plasmid otherwise identical to pHindIIIG. The transfection protocol is described in Methods.

erty suggested that cotransfection of E1A encoding DNA with a DHFR vector containing a regulated promoter would lead to an increase in the number of stable phenotypic transformants obtained. This is the observed result when a plasmid encoding the E1A region (pHindIIIG) is cotransfected with pEII-DHFR (Fig. 2).

Plasmids containing two mutants in the E1A region were tested for their ability to stimulate EII expression in this assay. Plasmid pEKpm975 (Montell et al. 1982) can encode the E1A 13S message (289-amino acid protein) but not the 12S message. It and a wild-type E1A region stimulate expression of pEII-DHFR to a similar level (Fig. 2). In contrast, plasmid pGhr1 does not stimulate as well as wild type. pGhr1 contains a frameshift mutation in the 13S message. This mutation in the Ad5 *hr*1 mutant has previously been characterized to be defective for transcription of early adenoviral promoters in lytic infection (Berk et al. 1979).

Stimulation of the *Drosophila* hsp70 promoter by E1A

The E1A region has been shown to stimulate expression of a human heat-shock gene (Nevins 1982). We constructed a vector containing one of the hsp70 promoters of *Drosophila* fused to DHFR (termed pHSD26) to test the ability of the E1A region to regulate expression of this promoter. Cotransfection of the E1A region with pHSD26 results in a dramatic increase in the number of stable phenotypic transformants obtained (Fig. 3). The

level of stimulation by E1A of the hsp70 constructs was comparable to that observed with the EII promoter.

Effects of an enhancer sequence on stimulation by E1A

Fusion of the SV40 72-bp enhancer region to a promoter increases transcription from the promoter in numerous instances. Insertion of this region 5′ to the hsp70 promoter (in p72HS-DHFR) dramatically increased its ability to transform stably DHFR-deficient CHO cells (Fig. 3). Interestingly, expression of this modified promoter is no longer increased by cotransfection with the E1A region.

The observation that expression of p72HS-DHFR is no longer regulated by the E1A region suggested the possibility that the 289 protein of E1A and enhancer elements may function by a similar mechanism. Insertion of the SV40 72-bp enhancer element 5′ to the EII promoter results in a significant increase in the number of stable phenotypic transformants obtained (Fig. 4). How-

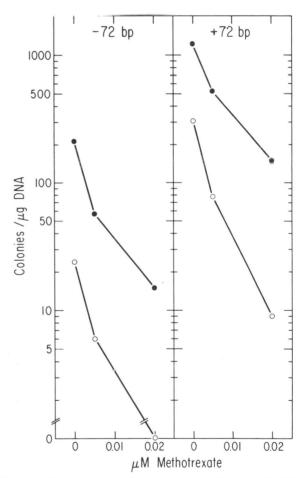

Figure 4 The effect of Ad5 E1A on expression of pEII-DHFR with and without the SV40 72-bp region. One μg of either pEII-DHFR or p72EII-DHFR was transfected with either 5 μg of pBR322 (○) or 5 μg of pEKpm975 (●). p72EII-DHFR contains the 72-bp enhancer region of SV40 in the same location and orientation as in the p72HS-DHFR. The transfection protocol was as described in Methods.

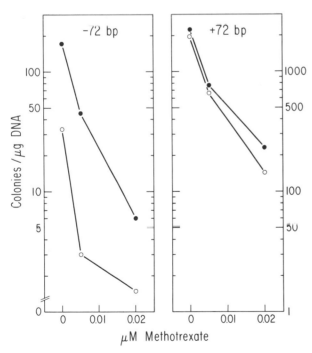

Figure 3 The effect of Ad5 E1A on pHSD26 and p72HS-DHFR. One μg of plasmid pHSD26 (−72 bp) or p72HS-DHFR (+72 bp) was transfected with either 5 μg of pBR322 (○) or 5 μg of plasmid pEKpm975 (●). The transfection protocol was exactly as described in Methods.

ever, this level is further increased by cotransfection with the E1A region. The level of stimulation of this promoter by E1A is similar in the presence or absence of the 72-bp enhancer region.

Effects of *rc-myc* on expression of the EII and hsp70 promoters

The E1A region and a rearranged mouse *c-myc* gene (*rc-myc*) are both capable of complementing the *c*-Ha-*ras* oncogene in transformation of primary cells (Land et al. 1983; Ruley 1983). In addition, E1A and *c-myc* proteins share a limited amino acid sequence homology (Ralston and Bishop 1983). We therefore tested the ability of a mouse *rc-myc* gene under control of the SV40 early promoter (Shen-Ong et al. 1982; Land et al. 1983) to stimulate expression from the adenoviral EII promoter (pEII-DHFR) and the *Drosophila* hsp70 promoter (pHSD26). Cotransfection of *rc-myc* with pEII-DHFR effected a moderate increase in the number of stable phenotypic transformants obtained (Fig. 5). Cotransfection of *rc-myc* with pHSD26 effected a larger increase in the number of transformants. As in the E1A cotransfection experiment, the number of transformants obtained was not affected by *rc-myc* when p72HS-DHFR was tested (Fig. 5C).

Discussion

The mechanism by the which the E1A region stimulates transcription has been investigated with vectors containing promoters from the adenoviral EII and *Drosophila* hsp70 transcription units. These promoters have been fused to a mouse DHFR cDNA and tested by transfection into DHFR-deficient CHO cells (Urlaub et al. 1983). In experiments not described here, similar constructs with the adenoviral major late promoter and SV40 late promoter were tested for stimulation of expression of DHFR by E1A. In all four cases, cotransfection with a segment containing E1A resulted in establishment of an increased number of colonies resistant to methotrexate. This is interpreted as a stimulation in the level of transcription from the inserted promoter; however, in most cases this has not been shown directly. Similar results have been reported by Weeks and Jones (1983) using transfection of mouse and human cells with a thymidine kinase gene, and also by others at this meeting.

The stimulation of expression assayed by transfection with the DHFR cDNA gene is almost certainly a reflection of the activity of the E1A-289 amino acid protein. Cotransfection with a plasmid containing a mutant E1A gene that only expresses the 289-amino acid mRNA stimulates expression at a level similar to the wild-type gene.

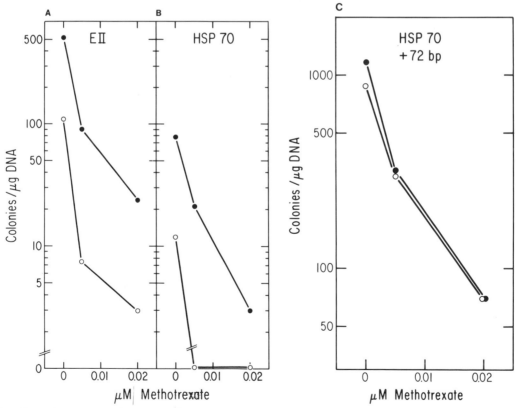

Figure 5 The effect of *rc-myc* on pEII-DHFR, pHSD26, and p72HS-DHFR. One µg of plasmid pEII-DHFR (*A*), pHSD26 (*B*), or p72HS-DHFR (*C*) was transfected with either 5 µg of pBR322 (○) or 4.6 µg of pBR322 and 0.4 µg of pSV2-*c-myc* (●). pSV2-*c-myc* contains a rearranged mouse *c-myc* gene under control of the SV40 early promoter (Land et al. 1983). The transfection protocol was exactly as described in Methods.

Cotransfection with a plasmid containing a mutant E1A gene with a frameshift alteration in the 289-amino acid coding sequences produces only a slight stimulation of expression. The latter mutant E1A gene, originally isolated in the AD5 *hr*1 mutant, has been shown to be defective for induction of synthesis of early adenoviral mRNAs (Berk et al. 1979).

Adenovirus infection of human cells has been shown to induce a small number of genes, one of which is the human hsp70 (Nevins 1982). However, no broad induction of cellular transcription is observed. This contrasts with the lack of specificity observed with cotransfection assay where most, if not all, promoters are stimulated. The specificity of stimulation by E1A could be explained in two ways: (1) the set of stimulated promoters may have a common and unique rate-limiting step for initiation of transcription; or (2) the stimulated promoters may be organized into a unique chromatin structure. The latter possibility could easily explain the cotransfection results but does not easily explain the observation that the E1A region can regulate the EII promoter in *trans* when both are stably integrated into the chromosomal DNA of a CHO cell line.

The constructs that are stimulated by E1A contain weak promoters. These promoters may be limited in activity by a rudimentary step in the initiation reaction. Modification of a component in this reaction could explain the observed specificity. It is perhaps interesting in this regard that deletion mutants of the EII promoter segment missing sequences beyond −50 are fully stimulated by cotransfection with E1A. This suggests that the E1A stimulation process must be capable of recognizing sequences very near the initiation site, perhaps part of the TATA recognition reaction.

Insertion of the 72-bp enhancer element of SV40 upstream of any of the promoters mentioned above enhances their activity for transformation of DHFR (−) cells. In the case of the *Drosophila* hsp70 promoter, insertion of the 72-bp element makes the promoter insensitive to further stimulation by E1A activity. This observation makes it unlikely that stimulation of transformation by cotransfection with E1A simply reflects an unsuspected property of E1A that either increases the frequency of integration of DNA segments or enhances the survival of transfected cells. The insensitivity of the "enhanced" hsp70 promoter to further stimulation by E1A activity also suggests that a common rate-limiting step in initiation is affected by both the insertion of a 72-bp enhancer element and stimulation by E1A. Do the E1A region and the SV40 72-bp enhancer region therefore function by the same molecular mechanism? Two observations argue that they do not: (1) E1A can function in *trans* whereas the enhancer region functions in *cis*. (2) The effects of the E1A region and the 72-bp enhancer region on the EII promoter appear additive (Fig. 4). Perhaps both the enhancer region and the E1A product facilitate, through separate molecular mechanisms, the kinetically slow reaction of promoter sequence recognition by RNA polymerase II. The observation that expression of the β-globin promoter becomes enhancer independent in E1A-containing cells is consistent with this model (Green et al. 1983; Treisman et al. 1983).

The effect of *rc-myc* on expression of pEII-DHFR and pHSD26

The E1A products and the *c-myc* gene have limited homologies in their primary protein structures (Ralston and Bishop 1983) and both complement the *c-Ha-ras* gene in transformation of primary cell lines (Land et al. 1983; Ruley 1983). Therefore, we were interested in determining whether *c-myc* could stimulate expression of the EII or hsp70 promoter-containing vectors. We have used a *c-myc*-expressing vector containing a rearranged mouse *c-myc* gene which is transcribed from the SV40 early promoter (Shen-Ong et al. 1982; Land et al. 1983). The number of stable phenotypic transformants obtained with a EII promoter construct (pEII-DHFR) was consistently increased by cotransfection with this vector. However, the level of stimulation of pEII-DHFR by *rc-myc* was consistently two- to threefold lower than that observed with the E1A region (compare Figs. 4 and 5). The number of stable phenotypic transformants obtained with the *Drosophila* hsp70 promoter construct (pHSD26) was consistently stimulated to a similar level by both E1A and *rc-myc* (compare Figs. 3 and 5). This does not appear to reflect the ability of *c-myc* generally to stimulate stable transfection frequency, as expression of the "enhancer" hsp70 promoter [enhanced by insertion of the 72-bp SV40 sequences (p72HS-DHFR)] was unaffected by *rc-myc*. These preliminary results suggest that the *c-myc* gene may encode activities that regulate transcription. This would also be consistent with the nuclear location of the *c-myc* protein (Abrams et al. 1982; Donner et al. 1982) and the recent observation that expression of the normal *c-myc* allele is suppressed in cells containing a rearranged *c-myc* allele (Stanton et al. 1983; A. Hayday, pers. comm.).

Acknowledgments

The authors wish to thank H. Land and L. Parada for donation of pSV2-*c-myc*, C. Montell for donation of pEKpm975, and K. Berkner for constructing pHindIIIG. R.E.K. is a fellow of the Jane Coffin Childs Memorial Fund for Medical Research. This work was supported by grants from National Science Foundation [PCM-7823230 (currently PCM-8200309)], from National Institutes of Health (No. PO1-CA26717) to P.A.S., and partially from Center for Cancer Biology at MIT (Core) grant (No. NIH-PO1-CA14051).

References

Abrams, H.D., L.R. Rohrschneider, and R.N. Eisenman. 1982. Nuclear location of the putative transforming protein of avian myelocytomatosis virus. *Cell* **29**: 427.

Berk, A.J., F. Lees, T. Harrison, J. Williams, and P.S. Sharp. 1979. Pre-early adenovirus 5 gene product regulates synthesis of early viral messengers RNAs. *Cell* **17**: 935.

Donner, P., I. Greiser-Wilke, and K. Moelling. 1982. Nuclear localization and DNA binding of the transforming gene product of avian myelocytomatosis virus. *Nature* **296**: 262.

Graham, F.L. and A.J. van der Eb. 1973. A new technique for the assay of infectivity of human adenovirus 5 DNA. *Virology* **52:** 456.

Green, M.R., R. Treisman, and T. Maniatis. 1983. Transcriptional activation of cloned human β-globin genes by viral immediate early gene products. *Cell* **35:** 137.

Halbert, D.N., D.J. Spector, and H.J. Raskas. 1979. *In vitro* translation products specified by the transforming region of adenovirus type 2. *J. Virol.* **31:** 621.

Hearing, P. and T. Shenk. 1983. The adenovirus type 5 EIA transcriptional control regions contains a duplicated enhancer element. *Cell* **33:** 695.

Ho, Y.S., R. Galos, and J. Williams. 1982. Isolation of type 5 adenovirus mutants with a cold-sensitive host range phenotype: Genetic evidence of an adenovirus transformation maintenance function. *Virology* **122:** 109.

Houweling, A., P.J. van den Elsen, and A.J. van den Elsen. 1980. Partial transformation of primary rat cells by the leftmost 4.5% fragment of adenovirus 5 DNA. *Virology* **105:** 537.

Jones, N. and T. Shenk. 1979. An adenovirus 5 early gene function regulates expression of other early viral genes. *Proc. Natl. Acad. Sci.* **76:** 3665.

Karch, F., I. Torok, and A. Tissières. 1981. Extensive regions of homology in front of two hsp 70 heat shock variant genes in *Drosophila melanogaster. J. Mol. Biol.* **148:** 219.

Kaufman, R.J. and P.A. Sharp. 1982a. A construction of a modular dihydrofolate reductase cDNA gene. Analysis of signals utilized for efficient expression. *Mol. Cell. Biol.* **2:** 1304.

———. 1982b. Amplification and expression of sequences cotransfected with a modular dihydrofolate reductase complimentary DNA gene. *J. Mol. Biol.* **159:** 601.

Land, H., L.F. Parada, and R.A. Weinberg. 1983. Tumorigenic conversion of primary embryo fibroblasts requires at least two cooperating oncogenes. *Nature* **304:** 596.

McDougall, J.K., A.R. Dunn, and P.H. Gallimore. 1974. Recent studies on the characteristics of adenovirus-infected and transformed cells. *Cold Spring Harbor Symp. Quant. Biol.* **39:** 591.

Montell, C., E.F. Fisher, M.H. Caruthers, and A.J. Berk. 1982. Resolving the function of overlapping viral genes by site-specific mutagenesis at a mRNA splice site. *Nature* **295:** 380.

Murray, M.J., J.M. Cunningham, L.F. Parada, F. Dautry, P. Lebowitz, and R.A. Weinberg. 1983. The HL-60 transforming sequence: A *ras* oncogene coexisting with altered myc genes in hematopoietic tumors. *Cell* **33:** 749.

Nevins, J.R. 1981. Mechanism of activation of early viral transcription by the adenovirus E1a gene product. *Cell* **26:** 213.

———. 1982. Induction of the synthesis of a 70,000 dalton mammalian heat-shock protein by the adenovirus E1a product. *Cell* **29:** 913.

Parada, L.F., C. Tabin, C. Shih, and R.A. Weinberg. 1982. Human EJ bladder carcinoma oncogene is homologue of Harvey sarcoma ras gene. *Nature* **297:** 474.

Perricaudet, M., G. Akusjarvi, A. Virtanen, and V. Peterson. 1979. Structure of two spliced mRNAs from the transforming region of human subgroup C adenoviruses. *Nature* **281:** 694.

Ralston, R. and J.M. Bishop. 1983. The protein products of the oncogenes *myc, myb,* and adenovirus EIA are structurally related. *Nature* **306:** 803.

Rassoulzadegan, M., A. Cowie, A. Carr, N. Glaichenhaus, R. Kamen, and F. Cuzin. 1982. The roles of individual polyoma virus early proteins in oncogenic transformation. *Nature* **300:** 713.

Rassoulzadegan, M., Z. Naghashfar, A. Lowie, A. Carr, M. Grisoni, R. Kamen, and F. Cuzin. 1983. Expression of the large T protein of polyoma virus promotes the establishment in culture of "normal" rodent fibroblast cell lines. *Proc. Natl. Acad. Sci.* **80:** 4354.

Ruley, H.E. 1983. Adenovirus early region IA enables viral and cellular transforming genes to transform primary cells in culture. *Nature* **304:** 602.

Shen-Ong, G.L.C., E.J. Keath, S.P. Piccoli, and M.D. Cole. 1982. Novel myc oncogene RNA from abortive immunoglobulin-gene recombination in mouse plasmacytoma. *Cell* **31:** 443.

Stanton, L.W., R. Watt, and K.B. Marev. 1983. Translocation, breakage and truncated transcripts of c-myc oncogene in murine plasmacytomas. *Nature* **303:** 401.

Taparowsky, E., Y. Suard, O. Fasano, K. Shimizu, M. Goldfarb, and M. Wigler. 1982. Activation of the T24 bladder carcinoma transforming gene is linked to a single amino acid change. *Nature* **300:** 762.

Treisman, R., M.R. Green, and T. Maniatis. 1983. *Cis* and *trans* activation of globin gene transcription in transient assays. *Proc. Natl. Acad. Sci.* **80:** 7428.

Urlaub, G., E. Kas, A.M. Carothers, and L.A. Chasin. 1983. Deletion of the diploid dihydrofolate reductase locus from cultured mammalian cells. *Cell* **33:** 405.

van den Elsen, P.J., S. de Pater, A. Houweling, J. van der Veer, and A.J. van der Eb. 1982. The relationship between region E1a and E1b of human adenoviruses in cell transformation. *Gene* **18:** 175.

Weeks, D.L., and N.C. Jones. 1983. EIA control of gene expression is mediated by sequences 5′ to the transcriptional starts of the early viral genes. *Mol. Cell. Biol.* **3:** 1222.

Transcriptional Activation of a Cloned Human β-Globin Gene by *Cis*- and *Trans*-acting Viral Control Elements

R. Treisman, M.R. Green, and T. Maniatis

Harvard University, Department of Biochemistry and Molecular Biology, Cambridge, Massachusetts 02138

DNA tumor virus genes can be activated transcriptionally by both *cis*- and *trans*-acting viral regulatory elements (for reviews, see Tooze 1981; Khoury and Gruss 1983). Expression of papovaviral early genes and adenoviral immediate early genes is dependent on the presence in *cis* of a transcriptional enhancer sequence (Khoury and Gruss 1983). In contrast, adenoviral and herpesviral early and late genes are activated by *trans*-acting products of viral immediate early genes (Berk et al. 1979; Jones and Shenk 1979; Watson and Clements 1980; Tooze 1981). Although enhancer elements, which act in a largely orientation and position independent manner, were first identified in DNA viruses (Banerji et al. 1981; Benoist and Chambon 1981; Gruss et al. 1981; Fromm and Berg 1982; for reviews, see Gluzman and Shenk 1983; Khoury and Gruss 1983) sequences with similar properties have also been isolated from cellular DNA (Conrad and Botchan 1982). Recently, enhancer elements were shown to be involved in the B-cell-specific activation of the mouse heavy-chain (Banerji et al. 1983; Gillies et al. 1983) and possibly the κ light-chain (Queen and Baltimore 1983) immunoglobulin genes. Interestingly, the activity of enhancers is not restricted to the genes with which they are normally associated. For example, both the SV40 enhancer (Banerji et al. 1981) and the immunoglobulin heavy-chain gene enhancer (Banerji et al. 1983) can activate the rabbit β-globin gene. Similarly, Wasylyk et al. (1983) have shown that the SV40 enhancer can act on a variety of different genes.

In contrast to enhancers, which act in *cis*, viral immediate early gene products act in *trans*. The transcriptional regulatory properties of viral immediate-early gene products were identified in studies of adenoviruses (Berk et al. 1979; Jones and Shenk 1979) and herpesviruses (for review, see Tooze 1981). During adenovirus infection of permissive (human) cells, the earliest transcripts detected (immediate early) map to the E1A region of the genome (Lewis and Mathews 1980). Analysis of E1A mutants revealed that a product of this gene is required for the accumulation of RNAs from all of the other adenoviral transcription units (Berk et al. 1979; Jones and Shenk 1979). The E1A effect on RNA accumulation is probably mediated at the transcriptional level (Nevins 1981). Transcription of the E1A gene is stimulated by but does not require functional E1A gene products (Berk et al. 1979; Nevins 1981). The E1A gene product could act directly on promoter sequences or indirectly by interacting with a cellular component.

The evidence obtained to date indicates that the activity of the E1A gene product is not promoter specific. First, E1A gene products activate several adenoviral transcription units whose promoter sequences differ significantly (Baker and Ziff 1981). Second, the E1A mutants can be complemented by the immediate-early gene product of the unrelated herpesvirus, pseudorabies virus (Feldman et al. 1982). Third, certain cellular genes such as the HeLa cell 70-kD heat-shock gene, are activated in the presence of the E1A gene product (Nevins 1982). Models for transcriptional activation by the E1A gene product have been proposed that involve the inactivation of cellular factors that repress viral gene expression (Katze et al., 1981, 1983; Nevins, 1981). However, an equally likely possibility is that the E1A protein itself or a cellular protein activated by E1A acts as a positive regulator of transcription.

The interactions of enhancers or immediate early gene products with cellular genes may provide useful models for the study of mechanisms involved in differential gene expression during development because enhancer sequences have been implicated in tissue-specific gene expression and immediate-early gene products can act on cellular genes. In this paper, we examine the interactions of both *cis*- and *trans*-acting viral regulatory elements with cloned human globin genes. These studies were prompted initially by the need to develop assays for the analysis of the transcription of mutant globin genes. In the experiments presented here, we use transient assays in which the cloned genes are introduced into recipient cells by calcium phosphate coprecipitation and transcription is analyzed 50 hours later. As recipient cells, we used HeLa cells, COS cells (which express SV40 large T antigen; Gluzman 1981), or 293 cells (which express Ad5 gene products; Graham et al. 1978). Previous work has shown that the transcription of the rabbit (Banerji et al. 1981) and human (Humphries et al. 1982; Treisman et al. 1982) β-globin gene is dependent on linkage to an enhancer sequence when carried on both replicating and nonreplicating plasmids. In contrast, the human α-globin gene is efficiently transcribed and unaffected by the enhancer sequence when carried on a replicating vector (Mellon et al. 1981; Humphries et al. 1982). In this paper, we show that the viral immediate-early gene products of adenovirus and pseudorabies virus directly or indirectly stimulate the transcription of the β-globin gene in the absence of a *cis*-linked enhancer. Furthermore, our experiments show that these *trans*-acting transcriptional factors can be studied using transient expression systems. Using this approach, we have identified the sequences within the β-globin promoter that are required for the viral gene products to act. Unexpectedly, we find that only a limited region of the β-globin promoter that includes the TATA box is necessary for accurate transcription in the presence of these viral immediate-early transcriptional regulatory proteins. We conclude that enhancers and viral immediate early gene products activate β-globin transcription by different mechanisms.

Effect of the SV40 enhancer sequence on globin gene transcription in HeLa cells

To examine the effect of linkage to the SV40 enhancer on the transcription of the human α- and β-globin genes, we constructed the plasmids shown in Figure 1, and analyzed the transcription following transfection into HeLa cells where no plasmid replication occurs. To quantitate the amount of correctly initiated globin RNA produced, total cellular RNA was analyzed by S1 nuclease mapping. The hybridization probes used in this analysis generate nuclease-resistant DNA fragments 40 and 70 nucleotides in length when hybridized to authen-

tic human α- and β-globin mRNA, respectively (Treisman et al. 1983b; data not shown). Analysis of the transcripts produced by cotransfected β- or α-globin reference plasmids showed that transfection efficiency and RNA recovery were comparable in each case (data not shown).

As shown in Figure 2A, α-globin transcripts are detected in HeLa cells in the absence of a linked enhancer sequence; linkage to the enhancer sequence increases the amount of correctly initiated RNA produced 5- to 10-fold (Fig. 2A, lanes 1 and 2). However, as observed previously in the case of the rabbit β-globin gene (Banerji et al. 1981; DeVilliers and Schaffner 1981), transcripts of the human β-globin gene are not detected in HeLa

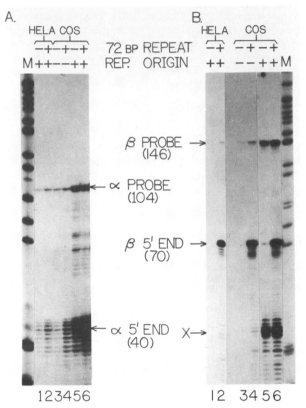

Figure 2 S1 nuclease analysis of α- and β-globin gene transcription in HeLa and COS cells. The presence of an intact SV40 replication origin and/or 72-bp enhancer element is indicated above each lane. (*A*) Analysis of α-globin gene transcription in HeLa (lanes *1* and *2*) and COS (lanes *3–6*) cells with the *Nco*I + *Hae*II probe. Total cellular RNA (3 μg or 30 μg) was used for each assay. (Lane *1*) Plasmid πSVHSα1, 30 μg; (lane *2*) plasmid πSVHPα1, 30 μg; (lane *3*) plasmid πSVHSα1Δ, 30 μg; (lane *4*) plasmid πSVHPα1Δ, 30 μg; (lane *5*) plasmid πSVHSα1, 3 μg; (lane *6*) plasmid πSVHPα1, 3 μg. (*B*) Analysis of β-globin gene transcription in HeLa (lanes *1* and *2*) and COS (lanes *3–6*) cells with the *Mst*II + *Hae*III probe. In each assay, 30 μg total cellular RNA was used. (Lane *1*) Plasmid πSVHSβΔ128; (lane *2*) plasmid πSVHPβΔ128; (lane *3*) plasmid πSVHSβΔ128Δ; (lane *4*) plasmid πSVHPβΔ128Δ; (lane *5*) plasmid πSVHSβΔ28Δ; (lane *6*) plasmid πSVHPβΔ128Δ. All probe and product lengths are shown on the figure. Primer extension experiments indicate that the additional apparent β-globin 5′ ends apparently mapping within the first exon (products X) represent a 3′ splice site (G.C. Grosveld and R. Flavell, pers. comm.).

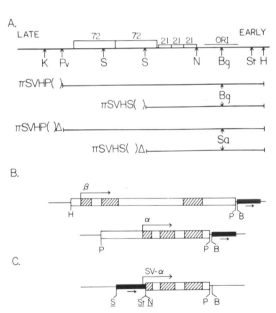

Figure 1 Plasmid structures. (*A*) SV40 sequences carried on miniplasmid (Seed 1983) vectors. The SV40 origin of replication region is shown with relevant restriction sites, with the 72-bp and 21-bp repeated sequences and replication origin indicated. Below are shown the extent of SV40 sequences present in the vectors used in this study; plasmids are named according to the extent of SV40 sequence present and the type of insert. (*B*) Structure of πSVβΔ128 and πSvα series of plasmids. Globin DNA sequences are shown as open boxes, with the exons shaded. SV40 sequences are shown as solid blocks with arrows pointing in the direction of early transcription, πVX vector (Seed 1983) sequences are shown as thin lines. (*C*) Structure of SV40–α-globin fusion genes. Symbols are as in *B*; vector sequences are pBRd (DiMaio et al. 1982). (K) *Kpn*I; (Pv) *Pvu*II; (S) *Sph*I; (N) *Nco*I; (Bg) *Bgl*I; (St) *Stu*I; (H) *Hin*dIII; (P) *Pst*I; (B) *Bam*HI; (Sa) *Sac*II. Underlined symbols indicate restriction sites destroyed in the plasmid construction.

cells unless the plasmid contains the SV40 enhancer (Fig. 2B, lanes 1 and 2). Linkage to the enhancer sequence increases the amount of correctly initiated β-globin RNA produced at least 100-fold. On the basis of these and other experiments, we estimate that the level of α-globin RNA produced by plasmids without an enhancer is comparable to the level of β-globin RNA produced by plasmids with an enhancer.

Effect of DNA replication on globin gene transcription in COS cells

Previous work demonstrated that the human α-globin gene is efficiently transcribed when introduced into COS cells on a plasmid that can replicate to high copy number (Mellon et al. 1981). In contrast, a β-globin gene carried on both replicating or nonreplicating plasmids requires an enhancer in cis for transcription to be detectable (Banerji et al. 1981; Humphries et al. 1982; Treisman et al. 1982). To compare the relative effects of transcription enhancement and plasmid replication on the amount of globin RNA produced in transient assays, we compared the amount of correctly initiated globin RNA produced in COS cells by plasmids that contain intact or inactivated SV40 replication origins. All plasmids containing intact SV40 replication origins replicated equally efficiently in COS cells; however, replication of those plasmids containing deleted replication origins was not detected (data not shown).

When the α-globin gene is introduced into COS cells on nonreplicating plasmids, the effect of the enhancer on transcription is similar to that observed in HeLa cells: α-globin RNA is detected in the absence of an enhancer sequence, and linkage to the enhancer results in a 5- to 10-fold increase in the amount of RNA produced (Fig. 2A, lanes 3 and 4; plasmids). As previously reported, a large amount of α-globin RNA is produced when the α-globin gene is introduced into COS cells on replicating plasmids (Mellon et al. 1981; Humphries et al. 1982); in some experiments, the enhancer also slightly increases the amount of correctly initiated α-globin RNA produced (Fig. 2A, compare lanes 5 and 6). Plasmid replication results in a 50-fold increase in the amount of α-globin RNA produced (Fig. 2A, compare lanes 3 and 4 with 5 and 6).

As observed in HeLa cells, transcription of the β-globin gene on nonreplicating plasmids in COS cells is not detected in the absence of an enhancer (Fig. 2B, lanes 3 and 4). When the β-globin gene is introduced into COS cells on replicating plasmids, an enhancer is also required for transcription (Fig. 2B, lanes 5 and 6), in agreement with previous observations (Humphries et al. 1982). In addition to correctly initiated β-globin RNA, replicating β-globin plasmids produce large quantities of transcripts initiated at positions 5′ to the mRNA cap site (Fig. 2B, lanes 5 and 6, 141 nucleotide products). Comparison of the amount of correctly initiated β-globin RNA produced in COS cells by replicating and non-replicating β-globin plasmids containing the enhancer shows that plasmid replication leads to essentially no

increase in the amount of correctly initiated β-globin RNA produced (Fig. 2B, compare lanes 4 and 6).

We conclude that replication of globin plasmids in COS cells substantially increases α-globin transcription irrespective of whether the plasmid contains an enhancer sequence. However, replication does not significantly increase the amount of β-globin RNA produced and does not relieve the requirement of the β-globin gene for a cis-linked enhancer sequence.

Efficient transcription of both α- and β-globin genes does not require a cis-linked enhancer sequence in 293 cells

As reviewed in the introduction, previous studies concerning the mechanism of action of viral immediate-early proteins suggested that these proteins do not appear to act in a promoter-specific manner. Therefore, we decided to test whether such gene products might also be capable of activating globin gene transcription. The α- and β-globin genes were transfected into 293 cells (Graham et al. 1977), which constitutively express the adenovirus type 5 (Ad5) immediate-early region E1A proteins. As shown in Figure 3, transcripts of the endogenous α- or β-globin genes are not detected in mock-transfected 293 cells (Fig. 3A, B, lanes 1 and 4); DNA blotting experiments confirmed that the endogenous β-globin gene in 293 cells is intact (data not shown). In transfected 293 cells, β-globin transcription is readily detected in the absence of an enhancer sequence (Fig. 3A, lane 2); moreover, transcription is not increased by the enhancer in these cells (Fig. 3A; compare lanes 2 and 3). Similarly, the enhancer has no effect on α-globin gene transcription in 293 cells (Fig. 3B, lanes 5 and 6). Although Figure 3 shows an experiment in which 293 cells were transfected with plasmids carrying both α- and β-globin genes, similar results were obtained when separate plasmids carrying each gene, with or without linked SV40 sequences, were used (see below). We also observed enhancer-independent transcription of the β-globin gene in cell lines into which Ad5 early-region 1 sequences were introduced by cotransformation with the herpes simplex virus thymidine kinase gene (Grodzicker and Klessig 1980; data not shown).

The SV40 enhancer is not required for activity of the SV40 early promoter in 293 cells

The results described above suggest that 293 cells contain factors that are specific for globin gene transcription or that bypass the requirement for an enhancer sequence for all enhancer-dependent genes. To distinguish between these two possibilities, we examined the activity of the SV40 early promoter in 293 cells: the SV40 enhancer sequence is normally required for activity of this promoter (Benoist and Chambon 1981; Gruss et al. 1981; Fromm and Berg 1982). To eliminate the effects of autoregulation of the promoter by large T antigen (for review, see Tooze 1981), an SV40 early-region gene product, we constructed fusion genes in which the large T antigen protein-coding sequences were replaced by those of the α-globin gene. These genes comprise frag-

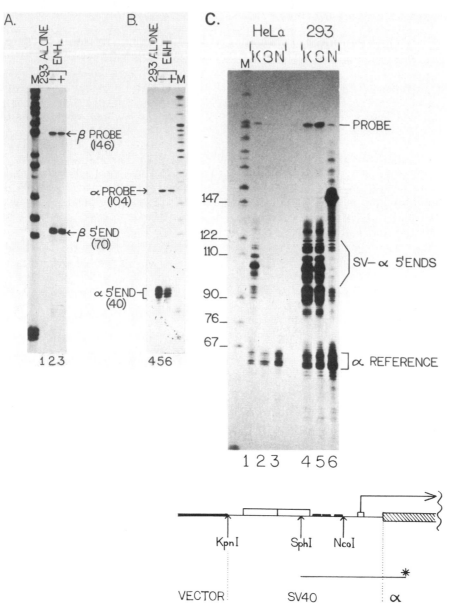

Figure 3 Transcription of the human α- and β-globin genes and the SV40 early region in 293 cells. The presence or absence of an intact enhancer sequence on the transfected plasmids is indicated. The β-globin *Mst*II + *Hae*III (A) or the α-globin *Nco*I + *Hae*II (B) probes were used. (Lanes *1* and *4*) 40 μg total cellular RNA from mock-transfected 293 cells. (Lanes *2* and *5*) 40 μg total cellular RNA from 293 cells transfected with plasmid πSVHRαβ + . (Lanes *3* and *6*) 40 μg total cellular RNA from 293 cells transfected with plasmid πSVHPαβ + . Nuclease-resistant product lengths are indicated. (C) S1 nuclease analysis of SV40–α-globin fusion gene transcription in HeLa and 293 cells. The *Bss*HIII + *Sph*I probe shown below the figure was used. Total cellular RNA (40 μg) was used in each assay. (Lanes *1–3*) HeLa cells; (lanes *4–6*) 293 cells. (Lanes *1* and *4*) Plasmid pSVKα; (lanes *2* and *5*) plasmid pSVSα; (lanes *3* and *6*) plasmid pSVNα. K,S, and N indicate that the SV40 sequences extend to the *Kpn*I, *Sph*I, and *Nco*I sites, respectively, as shown below the figure.

ments of the SV40 promoter containing various extents of 5′-flanking sequence joined, at a point some 40 nucleotides 3′ to the early mRNA cap sites, to α-globin sequences extending from the translational initiation codon to the 3′ end of the gene (Fig. 1).

The transcriptional analysis of the fusion genes in HeLa and 293 cells is shown in Figure 3C. The probe used in this assay is complementary to α-globin mRNA sequences to the 3′ side of the α-globin translational

initiation codon; transcripts of the cotransfected α-globin reference plasmid therefore generate nuclease-resistant DNA fragments 60 nucleotides in length, which also appear on the gel (α-reference products in Fig. 3C). In HeLa cells, plasmid pSVKα, which contains an intact enhancer sequence, produces a large amount of RNA that generates S1 nuclease-resistant products of the length expected for transcripts initiated at the normal SV40 early mRNA cap sites (110-nucleotide SV-α products in Fig. 3C, lane 1). The plasmid pSVSα, in which the truncated SV40 promoter contains the repeated 21-bp element but lacks an intact enhancer sequence, exhibits dramatically reduced promoter activity in HeLa cells (compare Fig. 3C, lanes 1 and 2); a further truncation which also removes the 21-bp repeats (plasmid pSVNα) completely abolishes transcription in HeLa cells (Fig. 3C, lane 3). In contrast, in 293 cells, transcription is initiated efficiently at heterogeneous positions centered on the normal SV40 early mRNA cap sites regardless of whether the SV40 promoter contains an intact enhancer sequence (compare plasmids pSVKα and pSVSα; Fig. 3C, lanes 4 and 5). However, a truncation that removes both the 72-bp and 21-bp repeated elements (plasmid pSVNα) results in total inactivation of the promoter in 293 cells (Fig. 3C, lane 6). This truncation also causes an increase in the amount of initiation at positions 5′ to the SV40 early mRNA cap sites, which generates a 150-nucleotide product that maps the point of divergence between the probe and the template (Fig. 3C, lane 6). We conclude that 293 cells contain a trans-acting factor(s) capable of relieving the enhancer requirement of both the β-globin and SV40 early promoters.

Adenovirus infection of HeLa cells eliminates the enhancer requirement for β-globin transcription

The results discussed above, together with the known properties of the E1A protein, suggest that the factor that relieves the enhancer requirement for β-globin transcription in 293 cells is an E1A protein. However, the possibility remains that the phenomenon we observe is due to the presence of other factors in the 293 cell line. Therefore, to determine whether enhancer-independent transcription can be observed in other cell types in the presence of E1A, HeLa cells were infected with Ad2 and subsequently transfected with β-globin plasmids that either contain or lack the SV40 enhancer. To maximize production of E1A RNAs and proteins and to maintain the infection in the early phase, the viral infection was carried out in the presence of the DNA synthesis inhibitor cytosine arabinoside (Gaynor et al. 1982). With this protocol, the amount of E1A RNA produced in virus-infected HeLa cells between 8 and 36 hours postinfection is equivalent to that present in 293 cells (data not shown).

RNA was prepared 40 hours after transfection and correctly initiated β-globin RNA was assayed by S1 nuclease mapping. In mock-infected cells maintained in the presence of cytosine arabinoside, β-globin RNA is only detectable when the β-globin gene is linked to an enhancer (Fig. 4A, compare lanes 3 and 4). In contrast, when HeLa cells are infected with Ad2 prior to transfection, production of correctly initiated β-globin RNA is not dependent upon a linked enhancer (Fig. 4A, lane 6). Furthermore, in Ad2-infected HeLa cells, which contain levels of E1A gene products comparable to those present in 293 cells, the enhancer does not increase the level of accumulated β-globin RNA (Fig. 4A, lanes 5 and 6). Control experiments show that the endogenous HeLa cell α- and β-globin genes are not transcriptionally ac-

tivated during adenovirus infection (data not shown). We conclude that the enhancer-independent transcription of transfected β-globin genes in 293 cells is due to an adenoviral gene product.

β-Globin transcription is activated in *trans* by a cotransfected adenovirus E1A gene

The virus infection experiments described above demonstrate that adenoviral gene product(s) synthesized at the early stage of infection directly or indirectly relieves the enhancer requirement for β-globin transcription. To prove that a product of early region 1A is responsible for β-globin transcriptional stimulation, we carried out cotransfection experiments in which HeLa cells were simultaneously transfected with separate plasmids containing the β-globin gene and the Ad5 E1A gene. In addition, we included in the transfection mix a reference plasmid, containing the α-globin gene and a linked enhancer, to allow evaluation of transfection efficiency and RNA recovery. The amount of α-globin RNA produced provides a valid quantitative reference for the comparison of different experiments that all include, or all lack, a cotransfected viral immediate-early gene. However, the level of α-globin transcription does not allow quantitative comparison of experiments that include viral immediate-early gene plasmids to experiments that lack them, since the viral gene products may stimulate transcription of the reference gene as well as the test gene. This possibility is supported by the observation that in some cotransfection experiments transcription of the α-globin reference gene is apparently stimulated by a cotransfected viral immediate-early gene plasmid.

As shown in Figure 4B, the β-globin gene plasmid lacking an enhancer does not produce detectable levels of β-globin RNA (Fig. 4B, lane 2). However, cotransfection of the same β-globin plasmid with the E1A gene plasmid results in readily detectable levels of steady-state β-globin RNA (Fig. 4B, lane 3). The amount of β-globin RNA produced in this cotransfection experiment is significantly less than that produced when the β-globin plasmid contains an enhancer (Fig. 4B, compare lanes 1 and 3). This difference is most likely due to the fact that activation of the β-globin gene in the cotransfection experiments depends upon transcription of the E1A gene followed by protein synthesis to produce the E1A gene product, resulting in a slower rate of accumulation of β-globin RNA. In any case, the observation that the amount of β-globin RNA produced from plasmids lacking an enhancer increases in the presence of the E1A plasmid strongly suggests that the *trans*-acting factor that activates β-globin transcription in 293 cells (Treisman et al. 1983a) and in adenovirus-infected HeLa cells (Fig. 4A) is in fact an E1A gene product.

As mentioned in the introduction, the immediate-early gene of pseudorabies virus, a herpesvirus, can complement Ad5 E1A mutants in a virus coinfection experiment, suggesting that the immediate-early proteins of these two unrelated viruses act through a common mechanism (Feldman et al. 1982). Moreover, during such mixed infections, the products of the adenoviral early genes ac-

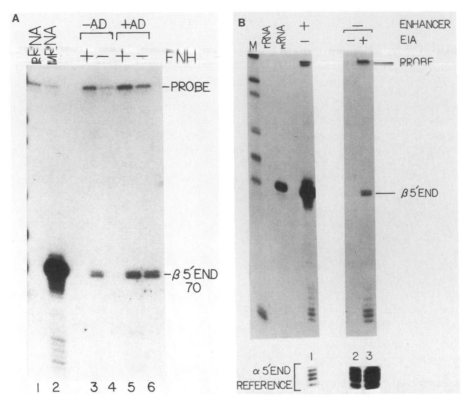

Figure 4 Transcriptional activity of the human β-globin gene in adenovirus-infected HeLa cells. HeLa cells maintained in the presence of cytosine arabinoside were either infected with Ad2 (+AD) or mock-infected (−AD). Then 8 hr later the cells were transfected with plasmids containing the β-globin gene with or without a linked SV40 enhancer sequence. Transfections included a human α-globin plasmid (πSVHPα2) as an internal reference. Total cellular RNA was prepared 48 hr postinfection and 40 μg analyzed for β-globin RNA by 5′ S1 nuclease mapping using the *Mst*II–*Hae*III [³²P]DNA probe (−76 to +70). This probe generates a 70-nucleotide S1 nuclease-resistant [³²P]DNA product with β-globin mRNA. (Lane *1*) rRNA; 40 μg HeLa cell RNA. (Lane *2*) mRNA; 40 μg HeLa cell RNA plus human β-globin RNA. (Lanes *3* and *4*) Mock-infected HeLa cells maintained in the presence of cytosine arabinoside transfected with β-globin plasmids containing (lane *3*) and lacking (lane *4*) the enhancer. (Lanes *5* and *6*) Ad2-infected HeLa cells transfected with β-globin plasmids containing (lane *5*) and lacking (lane *6*) the enhancer. The positions of the full-length probe and S1 nuclease-resistant product from β-globin mRNA are indicated. (Reprinted, with permission, from Green et al. 1983.) (*B*) Cotransfection of the human β-globin and Ad5 E1A genes in HeLa cells. HeLa cells were transfected with plasmids containing the β-globin gene with or without a linked SV40 enhancer as indicated. Transfections either included or lacked the Ad5 E1A plasmid, pH3G, as indicated. Total cellular RNA was prepared 48 hr following the transfection and 40 μg analyzed for β-globin RNA as in the legend to Fig. 1. (Lane M) [³²P]DNA markers from a *Msp*I digest of pBR322 DNA; (lane rRNA) 40 μg HeLa cell RNA; (lane mRNA) 40 μg HeLa cell RNA plus human β-globin mRNA. (Lane *1*) HeLa cells transfected with the β-globin plasmid containing the enhancer; (lanes *2* and *3*) HeLa cells transfected with the β-globin plasmid lacking the enhancer without (lane *2*) or with (lane *3*) cotransfection of pH3G. The positions of the full-length probe and S1 nuclease-resistant product from β-globin mRNA are indicated. Also shown are the S1 nuclease-resistant products generated by transcripts of the α-globin reference gene. (Reprinted, with permission, from Green et al. 1983.)

cumulate at greater rates and to higher levels, suggesting that the pseudorabies virus immediate-early gene product is more effective at activating adenoviral gene transcription than the Ad5 E1A gene product itself. We therefore considered it possible that the pseudorabies virus immediate-early gene product might be more effective than E1A gene products in stimulating β-globin transcription in cotransfection experiments.

To test this possibility, HeLa cells were transfected with β-globin plasmids together with the plasmid pIE, which contains the pseudorabies virus immediate-early gene (a gift from T. Ben Porat). Similar to the result obtained with the E1A gene, cotransfection of plasmids containing the β-globin gene lacking an enhancer and the pseudorabies virus gene results in readily detectable levels of β-globin RNA (Green et al. 1983). Furthermore, the level of transcriptional stimulation of the β-globin

gene by the cotransfected pseudorabies viral gene appears to be greater than that obtained with the cotransfected E1A gene, but still considerably less β-globin RNA is produced compared with plasmids that contain the enhancer. This result is consistent with the virus coinfection studies (Feldman et al. 1982). It is possible that the pseudorabies viral gene product is intrinsically more active, or that during the course of the cotransfection experiment it is produced in larger quantities than the adenoviral E1A gene product.

Identification of sequences within the β-globin promoter required for transcription in the presence of viral immediate-early gene products

To identify the sequences required for β-globin transcription mediated by *cis*- and *trans*-acting viral factors, we analyzed the transcriptional activity of deletion and point mutants of the β-globin promoter in HeLa and 293 cells. HeLa cells provide information regarding the sequence requirements for enhancer-dependent transcription, whereas 293 cells provide an assay for E1A-mediated transcription. Deletion mutants containing 75, 44, 36, and 25 bp of 5′-flanking sequence were constructed (Green et al. 1983). All four deletions remove the CCAAT box (Efstratiadis et al. 1980); however, all but the − 25 deletion contain the TATA box. Each mutant was subcloned into vectors that either contain or lack an intact enhancer sequence, and their transcription in HeLa and 293 cells was compared with that of a β-globin gene containing 128 bp of 5′-flanking sequence.

The β-globin gene containing only 128 bp of 5′-flanking DNA is transcribed in HeLa cells when linked to an enhancer (Fig. 5A, lane 3; Treisman et al. 1983b). In contrast, very little β-globin RNA is detected following transfection of each of the deletion mutants into HeLa cells (Fig. 5A, lanes 4–7). We conclude that in HeLa cells, the sequences between − 75 and − 128 are necessary for the transcription of the human β-globin gene linked to an enhancer sequence, in agreement with previous studies on the rabbit β-globin gene (Grosveld et al. 1982; Dierks et al. 1983). As expected, in HeLa cells β-globin transcripts were not detected when the plasmids lacked an enhancer sequence (data not shown).

The effect of promoter deletions on β-globin gene transcription in 293 cells is in striking contrast to that ob-served in HeLa cells. The analysis of the the β-globin deletion mutants in 293 cells is shown in Figure 5B. 293 cells were transfected with the same calcium phosphate precipitates used for the HeLa cell experiment described above (Fig. 5A). In 293 cells, the − 75, − 44, and − 36 deletions decrease transcription only slightly (Fig. 5B, lanes 3–6). However, the − 25 deletion, which lacks the TATA box, produces no correctly initiated RNA (Fig. 5B, lane 7). Exactly the same results were obtained when these deletion mutants were analyzed in 293 cells using plasmids lacking the enhancer (data not shown).

In addition to accurately transcribed β-globin RNA, a significant amount of RNA with 5′ ends mapping upstream of the β-globin gene is produced in 293 cells (Fig. 5B). For the − 128 β-globin gene, these upstream transcripts generate nuclease-resistant products that are the same size as the [^{32}P]DNA probe (Fig. 5B, lane 3). In the case of the various deletion mutants, such readthrough transcripts generate S1 nuclease-resistant products that map the deletion end point with respect to the ^{32}P-labeled 5′ terminus of the probe. The amount of this upstream transcription appears to increase with more extensive deletions (Fig. 5B), suggesting that in 293 cells the upstream elements of the β-globin promoter allow preferential transcription initiation at the β-globin mRNA cap site.

To obtain additional information regarding the β-globin sequences required for transcriptional activity by cis-

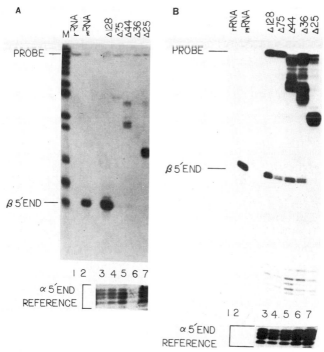

Figure 5 Transcriptional activity of β-globin promoter deletion mutants in HeLa and 293 cells. HeLa (*A*) or 293 (*B*) cells were transfected with 15 μg β-globin plasmids containing the indicated extents of 5′-flanking sequences. In all cases, the plasmids contain the enhancer. Each transfection included 5 μg of the α-globin plasmid πSVHPα2 as an internal reference. Total cellular RNA was prepared 48 hr following the transfection, and 40 μg were analyzed for β-globin RNA as described in the legend to Fig. 1. (Lane M) [^{32}P]DNA markers from an *Msp*I digest of pBR322 DNA. (Lane *1*) rRNA; 40 μg Hela cell RNA. (Lane *2*) mRNA; 40 μg HeLa cell RNA plus human β-globin mRNA. (Lanes *3–7*) HeLa cells or 293 cells transfected with β-globin plasmids containing, respectively, 128, 75, 44, 36, and 25 bp of β-globin sequence 5′ to the mRNA cap site. The positions of the full-length probe and S1 nuclease-resistant products of β-globin mRNA are indicated. Also shown are the S1 nuclease-resistant products generated by transcripts of the α-globin reference gene. (Reprinted, with permission, from Green et al. 1983.)

and *trans*-acting viral sequences, we analyzed the transcription of two β-thalassemia genes that contain single-base change mutations in the β globin promoter. The first gene, containing a C → G transversion at position −87, produces 10-fold less RNA than a normal β-gene when introduced into HeLa cells on plasmids containing an enhancer (Treisman et al. 1983b). In contrast to the 10-fold decrease in transcription observed in HeLa cells (Treisman et al. 1983b), the −87 mutant is expressed approximately at the wild-type level in 293 cells (Green et al. 1983). Furthermore, the presence of the enhancer does not increase the amount of RNA produced by the mutant or wild-type genes in 293 cells consistent with the results presented above and previously (Treisman et al. 1983a).

We have also examined the transcription of a second β-thalassemia gene that contains an A → G transition in the TATA box sequence at position −28 (Orkin et al. 1983). This gene produces about fivefold less β-globin RNA than the normal β-globin gene when introduced into HeLa cells on a plasmid containing an enhancer (Fig. 6, lanes 1 vs. 2), consistent with the previously reported data (Orkin et al. 1983). As expected, transcription is not detectable from the wild-type or mutant gene in HeLa cells if the plasmid lacks the enhancer (Fig. 6, lanes 3 and 4). In 293 cells, the wild-type gene produces at least 10-fold more RNA than the mutant gene, regardless of the presence of the enhancer (Fig. 6, compare lanes 5 and 7 with 6 and 8). Therefore, in contrast to the −87 mutant, a single-base change in the TATA box has a significant impact on transcriptional activity in 293 cells. These results in conjunction with the deletion mutant analyses suggest that the β-globin TATA box, but not the upstream promoter sequences, is required for transcription in the presence of viral immediate-early gene products.

Discussion

We have used transient expression assays to analyze the requirements for transcription of cloned human α- and β-globin genes introduced into cultured nonerythroid mammalian cells. We find that the β-, but not α-, globin gene requires linkage to the SV40 enhancer sequence for transcription to be detected in both HeLa and COS cells. In contrast, neither the globin genes nor the SV40 early promoter require a *cis*-linked enhancer for efficient expression in the presence of adenovirus immediate-early proteins. These gene products can be provided by a stably integrated constitutively expressed viral gene, or introduced into cells by viral infection or by transfection of plasmids carrying the viral gene. The sequence requirements for enhancer-dependent β-globin gene transcription and for transcription in the presence of viral immediate-early proteins are significantly different, indicating that different activation mechanisms operate in each case.

The effect of the SV40 enhancer on globin gene transcription

Linkage of the human β-globin gene to the SV40 enhancer sequence results in an increase of at least 100-

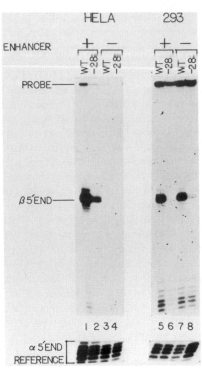

Figure 6 Transcriptional activity of a −28 β-globin point mutant in HeLa and 293 cells. HeLa cells or 293 cells were transfected with either a wild-type β-globin gene plasmid or a β-globin gene plasmid with a single-base mutation at position −28 described by Orkin et al. (1983). These plasmids either contained or lacked the enhancer as indicated. Total cellular RNA was prepared 48 hr following the transfection and 40 μg analyzed for β-globin RNA as described in the legend to Fig. 1. (Lanes 1 and 2) HeLa cells transfected with wild-type (lane 1) or the −28 mutant (lane 2) β-globin plasmids containing the enhancer. (Lanes 3 and 4) HeLa cells transfected with the wild-type (lane 3) or the −28 mutant (lane 4) β-globin plasmids lacking the enhancer. (Lanes 5 and 6) 293 cells transfected with the wild-type (lane 5) or the −28 mutant (lane 6) β-globin plasmids containing the enhancer. (Lanes 7 and 8) 293 cells transfected with the wild-type (lane 7) or the −28 mutant (lane 8) β-globin plasmids lacking the enhancer. The positions of the full-length probe and S1 nuclease-resistant product from β-globin mRNA are indicated. Also shown are the S1 nuclease-resistant products generated by transcripts of the α-globin reference gene. (Reprinted, with permission, from Green et al. 1983.)

fold in the amount of correctly initiated β-globin RNA synthesized in HeLa cells, in agreement with previous reports (Banerji et al. 1981; De Villiers and Schaffner 1981; Humphries et al. 1982; Treisman et al. 1982). A similar increase in β-gene transcription is observed when the gene is introduced into COS cells on a nonreplicating vector. In contrast, linkage of the enhancer to the human α-globin gene results in only a 5- to 10-fold increase in the synthesis of correctly initiated α-globin RNA. Other genes respond to the enhancer either only weakly (Pelham 1982; M. Poritz and R. Treisman, unpubl.) or in a strongly position-dependent manner (Pelham 1982; Picard and Schaffner 1983). It is unlikely that the weak response of the α-globin gene to the enhancer is due to the presence of an enhancer on the α-globin gene fragment itself, since the presence of α-globin gene fragments in *cis* to the β-globin gene in a number of different configurations does not activate transcription of the β-globin gene (Humphries et al. 1982; R. Treisman, unpubl.). Alternatively, the α-globin may either be incapable of responding to the enhancer, or the effect of the enhancer may be attenuated by sequences within or near the gene. A precedent for the latter possibility is the observation that certain DNA sequences placed between the SV40 enhancer and a promoter may block transcription enhancement (Banerji et al. 1981; De Villiers et al. 1982; Wasylyk et al. 1983). In some cases, these effects are due to the presence of promoter sequences within the interposed DNA segments (De Villiers et al. 1982; Wasylyk et al. 1983). In the case of blocking effects due to the rabbit β-globin gene promoter, the upstream sequences of the promoter are required for the blocking effect, since a single-base change at −89 relieves the block (De Villiers et al. 1982). The blocking effect therefore requires at least some of the sequences that are required for transcription in the presence of a *cis*-linked enhancer. The mechanism by which enhancers stimulate transcription is not understood. The observations that enhancers can stimulate transcription over long distances, in *cis*, and in an orientation-independent manner, has led to the proposal that the enhancer may provide a bidirectional entry site for RNA polymerase II or some other component of the transcriptional machinery (Moreau et al. 1981; Wasylyk et al. 1983). We are currently investigating which sequences determine the response of a particular globin gene to the enhancer sequence by constructing and analyzing the transcription of α–β-globin gene hybrids.

The effect of DNA replication on globin gene transcription

We also examined the effect of plasmid replication on the amount of α- and β-globin RNA produced in transient assays. Each plasmid containing an intact SV40 origin replicates equally efficiently in COS cells regardless of whether an enhancer is present: enhancer-dependent transcription therefore does not interfere with efficient replication. In the case of the α-globin gene, plasmid replication increases transcription by a factor of about 50. The enhancer has little effect on transcription of the α-globin gene carried on replicating plasmids; similar observations have been made with the α-globin gene carried on a different vector (Humphries et al. 1982) and in the case of the sea urchin histone *H2A* gene (T. Gerster and W. Schaffner, pers. comm.). In contrast to the α-globin gene, however, plasmid replication does not affect transcription of the β-globin gene carried on plasmids containing an intact enhancer sequence. Possibly some factor required for enhancer-dependent β-globin gene expression in these cells is limiting; alternatively, replication per se may interfere with enhancer-dependent transcription. Replication of β-globin plasmids lacking an intact enhancer appears to increase slightly the amount of correctly initiated β-globin RNA produced, although the sensitivity of our assay was not sufficient to quantitate the increase. At present therefore, we cannot say whether the increase in transcription observed

upon replication of α globin plasmids is due to a fundamental difference in the properties of the α- and β-globin gene promoters.

The effect of viral immediate early gene products on globin gene transcription

To examine the possible effect of adenoviral E1A gene products on globin gene transcription, we initially performed transient assays in 293 cells, which constitutively produce Ad5 E1A proteins. These proteins are known to act in *trans* to activate transcription from both adenovirus (Berk et al. 1979; Jones and Shenk 1979) and certain cellular (Nevins 1982) promoters. In contrast to the situation in HeLa and COS cells, neither the α- nor the β-globin gene requires linkage to the SV40 enhancer for transcripts to be detected in 293 cells; moreover, a *cis*-linked SV40 enhancer sequence does not affect transcription of either gene in these cells. Since the SV40 early promoter also does not require an enhancer for activity in 293 cells, we conclude that the factor present in these cells does not specifically activate globin genes, but rather circumvents the constraints on promoter activity that render an enhancer sequence necessary for efficient transcription of a transfected gene. Two observations demonstrate that the enhancer-independent β-globin gene transcription that we observe in 293 cells is due to the presence of the adenoviral E1A gene products constitutively produced by this cell line. First, we were able to reproduce the effect by transfecting adenovirus-infected HeLa cells with β-globin plasmids. Second, we observed β-globin transcription in the absence of a linked enhancer when β-globin plasmids were cotransfected together with a plasmid carrying the entire Ad5 E1A transcription unit. We have made similar observations in the case of the immediate-early gene of a herpesvirus, pseudorabies virus (data not shown).

The level of β-globin RNA is less in the cotransfection experiments than that observed in 293 cells or in virus-infected HeLa cells. We feel that this is most likely a consequence of the cotransfection protocol. In 293 cells and virus-infected HeLa cells, high levels of viral immediate-early gene products are present prior to introduction of the globin genes. In the cotransfection experiment, the viral immediate-early gene must be expressed and its products must accumulate. The stimulation of globin gene transcription must therefore take place in the relatively short time-frame of the transient assay. Thus, even if the viral immediate-early gene product is fully active, globin RNA does not begin to accumulate until late stages of the experiment. However, we cannot rule out the possibility that in 293 cells and virus-infected HeLa cells other viral gene products may contribute to the high level of β-globin transcription.

Sequence requirements for enhancer-dependent and E1A-dependent β-globin gene transcription

To determine whether the sequences necessary for initiation of transcription at the β-globin mRNA cap site in the presence of E1A product are the same as those required for enhancer-dependent transcription, we carried out transient assays in HeLa and 293 cells with a series of β-globin deletion and point mutants. Our results strongly suggest that the mechanisms by which enhancers and viral immediate-early gene products act are different. Previous studies have shown that accurate and efficient transcription of the rabbit β-globin gene introduced into HeLa cells on plasmids containing the SV40 enhancer sequence requires at least 109 bp of 5′-flanking sequence (Grosveld et al. 1982; Dierks et al. 1983). Consistent with these observations, we find that 5′ deletions with end points between −75 and −36 dramatically decrease the level of human β-globin RNA produced in HeLa cells. In contrast, we find that β-globin transcription in the presence of viral immediate-early gene products requires no more than 36 bp of 5′-flanking sequence. Moreover, deletions that remove the TATA box, leaving 25 nucleotides 5′ to the mRNA cap site, severely affect promoter activity, as do point mutations that alter the TATA box but retain upstream sequences. Further analysis of these differences in sequence requirements for *cis*- and *trans*-activation of transcription could provide important clues regarding the mechanisms of enhancer activity and the means by which viral immediate-early gene products can act on a variety of viral and cellular promoters.

The sequences required for transcription of the human β-globin gene in the presence of viral immediate-early gene products appear to be the same as those required for rabbit (Grosveld et al. 1981) and human (A. Krainer, unpubl.) β-globin gene transcription in whole-cell extracts. Similarly, we find that the SV40 early promoter requires the 21-bp repeat sequences located 5′ to the TATA homology for activity in the presence of viral immediate-early gene products; these sequences are also required for transcription in vitro (Myers et al. 1981; A. Krainer, unpubl.). Unlike the β-globin TATA box, the SV40 TATA homology is not sufficient for maximal transcription in vitro in the absence of its linked upstream element. The 21-bp repeat sequences are thought to interact with a cellular transcription factor that is required for the in vitro transcription of SV40 but not the β-globin gene (Dynan and Tjian 1983, and pers. comm.). Thus, when each promoter is considered individually, the minimal sequence requirements for in vitro transcription and in vivo transcription in the presence of viral immediate-early gene products are the same. It will be interesting to test whether other genes whose transcriptional activity in vitro is dependent upon upstream sequences, such as the human α-globin gene (A. Krainer, unpubl.), also require upstream promoter sequences for transcription in the presence of viral immediate-early gene products. It is possible that an understanding of the basis for the reduced sequence requirements for β-globin transcription in vitro may also provide insights into the mechanism of action of viral immediate-early proteins.

As with enhancers, the mechanism by which viral immediate-early proteins act to increase the activity of both viral and cellular promoters remains unclear. However, a number of mechanisms can be envisaged. For example, the proteins could directly interact with the promoter

in a way that enables a functional transcriptional complex to form in the absence of an enhancer. Our data indicate that in the case of the β-globin gene, a 36-bp region of the promoter containing the TATA box is sufficient for such an interaction. Alternatively, viral immediate-early gene products might allow a modification of the template that would facilitate transcription initiation (Gaynor and Berk 1983) or they might interact directly with RNA polymerase II or another transcription factor to alter its activity. Unfortunately, little additional information relevant to these possibilities is available. The adenoviral E1A gene encodes a complex set of related phosphoproteins, but there is no evidence that they interact with DNA or cellular transcription factors (for review, see Tooze 1981; Rowe et al. 1983 and references therein). However, there is some evidence that ICP4, an immediate-early protein of herpes simplex virus that is required for the transcriptional activation of other viral genes (Tooze 1981), can bind to DNA in the presence of an uncharacterized cellular factor (Freeman and Powell 1982). It is not known whether this binding is relevant to the regulatory properties of ICP4.

An alternative to a role in positive activation of transcription is the possibility that an E1A protein inactivates a nonspecific cellular repressor of transcription (Katze et al. 1981, 1983; Nevins 1981). According to this model, transfected β-globin and SV40 genes would also be subject to this negative control, which could be bypassed either by a *cis*-linked enhancer or by *trans*-acting viral immediate-early gene products. Although this model cannot be ruled out, the fact that E1A gene products can relieve the requirement for the upstream promoter sequences of the β-globin gene suggests that these viral proteins are more likely to be positive regulators of transcription.

Viral immediate-early proteins can stimulate transcription from both viral and cellular promoters but not all endogenous cellular genes are activated. For example, the endogenous α- and β-globin genes in 293 cells (Triesman et al. 1983a) and in HeLa cells are not activated by viral immediate-early gene products, but the endogenous 70-kD heat-shock protein gene in HeLa cells is expressed in the presence of E1A gene products (Nevins 1982). The reasons for the different responses of the endogenous globin and heat-shock genes to the E1A products are not clear; it is possible that viral immediate-early proteins can activate only those genes with promoters that are in a chromatin configuration that allows a functional interaction with regulatory proteins. Consistent with this possibility, the *Drosophila* heat-shock promoter is hypersensitive to digestion by DNase I even prior to heat shock (Wu 1980). In addition, when cloned genes are introduced into cells by transfection, their promoters are accessible to enzymatic and chemical reagents (Weintraub 1983). This increased accessibility is reflected in the increased transcriptional activity of such genes relative to their endogenous counterparts. For example, globin genes stably (Mantei et al. 1979; Wold et al. 1979) or transiently (for review, see Banerji and Schaffner 1983) introduced into cultured cells are transcribed, whereas transcripts from the endogenous globin genes (which are relatively insensitive to DNase I digestion; Treisman et al., unpubl.) cannot be detected. Similarly, the human growth hormone gene stably introduced into mouse L cells by cotransformation is responsive to glucocorticoid stimulation whereas the endogenous mouse growth hormone gene is not (Robins et al. 1982).

It is tempting to speculate that cellular proteins with properties similar to those of the viral immediate-early gene products are involved in the activation of genes during cellular differentiation or transformation. A role for such proteins in cellular transformation is suggested by the fact the E1A gene can complement the Ha-*ras* cellular oncogene in the transformation of primary rat fibroblasts (Land et al. 1983; Ruley 1983). Since neither the E1A gene nor the Ha-*ras* gene alone is capable of transforming these cells, and the E1A gene product appears to be a general transcriptional activator, the observed E1A complementation in the transformation assay could result from E1A-dependent transcriptional activation of one or more cellular genes. Interestingly, the activated *c-myc* gene is also capable of complementing the Ha-*ras* gene in the transformation assay. It is therefore possible that *c-myc* and E1A genes have at least one common function. We are currently determining whether *c-myc* and other other cellular oncogenes are active in our transcription assay.

Acknowledgments

We thank E. Greene for technical assistance. R.T. was supported by a Travelling Fellowship from the Imperial Cancer Research Fund and more recently by a special fellowship from the Leukemia Society of America, M.G. was supported by a fellowship from the Helen Hay Whitney Foundation. This work was funded by a grant to T.M. from the NIH.

References

Baker, C.C. and E.B. Ziff. 1981. Promoters and heterogeneous 5′ termini of the messenger RNAs of adenovirus serotype 2. *J. Mol. Biol.* **149**: 189.

Banerji, J. and W. Schaffner. 1983. Transient expression of cloned genes in mammalian cells. In *Genetic engineering - principles and methods* (ed. J.K. Setlow and A. Hollaender). Plenum Press, New York. (In press.)

Banerji, J., S. Rusconi, and W. Schaffner. 1981. Expression of a β-globin gene is enhanced by remote SV40 DNA sequences. *Cell* **27**: 299.

Benoist, C. and P. Chambon. 1981. *In vivo* sequence requirements for the SV40 early promoter region. *Nature* **290**: 304.

Berk, A.J., F. Lee, T. Harrison, J. Williams, and P.A. Sharp. 1979. Pre-early adenovirus 5 gene product regulates synthesis of early viral messenger RNAs. *Cell* **17**: 935.

Conrad, S. and M. Botchan. 1982. Isolation and characterization of human DNA fragments with nucleotide sequence homologies with the simian virus 40 regulatory region. *Mol. Cell. Biol.* **2**: 949.

De Villiers, J. and W. Schaffner. 1981. A small segment of polyoma virus DNA enhances transcription of a cloned rabbit β-globin gene over a distance of at last 1400 base pairs *Nucleic Acids Res.* **9**: 6251.

De Villiers, J., L. Olson, J. Banerji, and W. Schaffner. 1983.

Analysis of the transcriptional enhancer effect. *Cold Spring Harbor Symp. Quant. Biol.* **47**: 911.

Dierks, P., A.V. Ooyen, M.D. Cochran, C. Dobkin, J. Reiser, and C. Weissmann. 1983. Three regions upstream from the cap site are required for efficient and accurate transcription of the rabbit β-globin gene in mouse 3T6 cells. *Cell* **32**: 695.

DiMaio, D., R. Treisman, and T. Maniatis. 1982. Bovine papillomavirus vector that propagates as a plasmid in both mouse and bacterial cells. *Proc. Natl. Acad. Sci.* **79**: 4030.

Dynan, W.S. and R. Tjian. 1983. Isolation of transcription factors that discriminate between different promoters recognized by RNA polymerase II. *Cell* **32**: 669.

Efstratiadis, A., J.W. Posakony, T. Maniatis, R.M. Lawn, C. O'Connell, R.A. Spitz, J.K. DeRiel, B.G. Forget, S.M. Weissman, J.L. Slightom, A.E. Blechl, O. Smithies, F.E. Baralle, C.C. Shoulders, and N.J. Proudfoot. 1980. The structure and evolution of the human β-globin gene family. *Cell* **21**: 653.

Feldman, L.T., M.J. Imperiale, and J.R. Nevins. 1982. Activation of early adenovirus transcription by the herpesvirus immediate early gene: Evidence for a common cellular control factor. *Proc. Natl. Acad. Sci.* **79**: 4952.

Freeman, M.J. and K.L. Powell. 1982. DNA-binding properties of a herpes simplex virus immediate early protein. *J. Virol.* **44**: 1084.

Fromm, M. and P. Berg. 1982. Deletion mapping of DNA regions required for SV40 early region promoter function *in vivo*. *J. Mol. Appl. Genet.* **1**: 457.

Gaynor, R.B. and A.J. Berk. 1983. Cis-acting induction of adenovirus transcription. *Cell* **33**: 683.

Gaynor, R.B., A. Tsukamoto, C. Montell, and A.J. Berk. 1982. Enhanced expression of adenovirus transforming proteins. *J. Virol.* **44**: 276.

Gillies, S.D., S.L. Morrison, V.T. Oi, and S. Tonegawa. 1983. A tissue-specific transcription enhancer element is located in the major intron of a rearranged immunoglobulin heavy chain gene. *Cell* **33**: 717.

Gluzman, Y. 1981. SV40-transformed simian cells support the replication of early SV40 mutants. *Cell* **23**: 175.

Gluzman, Y. and T. Shenk, eds. 1983. *Enhancers and eukaryotic gene expression*. Cold Spring Harbor Laboratory, Cold Spring Harbor, New York.

Graham, F.L., J. Smiley, W.C. Russel, and R. Nairn. 1978. Characteristics of a human cell line transformed by DNA from human adenovirus type 5. *J. Gen. Virol.* **36**: 59.

Green, M.R., R.H. Treisman, and T. Maniatis. 1983. Activation of globin gene transcription in transient assays by *cis* and *trans*-acting factors. *Cell* **35**: 137.

Grodzicker, T. and D.F. Klessig. 1980. Expression of unselected adenovirus genes in human cells co-transformed with the HSV-1 tk gene and adenovirus 2 DNA. *Cell* **21**: 453.

Grosveld, G.C., E. deBoer, C.K. Shewmaker, and R.A. Flavell. 1982. DNA sequences necessary for transcription of the rabbit β-globin gene *in vivo*. *Nature* **295**: 120.

Grosveld, G.C., C.K. Shewmaker, P. Jat, and R.A. Flavell. 1981. Localization of DNA sequences necessary for transcription of the rabbit β-globin gene *in vitro*. *Cell* **25**: 215.

Gruss, P., R. Dhar, and G. Khoury. 1981. Simian virus 40 tandem repeated sequences as an element of the early promoter. *Proc. Natl. Acad. Sci.* **78**: 943.

Humphries, R.K., T. Ley, P. Turner, A.D. Moulton, and A.W. Nienhuis. 1982. Differences in human α-, β, and δ-globin gene expression in monkey kidney cells. *Cell* **30**: 173.

Jones, N. and T. Shenk. 1979. An adenovirus 5 early gene product function regulates expression of other early viral genes. *Proc. Natl. Acad. Sci.* **76**: 3665.

Katze, M.G., H. Persson, and L. Phillipson. 1981. Control of adenovirus early gene expression: Post-transcriptional control mediated by both viral and cellular gene products. *Mol. Cell. Biol.* **1**: 807.

Katze, M.G., H. Persson, B.M. Johansson, and L. Phillipson. 1983. Control of adenovirus gene expression: Cellular gene products restrict expression of adenovirus host range mutants in nonpermissive cells. *J. Virol.* **46**: 50.

Khoury, G. and P. Gruss. 1983. Enhancer elements. Mini-review. *Cell* **33**: 313.

Land, H., L.F. Parada, and R.A. Weinberg. 1083. Tumorigenic conversion of primary embryo fibroblasts requires at least two cooperating oncogenes. *Nature* **304**: 596.

Lewis, J.B. and M.B. Mathews. 1980. Control of adenovirus early gene expression, a class of immediate early products. *Cell* **21**: 303.

Mantei, N., W. Boll, and C. Weissmann. 1979. Rabbit β-globin mRNA production in mouse L cells transformed with cloned rabbit β-globin chromosomal DNA. *Nature* **281**: 40.

Mellon, P., V. Parker, Y. Gluzman, and T. Maniatis. 1981. Identification of DNA sequences required for transcription of the human α1-globin gene in a new SV40 host vector system. *Cell* **27**: 279.

Moreau, P., R. Hen, B. Wasylyk, R. Everett, M.P. Gaub, and P. Chambon. 1981. The SV40 72 base pair repeat has a striking effect on gene expression both in SV40 and other chimeric recombinants. *Nucleic Acids Res.* **9**: 6047.

Myers, R.M., D.C. Rio, A.K. Robbins, and R. Tjian. 1981. SV40 gene expression is modulated by the cooperative binding of T antigen to DNA. *Cell* **25**: 373.

Nevins, J.R. 1981. Mechanism of activation of early viral transcription by the adenovirus E1A gene product. *Cell* **26**: 213.

———. 1982. Induction of the synthesis of a 70,000 dalton mammalian heat shock protein by the adenovirus E1A gene product. *Cell* **29**: 913.

Orkin, S.H., J.P Sexton, T.C. Cheng, S.C. Goff, J.V. Giardina, J.I. Lee, and H.H. Kazazian, Jr. 1983. ATA box transcription mutation in β-thalassemia. *Nucleic Acids Res.* **11**: 4727.

Pelham, H.R.B. 1982. A regulatory upstream promoter element in the *Drosophila* HSP 70 heat-shock gene. *Cell* **30**: 517.

Picard, D. and W. Schaffner. 1983. Correct transcription of a cloned mouse immunoglobulin gene in vivo. *Proc. Natl. Acad. Sci.* **80**: 417.

Queen, C. and D. Baltimore. 1983. Immunoglobulin gene transcription is activated by downstream sequence elements. *Cell* **33**: 741.

Robins, D.M., I. Paek, P.H. Seeburg, and R. Axel. 1982. Regulated expression of human growth hormone genes in mouse cells. *Cell* **29**: 623.

Rowe, D.T., S.P. Yee, J. Otis, F.L. Graham, and P.E. Branton. 1983. Characterization of human adenovirus type 5 region 1A polypeptides using antitumor sera and an antiserum specific for the carboxy terminus. *Virology* **127**: 253.

Ruley, H.E. 1983. Adenovirus early region 1A enables viral and cellular transforming genes to transform primary cells in culture. *Nature* **304**: 602.

Seed, B. 1983. Purification of genomic sequences from bacteriophage libraries by recombination and selection *in vivo*. *Nucleic Acids Res.* **11**: 2427.

Tooze, J., ed. 1981. *Molecular biology of tumor viruses*, 2nd edition, revised: *DNA tumor viruses*. Cold Spring Harbor Laboratory, Cold Spring Harbor, New York.

Treisman, R., M.R. Green and T. Maniatis. 1983a. *Cis-* and *trans*-activation of globin gene transcription in transient assays. *Proc. Natl. Acad. Sci.* **80**: 7428.

Treisman, R., S.H. Orkin, and T. Maniatis 1983b. Specific transcription and RNA splicing defects in five cloned β-thalassemia genes. *Nature* **302**: 591.

Treisman, R., B. Seed, P. Little, M.R. Green, N. Proudfoot, and T. Maniatis. 1982. An approach to the analysis of the structure and expression of mutant globin genes. In *Eukaryotic viral vectors* (ed. Y. Gluzman), p. 61. Cold Spring Harbor Laboratory, Cold Spring Harbor, New York.

Wasylyk, B., C. Wasylyk, P. Augereau, and P. Chambon. 1983. The SV40 72 bp repeat preferentially potentiates transcription starting from proximal natural or substitute promoter elements. *Cell* **32**: 503.

Watson, J. and J.B. Clements. A Herpes simplex virus type 1 function required for early and late viral RNA synthesis. *Nature* **285**: 329.

Weintraub, H. 1983. A dominant role for DNA secondary structure in forming hypersensitive structures in chromatin. *Cell* **32**: 1191.

Wold, B., M. Wigler, L. Lacy, T. Maniatis, S. Silverstein, and R. Axel. 1979. Introduction and expression of a rabbit β-globin gene in mouse fibroblasts. *Proc. Natl. Acad. Sci.* **76**: 5688.

Wu, C. 1980. The 5′ ends of *Drosophila* heat shock genes in chromatin are hypersensitive to DNAse I. *Nature* **286**: 854.

Author Index

Subject Index